DVD Contents

SECTION I
FOREFOOT

Hallux Valgus Correction with Modified Chevron Osteotomy
Glenn B. Pfeffer

Modified "Lapidus" Procedure—Tarsometatarsal Corrective Osteotomy and Fusion with First Metatarsophalangeal Joint Correction and Realignment
Andrew K. Sands

Proximal Long Oblique (Ludloff) First Metatarsal Osteotomy with Distal Soft Tissue Procedure
Mark E. Easley

Forefoot Reconstruction for Rheumatoid Disease
Glenn B. Pfeffer

SECTION II
MIDFOOT

Cavovarus Correction in Charcot-Marie-Tooth Disease
Glenn B. Pfeffer

Open Reduction and Internal Fixation of the Proximal Fifth Metatarsal (Jones' or Stress) Fracture
Mark E. Easley and James A. Nunley, II

SECTION III
HINDFOOT/ANKLE

Arthroscopic Ankle Arthrodesis
Carol Frey

Tibiotalocalcaneal Fusion with a Retrograde Intramedullary Nail
Alexej Barg, Beat Hintermann, and Markus Knupp

Osteochondral Lesion of the Ankle—OATS Procedure
Carol Frey

Arthroscopy of the Subtalar Joint
Carol Frey

Ligament Reconstruction for Chronic Medial Ankle Instability
Beat Hintermann

Intra-articular Calcaneus Fractures
Mark E. Easley

Anterior Ankle Impingement
Carol Frey

Triple Arthrodesis
Edmund H. Choi and Andrew K. Sands

SECTION IV
THE LEG

Peroneal Tendon Tears, Debridement, and Repair
Christina Kabbash and Andrew K. Sands

OPERATIVE TECHNIQUES

foot and ankle surgery

OPERATIVE TECHNIQUES

foot and ankle

surgery

Glenn B. Pfeffer, MD
Director, Foot and Ankle Center
Cedars-Sinai Medical Center
Los Angeles, California

Mark E. Easley, MD
Assistant Professor and Orthopaedic Surgeon
Duke University Medical Center
Durham, North Carolina

Carol Frey, MD
Assistant Clinical Professor
Orthopedic Surgery
University of California, Los Angeles
Los Angeles, California
Co-Director, Sports Medicine Fellowship
West Coast Sports Medicine Foundation
Director, Orthopedic Foot and Ankle Surgery
West Coast Center for Orthopedic Surgery
and Sports Medicine
Manhattan Beach, California

Beat Hintermann, MD
Associate Professor
University of Basel
Chairman
Clinic of Orthopaedic Surgery
Kantonsspital
Liestal, Switzerland

Andrew K. Sands, MD
Chief, Foot and Ankle Surgery
Director, Foot and Ankle Institute
St. Vincent's Hospital
New York, New York

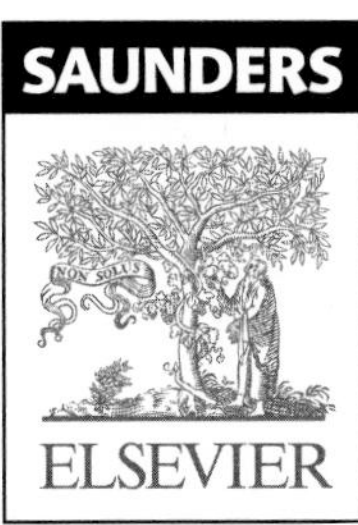

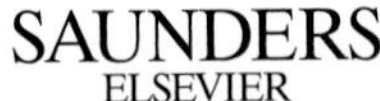

1600 John F. Kennedy Blvd.
Ste 1800
Philadelphia, PA 19103-2899

OPERATIVE TECHNIQUES: FOOT AND ANKLE SURGERY ISBN: 978-1-4160-3280-9

Notice

Knowledge and best practice in this field are constantly changing. As new research and experience broaden our knowledge, changes in practice, treatment and drug therapy may become necessary or appropriate. Readers are advised to check the most current information provided (i) on procedures featured or (ii) by the manufacturer of each product to be administered, to verify the recommended dose or formula, the method and duration of administration, and contraindications. It is the responsibility of the practitioner, relying on their own experience and knowledge of the patient, to make diagnoses, to determine dosages and the best treatment for each individual patient, and to take all appropriate safety precautions. To the fullest extent of the law, neither the Publisher nor the Editors assumes any liability for any injury and/or damage to persons or property arising out of or related to any use of the material contained in this book.

The Publisher

Library of Congress Cataloging-in-Publication Data
Foot and ankle surgery / [edited by] Glenn B. Pfeffer . . . [et al.].
p. ; cm. — (Operative techniques)
Includes index.
ISBN 978-1-4160-3280-9
1. Foot—Surgery—Handbooks, manuals, etc. 2. Ankle—Surgery—Handbooks, manuals, etc. I. Pfeffer, Glenn B. II. Series: Operative techniques.
[DNLM: 1. Foot—surgery—Atlases. 2. Foot Diseases—surgery—Atlases. 3. Foot Injuries—surgery—Atlases. 4. Orthopedic Procedures—methods—Atlases. WE 17 F687 2009]
RD563.F6438 2009
617.5′85—dc22 2009022703

Publishing Director: Kimberly Murphy
Design Direction: Steven Stave

Printed in China

Last digit is the print number: 9 8 7 6 5 4 3 2 1

To my wonderful sons, Daniel and William.

Glenn B. Pfeffer

To my wife, Mary,
and my three children, Ford, Benson, and Charlotte
for allowing me to share the free time I would have spent with them
to make my contribution to this text possible.

Mark E. Easley

Dick Frey was an athlete, scholar, scientist, war hero, and father.
I dedicate this book to my father, a great man.

Carol Frey

To my children Sabrina, and Mathias,
And my Mom and Dad
For their support, love, and care that have made this all possible.

Beat Hintermann

For Alec, Charlotte and James who put up with my long periods of time in the batcave.
For Mom and Dad.
For Eric, always generous with his time and patient with my many questions.
For S.T.H. from whom all knowledge flows.
And mostly for Betsy. I love you.
Thank you all.
With love and respect,

Andrew K. Sands

CONTRIBUTORS

Su-Young Bae, MD, PhD
Assistant Professor of Orthopaedic Surgery, Foot and Ankle Center, INJE University Sanggye Paik Hospital, Seoul, Korea
Charcot Neuroarthropathy of the Midfoot/Hindfoot

Alexej Barg, MD
Resident, Clinic of Orthopaedic Surgery, Kantonsspital Liestal, Liestal, Switzerland
Tibiotalocalcaneal Fusion with a Retrograde Intramedullary Nail; Exosectomy for Haglund's Disease

Gregory C. Berlet, MD
Chief, Division of Foot and Ankle Surgery, The Ohio State University, Columbus; Orthopedic Foot and Ankle Center, Westerville, Ohio
Turf Toe Repair: Capsular Repair of First Metatarsophalangeal Plantar Plate Rupture

Donald R. Bohay, MD, FACS
Associate Clinical Professor, Orthopaedic Surgery, College of Human Medicine, Michigan State University, East Lansing; Spectrum Health Hospitals Staff, Private Practice, and Orthopaedic Associates of Michigan, Grand Rapids, Michigan
Ankle Arthrodesis for Salvage of the Failed Total Ankle Arthroplasty

Edmund H. Choi, MD
House Staff, Kingsbrook Jewish Hospital, Brooklyn, New York
Modified "Lapidus" Procedure—Tarsometatarsal Corrective Osteotomy and Fusion with First Metatarsophalangeal Joint Correction and Realignment; Lateral Ankle Reconstruction with the Fourth Extensor Digitorum Communis Tendon; Triple Arthrodesis

James K. DeOrio, MD
Associate Professor and Orthopaedic Surgeon, Duke University Medical Center, Durham, North Carolina
Chronic Peroneal Tendon Subluxation-Dislocation

Matthew DeOrio, MD
Private Practice, The Orthopaedic Center, Huntsville, Alabama
Intra-articular Calcaneus Fractures

Jeroen De Wachter, MD
Resident, Clinic of Orthopaedic Surgery, Kantonsspital Liestal, Liestal, Switzerland
Single Medial Approach for Triple Arthrodesis

Mark E. Easley, MD
Assistant Professor and Orthopaedic Surgeon, Duke University Medical Center, Durham, North Carolina
Proximal Long Oblique (Ludloff) First Metatarsal Osteotomy with Distal Soft Tissue Procedure; Fifth Metatarsal Osteotomy for Correction of Bunionette Deformity; Metatarsal Lengthening; Open Reduction and Internal Fixation of Proximal Fifth Metatarsal (Jones' or Stress) Fracture; Ankle Arthrodesis Using Ring/Multiplanar External Fixation; Intra-articular Calcaneus Fractures; Chronic Peroneal Tendon Subluxation-Dislocation; Posterior Tibial Tendon Transfer for Footdrop

Carol Frey, MD
Assistant Clinical Professor, Orthopedic Surgery, UCLA, Los Angeles; Co-Director, Sports Medicine Fellowship, West Coast Sports Medicine Foundation, and Director, Orthopedic Foot and Ankle Center, West Coast Center for Orthopedic Surgery and Sports Medicine, Manhattan Beach, California
Hallux Rigidus: Cheilectomy with and without a Dorsiflexion Phalangeal Osteotomy; Morton's Neuroma; Deviated Lesser Toe/Metatarsal Shortening (Weil) Osteotomy; Arthroscopy of the Great Toe; Arthroscopic Ankle Arthrodesis; Osteochondral Lesion of the Ankle—OATS Procedure; Arthroscopy of the Subtalar Joint; Haglund's Deformity: Open and Arthroscopic Treatment; Tarsal Tunnel Syndrome; Anterior Ankle Impingement

Beat Hintermann, MD
Associate Professor, University of Basel, Basel; Chairman, Clinic of Orthopaedic Surgery, Kantonsspital, Liestal, Switzerland
Internal Fixation of the Sesamoid Bone of the Hallux; Midfoot Arthrodesis in Charcot Foot Deformity with "Charcot Screws"; Total Ankle Arthroplasty with a Current Three-Component Design (HINTEGRA Prosthesis); Salvage of Failed Total Ankle Arthroplasty; Rigid Fixation for Ankle Arthrodesis Using Double Plating; Tibiotalocalcaneal Fusion with a Retrograde Intramedullary Nail; Realignment Surgery for Valgus Ankle Osteoarthritis; Mosaicplasty with Bone-Periosteum Graft from the Iliac Crest for Osteochondral Lesions of the Talus; Lateral Ankle Ligament Reconstruction Using Plantaris Autograft; Ligament Reconstruction for Chronic Medial Ankle Instability; Exosectomy for Haglund's Disease; Osteotomies for the Correction of Varus Ankle; Lateral Calcaneal Lengthening Osteotomy for Supple Adult Flatfoot; Single Medial Approach for Triple Arthrodesis

Stefan G. Hofstaetter, MD
Resident, Department of Orthopaedics, Klinikum Wels-Grieskirchen, Wels, Austria
Ankle Arthrodesis Using Ring/Multiplanar External Fixation

Christina Kabbash, MD, PhD, MPH
Foot and Ankle Fellow, and Voluntary Staff, Attending, St. Francis Hospital, Hartford, Connecticut
Calcaneus Open Reduction and Internal Fixation with Extensile Lateral Incision; Peroneal Tendon Tears: Débridement and Repair

Robert Kilger, MD
Resident, Clinic of Orthopaedic Surgery, Kantonsspital Liestal, Liestal, Switzerland
Mosaicplasty with Bone-Periosteum Graft from the Iliac Crest for Osteochondral Lesions of the Talus

Markus Knupp, MD
Senior Attending Resident, Clinic of Orthopaedic Surgery, Kantonsspital Liestal, Liestal, Switzerland
Tibiotalocalcaneal Fusion with a Retrograde Intramedullary Nail; Realignment Surgery for Valgus Ankle Osteoarthritis; Osteotomies for the Correction of Varus Ankle

Hans-Peter Kundert, MD
Senior Consultant, Foot and Ankle Center, Hirslanden Clinic Zurich, Zurich, Switzerland
Scarf Osteotomy for Correction of Hallux Valgus; Lateral Calcaneal Lengthening Osteotomy for Supple Adult Flatfoot

André Leumann, MD
Resident, Clinic of Orthopaedic Surgery, Universitatsspital Basel, Basel, Switzerland
Mosaicplasty with Bone-Periosteum Graft from the Iliac Crest for Osteochondral Lesions of the Talus; Lateral Calcaneal Lengthening Osteotomy for Supple Adult Flatfoot

Roman Lusser, MD
Senior Attending Resident, Clinic of Orthopaedic Surgery, Kantonsspital Liestal, Liestal, Switzerland
Midfoot Arthrodesis in Charcot Foot Deformity with "Charcot Screws"

Marc Merian-Genast, MD
Private Practice, Regina Qu'Appelle Health Region, Regina, Saskatchewan, Canada
Chronic Peroneal Tendon Subluxation-Dislocation

James A. Nunley II, MD
Professor and Chairman, Division of Orthopaedic Surgery, Duke University Medical Center, Durham, North Carolina
Metatarsal Lengthening; Open Reduction and Internal Fixation of Proximal Fifth Metatarsal (Jones' or Stress) Fracture

Geert I. Pagenstert, MD
Attending Orthopaedic Surgeon, Department of Orthopaedic Surgery, Friedrich-Wilhelms-University Bonn, Bonn, Germany
Internal Fixation of the Sesamoid Bone of the Hallux; Realignment Surgery for Valgus Ankle Osteoarthritis; Mosaicplasty with Bone-Periosteum Graft from the Iliac Crest for Osteochondral Lesions of the Talus; Lateral Ankle Ligament Reconstruction Using Plantaris Autograft; Osteotomies for the Correction of Varus Ankle

Glenn B. Pfeffer, MD
Associate Professor, University of Basel, Attending Orthopaedic Surgeon, Department of Orthopaedic Surgery, University Hospital, Basel, Switzerland
Hallux Valgus Correction with Modified Chevron Osteotomy; Arthrodesis of the Great Toe Metatarsophalangeal Joint; Forefoot Reconstruction for Rheumatoid Disease; Revision Surgery through a Plantar Approach for Recurrent Interdigital Neuroma; Correction of Acquired Hallux Varus; Cavovarus Correction in Charcot-Marie-Tooth Disease; Painful Accessory Navicular Treated with Fusion; Modified Brostrom Procedure for Lateral Ankle Laxity; Salvage of a Failed Lateral Ligament Repair

Terrence M. Philbin, DO
Assistant Clinical Professor, The Ohio State University, Columbus; Director, Foot and Ankle Fellowship, Orthopedic Foot and Ankle Center, Westerville, Ohio
Turf Toe Repair: Capsular Repair of First Metatarsophalangeal Plantar Plate Rupture

Christian Plaass, MD
Resident, Clinic of Orthopaedic Surgery, Kantonsspital Liestal, Liestal, Switzerland
Rigid Fixation for Ankle Arthrodesis Using Double Plating; Mosaicplasty with Bone-Periosteum Graft from the Iliac Crest for Osteochondral Lesions of the Talus

Andrew K. Sands, MD
Chief, Foot and Ankle Surgery, and Director, Foot and Ankle Institute, St. Vincent's Hospital, New York, New York
Modified "Lapidus" Procedure—Tarsometatarsal Corrective Osteotomy and Fusion with First Metatarsophalangeal Joint Correction and Realignment; Open Reduction and Internal Fixation of Lisfranc/Tarsometatarsal Injuries; Painful Accessory Navicular: Augmented Kidner Procedure with Flexor Digitorum Longus Transfer; Open Reduction and Internal Fixation of the Cuboid Fracture/Nutcracker Injury; Lateral Ankle Reconstruction with the Fourth Extensor Digitorum Communis Tendon; Calcaneus Open Reduction and Internal Fixation with Extensile Lateral Incision; Triple Arthrodesis; Treatment of Distal Achilles (Insertional) Degeneration and Associated Calf Tightness Plus Calcaneal Tuber Exostosis; Achilles Tendon Reconstruction with Flexor Hallucis Longus Transfer Augmentation; Peroneal Tendon Tears: Débridement and Repair; Calf Lengthening for Equinus Contracture; Proximal Tibia Bone Graft; Anterior Leg Compartment Release for Exertional Compartment Syndrome

Lew C. Schon, MD
Attending Surgeon, and Director, Foot and Ankle Division, Orthopaedic Surgery, Union Memorial Hospital, Baltimore, Maryland
Charcot Neuroarthropathy of the Midfoot/Hindfoot

Aaron T. Scott, MD
Assistant Professor, Wake Forest University School of Medicine; Orthopaedic Surgeon, Wake Forest University Baptist Medical Center, Winston-Salem, North Carolina
Posterior Tibial Tendon Transfer for Footdrop

W. Bret Smith, DO
Moore Orthopaedics, Columbia, South Carolina
Turf Toe Repair: Capsular Repair of First Metatarsophalangeal Plantar Plate Rupture

Hans-Joerg Trnka, MD
Consultant, KH Göttlicher Heiland, Vienna, Austria
Proximal Long Oblique (Ludloff) First Metatarsal Osteotomy with Distal Soft Tissue Procedure

Victor Valderrabano, MD, PhD
Associate Professor, University of Basel, Attending Orthopaedic Surgeon, Department of Orthopaedic Surgery, University Hospital, Basel, Switzerland
Internal Fixation of the Sesamoid Bone of the Hallux; Realignment Surgery for Valgus Ankle Osteoarthritis; Mosaicplasty with Bone-Periosteum Graft from the Iliac Crest for Osteochondral Lesions of the Talus; Lateral Ankle Ligament Reconstruction Using Plantaris Autograft; Osteotomies for the Correction of Varus Ankle; Lateral Calcaneal Lengthening Osteotomy for Supple Adult Flatfoot

PREFACE

There is nothing more valuable to an orthopaedic surgeon than a detailed and well illustrated chapter on surgical technique. *Operative Techniques: Foot and Ankle Surgery* presents a wide spectrum of such techniques, each laid out in an easy to follow and visually elegant format. I have been privileged to work with eminent colleagues from around the world who have brought an unparalleled diversity of surgical experience to this project. Their contributions span the breadth of foot and ankle surgery, from the simplest excision to the most complex reconstruction. This text will be an invaluable addition to the libraries of both general orthopaedists and foot and ankle specialists.

On behalf of all of the authors we want to thank Berta Steiner, Bruce Robison, and Kim Murphy from Elsevier for their tireless guidance and support.

Glenn B. Pfeffer, MD

FOREWORD

Over the last ten years, there has been an explosion of knowledge related to the treatment of disorders that affect the foot and ankle. This is in large part due to the interest of dedicated foot and ankle surgeons. I have had the honor of knowing all of the authors of this textbook. Dr. Pfeffer has authored numerous textbooks on foot and ankle surgery. Dr. Mark Easley has been my partner for over 10 years and is an outstanding foot and ankle educator. Carol Frey has been an authority for over 20 years and Professor Hintermann has dedicated his life to the study of ankle and hindfoot arthritis. Andy Sands is a recent addition to a young cadre of outstanding foot and ankle surgeons.

As disorders of the foot and ankle become increasingly better investigated and better understood, this would seem to be an ideal time for a textbook that would be particularly useful to the practicing foot and ankle surgeon. This text authored by Pfeffer, Easley, Frey, Hintermann and Sands is not intended as a reference tome or a complete authoritative review relating to every disorder that affects the foot and ankle. Rather, this text fits the unique need that most practicing foot and ankle surgeons and those in their training have on a very frequent basis. I refer to this type of text as "just in time knowledge". It detailed technical information about a specific surgical procedure that one may be contemplating performing the next day or the next week. This will be particularly useful for someone who wants a review of the surgical techniques either during surgery or the day before. The text gives us a clear idea of the indications for a specific procedure, it identifies pitfalls of the surgical procedure, and best of all, this book is incredibly well illustrated. The photographs of the surgical procedures will lead the clinician through a complex procedure in a very orderly manner and I believe will greatly enhance our technical skills.

Although the field of foot and ankle surgery is incredibly large, these authors have chosen to provide us with a compendium of some of the more common surgical procedures with a well thought out, but abbreviated approach such that the material might be reviewed in a very short period of time. Yet there does not seem to be any material of critical value that has been left out. The techniques range from the simple excision of a neuroma to the complex reconstruction of an ankle malunion.

I am honored to have been given the opportunity to provide the foreword to the text. The authors are recognized authorities who have contributed significantly in the areas of their expertise. I believe that this text will provide much needed useful information on a just in time basis to the busy clinician.

James A. Nunley II, MD
Professor and Chairman
Division of Orthopaedic Surgery
Duke University Medical Center
Durham, North Carolina

CONTENTS

SECTION I
Forefoot 1

PROCEDURE 1
Hallux Valgus Correction with Modified Chevron Osteotomy 3
Glenn B. Pfeffer

PROCEDURE 2
Scarf Osteotomy for Correction of Hallux Valgus 21
Hans-Peter Kundert

PROCEDURE 3
Modified "Lapidus" Procedure—Tarsometatarsal Corrective Osteotomy and Fusion with First Metatarsophalangeal Joint Correction and Realignment 35
Andrew K. Sands and Edmund H. Choi

PROCEDURE 4
Proximal Long Oblique (Ludloff) First Metatarsal Osteotomy with Distal Soft Tissue Procedure 47
Mark E. Easley and Hans-Joerg Trnka

PROCEDURE 5
Hallux Rigidus: Cheilectomy with and without a Dorsiflexion Phalangeal Osteotomy 65
Carol Frey

PROCEDURE 6
Arthrodesis of the Great Toe Metatarsophalangeal Joint 75
Glenn B. Pfeffer

PROCEDURE 7
Forefoot Reconstruction for Rheumatoid Disease 87
Glenn B. Pfeffer

PROCEDURE 8
Fifth Metatarsal Osteotomy for Correction of Bunionette Deformity 101
Mark E. Easley

PROCEDURE 9
Turf Toe Repair: Capsular Repair of First Metatarsophalangeal Plantar Plate Rupture 111
W. Bret Smith, Terrence M. Philbin, and Gregory C. Berlet

PROCEDURE 10
Morton's Neuroma 121
Carol Frey

PROCEDURE 11
Revision Surgery through a Plantar Approach for Recurrent Interdigital Neuroma 127
Glenn B. Pfeffer

PROCEDURE 12
Deviated Lesser Toe/Metatarsal Shortening (Weil) Osteotomy 135
Carol Frey

PROCEDURE 13
Correction of Acquired Hallux Varus 143
Glenn B. Pfeffer

PROCEDURE 14
Arthroscopy of the Great Toe 153
Carol Frey

PROCEDURE 15
Metatarsal Lengthening 163
Mark E. Easley and James A. Nunley II

PROCEDURE 16
Internal Fixation of the Sesamoid Bone of the Hallux 181
Geert I. Pagenstert, Victor Valderrabano, and Beat Hintermann

SECTION II
Midfoot 193

PROCEDURE 17
Cavovarus Correction in Charcot-Marie-Tooth Disease 195
Glenn B. Pfeffer

PROCEDURE 18
Charcot Neuroarthropathy of the Midfoot/Hindfoot 217
Lew C. Schon and Su-Young Bae

PROCEDURE 19
Midfoot Arthrodesis in Charcot Foot Deformity with "Charcot Screws" 237
Roman Lusser and Beat Hintermann

PROCEDURE 20
Open Reduction and Internal Fixation of Lisfranc/Tarsometatarsal Injuries 245
Andrew K. Sands

PROCEDURE 21
Painful Accessory Navicular: Augmented Kidner Procedure with Flexor Digitorum Longus Transfer 257
Andrew K. Sands

PROCEDURE 22
Painful Accessory Navicular Treated with Fusion 267
Glenn B. Pfeffer

PROCEDURE 23
Open Reduction and Internal Fixation of Proximal Fifth Metatarsal (Jones' or Stress) Fracture 277
Mark E. Easley and James A. Nunley II

PROCEDURE 24
Open Reduction and Internal Fixation of the Cuboid Fracture/Nutcracker Injury 287
Andrew K. Sands

SECTION III
HINDFOOT/ANKLE 297

PROCEDURE 25
Total Ankle Arthroplasty with a Current Three-Component Design (HINTEGRA Prosthesis) 299
Beat Hintermann

PROCEDURE 26
Salvage of Failed Total Ankle Arthroplasty 325
Beat Hintermann

PROCEDURE 27
Ankle Arthrodesis for Salvage of the Failed Total Ankle Arthroplasty 341
Donald R. Bohay

PROCEDURE 28
Ankle Arthrodesis Using Ring/Multiplanar External Fixation 359
Mark E. Easley and Stefan G. Hofstaetter

PROCEDURE 29
Arthroscopic Ankle Arthrodesis 373
Carol Frey

PROCEDURE 30
Rigid Fixation for Ankle Arthrodesis Using Double Plating 381
Christian Plaass and Beat Hintermann

PROCEDURE 31
Tibiotalocalcaneal Fusion with a Retrograde Intramedullary Nail 395
Alexej Barg, Beat Hintermann, and Markus Knupp

PROCEDURE 32
Realignment Surgery for Valgus Ankle Osteoarthritis 407
Geert I. Pagenstert, Markus Knupp, Victor Valderrabano, and Beat Hintermann

PROCEDURE 33
Osteochondral Lesion of the Ankle—OATS Procedure 431
Carol Frey

PROCEDURE 34
Mosaicplasty with Bone-Periosteum Graft from the Iliac Crest for Osteochondral Lesions of the Talus 443
André Leumann, Victor Valderrabano, Robert Kilger, Christian Plaass, Geert I. Pagenstert, and Beat Hintermann

PROCEDURE 35
Arthroscopy of the Subtalar Joint 457
Carol Frey

PROCEDURE 36
Modified Brostrom Procedure for Lateral Ankle Laxity 471
Glenn B. Pfeffer

PROCEDURE 37
Lateral Ankle Ligament Reconstruction Using Plantaris Autograft 481
Geert I. Pagenstert, Victor Valderrabano, and Beat Hintermann

PROCEDURE 38
Salvage of a Failed Lateral Ligament Repair 497
Glenn B. Pfeffer

PROCEDURE 39
Lateral Ankle Reconstruction with the Fourth Extensor Digitorum Communis Tendon 509
Edmund H. Choi and Andrew K. Sands

PROCEDURE 40
Ligament Reconstruction for Chronic Medial Ankle Instability 521
Beat Hintermann

PROCEDURE 41
Exosectomy for Haglund's Disease 537
Alexej Barg and Beat Hintermann

PROCEDURE 42
Haglund's Deformity: Open and Arthroscopic Treatment 547
Carol Frey

PROCEDURE 43
Intra-articular Calcaneus Fractures 557
Matthew DeOrio and Mark E. Easley

PROCEDURE 44
Calcaneus Open Reduction and Internal Fixation with Extensile Lateral Incision 575
Christina Kabbash and Andrew K. Sands

PROCEDURE 45
Osteotomies for the Correction of Varus Ankle 589
Markus Knupp, Geert I. Pagenstert, Victor Valderrabano, and Beat Hintermann

PROCEDURE 46
Tarsal Tunnel Syndrome 603
Carol Frey

PROCEDURE 47
Anterior Ankle Impingement 615
Carol Frey

PROCEDURE 48
Lateral Calcaneal Lengthening Osteotomy for Supple Adult Flatfoot 621
Victor Valderrabano, André Leumann, Hans-Peter Kundert, and Beat Hintermann

PROCEDURE 49
Single Medial Approach for Triple Arthrodesis 629
Jeroen De Wachter and Beat Hintermann

PROCEDURE 50
Triple Arthrodesis 643
Edmund H. Choi and Andrew K. Sands

SECTION IV
THE LEG **653**

PROCEDURE 51
Treatment of Distal Achilles (Insertional) Degeneration and Associated Calf Tightness Plus Calcaneal Tuber Exostosis 655
Andrew K. Sands

PROCEDURE 52
Achilles Tendon Reconstruction with Flexor Hallucis Longus Transfer Augmentation 667
Andrew K. Sands

PROCEDURE 53
Peroneal Tendon Tears: Débridement and Repair 679
Christina Kabbash and Andrew K. Sands

PROCEDURE 54
Chronic Peroneal Tendon Subluxation-Dislocation 689
Marc Merian-Genast, James K. DeOrio, and Mark E. Easley

PROCEDURE 55
Posterior Tibial Tendon Transfer for Footdrop 699
Aaron T. Scott and Mark E. Easley

PROCEDURE 56
Calf Lengthening for Equinus Contracture 709
Andrew K. Sands

PROCEDURE 57
Proximal Tibia Bone Graft 721
Andrew K. Sands

PROCEDURE 58
Anterior Leg Compartment Release for Exertional Compartment Syndrome 729
Andrew K. Sands

INDEX **737**

SECTION I

FOREFOOT

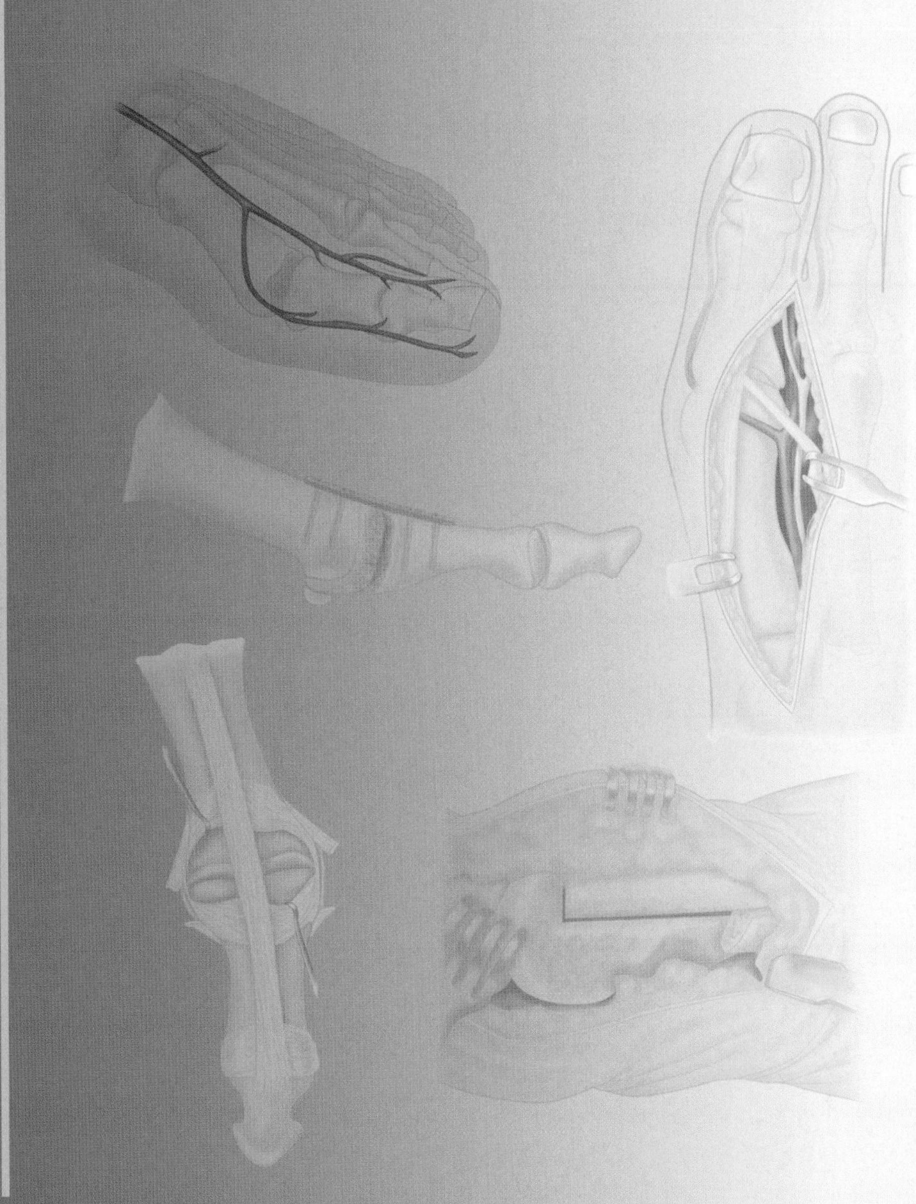

PROCEDURE 1

Hallux Valgus Correction with Modified Chevron Osteotomy

Glenn B. Pfeffer

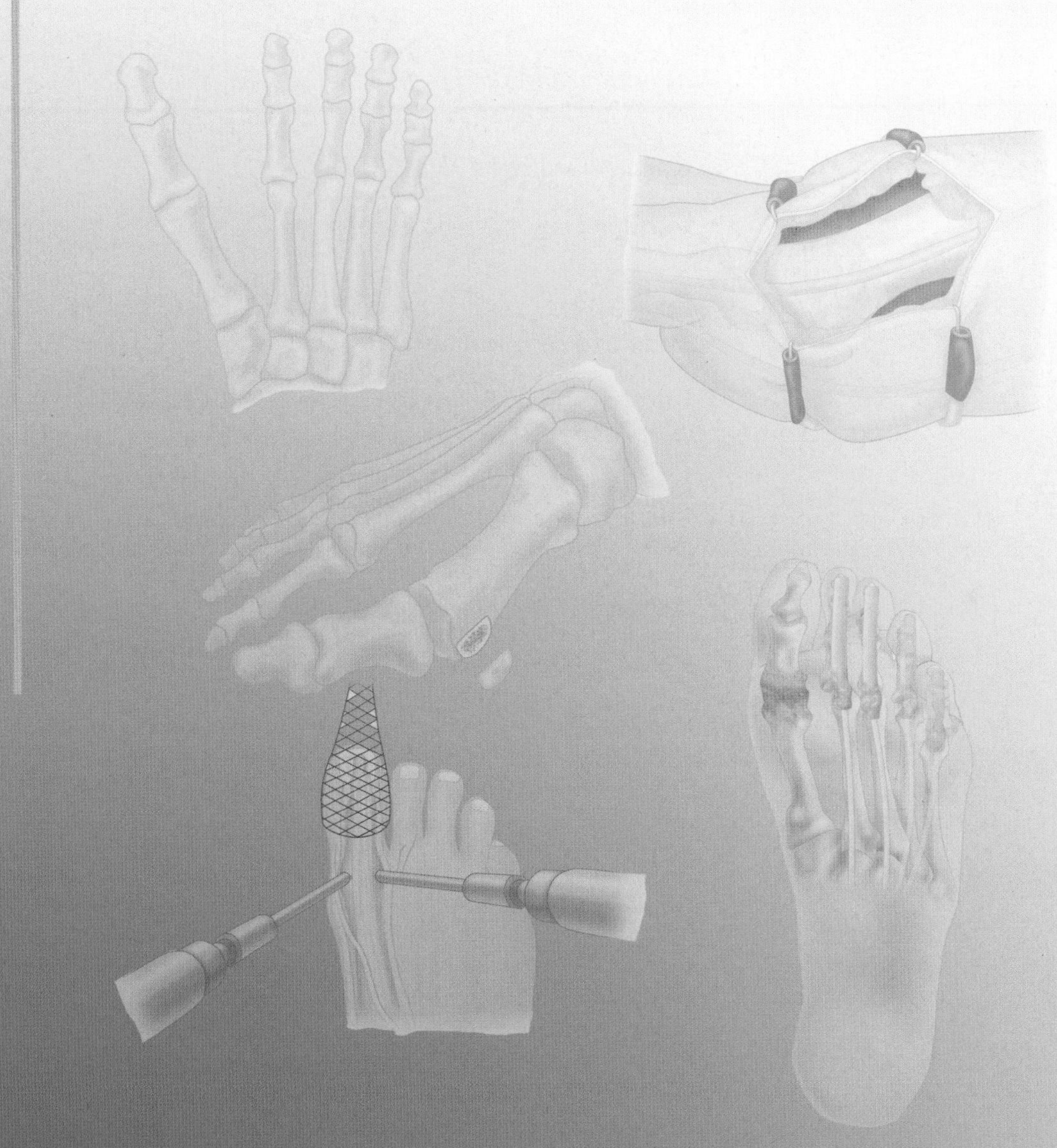

Indications

- Painful hallux valgus deformity
- Failure of shoe modification
- Symptoms that interfere with daily activities
- A mild to moderate deformity (hallux valgus angle <30°; intermetatarsal angle [IMA] <13–15°)
- Patients with a high distal metatarsal articular angle (DMAA) require a chevron osteotomy with the addition of a closing wedge.

PITFALLS

- *Arthritic changes of the joint are usually a contraindication to hallux valgus surgery.*
- *Compromised blood supply.*
- *Ulceration over the bunion prominence.*
- *An IMA of more than 13–15°.*
- *An extremely hypermobile first ray.*
- *Osteoporosis makes this specific procedure more difficult because of poor screw fixation.*
- *Patients with an excessively short first metatarsal may do better with a basilar opening wedge procedure (using an Arthrex low-profile plate) that does not further shorten the metatarsal.*
- *Avascular necrosis of the metatarsal head is a reported complication of the chevron osteotomy, but rarely occurs if the procedure is performed with precision.*
- *Hallux valgus deformity will recur, to some degree, without some postoperative modification of high-heeled, tight-fitting shoes.*

Controversies

- Hallux valgus correction with a proximal first metatarsal osteotomy is a much more powerful correction than a distal chevron. A proximal osteotomy (see Procedure 4) is a preferable procedure for moderate to severe bunion deformities. While it is possible to "push" the indications for a chevron, there is little point given the superb results of alternative procedures that involve a proximal osteotomy of the metatarsal base.
- A patient with metatarsus adductus will have a spuriously low IMA on radiographs. A proximal osteotomy is often required in these patients, in spite of a low IMA.
- Simultaneous bilateral bunionectomies are technically possible, but present a very difficult recovery for the patient, and are usually not recommend.
- The Acutrak 2 self-drilling/tapping screw negates the difficult step of drilling across the osteotomy.

Treatment Options

- Shoe modification, with lower heels (<2.5 inches) and a wider toe box. Stretch the shoes.
- A medial longitudinal arch support may be helpful in athletic shoewear.

Examination/Imaging

- Standing examination of the foot demonstrates a hallux valgus deformity (Fig. 1).
- The bunion prominence is usually erythematous from shoewear irritation.
- Examine the interphalangeal (IP) joint to determine if a hallux interphalangeus is present (valgus IP angle >10°). A closing wedge osteotomy of the proximal phalanx may be needed for these cases.
- Evaluate hypermobility of the first ray. A fusion of the metatarsal-cuneiform joint is rarely required.
- Pes planus may be present, but simultaneous surgery for this condition is rarely indicated.

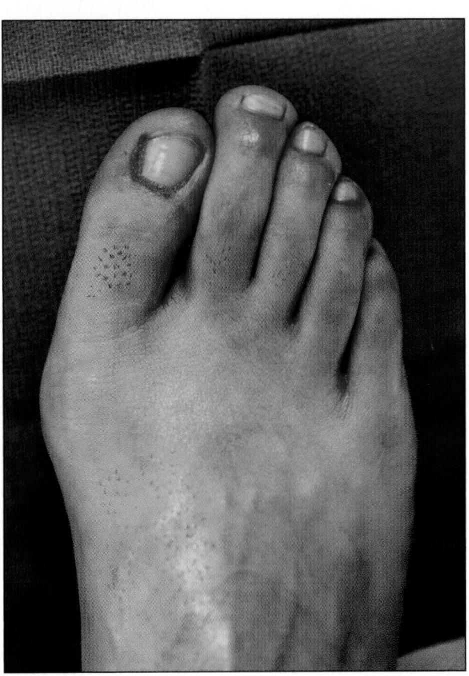

FIGURE 1

- Standing anteroposterior (AP) (Fig. 2A and 2B) and lateral (Fig. 3) radiographs of the foot.
  - Measure the first metatarsal–phalangeal angle and IMA (see Fig. 2B). Determine if metatarsus adductus is causing a spuriously low IMA.
  - Measure the DMAA, which may require correction if >10°.
  - Evaluate arthritic changes of the first metatarsophalangeal joint and the sesamoid-metatarsal articulation. Determine the station of the sesamoid (degree of subluxation from beneath the metatarsal head).

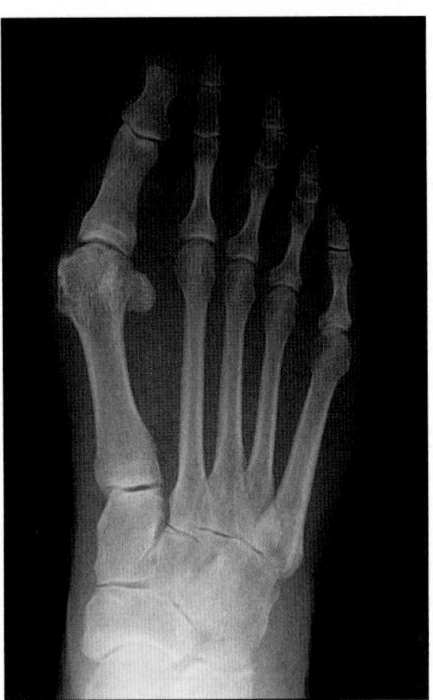

A

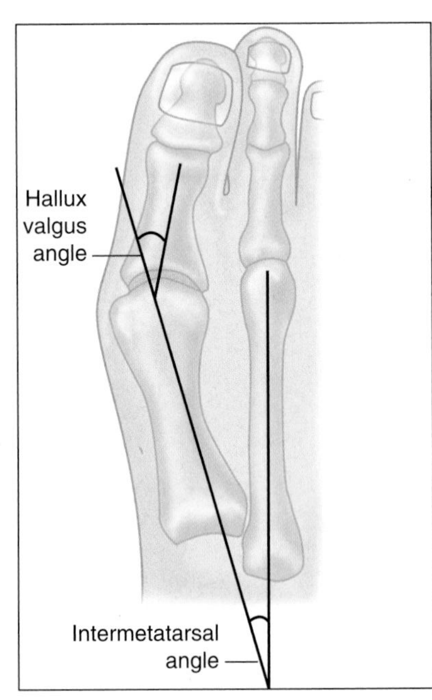

B

FIGURE 2

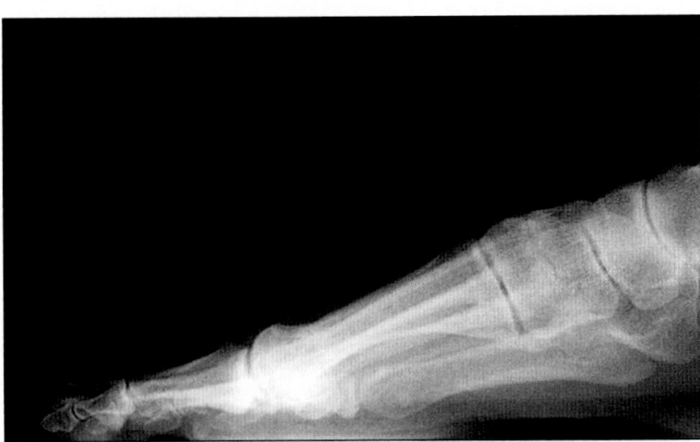

FIGURE 3

Surgical Anatomy

- Bones and tendons of the great toe (Fig. 4)
- Vascular supply to the great toe (Fig. 5A)
- Nerve supply to the first and second metatarsals and toes (Fig. 5B)

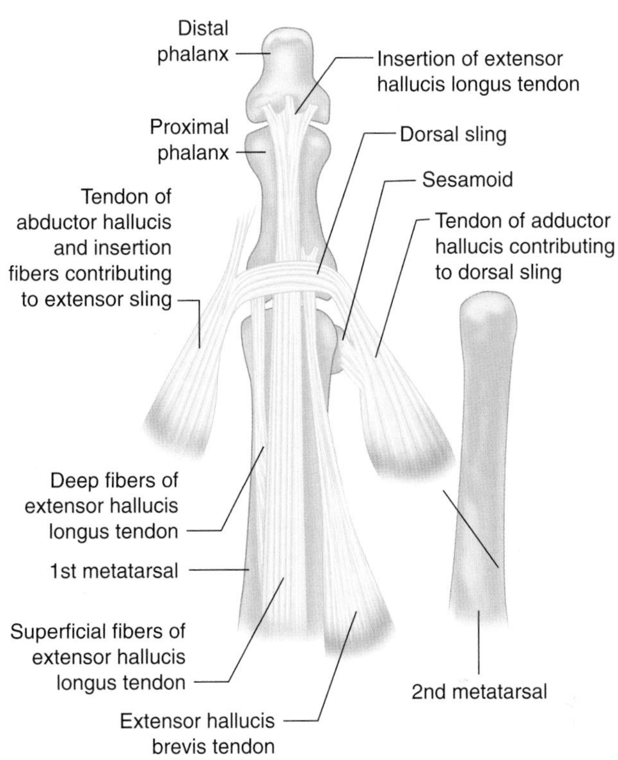

FIGURE 4

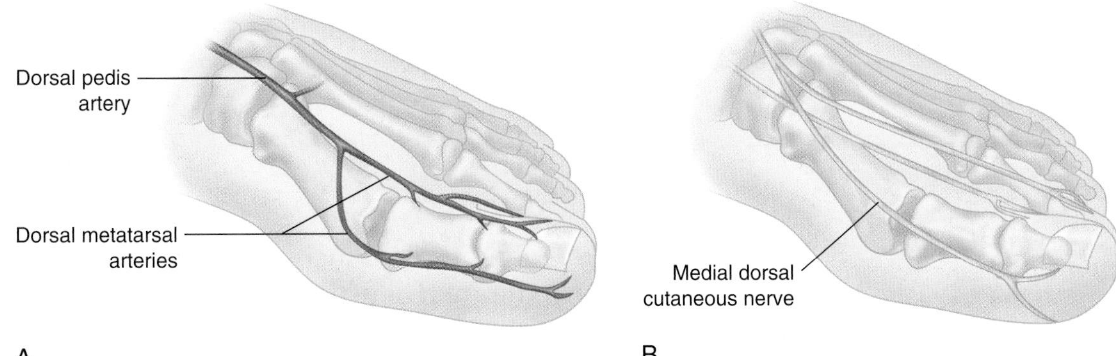

FIGURE 5

Positioning

- The patient is in the supine position.
- A bump under the contralateral hip will externally rotate the leg, which will improve the exposure to the medial side of the foot.
- An ankle or thigh tourniquet may be used.
- The procedure is performed on an outpatient basis under a regional block (femoral-sciatic or popliteal), to achieve maximal pain control postoperatively and reduce the amount of general anesthetic used.

Portals/Exposures

- Make a longitudinal incision over the medial eminence of adequate length to expose the metatarsal head and base of the proximal phalanx (Fig. 6A).
  - Isolate and protect the dorsal cutaneous sensory nerve (see Fig. 5B).
  - Identify the medial plantar sensory nerve so that it is not injured during the procedure.
- A 3-cm longitudinal incision in the first web space is usually required to release the lateral capsule and adductor tendon (Fig. 6B).

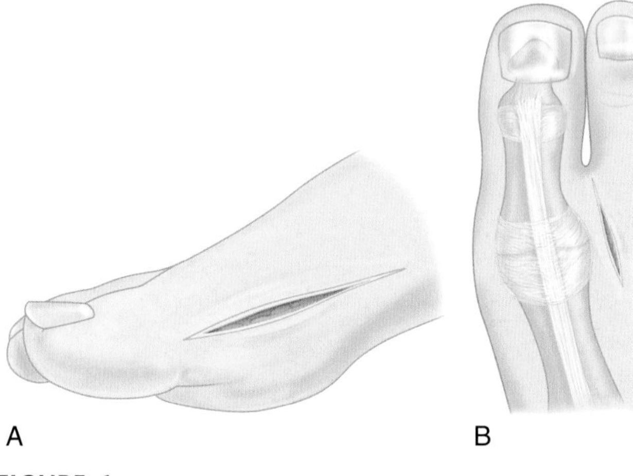

FIGURE 6

> **PEARLS**
>
> - *Document any arthritic changes that may not have been visible on radiographs. Mild arthritis can explain symptoms that do not resolve postoperatively.*

Procedure

Step 1

- Make a longitudinal incision in the capsule and expose the medial aspect of the metatarsal head. Keep the proximal and distal capsular attachments intact.
- Expose the sagittal groove (Fig. 7A and 7B).

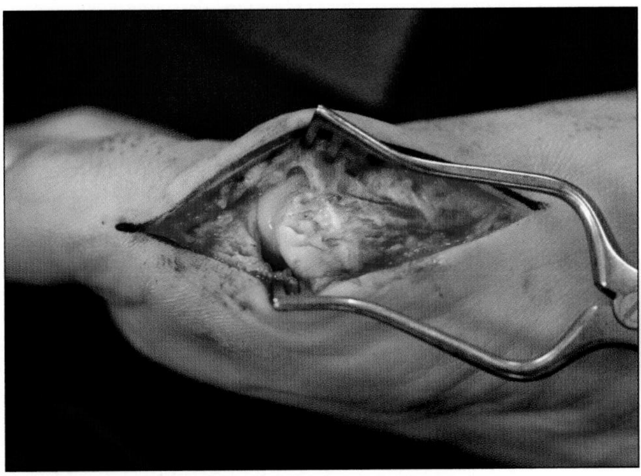
A

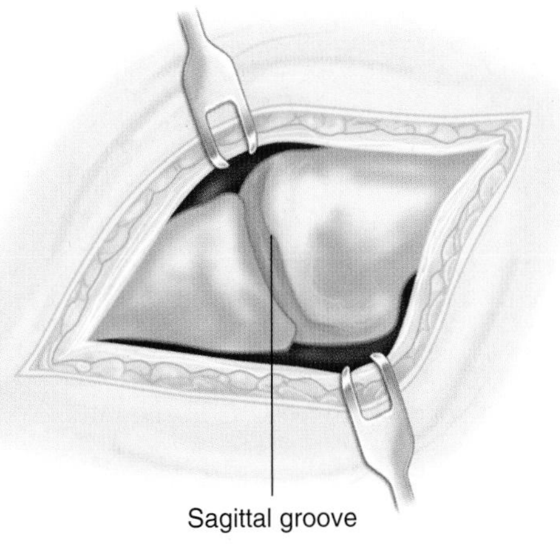

B

FIGURE 7

PEARLS

- *Only a small portion of the medial eminence has to be excised. The head will be shifted laterally and the medial portion will no longer be prominent, regardless of the amount resected.*
- *The wider the head after resection of the eminence, the more it can be shifted laterally, and the greater the correction of the IMA.*

- Inspect the joint and the medial sesamoid articulation for arthritic changes.

STEP 2

- Excise the medial eminence with a cut slightly medial to the sagittal groove (Fig. 8A and 8B). The cut is parallel to the medial metatarsal shaft, or angled slightly toward the medial border of the foot (Fig. 9). Do not skive into the cortical bone of the shaft.
- A micro-sagittal saw blade should be used for this case to minimize bone loss with each cut.

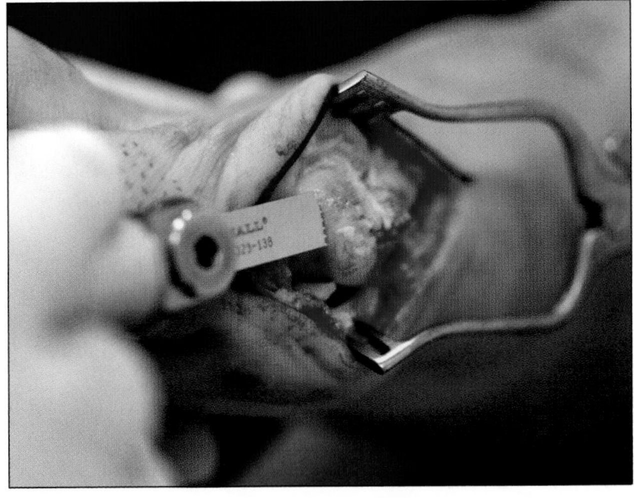
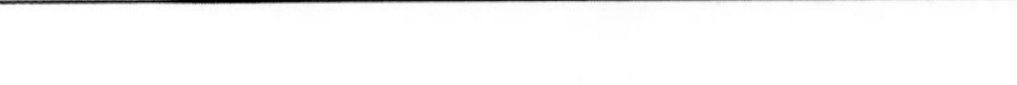
A

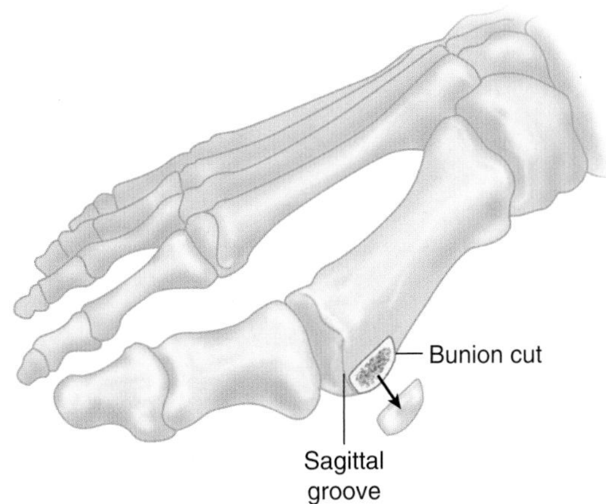

B

FIGURE 8

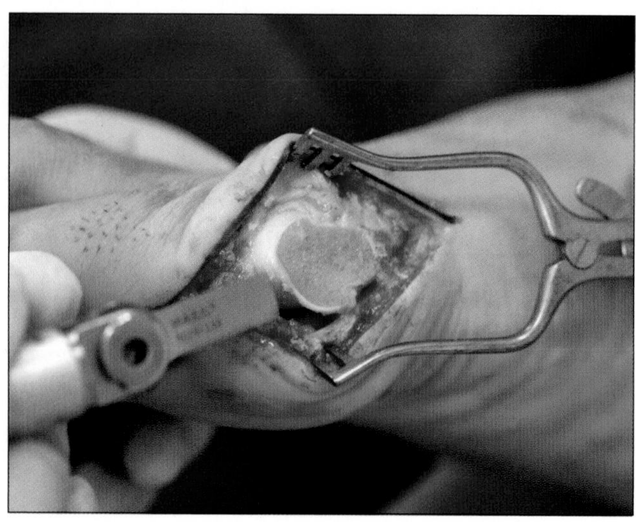

FIGURE 9

Step 3

- Deepen the incision in the first web space using blunt dissection with the tip of a finger. This approach will avoid damage to branches of the superficial peroneal nerve and first dorsal metatarsal artery.
- Expose the lateral capsule.

Step 4

- Place a Weitlander retractor or lamina spreader between the first and second metatarsals.
  - Locate the lateral sesamoid and incise the capsule with a horizontal cut just dorsal to the sesamoid (Fig. 10).

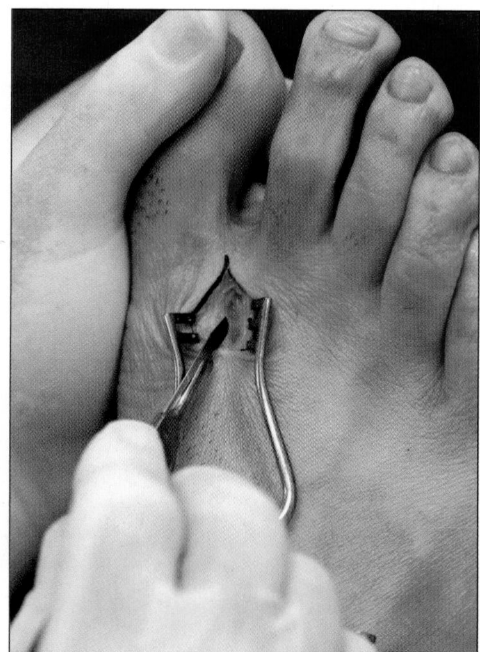

FIGURE 10

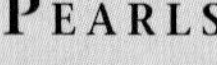

Pearls

- *Always inspect the lateral sesamoid for arthritic changes. Excise the sesamoid if advanced arthritis is present or it cannot be reduced beneath the metatarsal head. Excision of the sesamoid is rarely required, however, and will significantly increase the risk of a varus deformity.*

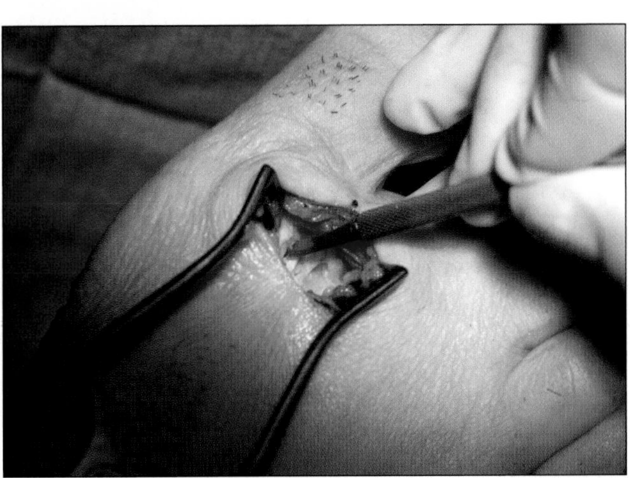

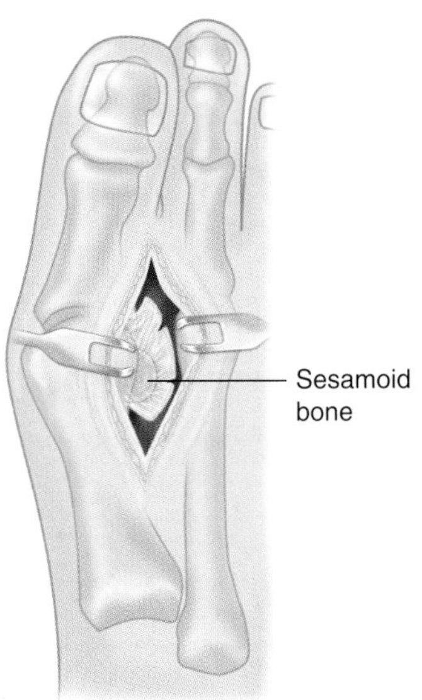

FIGURE 11 A B

- Free up the sesamoid proximally and distally so that it can later be reduced beneath the metatarsal head (Fig. 11A and 11B).

- The flexor hallucis longus runs just medial to the sesamoid, and care should be taken to not injure the tendon during this part of the procedure (see Fig. 4).
- Release the adductor attachment onto the sesamoid and proximal phalanx (Fig. 12A and 12B). Avoid further dissection of the lateral capsule, which can compromise blood supply to the metatarsal head (see Fig. 5A).

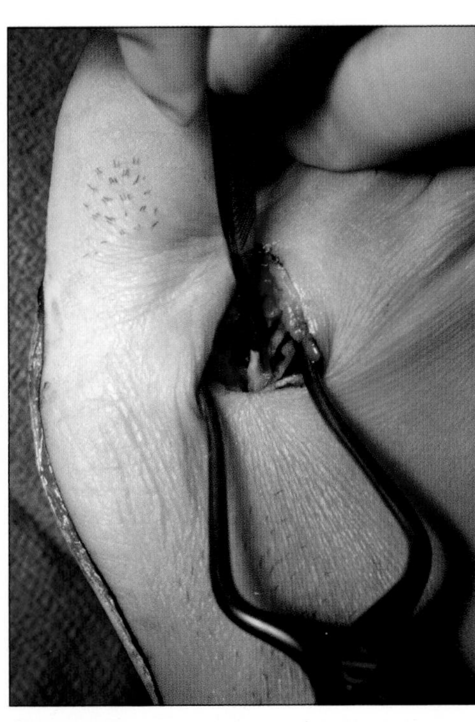

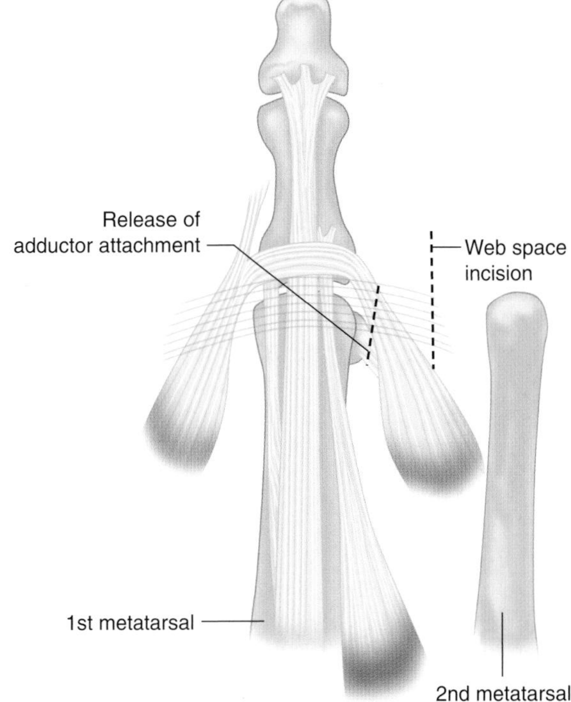

FIGURE 12 A B

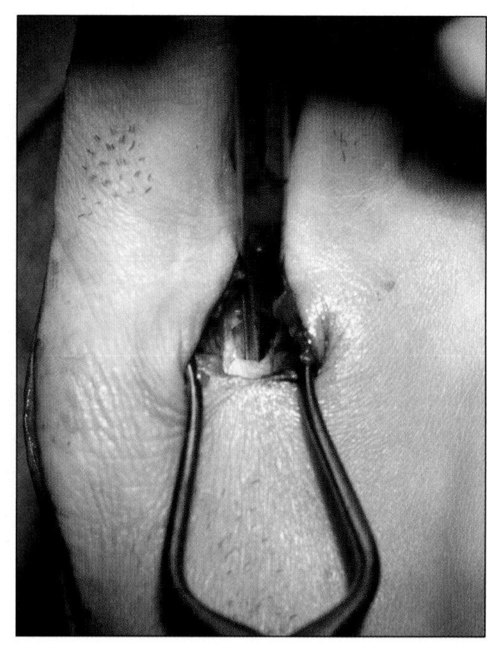
FIGURE 13

- Division of the transverse metatarsal ligament is usually not required (Fig. 13).

Step 5

- Perforate (chicken-hatch) the lateral capsule at the level of the joint (Fig. 14).
- While holding the metatarsal heads together, bring the toe into varus until the capsule ruptures. This usually occurs with a definitive pop (Fig. 15).

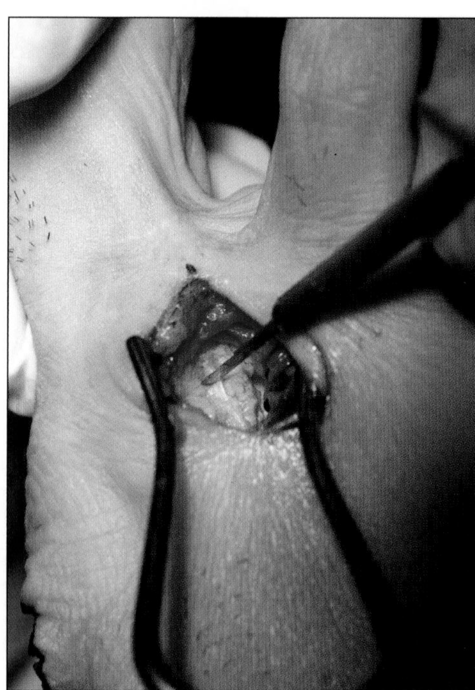
FIGURE 14

Pearls

- *A Kirschner wire placed into the metatarsal head under fluoroscopic guidance will help assure that the osteotomy cuts are parallel to the joint line. The wire and cuts can be angled slightly distally or proximally if lengthening or shortening of the metatarsal is needed.*
- *The long plantar arm prevents damage to the primary blood supply to the metatarsal head, which is plantar-lateral.*

Pitfalls

- *An osteotomy angle of less than 70° will produce either an excessively long plantar arm or a dorsal arm that does not leave sufficient bone for the compression screw.*
- *Avoid damaging the vascular leash that runs in the first metatarsal space by gently cutting through the lateral cortex.*

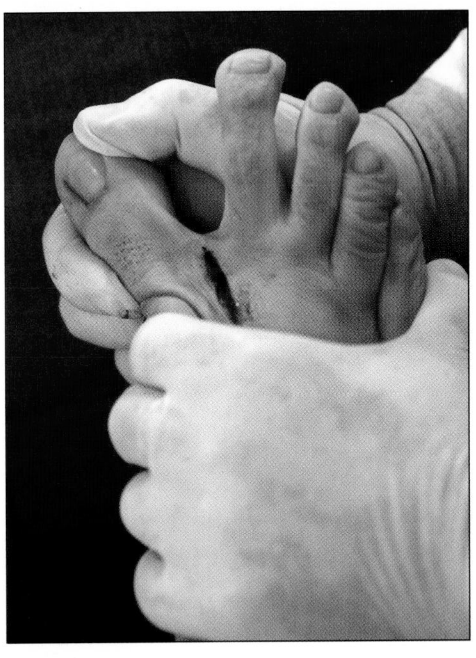

FIGURE 15

- At this point the lateral sesamoid should easily reduce when the first and second metatarsals are compressed together.

STEP 6

- With a marking pen, outline a V-shaped chevron osteotomy in the metatarsal head (Fig. 16A and 16B). The apex should be at least 1 cm proximal to the joint line. The plantar limb of the osteotomy is approximately twice the length of the short dorsal limb. The apex of the chevron is just dorsal to the longitudinal axis of the metatarsal.

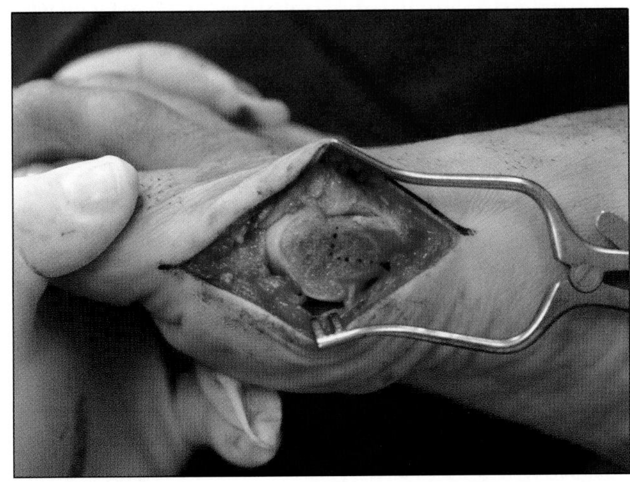

A

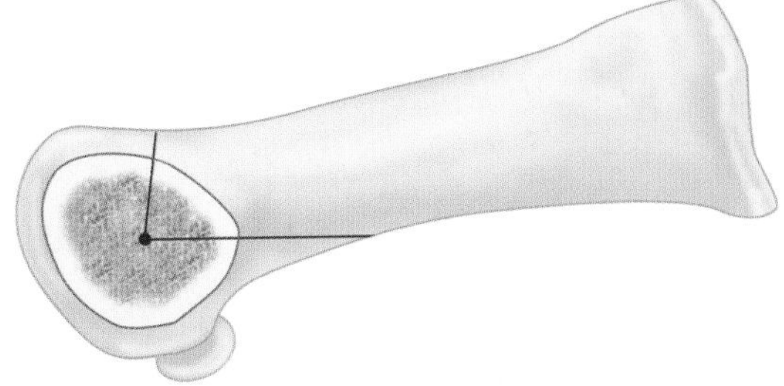

B

FIGURE 16

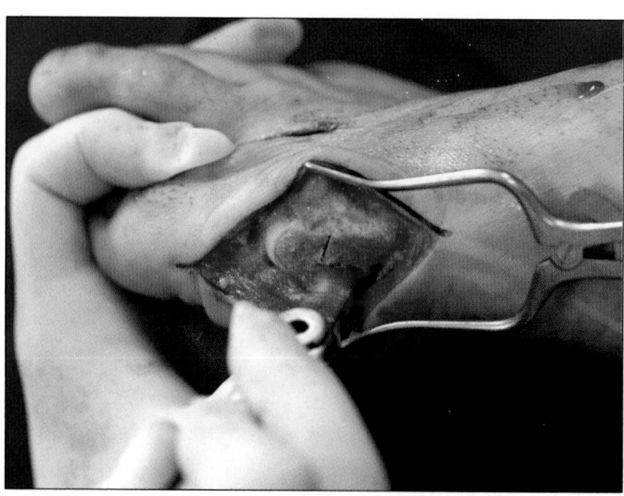

FIGURE 17

- The angle is between 70 and 80°. Under cool saline irrigation, use the micro-sagittal saw to cut through the head.
- The plantar arm should exit proximal to the sesamoid articulation (Fig. 17).
- Great care should be taken to protect the extensor hallucis longus and the dorsal and plantar sensory nerves.

Step 7

- The metatarsal head is stabilized while the metatarsal shaft is pulled medially with a small towel clip (Fig. 18A and 18B).
- The head can be displaced 5–10 mm, depending on the width of the metatarsal head.
- The micro-saggital saw may have to be reintroduced into the wound to cut small bony bridges that are preventing displacement of the head.
- If the DMAA is high, a small (1–3 mm) oblique wedge should be excised from the distal aspect of the dorsal metatarsal, prior to impacting the two pieces.

Step 8

- A 0.045-inch guide pin from the Acutrak 2 self-drilling cannulated screw set is placed across the osteotomy from dorsal-medial to plantar-lateral (Fig. 19). The pin should extend to, but not beyond, the articular surface. Measure the screw length using a depth gauge. The actual screw used is usually 2–4 mm shorter, to avoid penetration of the joint as the bone pieces compress.
- Check the pin and metatarsal head position by fluoroscan.

Pearls

- *The metatarsal head can be displaced up to one half of its width without the risk of an unstable construct. The exact amount of displacement, therefore, depends on the width of the head. A smaller head may only tolerate 3 mm of displacement, while the larger head of a man may be displaced up to a centimeter.*

Pitfalls

- *Avoid excessive pressure on the metatarsal head. The osteotomy can fracture into the joint through the apex of the cut.*

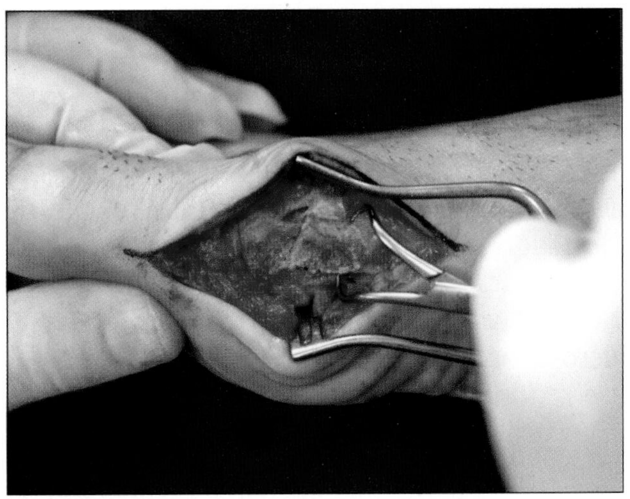

A

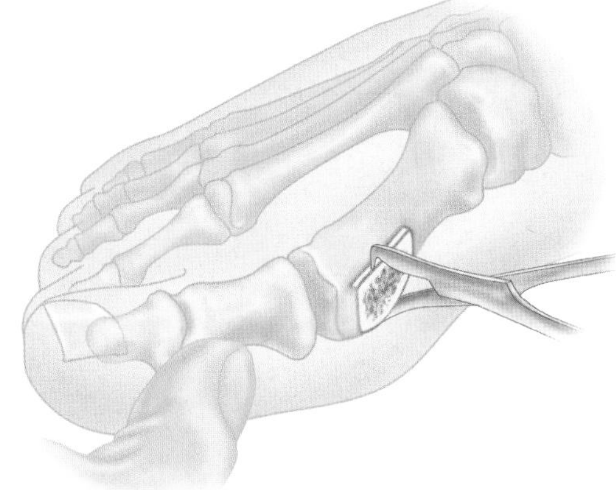

B

FIGURE 18

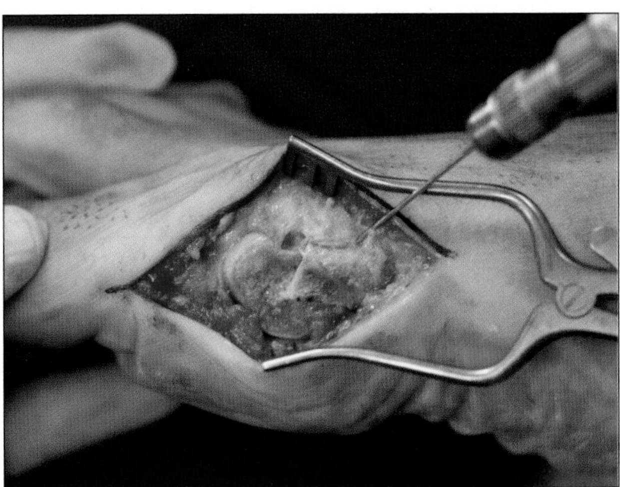

FIGURE 19

PEARLS

- *Before using the cannulated depth gauge, always inspect the joint to make sure that the pin does not breach the articular surface. Because of the curvature of the metatarsal head, the pin may appear to be in the correct position by fluoroscan, while actually penetrating into the joint (Fig. 20).*
- *Before placing the screw, make sure the metatarsal articular surface is not in a valgus position, which can occur because of an uncorrected DMAA, a poorly directed osteotomy, or lateral impaction.*

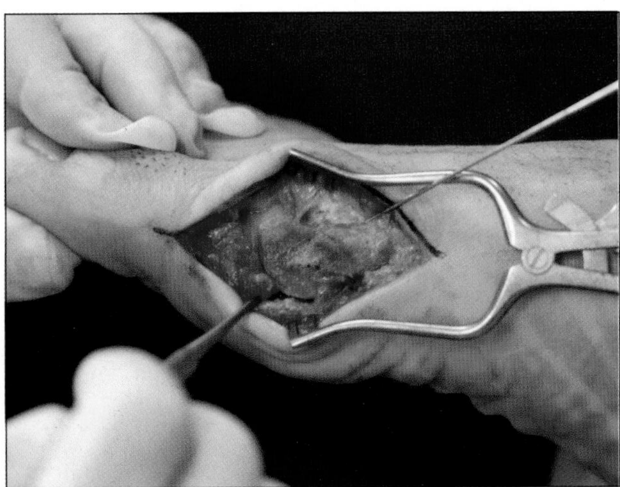

FIGURE 20

Step 9

- Drill *only* the hard dorsal cortex of the metatarsal. No further drilling is required for the self-drilling/tapping Acutrak screw system. Place an appropriately sized miniscrew (Fig. 21A and 21B and Fig. 22). Holding the osteotomy closed with a small towel clip during introduction of the screw will help obtain maximal compression.
- Smooth down the prominent medial metatarsal with a micro-reciprocating rasp (Fig. 23A and 23B).
- Excise redundant portions of the joint capsule (Fig. 24). Vertical cuts in the capsule, just proximal to the joint line, are used to tighten the capsule (Fig. 25A and 25B). Use an absorbable 2–0 suture. Derotate the toe out of pronation while the capsule is repaired. Place the joint through a range of motion.

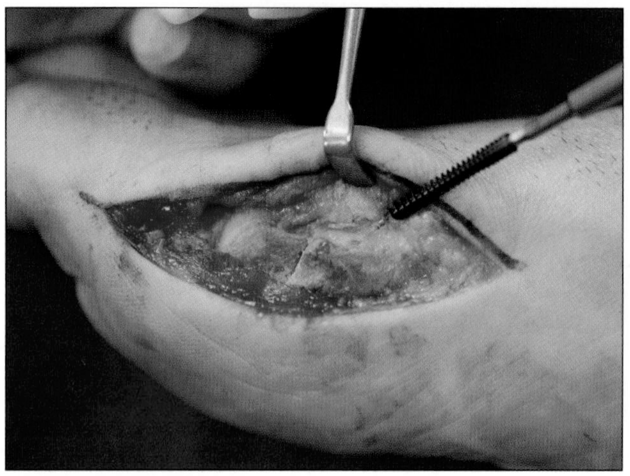

A

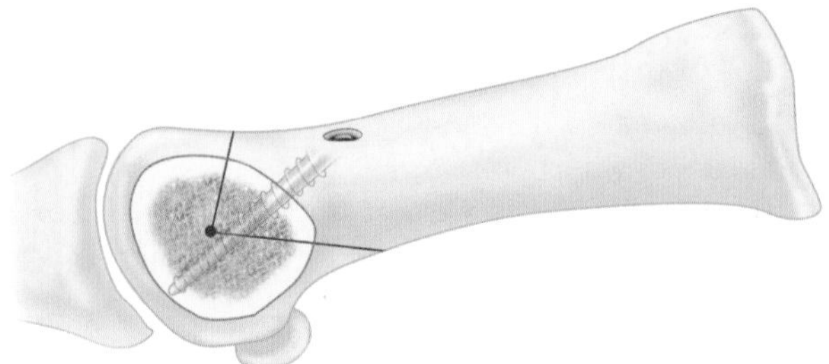

B

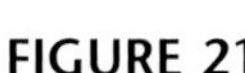

FIGURE 21

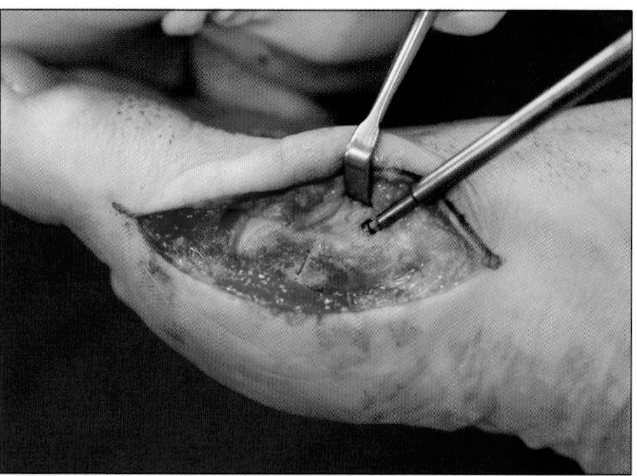

FIGURE 22

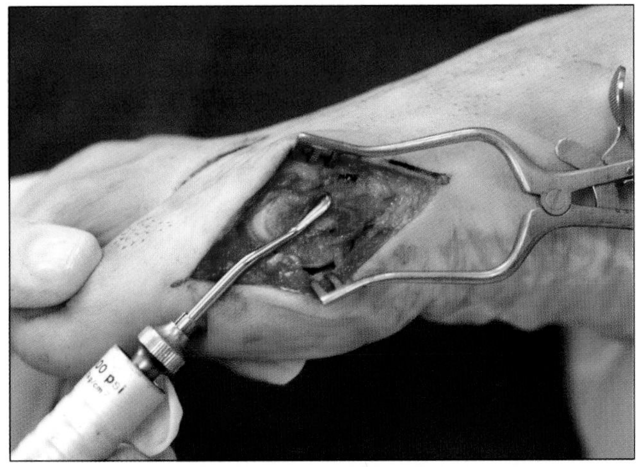

A

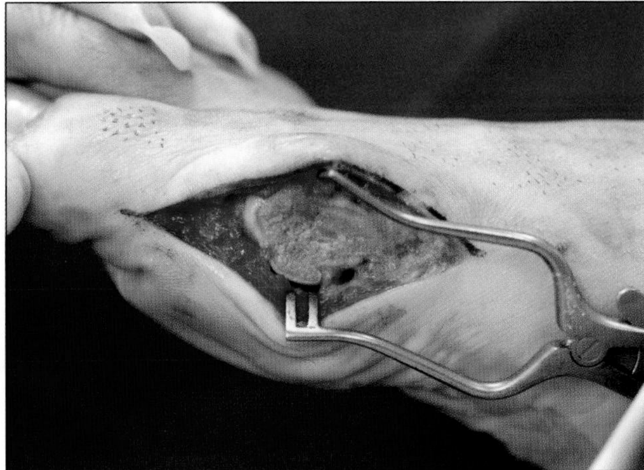

B

FIGURE 23

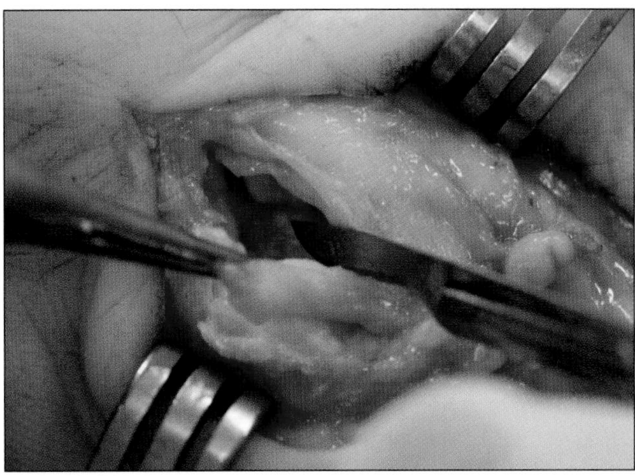

FIGURE 24

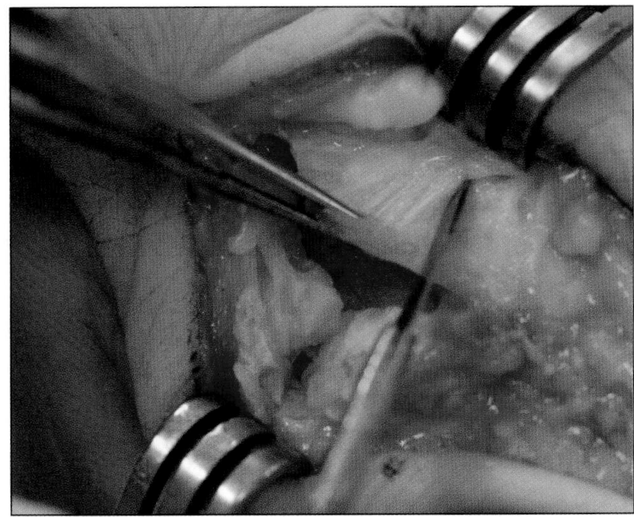

A

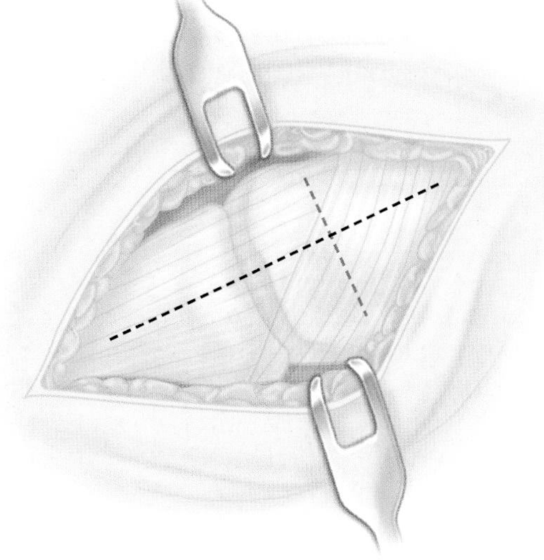

B

FIGURE 25

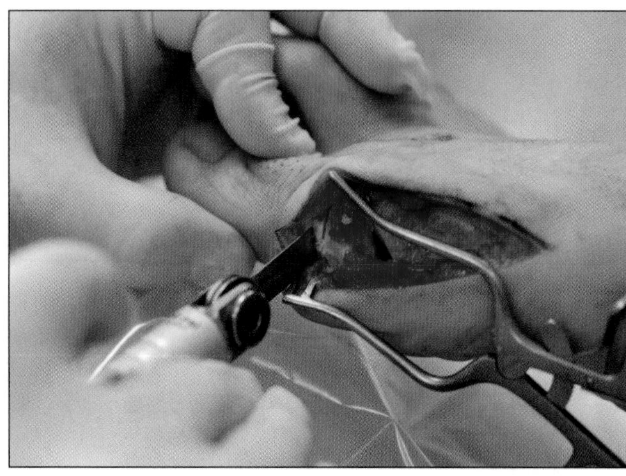

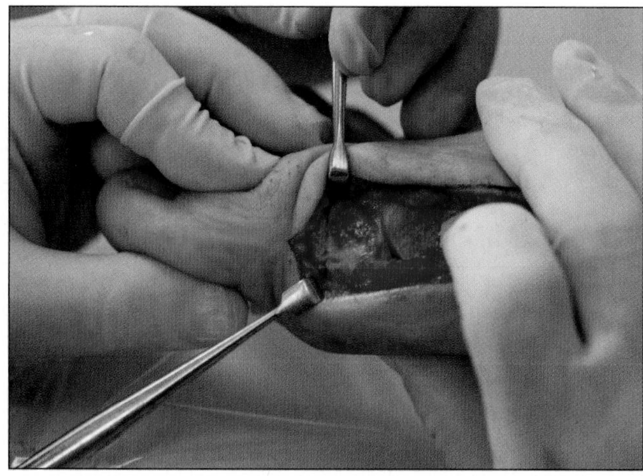

A B

FIGURE 26

- Release the tourniquet. Obtain meticulous hemostasis and close the skin with interrupted 3–0 nylon sutures.
- Apply a bunion spica splint, holding the toe in a slightly overcorrected position.

PEARLS

- *If hallux interphalangeus causes the great toe to impinge on the second toe, a closing wedge osteotomy of the proximal phalanx may be added (Fig. 26A and 26B). Keep the lateral cortex intact and only remove 1–2 mm of bone. Fix the osteotomy with a small screw or Kirschner wire.*

PITFALLS

- *Inadequate bony correction may lead a surgeon to overtighten the medial capsule, in an effort to bring the toe out of valgus. This can cause postoperative stiffness of the joint.*

Controversies

- Various capsular incisions are possible, including L-shaped with dorsal or plantar cuts, or Y-cuts. No capsular incision has been shown to be superior.

Postoperative Care and Expected Outcomes

- The patient remains non–weight bearing until the first clinic visit, 10–12 days postoperatively. At that time the sutures are removed and a spica wrap of Kling and Coban is applied, with slight abduction and supination of the toe (Fig. 27). AP and lateral radiographs in the dressing confirm the position. At this point the patient can use a postoperative shoe or cast boot to start weight bearing as tolerated. The superb fixation of the osteotomy allows early weight bearing.
- The patient starts range of motion (ROM) of the toe within the toe spica dressing.
- Every 7–10 days the dressing is changed. The radiographs are repeated at the third postoperative visit. The patient is allowed to apply an Ace bandage spica starting 4 weeks after surgery. If the toe is stiff, which is unusual, physical therapy can be started at this point.
- A shoe with a wide toe box is used at 6–10 weeks postoperatively, with regular shoes used after that point. The patient should use a spacer (silicone or cotton) in the first web space until 3 months after surgery. AP (Fig. 28A) and lateral (Fig. 28B) radiographs confirm an appropriate correction and healing of the osteotomy.

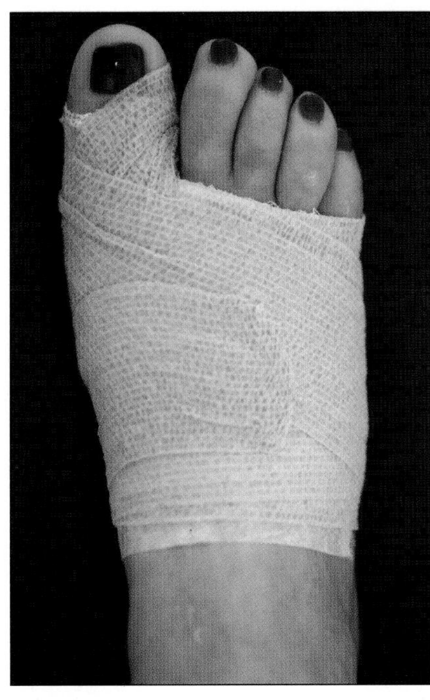

FIGURE 27

> **PEARLS**
>
> - *The rigid fixation obtained by the Acutrak screw allows early ROM, and markedly diminishes postoperative pain and swelling, compared to procedures that do not use rigid internal fixation.*

- Some recurrence of hallux valgus may occur, depending on the patient's ultimate postoperative shoewear. Hallux varus, avascular necrosis of the metatarsal head, and malunion are also known complications. Patients who have mild arthritic changes in the joint may also experience some chronic discomfort. These problems are unusual,

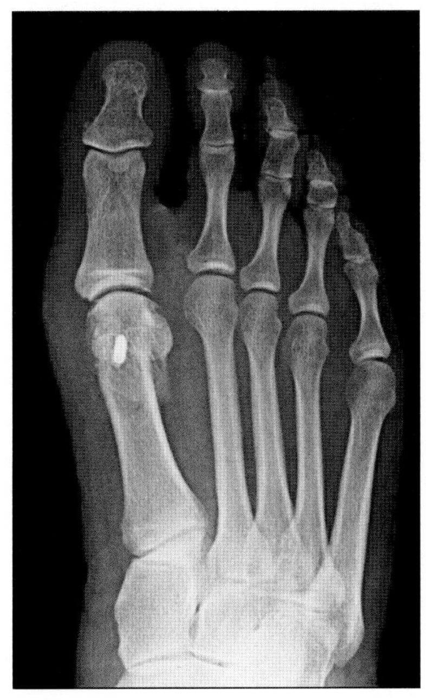

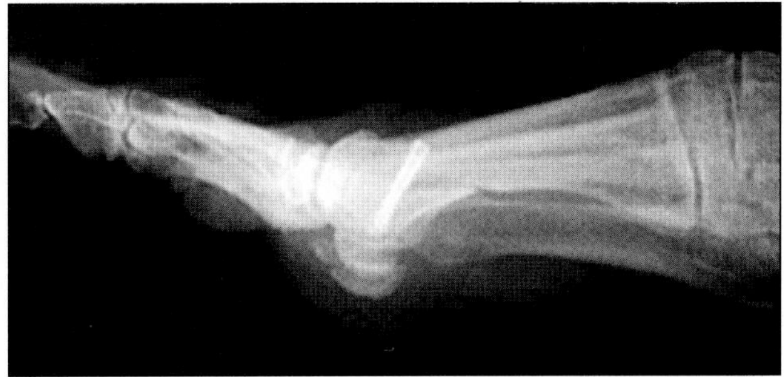

A B

FIGURE 28

however, with the vast majority of patients reporting long-term satisfaction. Persistent swelling and joint stiffness are probably the two most common complaints. Early ROM helps avoid both of these problems.

Evidence

Lin I, Bonar SK, Anderson RB, et al. Distal soft tissue release using direct and indirect approaches: an anatomic study. Foot Ankle Int. 1996;17:458–63.

(Level IV evidence)

Malal JJG, Shaw-Dunn J, Kumar CS. Blood supply to the first metatarsal head and vessels at risk with a chevron osteotomy. J Bone Joint Surg [Am]. 2007;89:2018–22.

This study confirms that a chevron with a long plantar limb will diminish risk of injury to the major blood supply to the head, which is plantar-lateral.

Mitchell LA, Baxter DE. A chevron-Aiken double osteotomy for correction of hallux valgus. Foot Ankle. 1991;12:7–14.

A series of patients with hallux valgus and concomitant hallux interphalangeus. (Level IV evidence)

Nery C, Barroco R, Ressio C. Biplanar chevron osteotomy. Foot Ankle Int. 2002;9:792–8.

Thirty-two patients with a DMAA of greater than 8° had a biplanar chevron osteotomy. The hallux valgus angle was improved from an average of 25° to 14°, the IMA from 12° to 8°, and the DMAA from 15° to 5°. (Level IV evidence)

Trnka HJ, Zembsch A, Easley ME, et al. The chevron osteotomy for correction of hallux valgus: comparison of findings after two and five years of follow-up. J Bone Joint Surg [Am]. 2000;82:1373–8.

This study followed 66 feet for 5 years after a chevron correction for hallux valgus. Between the 2-year and 5-year follow-up evaluations, there was only a minimal change in overall patient satisfaction, and the average score on the hallux-metatarsophalangeal-interphalangeal scale was unchanged. (Level IV evidence)

PROCEDURE 2

Scarf Osteotomy for Correction of Hallux Valgus

Hans-Peter Kundert

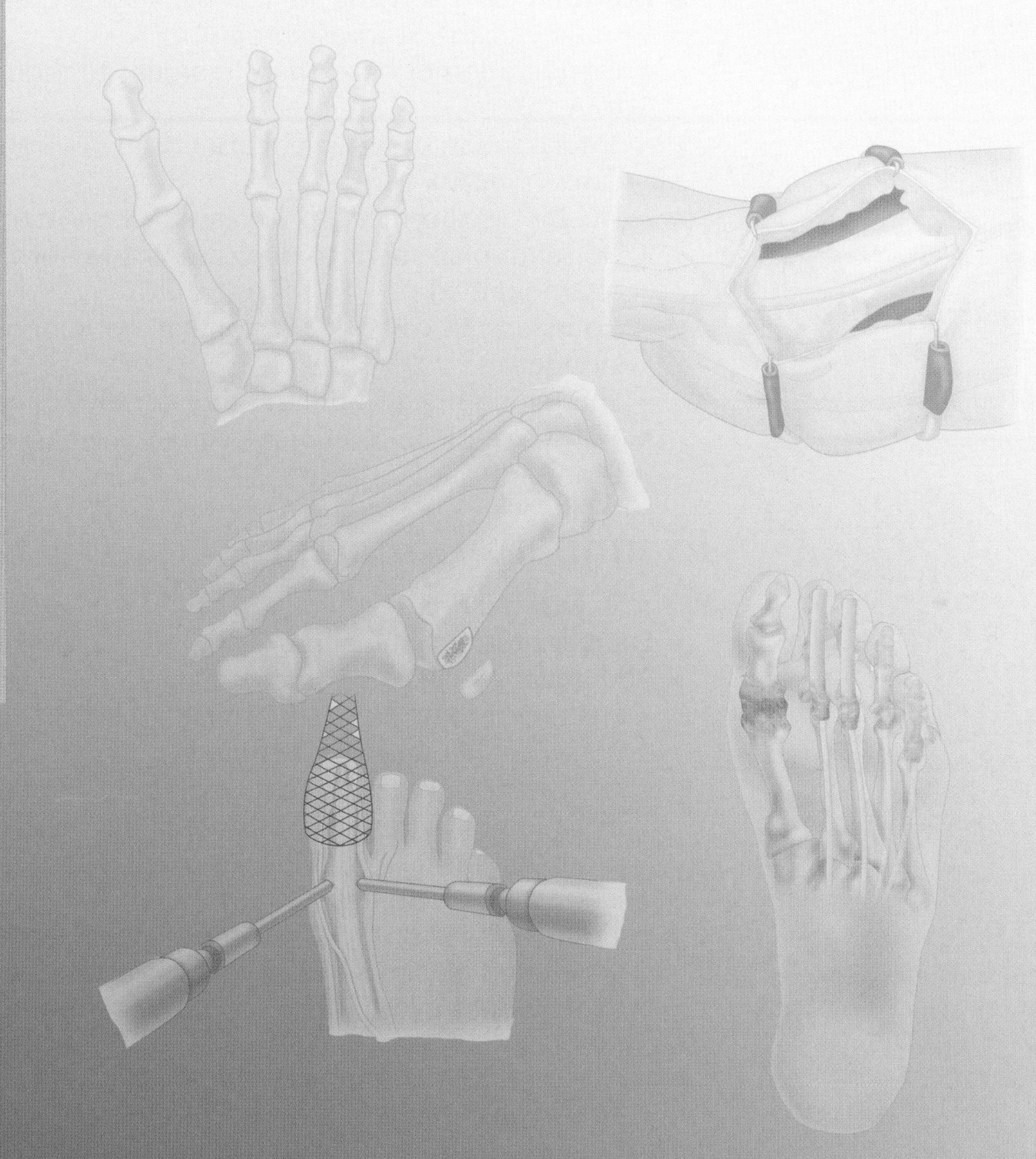

Indications

- Objective indications
  - Mild to moderate hallux valgus deformities with
    - Increased hallux valgus angle (HVA) up to 40°
    - Increased intermetatarsal angle (IMA) up to 20°
    - Increased distal metatarsal articular angle (DMAA) up to 10°
  - Bunionette deformity of fifth metatarsal (type 3, increased fourth-fifth IMA)
- **Modular corrections** are feasible via the great versatility of the Scarf osteotomy.
  - Lateralization of head-shaft fragment to reduce IMA
  - Medialization of first metatarsal head (1MTH) in cases of hallux varus
  - Plantar displacement to increase first ray load
  - Dorsal displacement to decrease first ray or sesamoid load
  - Elongation in cases of short metatarsal (congenital, iatrogenic)
  - Shortening in cases of long metatarsal
  - Transverse plane rotation to correct increased DMAA

Pitfalls

- *Severe hallux valgus deformity (HVA > 40°)*
- *Increased lateral slope of the distal metatarsal articular surface (DMAA > 10°)*
- *Hypermobile first tarsometatarsal joint (ligamentous laxity)*
- *Range of motion of first metatarsophalangeal (1MTP) joint less than 50°*
- *Symptomatic osteoarthritis of 1MTP joint*
- *Damage to cartilage of more than 60% of 1MTH*
- *Bad bone density (severe osteoporosis)*
- *Rheumatoid arthritis*

Controversies

- Other techniques exist for operative correction of mild to moderate hallux valgus deformities (Easley and Trnka, 2007).
  - Distal procedures: modified McBride distal soft tissue procedure, chevron osteotomy, resection arthroplasty
  - Proximal procedures: crescentic metatarsal osteotomy, Ludloff oblique osteotomy, closing wedge proximal osteotomy
  - Combined procedures: double/triple osteotomies

Examination/Imaging

Physical Examination

- Standard foot examination
- Additional specific assessment
  - Posture of foot, presence of plantar callosities, bursal or skin irritation at bunion
  - Appearance and alignment of great toe (medial deviation of first metatarsal, lateral deviation and pronation of hallux), evidence of splay foot and lesser toe deformities
  - Tightness of gastrocnemius-soleus (assessed with flexed and extended knee, foot maintained with talonavicular joint reduced to eliminate transverse tarsal or subtarsal motion)
  - Palpation and range of motion (active and passive) of hindfoot, midfoot, and forefoot joints
  - Clinical assessment of first ray hypermobility
  - Pedobarography or podoscopy

Radiographic Assessment

- Weight-bearing standard radiographs of both feet: anteroposterior (Fig. 1) and lateral views

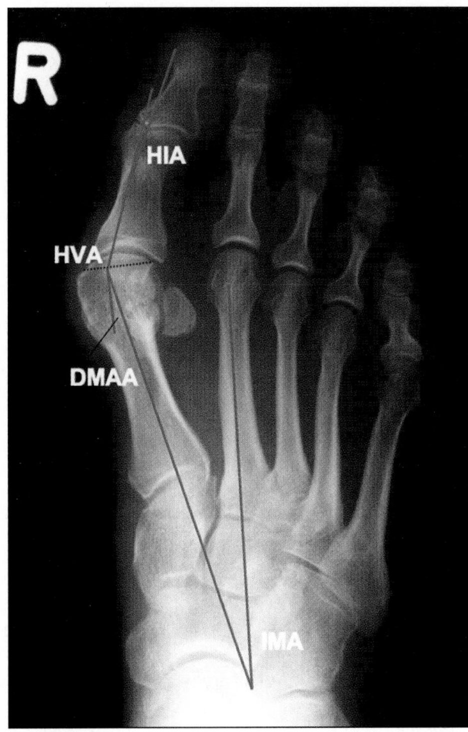

FIGURE 1

- Check associated problems to be corrected (Coughlin and Jones, 2007):
  - HVA, IMA, and DMAA
  - Hallux interphalangeal angle (HIA)
  - Articular shape (curved, chevron, or flat) and congruency of the 1MTP joint
  - Metatarsal index (length of first metatarsal in comparison to second metatarsal)
  - Evidence of pes planus (talonavicular coverage, calcaneal pitch angle, lateral talocalcaneal angle, talus–first metatarsal angle)

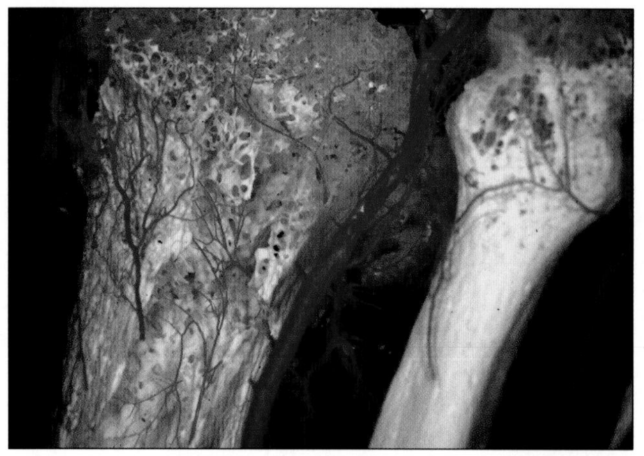
A

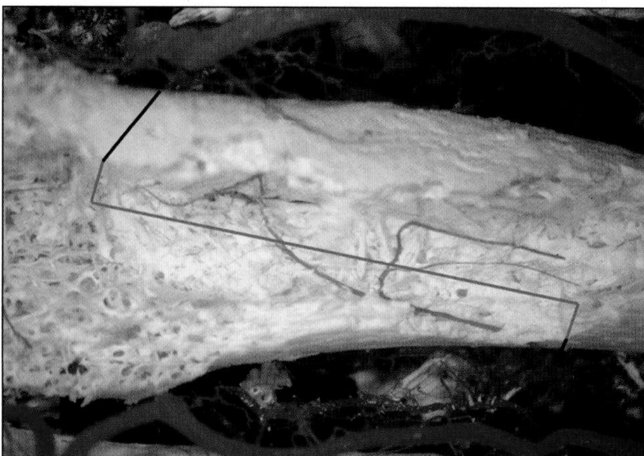
B

FIGURE 2

Surgical Anatomy

- Vascular network around first metatarsal and 1MTP joint (Fig. 2A and 2B)
  - Dorsal and plantar metatarsal artery
  - Superficial branch of the medial plantar artery
  - Extensive network on the dorsal and lateral capsular aspects
- Dorsal and plantar sensory nerve branches around first metatarsal
- Deep common nerve in first web space
- Lateral soft tissues to be released
  - Lateral suspensory and anterior fibular sesamoid ligaments
  - Adductor hallucis tendon
  - 1MTP joint capsule
  - First transverse intermetatarsal ligament

PEARLS

- *Exsanguination can be accomplished with a sterile rubber bandage that is left in the supramalleolar region, serving as an Esmarch-type ankle tourniquet (Fig. 3).*

Positioning

- Supine position
- Heel at the edge of table
- Standardized prepping and draping of the foot
- Tourniquet at the ipsilateral thigh

PEARLS

- *To perform an additional Akin osteotomy (proximal phalangeal variation of the great toe), the incision starts at the first interphalangeal joint.*

Portals/Exposures

- Make a medial longitudinal incision across the 1MTP joint, running from the proximal half of the proximal phalanx to the proximal part of the first metatarsal (Fig. 4).
- Expose the capsular structures, paying attention not to injure the plantar and dorsal sensory nerve branches (Fig. 5A and 5B).

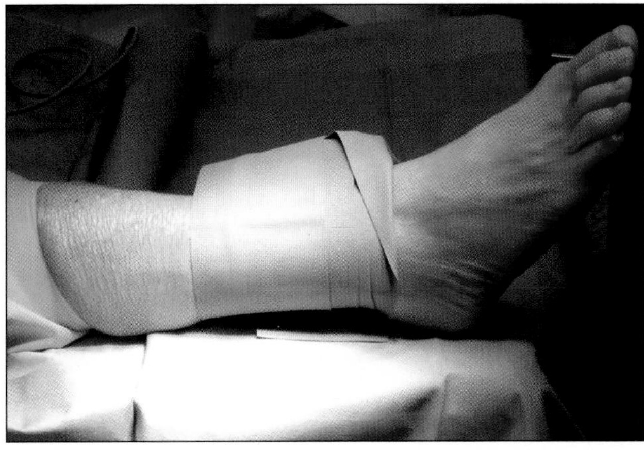

FIGURE 3

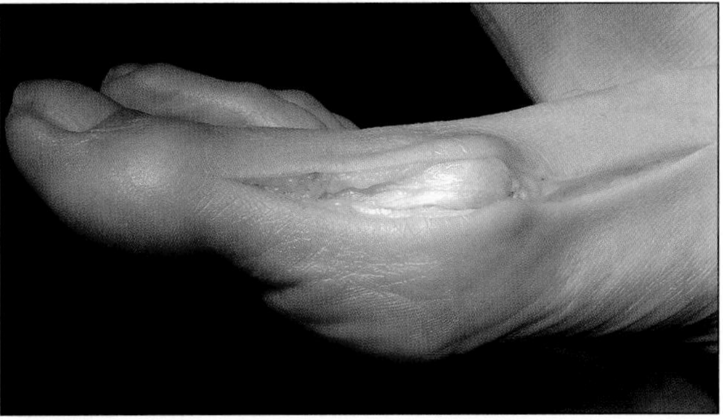

FIGURE 4

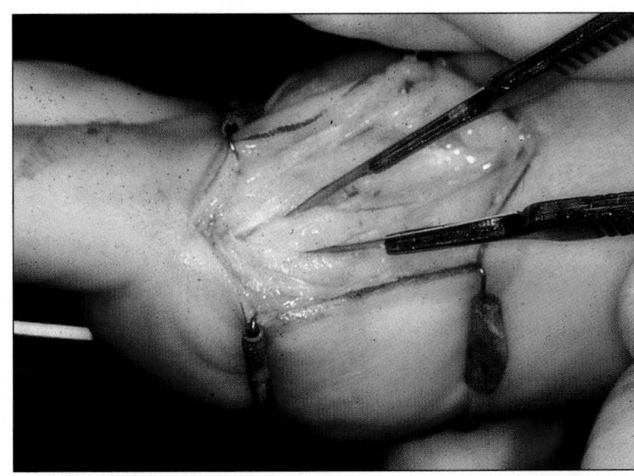

A

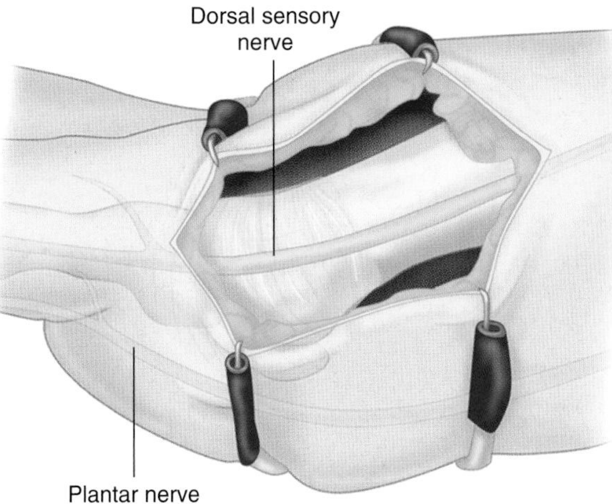

B

FIGURE 5

Pitfalls

- *When exposing the first metatarsal, even by blunt dissection, avoid detaching the dorsal and plantar neurovascular bundles in order to preserve blood supply to the 1MTH (i.e., to the distal fragment of the osteotomy).*

Instrumentation/ Implantation

- Flexible skin hooks facilitate exposure of soft tissues.

Pearls

- *Preliminary resection of the 1MTH bunion facilitates the correct positioning of the starting point of the Z-osteotomy.*

Procedure

Step 1

- The capsule of the 1MTP joint is incised longitudinally, removing a small ellipse of capsule, while taking care not to injure the dorsal and plantar sensory nerve branches (Fig. 6).
- The capsule and periosteum are reflected dorsally along the medial aspect of the base of the first phalanx, 1MTH, and shaft.
- Inspection of 1MTH cartilage is essential to the surgeon's decision to continue with a Scarf procedure. A great toe with an intraoperatively assessed level of damage to more than 60% of the cartilage at the 1MTH does not respond well to this joint-preserving type of osteotomy (Fuhrmann et al., 2009).

Step 2

- The Z-osteotomy is marked (Fig. 7).
- Place a 0.045-inch Kirschner guidewire at the upper one third of the medial surface of the 1MTH in a lateral direction and plantar declination of about 15°, aiming just slightly plantar to the fifth metatarsal head (Fig. 8A and 8B).
- The proper position of this guide pin is essential to formulate the displacement of the metatarsal head and shaft.
  - Directing the pin slightly proximally causes a small shortening.
  - Directing the pin less plantarward does not provide the desirable plantar displacement (offset of elevation) of the first metatarsal to decrease the postoperative load under the second metatarsal.

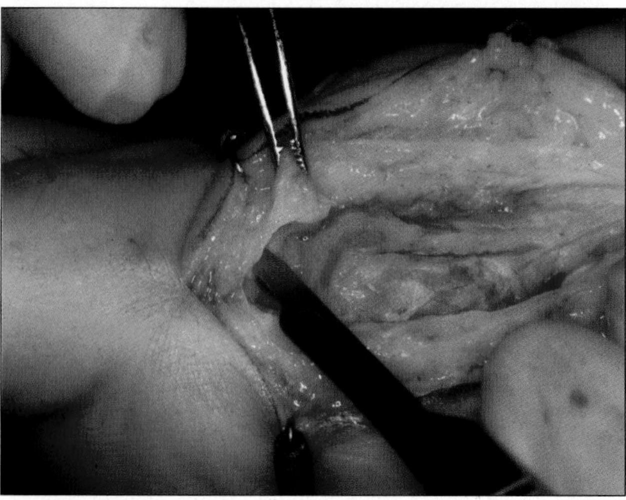

FIGURE 6

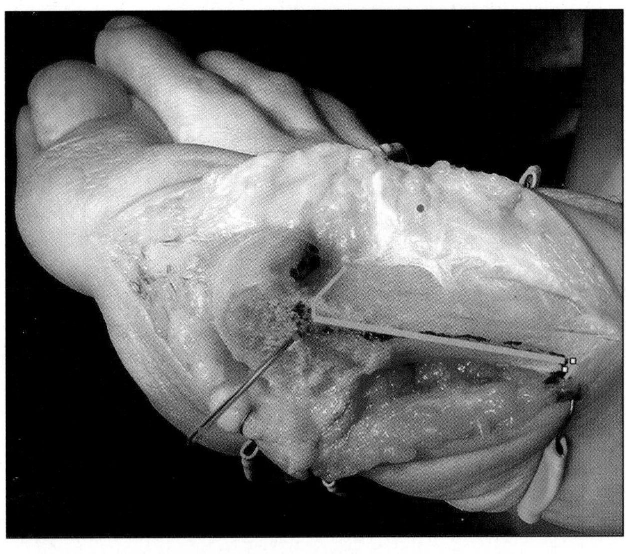

FIGURE 7

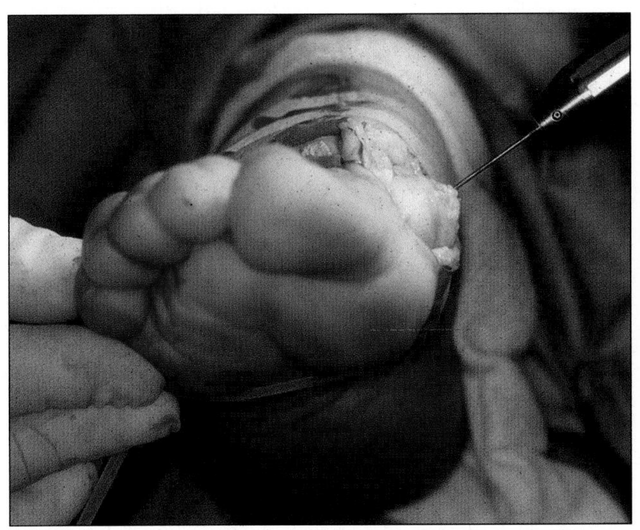

A

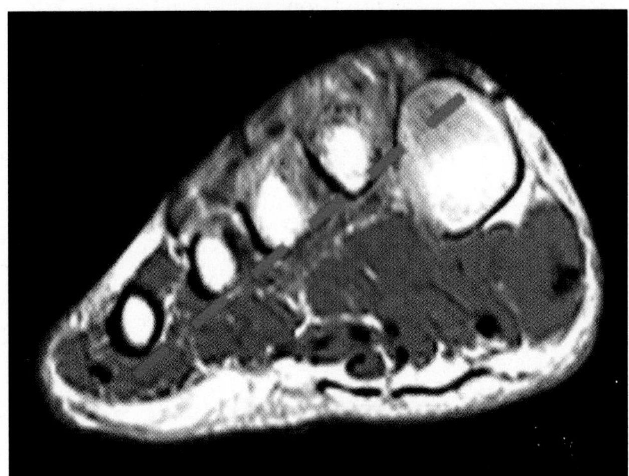

B

FIGURE 8

Pearls

- *Pulling the 1MTH toward medial, using a bone hook, helps to improve visualization and to assess tension of the structures to be released (Fig. 9).*

Pitfalls

- *Identify and protect the underlying common digital nerve when dissecting the intermetatarsal ligament.*
- *Avoid dissection of the oblique head of the adductor tendon, as this may inadvertently injure the lateral head of the FHB tendon.*

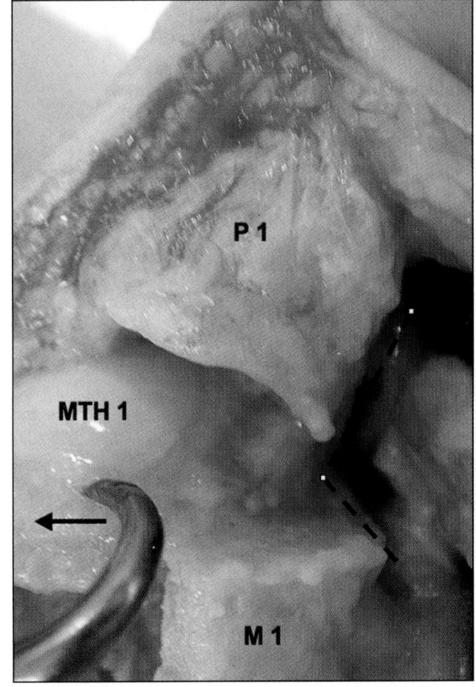

FIGURE 9

Controversies

- A transarticular release of the lateral sesamoid suspensory and anterior fibular sesamoid ligaments has been proposed (Stamatis et al., 2004; Weil, 2000), placing a self-retaining retractor between the medial plantar capsule and 1MTH and using a curved arthroscopic blade (Fig. 10). Using this technique, care should be taken to avoid additional damage to the cartilage. To enhance visualization of the lateral soft tissue structures to be released, detach the joint capsule dorsally from the base of the proximal phalanx, exerting a subluxation and slight axial traction of the great toe.
- In advanced deformities, the lateral release probably cannot be done adequately via the transarticular approach (Fuhrmann et al., 2009).

Pearls

- *Distal and proximal vertical cuts (1 and 3) of the Z-osteotomy should be limited to 2–3 mm in depth, to avoid cutting into the cancellous part of the metatarsal, thus limiting the risk of "troughing" or proximal stress fractures.*
- *Traction on the hallux during the final proximal cut facilitates its completion.*

Pitfalls

- *As the longitudinal cut is made through the shaft in a lateral direction, careful attention is paid to avoid burying the saw blade into the intermetatarsal space, thus preserving the vital structures in this area.*

Step 3

- Lateral soft tissue release is necessary for complete repositioning of the metatarsal head over the sesamoids.
  - Accomplished through the same medial incision
  - Dissection of the lateral sesamoid suspensory and anterior fibular sesamoid ligaments
  - Release of the adductor hallucis longus tendon at the insertion on the proximal phalangeal base and at the margin of the lateral sesamoid, preserving the most plantar fibers of the flexor hallucis brevis (FHB) tendon
  - Stepwise longitudinal capsular perforation just dorsal to the lateral sesamoid under slight varus stress to the great toe
- In contracted deformities, dissection of the transverse intermetatarsal ligament is necessary to release its tethering effect on the sesamoid complex.

Step 4

- Create the following three cuts (Fig. 11A and 11B):
  - Cut 1—vertical distally, transverse from medial to lateral, about 5 mm proximal to the margin of the dorsal cartilage, using a 7-mm-long narrow sagittal saw blade.
  - Cut 2—longitudinal, inclined from the distal dorsal one fourth to the proximal plantar one fourth of the metatarsal cortex, typically between 25 and 30 mm long, using a 9-mm-long medium sagittal saw blade. The larger the IMA, the longer the horizontal cut.
  - Cut 3—vertical proximally, transverse from medial to lateral, strictly parallel to cut 1, again using the 7-mm-long saw blade. Complete the plantar

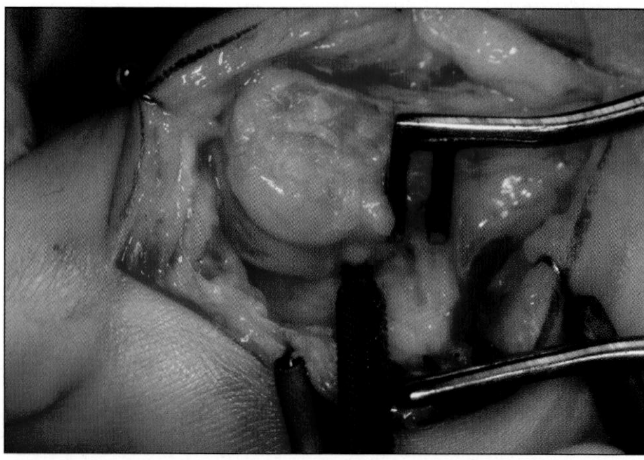

FIGURE 10

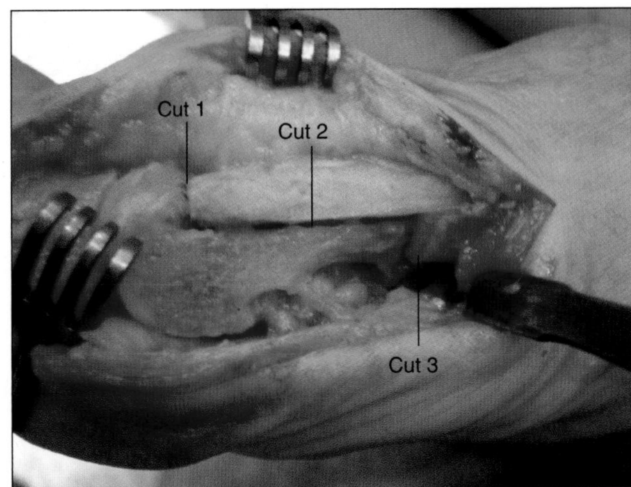

A

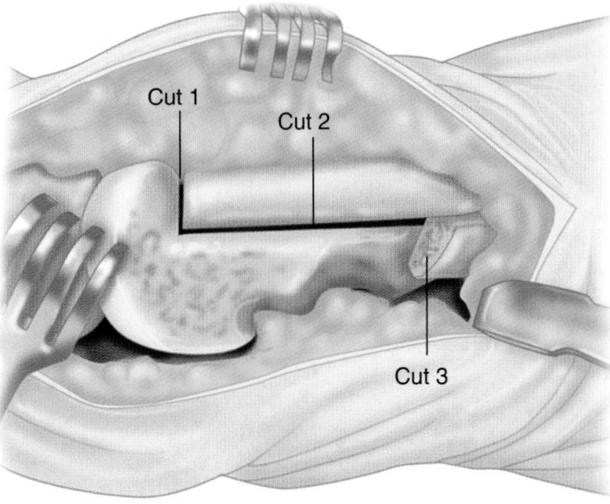

B

FIGURE 11

proximal cut at a 45° angle to form a locking mechanism once the bones are displaced and compressed.

Instrumentation/ Implantation

- Utilizing a Reese guide facilitates maintaining the same plane when performing the three osteotomies (Fig. 12).

Pitfalls

- *In osteoporotic bones, the squeezing effect of a reduction bone clamp may facilitate troughing. In these cases we recommend preliminary fixation with two Kirschner wires.*
- *Visual control of the position of the distal and proximal screws is mandatory as overlength might irritate the sesamoid apparatus or the flexor tendons, respectively.*

Step 5

- The 1MTH and shaft portions of the metatarsal are now mobile.
  - A small clamp is placed distally on the intact shaft and pulled medially by an assistant.
  - The free-floating 1MTH-shaft section is displaced laterally as much as possible until resistance is encountered. Any other corrective movements of the fragments must be applied during this maneuver.
  - Final corrections of the DMAA of up to 10° are feasible by alterating the distal cut, or by pivoting the proximal part of the plantar fragment to the lateral side.

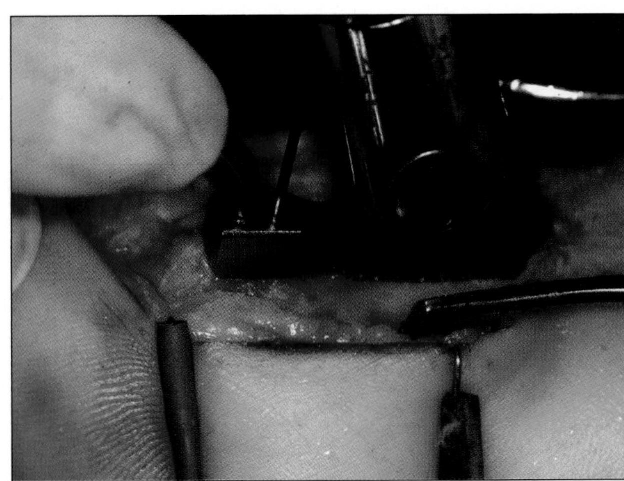

FIGURE 12

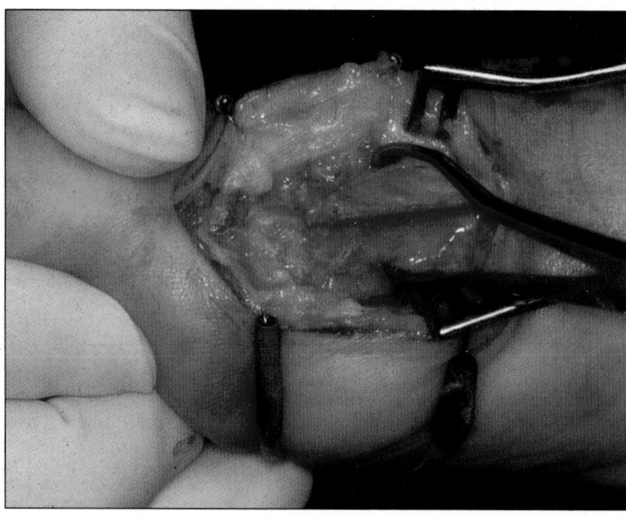

FIGURE 13

- While pushing the hallux in a proximal direction, a reduction bone clamp can be applied for preliminary stabilization of the osteotomy (Fig. 13).

■ The osteotomy is fixated with two screws (Figs. 14 and 15):
- One distally from the dorsomedial aspect into the 1MTH.
- One proximally from the dorsomedial aspect to the plantar lateral aspect.

Instrumentation/ Implantation

- Positioning of the drill holes can be facilitated using an awl to precisely perforate the cortex
- We use cannulated threaded-head BOLD screws (Herbert type) that are flush with the dorsal cortex (see Fig. 14). We advise not using compressive screws to avoid excessive interfragmentary pressure.

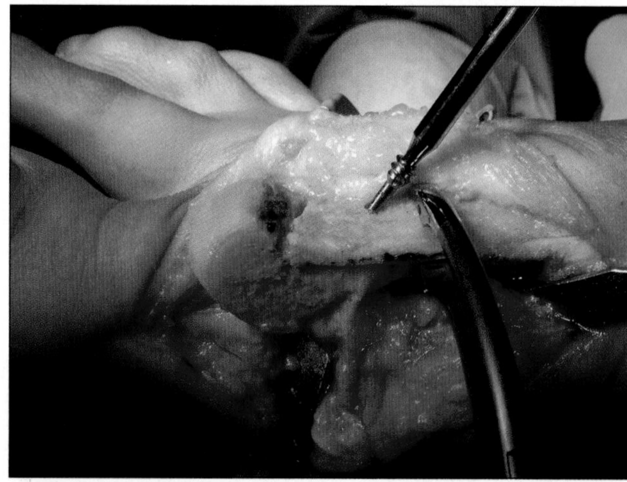

FIGURE 14

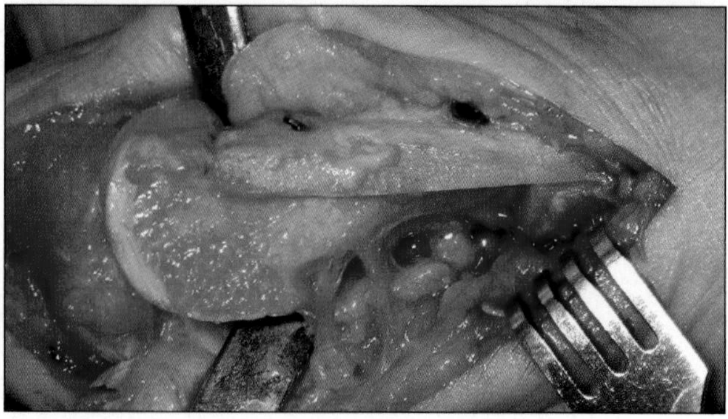

FIGURE 15

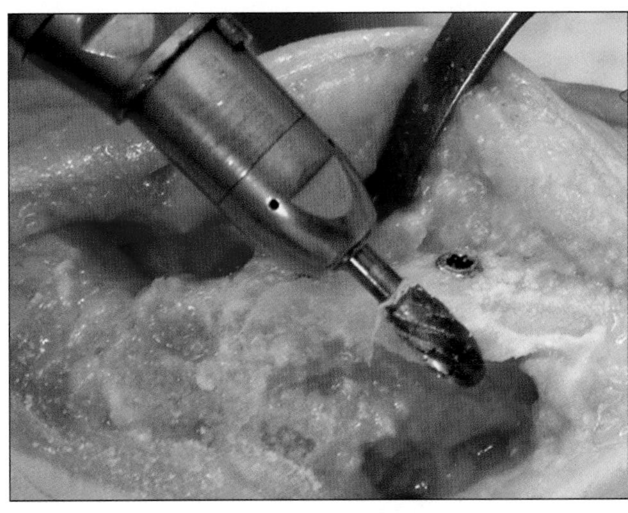

FIGURE 16

- Any redundant bone at the dorsomedial aspect of the 1MTH and shaft is removed and smoothed with a rotary burr (Fig. 16).
- A weight-bearing situation is simulated by applying the surgeon's hand or the lid of an instrument tray under the plantar aspect of the forefoot, with the foot remaining in a neutral position. If there is a remaining contact between the ends of the great toe and the second toe, an additional Akin osteotomy (proximal phalangeal variation of the great toe) is performed.

Pearls

- *In order to assess the tension of the capsular suture, we place a double-folded sponge into the first web space.*

Pitfalls

- *Although tensioning of the repair is important to correct the deformity, it should not cause a postoperative hallux varus. The final bandage should not be an additional attempt at correction.*

Step 6

- Closure and reefing of the joint capsule is accomplished with 2–0 absorbable sutures placed immediately medial to the tibial sesamoid and connected to the dorsal portion of the capsule in a continuous running "shoelace" fashion, producing a true locking effect (Fig. 17A and 17B) (Roukis, 2001).

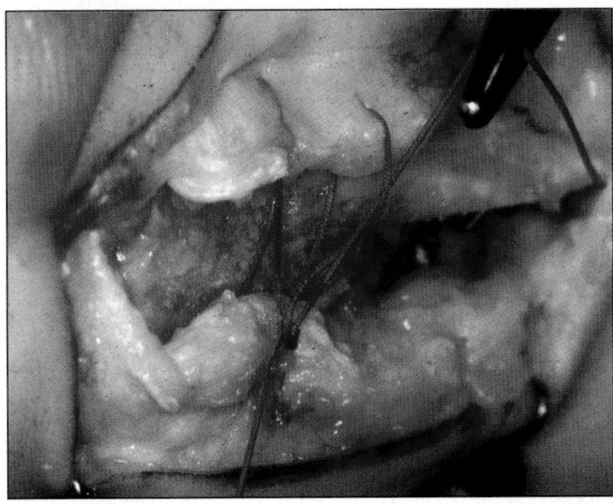

A

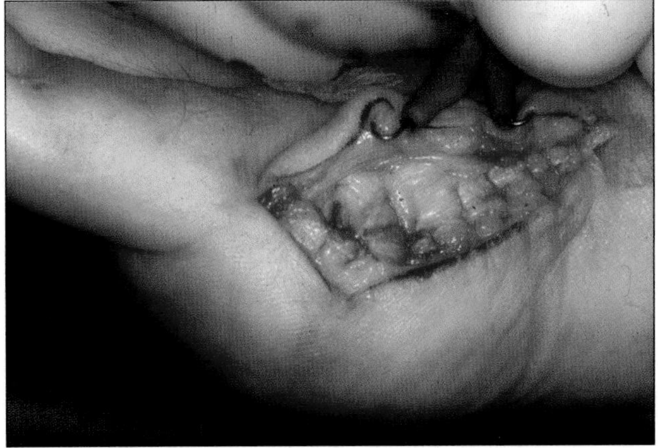

B

FIGURE 17

- After careful hemostasis and extensive irrigation, the wound is closed with 3–0 nonabsorbable sutures (Fig. 18) and augmented with adhesive Steri-Strips. We do not use suction drains regularly. We do not use postoperative local instillation of anesthetics or steroids.
- The forefoot is bandaged with the great toe in slight adduction, and the tourniquet is released (Fig. 19).

Controversies

- Anchor-enhanced capsulorrhaphy may help to prevent early capsular slippage in patients with weakened and overstretched medial capsular tissues (Gould et al., 2003).

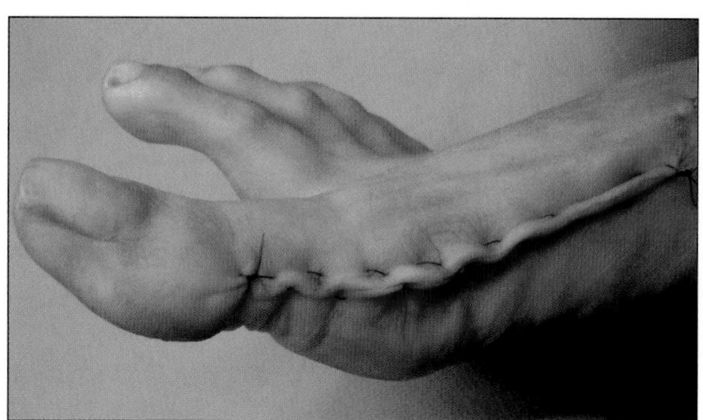

FIGURE 18

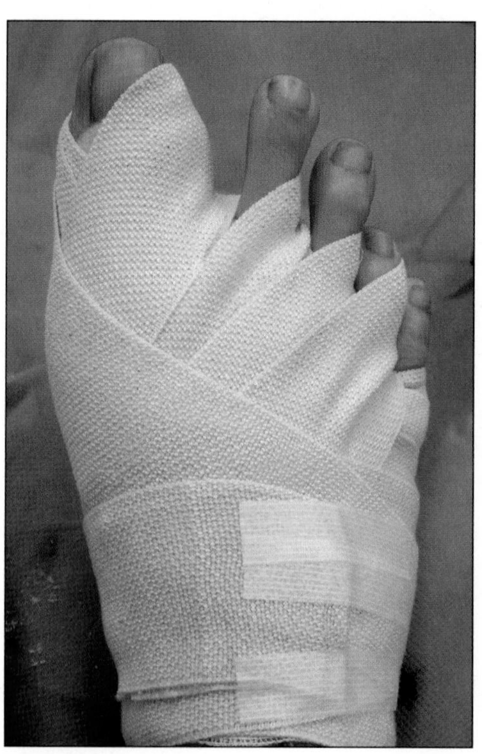

FIGURE 19

PITFALLS

- *Stress fractures proximally: lower the longitudinal cut to avoid.*
- *Troughing (i.e., an impaction of the two osteotomy fragments), resulting in functional elevation with or without rotation of the first ray (Fig. 21): limit the distal and proximal vertical Z-osteotomies to 2–3 mm in depth.*
- *Prominent hardware interfering with sesamoid bones: need to visualize the length of the distal implant.*
- *Avascular osteonecrosis of 1MTH: the vascular network must be preserved.*
- *Postoperative joint stiffness: prolonged postoperative foot rehabilitation is important.*
- *Hallux varus: lateral soft-tissue release and capsular suture must be balanced—do not excise the lateral sesamoid bone.*

Postoperative Care and Expected Outcomes

- The bandage is removed and reapplied daily. Sutures are removed 2 weeks after surgery.
- The patient is allowed to walk fully weight bearing from the beginning, using a forefoot relief shoe for 4 weeks; after that a comfortable walking shoe is recommended for another 4–6 weeks.
- The patient is instructed to increase the duration of walking activities according to the residual amount of pain and swelling.
- Four and 8 weeks following surgery, radiographs are taken to confirm maintenance of fixation and sufficient consolidation of the osteotomy (Fig. 20).
- The patient is instructed to actively exercise the great toe in plantar flexion as well as the hindfoot joints in rotation, and not to supinate the foot too much for rolling-off. Range-of-motion and strengthening exercises are to be continued for a total of 8 weeks.
- It sometimes takes several weeks until the strength and comfort of the great toe is sufficient to off-load the first ray of the foot, and 3–5 months for complete reduction of swelling, maximum range of motion, and recovery of full recreational and athletic activities.

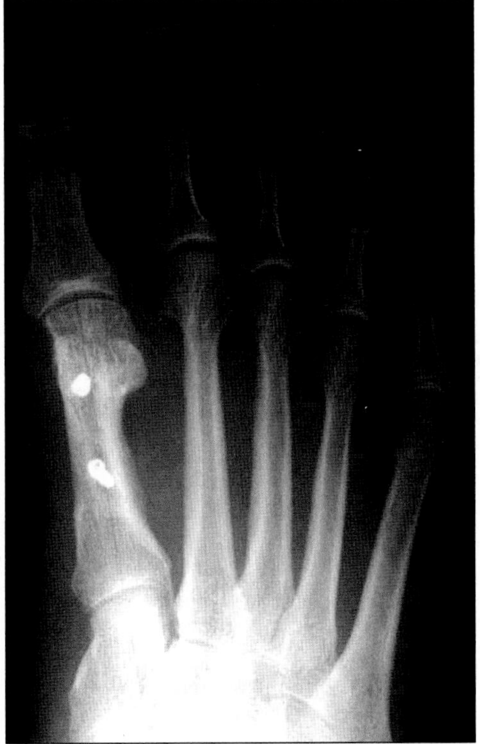

FIGURE 20

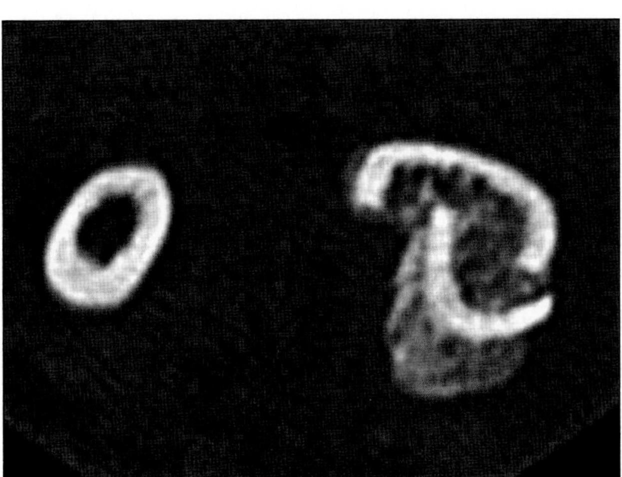

FIGURE 21

Evidence

Coetzee JC. Scarf osteotomy for hallux valgus repair: the dark side. Foot Ankle Int. 2003;24:29–33.

Twenty patients. Multiple potential pitfalls, the most common (35%) is "troughing" of the metatarsal with loss of height. 45% are unsatisfied at one year. (Level IV evidence [case series])

Coughlin MJ, Jones CP. Hallux valgus: demographics, etiology, and radiographic assessment. Foot Ankle Int. 2007;28:759–77.

A most comprehensive evaluation of physical examination and radiographic data, important for decision-making in bunion surgery, based on a postoperative follow-up study in 103 patients. (Level V evidence [expert opinion])

Deenik A, van Mammeren H, de Visser E, de Waal Malefijt M, Draijer F, de Bie R. Equivalent correction in Scarf and Chevron osteotomy in moderate and severe hallux valgus: a randomized controlled trial. Foot Ankle Int. 2009;29:1209–15.

136 feet, 66 scarf and 70 chevron osteotomies, classified as mild, moderate and severe according to IMA. Chevron osteotomy is at least as effective as Scarf osteotomy in correction of HVA and IMA. Scarf seems to have a higher incidence of CRPS, Chevron a higher incidence of avascular necrosis. There is no significant difference in secondary 1 MTP joint subluxation (19%) between the two groups. (Level I evidence [prospective randomized study])

Easley ME, Trnka HJ. Current concepts review: hallux valgus part II: operative treatment. Foot Ankle Int. 2007;28:748–58.

Overview of distal (simple bunionectomy, distal soft-tissue procedure, chevron osteotomy, Keller resection arthroplasty) and proximal first metatarsal procedures (crescentic osteotomy, proximal chevron osteotomy, opening and closing wedge osteotomies, Ludloff oblique osteotomy), Scarf osteotomy, first TMT joint arthrodesis, double/triple osteotomies and first MTP joint arthrodesis). Clinical, radiographic and biomechanical aspects are discussed. Levels of evidence and grades of recommendation are assessed, based on published articles on these different procedures. (Level V evidence [expert opinion])

Fuhrmann RA, Zollinger-Kies H, Kundert H-P. Long-term results of Scarf osteotomy in hallux valgus. Int Orthop. (submitted April 2009).

Multicenter study on 178 scarf osteotomies. At follow-up (mean 44.9 months) only 55% of the 1MTP joints were perfectly aligned. Patients with a HV angle exceeding 30° preoperatively presented with worse results compared to those with less than 30°. Range of 1MTP joint motion worsened in more than 20%, attributed to medial capsular tightening and inadequate joint congruity. Deterioration of obvious preoperative degenerative signs is possibly procedure-related, for which reason damage to the vascular network must be avoided when preparing the distal osteotomy region. Recurrency of hallux valgus deformity seems to be related to the underlying soft-tissue imbalance in splayfoot, rather than to inadequate intraoperative lateral release or to other deficiencies of the Scarf technique. (Level IV evidence [case series])

Gould LS, Ali S, Fowler R, Fleisig GS. Anchor enhanced capsulorrhaphy in bunionectomies using an L-shaped capsulotomy. Foot Ankle Int. 2003;24:61–6.

106 cases of proximal concentric shelf osteotomies/modified McBride procedures and Chevron procedures, performing the capsulorrhaphy with and wihout anchors. When comparing the correction of HV and IM angles, enhanced capsulorrhaphy seems to play a significant role in maintaining the surgical correction by preventing early capsular slippage. (Level IV evidence [case series])

Roukis TS. Unassisted locking-suture technique for bunionectomy capsular closure. J Foot Ankle Surg. 2001;40:116–7.

Description of a suture technique which maintains the original capsular apposition and ensures the strength of the closure. (Level V evidence [expert opinion, technique tip])

Stamatis ED, Huber MH, Myerson MD. Transarticular distal soft-tissue release with an arthroscopic blade for hallux valgus correction. Foot Ankle Int. 2004;25:13–8.

The use of a flexible curved arthroscopic Beaver blade allows for complete release of the lateral sesamoid ligament, lateral 1MTP capsule, and the adductor insertion onto the proximal phalanx. Lacerations of the lateral head of the FBH tendon occurred in 6% of the specimens. There were no injuries to the first web space neurovascular bundle, nor to the 1MTH cartilage. (Level V evidence [expert opinion, technique tip])

Weil LS. Scarf osteotomy for correction of hallux valgus. Foot Ankle Clin. 2000;5:559–80.

A comprehensive representation by one of the most expert DPM's, popularizing the use of the Scarf osteotomy especially in Europe since 1984. Scarf bunionectomy is a technically demanding procedure that has a long learning curve. Once mastered it provides a predictable and satisfying outcome for both surgeon and foot surgeon. (Level V evidence [expert opinion])

These and the favorable results from numerous other case series support a Grade B recommendation for the use of the Scarf osteotomy in the treatment of hallux valgus.

PROCEDURE 3

Modified "Lapidus" Procedure—Tarsometatarsal Corrective Osteotomy and Fusion with First Metatarsophalangeal Joint Correction and Realignment

Andrew K. Sands and Edmund H. Choi

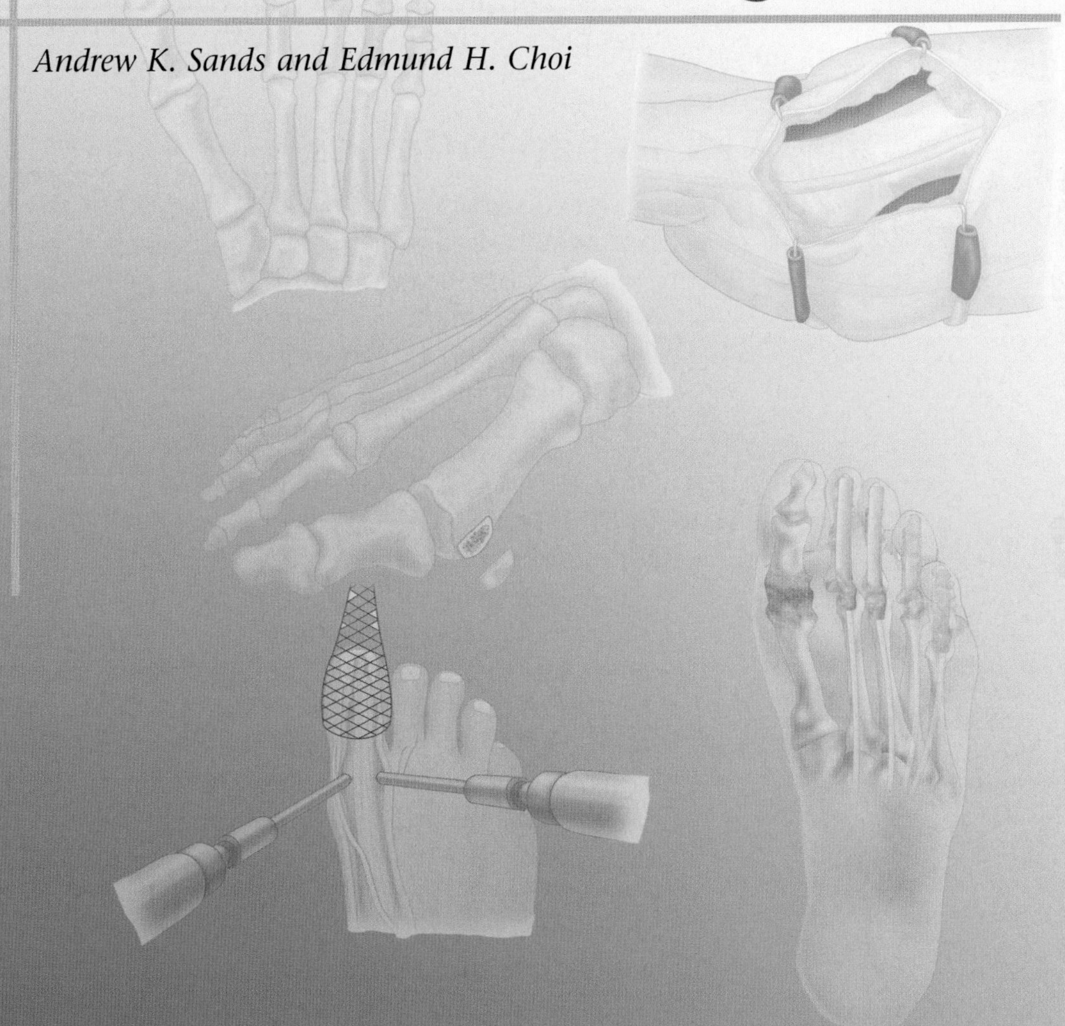

Tarsometatarsal Corrective Osteotomy and Fusion with First Metatarsophalangeal Joint Correction and Realignment

Indications

- Moderate to severe foot deformity, including
  - Hallux valgus with metatarsus primus varus
  - Hypermobility of the medial column
  - Pes planoabductovalgus (PPAV)

Examination/Imaging

Physical Examination

- Upon weight bearing, hallux valgus is observed toward a more severe deformity.
- Proper examination of the foot often will reveal associated hypermobility of the medial column and an equinus contracture of the gastrocnemius. There may also be flatfoot deformity (PPAV).

Treatment Options

- Several recent papers have questioned the existence and significance of hypermobility of the medial column. TMT fusion is important in the realignment and stabilization of the medial column. If hypermobility is not present or significant, then other metatarsal osteotomies can be used to correct the deformity. However, if a basal osteotomy is chosen, the medial column can be stabilized without a fusion by driving the screw across the osteotomy and through the first TMT joint (1TMT).

Imaging Studies

- Radiographs
  - Anteroposterior (AP), oblique, and lateral plane radiographs show the deformity, along with subluxation of the flexor complex/sesamoids.
  - On the AP view, the medial tarsometatarsal (TMT) joints will often show a gap between the first metatarsal (1MT) and second metatarsal (2MT), which may be indicative of hypermobility.
  - The oblique view may show lesser metatarsal overload with cortical hypertrophy (further indicating lack of proper weight bearing by the medial column/1MT).
  - The lateral view may show slight upward subluxation of the 1MT base on the medial cuneiform with dorsiflexion of the medial column (which can be seen at the TMT and calcaneonavicular joints).
- There is no indication for magnetic resonance imaging, computed tomography, or other imaging studies.

Surgical Anatomy

- The plane of approach is a dorsomedial one along the top of the foot (Fig. 1A and 1B). Care should be taken to avoid the sensory nerve (to the first web space) along with the dorsalis pedis artery.

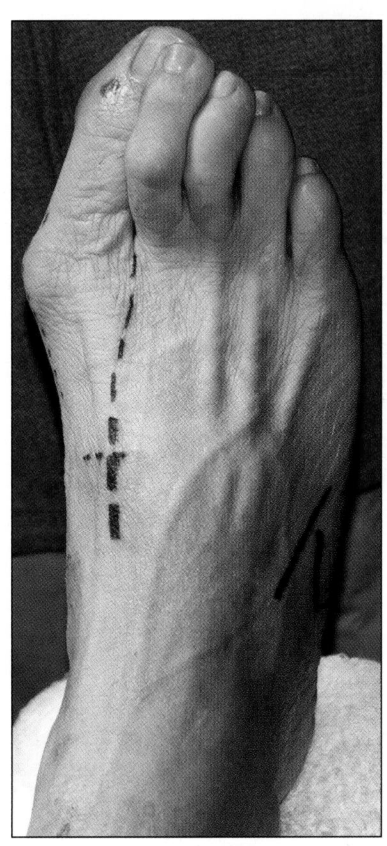

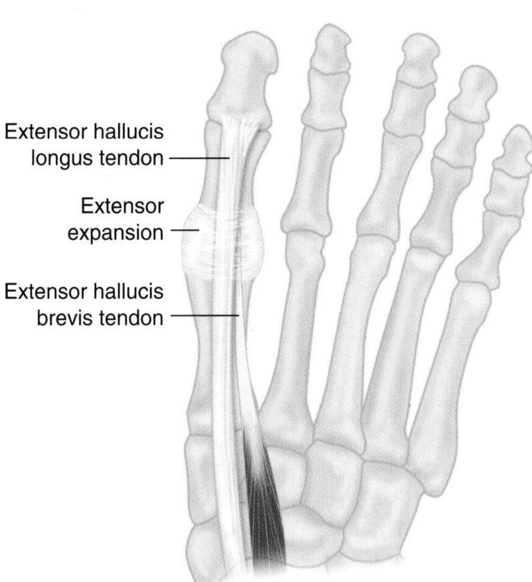

A B

FIGURE 1

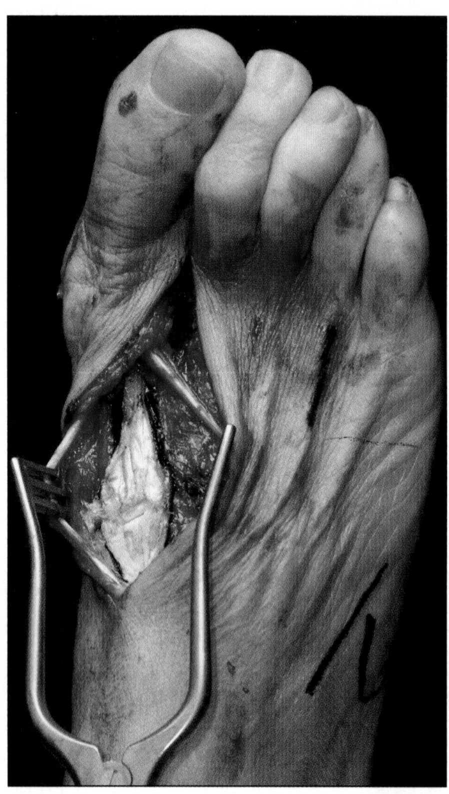

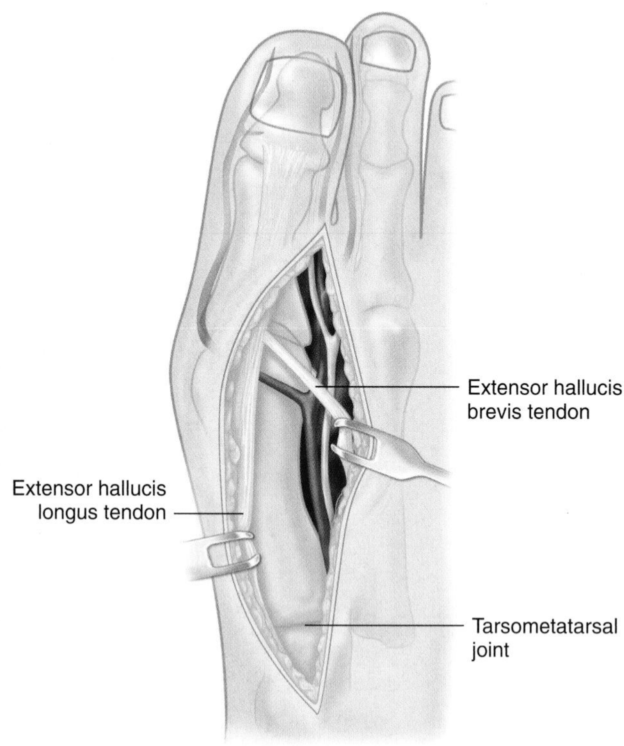

FIGURE 2 A B

> **PEARLS**
>
> - *Using the towel bump lifts the foot up off the operating room table and allows easier access to the foot. A firm towel bump can be made by using operating room towels.*
>   - *Fold five towels into thirds the long way, then into quarters to make squares. Stack five of these and wrap another long-thirds folded towel around the other five. Pull tightly on the wrapping towel to densely pack the interior. It should form a cube.*
>   - *Next wrap the whole cube in a Kerlex gauze or Coban (whichever is extra and available around the operating room from prefabicated packs).*
> - *Since the towel bump often falls off the table, it is helpful to clamp it to the drape with a large Kelly clamp.*

- The approach is made between the extensor hallucis longus (EHL) and extensor hallucis brevis (EHB) (Fig. 2A and 2B). Distally, the approach to the first metatarsophalangeal (1MTP) joint can be made medially or dorsally. The dorsal approach places the distal sensory nerve at risk. It allows access to the lateral aspect of the 1MTP joint (capsule and attached structures).
- The medial utility approach allows safe access to the 1MTP joint and the flexor complex/sesamoids.

Positioning

- Supine with ipsilateral bump under the buttock.
- A separate towel bump is used to elevate the foot off of the operating room table.

Portals/Exposures

- Two incisions are used: dorsomedial and straight medial.
- Dorsomedial incision
  - Start the incision at the interspace between the medial and intermediate cuneiform.

PEARLS

- *If just the 1MTP is being addressed, the dorsomedial incision can be on the medial side of the first web space, then down along the lateral aspect of the 1MTP joint.*
- *If a procedure is coincidently planned for the second toe (i.e., correction of lesser toe deformity), then the incision can be brought down the center of the web space and continued distally along the medial border of the second toe (for tendon transfer and interphalangeal releases).*

- The incision is brought distally to the first web space, and then deepened along the lateral capsule of the 1MTP. Firm thumb pressure along the capsule allows for blunt exposure of the capsule.
- The proximal part of the incision allows access to the 1TMT and intertarsal joints. If there is a significant amount of hypermobility, the intertarsal area can be fused as well to increase stability.

Procedure

STEP 1

- The dorsomedial incision is carried down between the EHL and EHB tendon, taking care to avoid the dorsalis pedis artery and sensory branch of the superficial peroneal nerve.
- The capsule and periosteum is marked, then incised axially (Fig. 3).
- The 1TMT is entered and the soft tissues are reflected medially and laterally, exposing the TMT and intertarsal area along with the medial base of the 2MT.

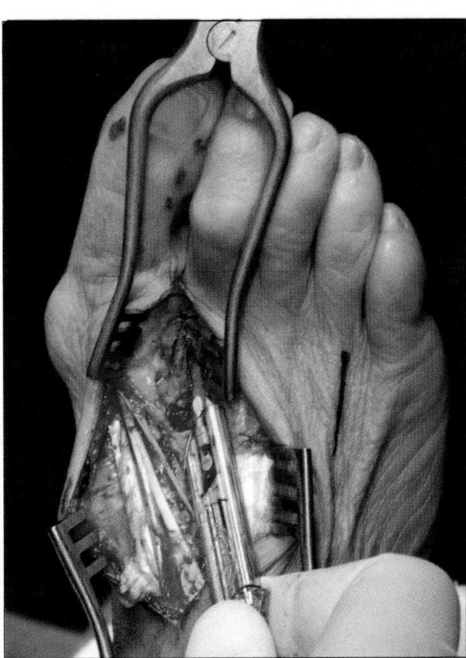

FIGURE 3

Pearls

- *Use a blue operating room marker to mark the capsule and periosteum. At the end of the case, it makes it much easier to find this layer to close over the fusion site and bone graft, which promotes bony healing.*
- *Pocket hole (see Procedure 20)*
  - *Make the pocket hole at least 2 cm distal to the 1TMT joint to make sure there is good leverage. Placing it too close to the joint does not allow good screw purchase and hold.*
  - *The pocket hole should have a near-vertical wall proximally and a slope going distally. This allows the screw head to slide down the slope before engaging the 1MT base, which prevents dorsal "blowout" of the base of the 1MT.*
  - *The pocket hole should be made with a round burr laid on its side. The slope portion should be slightly larger than the size of the screw head. The pocket hole is made prior to the osteotomy. Once the osteotomy is cut, the metatarsal becomes less stable and making the burr pocket hole is more difficult.*

Pitfalls

- *Care must be taken while cutting the 1TMT to not cut the shaft of the 2MT.*
- *Make sure to remove all of the waste cut from the depths of the 1TMT. If by-products of the cut are left in the depths of the cut, it will result in pathologic dorsiflexion at the 1TMT and upward displacement of the medial column.*

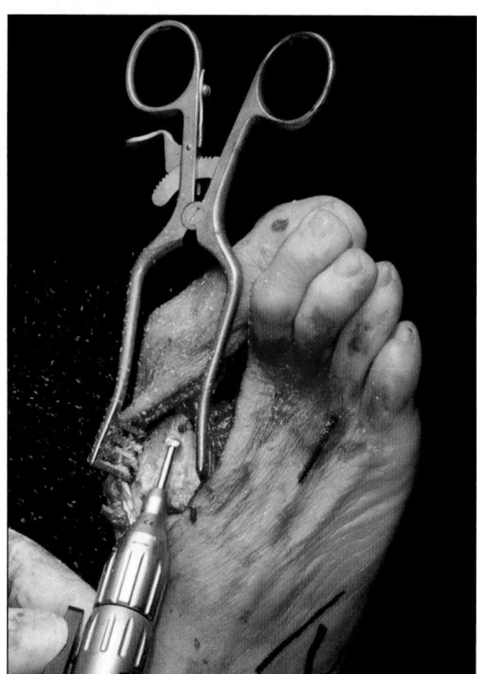

FIGURE 4

Step 2: Osteotomy

- The pocket hole is made on the dorsal base of the 1MT 2 cm distal to the joint before the osteotomy is cut (Fig. 4).
- The osteotomy is then cut using a straight saw (Fig. 5A). The depth of the joint and cut is 3 cm, and the blade should be that long.
- The osteotomy is made in a slightly lateral and plantar-based direction, which allows for correction at the TMT (Fig. 5B and 5C).
  - The first cut is made at the base of the 1MT.
  - The second cut, in the medial cuneiform, is lateral based to correct the intermetatarsal angle.
- The cut can be completed with a thin chisel. The TMT is then carefully distracted with a lamina spreader. A pituitary ronguer can be used to remove the waste of the cut.

Step 3: Preparing the Fusion

- The 1TMT is distracted gently with a lamina spreader and the soft tissue along the medial base of the 2MT is removed. The joint surfaces, medial base of the 2MT, and lateral area of the 1MT base are drilled with a 2-mm wire to prepare them for fusion (Fig. 6).

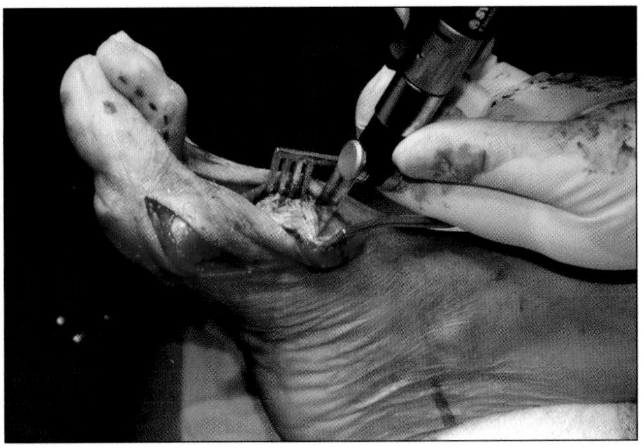

A

Intermetatarsal angle

1st metatarsal

1st cut

2nd cut

Medial cuneiform

B

Navicular

Medial cuneiform

Talus

1st metatarsal

Cut to correct 1st metatarsal elevation deformity by bringing 1st metatarsal plantar grade

1st cut

2nd cut

C

FIGURE 5

- Distally, the dissection is carried down along the lateral capsule. The capsule is then incised axially. The lateral tendons are not released as this destabilizes the joint and can lead to hallux varus complications

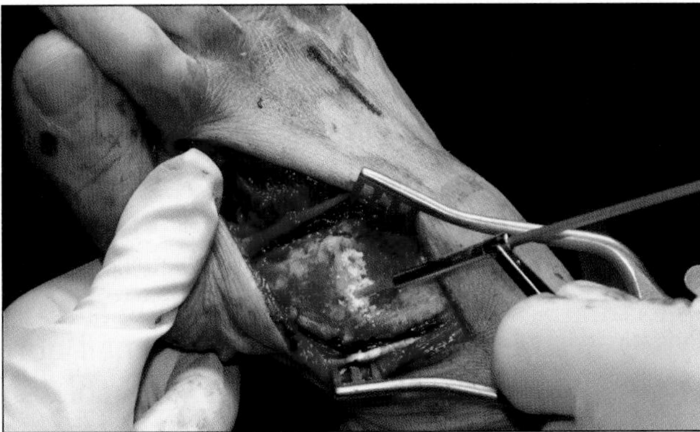

FIGURE 6

- The medial utility incision is made along the midaxial line, centered over the 1MTP joint.
  - The capsule and periosteum are reflected dorsally and plantarward. The adhesions between the flexor complex and the underside of the 1MT are released (Fig. 7A and 7B). These sometimes are vascular, and cautery can be used as long as the articular cartilage is protected.
  - The dorsal capsule is released along the shaft. This allows the MT head to shift back over the flexor complex/sesamoids when the osteotomy is reduced.
  - An elevator should be passed under the 1MT head from one incision to the other to make sure that the adhesions are released and that the head is correctable above the flexor complex.

PEARLS

- *When closing the 1MTP medial capsule, place a stitch in each of the two flaps and hold each with a clamp. Gently pull the superior arm distally and the inferior one proximally, shifting the capsule and further correcting the deformity at the 1MTP. Closure can then be completed with 0 braided absorbable suture.*

Instrumentation/ Implantation

- The drills should be long shaft. This allows them to be used without the drill chuck impacting the toes. Also, it is important to have the drill bit lay flat relative to the foot. Using a short drill bit would prevent the holes from being drilled horizontally as the drill bit forces the surgeon's hand upward away from the foot.
- The reduction of the osteotomy can be made using a pointed reduction clamp and then held with the clamp or Kirschner wires. Two small drill holes can be made to prevent the ends of the clamp from moving or sliding.

STEP 4: REDUCTION AND FUSION

- Reduction of the deformity
  - The flexor complex is grasped with a clamp and pulled medially while a thumb is used to push the metatarsal laterally over the sesamoids. At the same time, the osteotomy is reduced with a dental pick and pointed reduction clamp.
  - The reduced deformity can be provisionally fixed with Kirschner wires, but care must be taken to not place the wires in the path of the screws.
- The screws are then placed.
  - The first screw is placed from the pocket hole into the plantar medial aspect of the medial cuneiform (Fig. 8). The screw is placed in a lag fashion.
  - A second screw is then placed from the medial cuneiform to the plantar base of the 1MT.
  - A third screw is sometimes needed if there is excessive hypermobility or, as in the case of revision surgery, more stability is needed.
- The medial capsule of the 1MTP is then reefed and advanced and closed with 0 braided absorbable suture. Advance the superior capsule distally and the inferior capsule proximally to shift and straighten the hallux more.
- Bone grafting
  - Small burr holes should be made dorsomedial and dorsolateral along the TMT fusion. These "shear strain relief" holes are filled with morselized bone graft and serve as "spot welds."

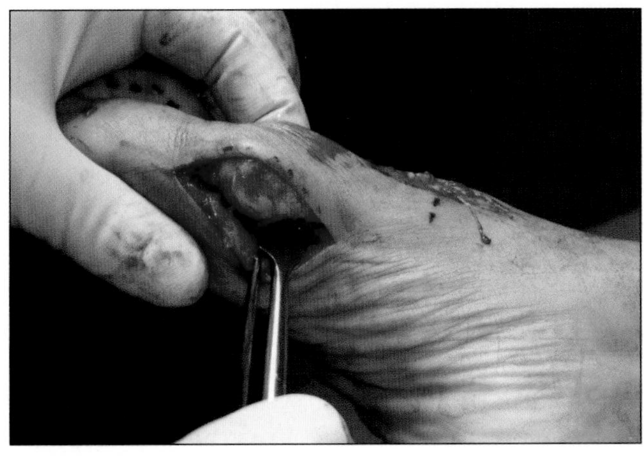

A

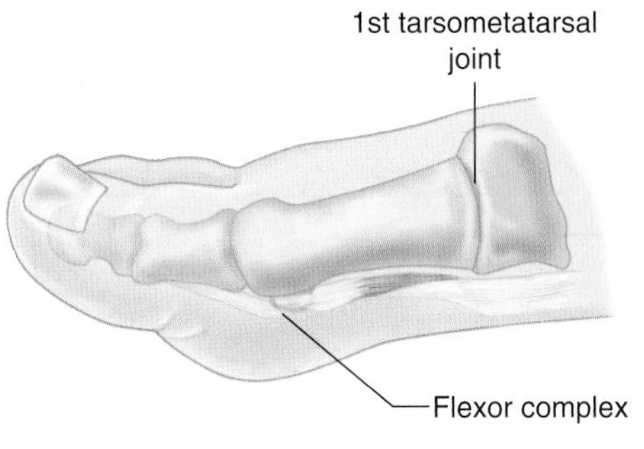

B

FIGURE 7

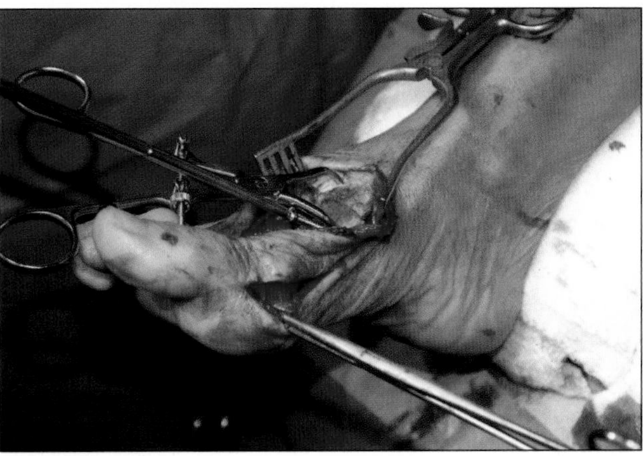

FIGURE 8

- These small areas heal quickly; they hold the rest of the joint from shearing up and down. This shearing causes fibrous tissue growth and nonunion.

- The blue-marked capsule/periosteum is then closed with 2–0 braided absorbable suture.

Postoperative Care and Expected Outcomes

- Since rigid internal fixation is holding the osteotomy, fancy dressings are not required. Bacitracin and Xeroform gauze are placed on the wounds. Sterile dressings and Webril wrap are placed. A three-sided plaster splint is placed and overwrapped with elastic bandages.

- The splint is left in place for 2 weeks. It is then removed in the office and the patient is placed into a cam boot. The boot can be removed for washing.
- Progression to full function is as follows:
  - Non–weight bearing for 6–8 weeks with two crutches or walker or scooter.
  - Weight bearing in cam boot with cane assistance as needed for another 6–8 weeks.
  - Running sneakers with medial-supported orthotic from then on (for 1 year).
- Patients may expect swelling and discomfort for 1 year with continuing improvement for 2 years.
- Patients can return to full sports, even marathon running.

Evidence

Bednarz PA, Manoli A. Modified Lapidus procedure for the treatment of hypermobile hallux valgus. Foot Ankle Int. 2000;21:816–21.

This study is a review of 26 patients who underwent a modified Lapidus procedure. Outcome was determined by patient satisfaction, pain relief, clinical joint stiffness and radiographic assessment. (Level IV evidence [case series])

Coetzee JC, Resig SG, Kuskowski M, Saleh KJ. Lapidus procedure as salvage after failed surgical treatment of hallux valgus. J Bone Joint Surg [Am]. 2003;85:60–5.

This study is a retrospective review of 24 patients with symptomatic recurrences of hallux valgus after previous procedures that were subsequently reated with a Lapidus procedure. Follow-up averaged 24 months. Outcome was determined by AOFAS scale, visual analog pain scale, and radiographic assessment. (Level IV evidence [case series])

Haas Z, Hamilton G, Sundstrom D, Ford L. Maintenance of correction of first metatarsal closing base wedge osteotomies versus modified Lapidus arthrodesis for moderate to severe hallux valgus deformity. J Foot Ankle Surg. 2007;46:358–65.

This study is a retrospective review of 57 feet with moderate to severe valgus deformity treated by either a modified Lapidus or a 1MT closing base wedge osteotomy. At 11 months postoperative, the radiographs were reviewed for both procedures. (Level IV evidence [case series])

Kopp FJ, Patel MM, Levine DS, Deland JT. The modified Lapidus procedure for hallux valgus: a clinical and radiographic analysis. Foot Ankle Int. 2005;26:913–7.

This study is a retrospective review of 32 patients treated with the modified Lapidus procedure. Follow-up averaged 42 months. Outcome was determined by radiographic results, postoperative questionnaires, and physical examination. (Level IV evidence [case series])

Manoli A 2nd, Hansen ST Jr. Screw hole preparation in foot surgery. Foot Ankle. 1990;11:105–6.

This is a technique review on the proper way to make the pocket hole.

McInnes BD, Bouche RT. Critical evaluation of the modified Lapidus procedure. J Foot Ankle Surg. 2001;40:71–90.

This study is a retrospective review of 34 patients treated with the modified Lapidus procedure by the senior author. Follow-up averaged 39 months. Outcome was determined by subjective questionnaire, physical examination, and radiographic assessment. (Level IV evidence [case series])

Patel S, Ford LA, Etcheverry J, Rush SM, Hamilton GA. Modified Lapidus arthrodesis: rate of nonunion in 227 cases. J Foot Ankle Surg. 2004;43:37–42.

This study is a retrospective review of 211 consecutive patients treated with a modified Lapidus procedure. For a minimum of 6 months' follow-up, the radiographic results were reviewed. (Level IV evidence [case series])

Shi K, Hayashida K, Tomita T, Tanabe M, Ochi T. Surgical treatment of hallux valgus deformity in rheumatoid arthritis: clinical and radiographic evaluation of modified Lapidus technique. J Foot Ankle Surg. 2000;39:376–82.

This study is a retrospective review of 21 rheumatoid hallux valgus deformities treated by a modified Lapidus procedure. Outcome was determined by subjective improvement of pain, footwear comfort, and radiographic assessment. (Level IV evidence [case series])

Thompson IM, Bohay DR, Anderson JG. Fusion rate of first tarsometatarsal arthrodesis in the modified Lapidus procedure and flatfoot reconstruction. Foot Ankle Int. 2005;26:698–703.

This study is a retrospective review of 182 patients who had either a modified Lapidus procedure or a TMT joint arthrodesis as part of a flatfoot reconstruction. At a follow-up of 6 months, the radiographic evidence of union was reviewed between the two procedures. (Level IV evidence [case series])

PROCEDURE 4

Proximal Long Oblique (Ludloff) First Metatarsal Osteotomy with Distal Soft Tissue Procedure

Mark E. Easley and Hans-Joerg Trnka

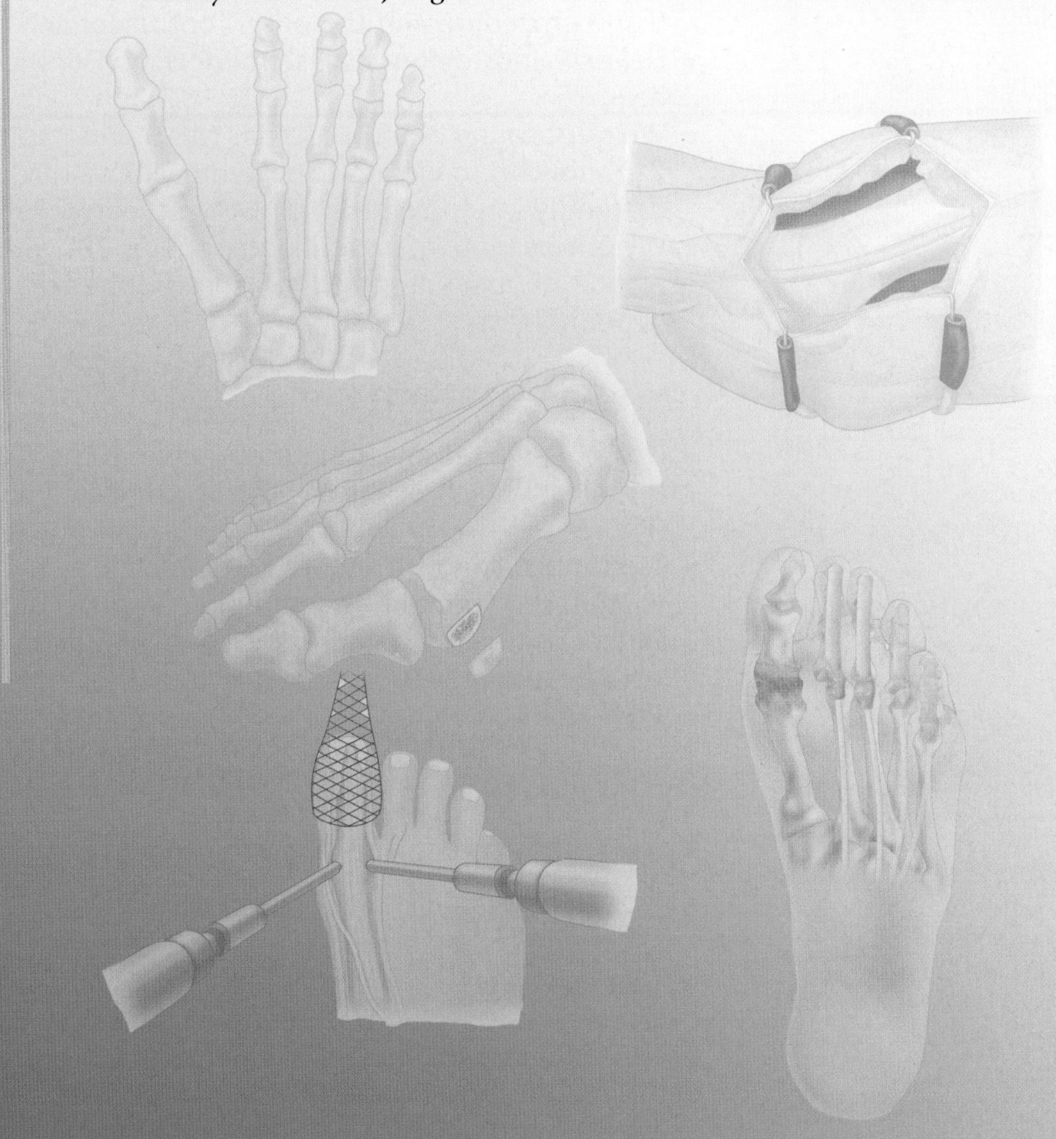

Indications

- Symptomatic moderate to severe hallux valgus (first-second intermetatarsal angle [1/2 IMA] >15°) failing nonoperative treatment

Examination/Imaging

- Relatively wide forefoot with a tender, prominent medial eminence (medial 1MT head). Figure 1 shows a patient in weight-bearing stance with one foot corrected with a Ludloff osteotomy and distal soft tissue procedure and the other foot uncorrected.
- Hallux valgus deformity (lateral deviation of the hallux)
- Weight-bearing anteroposterior (AP) radiograph (Fig. 2A) showing moderate to severe hallux valgus deformity (an increased 1/2 IMA exceeding 15°)
- Weight-bearing lateral radiograph (Fig. 2B) without plantar gapping at the 1TMT joint (suggestive of hypermobility)

Surgical Anatomy

- Dorsomedial sensory cutaneous nerve to the hallux (terminal branch of the superficial peroneal nerve) (Fig. 3A)
- Medial position of the 1MT head relative to the anatomically positioned sesamoid complex (Fig. 3B)
- Lateral capsule with important blood supply to the 1MT head (Fig. 3C)
- 1TMT joint

Positioning

- Supine position on the operating room table

Portals/Exposures

- Two exposures are typically required: (1) a dorsal first web space incision to perform the lateral release and (2) a longitudinal medial approach to perform the medial capsulotomy and first metatarsal osteotomy.
- **Dorsal First Web Space Incision**
  - A 3- to 4-cm incision is made between the distal first and second metatarsals. The superficial neurovascular structures are protected.
  - The enveloping fascia (inominate fascia) is split longitudinally and blunt dissection (with a finger)

Pitfalls

- *Contraindications to surgical correction of hallux valgus deformity: peripheral vascular disease, peripheral neuropathy*
- *Contraindication to surgical correction of hallux valgus correction with a metatarsal osteotomy: hallux rigidus (degenerative joint disease of the first metatarsophalangeal [1MTP] joint)*
- *Relative contraindications to the Ludloff osteotomy: narrow first metatarsal (1MT) (limited surface area for healing) and osteopenia (risk for poor fixation)*

Controversies

- Hypermobility of the first ray: some surgeons recommend a first tarsometatarsal (1TMT) joint arthrodesis (modified Lapidus procedure) in lieu of a metatarsal osteotomy.

Treatment Options

- One of over 130 corrective procedures for symptomatic hallux valgus; with moderate to severe deformity, a proximal osteotomy or modified Lapidus procedure is favored.

Pearls

- *Unlike many other 1MT osteotomies, periosteal stripping is not required and should be avoided.*

Pitfalls

- *Making the medial incision too plantar may limit exposure of the 1MT and lead to excessive skin retraction and potential skin necrosis at the dorsal wound margin.*

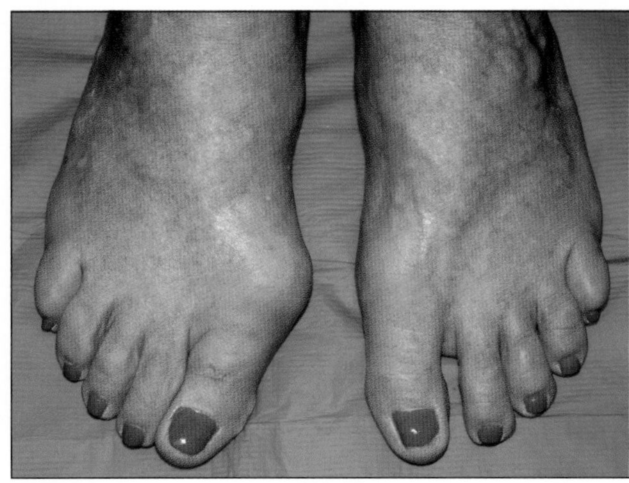

FIGURE 1

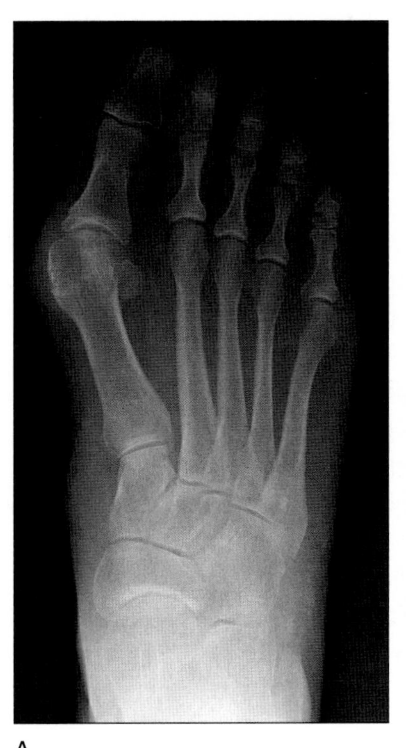

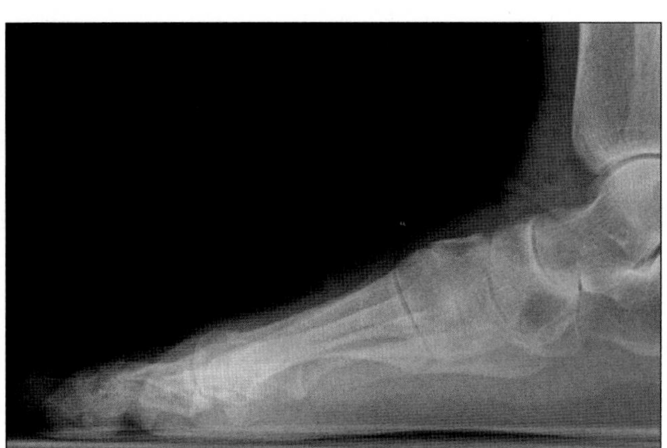

FIGURE 2 A B

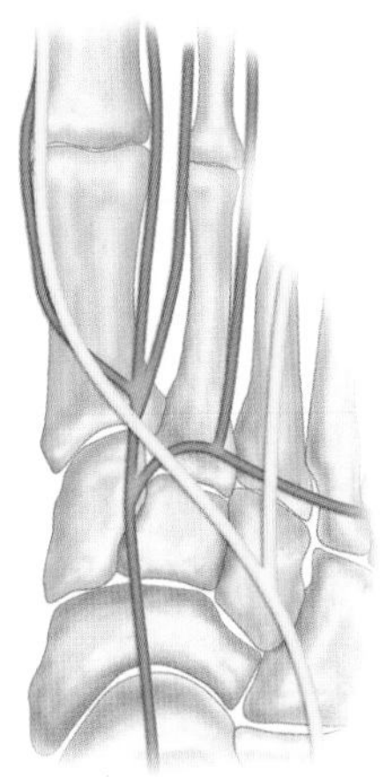

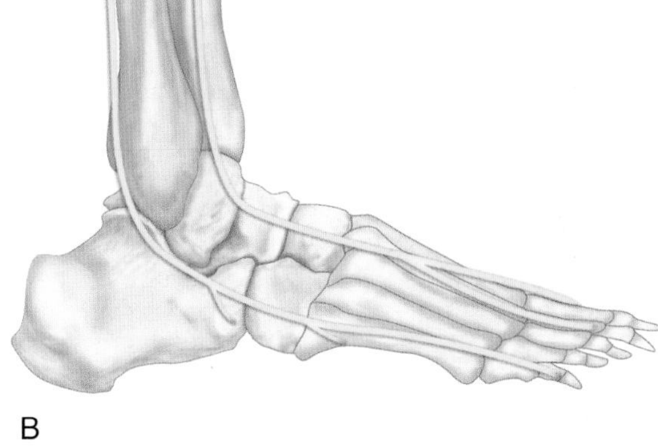

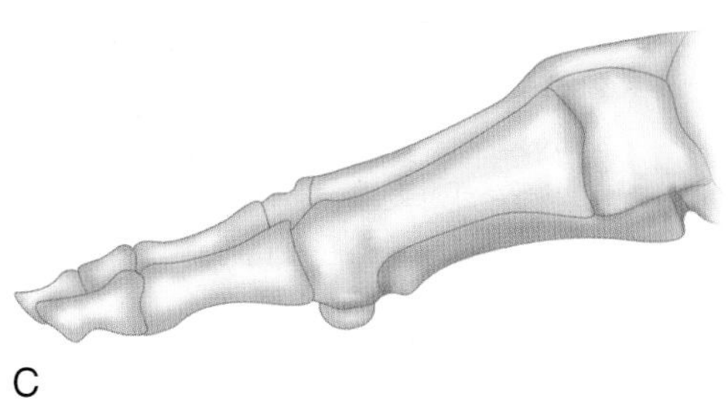

A B C

FIGURE 3

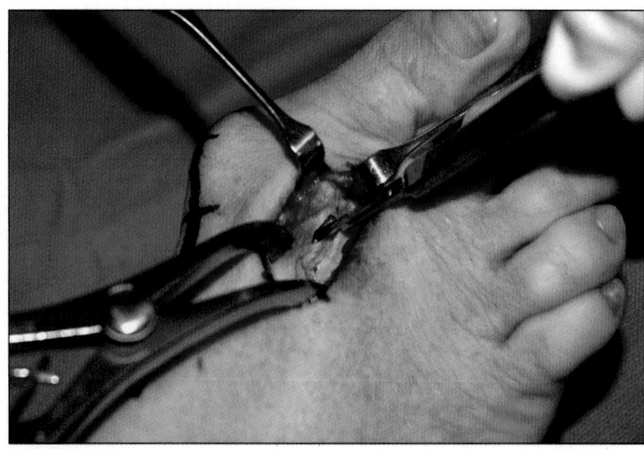

FIGURE 4

is performed to access the lateral aspect of the 1MTP joint. A lamina spreader may be placed between the first and second metatarsals to improve access to the first web space (Fig. 4).

- **Medial Midaxial Longitudinal Approach**
  - A longitudinal incision is made from the 1MTP joint to the 1TMT joint, directly over the 1MT (Fig. 5A). A tendency to make the incision slightly more dorsal than plantar will facilitate exposure of the 1MT for the osteotomy.
  - The dorsomedial cutaneous sensory nerve to the hallux and extensor hallucis longus (EHL) tendon must be identified and protected throughout the procedure (Fig. 5B).
  - The medial 1MTP joint capsule should be exposed but not violated during the surgical approach.

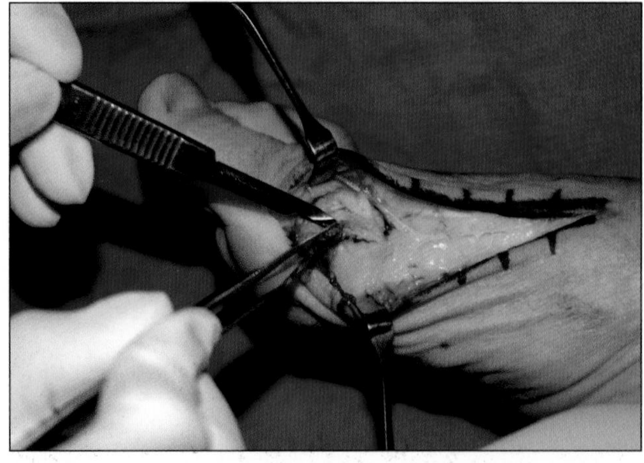

A

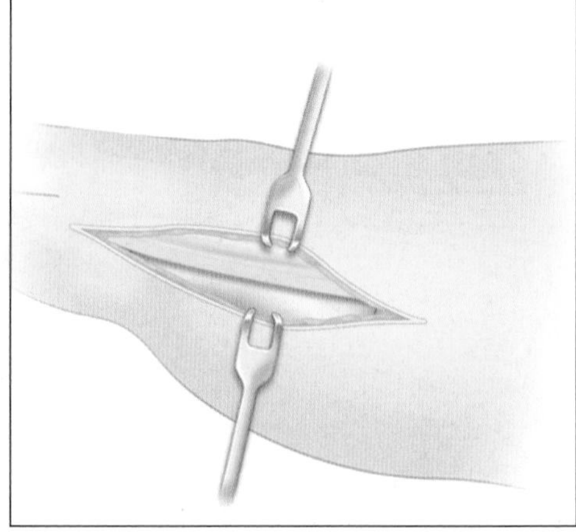

B

FIGURE 5

Procedure

Step 1: Lateral Release and Medial Capsulotomy

Lateral Release

- The ligament between the lateral capsule and lateral sesamoid is released sharply by introducing the scalpel blade directly into the articulation between the plantar metatarsal head and lateral sesamoid (Fig. 6). This maneuver can be performed from proximal to distal and, if carefully controlled, may be continued distally and slightly laterally to simultaneously release the adductor hallucis tendon from the base of the first proximal phalanx (Fig. 7A).
- Next, the adductor hallucis is directly released from the lateral sesamoid (Fig. 7B), thereby fully detaching both aspects of the adductor hallucis to the 1MTP joint and sesamoid complex (Fig. 7C).

Pearls

- *With long-standing hallux valgus deformity, an audible "pop" indicative of a successful release is typically experienced and desirable.*

Pitfalls

- *Fenestrate the lateral capsule distal to the metatarsal head in order to preserve the blood supply to the metatarsal head that courses through the proximal aspect of the lateral capsule, in the event a distal osteotomy is required in conjunction with the proximal Ludloff osteotomy (risk of 1MT head avascular necrosis).*
- *Avoid over-releasing the lateral capsule to limit the risk of hallux varus (multiple fenestrations and a varus stress of only 20° typically suffice).*

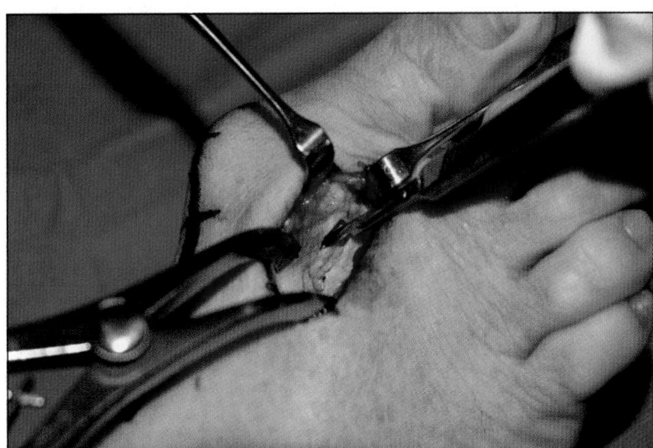

FIGURE 6

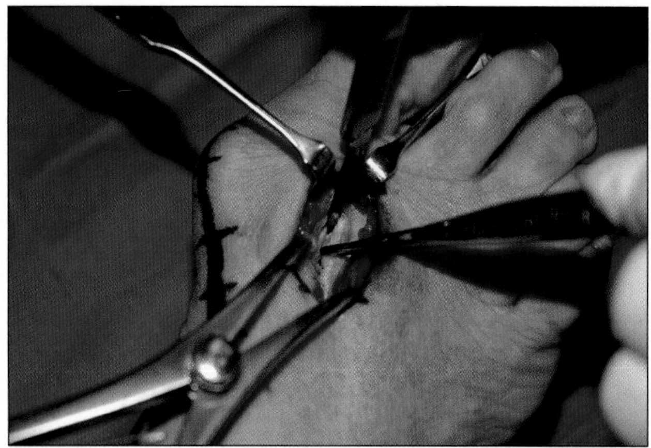
A

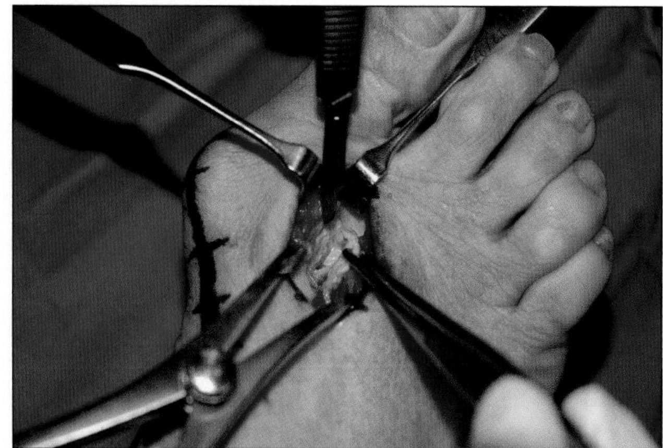
B

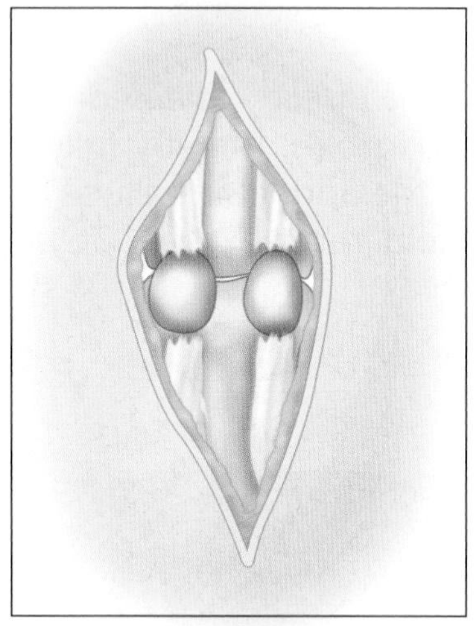
C

FIGURE 7

Controversies

- Alternatively, the lateral release may be performed through the medial approach, but this may not provide full visualization of the contracted lateral soft tissues.

- Then, the lateral capsule is weakened distal to the lateral metatarsal head by fenestrating it with multiple scalpel blade stab incisions (Fig. 8).
- Depending on surgeon preference, the transverse intermetatarsal ligament may be carefully elevated from the underlying common digital artery and nerve and divided while protecting these neurovascular structures; we do not routinely release this ligament.
- Finally, a varus stress is applied to the hallux while applying medially directed counterpressure on the 1MT to complete the lateral release (Fig. 9). Provided adequate multiple fenestrations were performed laterally, a varus stress of 20° is sufficient.

- **Medial Capsulotomy and Medial Eminence Resection**
- With the medial capsule fully exposed and the EHL tendon and the cutaneous nerve branch to the hallux protected, the medial capsulotomy is performed.
- We favor an L-shaped capsulotomy (Fig. 10A and 10B), but any one of a number of described techniques are applicable. Of import is that sufficient tissue remains at the time of closure to perform a satisfactory capsulorrhaphy.

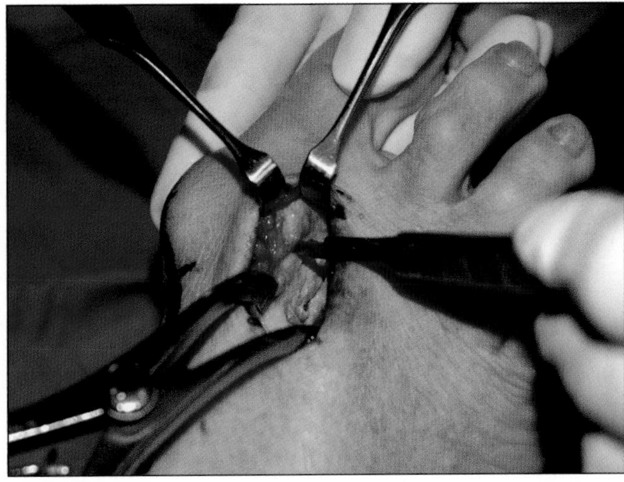

FIGURE 8

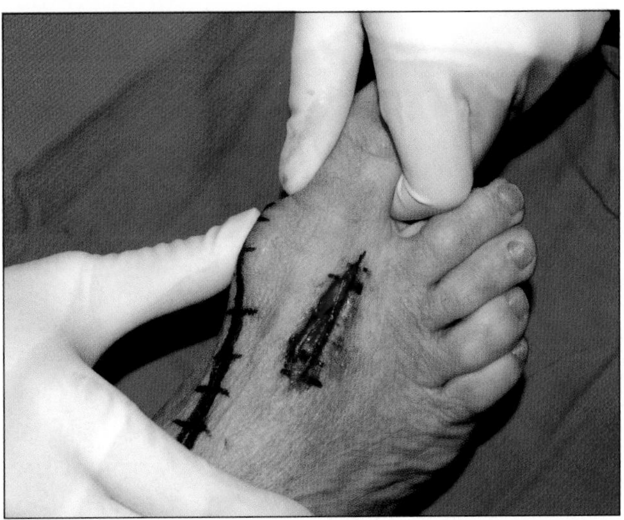

FIGURE 9

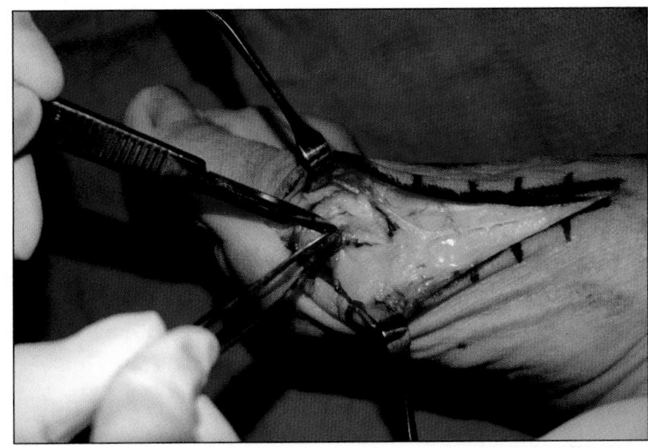

A

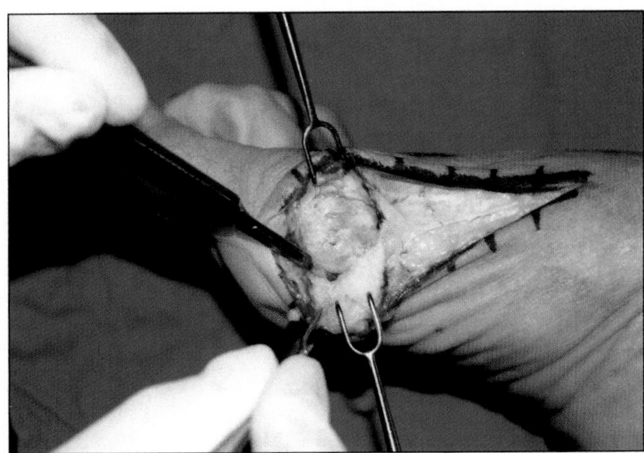

B

FIGURE 10

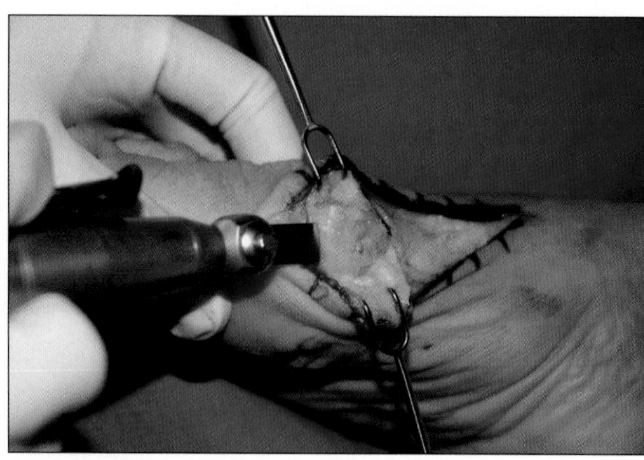

FIGURE 11

- The medial eminence may be resected at this point or immediately before capsulorrhaphy. The medial eminence is resected in line with the medial 1MT shaft (Fig. 11), immediately medial to the medial sulcus, avoiding over-resection (which may promote hallux varus).
- Also, the micro-sagittal saw must be held in the proper sagittal plane to avoid over-resection of the plantar aspect of the 1MT head, which articulates with the medial sesamoid.

Pearls

- *We recommend cooling the micro-sagittal saw blade with cool saline irrigation to limit heat that may create areas of osteonecrosis along the osteotomy.*
- *Hold the forefoot with the opposite hand while creating the 1MT osteotomy; this will provide greater stability and facilitate orienting the osteotomy properly*

Pitfalls

- *Do not make the osteotomy too short; a longer osteotomy typically leads to greater stability.*

Step 2: Proximal Oblique (Ludloff) First Metatarsal Osteotomy

- The 1MT is fully exposed. The sensory cutaneous terminal branch of the superficial peroneal nerve and the EHL tendon are protected.
  - With minimal periosteal stripping, a small blunt Hohmann retractor is positioned on the lateral side of the 1MT. To define the 1TMT joint, a small-diameter Kirschner wire may be placed in the joint and its position confirmed on intraoperative fluoroscopy.
  - Dissection plantar to the metatarsal may be kept to a minimum, but some exposure is required to define the exit point of the osteotomy and to create adequate access to place a second screw.
- With the 1MT exposed, the planned osteotomy is marked and/or scored (Fig. 12A and 12B). The desired osteotomy should originate at or just distal to the dorsal aspect of the 1TMT joint and extend obliquely and plantarward to a point just proximal to the metatarsal head–sesamoid complex. A long osteotomy provides the greatest surface area for healing and readily permits fixation with two screws.

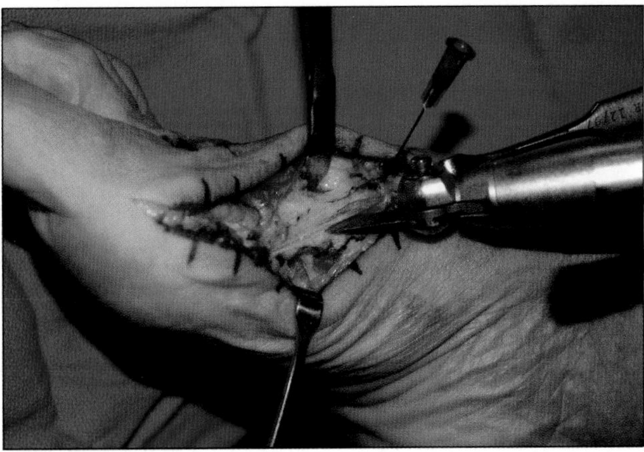

A

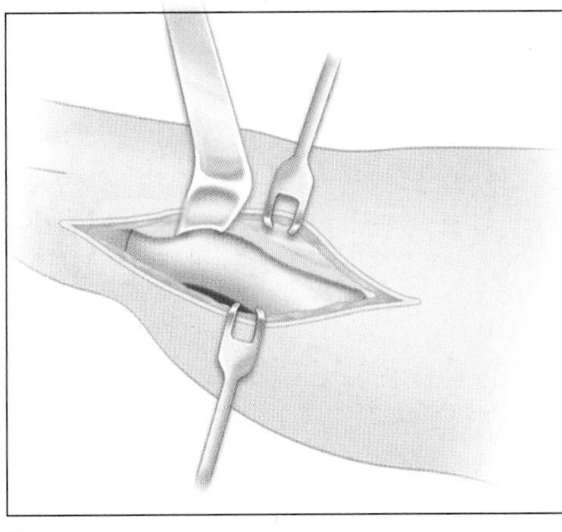

B

FIGURE 12

Instrumentation/ Implantation

- Micro-sagittal saw
- Small-fragment screws (solid or cannulated)
- Towel clip
- Small fluoroscopy unit

In our experience, a short osteotomy tends to be less stable than a long osteotomy.

- The greatest challenge with this osteotomy is achieving its ideal orientation and congruency.
  - The osteotomy must be made from the direct medial aspect of the 1MT, avoiding the tendency is to start the osteotomy too dorsally.
  - Staying in the same plane for the entire length of the osteotomy is facilitated by not allowing the saw blade to completely exit the osteotomy when it is advanced distally and plantarward.
  - To avoid a tendency to elevate the distal fragment during IMA correction, the saw blade may be inclined 10° in a plantarward direction, to promote slight plantar flexion of the distal fragment.
- With the ideal osteotomy marked/scored on the medial aspect of the 1MT and a small blunt Hohmann retractor protecting against accidental

overpenetration of the saw blade through the lateral cortex, the micro-sagittal saw is fully seated through the proximal aspect of the planned osteotomy. The distal corner of the saw blade is then retracted, leaving the proximal aspect of the blade within the osteotomy, and the saw blade is then fully seated through both cortices more distally than the initial cut. This process is repeated multiple times to advance the saw along the proximal two thirds of the planned osteotomy (Fig. 13).

- After completing the proximal two thirds of the osteotomy, the saw is removed and a small-fragment lag screw is inserted perpendicular to the completed portion of the osteotomy (Fig. 14).
  - The proximal two thirds of the osteotomy must be fully completed before inserting this screw, because access to the lateral cortex will be limited once the screw is in position.
  - This position of this screw should not violate the 1TMT joint, not fracture the thinner dorsal fragment, and be proximal enough to allow for insertion of a second screw across the more distal aspect of the osteotomy.
  - When using a fully threaded solid screw, the proximal (dorsal) cortex will need to be overdrilled to create a lag effect. We routinely use a dual-pitch or partially threaded cannulated screw.
  - With compression of the proximal osteotomy confirmed, the screw is temporarily released a few turns to allow completion of the osteotomy.
- The micro-sagittal saw is reintroduced into the osteotomy, and in a manner similar to that described above, the distal portion of the osteotomy is completed (Fig. 15). The plantar soft tissues must be protected as the saw blade exits the plantar cortex. A tendency may be to advance the saw blade too distally, potentially creating an exit point in the metatarsal head or one that violates the sesamoid complex, and therefore it is essential that the target remains the planned exit point of the scored/marked osteotomy.
- The IMA is corrected by rotating the distal fragment on the proximal fragment, pivoting about the screw that has been inserted across the proximal aspect of the osteotomy (Fig. 16A and 16B).

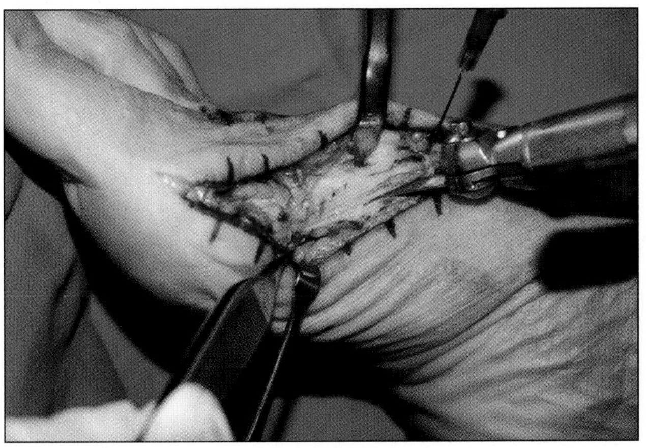

FIGURE 13

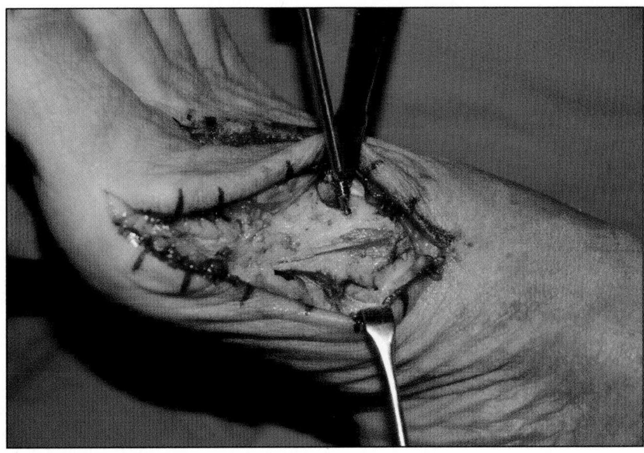

FIGURE 14

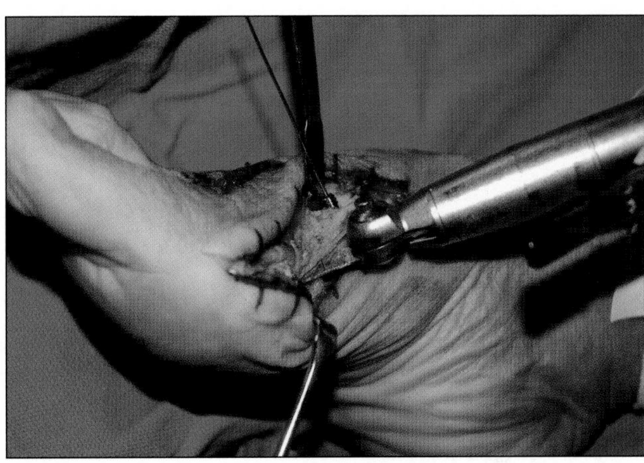

FIGURE 15

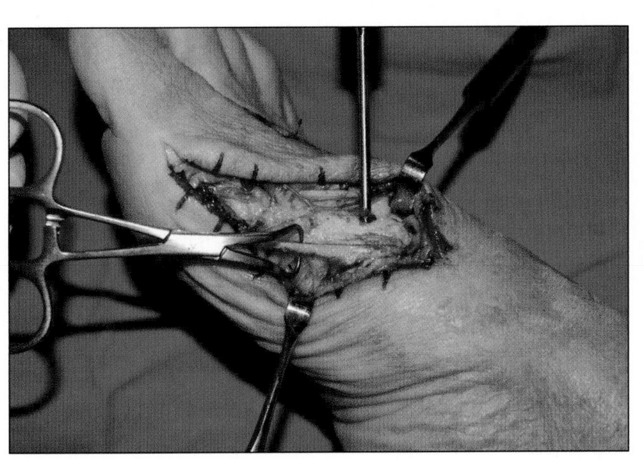

A

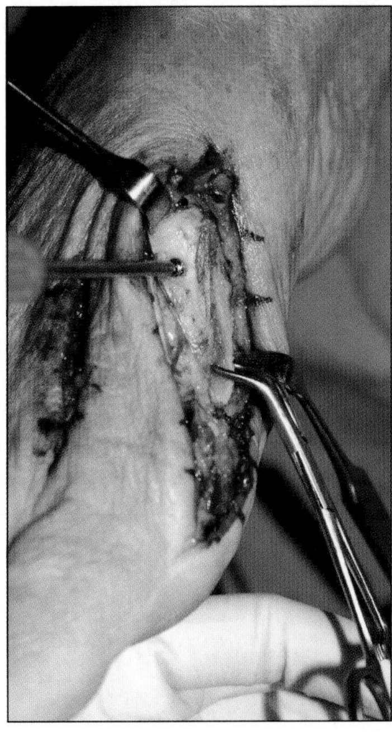

B

FIGURE 16

- Occasionally the soft tissues at the proximal-most and distal-most aspects of the osteotomy need to be carefully released to permit the osteotomy to mobilize. A towel clip attached to the distal aspect of the proximal fragment provides stability as manual pressure is applied to the medial 1MT head. With desired correction, the proximal screw is secured and the towel clip positioned to temporarily prevent loss of correction (see Fig. 16). IMA correction is confirmed with intraoperative fluoroscopy (Fig. 17A and 17B).
- With over- or undercorrection of the IMA, the proximal screw and towel clip may be readily released, further correction can be made, and the screw and towel clip again secured.

■ A second lag screw is placed over the distal aspect of the metatarsal (Fig. 18).
  - We prefer to direct this screw from plantar to dorsal. With the plantar soft tissues retracted and retraction of the dorsal soft tissues released, the plantar screw can be safely inserted. If the screw is placed obliquely from medial to lateral, its compression may promote loss of correction as the distal fragment is pulled medially. Therefore, the distal screw should be directed as much as is possible from plantar to dorsal while remaining perpendicular to the osteotomy.
  - This screw should be started centrally on the distal aspect of the plantar fragment, avoiding the risk of medial or distal fracture as the screw is compressed. Also, the screw should not penetrate the dorsal cortex of the distal fragment more than a millimeter or two since this may create symptomatic hardware postoperatively.
  - We recommend intraoperative fluoroscopy to confirm satisfactory correction of the IMA (Fig. 19).

Pearls

- *Even without complete repair of the medial capsule, the hallux position should be nearly anatomic with appropriate correction of the IMA.*

Pitfalls

- *The operation is not over until the hallux is properly positioned; greater tightening of the medial capsulorrhaphy is rarely the solution.*
- *If the IMA is undercorrected; the proximal osteotomy will need to be repositioned.*
- *If the DMAA is increased, a supplemental distal, medial closing wedge 1MT osteotomy must be added.*

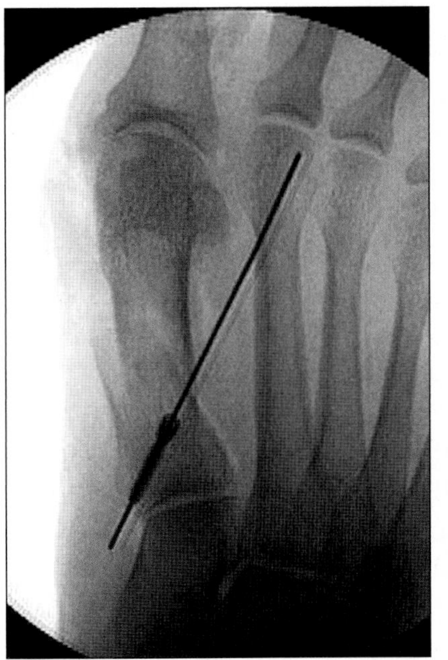
A

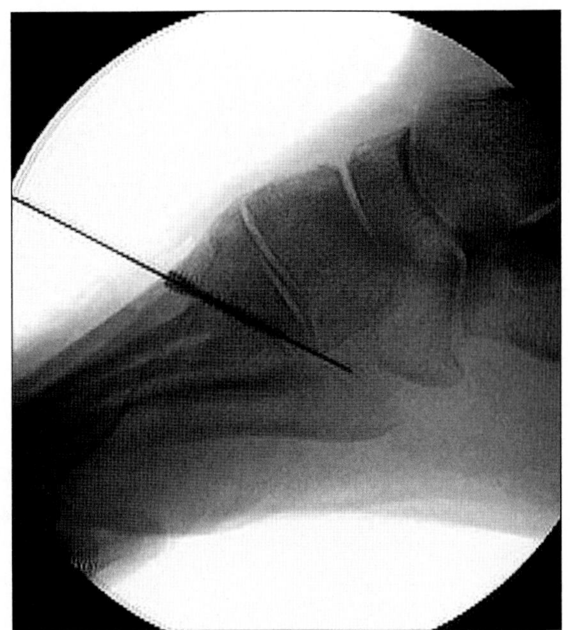
B

FIGURE 17

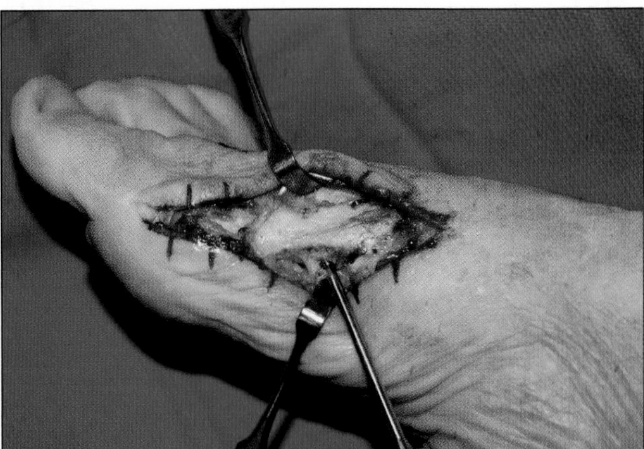

FIGURE 18

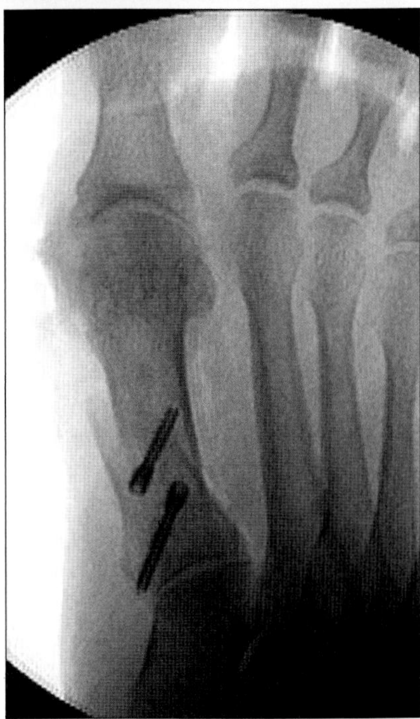

FIGURE 19

Step 3: Medial Capsulorrhaphy and Closure

- Typically, distal and proximal prominences remain on the medial aspect of this osteotomy upon completion of the IMA correction. These should be removed with the micro-sagittal saw (Fig. 20A and 20B). While protecting the sensory cutaneous nerve to the hallux, the medial capsule is repaired, typically with imbrication (Fig. 21). We use a combination of absorbable and nonabsorbable suture to close the capsule.
- In order to rebalance the hallux on the first metatarsal head, slight supination and varus is applied to the hallux during the medial capsulorrhaphy. Intraoperative fluoroscopy confirms that the hallux is balanced in an anatomic position and that the metatarsal head is properly repositioned on the sesamoid complex (Fig. 22).
- We deem a minimal amount of varus positioning optimal as this tends to correct to an anatomic position; however, a true varus positioning of the hallux should be avoided.
  - In the event that overcorrection has occurred, either the IMA is overcorrected (necessitating repositioning of the 1MT osteotomy) or the lateral capsule has been over-released.
  - With over-release of the lateral capsule, one option is to attach the residual adductor hallucis tendon to the distal lateral capsular tissues.
- If the metatarsal head, sesamoid, and hallux relationship is not anatomic, then the IMA correction is inadequate, the capsular closure is not appropriate, or the patient has an increased distal metatarsal articular angle (DMAA). The surgeon should not leave the operating room until the hallux is properly positioned.
  - Rarely is the problem related to an inappropriate medial capsular closure.
  - If the IMA proves to be undercorrected, then the proximal osteotomy will need to be realigned to achieve appropriate IMA correction.

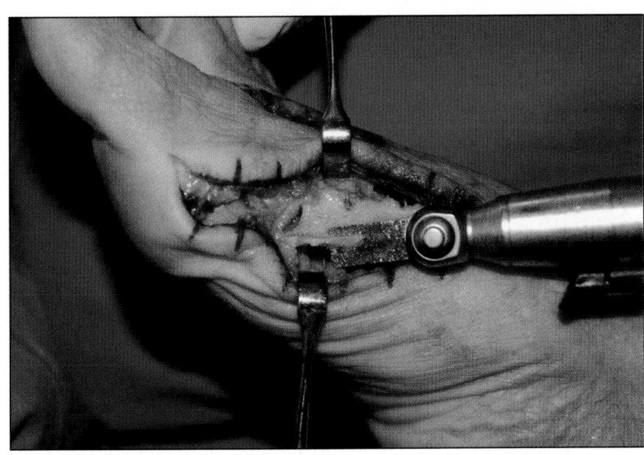
A

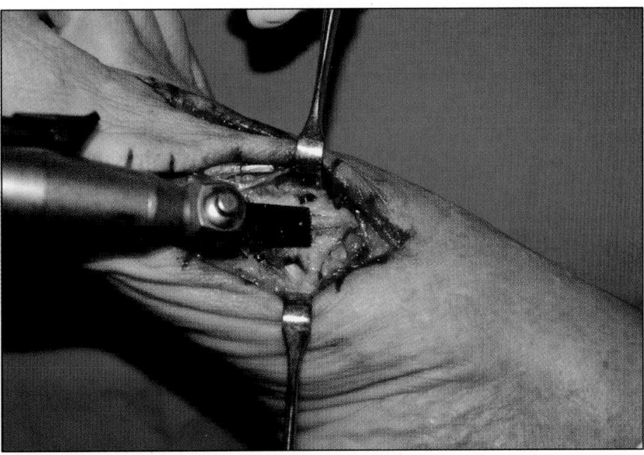
B

FIGURE 20

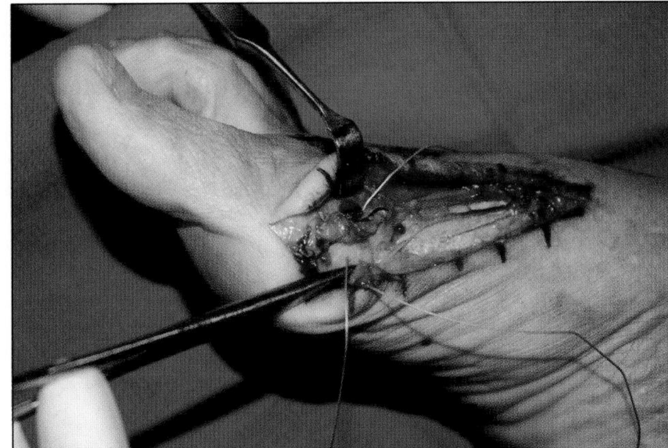

FIGURE 21

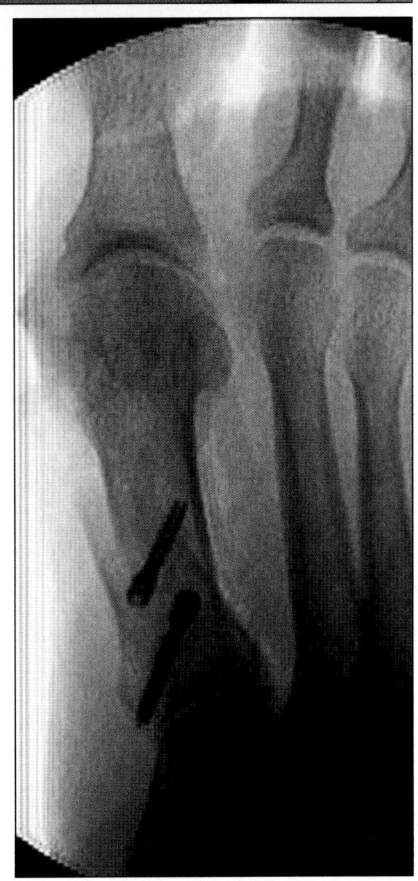

FIGURE 22

- With an increased DMAA, a supplemental distal 1MT osteotomy is warranted, either a medial closing wedge osteotomy (Reverdin) or a biplanar distal chevron osteotomy, to re-establish the proper alignment of the 1MT's articular surface on the 1MT shaft. Because of the potential need for a distal osteotomy in addition to a proximal correction, the lateral capsular release must always be performed judiciously in order to prevent compromising the blood supply to the 1MT head.

- Occasionally, deeper soft tissues may be repaired over the osteotomy and at the 1TMT joint, but typically the only layers that can be closed are the subcutaneous tissue and the skin. The sensory nerve to the hallux must be protected during this closure. The dorsal first web space incision is closed as well (Fig. 23).
- A sterile dressing is applied to the wounds.

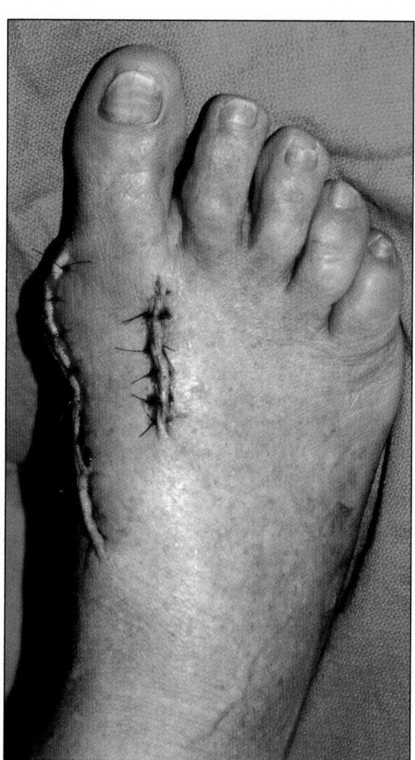

FIGURE 23

PEARLS

- *Edema will persist for a minimum of 6 months.*
- *Routine bunion strapping may not be required; postoperative radiographs determine hallux position and guide the need for bunion strapping.*

Postoperative Care and Expected Outcomes

- Bunion strapping and surgical dressing are applied.
- Weekly follow-up is scheduled for 1MTP joint manipulation, bunion strapping, and radiographs to assess 1MTP joint position and healing.
- Bunion strapping is recommended for 6 weeks and a toe spacer for an additional 4–6 weeks to unload the medial capsulorrhaphy while it heals.
- Protective weight-bearing status, with heel weight bearing only and limiting weight bearing on the forefoot, should be maintained until there is radiographic evidence for healing of the osteotomy (typically 6 weeks).
- Figure 24 shows the final follow-up of a proximal 1MT osteotomy 7 years postoperatively in a clinical view (Fig. 24A) and a weight-bearing lateral

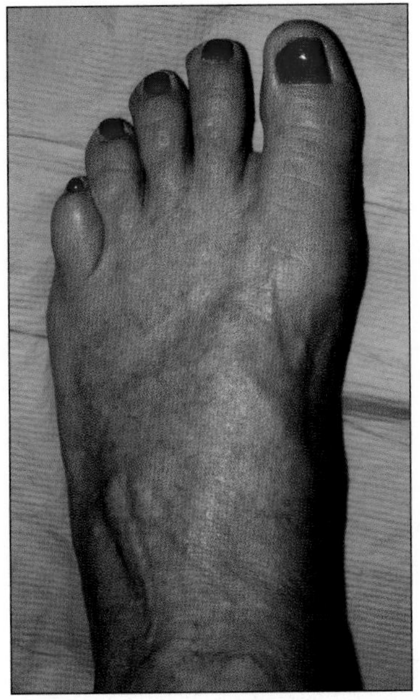

A

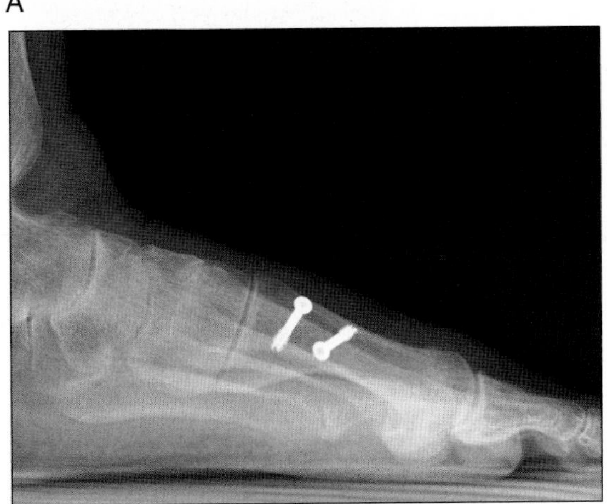

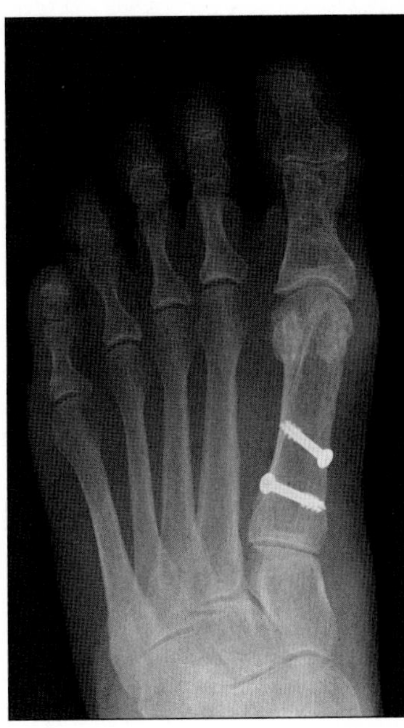

FIGURE 24 B C

radiograph (Fig. 24B). In a weight-bearing AP radiograph (Fig. 24C), note the ideal 1MT head position centered over the sesamoid complex.

PITFALLS

- *Postoperative callus formation at the osteotomy site (Fig. 25A) indicates inadequate fixation, motion at the osteotomy site, and potential for loss of correction. We recommend casting and protective weight bearing until there is radiographic evidence for healing (typically 8–10 weeks from time of surgery). Note the relatively short osteotomy (lacking stability) in Figure 25B. After casting and delaying weight bearing, callus consolidation is achieved with minimal loss of correction (Fig. 25C). On follow-up at 1 year, there is satisfactory maintenance of correction and healing with callus resorption (Fig. 25D).*

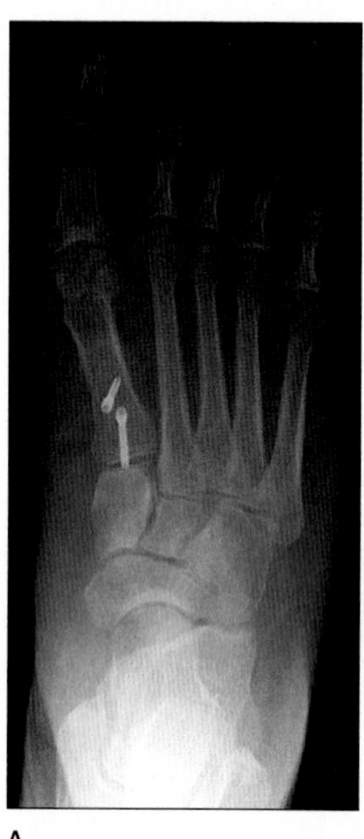
A

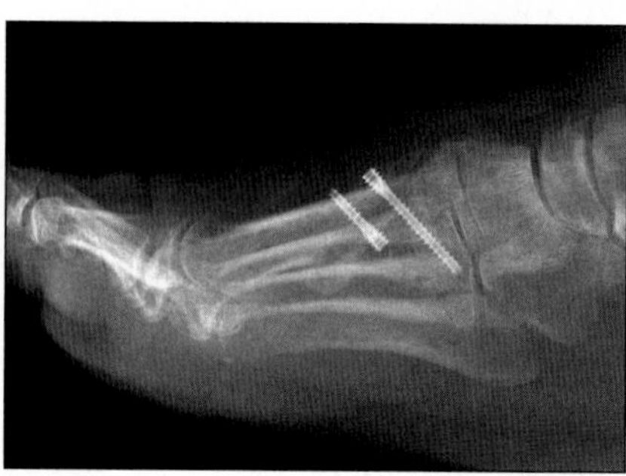
B

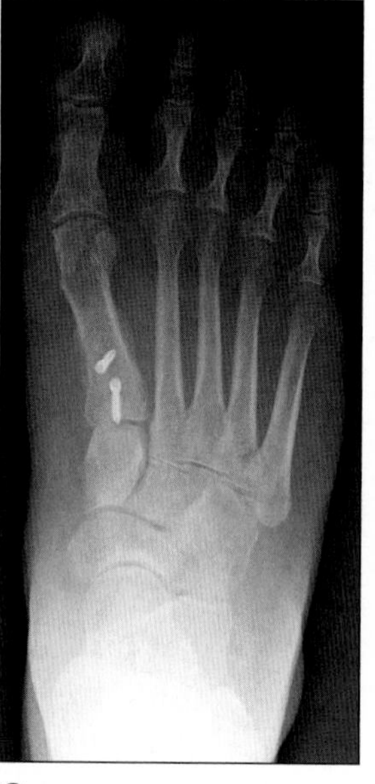
C

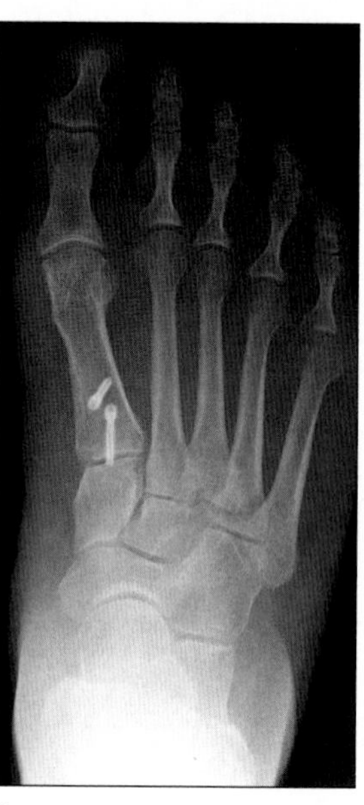
D

FIGURE 25

Evidence

Chiodo CP, Schon LC, Myerson MS. Clinical results with the Ludloff osteotomy for correction of adult hallux valgus. Foot Ankle Int. 2004;25:532–6.

Peer-reviewed article on the clinical results of the Ludloff osteotomy (Grade B recommendation). (Level IV evidence)

Nyska M, Trnka HJ, Parks BG, et al. The Ludloff metatarsal osteotomy: guidelines for optimal correction based on a geometric analysis conducted on a sawbone model. Foot Ankle Int. 2003;23:34–9.

Biomechanical study that provides a better understanding of how to perform the Ludloff osteotomy.

Trnka HJ, Hofstaetter SG, Hofstaetter JG, Gruber F, Adams SB Jr, Easley ME. Intermediate-term results of the Ludloff osteotomy in one hundred and eleven feet. J Bone Joint Surg Am. 2008;90:531–9.

Peer-reviewed article on the clinical results of the Ludloff osteotomy (Grade B recommendation). (Level IV evidence)

Trnka HJ, Hofstaetter SG, Easley ME. Intermediate-term results of the Ludloff osteotomy in one hundred and eleven feet. Surgical technique. J Bone Joint Surg Am. 2009;91(Suppl 2):156–68.

Detailed surgical technique of the Ludloff osteotomy.

PROCEDURE 5

Hallux Rigidus: Cheilectomy with and without a Dorsiflexion Phalangeal Osteotomy

Carol Frey

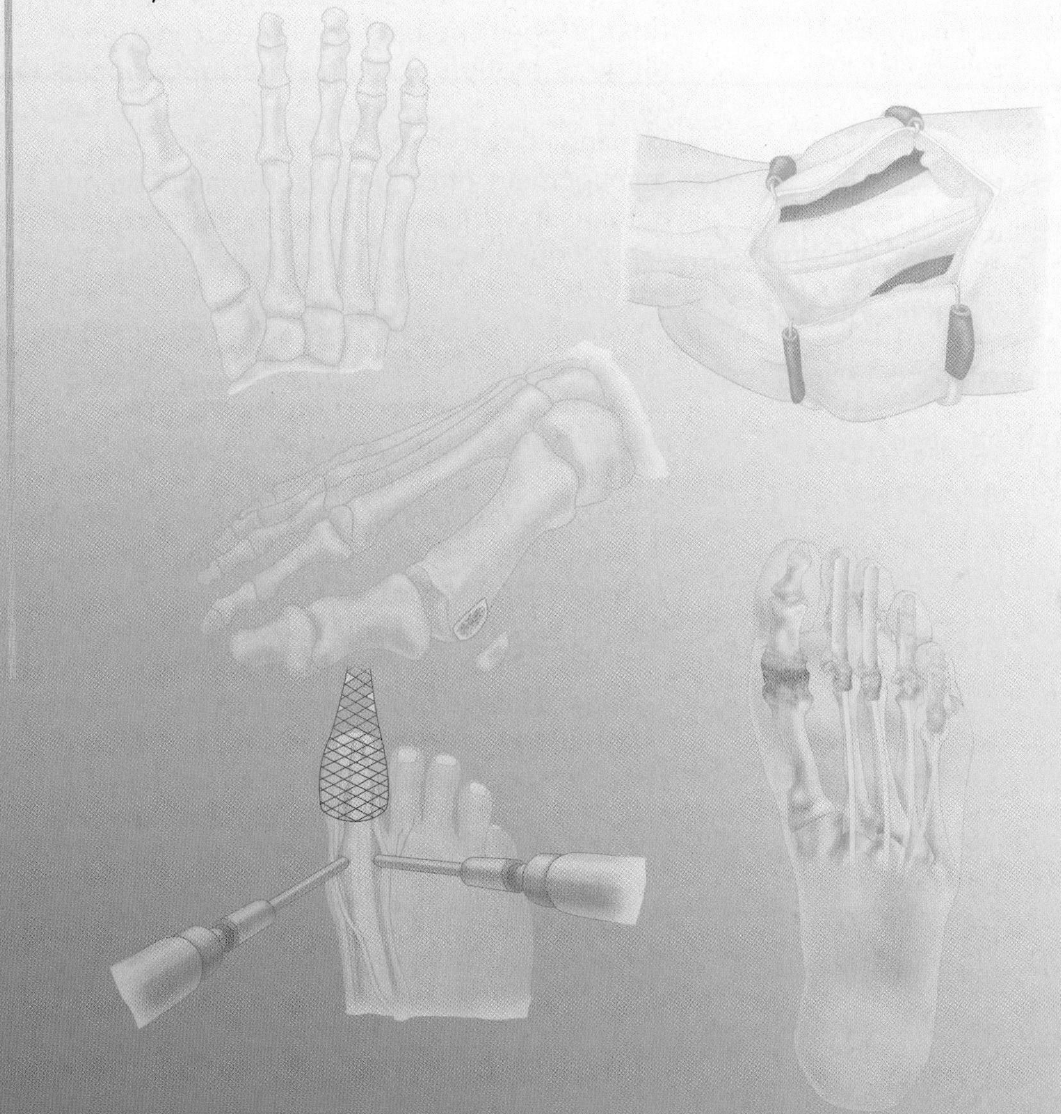

Cheilectomy with and without a Dorsiflexion Phalangeal Osteotomy

PITFALLS

- *In cases of grade III hallux rigidus, the patient must accept higher failure rate.*
- *Cheilectomy is not indicated where there is pain in all ranges of motion.*

Controversies

- The cheilectomy requires early range of motion and the proximal phalanx osteotomy needs some immobilization time to heal. Thus, rehabilitation in combined cases is at odds.

Indications

- Cheilectomy is indicated in patients with mild to moderate (grade I and II) hallux rigidus (the procedure of choice in this group).
- Cheilectomy is also indicated in grade III hallux rigidus when the patient wishes to preserve range of motion of the metatarsophalangeal (MTP) joint.
- Phalangeal osteotomy is indicated in the management of grade I and II hallux rigidus in patients in whom more dorsiflexion is required than can be obtained by cheilectomy alone (~10% of patients).
- Phalangeal osteotomy is usually combined with a cheilectomy.
- Surgical options depend on the degree of involvement of the great toe, as well as the functional needs of the patient.
  - With grades I and II disease, the osteophytes should be removed, a cheilectomy performed, and the joint preserved.
  - A dorsal closing wedge osteotomy of the proximal phalanx, also referred to as a Moberg procedure, helps improve dorsiflexion in a patient who has satisfactory plantar flexion at the MTP.
  - Patients with grade III disease can benefit from resection arthroplasty, fusion, and, in some rare cases, joint replacement.
  - A dorsiflexion phalangeal osteotomy is usually added in a younger and more active patient with grade I and II hallux rigidus.

Examination/Imaging

PHYSICAL EXAM

- There will be swelling around the great toe and prominent dorsal osteophytes (Fig. 1).
- There may be an associated bursitis.
- The interphalangeal joint of the great toe may have compensatory hyperextension with an associated underlying plantar callus.

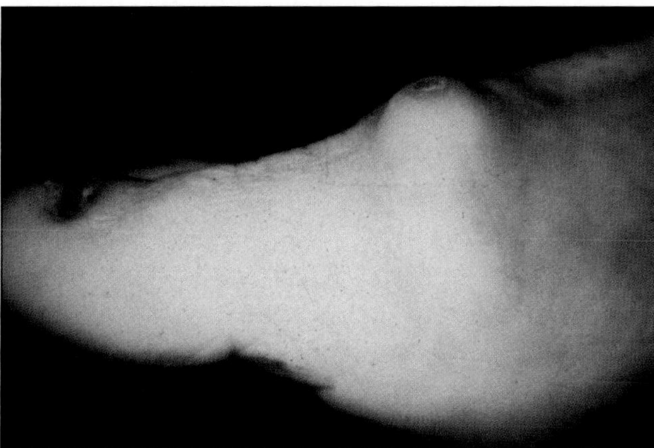

FIGURE 1

- Compare range of motion of the hallux MTP to the opposite side. Normal is 30° of plantar flexion and 90° of dorsiflexion. Dorsiflexion is limited with hallux rigidus.
- Axial load, sagittal motion, and dorsiflexion often reproduce the pain.
- Systemic conditions such as gout or rheumatoid arthritis must be ruled out. Look for other features of systemic arthropathy.
- Pain may be over the osteophyte or with range of motion.

Imaging Studies

- Weight-bearing anteroposterior (AP), lateral, and oblique radiographs are recommended. The radiographs may show joint space narrowing, particularly on the AP view, where there may be bone overlap from the osteophytes. The lateral view provides a better assessment of the joint space (Fig. 2); osteophytes can be identified on the margins of the metatarsal and proximal phalanx of the great toe.

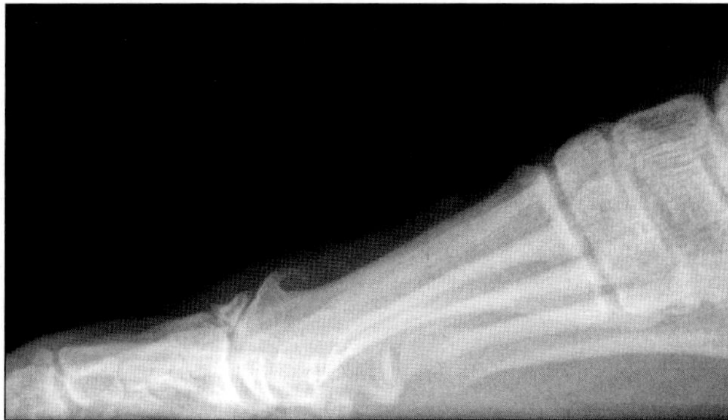

FIGURE 2

Treatment Options

- Shoe modifications and orthotic devices can be used to reduce the movement that causes pain.
  - Shoe modifications include a rocker sole, stable sole, graphic midsole, or steel shank.
  - Avoid high-heeled shoes, which put the toe into the painful plantar flexed position.
  - Avoid excessive pushoff.
  - Orthotic devices fashioned with a Morton's extension will help decrease motion at the MTP and make the patient more comfortable.
- Stretch the Achilles tendon to improve dorsiflexion at the ankle.
- Additional options include
  - Anti-inflammatory medication
  - Manipulation and injection of the great toe MTP

- Plain radiographs may show flattening of the distal metatarsal articular surface, narrowing of the joint space, osteophytes surrounding the articular surface, sclerosis, and cyst formation in the subchondral regions.
- Radiographic changes are categorized as follows (Fig. 3):
  - Grade I: mild to moderate osteophyte formation but good preservation of the MTP joint space.
  - Grade II: moderate osteophyte formation with joint space narrowing and subchondral sclerosis.
  - Grade III: marked osteophyte formation and loss of the visible joint space, with or without subchondral cyst formation.
- Magnetic resonance imaging is indicated if the patient has significant loss of motion of the MTP, yet the radiographs are normal. In this case the patient should be evaluated for chondral and capsular injuries to the great toe MTP.

Surgical Anatomy

- Figure 3 shows the anatomy of the great toe.

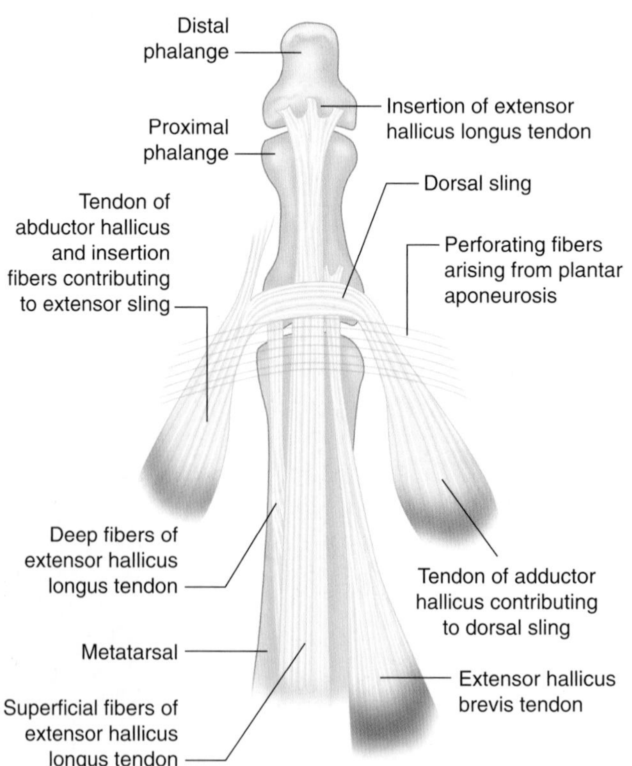

FIGURE 3

Instrumentation

- The cheilectomy and proximal phalanx osteotomy are usually performed under regional anesthesia with intravenous sedation.
- A pneumatic ankle tourniquet is applied over several layers of soft roll or cast padding.

Pearls

- *Do not enter the sheath of the EHL; this will decrease the risk of postoperative adhesions.*

Positioning

- The patient should be placed supine with the surgeon seated with his or her back to the patient and facing the foot.

Portals/Exposures

- A dorsal longitudinal incision is made over the dorsomedial aspect of the first MTP and just medial to the extensor hallucis longus (EHL) tendon (Fig. 4).
- Care must be taken to avoid the dorsal cutaneous sensory nerve to the hallux.

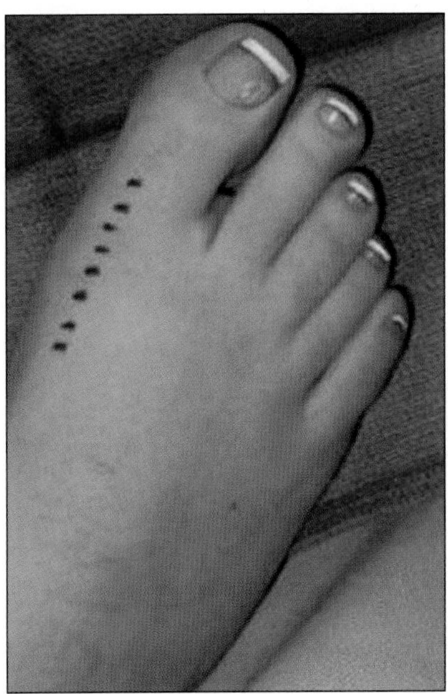

FIGURE 4

Procedure

Step 1

- The extensor hood is divided, and the capsule of the first MTP (1MTP) is entered through a straight incision medial to the EHL, exposing the first metatarsal (1MT) head and dorsal osteophytes (Fig. 5).
- Using sharp and blunt dissection, the capsule is elevated off of the 1MT head and base of the proximal phalanx.
- The EHL is retracted in a lateral direction.
- Two small Hohmann retractors are used to retract the capsule and EHL tendon.

Step 2

- The great toe is plantar flexed about 45–60° and the condition of the cartilage on the 1MT head and the base of the proximal phalanx is inspected.
- The dorsal osteophytes are revealed and the osteotomy is begun.
- One third of the MT head can safely be removed.
- Care must be taken to remove the dorsal, lateral, and medial osteophytes using a micro-sagittal saw (Fig. 6A and 6B). Figure 6C shows the 1MTP head after the removal of the osteophytes.
- The metatarsal head is inspected for chondromalacia. Any area with complete loss of cartilage and exposed bone can be drilled to promote the formation of fibrous cartilage.

Pearls

- *The amount of MT head removal is dependent on the amount that is required to regain 90° of dorsiflexion and also adequately remove all of the osteophytes.*
- *Any areas of cartilage damage with exposed bone should be drilled or microfractured, to facilitate the growth of fibrocartilage.*

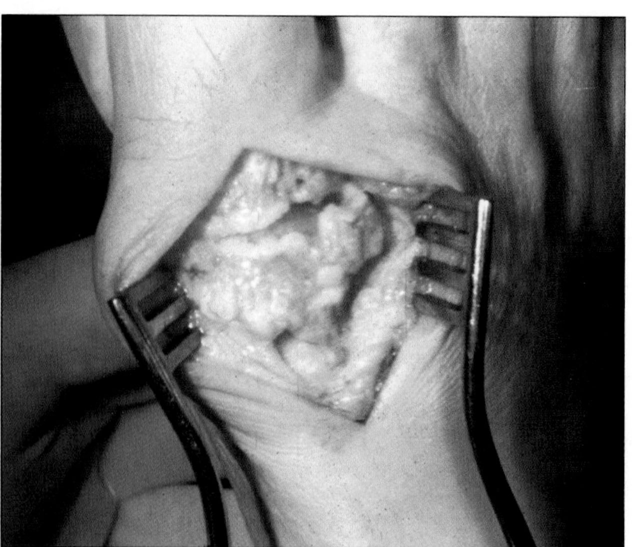

FIGURE 5

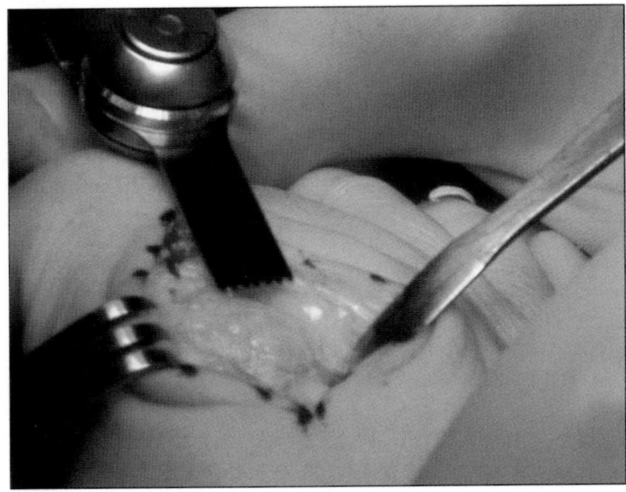

A

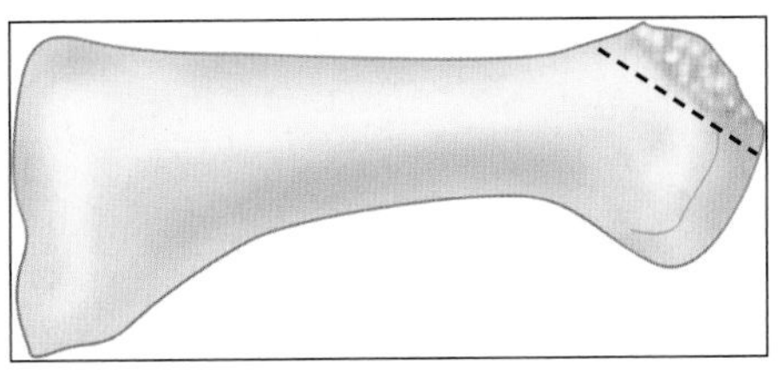

B

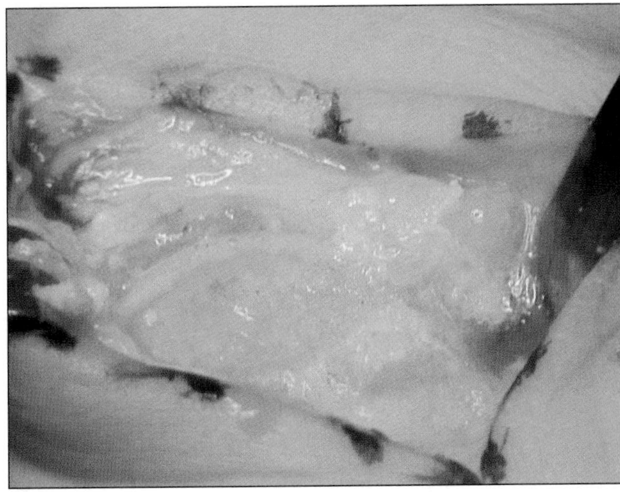

C

FIGURE 6

- The saw is used in a distal-to-proximal direction. The line of resection should not excavate into the shaft of the 1MT. Therefore, it is angled upward.
- A micro-reciprocating rasp is utilized to reshape the metatarsal head to its original contour and to remove any areas of prominent bone and ridges that may remain (Fig. 7). The rasp is an efficient tool to use in the lateral and medial gutter.
- Marginal osteophytes on the base of the proximal phalanx are removed with a rongeur.

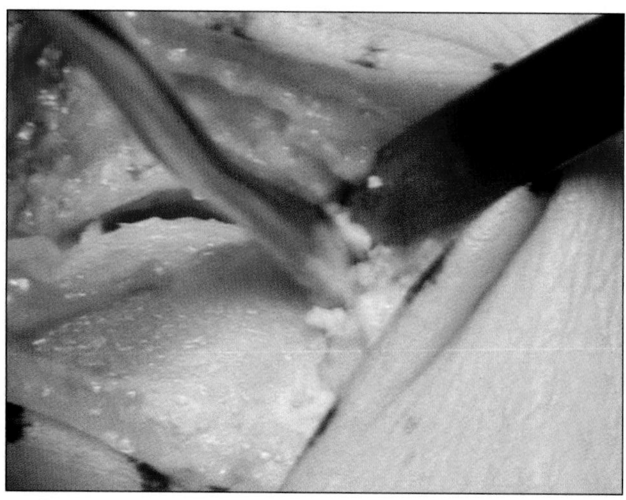

FIGURE 7

Pearls

- *The patient should have normal motion in plantar flexion.*
- *Some plantar flexion is sacrificed to improve dorsiflexion.*
- *The hallux is placed in a position of dorsiflexion.*

Pitfalls

- *When the Moberg procedure is utilized, the patient may develop arthritis in the interphalangeal joint of the great toe, as it tries to compensate for the expected loss of plantar flexion.*

Step 3

- The joint is irrigated and the range of motion is checked.
- The MTP should regain about 90° of dorsiflexion on the operating room table. Usually half of this is lost once the patient begins range-of-motion exercises postoperatively.
- If the patient has less than 45° of dorsiflexion at the conclusion of the cheilectomy, a Moberg procedure is recommended.

Step 4

- The Moberg procedure is added for a patient who has not regained a significant amount of dorsiflexion of the MTP after a cheilectomy.
- The approach for the Moberg procedure is through a distal extension of the dorsal medial incision used for the cheilectomy. If the procedure was to be done alone, the MTP joint capsule would not be opened.
- A micro-sagittal saw is used to create a dorsally based wedge osteotomy (Fig. 8A).
  - The first cut is made in the metaphyseal flare of the proximal aspect of the proximal phalanx of the great toe. The cut goes through the dorsal cortex and up to but not through the plantar cortex. The first cut is parallel to the MTP joint surface. Approximately 2 mm of the plantar surface is kept intact.
  - The wedge is created by making a second cut 1–3 mm distal to the first and angled to make a dorsally based wedge. The second cut meets up with the first at the plantar cortex.
  - The wedge is removed.

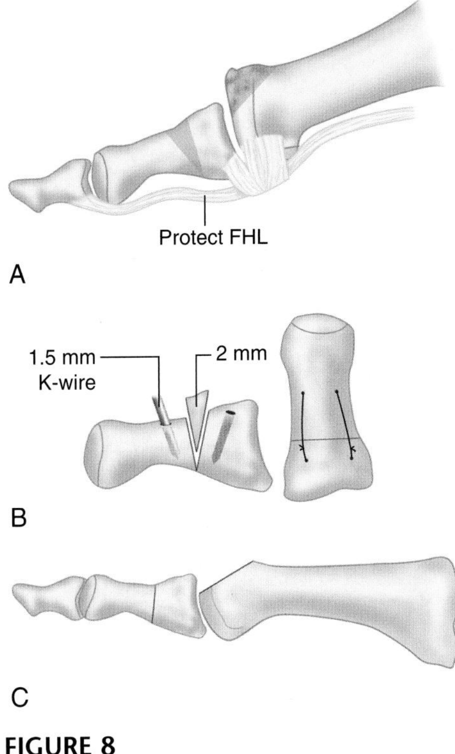

FIGURE 8

- Manual pressure is used to place the hallux in the desired position of dorsiflexion and lifted slightly above horizontal (Fig. 8B).
- To close down the wedge and hold it in position, 0.045-inch Kirschner wires are placed from proximal to distal in a crossed pattern (Fig. 8C). (A small dorsal staple may be used instead of the Kirschner wires.) A drill hole can be made on either side of the osteotomy and a wire suture or Fiberwire can be used to close the osteotomy. The knot should be placed to the lateral side, so as not to rub on shoes.

Controversies

- Rehabilitation planning is at odds with a Moberg procedure, where some immobilization is required for proper healing, and a cheilectomy, where early range of motion encourages good results.

Postoperative Care and Expected Outcomes

- Over 95% of patients with grade I and II hallux rigidus should expect good to excellent results with cheilectomy.
- The cheilectomy is not a difficult operation, and the results are largely dependent on the proper selection of patients for this procedure.

Evidence

Coughlin MJ, Shurnas PS. Hallux rigidus: demographics, etiology, and radiographic assessment. Foot Ankle Int. 2003;24:731–43.

Hallux rigidus was not found to be associated with first ray hypermobility, long 1MT, Achilles or gastrocnemius tightness, elevatus, abnormal foot posture, symptomatic hallux valgus, shoewear, occupation, or adolescent onset. It was associated with bilateral involvement in those with a family history, hallux valgus interphalangeus, history of trauma in unilateral cases, and females. (Level II evidence)

Coughlin MJ, Shurnas PS. Hallux rigidus: grading and long-term results. J Bone Joint Surg [Br]. 2003;85:2072–88.

This report evaluates the long-term results of surgical treatment for hallux rigidus in 114 patients. The mean follow-up period was 9.6 years for cheilectomy and 6.7 years for fusions. The authors report a significant improvement in range of motion in the cheilectomy group and a significant improvement in pain in both groups. Ninety-seven percent of all patients had good to excellent results reported. A five-grade clinical and radiographic system was used in this study. (Level II evidence)

Solan MC, Calder JDF, Bendall SP. Manipulation and injection for hallux rigidus. J Bone Joint Surg [Br]. 2001;83:706–8.

Patients with mild (grade I) hallux rigidus had symptomatic relief with the injections for a median of 6 months, and only one third eventually required surgery. Patients with moderate (grade II) changes required surgery two thirds of the time, and those with severe (grade III) changes had little symptomatic relief. All of the grade III patients eventually required surgery. (Level II evidence)

PROCEDURE 6

Arthrodesis of the Great Toe Metatarsophalangeal Joint

Glenn B. Pfeffer

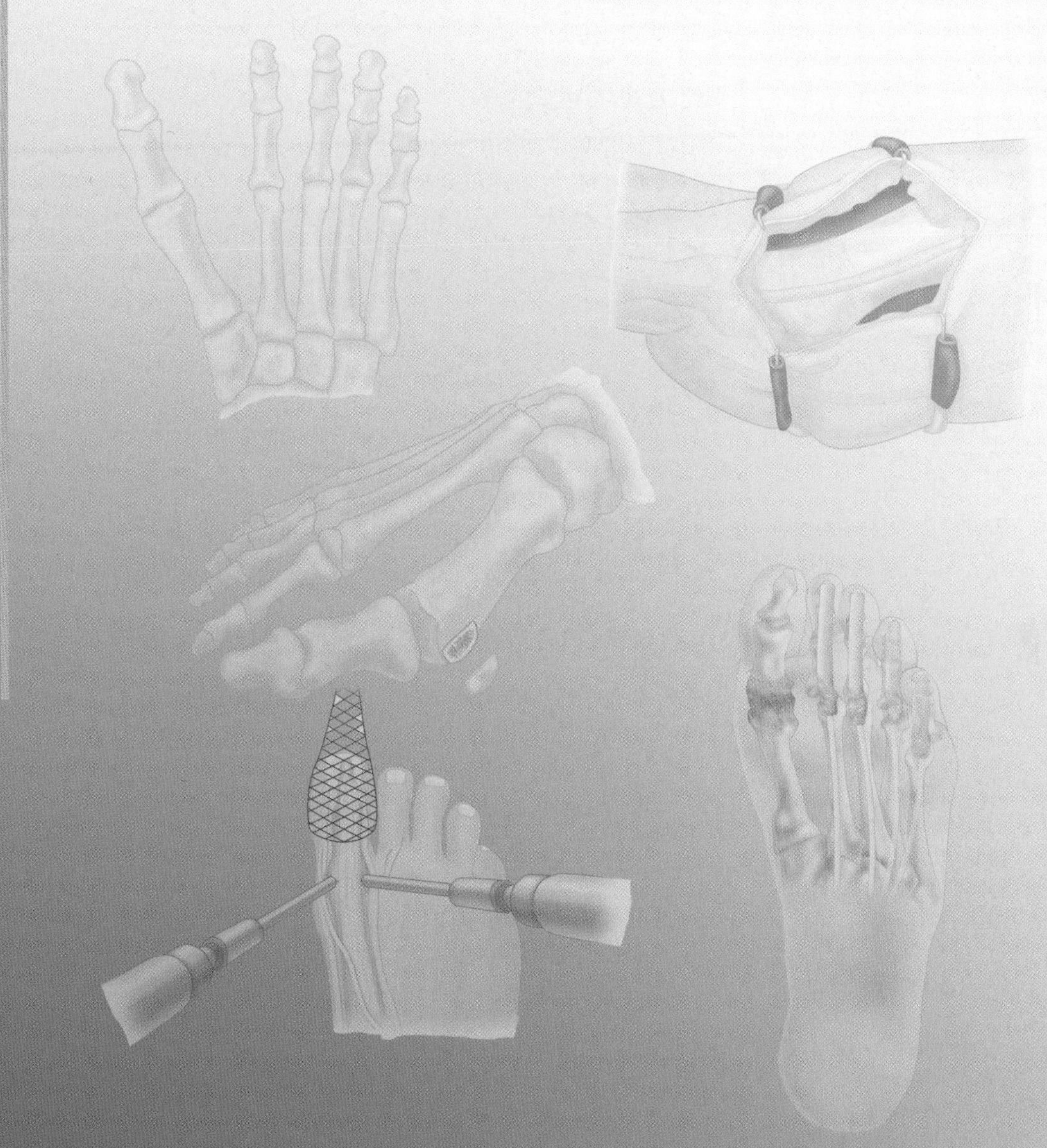

Indications

- Chronic joint pain from advanced arthritis
- Severe deformity that limits activity or shoewear

Pitfalls

- *High-heeled shoes will be limited after surgery to approximately 2 inches, which may be unacceptable to some patients.*
- *Infection, inadequate blood supply, and severe osteopenia are contraindications to the procedure.*

Controversies

- Arthrodesis is the most commonly performed procedure for advanced symptomatic arthritis or severe deformity of the great toe. The end result is highly predictable, alleviates symptoms, and restores excellent function.
- Unreliable surgical options include resection arthroplasty, hemiarthroplasty, or total joint arthroplasty.
- Concomitant arthritic changes of the interphalangeal joint are not an absolute contraindication to metatarsophalangeal (MTP) fusion.
- A first MTP fusion will cause the intermetatarsal angle to narrow by approximately 4°. A simultaneous osteotomy of the first metatarsal base is therefore rarely needed.
- A sesmoid may be arthritic, but rarely has to be excised at the time of the fusion.

Treatment Options

- A medial longitudinal arch support may decrease pressure on the great toe.
- A stiff-soled shoe will decrease motion of the great toe during ambulation. Patients have often tried this approach on their own, prior to seeking consultation.
- A rocker sole, which stiffens the shoe sole and takes stress off of the forefoot, can be added to a walking shoe by a pedorthist or orthotist. Although highly effective, all of the patient's shoes will require this modification.
- A cortisone injection may improve symptoms for a short period of time.

Examination/Imaging

- There is limited and painful motion of the great toe.
- Large dorsal osteophytes are often present.
- An incision from a previous surgery may dictate the operative approach.
- Standing anteroposterior (AP) (Fig. 1A) and lateral (Fig. 1B) radiographs should be taken. Oblique views often provide the best visualization of the joint.
- Arthritic changes in the sesamoid may be present, but rarely have to be addressed operatively.

Surgical Anatomy

- Anatomy of the MTP joint of the great toe (Fig. 2)

Positioning

- The patient is supine.
- A small bump under the ipsilateral hip will help bring the foot into an upright position.
- An ankle or thigh tourniquet is used.

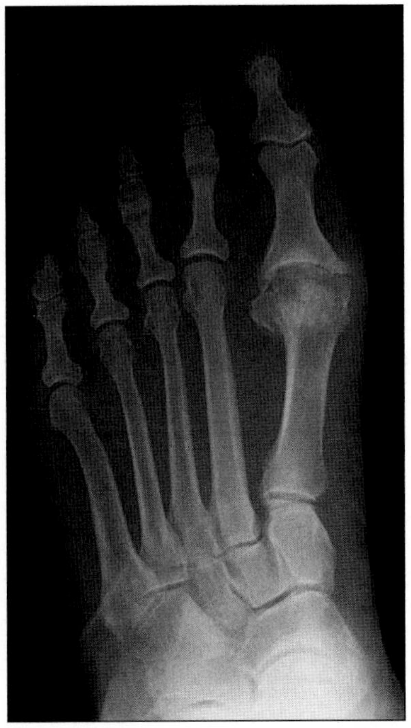

A

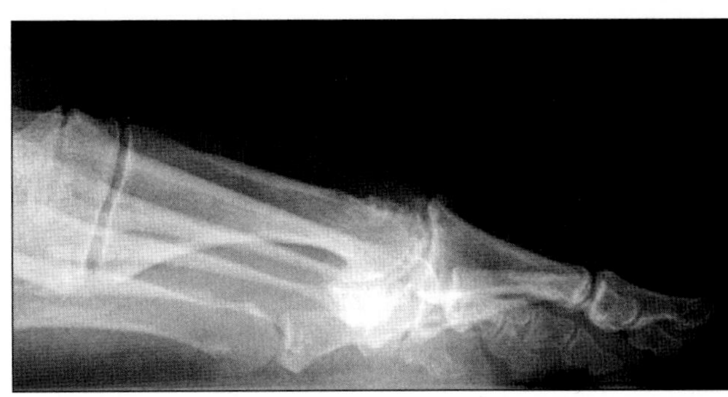

B

FIGURE 1

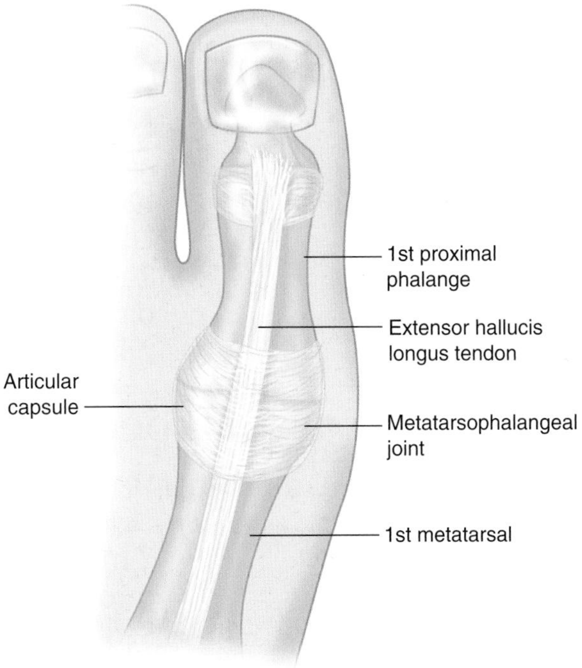

1st proximal phalange

Extensor hallucis longus tendon

Articular capsule

Metatarsophalangeal joint

1st metatarsal

FIGURE 2

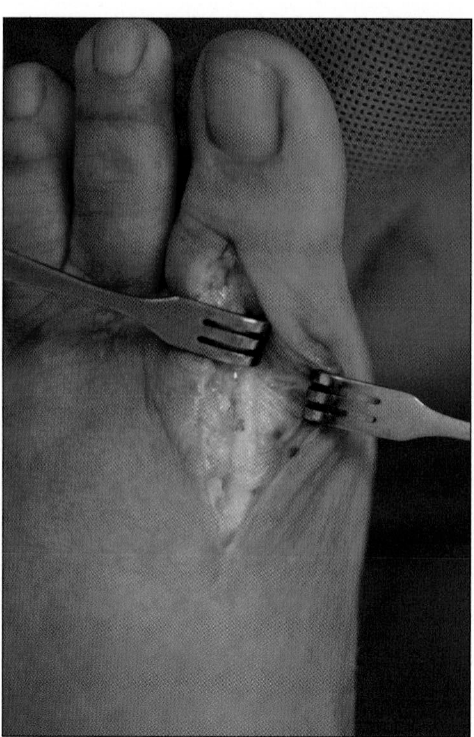

FIGURE 3

Portals/Exposures

- Make a 5-cm longitudinal incision over the dorsal aspect of the great toe, just medial to the extensor hallucis longus (EHL) (Fig. 3).
- Loupe magnification may be helpful.
- The procedure is performed under a femoral/sciatic or popliteal block, to help maximize postoperative pain control.

Procedure

Step 1

- Divide the dorsal capsule with a longitudinal incision 2 mm medial to the EHL. Retract the tendon laterally throughout the case.
- Remove any loose bodies that often sit on the dorsum of the joint.
- Elevate the capsule medially and laterally, while protecting the EHL tendon (Fig. 4A). Divide the collateral ligaments, mobilize the plantar plate, and expose the entire metatarsal head and base of the proximal phalanx (Fig. 4B).
- Use a small dental rongeur to remove osteophytes.

Pearls

- *Hyperflexion of the MTP will help expose the metatarsal head during the initial approach.*
- *Injury to the tendon can occur if the EHL is forcefully retracted while the joint is hyperflexed.*

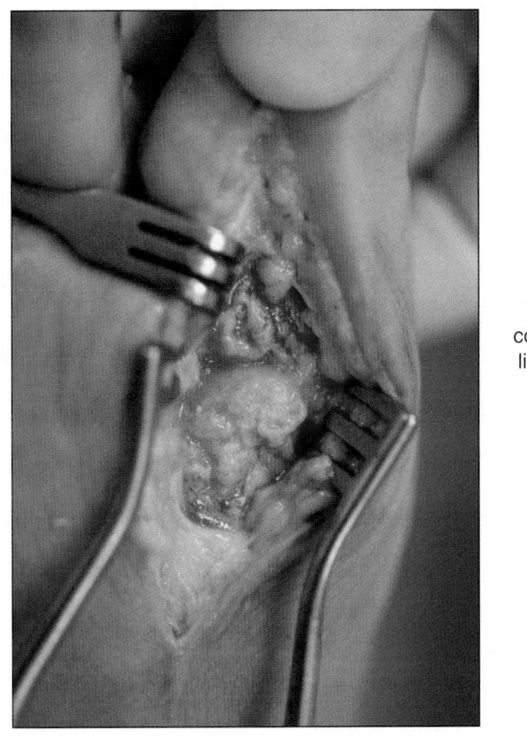

A

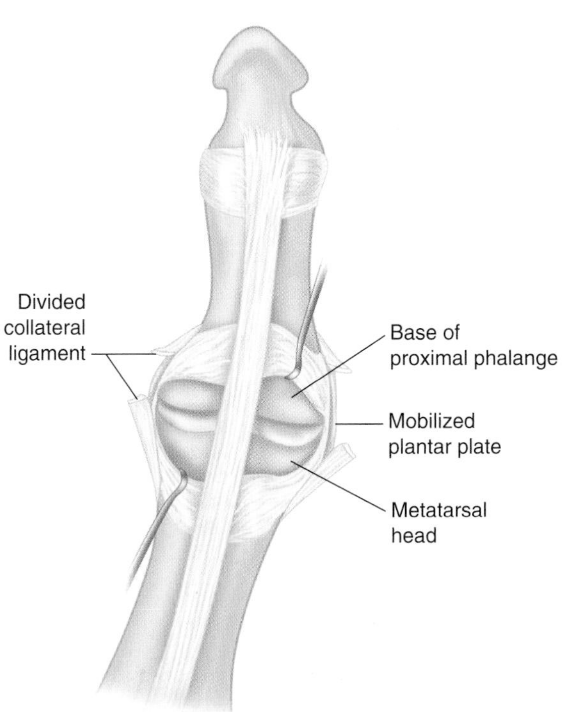

B

FIGURE 4

Step 2

- Use a micro-sagittal saw to remove the articular surfaces (Fig. 5). Only 1–2 mm of bone is removed with these initial cuts, which are perpendicular to the long axis of the metatarsal and to the proximal phalanx.
- Place a pin from the Stryker great toe reamer set into the central metatarsal head and several inches down the shaft. It is important to be central on the head.

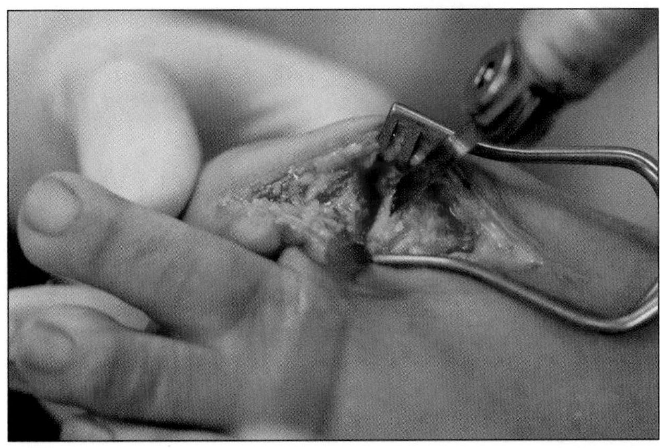

FIGURE 5

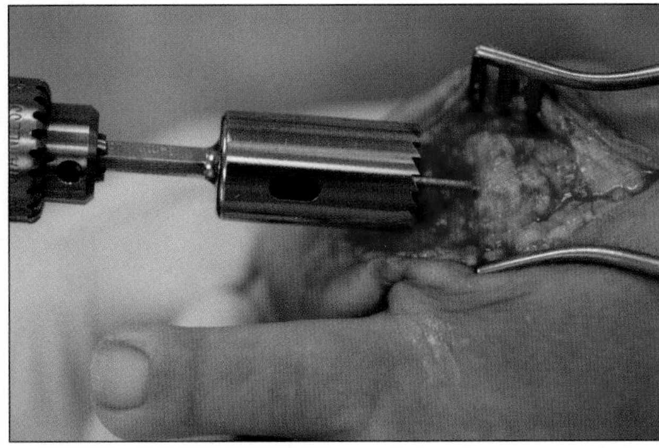

FIGURE 6

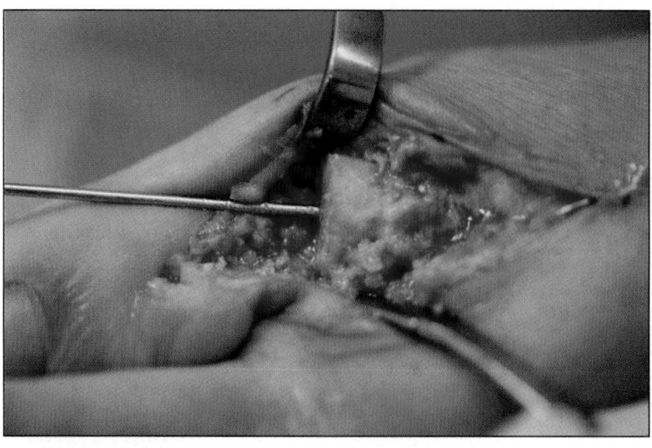

FIGURE 7

PEARLS

- *A goal of surgery is to end up with a great toe that is within 1 cm of overall length of the second toe.*
- *Attempt to preserve the weight-bearing function of the first metatarsal head by maintaining adequate length.*
- *Use cool water lavage on the bone surfaces while reaming, to avoid heating the bone.*
- *The fusion surfaces can be drilled with a small Kirschner wire (K-wire) to maximize surface area and remove small portions of sclerotic bone.*

PITFALLS

- *Protect the EHL during reaming. The tendon can easily be cut by the sharp edge of the reamers.*

- Ream the head with the appropriately sized barrel-shaped reamer, while holding the joint in maximal plantar flexion (Fig. 6). Carefully protect the tendon. The chosen reamer should be approximately equal to the width of the metatarsal shaft (Fig. 7).
- The concave-shaped reamer should then be used to remove the remaining cartilage and sclerotic bone (Fig. 8). Minimize bone resection (Fig. 9).

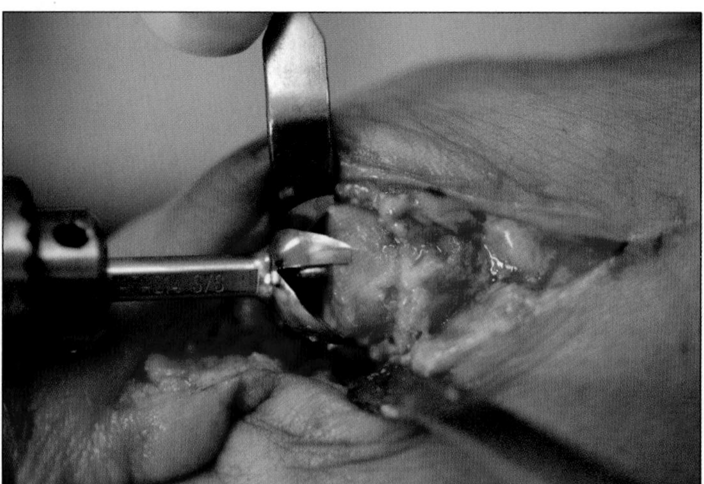

FIGURE 8

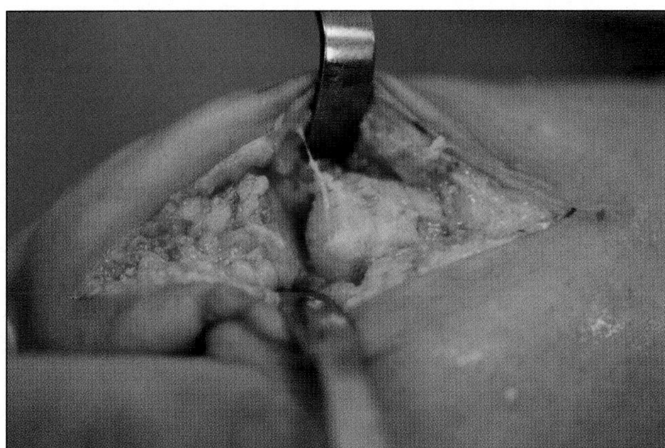

FIGURE 9

- Remove the pin and drill it into the central longitudinal axis of the proximal phalanx. Use the convex-shaped reamer to prepare the fusion site (Fig. 10).
  - This reamer should be the same size as the one used for the metatarsal. This reamer has the sharpest edges and can most easily damage the EHL.

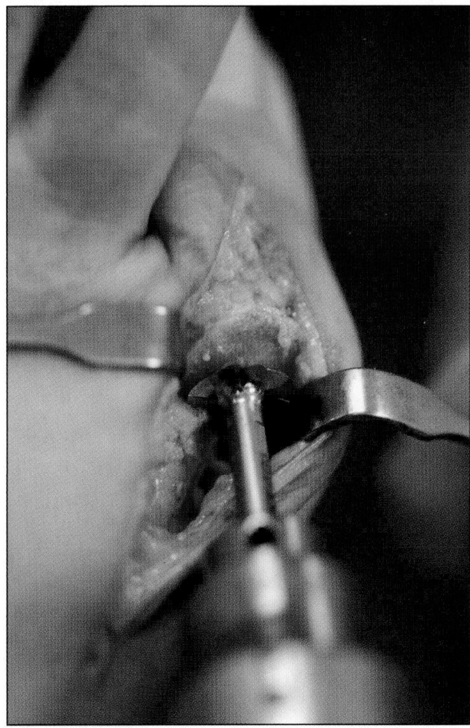

FIGURE 10

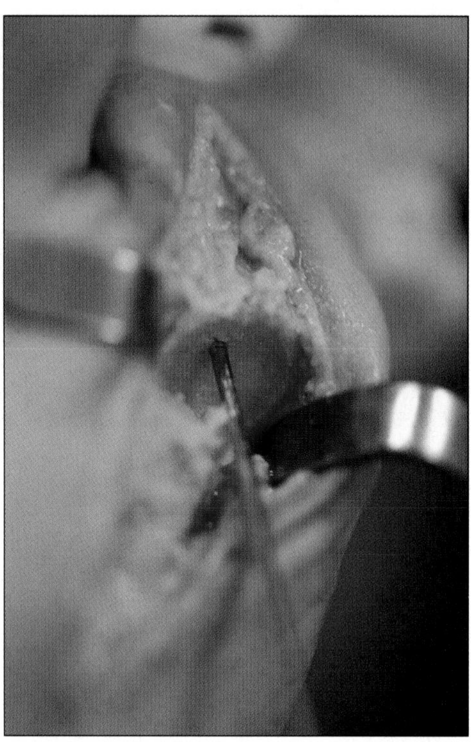

A

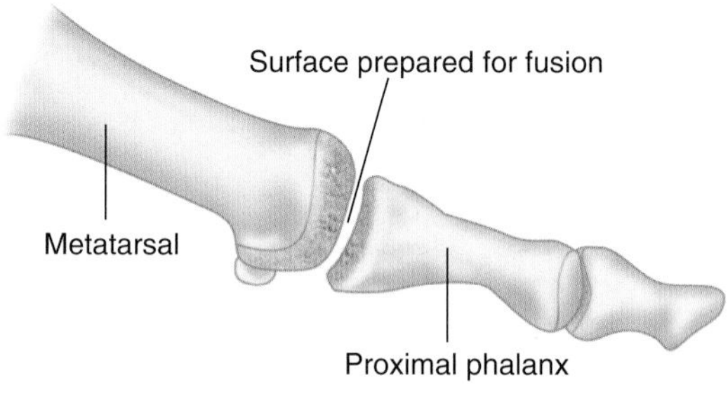

B

FIGURE 11

- Ream into the proximal phalanx until the reamer is completely seated into the bone (Fig. 11A). Otherwise a gap will occur circumferentially when the concave metatarsal is seated into the convex phalanx. Remove the proximal phalanx pin (Fig. 11B).

Controversies

- Flat cuts are another option for fusion. Perfect bone apposition and fusion position are much more difficult with this approach, often requiring multiple cuts. Spherical reaming allows meticulous positioning of the fusion in a stable construct.
- The toe reamer technique is not appropriate for a patient with a failed implant. These patients require a graft both to fill the defect and to preserve as much length as possible.

Step 3

- Accurate positioning of the toe is essential.
  - The great toe should be positioned in sufficient valgus so that it neither impinges on the second toe nor creates a gap between the toes.
  - The great toe should be in 10° of dorsiflexion relative to the floor, which usually correlates with 5 mm elevation off of the weight-bearing surface (Fig. 12A). A rigid plate, such as the top of an instrument box, can be used to simulate a weight-bearing position of the foot (Fig. 12B).
  - If the toe is fused in too much dorsiflexion, it will rub on the top of the shoe; if it is fused in too much plantar flexion, normal toeoff will be compromised.
- The *radiographic bone angles* are usually 10–20° of valgus and 20–25° of dorsiflexion. A short toe commonly requires less valgus.
- The toe should be in neutral rotation, which can be judged by the position of the nail.

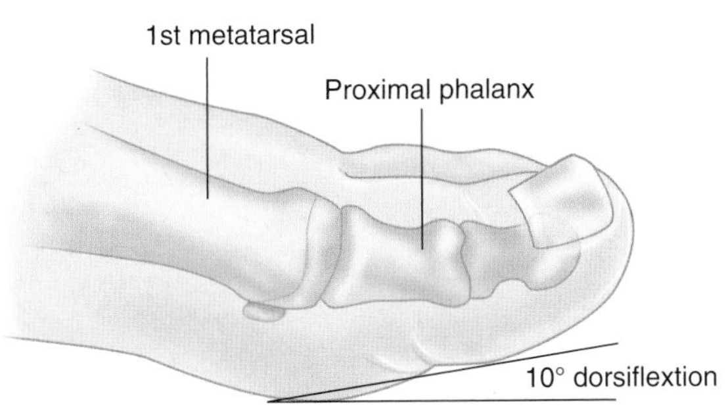

A

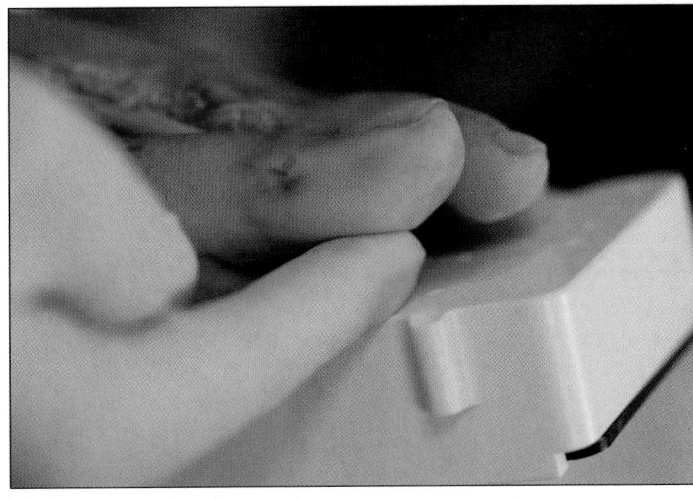
B

FIGURE 12

- Place a temporary percutaneous 0.62-inch K-wire across the fusion site (Fig. 13). Use a 4- to 6-hole low-profile plate for fixation. A Leibinger maxillofacial plate is an excellent option (Fig. 14A and 14B). The Arthrex toe fusion plate is another good option, especially for a revision fusion.

Pearls

- *There is great variation in first metatarsal declination, depending on the degree of pes planus or cavus of the foot. For this reason, there is no definitive phalangeal-metatarsal bone fusion angle. Intraoperative fluoroscopy should be used to evaluate the bony position of the fusion, but the external posture of the toe is what counts. An oblique 4-0 lagged screw can be added to the fusion construct, if needed.*
- *Two crossed screws may be used instead of the dorsal plate in patients who have excellent bone stock.*

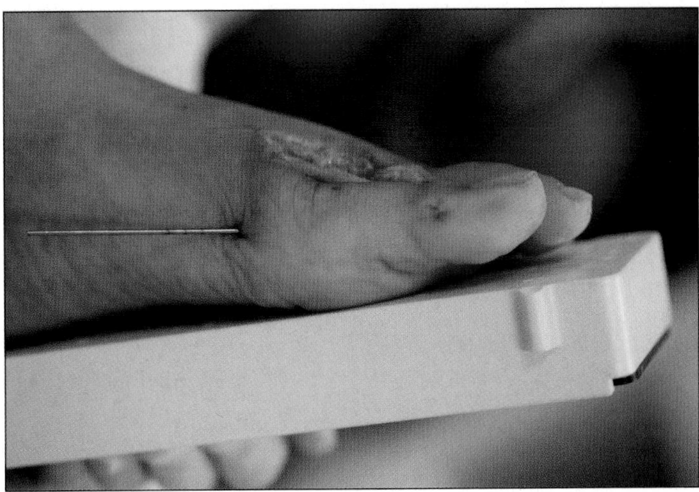

FIGURE 13

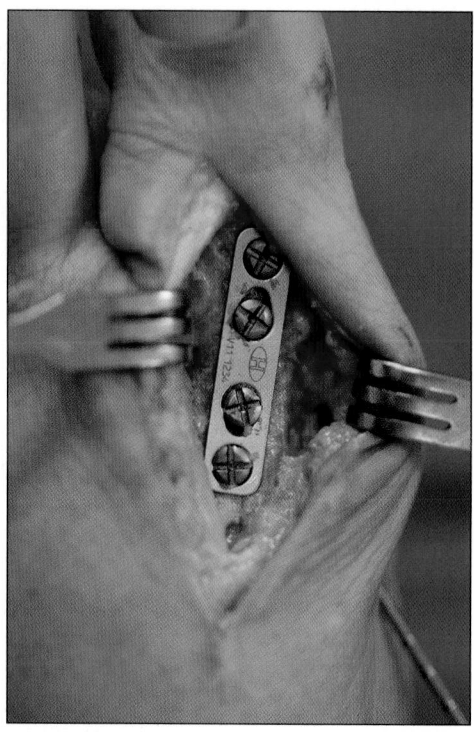
A

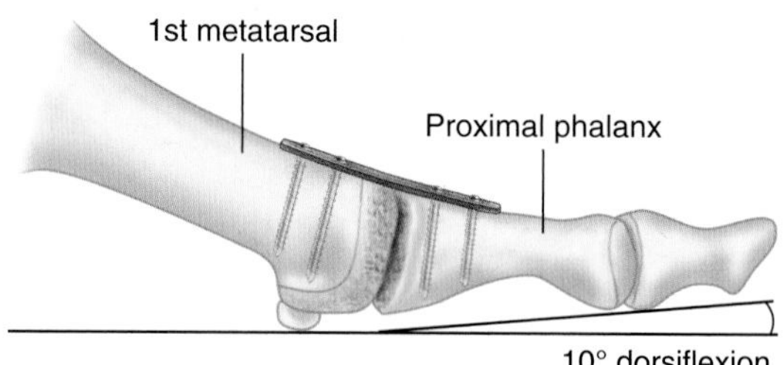

B

FIGURE 14

PITFALLS

- *A plantar shelf of bone can prevent the metatarsal head from seating into the proximal phalanx. It can also block the appropriate position of fusion.*
- *The plate should be exactly contoured. Otherwise, the fusion angle can change as the screws are tightened. Always assess the position of the fusion after each screw is placed.*
- *There is little leeway in positioning the fusion. The end result must allow the patient to walk comfortably in flats or a small heel. The toe should not be placed in excessive dorsiflexion to accommodate a woman who wishes to wear higher heels.*

  - Contour the plate to the dorsal surface of the bone. A very slight dorsal bend is all that is usually needed. Check the screw lengths and fusion position by fluoroscopy.
  - The percutaneous K-wire can be left in for 3 weeks to obtain increased stability, or an oblique 4-0 cannulated screw can be added.
- Close the capsule with interrupted 3-0 Vicryl sutures. Deflate the tourniquet and obtain hemostasis.

Postoperative Care and Expected Outcomes

- Place a sterile toe spica dressing (see Procedure 1).
- The patient is non–weight bearing until the first postoperative visit 12 days after the procedure. At that point, the sutures are removed and AP and lateral radiographs are taken. The patient is placed in a rigid postoperative shoe and is allowed to bear weight on the heel or lateral side of the foot. A RollerAid can help with ambulation, by allowing the patient to bear weight on a flexed knee.

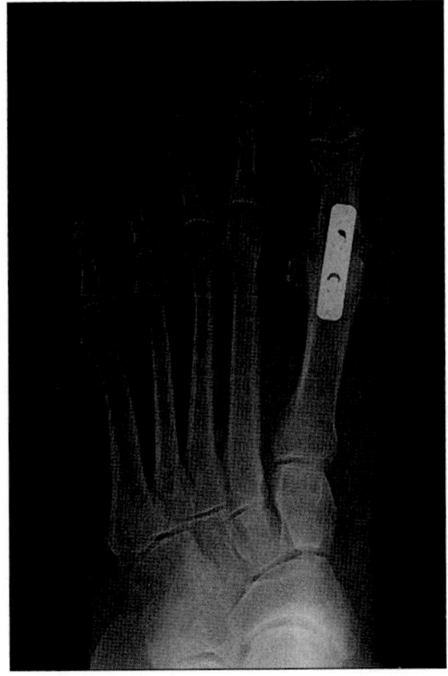

A

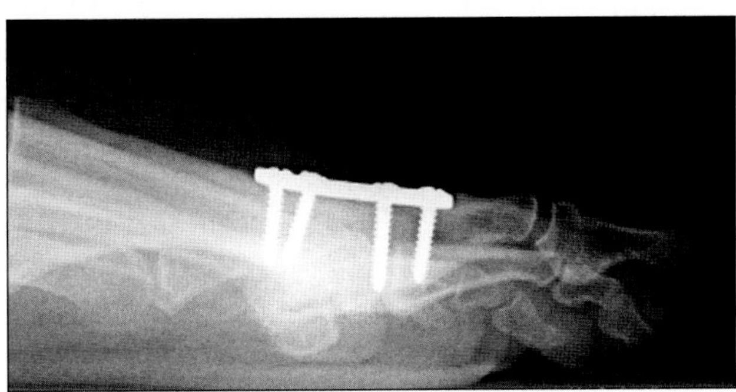

B

FIGURE 15

- By 8 weeks after the procedure, the fusion has invariability healed and the patient is allowed to start normal weight bearing in a walking shoe. AP (Fig. 15A) and lateral (Fig. 15B) radiographs should be taken to document the fusion. Oblique views may be helpful if a delayed union is suspected. If the fusion is slow to heal, a weight-bearing cast boot can be used for several weeks.
- Patients can expect an excellent result and return to painless activity. Most patients will be able to golf, ski, play doubles tennis, swim, and use an elliptical trainer. Running, soccer, football, and basketball are usually not possible, although the addition of a rocker sole on an athletic shoe may allow some degree of participation in these sports.
- It is unlikely that symptomatic arthritis will develop in adjacent joints.

Evidence

Coughlin MJ, Abdo RV. Arthrodesis of the first metatarsophalangeal joint with a Vitallium plate fixation. Foot Ankle Int. 1994;15:18-28.

Excellent results were obtained with toe reamers, a cup-and-ball construct, and use of a rigid low-profile plate. (Level IV evidence)

Goucher NR, Coughlin MJ. Hallux metatarsophalangeal joint arthrodesis using dome-shaped reamers and dorsal plate fixation: a prospective study. Foot Ankle Int. 2006;27:869-76.

Fifty-four patients who underwent fusion of the great toe were studied prospectively. There was a 96% satisfaction rate in 49 patients. There was an 8% nonunion rate. This is an excellent study. (Level IV evidence)

Raikin SM, Ahmad J, Pour AE, Abidi N. Comparison of arthrodesis and metallic hemiarthroplasty of the hallux metatarsophalangeal joint. J Bone Joint Surg [Am]. 2007;89:1979-85.

A study of 46 patients who had either fusion or metallic hemiarthroplasty of the great toe. After a mean of 79 months' follow-up, the authors concluded that arthrodesis is a preferable procedure for patients with arthritis of the MTP joint. (Level III evidence)

Vertullo CJ, Nunley James A. Participation in sports after arthrodesis of the foot or ankle. Foot Ankle Int. 2002;23:625-8.

This paper reports on the responses of orthopedic foot and ankle surgeons and professional trainers about return to sports after various fusion procedures in the foot and ankle. Golf, skiing, and tennis were recommended sports activities after an MTP fusion. (Level V evidence)

PROCEDURE 7

Forefoot Reconstruction for Rheumatoid Disease

Glenn B. Pfeffer

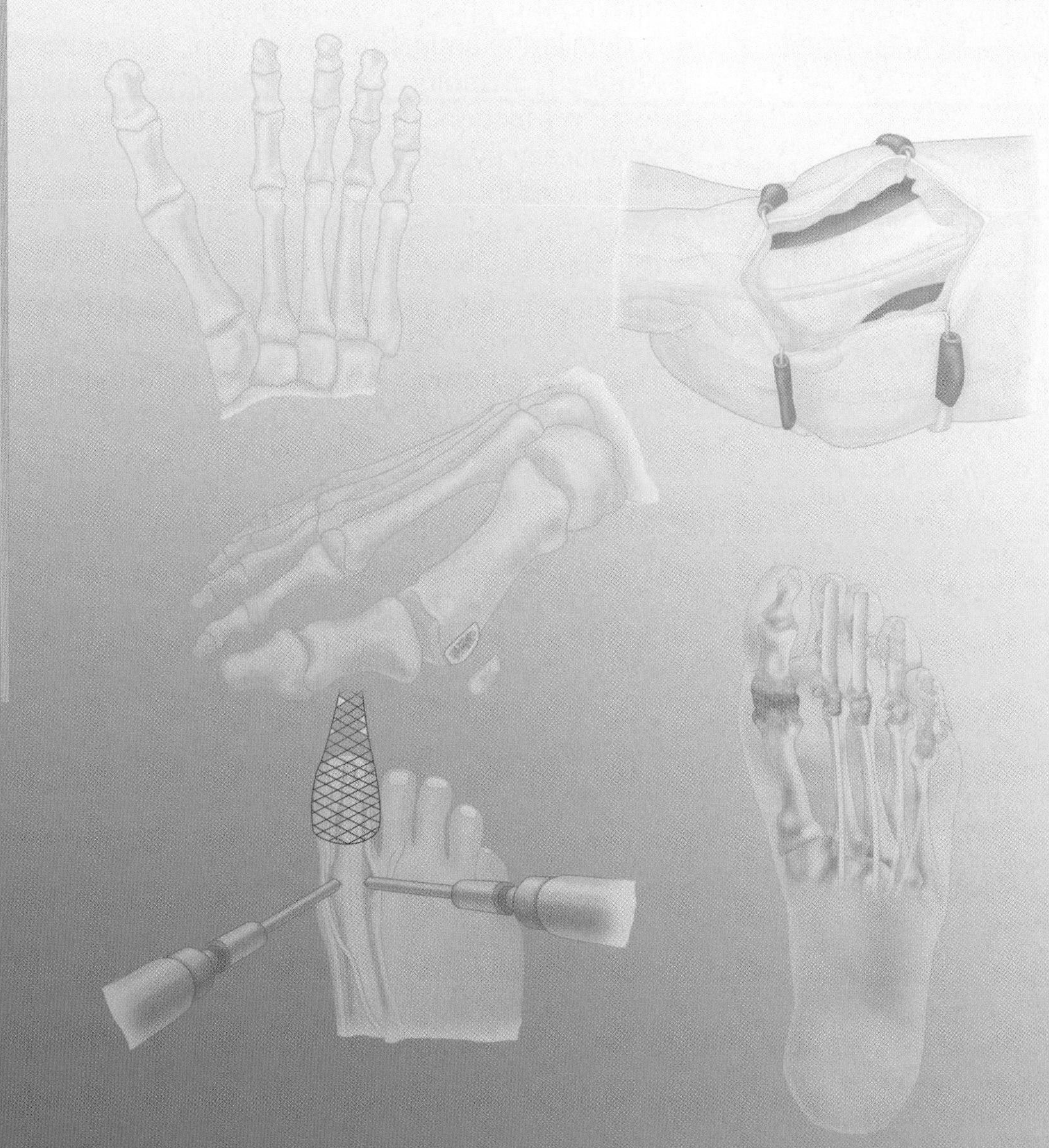

PITFALLS

- *Active infection or ulceration should be eradicated prior to surgery.*
- *Severe skin fragility may preclude operative intervention.*
- *Medications that interfere with bone and wound healing, especially methotrexate and tumor necrosis factor antagonists, should be stopped 2 weeks prior to surgery. They can be started again when the wounds have healed.*
- *Cervical spine stability should be established preoperatively (flexion and extension views may be required).*
- *Patients on prednisone will often need perioperative supplementation.*
- *A preoperative physical therapy evaluation is very helpful, both to determine a patient's ability to ambulate after surgery and to provide training with ambulatory aids.*

Controversies

- New medical management has altered the previously inevitable progression of autoimmune disease. While patients with extensive forefoot involvement require the reconstruction discussed in this procedure, others may benefit from a more limited procedure (e.g., isolated great toe fusion, single MTP synovectomy, or a metatarsal osteotomy to reduce a dislocated joint).

Indications

- Chronic pain and deformity of the forefoot from rheumatoid arthritis
- Recurrent ulceration
- Failure of nonoperative measures, including shoe modification and orthotics

Examination/Imaging

- All patients require a comprehensive preoperative history and physical examination.
- A detailed examination of the foot and ankle is required, including skin condition, joint stability, tendon function, neurovascular status, and gait.
- Specifically evaluate the function of the posterior tibial tendon.
- Synovitis, subluxation, or dislocation of the metatarsophalangeal (MTP) joints should be documented. If dislocated, determine if the joints are passively reducible.
- The most common symptomatic deformity includes hallux valgus, claw toes, dislocations of the lesser MTP joints, and metatarsalgia from pressure on the metatarsal heads (Fig. 1A and 1B).
- Radiographs should include standing anteroposterior (Fig. 2A) and lateral (Fig. 2B) views of the foot. Oblique views of the foot will help visualize arthritic changes of the MTP and midfoot joints. Standing views of the ankle can be obtained to make sure there is no medial laxity of the joint.
- Magnetic resonance imaging is helpful in detecting early joint involvement.

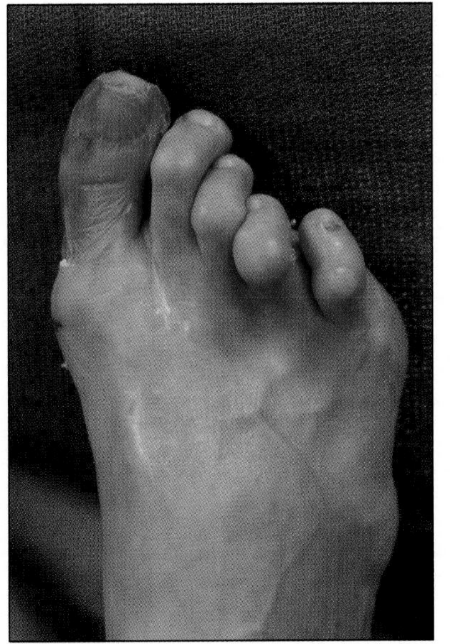

A

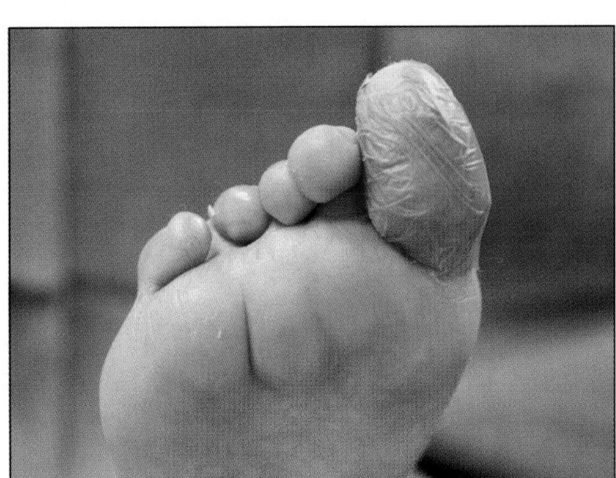

B

FIGURE 1

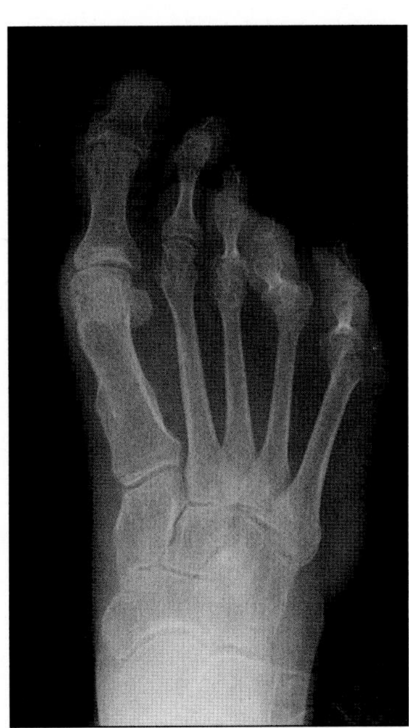

A

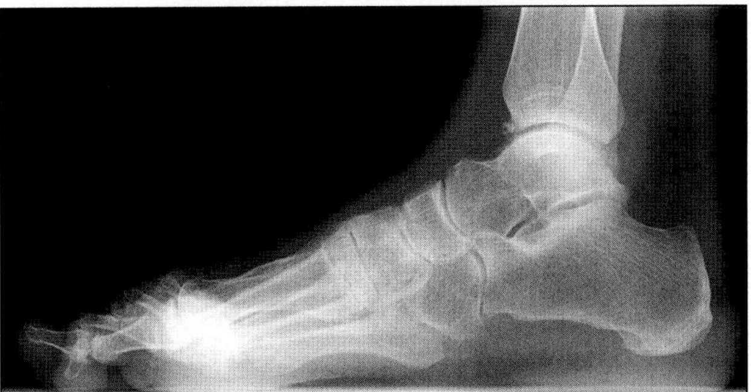

B

FIGURE 2

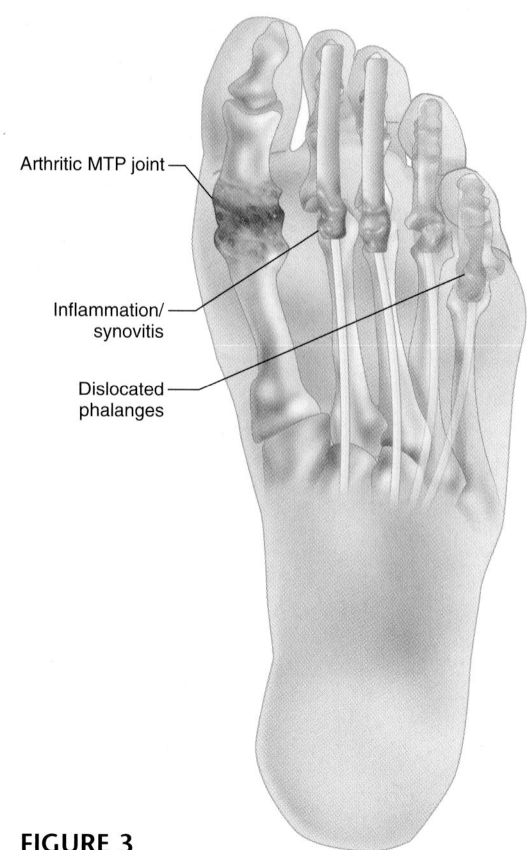

FIGURE 3

Surgical Anatomy

- Arthritic change of the great toe MTP. Erosion of the lesser metatarsal head often associated with MTP dislocation (Fig. 3).

Positioning

- Place the patient supine.
- A small bump under the ipsilateral hip may help position the foot. Place the foot 1 inch from the end of the table, which allows the surgeon to have easy access to the forefoot from all sides.
- A well padded ankle or thigh tourniquet is used.
- In most cases the procedure can be done on an outpatient basis, using a femoral-sciatic or popliteal block for postoperative pain control.

Portals/Exposures

- Three longitudinal incisions are used to gain access to all of the MTP joints (Fig. 4).
- The first is 5–6 cm over the dorsal aspect of the great toe and first metatarsal.
- The other two are 3–4 cm in the second and fourth intermetatarsal spaces.

Treatment Options

- Extra-depth shoes with rocker soles
- Cushioned plastizote orthotic inserts
- Metatarsal pads (Hapad)
- Silicone toe-caps for painful toe deformities (Silipos)
- A Budin splint (Alimed) can help reduce a passively correctable claw toe
- Medical management
- Physical therapy
- Corticosteroid injection into a symptomatic joint

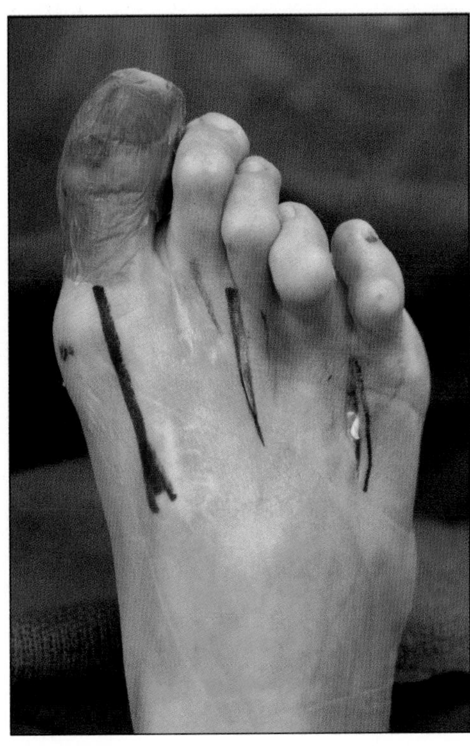

FIGURE 4

Procedure

Step 1

- Start with a longitudinal incision in the second intermetatarsal space using a #15 blade. Loupe magnification can be helpful.
- Use blunt dissection to locate the extensor tendons. Divide the extensor digitorum longus (EDL) and excise a 3- to 5-mm segment (Fig. 5).

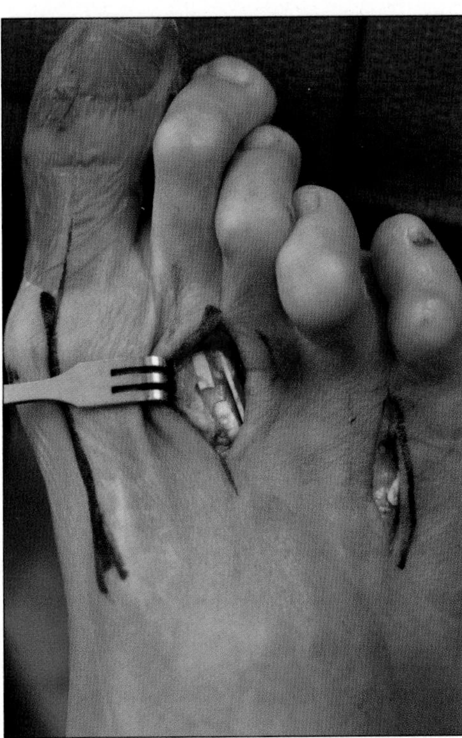

FIGURE 5

Pearls

- *Careful soft tissue technique is required to avoid skin injury. Gentle skin retraction with double hooks or small Weitlander retractors is best. Avoid squeezing the skin edges with a pickup, and minimize the use of self-retaining retractors.*

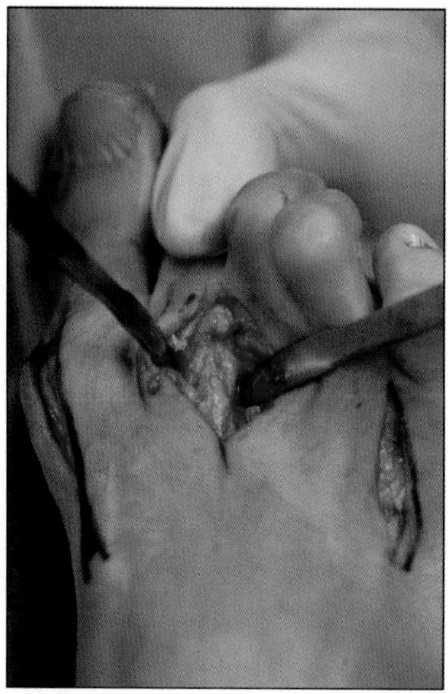

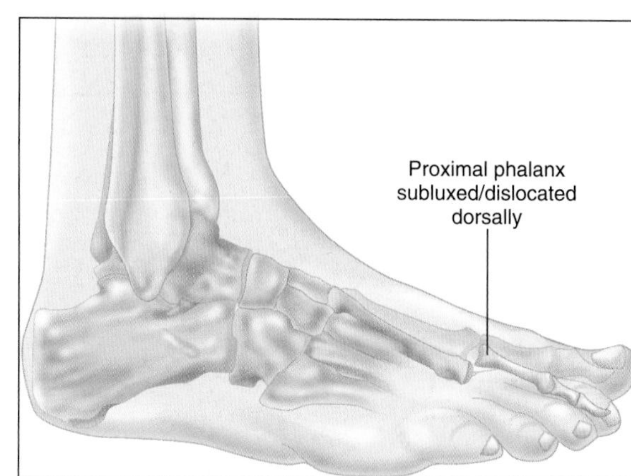

FIGURE 6 A B

Controversies

- Transverse plantar or dorsal incisions can be used. Longitudinal incisions provide the greatest ease of access with few skin problems.

A Z-lengthening of the tendon is another option.

- Locate the dorsal aspect of the proximal phalanx at the MTP joint, which is often subluxed or dislocated dorsally (Fig. 6A and 6B).
- Divide the capsule longitudinally and carefully expose the metatarsal head. Protect the neurovascular bundle, which may be displaced, especially when the MTP joint is dislocated.
- Divide the collateral ligaments and free up the plantar plate with a small elevator.
- Using a micro-sagittal blade, divide the metatarsal obliquely, usually at the neck for distal—dorsal to plantar—proximal. The cut is made approximately 30° to the longitudinal axis of the metatarsal, in order to avoid a sharp plantar bone prominence (Fig. 7).

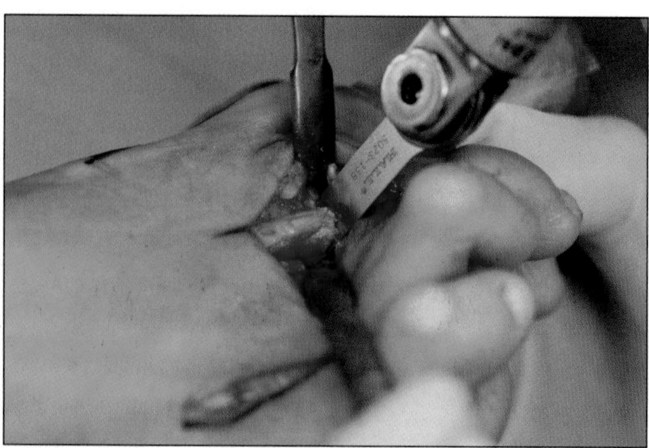

FIGURE 7

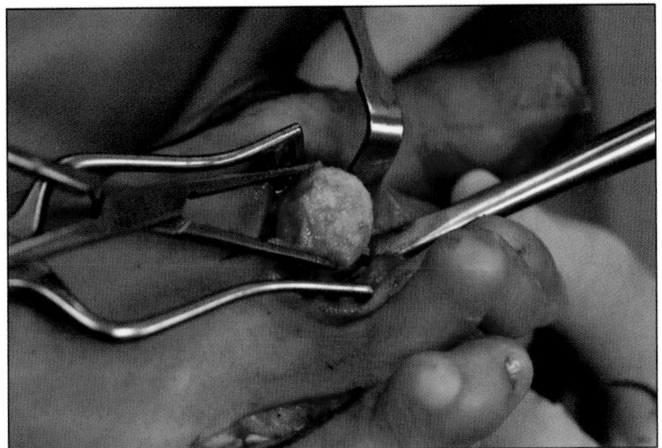

FIGURE 8

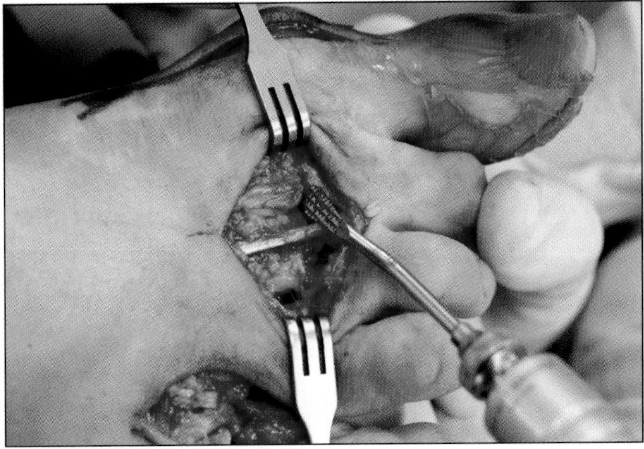

FIGURE 9

- Grasp the distal metatarsal head with a towel clip and carefully excise it using sharp dissection. Stay close to the bone to avoid injury to adjacent structures (Fig. 8).
- Use a micro-reciprocating rasp to smooth down the bone edges (Fig. 9). Be careful, as this instrument will rapidly remove the osteoporotic bone of a patient with rheumatoid arthritis.

PEARLS

- *If the toe is deviated laterally, another option is to divide the deforming force of the extensor digitorum brevis and Z-lengthen the EDL.*
- *An irreducible MTP joint may make it impossible to expose the distal-most aspect of the metatarsal. If so, the metatarsal osteotomy will have to be performed proximal to the neck. In this case, excision of the distal metatarsal can be very difficult and time consuming. Careful traction on the toe by an assistant will help expose the metatarsal.*
- *It is essential to adequately decompress the MTP space. Resect as much of the metatarsal as needed to leave a 1- to 1.5-cm, finger-sized gap between the base of the proximal phalanx and the cut distal metatarsal.*
- *The level of the second metatarsal cut usually dictates the level of the other metatarsal cuts and, ultimately, the great toe MTP fusion. It is for this reason that the second MTP is addressed first. Rarely, a more severely dislocated and contracted third MTP joint should be addressed first, which in turn will affect the level of the other bone cuts.*

PITFALLS

- *Avoid penetration of the saw blade beyond the plantar border of the metatarsal. The neurovascular bundle lies just beyond.*
- *Neither resection of the proximal phalangeal base nor syndactilization of the toes is required in this procedure. Leaving the base of the proximal phalanx intact increases the stability of the reconstruction and minimizes recurrent postoperative deformity.*

STEP 2

- Once the second MTP is adequately decompressed, make cuts in the adjacent metatarsals from medial to lateral. Each cut should be more proximal than the next, creating a gentle arc. Each metatarsal must be shortened sufficiently to decompress the MTP space.
- The cut in the fifth metatarsal neck is angled slightly to avoid any bony prominence on the lateral border of the foot (Fig. 10A and 10B).
- Use the micro-reciprocating rasp sequentially on each metatarsal.

PITFALLS

- *When performing the osteoclasis, be careful not to rupture the fragile plantar skin of the toe.*

STEP 3

- At this point, the toe deformities should be corrected sequentially. Closed osteoclasis is easy and efficient, and usually possible because of osteoporotic bone. Gently hold the toe on each side of the proximal interphalangeal (PIP) joint, and forcibly straighten it.
- An open procedure may be required in a younger patient with good bone stock.
  - In such a case, make a transverse incision on the toe a few millimeters proximal to the level of the PIP joint.
  - Divide the extensor tendon transversely. Divide the collateral ligaments with a #15 blade, while keeping the toe hyperflexed to keep the neurovascular bundle out of the way.
  - Remove approximately 5 mm of the distal aspect of the proximal phalanx to adequately decompress the PIP joint. A small rongeur easily removes the necessary bone, and is safer than a power saw (Fig. 11A and 11B).
  - When the toe is extended into neutral position, the cut end of the proximal phalanx and the middle phalanx should not rub.

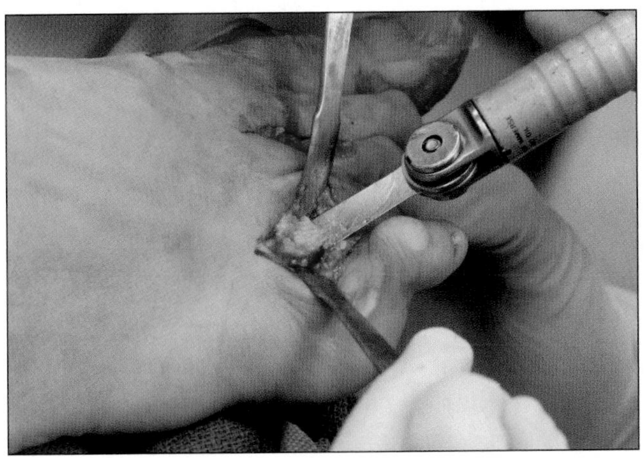

A

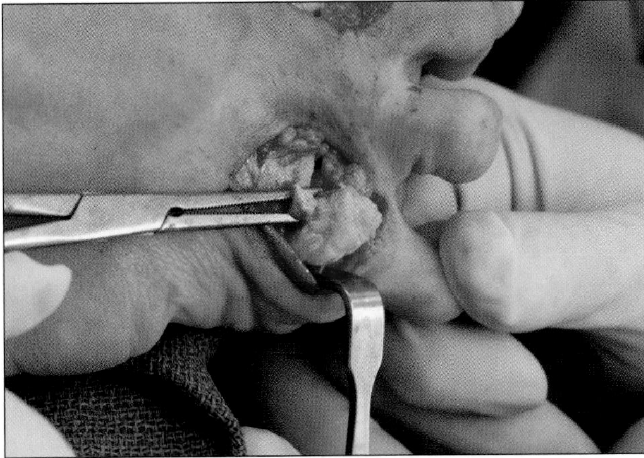

B

FIGURE 10

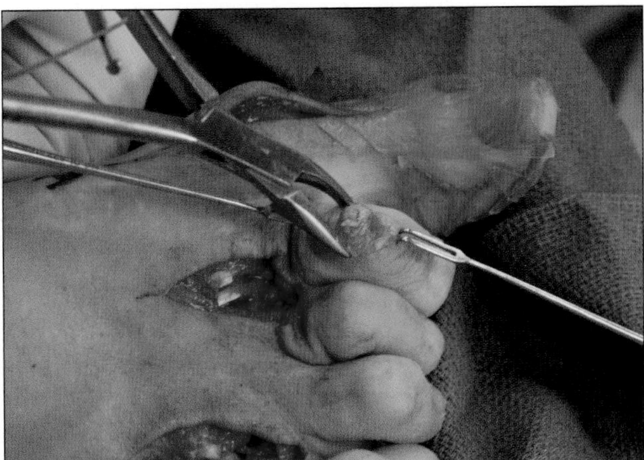

A

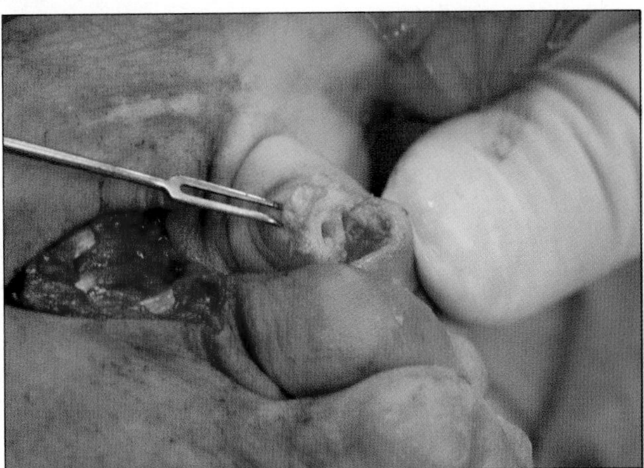

B

FIGURE 11

- Starting in the PIP space, insert a 0.062 Kirschner wire (K-wire) in a retrograde fashion out the tip of the toe, exiting just below the nail.
  - Run the K-wire out the base of the proximal phalanx into the metatarsal shaft (Fig. 12). The metatarsal and phalanx should be aligned longitudinally.
  - Drive the wire into the bone at the base of the metatarsals, to gain adequate fixation and minimize postoperative motion (Fig. 13). Fluoroscopic guidance can be helpful.
  - Bend the pin and apply a cap. Place two 3-0 Vicryl sutures into the extensor of each toe. Excise redundant skin.
- If a Z-plasty of the EDL has been performed, repair the tendon with a simple absorbable suture after the K-wire has been placed.

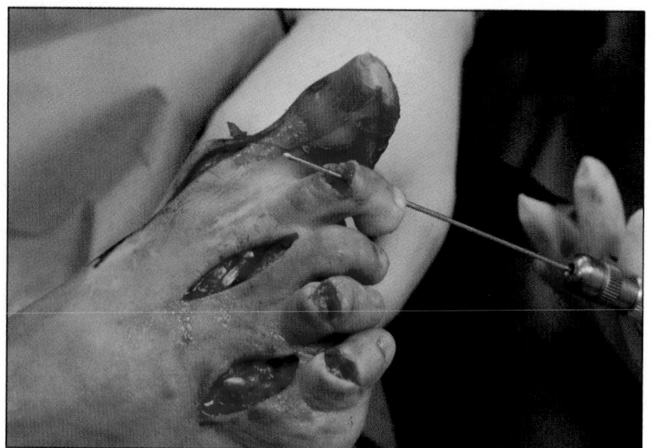

FIGURE 12

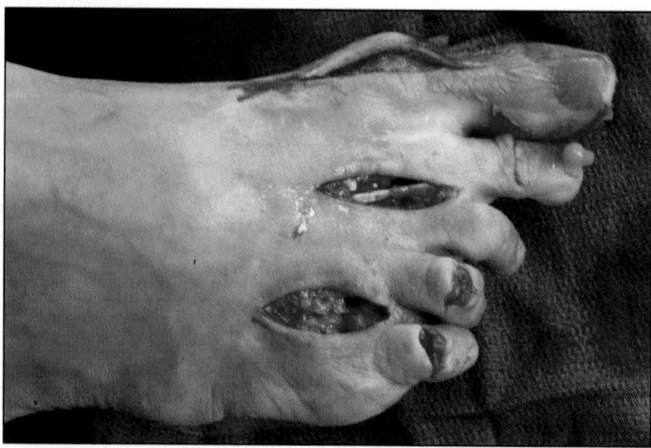

FIGURE 13

> **Pearls**
>
> - *Occasionally a toe will have poor arterial flow after the tourniquet is deflated. Shifting the toe either proximally or distally on the pin can resolve this problem. Slight rotation of the toe can also help. If not, apply warm saline-soaked sponges to the forefoot for several minutes. Nitro paste on the plantar aspect of the foot can also be used. If there is no resolution, pulling the pin of the affected toe will invariably restore good circulation.*

Step 4

- Fuse the great toe MTP joint, if required (see Procedure 6). Fusion is almost always required (Fig. 14A and 14B).
  - The first and second metatarsals should be cut at approximately equal levels.
  - Ideally, at the end of the procedure the tips of the first and second toes will be within 1 cm of each other in length.
- A fusion is almost always possible, even in a patient with severe osteoporosis. A resection arthroplasty (modified Keller) of the base of the proximal phalanx is an option, especially if there is involvement and loss of motion of the interphalangeal joint. An arthrodesis, however, will always produce a better result.
- Drop the tourniquet and obtain meticulous hemostasis. Carefully close the skin in layers. Apply a bulky dressing and a posterior splint.

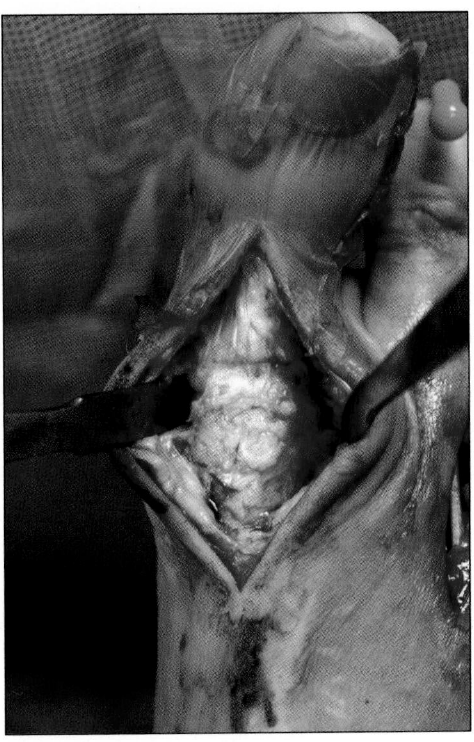

A

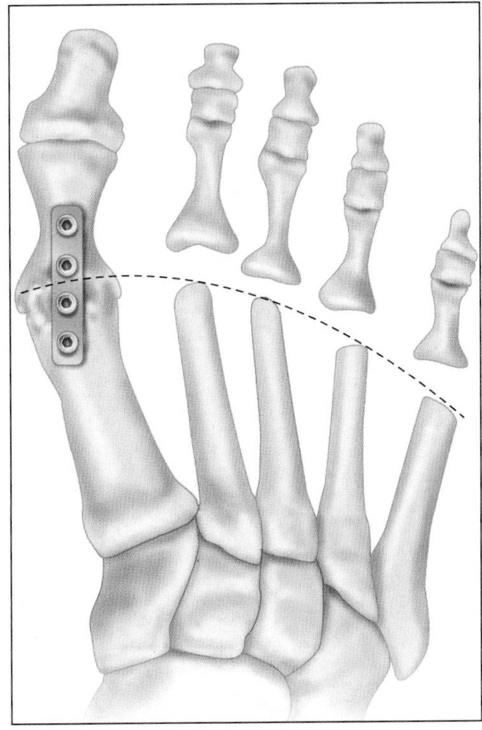

B

FIGURE 14

Postoperative Care and Expected Outcomes

- Most surgeries can be done on an outpatient basis, unless there is a medical indication for postoperative hospitalization.
- The first office visit is at 10–12 days after surgery. Until that time, no weight bearing should be allowed on the operated foot. Radiographs are taken (Fig. 15).
- Once the wound is healed and the sutures are removed, the patient can start to bear weight on the heel, as able. A non–weight-bearing cast may be required in a patient who has poor fixation of the first MTP fusion.
- The pins are pulled in the office 3 weeks after surgery. One-quarter inch paper tape is used to hold them in position for an additional 9 weeks. The tape extends from the plantar aspect of the toe, onto the dorsum of the foot. Keep the PIP and MTP joint in neutral position.
- By 8 weeks after surgery, or once radiographs confirm a successful fusion of the great toe (Fig. 16), the patient can return to normal shoewear, as tolerated. Swelling may persist for 6 months.

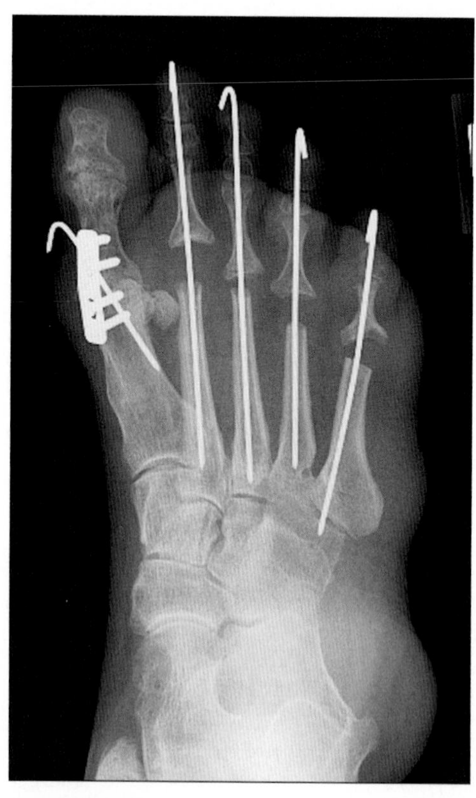

FIGURE 15

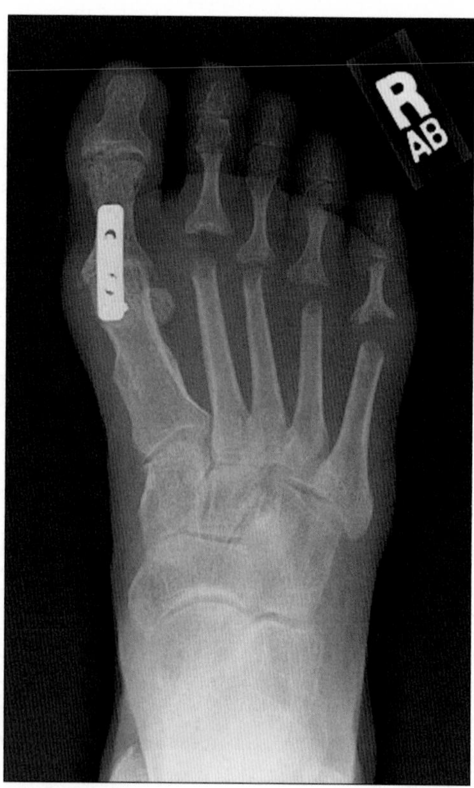

FIGURE 16

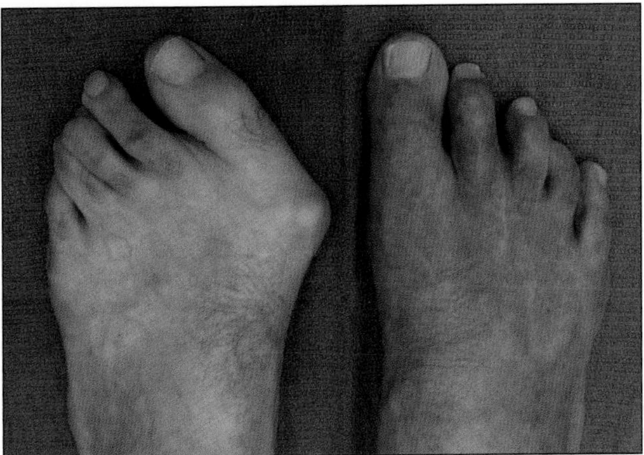

FIGURE 17

- A patient can expect to have an excellent result, with the elimination of forefoot pain and an improvement in function and shoewear (Fig. 17). Right foot has had surgery.

Evidence

Coughlin M. Rheumatoid forefoot reconstruction. J Bone Joint Surg [Am]. 2000;82:322-41.

This study showed 96% good to excellent results and 100% fusion rate at an average follow-up of 6.2 years. (Level IV evidence)

Jeng C, Campbell J. Current concepts review: the rheumatoid forefoot. Foot Ankle Int. 2008;29:959-68.

An excellent review of this topic.

Mann R, Schakel M. Surgical correction of rheumatoid forefoot deformities. Foot Ankle Int. 1995;16:1-6.

A retrospective study of metatarsal head resection and arthrodesis of the great toe MTP. Excellent results were obtained in 90% of patients. (Level IV evidence)

PROCEDURE 8

Fifth Metatarsal Osteotomy for Correction of Bunionette Deformity

Mark E. Easley

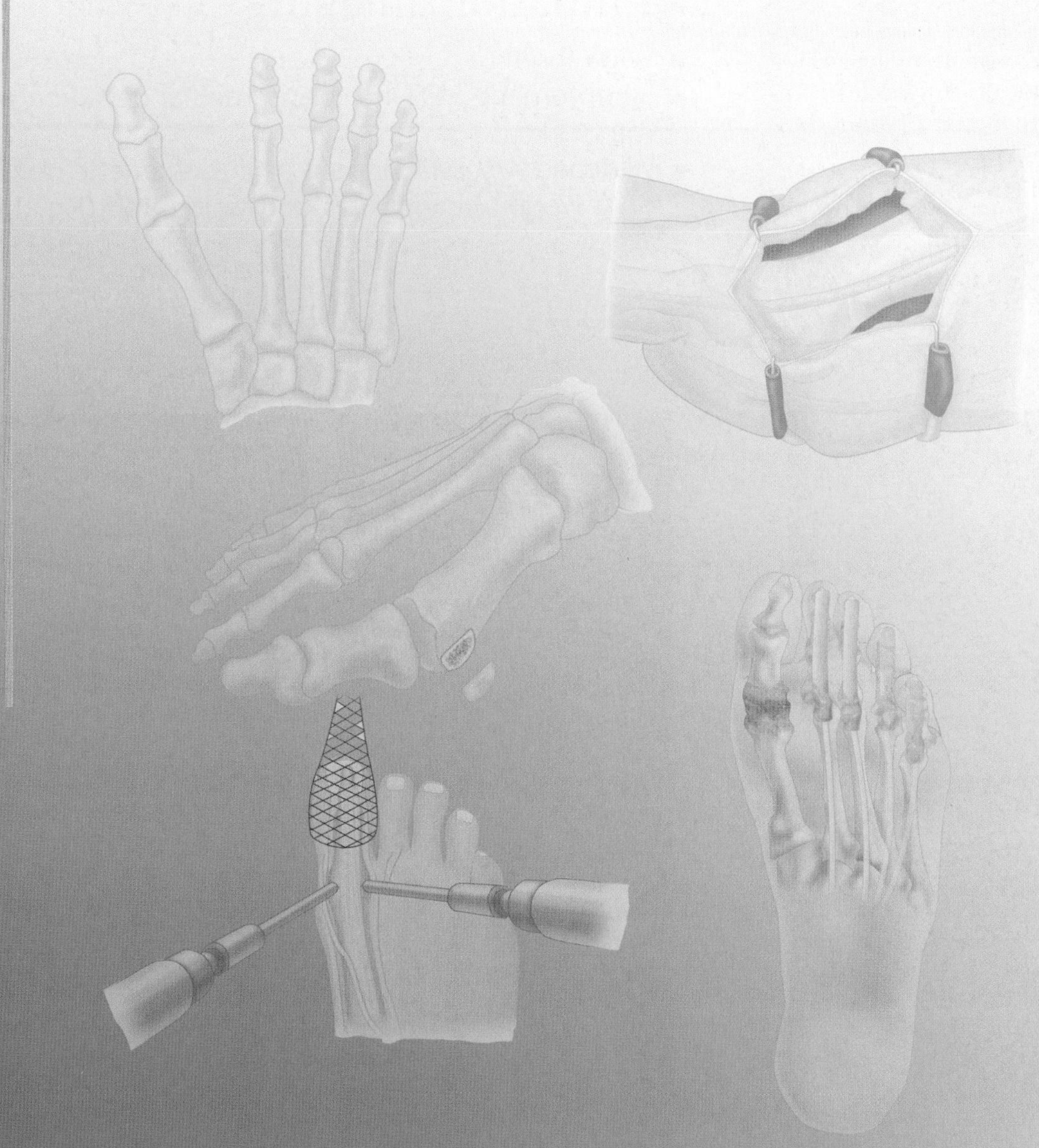

Indications

- Wide forefoot with symptomatic fifth metatarsal (5MT) head and medial deviation of fifth toe
- Failure of nonoperative treatment (shoe modifications)
- Weight-bearing anteroposterior (AP) foot radiograph demonstrating a widened fourth-fifth intermetatarsal angle (4/5 IMA)

Treatment Options

- Distal 5MT osteotomy typically reserved for prominent 5MT head without increased 4/5 IMA (type I deformity)
  - Minor increase in 4/5 IMA (Fig. 2A)
  - Readily corrected with a distal chevron osteotomy (Fig. 2B)

Examination/Imaging

- Wide forefoot
- Symptomatic 5MT head and medial deviation of fifth toe
- Widened 4/5 IMA (type II or III bunionette deformity) on a weight-bearing AP foot radiograph (Fig. 1)

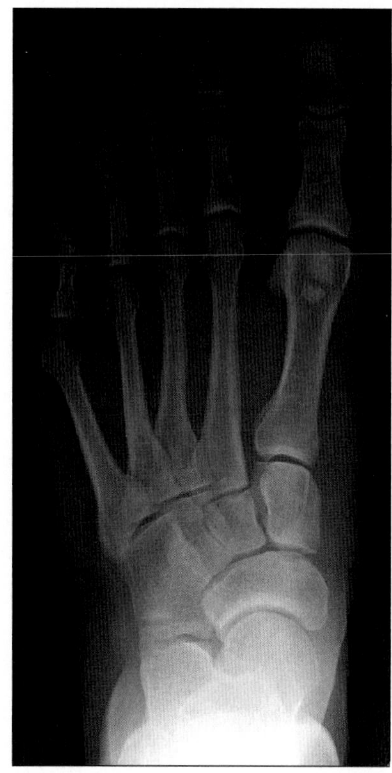

FIGURE 1

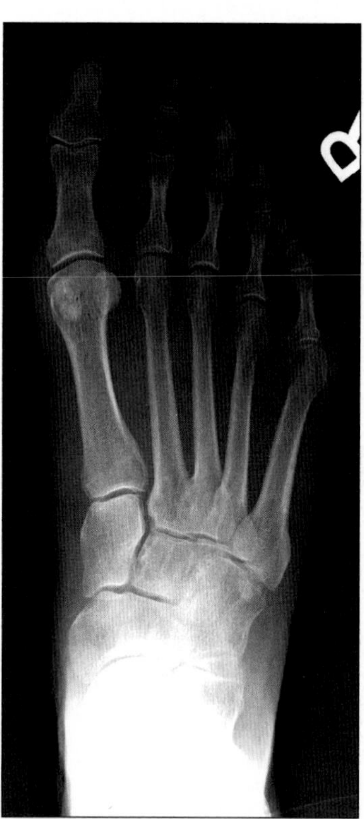

A

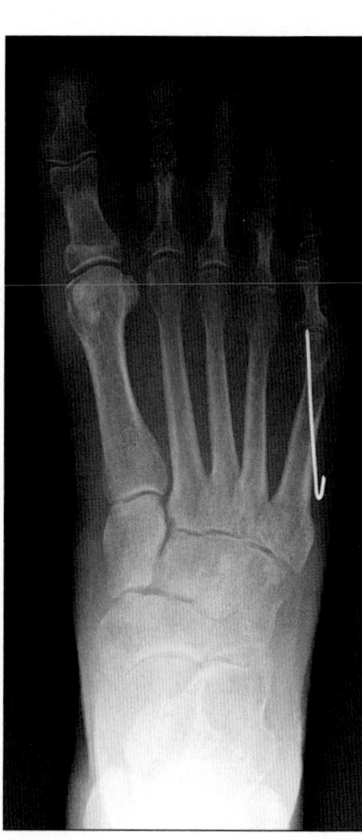

B

FIGURE 2

Surgical Anatomy

- Essentially a mirror image of a bunion deformity
- Widened 4/5 IMA, prominent 5MT head, medial deviation of the fifth toe (Fig. 3)
- Ligamentous attachments between fourth and fifth metatarsal bases (difficult to mobilize fracture that proximally)
- Watershed area of poor vascular supply at 5MT base (Fig. 4)
    - Commonly associated with Jones fracture
    - Osteotomy should be distal to this watershed area
- Sural nerve courses on dorsolateral aspect of 5MT

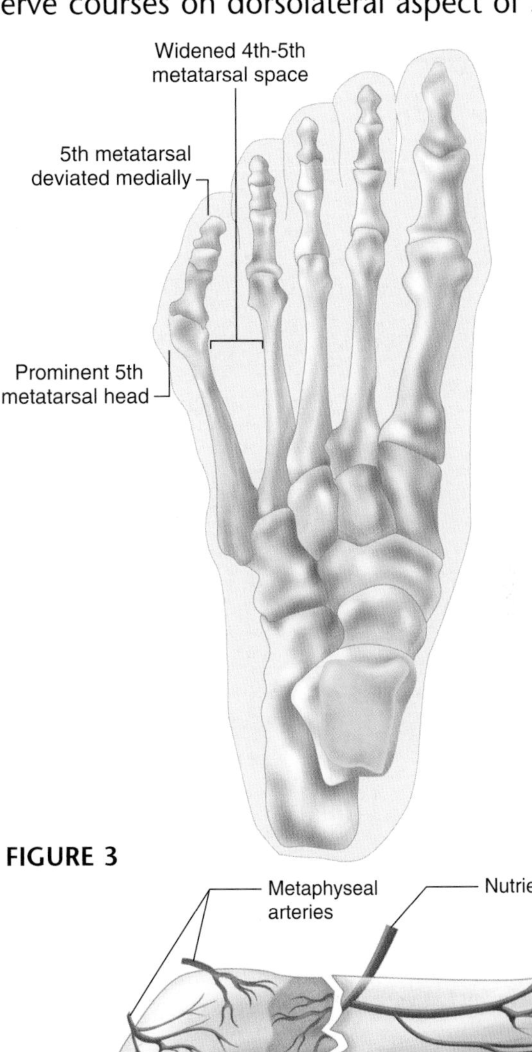

FIGURE 3

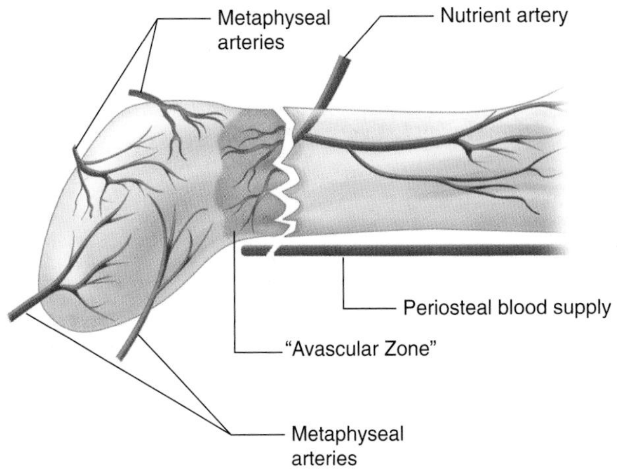

FIGURE 4

Positioning

- Supine position with bolster under ipsilateral hip to provide optimal exposure to lateral foot

Pitfalls

- *Avoid injuring the sural nerve.*
- *An incision too plantar will make screw insertion more difficult.*

Portals/Exposures

- A longitudinal lateral incision is made over the dorsolateral aspect of the 5MT extending from the fifth metatarsophalangeal (5MTP) joint to the junction of the middle and distal thirds of the 5MT (Fig. 5A).
- The sural nerve is at risk and should be retracted dorsally and medially if within the operative field (Fig. 5B).
- The lateral 5MTP joint capsule should be identified but not violated during the exposure (see Fig. 5B).

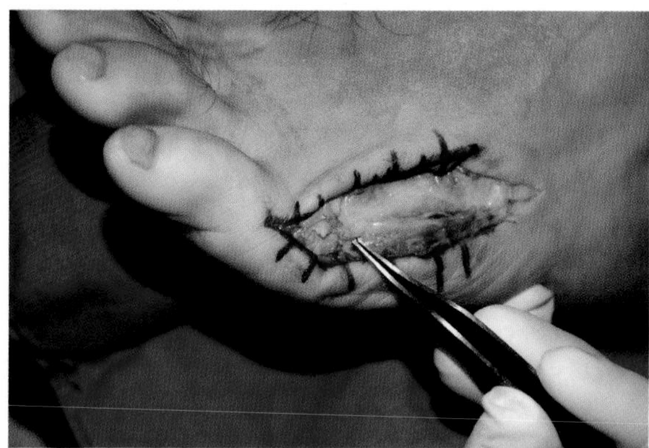

A

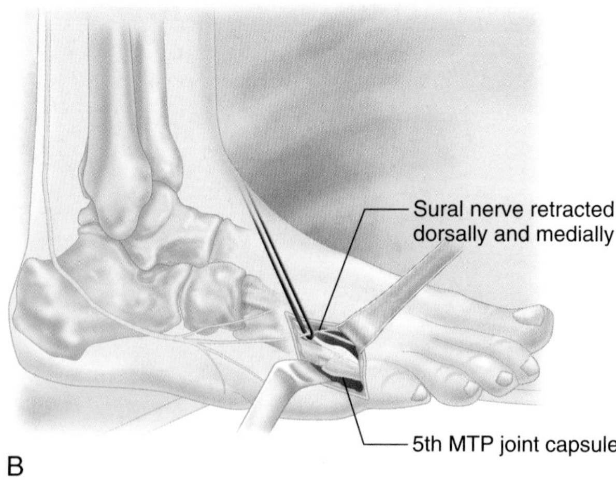

B

FIGURE 5

Pearls

- *A longer osteotomy will provide a greater surface area for healing and permit fixation with two screws.*

Pitfalls

- *To ensure the osteotomy will mobilize adequately, plan the osteotomy to originate just distal to the stout ligamentous attachments of the proximal 5MT.*
- *Extending the osteotomy too close to the 5MTP joint may violate the lateral capsule and make capsular closure difficult.*

Procedure

Step 1

- An L-shaped lateral capsulotomy is performed in the 5MTP joint capsule (Fig. 6). The sural nerve is in close proximity, and must be carefully retracted dorsally. Through the joint, a medial capsulotomy can be performed to improve the fifth toe alignment, similar to a lateral release performed for hallux valgus correction.
- The lateral eminence is resected in line with the 5MT shaft (Fig. 7).
- The lateral metatarsal is scored (with the saw blade) to mark the planned oblique osteotomy.
- Intraoperative fluoroscopy may be used to determine the proximal extent of the osteotomy to avoid encroaching on the watershed area of the proximal 5MT and to avoid the relatively immobile aspect of the 5MT bound by tight ligamentous attachments to the fourth metatarsal.

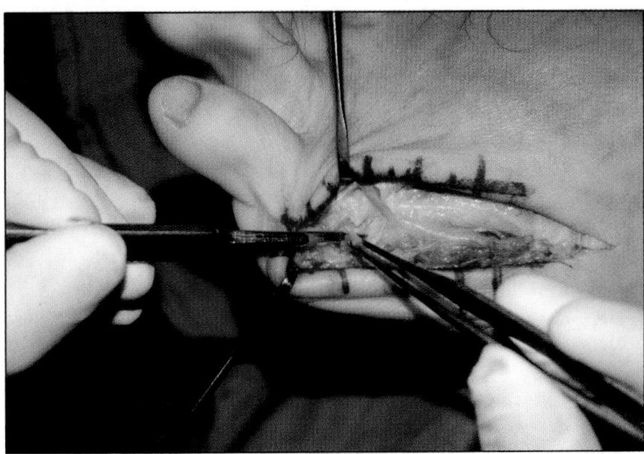

FIGURE 6

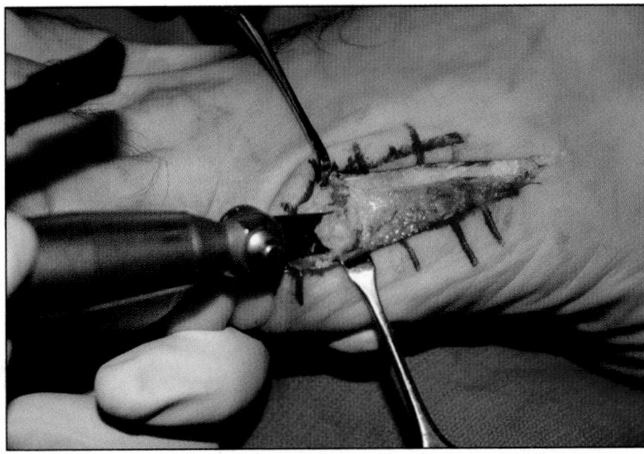

FIGURE 7

Pearls

- *Minimal periosteal stripping is required.*
- *To create a congruent osteotomy, only the distal corner of the saw blade exits the osteotomy each time the saw blade is advanced along the course of the planned osteotomy.*
- *If elevation of the 5MT is desired with correction of lateral deviation, the saw blade can simultaneously be angled dorsally.*

Pitfalls

- *This is a diaphyseal osteotomy, and the heat generated by the saw blade should be kept to a minimum (consider using cool saline irrigation).*

Instrumentation/ Implantation

- Micro-sagittal saw
- Mini-fragment set (cannulated or solid screws)
- Towel clip

Step 2

- The majority of the periosteum may be left intact, which may aid in healing this diaphyseal osteotomy.
- The micro-sagittal saw should be passed through both cortices over the proximal-dorsal two thirds of the osteotomy (Fig. 8). The osteotomy should not be completed at this stage in order to maintain control of both fragments throughout the procedure.
- A mini-fragment screw is inserted from dorsal to plantar across the completed proximal portion of the osteotomy.
  - When using solid screws, a standard lag technique is employed.
  - After compression is confirmed for either solid or cannulated (dual-pitch or partially threaded) screws, the screw is then slightly released to allow for repositioning of the saw blade to complete the osteotomy (Fig. 9).
  - The saw blade never completely exits the osteotomy as it is advanced to maintain a congruent cut the entire length of the osteotomy (Fig. 10).
- The distal portion of the osteotomy is completed with control of the osteotomy being maintained with the proximal lag screw in place.
- With a towel clip carefully securing the distal aspect of the proximal fragment and medially directed pressure applied on the distal fragment at the 5MT head, the 4/5 IMA is corrected.
  - The proximal screw is tightened to secure the osteotomy.
  - The towel clip can be repositioned to temporarily block any potential loss of reduction.
- Intraoperative fluoroscopy in the AP plane confirms an adequate reduction. If inadequate, the proximal screw is slightly loosened and the reduction maneuver is repeated, and the screw is again tightened.
- With a satisfactory reduction, a second screw is placed across the distal aspect of the osteotomy. We prefer to place this screw from a plantar to dorsal direction (Fig. 11).

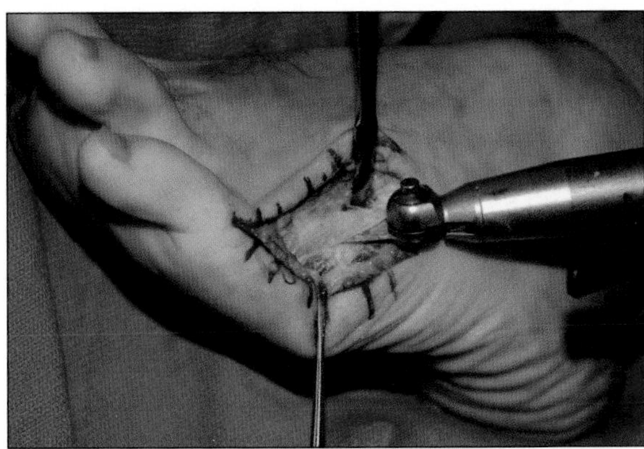

FIGURE 8

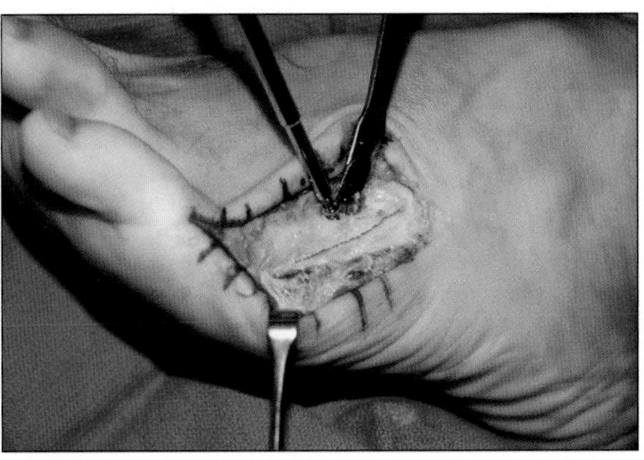

FIGURE 9

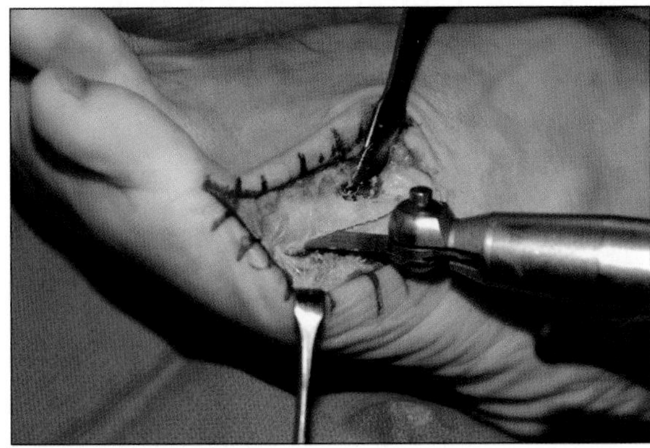

FIGURE 10

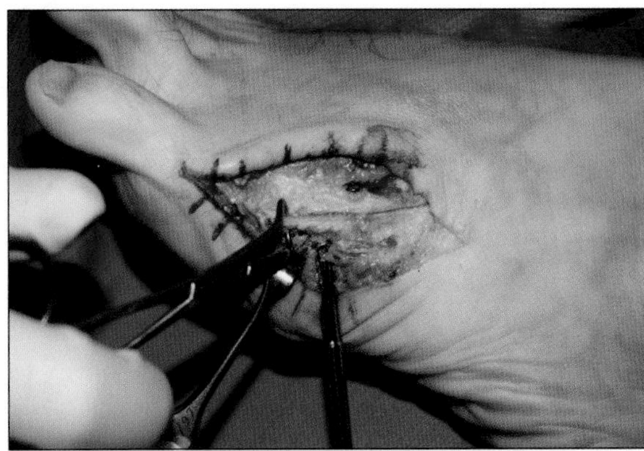

FIGURE 11

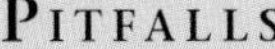

PITFALLS

- *If correction of the bunionette deformity requires considerable tension on the lateral capsular repair, then most likely the 4/5 IMA is undercorrected.*

STEP 3

- The lateral prominences, both distal (Fig. 12A) and proximal (Fig. 12B), are resected even with the realigned metatatarsal using a micro-sagittal saw to limit the risk of a pressure area with shoewear.

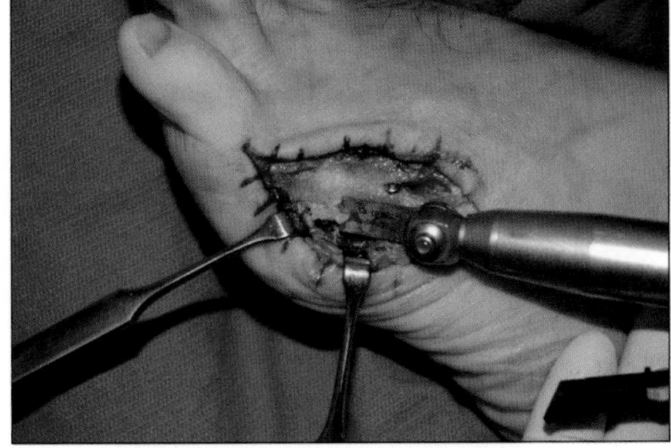

A

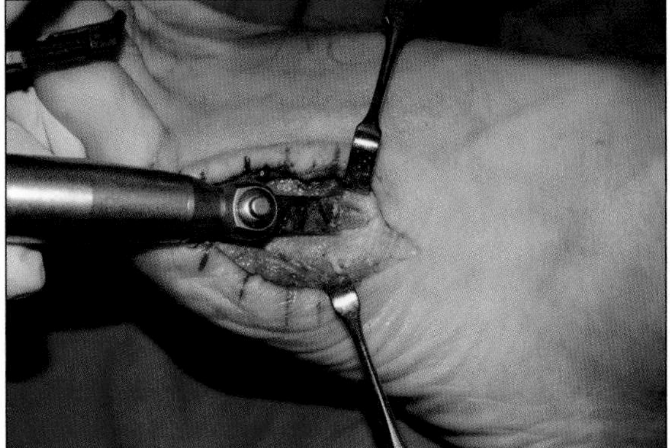

B

FIGURE 12

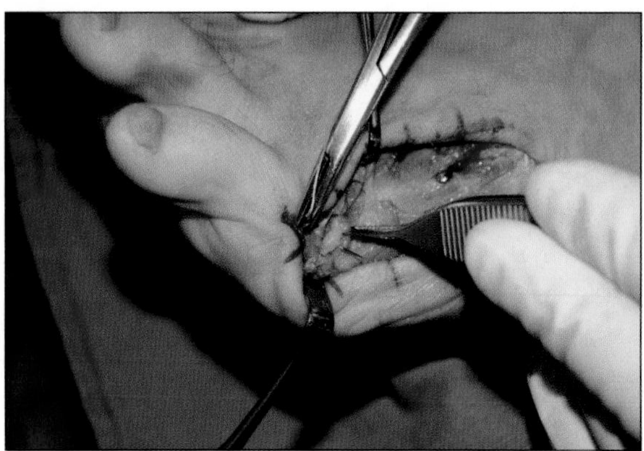

FIGURE 13

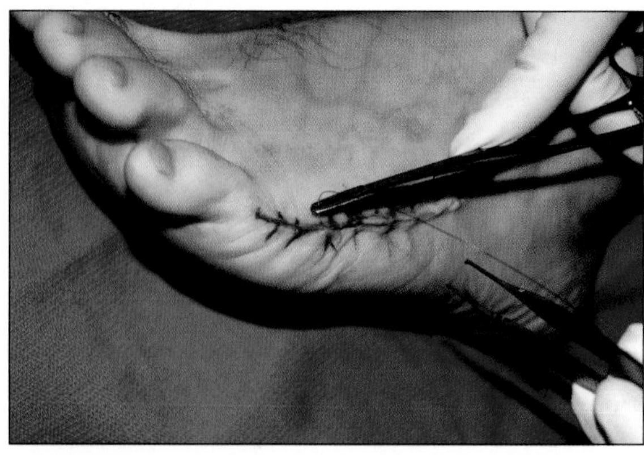

FIGURE 14

- The lateral capsulotomy is imbricated at its new resting tension (Fig. 13). A surgical sponge can be placed between the fourth and fifth toes to relax any tension on the lateral capsule during closure.
- The subcutaneous tissue and skin are reapproximated to a tensionless closure (Fig. 14).

PITFALLS

- *Since this is a diaphyseal osteotomy, a delay in healing is occasionally observed; protected weight bearing on the forefoot should be maintained until there is radiographic evidence for healing.*

Postoperative Care and Expected Outcomes

- The fifth toe is supported in a "reverse" bunion dressing, maintaining slight valgus alignment, and the foot and ankle are supported in a splint.
- With stable fixation and adequate wound healing, a walking boot or postsurgical shoe will allow heel weight bearing at 10–14 days.
- A toe spacer may be maintained between the fourth and fifth toes for 6–8 weeks, analogous to a bunion procedure (Fig. 15).

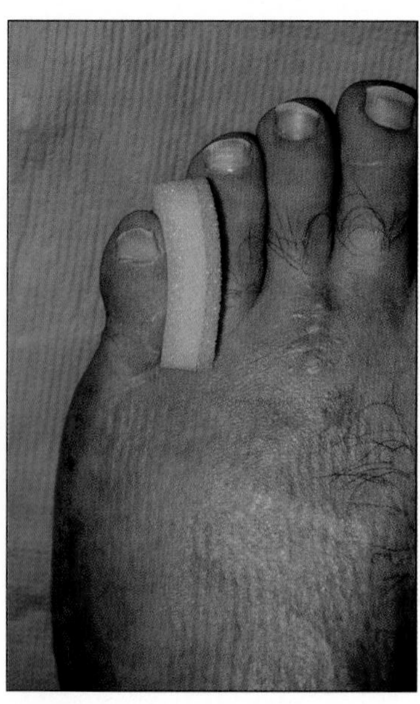

FIGURE 15

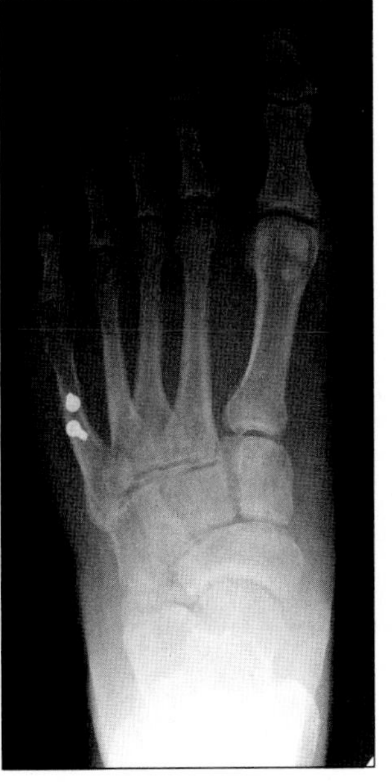
A

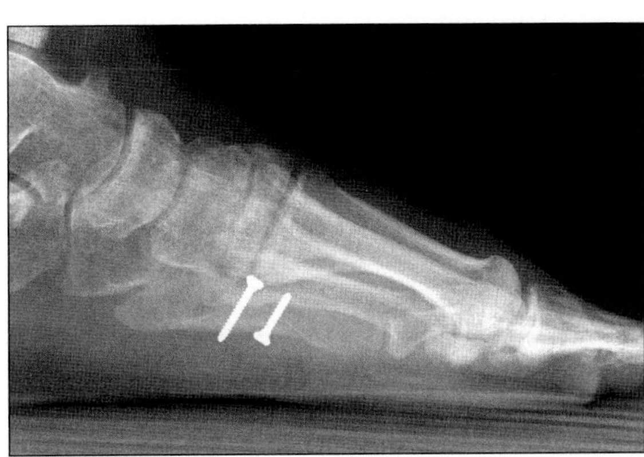
B

FIGURE 16

- Full weight bearing on the forefoot may be initiated with radiographic evidence of healing of the osteotomy (typically 5–6 weeks); protected weight bearing is maintained if there is any delay in healing.
- Anteroposterior (Fig. 16A) and lateral (Fig. 16B) radiographs at final follow-up will demonstrate correction of the 4/5 IMA and healing of the osteotomy.

Evidence

Cohen BE, Nicholson CW. Bunionette deformity. J Am Acad Orthop Surg. 2007;15:300-7.

Koti M, Maffulli N. Bunionette. J Bone Joint Surg [Am]. 2001;83:1076-82.

Radl R, Leithner A, Koehler W, Scheipl S, Windhager R. The modified distal horizontal metatarsal osteotomy for correction of bunionette deformity. Foot Ankle Int. 2005;26:454-7.

Vienne P, Oesselmann M, Espinosa N, Aschwanden R, Zingg P. Modified Coughlin procedure for surgical treatment of symptomatic tailor's bunion: a prospective followup study of 33 consecutive operations. Foot Ankle Int. 2006;27:573-80.

Weitzel S, Trnka HJ, Petroutsas J. Transverse medial slide osteotomy for bunionette deformity: long-term results. Foot Ankle Int. 2007;28:794-8.

Grade B recommendation for the oblique 5MT osteotomy for bunionette correction, since there is only Level IV and Level V evidence to support this technique.

PROCEDURE 9

Turf Toe Repair: Capsular Repair of First Metatarsophalangeal Plantar Plate Rupture

W. Bret Smith, Terrence M. Philbin, and Gregory C. Berlet

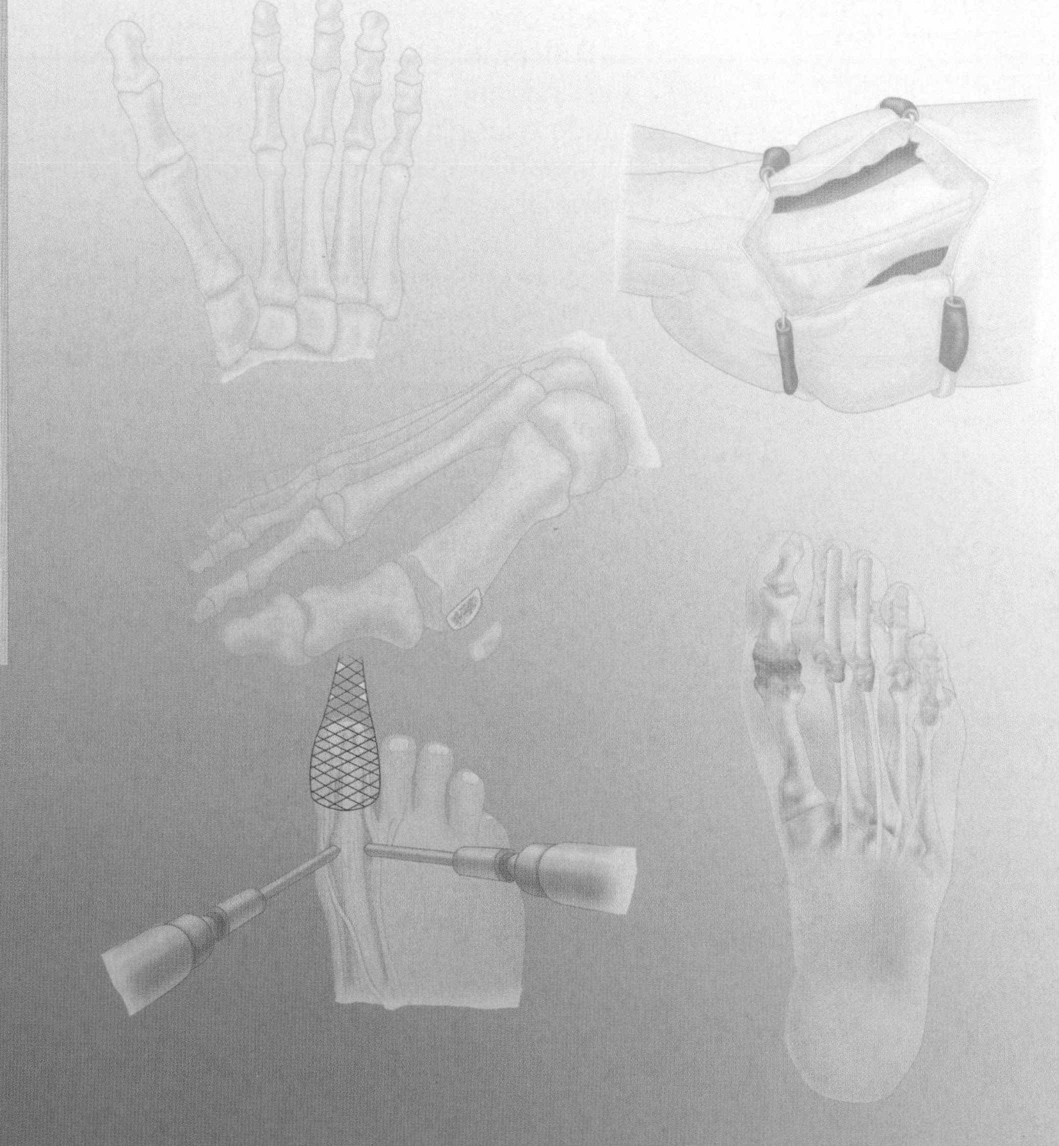

Capsular Repair of First Metatarsophalangeal Plantar Plate Rupture

PITFALLS

- *Associated injuries: articular cartilage and subchondral bone bruising, sesamoid fracture, and diastasis of bipartite sesamoid.*

Indications

- "Turf toe" is a capsular-ligamentous injury of the first metatarsophalangeal (1MTP) joint typically caused from a hyperextension force while playing on hard surfaces (Fig. 1A and 1B).
  - Grade one: stretching of the capsular-ligamentous 1MTP complex, localized tenderness, minimal swelling, and no ecchymosis
  - Grade two: partial tear, diffuse tenderness, moderate swelling, ecchymosis, and pain with range of motion
  - Grade three: complete tear, severe pain to palpation, marked swelling and ecchymosis, and a positive Lachman's test
- Surgical indications include a large capsular avulsion with an unstable joint, progressive diastasis of a bipartite sesamoid or sesamoid fracture, sesamoid retraction, traumatic bunion or progressive hallux valgus, a positive Lachman's test, a chondral injury, and symptomatic loose body.

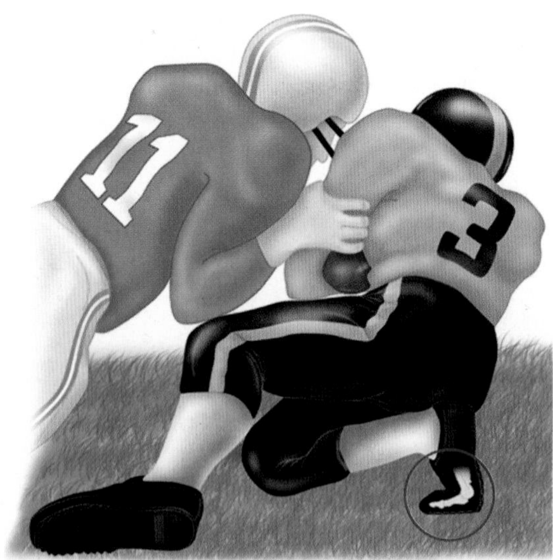

A

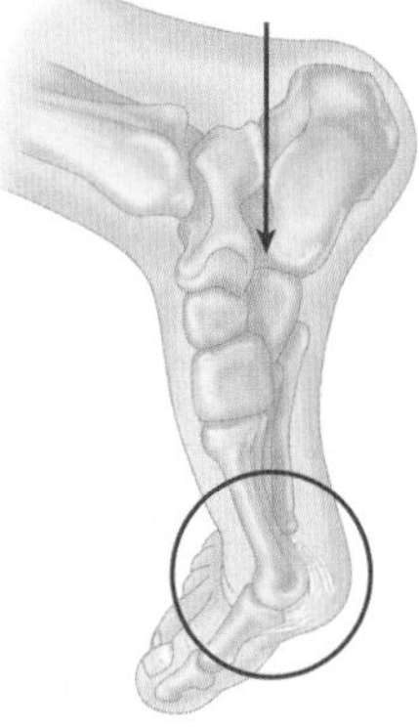

B

FIGURE 1

Treatment Options

- Nonoperative treatment consists of rest, ice, compression, and elevation. Initially, a walking boot is utilized to provide a more comfortable gait.
- A short-leg walking cast with a toe spica extension in plantar flexion is used in patients with severe soft tissue injury.
- As the athlete improves, range-of-motion exercises, taping regimens, and a carbon fiber insert or Morton's extension is necessary with return to play.

Examination/Imaging

- Physical examination of the injured hallux metatarsophalangeal (MTP) joint should include inspecting the joint for edema and ecchymosis, assessing range of motion (compare to contralateral hallux), and a great toe Lachman's test.
- Plain radiographs
  - Weight-bearing anteroposterior, lateral, and sesamoid axial views should be taken, with contralateral comparison views.
  - Evaluate the radiographs for capsular avulsions, chondral injuries, and sesamoid fractures.
  - Proximal migration of the sesamoids (Fig. 2) is consistent with a complete rupture of the plantar plate (Fig. 3A and 3B). The difference in the distance from the distal pole of the sesamoids to the MTP joint should be less than 3 mm compared to the contralateral hallux.

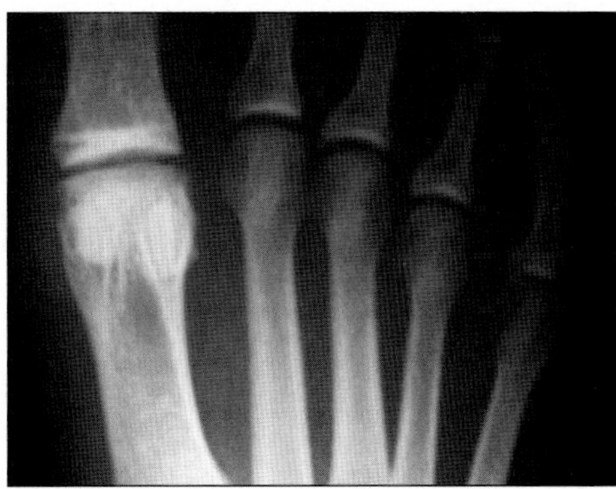

FIGURE 2

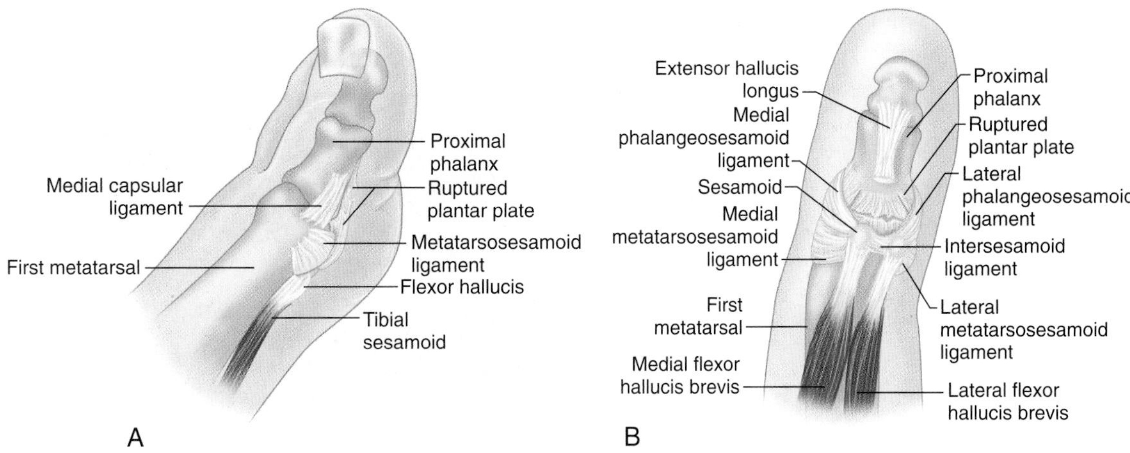

FIGURE 3

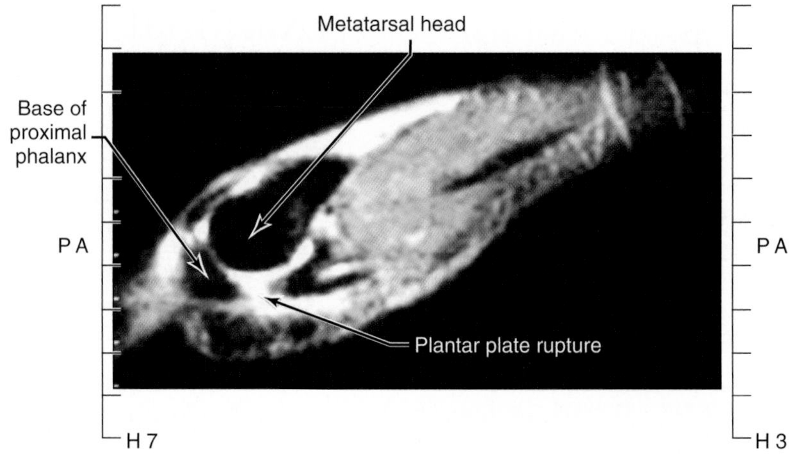

FIGURE 4

- Dorsiflexion stress lateral views taken bilaterally can be helpful in uncovering ligamentous rupture when other plain radiographs are inconclusive.
- Magnetic resonance imaging is the best modality to evaluate all the associated injuries of a turf toe (Fig. 4).

Surgical Anatomy

- Key components of anatomy to understand:
  - Plantar digital nerve
  - Capsular-ligamentous complex
- The medial plantar digital nerve runs parallel to the plantar aspect of the great toe at the inferior edge of the abductor hallucis tendon (Fig. 5).

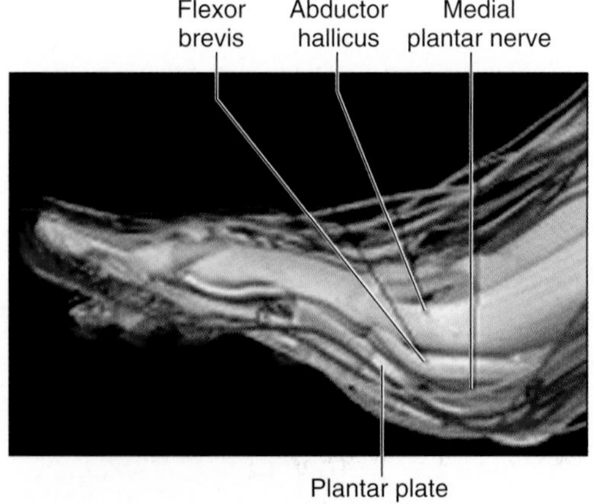

FIGURE 5

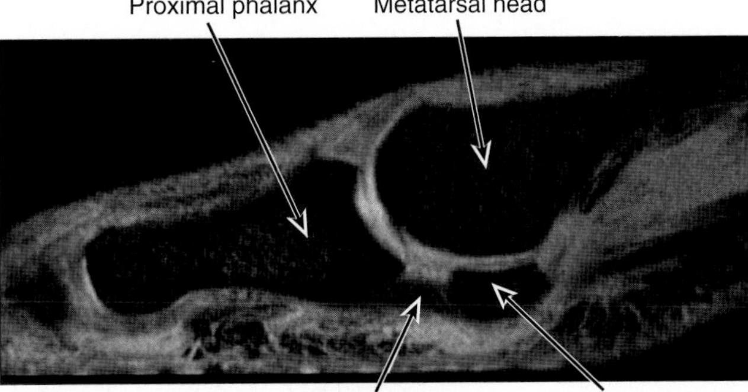

FIGURE 6

- Capsular-ligamentous complex (Fig. 6)
  - Motion of the joint consists of rotation and translation.
  - Anatomic restraints guide the motion of the 1MTP as the joint articulation provides little of the overall stability.
  - Most of the stability comes from the capsular-ligamentous complex.
    - The complex is a confluence of structures including the plantar plate, collateral ligaments, flexor hallucis brevis (FHB), adductor hallucis, and abductor hallucis.
    - The FHB is a split tendon that envelops the sesamoids before inserting into the base of the proximal phalanx.
    - The plantar plate is a strong fibrous structure firmly attached to the proximal phalanx and loosely attached to the metatarsal neck through the joint capsule. It blends with the sesamoids and tendons of the FHB to provide structural support.

Positioning

- Supine position
- Bump under contralateral side to facilitate external rotation of operative extremity
- Thigh tourniquet (ankle tourniquet will impact excursion of the long toe flexors, particularly the flexor hallucis longus)
- Fluoroscopic imaging available on same side as operative extremity

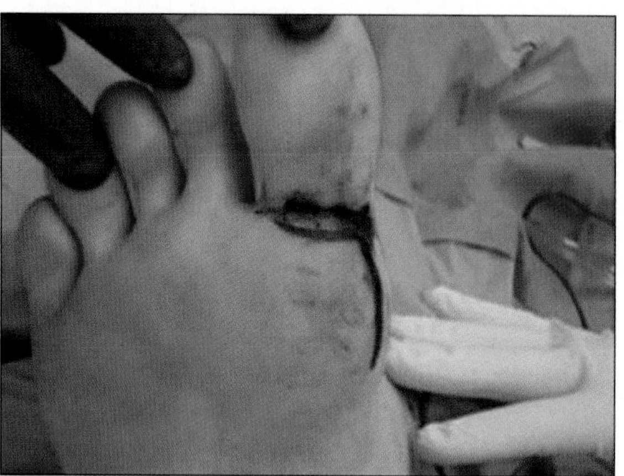

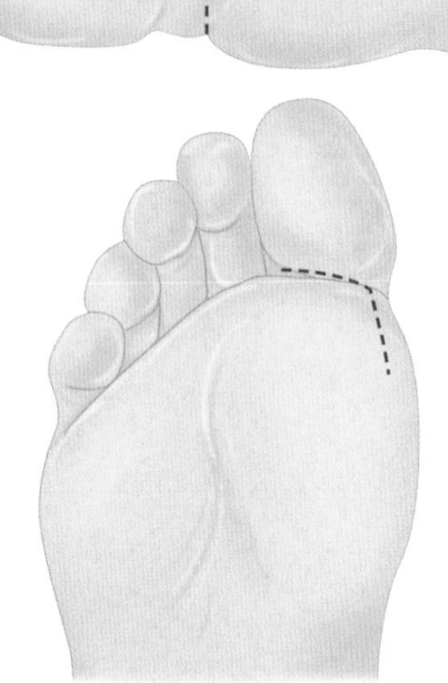

A B

FIGURE 7

Pearls

- *A J-shaped incision allows for extensile exposure and is recommended.*

Pitfalls

- *The plantar digital nerve is the structure most at risk with a surgical approach.*

Portals/Exposures

- Medial, medial and plantar, and J-shaped incisions have been described
- L-shaped or J-shaped incision (Fig. 7A and 7B)
  - The longitudinal arm parallels the plantar aspect of the great toe at the junction of the plantar and dorsal skin.
  - The transverse arm is then extended across the proximal toe crease.
- The plantar digital nerve is the first structure to be identified on the surgical approach to avoid injury.

Pearls

- *Plantar flexion of the 1MTP joint can assist in visualization.*

Pitfalls

- *Intra-articular loose bodies can be missed, leading to late dysfunction.*

Procedure

Step 1: Examination of Plantar Plate Rupture

- After completion of the exposure, the defect in the plantar plate should be visible (Fig. 8A and 8B). The location of the defect will determine the repair technique.
- Prior to repair, a thorough inspection of the 1MTP joint is completed. Any intra-articular pathology, such as osteochondral injuries, can be addressed at this time.

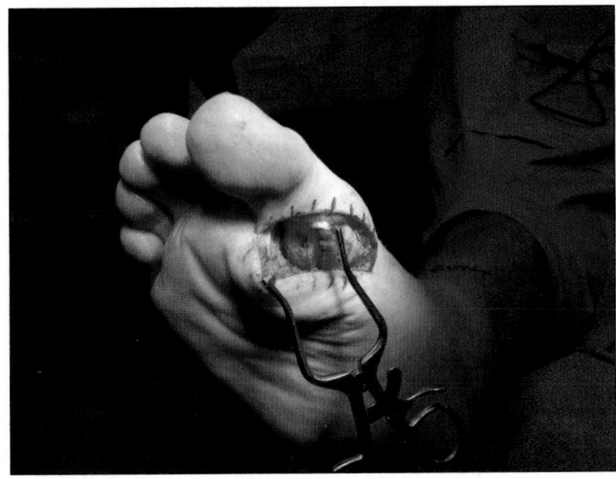

A

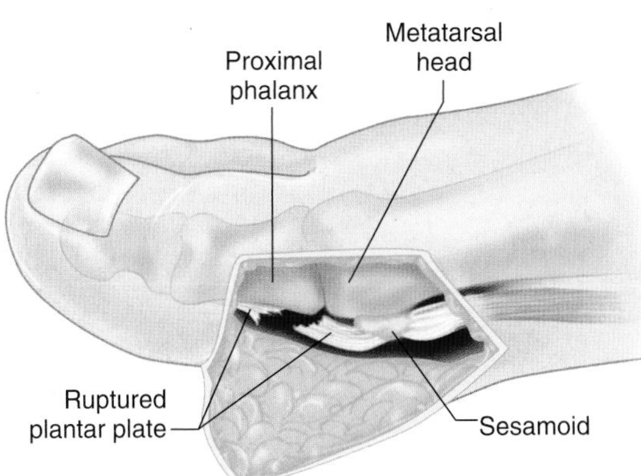

B

FIGURE 8

Pearls

- *Preservation of the soft tissue envelope of the plantar plate is essential to allow for primary repair.*

Pitfalls

- *Overtensioning of the repair must be avoided. Greater than 10° of static plantar flexion with the repair may lead to late problems with range of motion.*

Step 2: Primary Repair

- Having completed an examination of the joint, it is now time to repair the plantar complex. Identification of the proximal remnant of tissue, distal to the sesamoid, is essential.
- Next, identification of the distal remnant of the FHB tendon is completed.
- High-strength 0 suture is then used to approximate the two sides of the ruptured tissue for primary repair (Fig. 9A and 9B).
- A figure-of-8 suture technique is used for tensioning the repair.

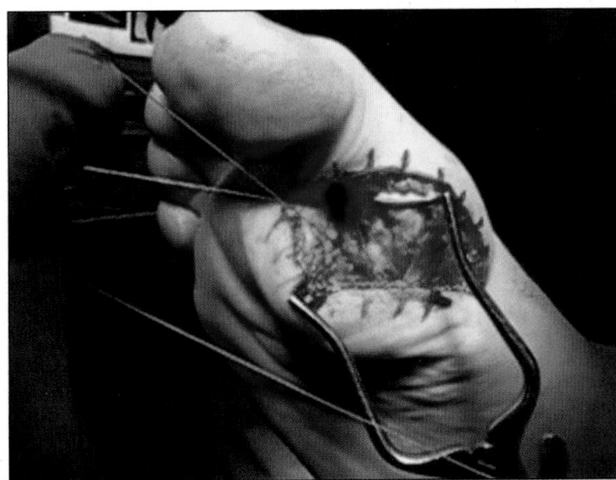

A

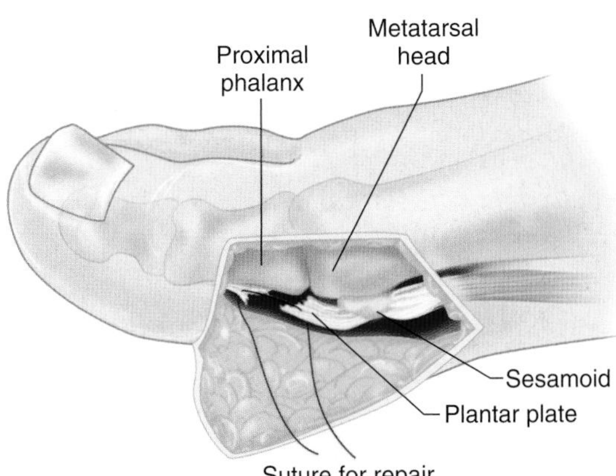

B

FIGURE 9

Controversies

- Nonabsorbable sutures may also be used for the repair.

Step 3: Distal Rupture

- Occasionally the plantar plate ruptures near the distal insertion of the FHB at the phalanx. In these situations, not enough tissue is available for suture repair.
- Drill holes or suture anchors (preferred) may be used for repair. The suture anchor is placed in the base of the proximal phalanx at the insertion site of the FHB.
- The proximal stump of tissue from the plantar plate is then secured by the suture anchor to the base of the phalanx.

Pearls

- *Good visualization of the joint will allow for identification of the insertion site of the FHB.*

Pitfalls

- *Careful drilling of bone tunnels must be done to assure that fracture of the phalanx does not occur.*

Step 4: Sesamoid Diastasis

- In the event of injury to the sesamoid in conjunction with a plantar plate rupture, several options are available.
- In the event of acute injury, primary repair of the sesamoid may be considered utilizing suture and bone grafting techniques. More likely these may be chronic injuries that are not amenable to primary repair of the sesamoid.
- If possible, only the distal pole of the sesamoid is excised. The remaining soft tissue of the plantar plate is then repaired to the proximal pole using drill holes or suture anchors.

Step 5: Closure

- The wound is copiously irrigated and hemostasis is confirmed. The subcutaneous layer is then closed using 2-0 absorbable sutures in an interrupted fashion.
- Skin is closed using interrupted 3-0 nonabsorbable sutures.
- The patient is then placed in a nonadherent sterile surgical bunion dressing with the toe in 5–10° of plantar flexion.
- A well-padded Jones dressing with a posterior splint is then applied with the ankle at neutral.

Pearls

- *A custom fabricated orthosis can be manufactured that will protect the patient from excessive dorsiflexion forces. The splint is usually fabricated at around week 3 postoperatively.*

Pitfalls

- *Early excessive dorsiflexion and active plantar flexion must be avoided to protect the repaired tissue.*

Postoperative Care and Expected Outcomes

- The operative dressing is removed approximately 7–10 days postoperatively. A splint is fabricated for the patient and used for protection (Fig. 10).
- The patient is allowed protected passive plantar flexion under the guidance of physical therapy. Active and passive dorsiflexion, as well as active plantar flexion, are avoided at this time. The patient

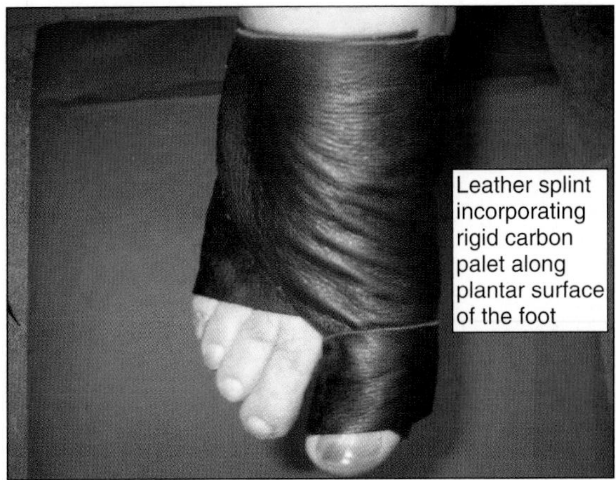

FIGURE 10

is also placed in a removable cast boot. The patient is to continue non–weight bearing for 4 weeks.

- Range of motion is increased at 6 weeks postoperatively, and progressive protected ambulation in the cast boot is encouraged.
- At approximately 2 months postoperatively, the patient is transitioned into an accommodative athletic shoe with an insole plate to prevent excessive dorsiflexion. Active range of motion is started at that time.
- At 3–4 months, the patient is allowed to return to sports conditioning with continued taping and shoewear modifications.
- It is expected to take 6–12 months for the patient to return to a preinjury level of function.

Evidence

Anderson RB. Turf toe injuries of the hallux metatarsophalangeal joint. Tech Foot Ankle Surg. 2002;1:102-11.

Grade-C recommendation. Paper outlines the mechanism, pathoanatomy, and surgical repair techniques of turf toe. (Level III evidence)

Clanton TO, Butler JE, Eggert A. Injuries to the metatarsophalangeal joints in athletes. Foot Ankle. 1986;7:162-76.

Grade-C recommendation. Articles reviews the injury patterns and treatment of turf toe injuries. (Level III evidence)

Frey C, Andersen GD, Feder K. Plantarflexion injury to the metatarsophalangeal joint ("Sand Toe"). Foot Ankle Int. 1996;17:576-81.

Grade-C recommendation. Article discusses the plantar flexion injury to the MTP joint with an overview of anatomy and treatment. (Level III evidence)

Jahass MH. Classic article: Foot & Ankle 1:15, 1980: Traumatic dislocations of the first metatarsophalangeal joint. Foot Ankle Int. 2006;27:401-6.

Grade-C recommendation. Classic article that describes traumatic dislocation of the 1MTP joint with treatment options. (Level III evidence)

Mullen JE, O'Malley MJ. Sprains—residual instability of subtalar, Lisfranc joints, and turf toe. Clin Sports Med. 2004;23:97-121.

Grade-C recommendation. Overvew article that discusses athletic sprain injuries to the hindfoot and forefoot. (Level III evidence)

Tewes DP, Fischer DA, Fritts HM, Guanche CA. MRI findings of acute turf toe. Clin Orthop Rel Res. 1994;(304):200-3.

Grade-C recommendation. Case report and review of anatomy of the turf toe injury utilizing MRI. (Level III evidence)

Watson TS, Anderson RB, Davis WH. Periarticular injuries to the hallux metatarsophalangeal joint in athletes. Foot Ankle Clin. 2000;5:687-713.

Grade-C recommendation. Overview article dealing with both nonoperative and operative treatment of turf toe injuries. (Level III evidence)

Yao L, Cracchiolo A, Farahani K, Seeger LL. Magnetic resonance imaging of plantar plate rupture. Foot Ankle Int. 1996;17:33-6.

Grade-C recommendation. Article discusses the radiographic anatomy of the plantar plate structure in both control patients and those with pathology. (Level III evidence)

PROCEDURE 10

Morton's Neuroma

Carol Frey

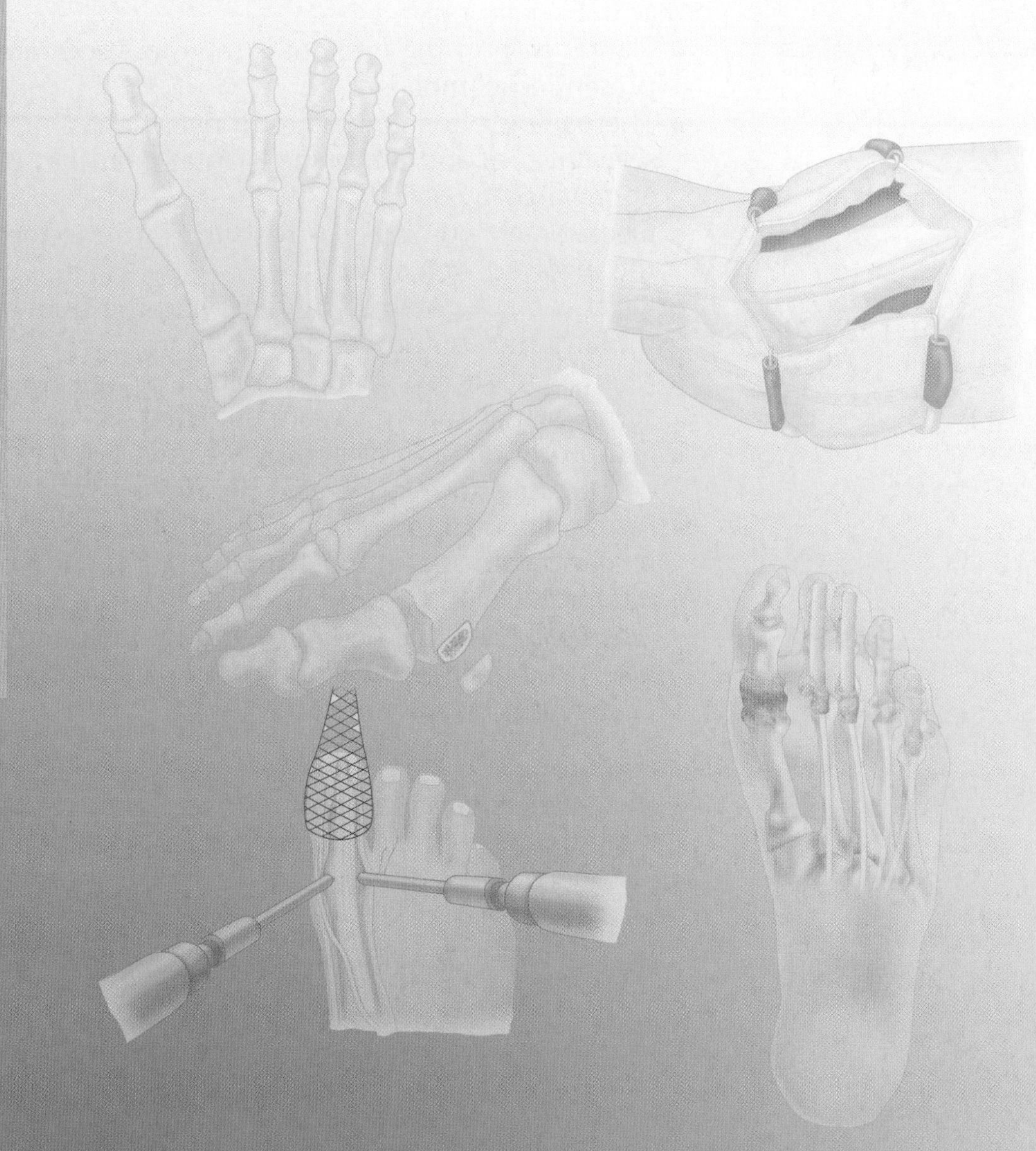

> **PITFALLS**
>
> - *Multiple neuromas may be present in the same foot or bilaterally.*
> - *Electromyographic studies may be indicated to rule out neuropathy from other causes.*
> - *Ninety percent of Morton's neuromas are single and occur in the third web space.*

Indications

- Failure of conservative treatment, as outlined below.
- Response to a diagnostic injection of local anesthetic agent.
- Other causes of metatarsalgia must be excluded, such as avascular necrosis, synovitis, ganglion cysts, and bone pathology.

Examination/Imaging

Physical Examination

- Plantar pain in the forefoot is the most common presenting complaint.
- The patient often complains of dyesthesias into the relevant toes and a burning plantar pain that is aggravated by activity.
- Occasionally numbness is reported into the toes of the involved web space.
- Relief is often obtained by removing the shoe and rubbing the ball of the foot.
- Many patients report the sensation of walking on a stone or that their socks are bunched.
- Symptoms are aggravated by wearing tight, compressive, or high-heeled shoes.
- Pain isolated to the plantar aspect of the foot, in the involved web space, is consistent with an interdigital neuroma (Fig. 1). Applying direct pressure to the web space and then compressing the metatarsal heads together can reproduce the pain. A clunk may or may not be present.

Imaging Studies

- Weight-bearing anteroposterior, lateral, and oblique radiographs are recommended to exclude bone disorders.

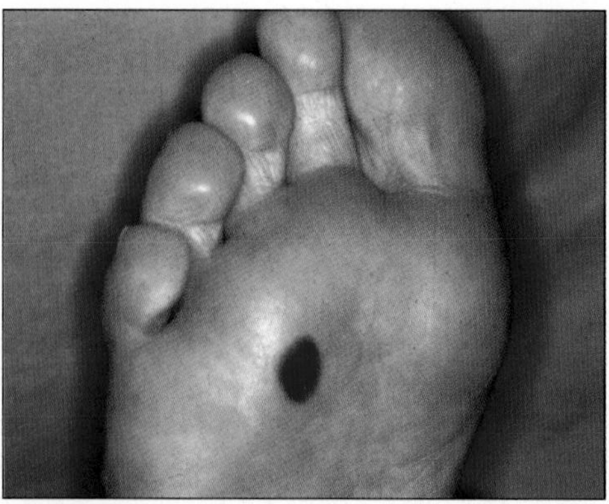

FIGURE 1

Treatment Options

- Injection of local anesthetic agent and cortisone
  - A mixture of 1–2 ml of lidocaine without epinephrine and 1 ml (10 mg/ml) of corticosteroid is recommended.
  - This mixture is injected just proximal to the metatarsal heads.
- Orthotic devices with small metatarsal pad proximal to the involved web space
- Anti-inflammatory medications
- Stretching the Achilles tendon
- Rocker-sole or rigid-sole shoe with high, wide toe box and soft upper
- Rocker-sole sandals

Pearls

- *The surgeon should be comfortable and seated. The back of the surgeon should be toward the head of the patient for the dorsal approach.*
- *The prone position is used for the plantar approach for a recurrent interdigital neuroma resection.*

- Magnetic resonance imaging may be recommended to exclude diagnoses such as avascular necrosis, ganglion cysts, or capsular and other soft tissue disorders, but are only rarely indicated.

Surgical Anatomy

- The metatarsophalangeal (MTP) joint and the interphalangeal joints of the foot are innervated by the plantar interdigital nerves.
  - The medial plantar nerve divides into digital branches that provide the main articular branches to the plantar aspect of the MTP joints of the first, second, and third toes and the medial aspect of the fourth toe.
  - The lateral plantar nerve divides into digital branches that provide the main articular branches to the plantar aspect of the fifth toe and the lateral aspect of the fourth toe.
- Morton's neuroma is not a true neuroma. It is a perineural fibrosis of the plantar interdigital nerve as it passes between the metatarsal heads (Fig. 2). The third web space is the most commonly involved.

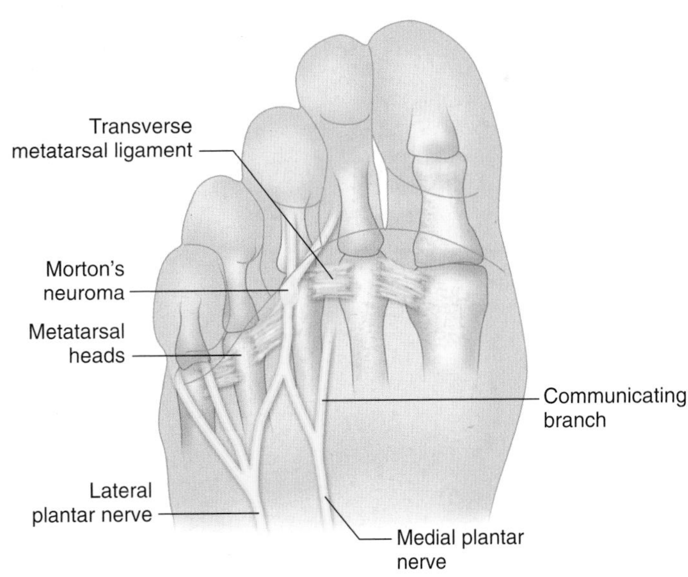

FIGURE 2

Positioning

- Supine for the dorsal approach for a primary interdigital neuroma resection

PEARLS

- *If a deeper bursa or ganglion off of an adjacent MTP joint is present, it is dissected and removed at this time.*

Instrumentation

- Foot tray
- Sharp Senn retractors
- Smooth lamina spreader
- Dissecting scissors
- #15 blade on a scalpel

PEARLS

- *Care should be taken to decrease any dissection or trauma to the plantar fat pad.*
- *Care should be taken to make sure that the proximal nerve transection does not retract under a metatarsal, but rather into soft tissue.*

PITFALLS

- *The intrinsic tendons of the foot can be mistaken for a neuroma and transected, especially the lumbrical tendon.*

Portals/Exposures

- A dorsal longitudinal incision is made in the involved web space between the toes and extends proximally to about the level of the metatarsal head and neck (Fig. 3).
- The dorsal sensory nerves are retracted.
- The superficial dorsal interosseous fascia is transected.
- The metatarsal heads are exposed.
- A smooth lamina spreader or Senn retractor may be used to separate the metatarsal heads (Fig. 4). This places the intermetatarsal ligament under tension. There may or may not be a bursa overlying this ligament. It should be dissected if present.
- A Freer elevator is passed under the ligament to protect the interdigital nerves and vessels.
- The ligament is transacted with small dissecting scissors or a #15 blade. The underlying structures are protected with a Freer elevator or hemostats.

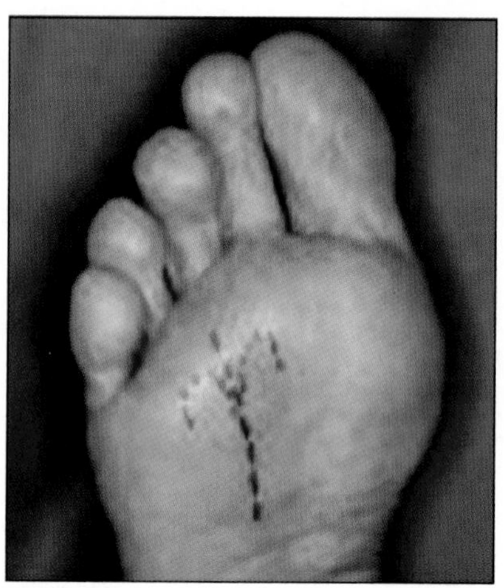

FIGURE 3

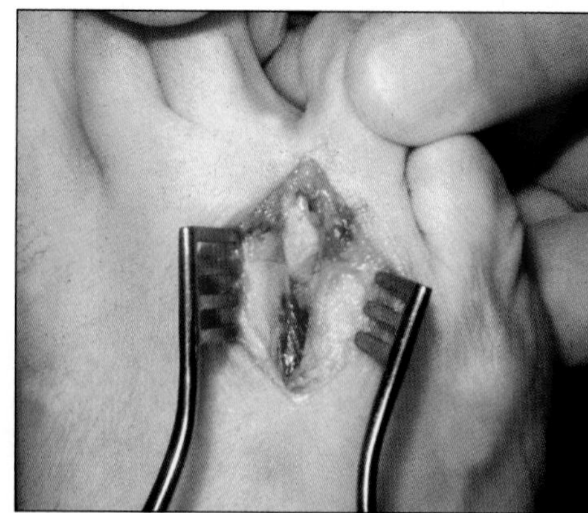

FIGURE 4

Procedure

STEP 1

- Pressure is applied to the plantar aspect of the foot in the area of the web space. The neuroma should pop into view (Fig. 5).
- A mosquito clamp is placed under the nerve to improve visualization.
- The nerve is dissected free of the neighboring vessels.
- The nerve should be exposed distally, after the bifurcation, and proximally.
- Gentle traction is applied to the nerve.
- A neurectomy is performed proximal to the metatarsal heads, in an area where the nerve may retract into soft tissues (Fig. 6).
- The neuroma and surrounding nerve material may be sent to pathology at this time (Fig. 7).

STEP 2

- The tourniquet is released and hemostasis obtained.
- The wound is closed in routine fashion.
- A compressive dressing is applied.

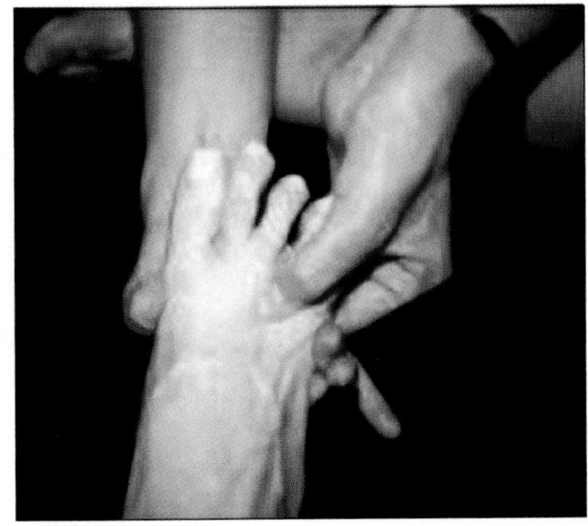

FIGURE 5

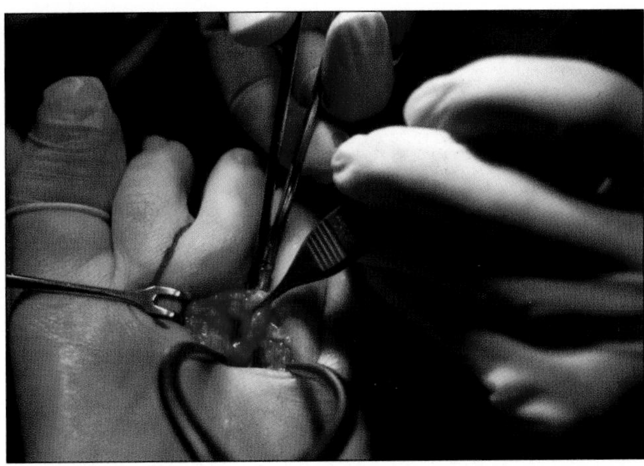

FIGURE 6

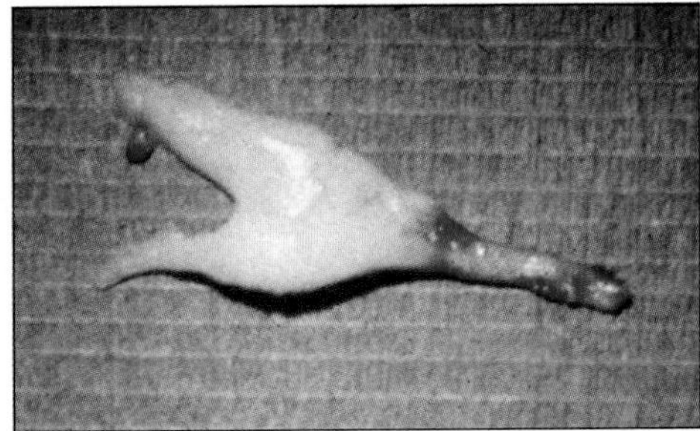

FIGURE 7

PEARLS

- *Swelling may be present postoperatively for 3–6 months.*

Postoperative Care and Expected Outcomes

- Weight bearing as tolerated in a postoperative shoe for 4 weeks.
- Elevation to decrease swelling.
- Sutures removed at 2 weeks.
- May resume activities as tolerated at 3–4 weeks.
- Patient is advised to wear a stable sole or rocker-sole sandal/shoe after discontinuing the postoperative shoe.

Evidence

Friscia DA, Strom DE, Parr JW, et al. Surgical treatment for primary digital neuroma. Orthopaedics. 1991;14:669-72.

Most common complication is recurrence. Recurrence is most likely the result of failure to resect the nerve in the first place, or insufficient proximal resection with a resultant stump neuroma. (Level II evidence)

Johnson JE, Johnson KA, Unni KK. Persistent pain after excision of an interdigital neuroma. J Bone Joint Surg [Br]. 1988;70:651-7.

The third web space is the most commonly involved (80–85% of the time). The second web space represents approximately 15–20% of cases. Neuroma is never present in the first or fourth web space. (Level II evidence)

Okafor B, Shergill G, Angel J. Treatment of Morton's neuroma by neurolysis. Foot Ankle Int. 1997;18:284-7.

Thirty-five patients with Morton's neuroma were reviewed at a mean of 21.4 months follow-up after a neurolysis. Seventeen of 35 patients had complete relief and 12 of 35 had only minimal discomfort after surgery. (Level II evidence)

PROCEDURE 11

Revision Surgery through a Plantar Approach for Recurrent Interdigital Neuroma

Glenn B. Pfeffer

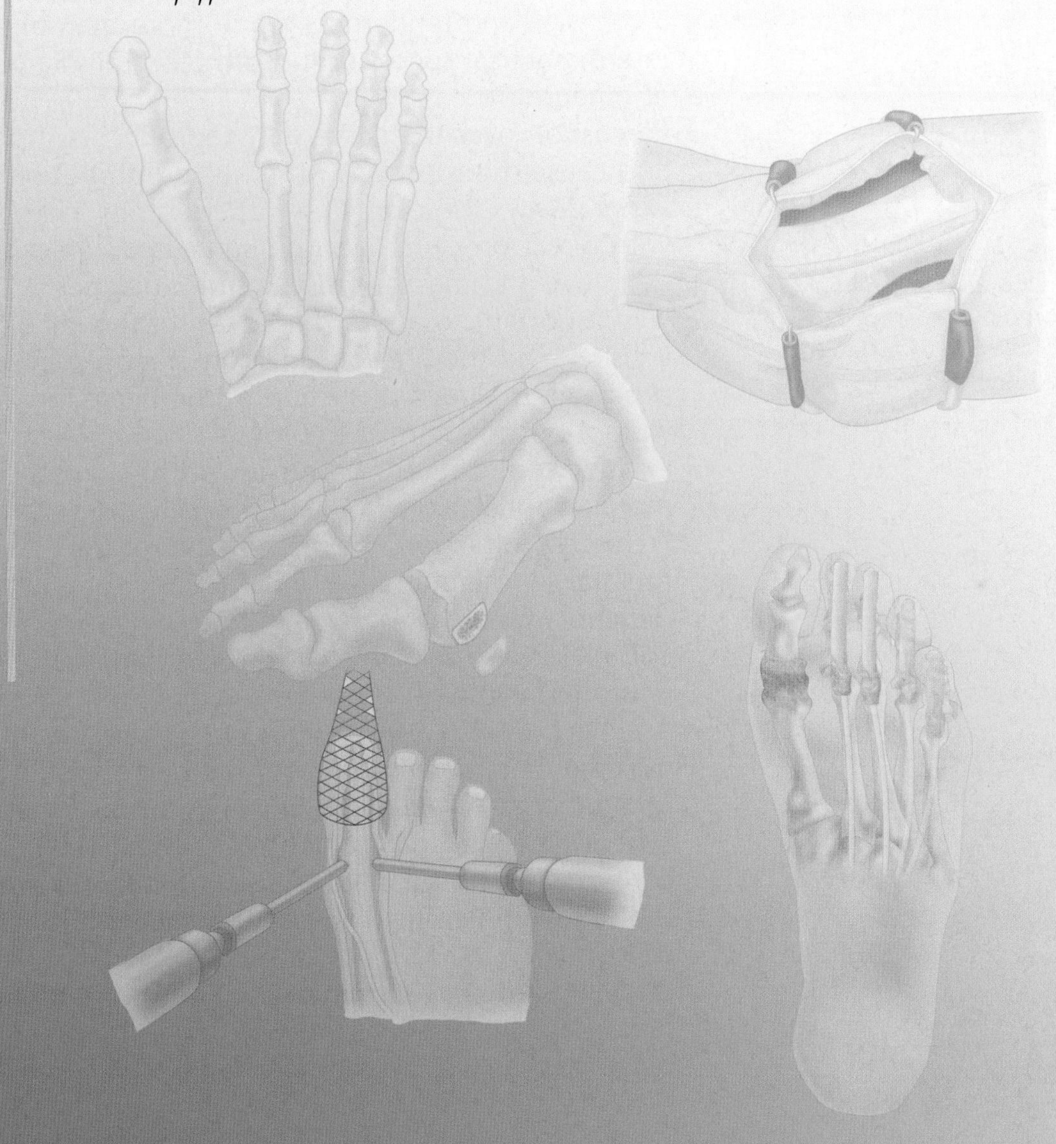

Pitfalls

- *The incidence of continued forefoot pain after primary interdigital neuroma excision is approximately 10%.*
- *Is the pain from an inadequate excision, a recurrent neuroma, or another undiagnosed condition?*

Treatment Options

- One cortisone injection, given through a dorsal approach
- A cushioned orthotic pad (Hapad) with pressure relief over the neuroma stump
- Shoewear with a wide toe box; the addition of a rocker sole
- A program of physical therapy for desensitization
- A plantar Lidoderm patch
- Gabapentin or an equivalent medication

Indications

- Recurrent or persistent pain in the intermetatarsal space following excision of a Morton's neuroma.
- Exclusion of other sources of forefoot pain.
- Transient relief from a focal injection of lidocaine.

Examination/Imaging

- A patient will have focal pain on the plantar aspect of the foot, over the stump of the nerve, usually in the second or third intermetatarsal space.
- If the pain and tenderness are in more than one intermetatarsal space, or in both feet, the diagnosis of a neuroma is unlikely.
- Percussion over the nerve may reproduce symptoms and cause dysesthesias in the nerve distribution. This is not always the case. Often there is only deep pain with direct pressure over the nerve end, which is less definitive and may be from another diagnosis.
- It is important to assess the length of the initial incision. Did the previous incision extend sufficiently proximal to allow transaction of the nerve in a non–weight-bearing part of the foot?
- Exclude subluxation or synovitis of the adjacent metatarsophalangeal joints (especially the second), Freiberg's infraction, a stress fracture of the metatarsal, metatarsalgia, inflammatory or degenerative arthritis, tarsal tunnel syndrome, and complex regional pain syndrome. An adjacent neuroma, although possible, is highly unusual.
- An injection of 0.5 ml of lidocaine in the area of maximal pain at the stump of the nerve should provide near-complete relief of symptoms for at least 1 hour. Use a 25-gauge needle. Without this confirmation of the diagnosis, it is highly unlikely that a revision surgery will have a successful outcome.
- Standing anteroposterior/lateral and both oblique radiographs of the forefoot will help *exclude* other diagnoses, as will magnetic resonance imaging. Ultrasonography may have a diagnostic role.

Surgical Anatomy

- A stump neuroma will be found proximal to the metatarsal head (Fig. 1).

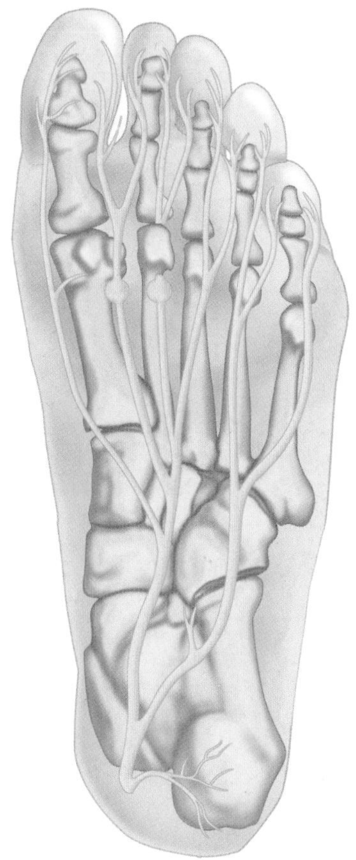

FIGURE 1

Positioning

- Prone
- An ankle resected at first surgery or thigh tourniquet

PEARLS

- *The surgery may be performed in the supine position, with the operating room table in a slight Trendelenburg position, if the patient is not able to tolerate a prone position.*

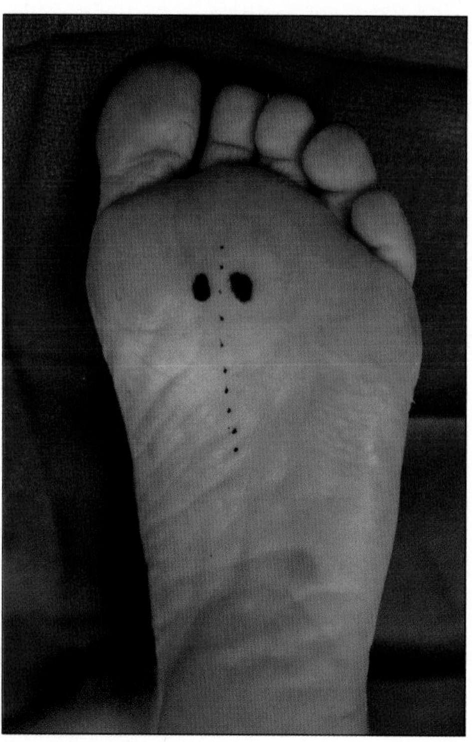

A

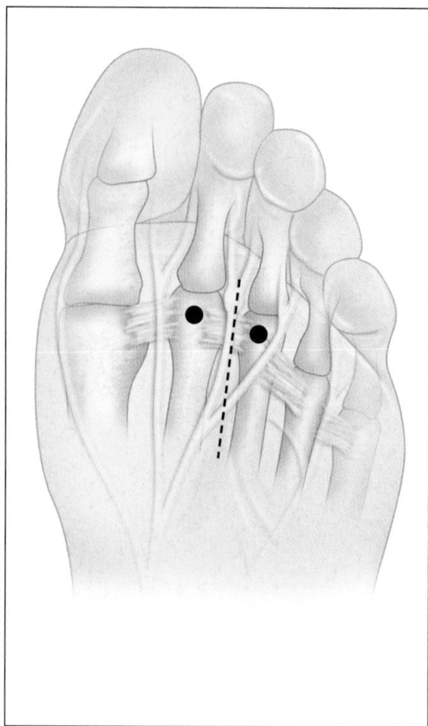

B

FIGURE 2

Controversies

- Performing the surgery in the supine position, with the table in slight Trendelenburg position.

Pearls

- *If the patient has already had a plantar incision for the original surgery, curve the new incision as far back as necessary to place the nerve stump off of the weight-bearing aspect of the foot.*

Instrumentation

- Loupe magnification

Portals/Exposures

- The plantar longitudinal incision should begin 1 cm distal to the area of maximal pain, which is usually just proximal to the metatarsal heads.
- The incision is centered between the metatarsal heads (Fig. 2A and 2B).
- Extend the incision proximally into a non–weight-bearing area, where the nerve will be divided. This excellent exposure is not possible with a transverse or dorsal incision.

Procedure

Step 1

- Identify the plantar fascia. At the most proximal aspect of the incision, carefully divide the fascia longitudinally with a #15 blade (Fig. 3).
- Identify a normal portion of the common digital nerve in an area that is free of scar tissue from the previous surgery (Fig. 4). Tag the nerve with a small rubber dam cut from a Penrose drain.

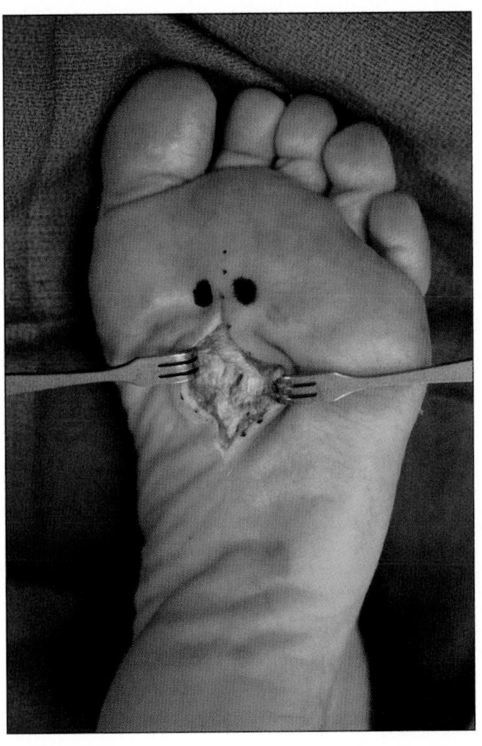
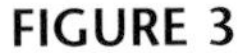

FIGURE 3

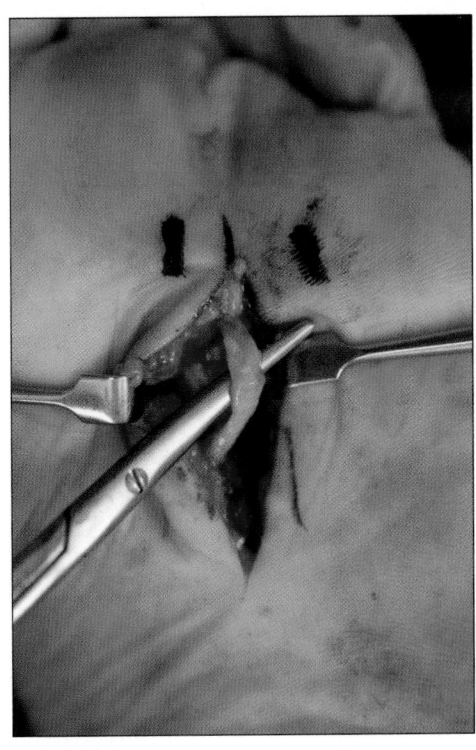

FIGURE 4

STEP 2

- Identify the distal pathology. Often the distal nerve end will be scarred down to the transverse metatarsal ligament or plantar plate (Fig. 5A and 5B). A stump neuroma may be present more proximally. In either case, sharply transect the nerve in a non–weight-bearing aspect of the foot.

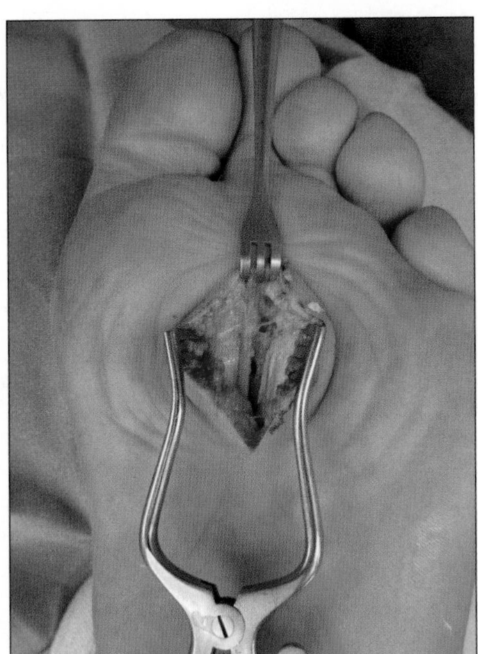

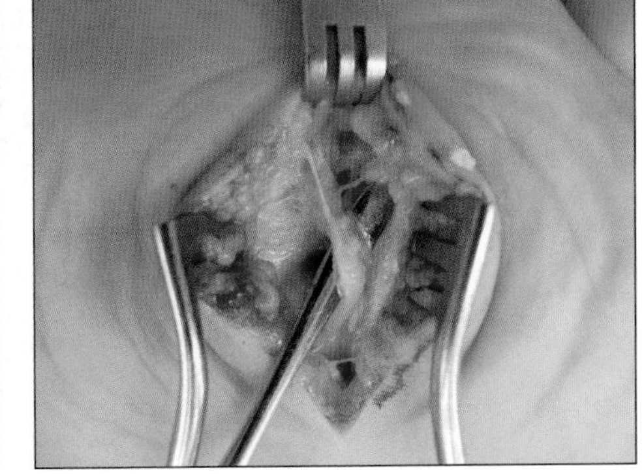

FIGURE 5 A B

Controversies

- A painful, hypertrophic scar may develop after a plantar incision, but is extremely rare.
- The neuroma is plantar, and should almost always be operated on from a plantar approach.
- It is very rare to have a problem with a plantar incision.
- The nerve cannot be exposed adequately from a dorsal incision.
- In the extremely rare situation in which there is a concomitant problem with the metatarsophalangeal joint (e.g., synovitis or instability), an additional dorsal incision can be used.

  - Place gentle traction on the nerve and sharply divide it in the most proximal aspect of the incision.
  - Cut down on a wet tongue depressor (Fig. 6). Allow the nerve to retract into normal tissue.
- In a salvage situation, an intrafascicular dissection of the common digital nerve will allow its branches to be separated proximally. In this way the neuroma can be dissected back to a non–weight-bearing aspect of the arch, while preserving innervation to the adjacent web space (Fig. 7).
- Make sure that the incision extends into the *non-weight-bearing* aspect of the arch (Fig. 8A and 8B).
- In a patient with pes planus, where the nerve end will still have direct pressure on it, bury the stump in the deep muscles of the foot using a 6-0 nonabsorbable epineural suture.
- Make sure there is no tension on the nerve as the foot and ankle are placed through a full range of motion.

Step 3

- Drop the tourniquet. Obtain meticulous hemostasis, and close the wound with one layer of 3-0 nylon (Fig. 9). If necessary, alternate simple and horizontal mattress sutures to assure excellent apposition of the

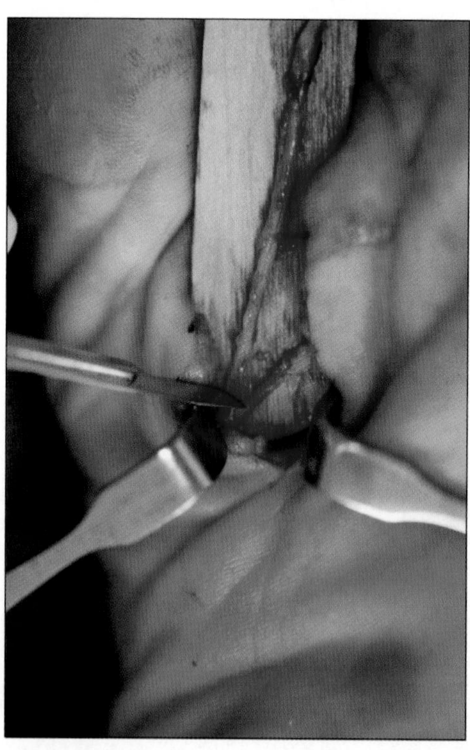

FIGURE 6

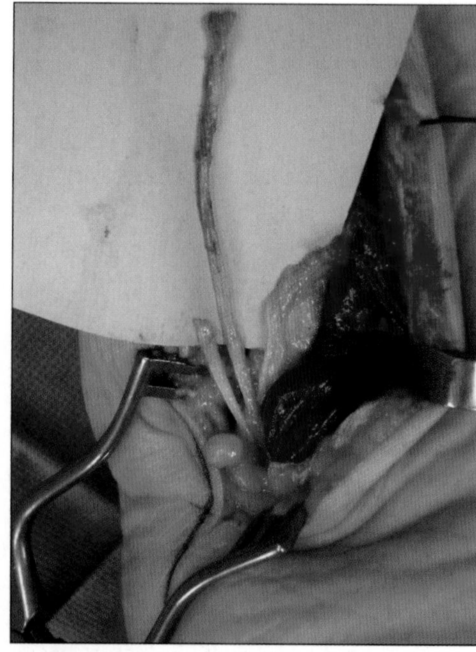

FIGURE 7

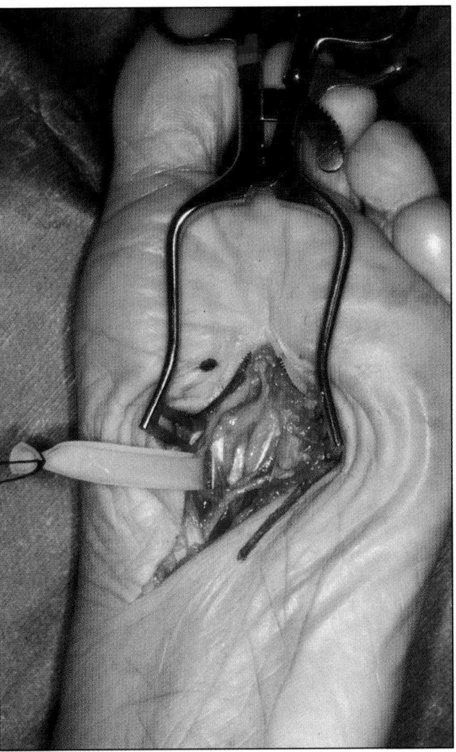

A

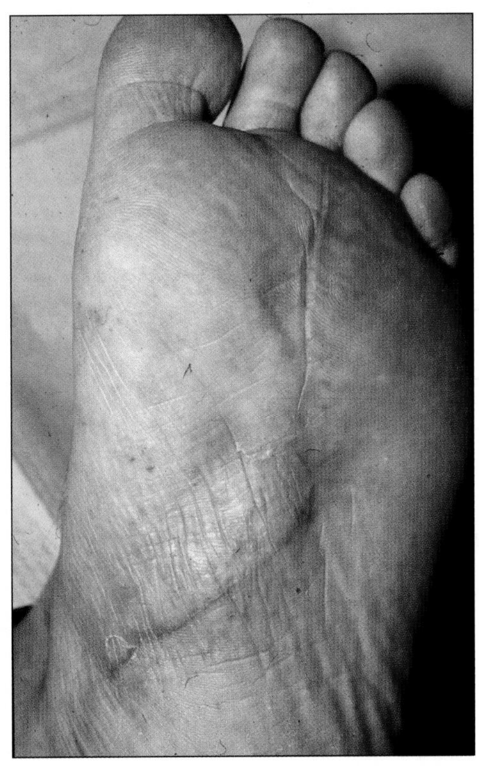

B

FIGURE 8

skin edges. Subcutaneous sutures should not be used in most cases.

- Apply a bulky sterile dressing. A posterior plaster splint may be added to further protect the wound.

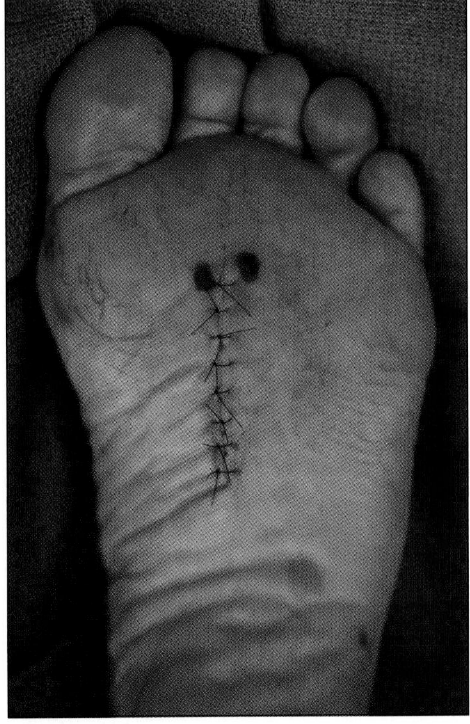

FIGURE 9

PEARLS

- *Never dissect directly onto a scarred nerve. Identify a more proximal portion of the nerve in normal tissue and begin your distal dissection from this point.*

PITFALLS

- *The common digital nerve lies directly beneath the plantar fascia, superficial to the arteries. Careful dissection is required. If the intrinsic muscles are reached, the dissection is too deep.*

PEARLS

- *If the proximal portion of the nerve is transected in a non–weight-bearing aspect of the arch, especially in a patient with a cavus foot, there is no need to bury the nerve.*

Controversies

- Numerous techniques have been tried to prevent a painful stump neuroma from developing. No one technique has proven superior.

Pearls

- *A small dehiscence of the wound should be treated with several weeks of moist dressing changes. Excellent healing will occur.*

Postoperative Care and Expected Outcomes

- The patient is kept non–weight bearing until the wound is completely healed. The sutures are usually removed 2-3 weeks after surgery.
- Steri-Strips should be used for an additional 2 weeks to prevent the incision from spreading apart.
- Once the sutures are removed, the patient can start to bear weight in a cast boot until 4 weeks postoperatively. Immobilization helps achieve appropriate wound healing.
- Most patients will experience significant improvement, although up to 25% will continue to experience some discomfort.

Evidence

Akermark C, Crone H, Saartok T, Zuber Z. Plantar versus dorsal incision in the treatment of primary intermetatarsal Morton's neuroma. Foot Ankle Int. 2008;29:136-41.

An excellent study of 125 patients among whom one group had a dorsal approach and the other a plantar approach for a primary neuroma excision. Both had similar outcomes, although the dorsal incision group had more complications. There were no significant problems with the plantar incisions. The authors concluded that a plantar approach is preferable. (Level IV evidence)

Beskin JL, Baxter DE. Recurrent pain following interdigital neurectomy—a plantar approach. Foot Ankle. 1988;9:34-9.

Supports a plantar approach for recurrent neuroma. (Level IV evidence)

Coughlin MF, Schenck RC, Shurmas PJ, Bloome D. Concurrent interdigital neuroma and MTP joint instability: long-term results of treatment. Foot Ankle Int. 2002;23:1018-25.

A study that presents a comprehensive approach to the differential diagnosis of primary neuroma pain in the forefoot. (Level III evidence)

Johnson J, Johnson K, Unni K. Persistent pain after excision of an interdigital neuroma. J Bone Joint Surg [Am]. 1988;70:651-7.

A study of 33 feet with persistent pain following excision of an interdigital neuroma. The revision surgery was performed through a plantar longitudinal incision. Only one patient had a minor problem with an intermittent callus at the proximal edge of the scar. (Level IV evidence)

PROCEDURE 12

Deviated Lesser Toe/ Metatarsal Shortening (Weil) Osteotomy

Carol Frey

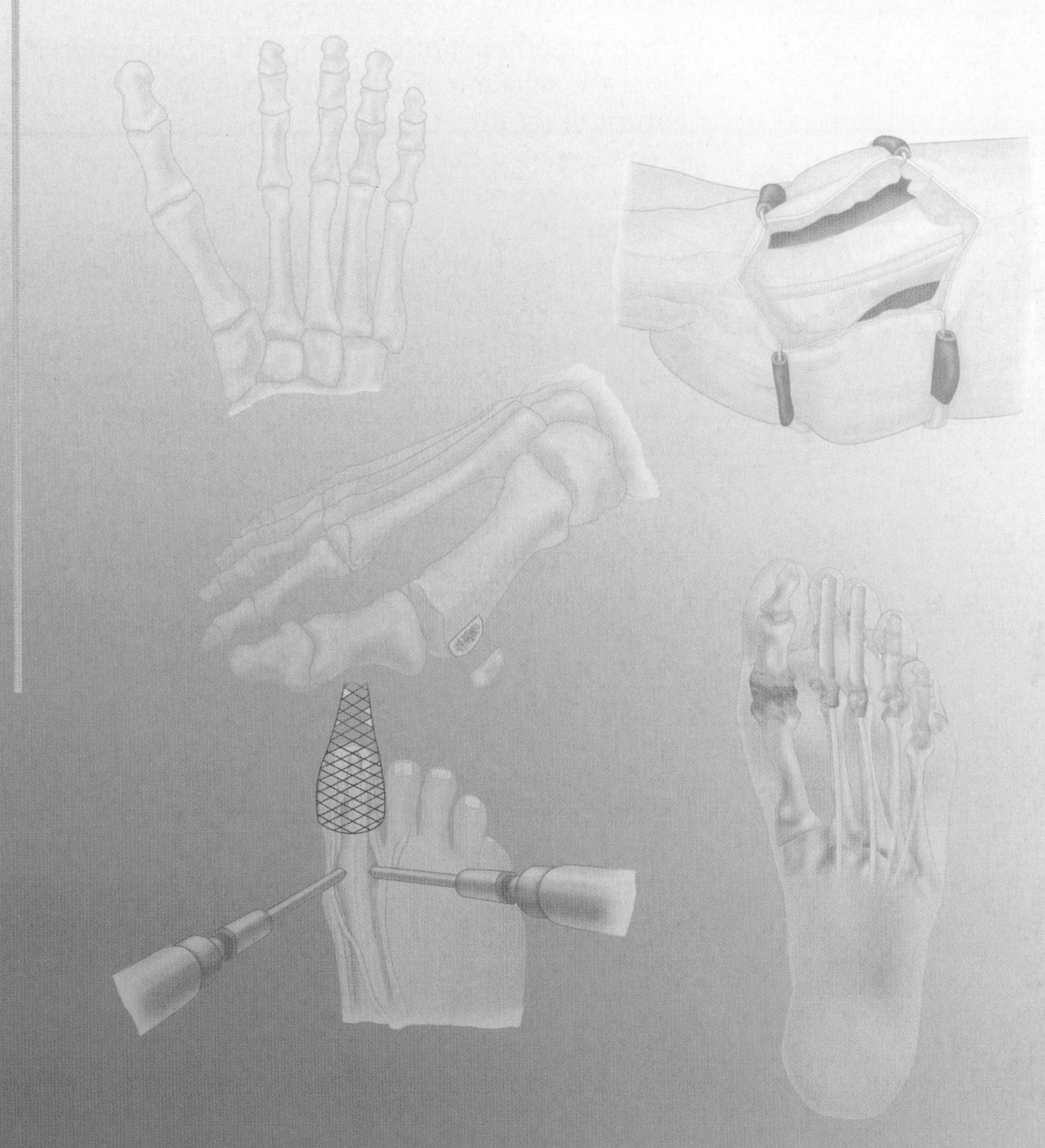

Pitfalls

- *Fixed deformities are rarely managed successfully with nonsurgical treatment.*

Controversies

- Involvement of more than one lesser metatarsal
- Synovitis of the lesser MTP without deformity

Treatment Options

- Anti-inflammatory medication
- Orthotic devices, rocker-sole or rigid-sole shoe (to decrease flexion at the MTP with gait), shoe with a high, wide toe box and soft upper
- Injections
- Splints and taping techniques

Indications

- Lesser metatarsophalangeal (MTP) joint dislocation
- Lesser MTP joint subluxation
- Rigid hammer toe
- Long second, third, or fourth metatarsal
- Most commonly indicated for a single metatarsal
- Hammer toe that is irreducible even with complete sequential release of soft tissues

Examination/Imaging

- The patient will often complain of pain, swelling, and occasionally a feeling of instability at the MTP joints, most likely the second.
- The toe may begin to sublux out of position; this is especially noted when the patient is standing. This is commonly seen as a crossover toe deformity as the second toe drifts over the great toe. Hallux valgus is an associated deformity.
- The patient will have pain on the dorsal and plantar aspects of the foot, unlike with a Morton's neuroma, which has pain only on the plantar aspect of the foot.
- Standing, oblique, and lateral radiographs of the foot are recommended.
  - The standing anteroposterior radiograph of the foot in Figure 1A shows a long second metatarsal with subluxation of the second and third MTP joints.
  - The oblique-view radiograph of the forefoot in Figure 1B shows a dislocation of the third MTP joint.
- A Lachman's test is recommended. Figure 2 shows a positive Lachman's test of the second MTP joint (Fig. 2A), which indicates subluxation of the joint (Fig. 2B).

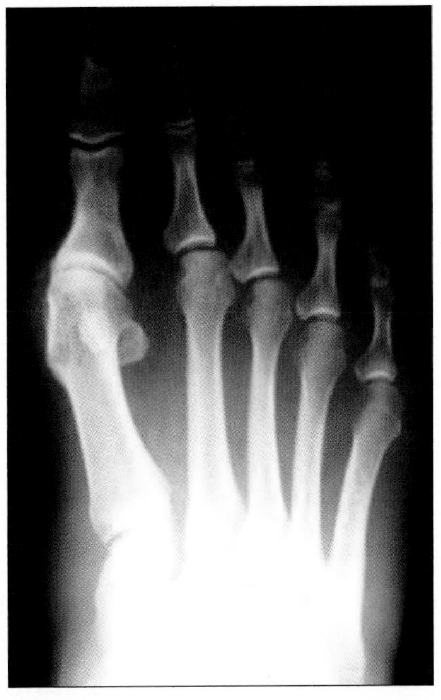

A

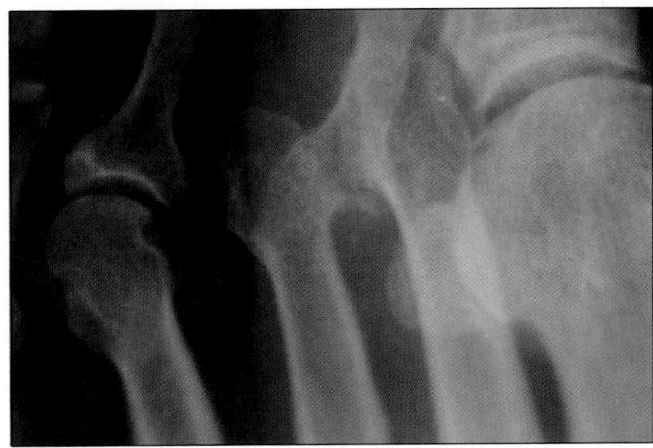

B

FIGURE 1

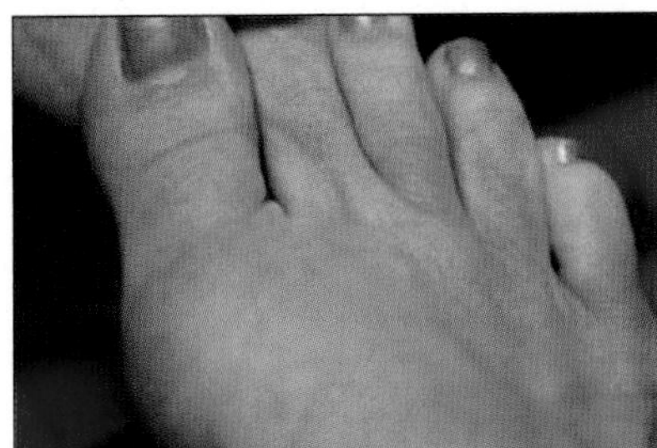

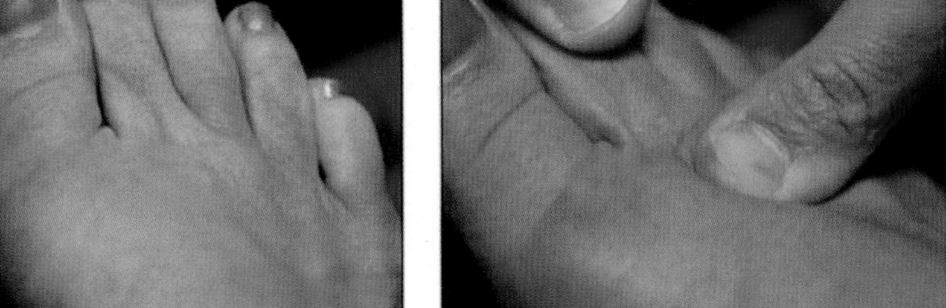

A B

FIGURE 2

Surgical Anatomy

- The tendon of the extensor digitorum longus (EDL) forms the central dorsal structure of the toe (Fig. 3A) It divides into three slips over the proximal phalanx. The middle slip inserts distally on the base of the middle phalanx. The two lateral slips insert at the base of the distal phalanx (Fig. 3B).
- An extensor sling anchors the central part of the EDL to the plantar aspect of the MTP joint and to the base of the proximal phalanx.
- The extensor digitorum brevis is located more lateral and deep to the EDL.
- The flexor digitorum longus inserts into the distal phalanx and the flexor digitorum brevis inserts into the middle phalanx.
- The tendons of the interosseous muscles are dorsal to the intermetatarsal ligament, and the tendons of the lumbrical muscles are plantar to the ligament.
- Stability of the MTP joint is mostly provided by the plantar aponeurosis and the plantar capsule where they combine to form the plantar plate. The plantar plate is the major structure to resist dorsiflexion of the MTP joint.

Positioning

- Supine position with the surgeon seated and facing the foot.

Portals/Exposures

- Begin with a dorsal approach at the MTP joint with an angled or straight longitudinal incision that begins within the intermetatarsal space (Fig. 4).
- Expose the extensor tendons.
- The capsule is opened and the metatarsal head and neck are exposed.
- Small Hohmann retractors protect the soft tissues.

Procedure

Pearls

- *When shortening the second metatarsal, try to match the length of the third metatarsal. This length helps to decrease the risk of transfer metatarsalgia.*

Step 1

- The toe is now plantar flexed to 90° (Fig. 5) and an oblique osteotomy is performed from distal dorsal to proximal plantar, starting at the dorsal edge of the metatarsal articular surface. The cut starts in the cartilage of the head (about 2 mm from the dorsal border) and should be about 2.5 cm long.

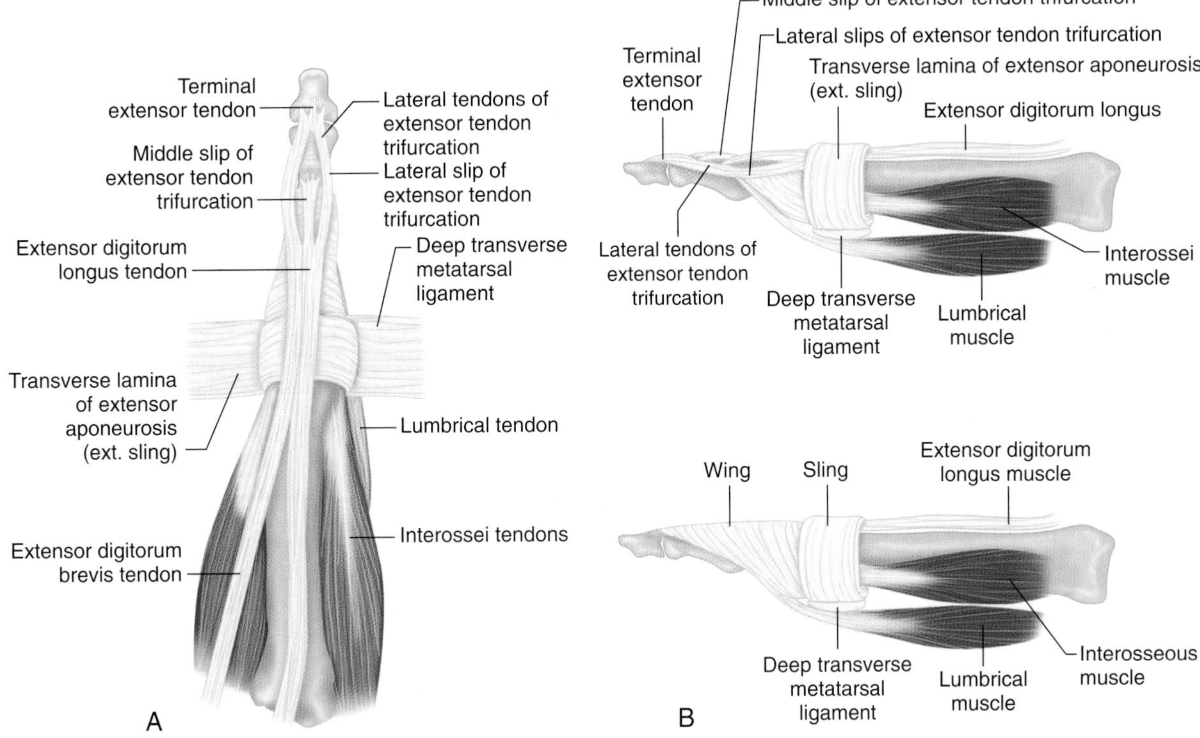

FIGURE 3

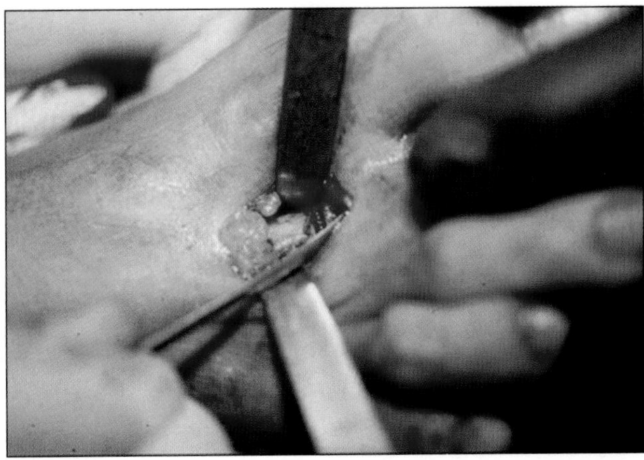

FIGURE 4

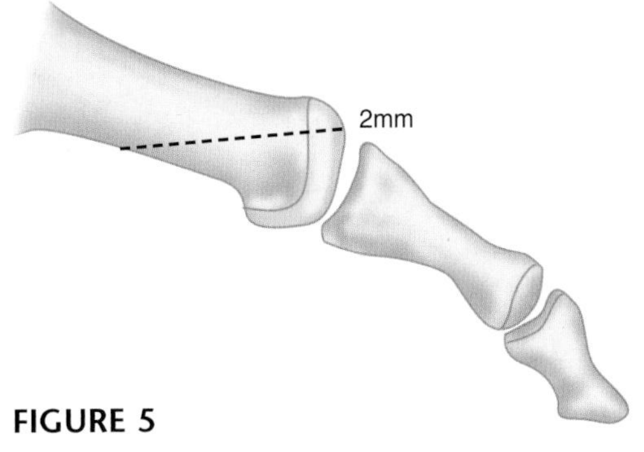

FIGURE 5

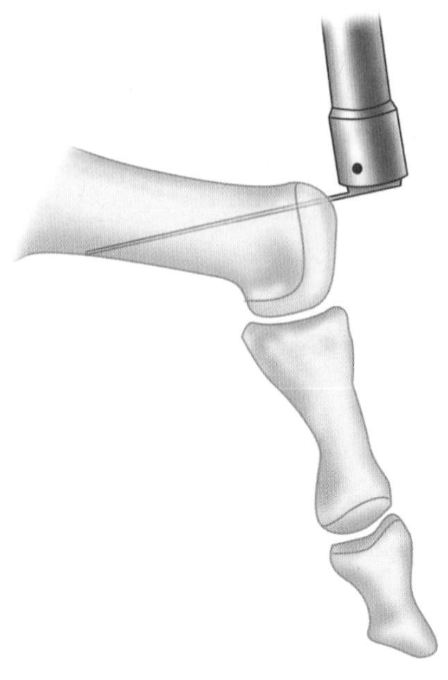

FIGURE 6

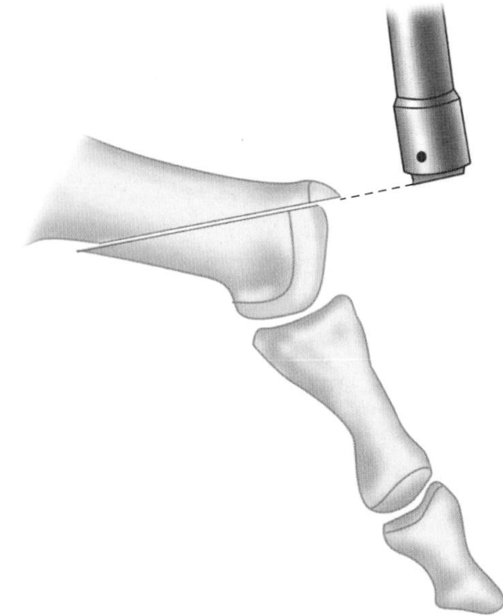

FIGURE 7

PEARLS

- *Temporary fixation may be obtained with a 0.045-inch Kirschner wire.*
- *A twist-off screw may be useful.*
- *With the ankle held at 90°, the toe should rest in a neutral position at the MTP joint.*
- *Rarely, a flexor tendon transfer into the extensor hood must be added to prevent dorsal subluxation at the MTP joint.*

PITFALLS

- *After fixation and before closure of the capsule, make sure that the MTP joint is reduced. This can be confirmed by fluoroscopy if necessary.*

- The saw blade is positioned in a plane parallel to the plantar surface of the foot (Fig. 6). This is usually an angle of about 25–30°.
- The osteotomy is proximally displaced approximately 6–8 mm (Fig. 7). In the case of dislocation, the shortening should be about equal to the initial proximal displacement of the proximal phalangeal base.

STEP 2

- 2.0-mm cortical screws are recommended for fixation (Fig. 8).
- The screw is oriented in a proximal-to-distal direction.
- The MTP capsule is closed, followed by routine closure of the skin.
- Intraoperative radiography will show decompression of the subluxated second MTP joint (Fig. 9A). With time, the fluid in the second MTP joint is absorbed and the joint assumes a reduced position (Fig. 9B).

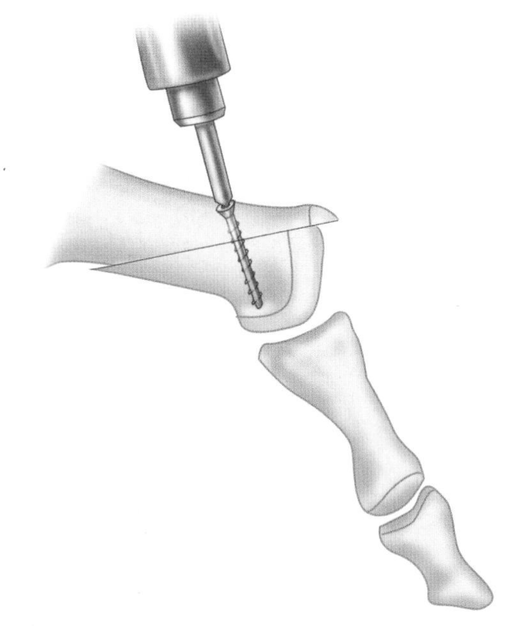

FIGURE 8

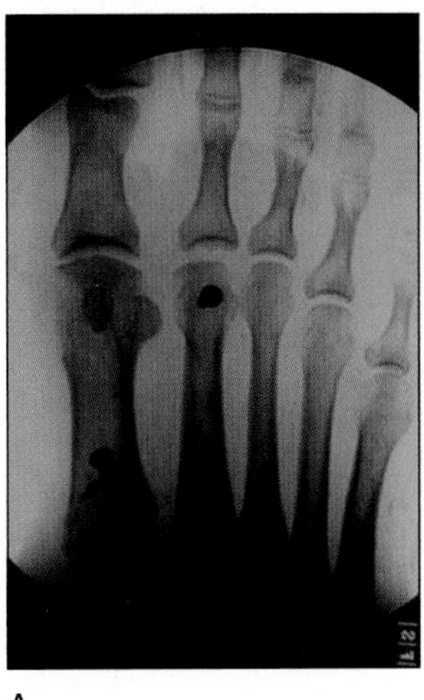

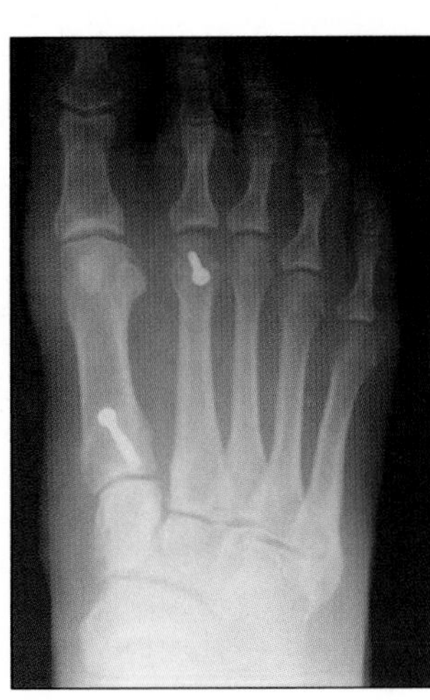

A B

FIGURE 9

Instrumentation/ Implantation

- Micro-sagittal saw
- Small Hohmann retractors
- 2.0-mm cortical screws
- 0.045-inch Kirschner wires
- Standard foot tray

Postoperative Care and Expected Outcomes

- Patient is immobilized in rigid postoperative shoe for 4–6 weeks.
- The sutures are removed at 2 weeks.
- Patient should have the toe taped in a neutral position for 4–6 weeks.
- Plantar-flexion exercises can begin once the osteotomy is clinically healed.

PEARLS

- *The patient's foot should be taped in a neutral position for at least 6 weeks to prevent dorsal displacement and contracture at the MTP.*
- *The patient should be instructed in plantar-flexion exercises as early as the osteotomy healing will allow, to decrease dorsal displacement and contracture at the MTP.*
- *Reduced voluntary control of the toe is expected to some degree after this procedure.*

PITFALLS

- *The screw may be painful in approximately 20% of patients, thus necessitating removal.*
- *If too much shortening is undertaken, the toe may become flail.*
- *A delay in wound healing is present in approximately 20% of the patients who undergo this procedure, especially if performed for a dislocated lesser MTP.*
- *There may be vascular compromise after correction of a severe deformity. This can be expected in less than 5% of patients.*

Evidence

Hofstaetter SG, Hofstaetter JG, Petroutsas JA, Gruber F, Ritschle P, Trnka HJ. The Weil osteotomy: a seven year follow-up. J Bone Joint Surg [Br]. 2005;87:1507-11.

The authors reported a prospective study of 1- and 7-year results of Weil osteotomy for the treatment of subluxed and dislocated MTP joints in 25 feet. Good to excellent results were reported in 84% after 1 year and 88% after 7 years. Floating toes and restricted motion at the MTP joint were reported in some patients. (Level II evidence)

Melamed EA, Schon LC, Myerson MS, Parks BG. Two modifications of the Weil osteotomy: analysis on sawbone models. Foot Ankle Int. 2002;23:400-5.

The authors noted that, with bone slice resection of the second metatarsal, there is shortening and mild plantar displacement of the head. With the use of a bone wedge excision, there is moderate shortening and essentially no plantar displacement of the head noted. (Level III evidence)

Trnka HJ, Gebhard C, Muhlbauer M, Ivanic C, Ristschl P. The Weil osteotomy for treatment of dislocated lesser metatarsophalangeal joints: good outcome in 21 patients with 42 osteotomies. Acta Orthop Scand. 2002;73:190-4.

This is a retrospective study of 60 Weil osteotomies for correction of dislocated lesser MTP joints in 31 patients. The average follow-up was 30 months. Excellent results were reported in 21 patients (42 osteotomies). A major complication was plantar penetration of the hardware in 10 cases. (Level II evidence)

PROCEDURE 13

Correction of Acquired Hallux Varus

Glenn B. Pfeffer

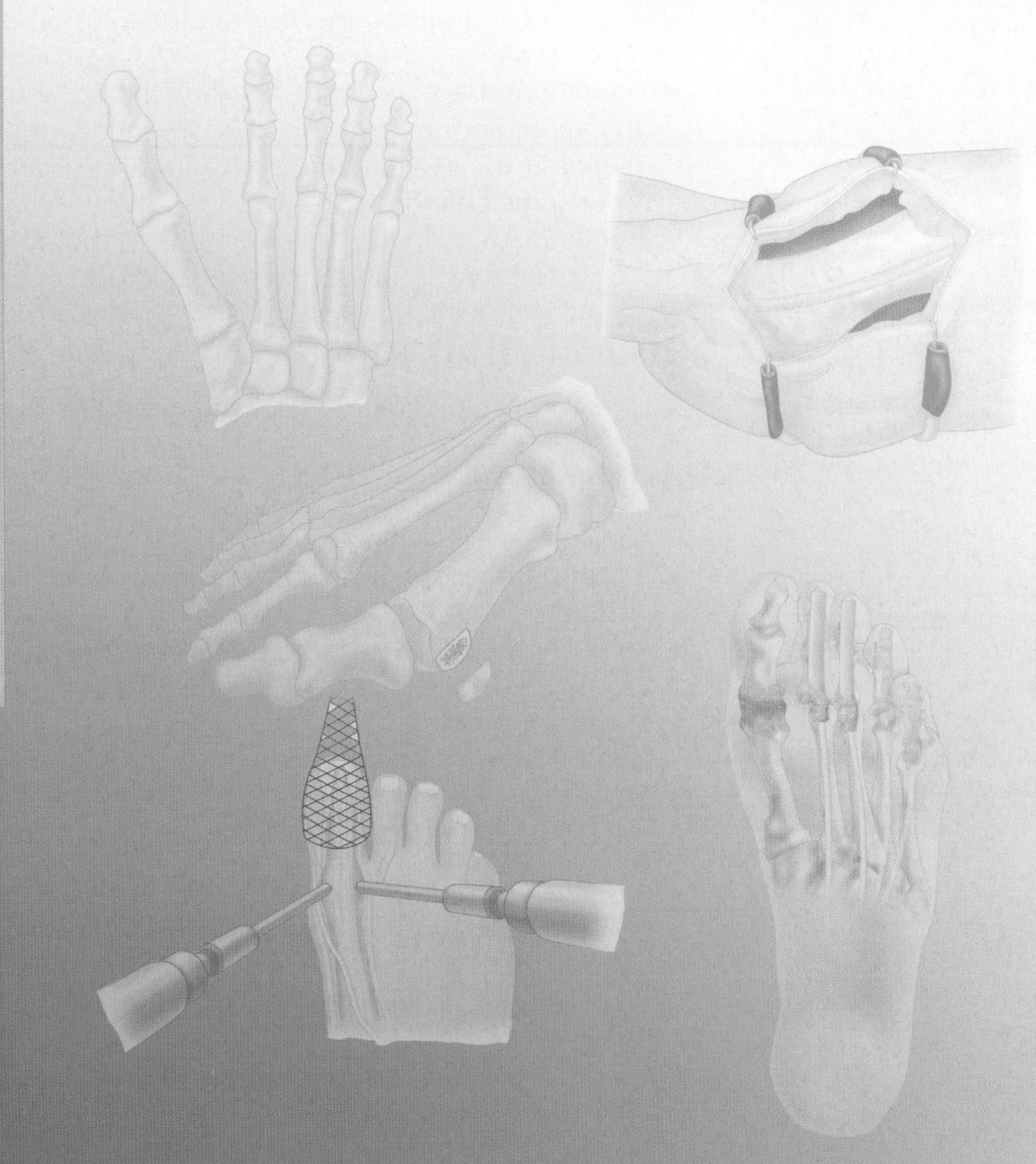

PITFALLS

- *Hallux varus must be reducible. Malunion of the metatarsal or proximal phalanx may preclude a simple soft tissue correction. A negative intermetatarsal angle may require correction. Consider a fusion for an arthritic joint.*

Controversies

- Correction using an endobutton is a new procedure with no long term follow-up.

Treatment Options

- Stretching out the shoe toe box can diminish irritation of the toe.
- Several other procedures exist for the correction of hallux varus, all of which require fusion of the adjacent IP joint, bony procedures, or compromise of one of the local extensor tendons (Johnson and Spiegel, 1984; Lau and Myerson, 2002). Another option is a reconstruction of the lateral collateral ligament with an allograft.

Indications

- Symptomatic deformity
- Difficulty with shoewear
- Flexible deformity
- Non-arthritic first metatarsophalangeal (MTP) joint

Examination/Imaging

- Weight-bearing examination of the toe (Fig. 1).
- Flexible great toe interphalangeal (IP) and MTP joints. A fixed deformity may require a fusion of either joint.
- Standing anteroposterior (AP), lateral, and both oblique radiographs of the foot. Oblique views are helpful in the evaluation of the joint and sesamoids for arthritic changes (Fig. 2).
- Standing AP and lateral radiographs of the normal foot (helpful as in intraoperative template).

Surgical Anatomy

- Lateral collateral ligaments of the great toe (Fig. 3)

Positioning

- Supine
- A bump under the ipsilateral hip may be helpful to position the foot.
- An ankle tourniquet can be used, but a thigh tourniquet is preferable so that no pressure is placed on the long extensors and flexors as the toe is balanced during the procedure.

Portals/Exposures

- A medial incision over the first MTP joint (Fig. 4).
  - Expose the capsule, in preparation for a vertical capsulotomy.
  - Locate and protect the dorsal and plantar sensory nerves.
- A 3- to 4-cm incision in the first intermetatarsal space.

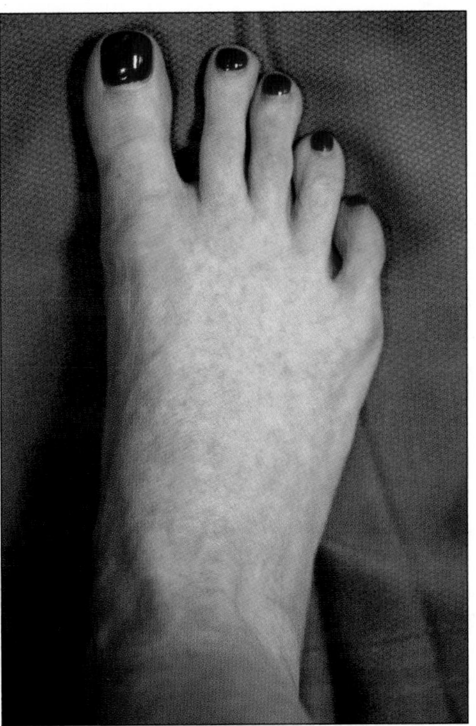

FIGURE 1

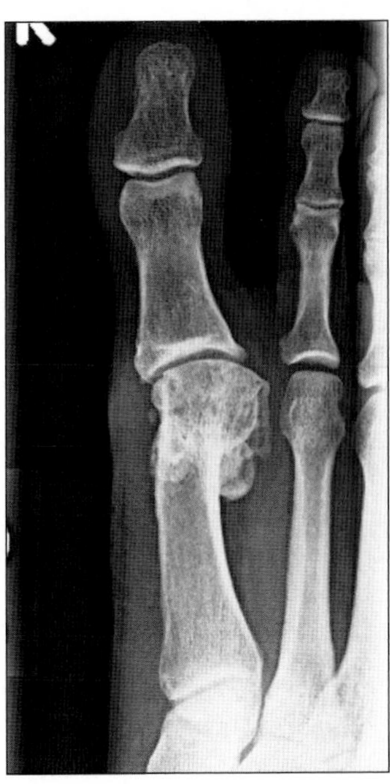

FIGURE 2

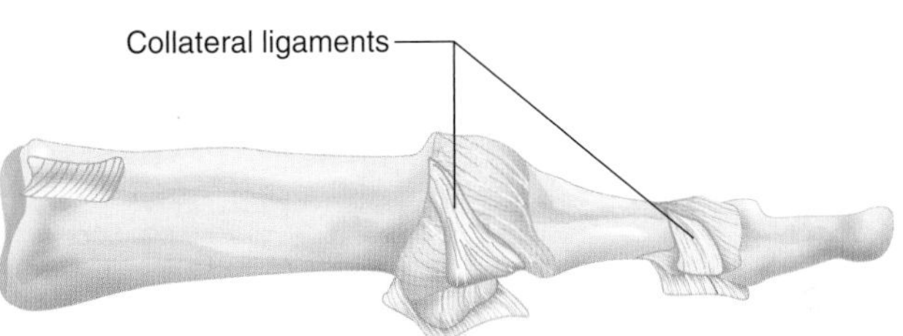

FIGURE 3

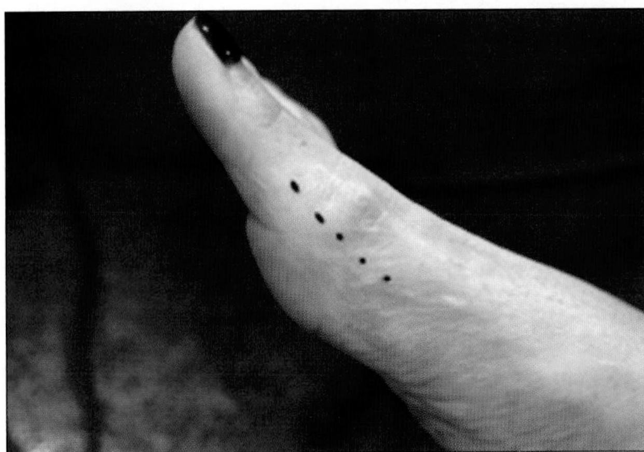

FIGURE 4

PEARLS

- *The plantar medial sensory nerve can easily be injured during the dissection and capsulotomy. It must be clearly identified, dissected free, and protected.*

PITFALLS

- *Previous incisions may preclude the use of two incisions. Sometimes a single dorsal-lateral incision has been used for a bunionectomy. Correction through this single incision is more difficult, but possible, if it is extended proximally and distally, and medial and lateral flaps are created.*

Procedure

STEP 1

- Make a vertical incision in the medial capsule, starting at the tibial sesamoid inferiorly and extending to the dorsal capsular attachment (Fig. 5).
- The incision should be 1 cm proximal to the joint line, which allows the joint to remain covered as the toe is brought into a corrected varus position (Fig. 6A and 6B).

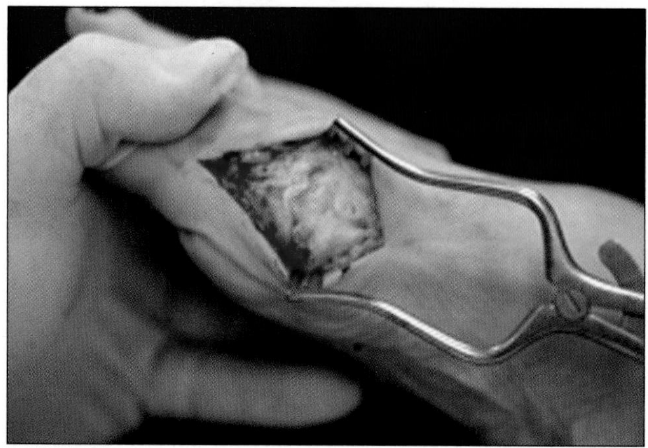

FIGURE 5

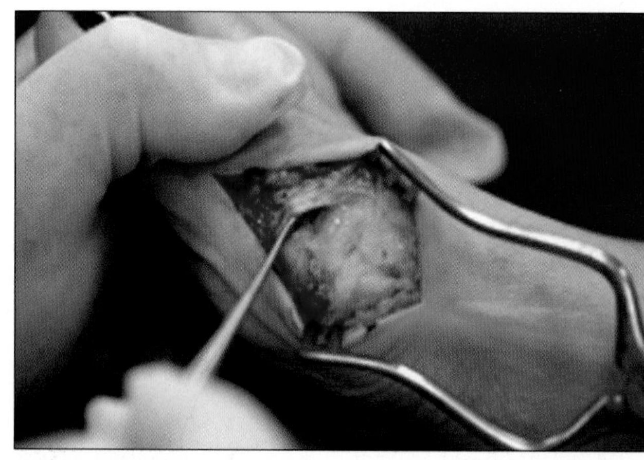

A

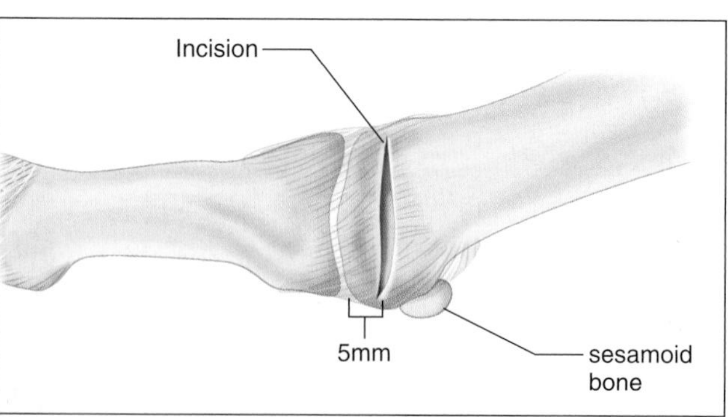

B

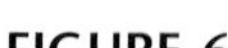

FIGURE 6

Instrumentation

- The repair requires the use of the Arthrex Mini Tightrope Endobutton implant with 2-0 Fiberwire.

Step 2

- The abductor hallucis tendon is located at its insertion on the base of the proximal phalanx. A complete release of the tendon is usually required (Fig. 7).

Step 3

- Deepen the incision in the first web space. Expose the lateral capsule. Protect the plantar neurovascular bundle.
- Divide the capsule with a vertical incision. Create distal and proximal capsular flaps that can be repaired after correction of the varus (Fig. 8).

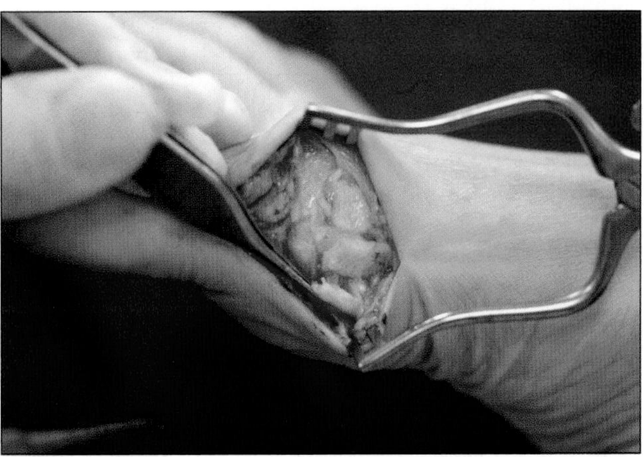

FIGURE 7

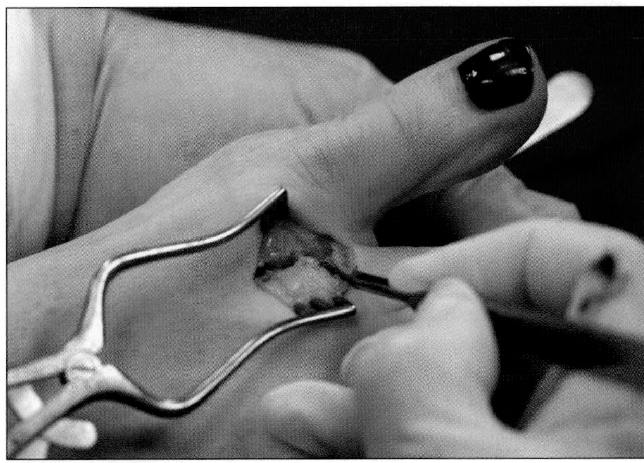

FIGURE 8

Pearls

- *A release of the medial capsule is a key step in balancing out the joint. A wide release is essential.*

Pearls

- *An excision of the tibial sesamoid may be required if it blocks reduction of the toe. This is rarely required, however, with adequate soft tissue release.*

Step 4

- Place a 1.2-mm guidewire across the base of the proximal phalanx from medial to lateral.
  - The medial entry point is 1 cm distal to the joint line, in the concave portion of the proximal phalanx. The pin should exit just plantar to the longitudinal axis of the phalanx, approximately 5 mm from the joint line (Fig. 9).
  - The goal is to have the Fiberwire, as best possible, anatomically recreate the location of the lateral collateral ligament.
- Overdrill the pin with a cannulated Arthrex 2.7-mm drill bit (Fig. 10).

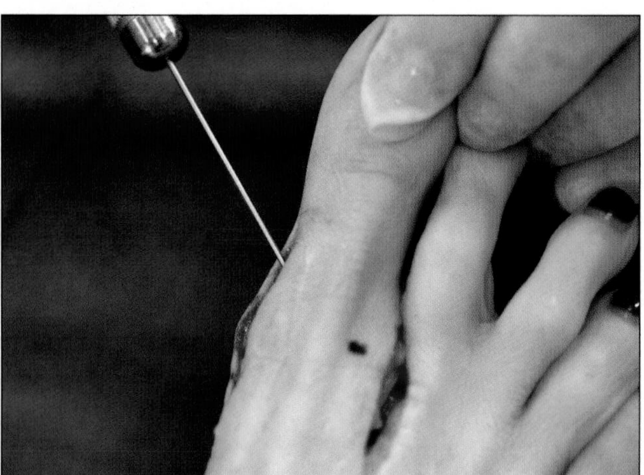

FIGURE 9

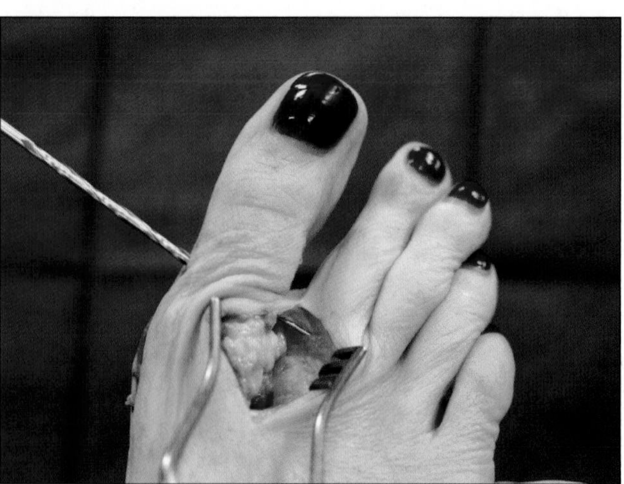

FIGURE 10

Step 5

- Pass the 1.6-mm guide pin with the attached suture through the tunnel in the proximal phalanx.
  - The Arthrex Endobutton and Fiberwire are passed from medial to lateral (Fig. 11).
  - The phalanx can be externally rotated to help expose the lateral portion of the tunnel, allowing the Endobutton to be pulled out (Fig. 12).

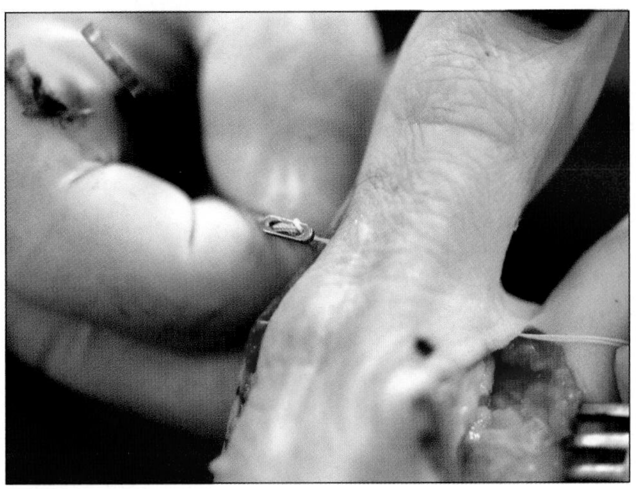

FIGURE 11

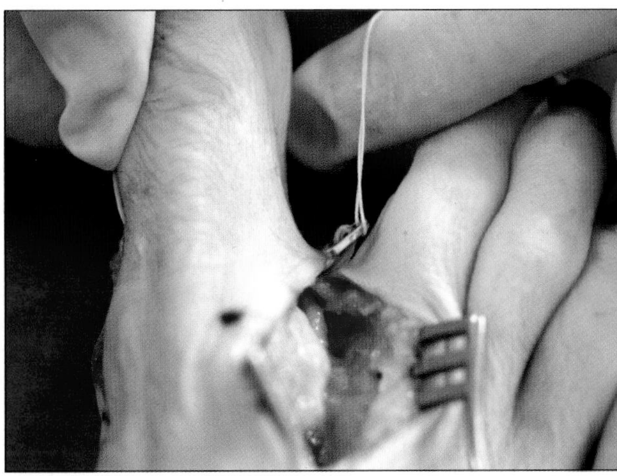

FIGURE 12

Step 6

- A similar approach is taken to the metatarsal tunnel. The medial entry site is 1–2 cm proximal to the joint line, and the exit site laterally is 5 mm (Fig. 13).

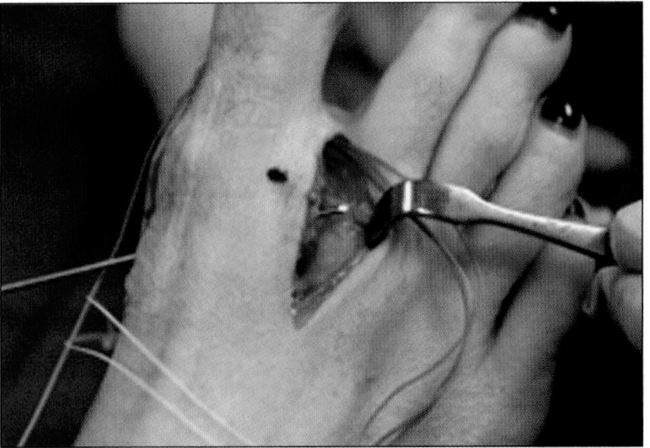

FIGURE 13

Pearls

- *The intermetatarsal plantar neurovascular bundle may be more dorsal than expected, and vulnerable to injury. This distorted anatomy results from previous bunion surgery in which the adductor attachment and the transverse metatarsal ligament were released.*

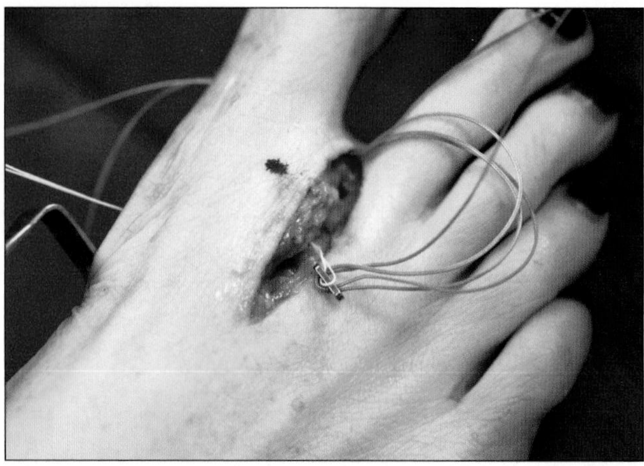

A

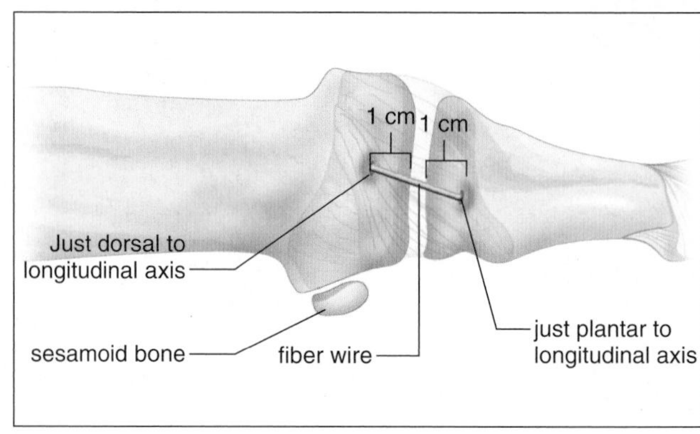

B

FIGURE 14

- As opposed to the tunnel in the proximal phalanx, the metatarsal tunnel is angled dorsally. It should exit laterally, just dorsal of the longitudinal axis, to recreate the origin of the lateral collateral ligament.
- The Endobutton is then passed from lateral to medial (Fig. 14A and 14B).

PEARLS

- *The lateral capsular reefing is an important part of the procedure as it reinforces the repair and may stabilize the joint if the Fiberwire construct loosens over time.*

Step 7

- The lateral vertical capsular flaps are repaired with several figure-of-8 sutures using 2-0 absorbable suture (Fig. 15).

Step 8

- The Fiberwire and Endobutton are tightened (Fig. 16). Six half-hitches with a long tail allow the knot to be adequately buried.
- Reduction of the joint is confirmed by fluoroscopy (Fig. 17). The proximal Endobutton should be turned parallel to the metatarsal, which usually creates the least prominent position.
- The white pull-through suture is cut and removed.

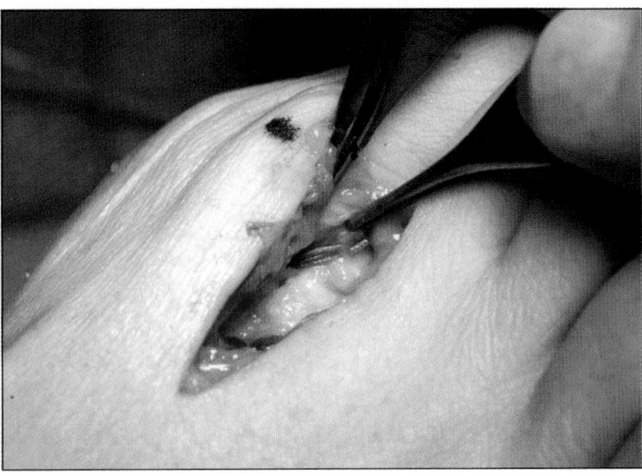

FIGURE 15

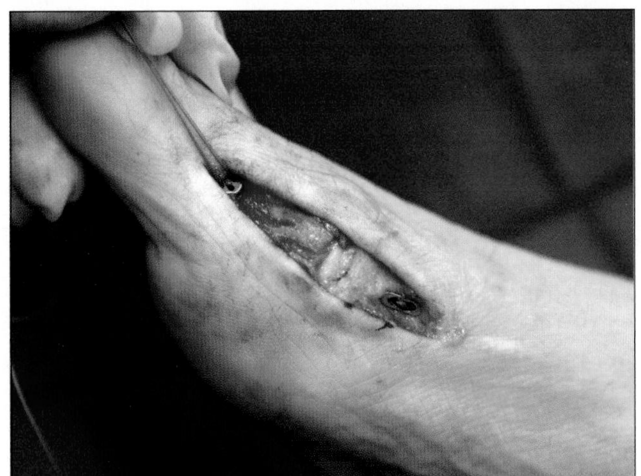

FIGURE 16

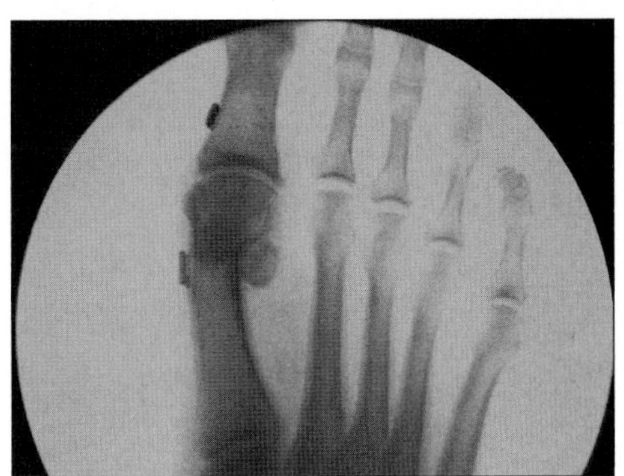

FIGURE 17

Postoperative Care and Expected Outcomes

- A bunion spica dressing is applied that holds the hallux in a valgus position, without bandages between the first and second toes.
- The patient should be non–weight bearing for 2 weeks. At 2 weeks postoperatively, weight bearing is begun in a postoperative shoe. Range-of-motion exercises can be started as early as 2 weeks after surgery. Normal shoewear can be used at 6 weeks after surgery

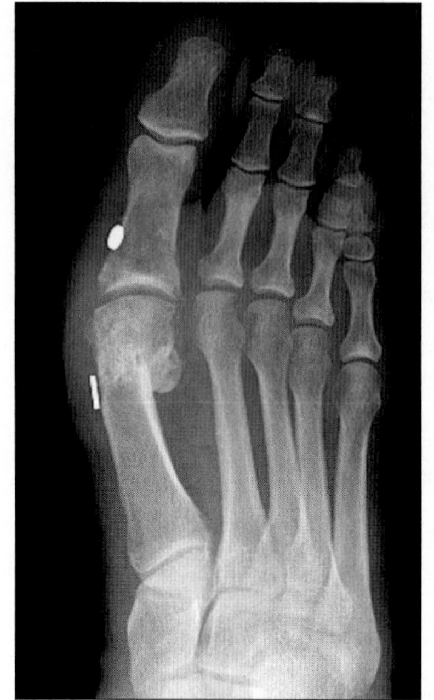

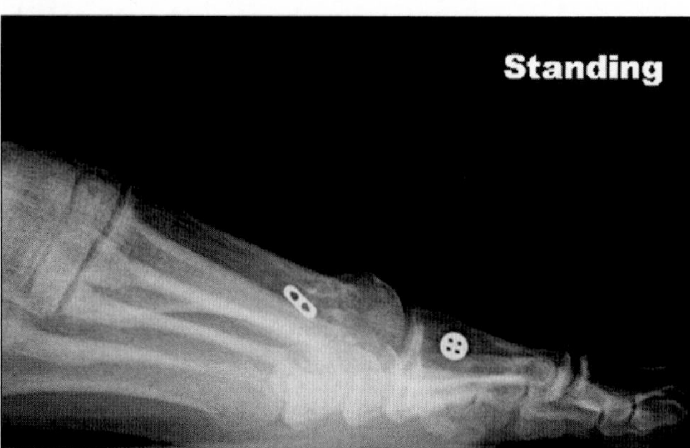

A B

FIGURE 18

- Standing AP (Fig. 18A) and lateral (Fig. 18B) radiographs 3 months postoperatively.
- Potential complications include stiffness of the joint. Overcorrection of the hallux should also be avoided.

Evidence

There are no long term published data on this procedure. Follow-up of my patients at 1 year demonstrates excellent results.

Johnson KA, Spiegel PV. Extensor hallucis longus transfer for hallux varus deformity. J Bone Joint Surg [Am]. 1984;66:681-6.

A retrospective review of a technique that uses the extensor hallucis longus passed beneath the transverse metatarsal ligament into the base of the proximal phalanx. (Level IV evidence [case series])

Lau JT, Myerson MS. Modified split extensor hallucis longus tendon transfer for correction of hallux varus. Foot Ankle Int. 2002;23:1138-40.

A retrospective case series of a technique that used a split extensor hallucis longus tendon. (Level IV evidence)

PROCEDURE 14

Arthroscopy of the Great Toe

Carol Frey

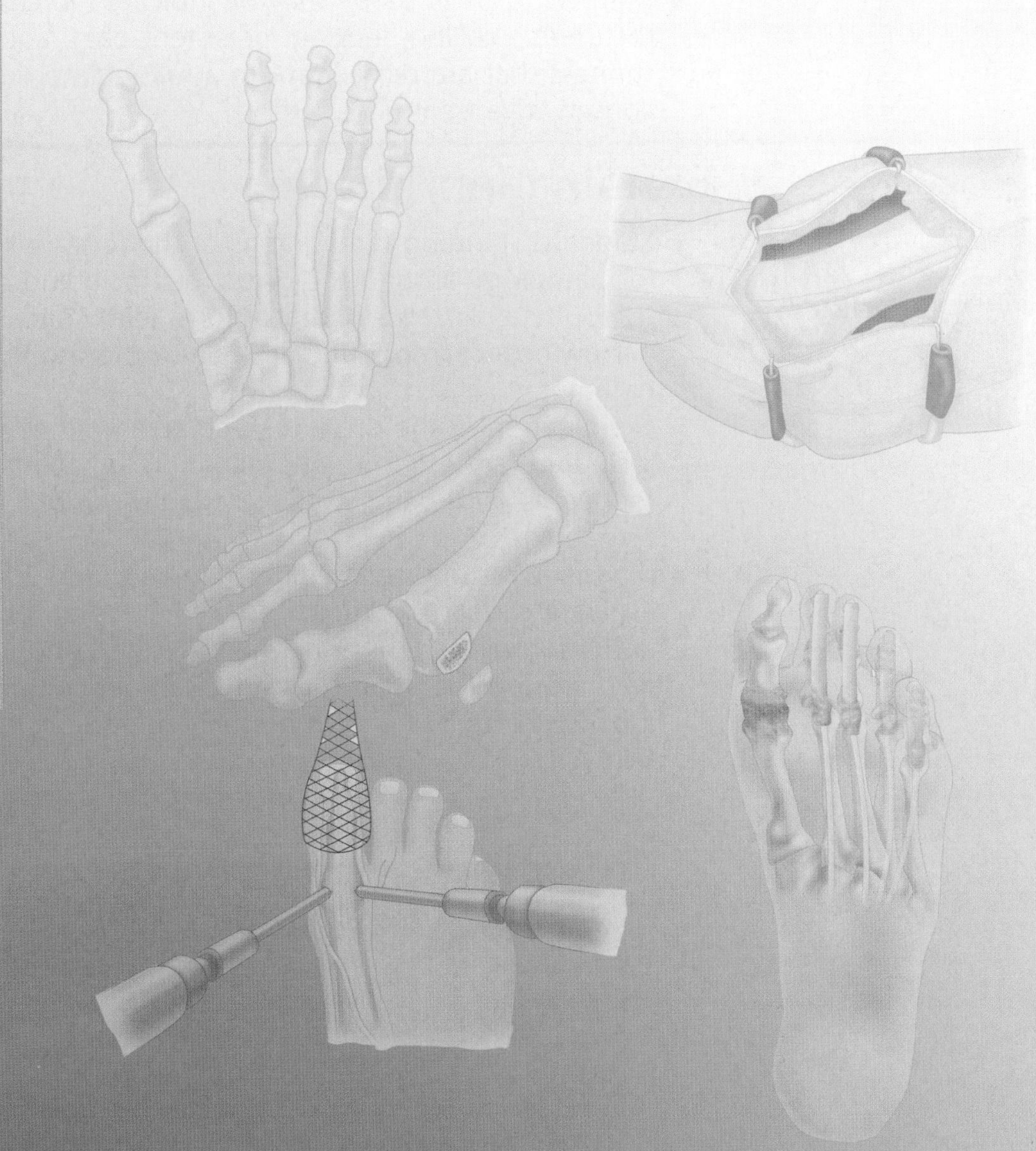

Controversies

- Arthrodesis of the great toe is possible with arthroscopic technique.
- Arthroscopy of the great toe is a relatively new application, and therefore indications are still developing and few long-term clinical studies have been published.

Treatment Options

- Anti-inflammatory medications
- Stable-sole or rocker-sole shoe
- Orthotic device with a sesamoid pad or Morton's extension
- Stretching the Achilles tendon

Indications

- Osteophytes
- Hallux rigidus
- Chondromalacia
- Osteochondral lesions
- Loose bodies
- Arthrofibrosis
- Synovitis secondary to hyperextension and hyperflexion injuries to the great toe
- Diagnostic arthroscopy may be indicated in cases of recurrent swelling, locking, persistent pain, and stiffness that are recalcitrant to a full regimen of conservative treatment.

Examination/Imaging

- Standard standing radiographs of the foot looking for pathology around the great toe, including osteophytes, osteochondral lesions, joint space narrowing, sesamoid fractures, and other bone pathology.
- Examination of the great toe and sesamoid complex, including range of motion, palpation for points of tenderness and pain, swelling, crepitus, and osteophytes.
- Magnetic resonance imaging may be ordered to evaluate cartilage pathology, osteochondral lesions, and sesamoid lesions and when there is continued pain around the great toe and sesamoid complex in a patient presenting with normal radiographs (Fig. 1).

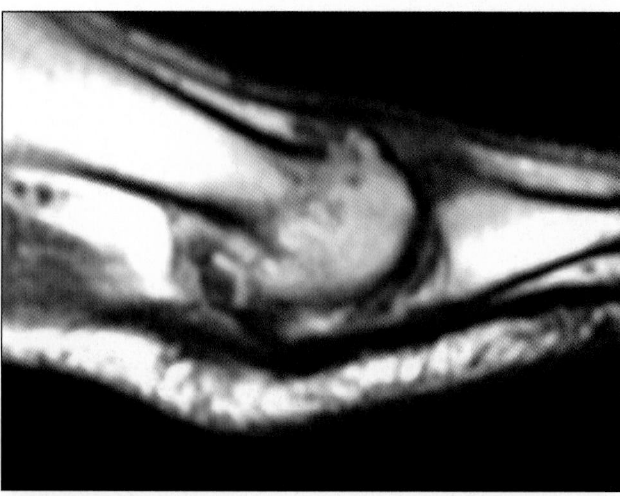

FIGURE 1

- Marked degenerative changes of the first metatarsophalangeal (1MTP) joint are noted.
- Edema is noted in both bones, and there is narrowing of the joint space, and large dorsal and plantar osteophytes.

Surgical Anatomy

- Minimal stability is provided by the shallow ball-and-socket articulation between the proximal phalanx (PP) and the metatarsal (MT) head.
- Soft tissues, including the capsule, ligaments, muscles, and tendons, provide most of the support to the 1MTP (Fig. 2).
- The extensor hallucis longus tendon divides the dorsum of the 1MTP in half.
- Anatomic structures at risk with portal placement for arthroscopy of the 1MTP are shown in Figure 3.
  - The branches of the deep peroneal nerve innervate the lateral half and the branches of the superficial peroneal nerve innervate the medial half of the joint.
  - The terminal branches of the saphenous nerve innervate the medial aspect of the great toe.

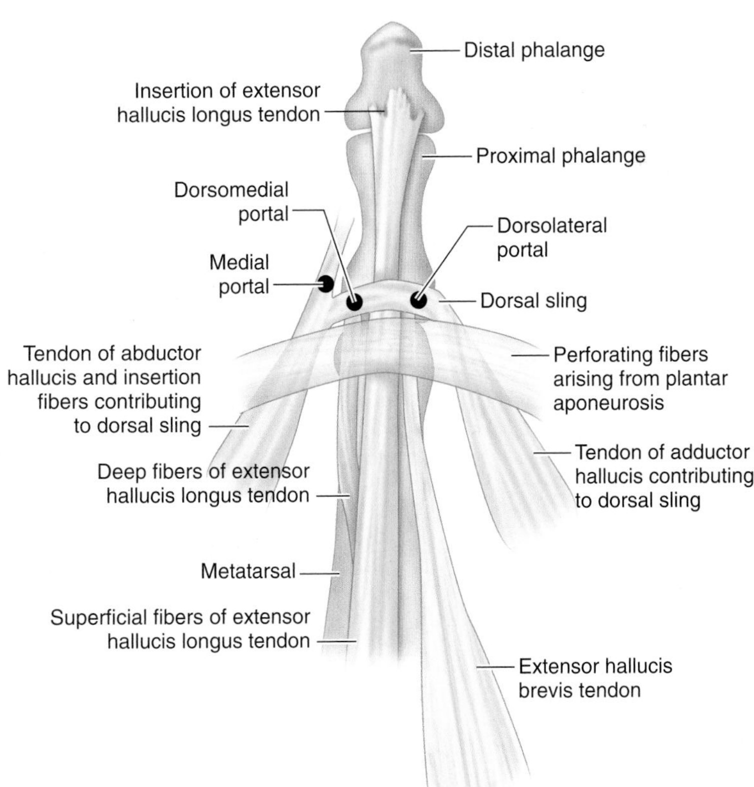

FIGURE 2

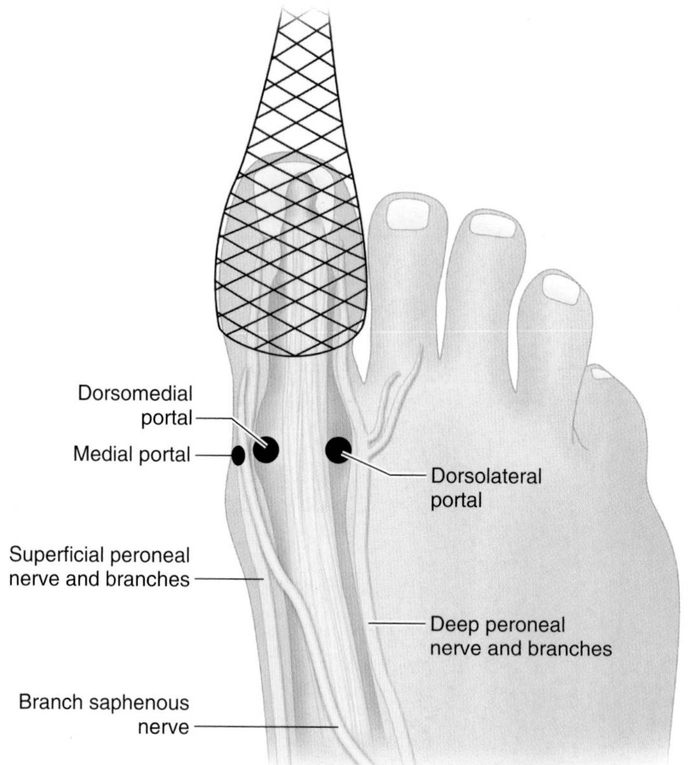

FIGURE 3

- On the plantar aspect of the 1MTP, the sesamoid are within the medial and the lateral portions of the flexor hallucis brevis (FHB) tendon.
- The FHB sends fibers to the plantar plate and subsequently attaches to the proximal aspect of the proximal phalanx.
- The plantar plate is a strong fibrous structure that inserts on either side of the MTP joint.
- The flexor hallucis longus tendon is both superficial and between the two heads of the FHB tendon.
- Biomechanically, the instant centers for motion of the 1MTP fall within the MT head.
  - Motion occurs between the MT head and the PP by sliding action at the joint surface.
  - In full extension or flexion, this sliding action gives way to compression of the dorsal or plantar articular surfaces of the MT head and PP.

Positioning

- Supine
- General, spinal, epidural, or local anesthesia can be used.
- A sterile finger trap is placed on the toe to suspend the lower extremity, with traction applied at the level of the ankle, if necessary. This will distract the 1MTP and improve visualization (Fig. 4).

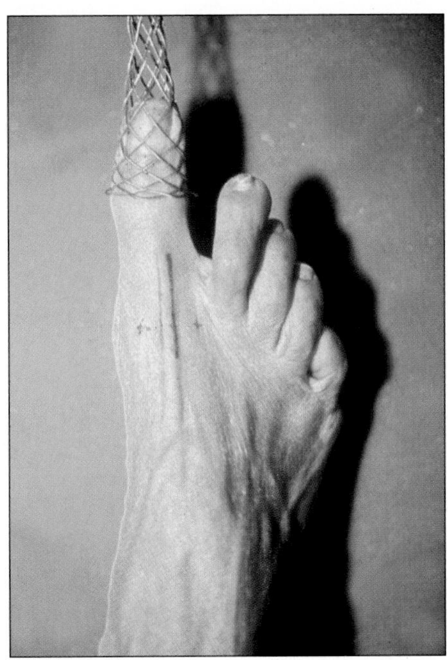

FIGURE 4

Portals/Exposures

- The dorsal medial, dorsal lateral, and straight medial portals are the most commonly used portals for arthroscopy of the 1MTP (Fig. 5).

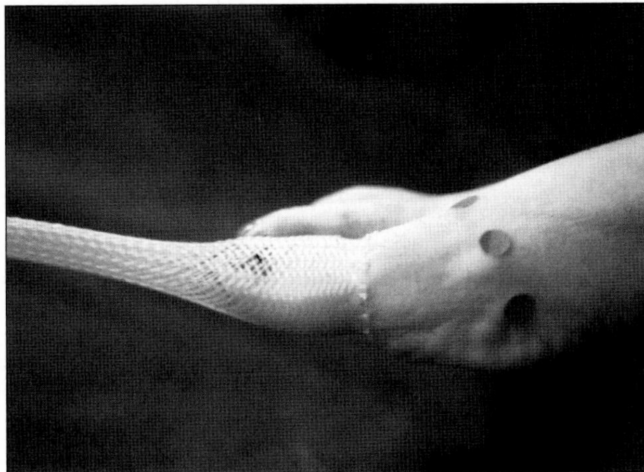

FIGURE 5

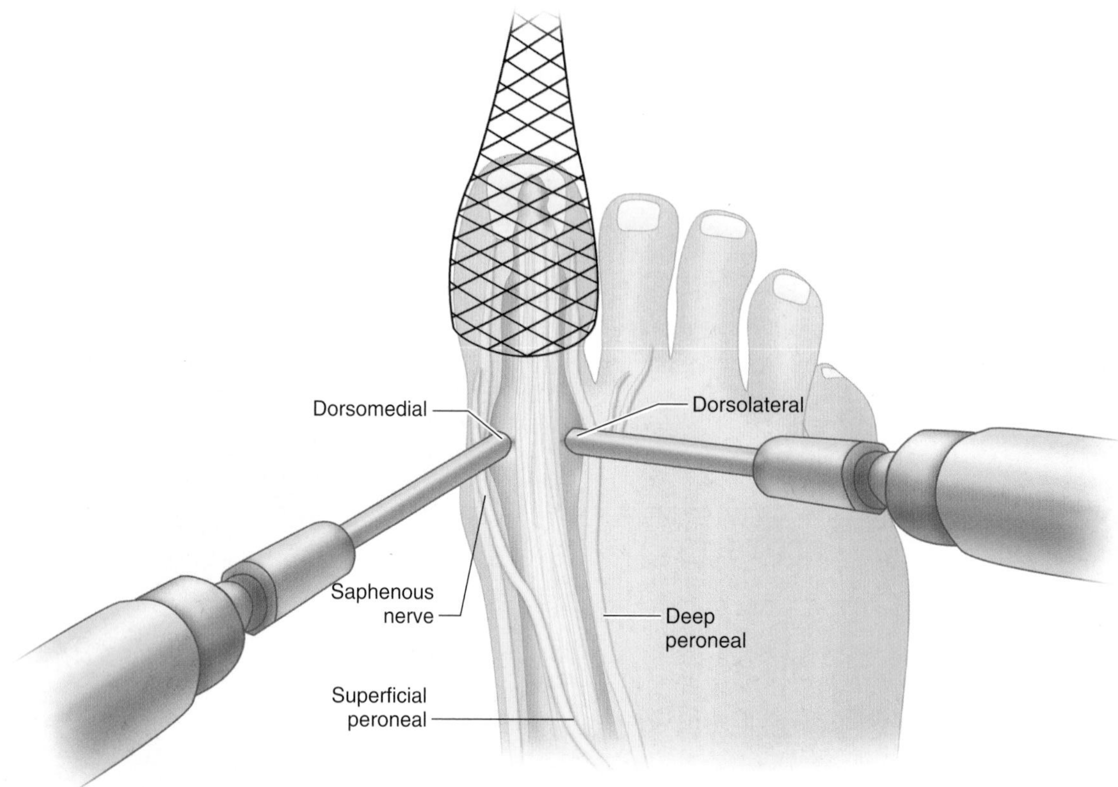

FIGURE 6

- The dorsal medial and dorsal lateral portals are placed at the joint line and on either side of the extensor hallucis longus tendon (Fig. 6).
- The straight medial portal is placed through the medial capsule midway between the dorsal and the plantar aspect of the joint, under direct visualization.

> **PEARLS**
>
> - *Use of the interchangeable cannula allows rotation of the videoarthroscope and instrumentation so that the entire joint and its pathology can be fully evaluated and treated.*
> - *The 10-point arthroscopic examination described above is performed through the dorsal lateral portal. The dorsal medial portal provides superior visualization of the dorsal aspect of the metatarsal head and proximal phalanx.*
> - *The medial and lateral sesamoid are well visualized from the medial portal.*

Procedure

Step 1: Arthroscopic Examination

- The dorsal medial and dorsal lateral portals are established first.
- The joint line is palpated just medial or lateral to the extensor hallucis longus tendon.
- An 18-gauge spinal needle is used to inflate the MTP joint with 5 ml of normal saline.
- A 4-mm longitudinal incision is made, the subcutaneous tissue is spread with a mosquito clamp to prevent neurovascular injury, and the joint is entered with an interchangeable cannula with a semiblunt trochar.
- Once visualization of the joint is accomplished through the initial portal, the remaining two portals can be established with a spinal needle under direct vision.

Instrumentation/ Implantation

- No. 11 blade
- Straight mosquito clamp
- 20-ml syringe
- 18-gauge spinal needle
- CHIP [Micro CHIP]
- CHP camera with compatible light source
- Video/TV monitor
- 1.9-, 2.2-, or 2.7-mm oblique, wide-angle 30° videoarthroscope
- 2.0-mm instrumentation: baskets, grasper, probe, curette
- Sterile toe trap
- Coban to hold toe in toe trap
- Shoulder holder or IV stand to suspend toe traction
- 7- to 15-pound sandbag
- Small hand drill
- Kirschner wires
- Tourniquet
- Small radiofrequency wand

- Intra-articular examination includes visualization of 10 major areas: the lateral gutter, lateral corner of the MT head, central portion of the MT head, medial corner of the MT head, medial gutter, medial portion of the PP, central portion of the PP, lateral portion of the PP, medial sesamoid, and lateral sesamoid.
  - The arthroscope is placed in the anteromedial portal (Fig. 7). The metatarsal head is on the left side and the base of the proximal phalanx is on the right side. Between the two structures is the plantar capsule and synovium. A loose osteophyte is seen in the middle frame of the picture locked between the two bones.
  - The arthroscope is placed into the medial portal (Fig. 8). The metatarsal head is on the left and the medial sesamoid is seen on the plantar aspect of the metatarsal head.

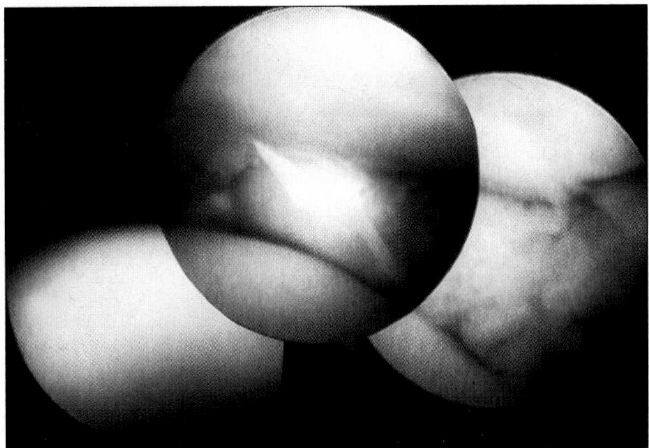

FIGURE 7

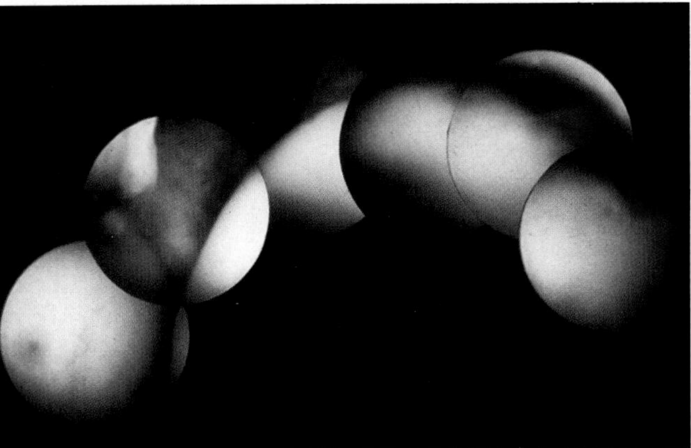

FIGURE 8

Step 2: Removal of Dorsal Osteophytes

- The most common indications for arthroscopy of the great toe include treatment of hallux rigidus with a dorsal osteophyte and chondromalacia.
- Dorsal osteophytes may be removed if they are mild to moderate in size. If the osteophyte is large, an open cheilectomy is recommended.
- The best placement of instruments for an arthroscopic cheilectomy is with the arthroscope in the dorsal lateral portal and the shaver and burr placed in the dorsomedial or medial portal.
- Remove the osteophyte from distal to proximal and medial to lateral.
- Up to one third of the articular surface may be removed with this technique.
- With an arthroscopic cheilectomy, it is usually not necessary to remove as much bone as with an open procedure.
- The finger trap is removed prior to removal of the osteophytes because traction may cause the capsule to pull tight against the osteophytes.

Pearls

- *In the case of hallux rigidus, the patient is heel walking postoperatively but begins gentle range of motion 1–2 days postoperatively.*

Step 3: Treatment of Chondromalacia

- In the case of chondromalacia or osteochondral lesions, the pathology may be evaluated, loose fragments excised, and bone drilled or abraded to a bleeding surface with stable cartilage margins.

Pearls

- *In the case of osteochondral lesions, the patient is kept non–weight bearing for 2 weeks postoperatively.*
- *Early range of motion is begun approximately 5 days postoperatively.*

Step 4: Sesamoids

- To evaluate the sesamoid compartment, it is helpful to release the toe traction and place the great toe into plantar flexion.
- For evaluation and surgery of the medial sesamoid, the dorsolateral portal is utilized for the arthroscope and the instruments are placed into the medial portal.
- For evaluation and surgery of the lateral sesamoid, the arthroscope is placed through the dorsomedial portal and the instruments are placed into the dorsolateral portal.

Postoperative Care and Expected Outcomes

Pearls

- *Arthroscopy of the great toe is considered an advanced arthroscopic technique and should only be undertaken by experienced arthroscopic surgeons.*

- Small portal wounds are closed with interrupted nylon sutures.
- To prevent fistula formation, a bulky compression dressing is applied for 4–7 days.
- Direct weight bearing is avoided.

- Sutures are removed at 7–10 days after surgery and the patient is started on a range-of-motion and strengthening program.
- A stable postoperative shoe or short cam walker is used until resolution of postoperative swelling and pain.
- Reports indicate 83% good results when this technique is used for various types of pathology.
- The few available reports in the literature indicate favorable outcomes with the procedure.

Evidence

Bartlett DH. Arthroscopic management of osteochondritis dissecans of the first metatarsal head. Arthroscopy. 1988;4:51.

The author reports his technique of 1MTP joint operative arthroscopy and the successful treatment of osteochondritis dissecans of the first metatarsal head. (Level III evidence)

Frey CC, van Dijk NC. Arthroscopy of the great toe. In Chow JCY (ed). Advanced Arthroscopy. New York: Springer-Verlag, 2001:675-82.

The authors describe their indications and technique for great toe arthroscopy. Four case reports are presented, as well as intraoperative photographs, outcomes, and pearls. (Level III evidence)

Lundeen RD. Arthroscopic approaches to the joints of the foot. J Am Podiatr Med Assoc. 1987;77:451-6.

The author reports on the performance of 11 great toe arthroscopies but does not give clinical results. (Level II evidence)

PROCEDURE 15

Metatarsal Lengthening

Mark E. Easley and James A. Nunley II

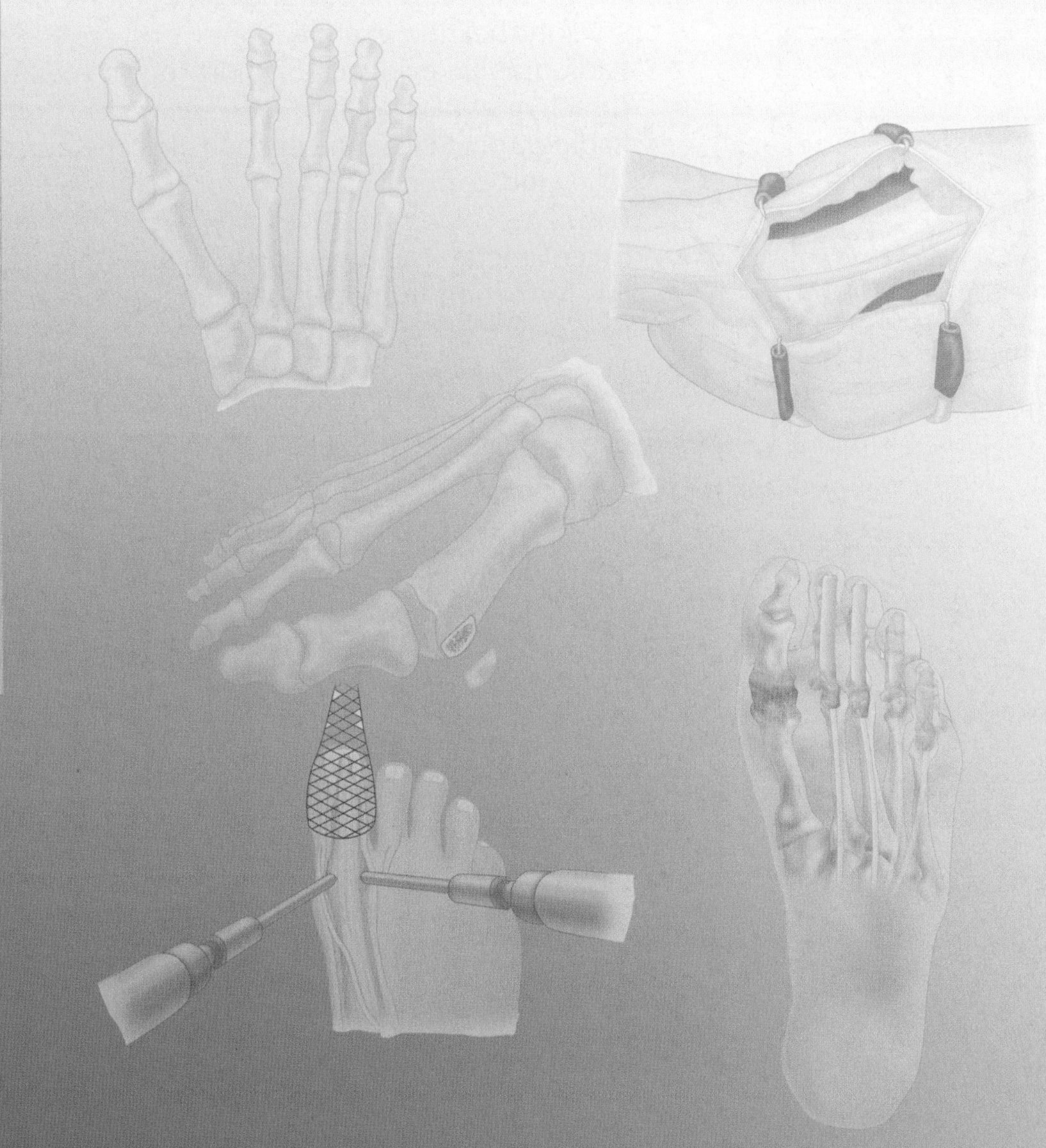

Figures from Mather R III, Hurst J, Easley M, Nunley JA. First metatarsal lengthening. Tech Foot Ankle Surg. 2008;7:25–30.

PITFALLS

- *Contraindicated for a dorsiflexion malunion of the first metatarsal, unless an adjunctive procedure can be performed to plantar flex the first ray*
- *Contraindicated in patients noncompliant with a protective weight-bearing status, pin care, and proper distraction (metatarsal lengthening) protocol*

Controversies

- Metatarsal lengthening of shortened metatarsal versus shortening of adjacent metatarsals; we advise against shortening physiologically normal anatomy when possible.

Indications

- Relatively short metatarsal (brachymetatarsalgia) (Fig. 1)
- Overload/transfer metatarsalgia to an adjacent metatarsal head
- Short first metatarsal following corrective surgery for hallux valgus

Examination/Imaging

- Short metatarsal clinically and radiographically, based on weight-bearing examinations
  - Radiographic evidence of short fourth metatarsal (brachymetatarsalgia)
  - Radiographic evidence of short first metatarsal following corrective surgery for hallux valgus (Fig. 2)
- Adjacent metatarsal heads may have tenderness and callus formation from overload.

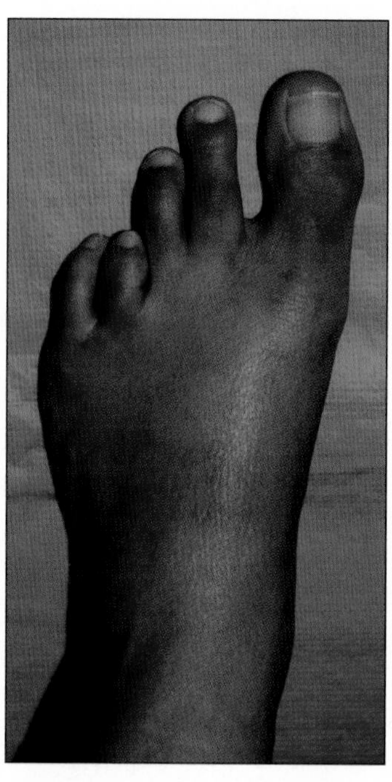

FIGURE 1

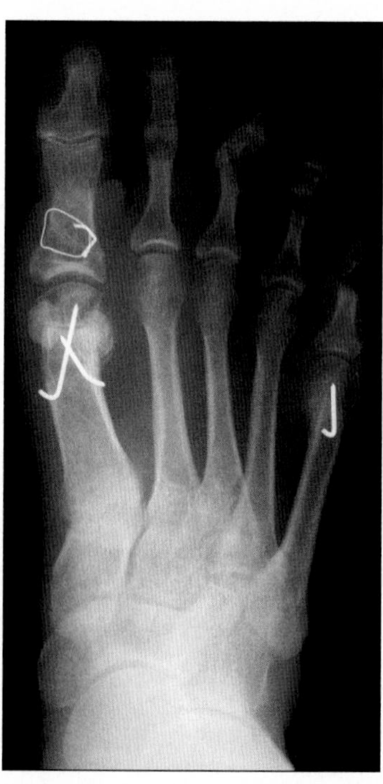

FIGURE 2

Treatment Options

- Shortening of all metatarsals experiencing overload
- Acute lengthening with interpositional structural auto- or allograft bone

Surgical Anatomy

- Determine associated elevation of the affected metatarsal head.
- Determine the amount of metatarsal shortening (i.e., the amount of lengthening required).
- Assess prior surgical scars for preoperative planning.
- Identify exact location of tarsometatarsal (TMT) joints for planning of pin placement.
  - Adjust the external fixator relative to the first metatarsal (Fig. 3A).
  - Define the location of the first metatarsophalangeal (MTP) joint (Fig. 3B).
  - Define the location of the first TMT joint (Fig. 3C).

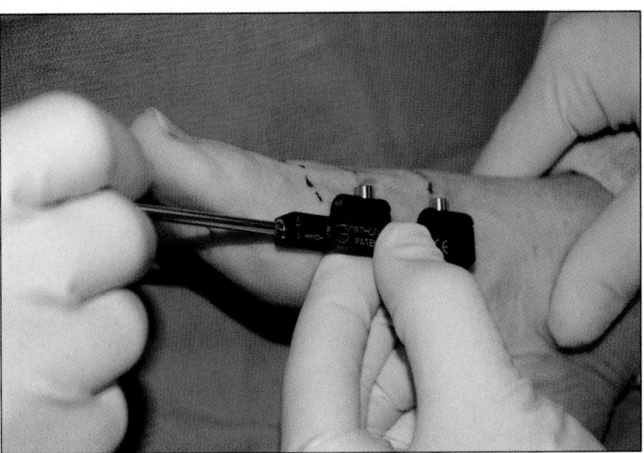

A

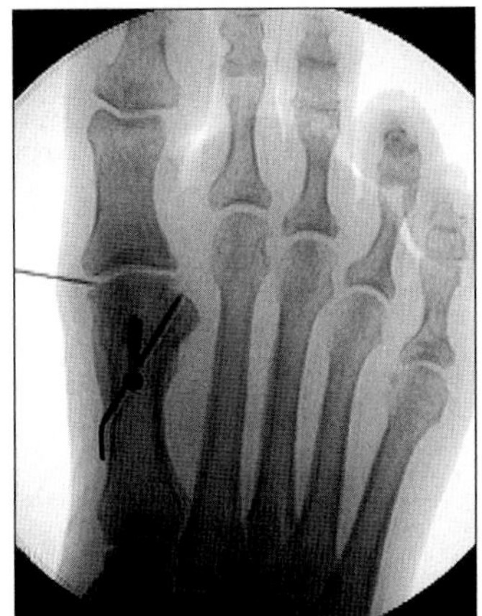

B

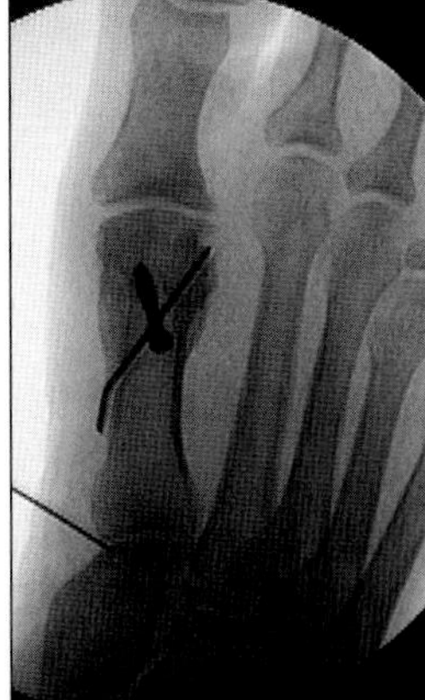

C

FIGURE 3

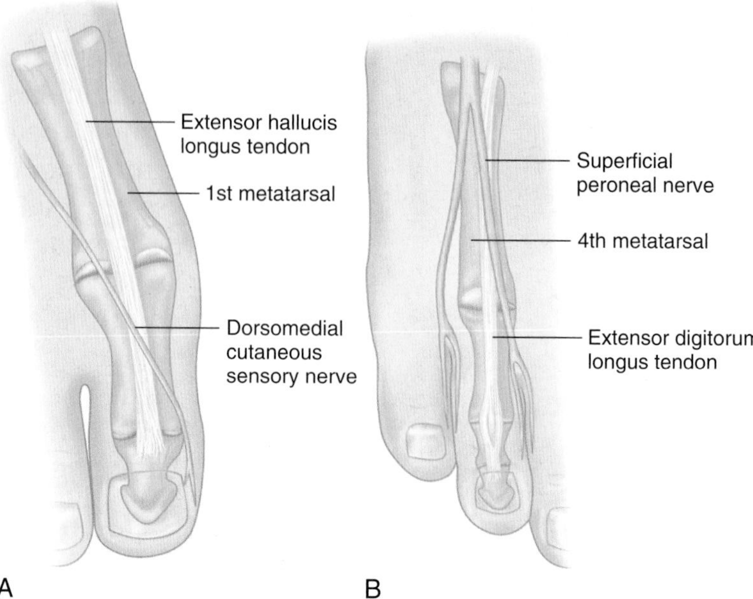

FIGURE 4

- At-risk structures include the following:
  - First metatarsal (1MT): the dorsomedial cutaneous sensory nerve to the hallux and the extensor hallucis longus tendon (Fig. 4A)
  - Fourth metatarsal (4MT): lateral branch of the superficial peroneal nerve and the extensor digitorum longus tendons (Fig. 4B)
- Assess associated MTP joint deformity (claw toe or varus/valgus deviation); this associated deformity will not be corrected with metatarsal lengthening unless an adjunctive procedure is performed.

Positioning

- Supine position
- Foot on edge of operating table to allow easy access to fluoroscopy unit
- For 4MT lengthening: bump under ipsilateral hip
- For 1MT lengthening: no bump under ipsilateral hip because access to medial foot is needed

Pearls

- *After making the skin incision, use a hemostat to spread the soft tissues down to the periosteum.*

Pitfalls

- *Skin tension at the pin sites is undesirable; only make the skin incision when the exact location for a particular pin has been determined.*

Portals/Exposures

- Four pins are placed through small stab incisions under fluoroscopic guidance.
- The surgical approach for the metatarsal corticotomy is performed between the two pins closest to the proposed corticotomy.
- The incision for the osteotomy is made in line with the respective metatarsal and, if possible, should avoid the pin sites.

Pearls

- *Place the first pin while simultaneously determining the ideal external fixator position for placing the subsequent pins.*
- *The external fixator must be placed in line with the desired axis of lengthening.*
- *Placing the first (and thus second) pin slightly plantar in the medial 1MT typically avoids 1MT dorsiflexion during distraction.*

Procedure

Step 1: Percutaneous Placement of First (Distal) Pin

- The external fixator is typically a monorail device.
- The four pins are placed in the same plane, within the bone to be lengthened, while avoiding the adjacent joints.
- The pins must be perpendicular to the bone and achieve a bicortical purchase in the affected metatarsal.
- The distal pins must be separated adequately from the proximal pins to allow for the osteotomy to be performed safely.
- We typically place the distal-most pin first; it must be as distal as possible in the metatarsal to be lengthened without violating the MTP joint.
- The first pin determines monorail external fixator alignment; we recommend holding the external fixator in the ideal position to determine optimal first pin placement (Fig. 5A).
- Fluoroscopic guidance is needed to ensure that, following first pin placement, the other pins can be placed in proper position in the involved metatarsal while avoiding the adjacent joints (Fig. 5B and 5C).

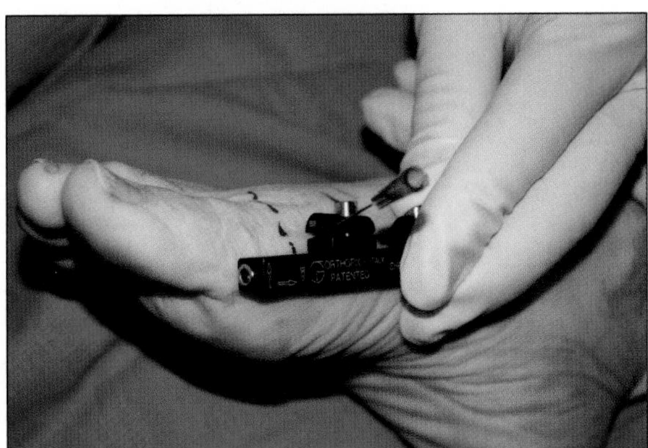

A

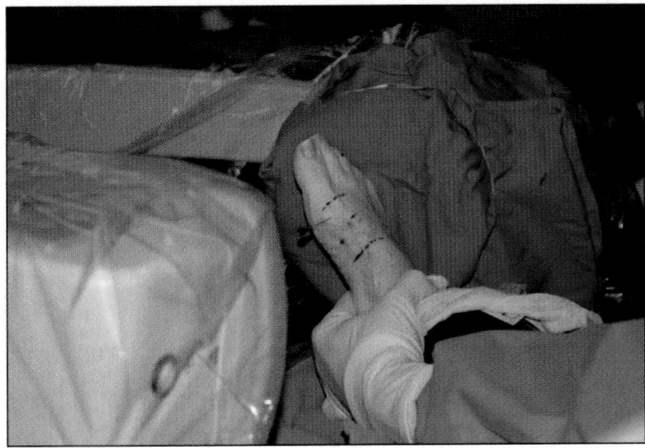

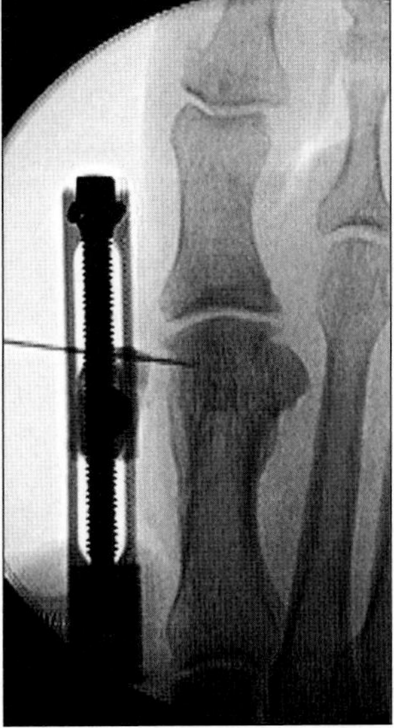

FIGURE 5 B C

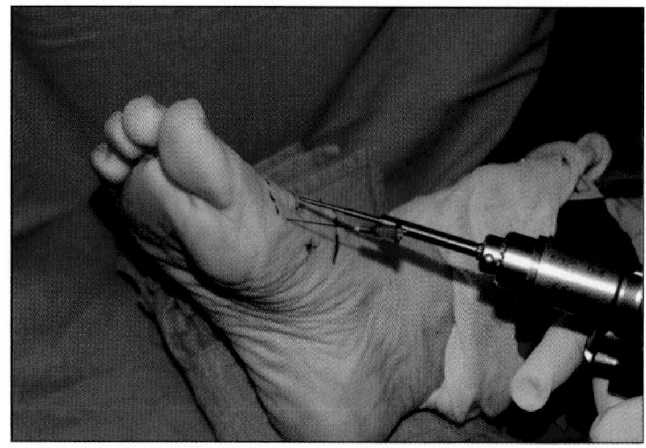
A

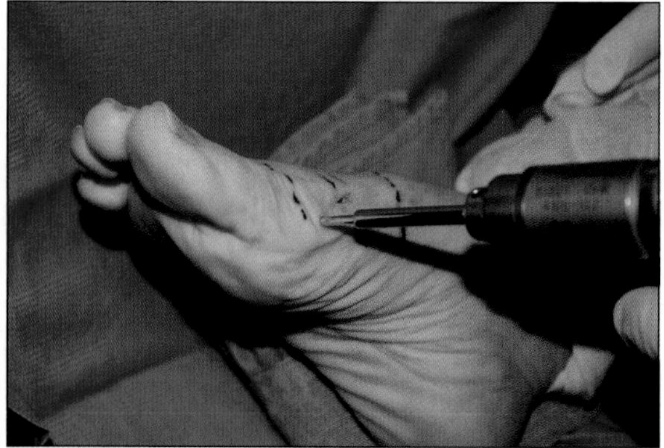
B

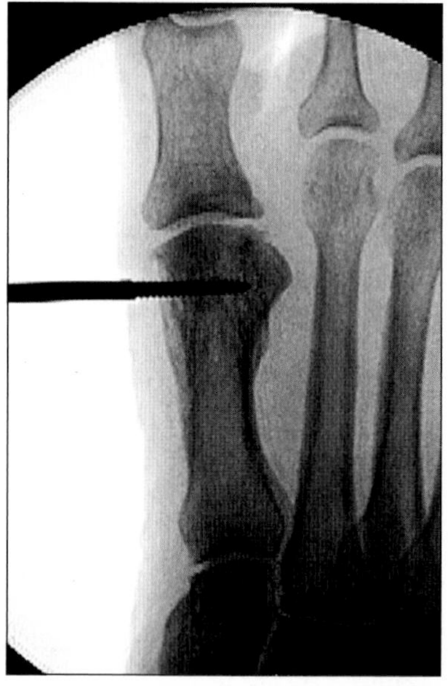
C

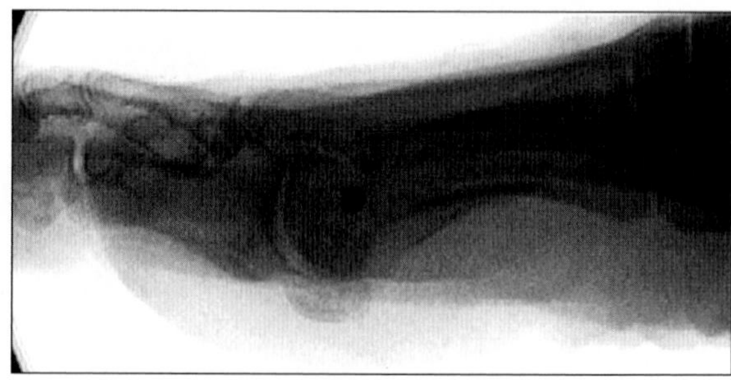
D

Pitfalls

- *Poor first pin positioning generally leads to difficulties with proper monorail external fixator position.*
- *Fluorscopic guidance assures bicortical pin positioning and that the subsequent pins are placed in the proper and safe positions.*
- *If a tapered pin system is used, the pin should be driven to its proper position in the bone and not reversed or it will lose purchase.*

- 1MT lengthening
  - Place first pin at site determined clinically and fluoroscopically (Fig. 6A).
  - Drive first pin using adapter and power drill (Fig. 6B).
  - Anteroposterior (AP) fluoroscopic view of first pin in proper position (Fig. 6C).
  - Lateral fluoroscopic view of first pin in proper position (Fig. 6D).

Instrumentation/ Implantation

- Pin driver that easily slides over the pin without the need for tightening with a chuck
- Small-diameter self-tapping/ drilling pins (typically 2.5-mm or 3.0-mm pins)
- Monorail external fixation system

- 4MT lengthening
  - Determining proper first pin positioning for 4MT (Fig. 7B).
  - Initial pin inserted for 4MT lengthening (Fig. 7A).
- The external fixator must be adjusted to the proper setting that will still allow some mild compression and adequate distraction to appropriately lengthen the metatarsal (i.e., do not complete the initial external fixator position with the fixator in its fully distracted setting).

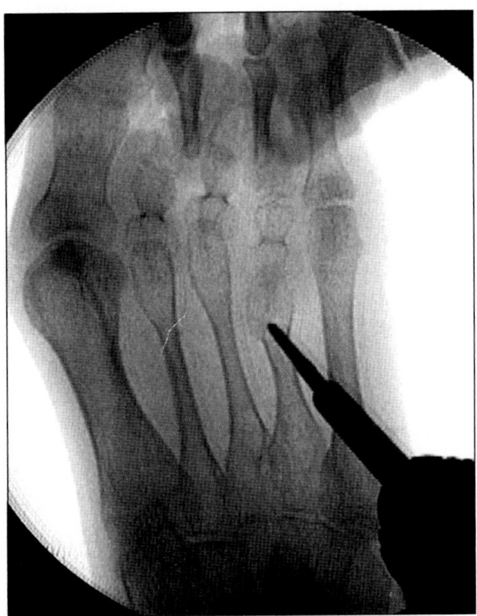

A

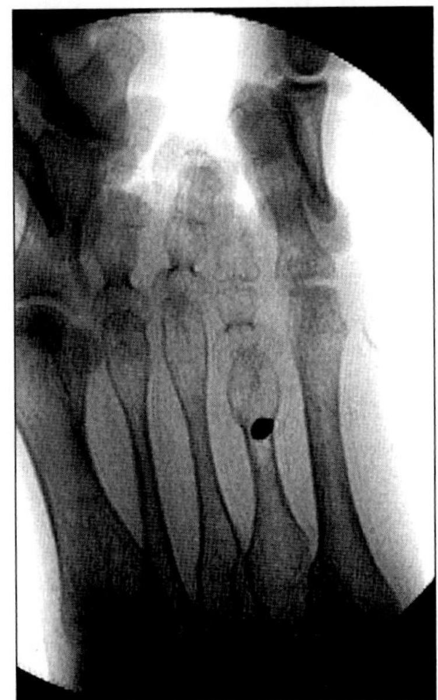

B

FIGURE 7

Pearls

- *If necessary, the proximal pin may be placed in the corresponding cuneiform, such that the two proximal pins safely straddle the TMT joint without either pin violating the joint (Fig. 11).*

Pitfalls

- *If the proximal pin is not placed in proper alignment, the two intermediate pins may not achieve bicortical purchase in the metatarsal*
- *If the other three pins are not aligned with the first, the monorail external fixator cannot be properly secured to the pins. If a tapered pin system is used, the pin should be driven to its proper position in the bone and not reversed or it will lose purchase.*

Instrumentation/ Implantation

- Pin driver that easily slides over the pin without the need for tightening with a chuck
- Small-diameter, self-tapping/ drilling pins (typically 2.5-mm or 3.0-mm pins)
- Monorail external fixation system

Step 2: Inserting Remaining Pins

- Percutaneous insertion with fluoroscopic guidance is used for placement of the remaining pins.
- With the monorail external fixator loosely attached to the first pin, the proximal-most pin is placed through a small stab incision, using the monorail external fixator as a guide.
  - Ideally, the proximal pin is in the bone immediately proximal to the respective TMT joint.
  - Before securing the proximal pin, fluoroscopic guidance must confirm that the other two intermediate pins can be placed with bicortical purchase through the monorail external fixator and will allow for adequate surface on the metatarsal to safely create the corticotomy. Figure 8A shows the fluoroscopic determination of proper external fixator and residual pin positions for 4MT lengthening, based on the external fixator loosely secured to the first pin.
- After placing the proximal pin, the two intermediate pins are placed, again using the monorail external fixator as a guide. Figure 8B shows a fluoroscopic view of four pins and external fixator in place for 4MT lengthening.
- The monorail is secured to the four pins to assure proper alignment and that no skin impingement occurs.
- 1MT lengthening: proximal pin placement
  - Determine proper proximal pin location (Fig. 9A).
  - Confirm proper location for pin using fluoroscopy (Fig. 9B and 9C).
  - Insert second pin in proximal 1MT (Fig. 9D).
  - Figure 9E shows the proximal pin inserted and external fixator attached (note slight relative plantar flexion of the external fixator relative to the 1MT).
- Placing the residual pins in the 1MT
  - Insert third pin (Fig. 10A).
  - Insert fourth pin and secure external fixator (Fig. 10B).
  - Figure 10C shows a fluoroscopic view of all four pins in the 1MT.
  - An additional "floating pin" can be inserted to further stabilize the external fixator to the pins, avoiding eccentric compression about the two distal pins (Fig. 10D).

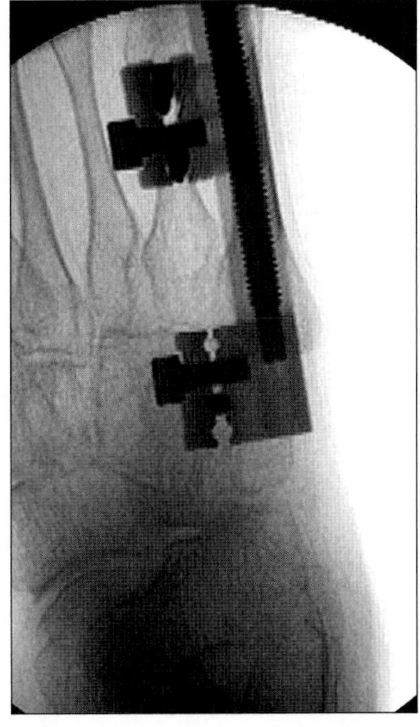
A

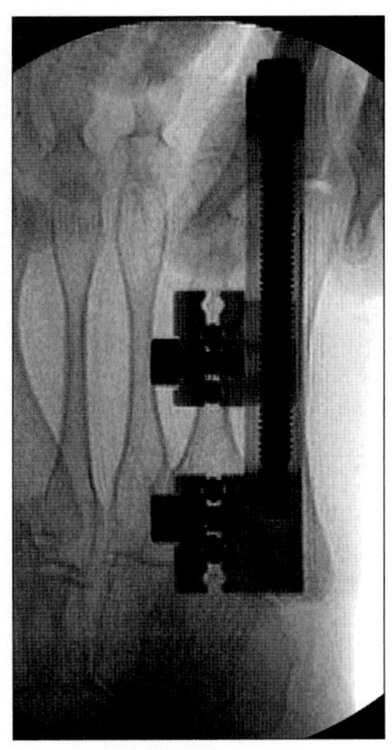
B

FIGURE 8

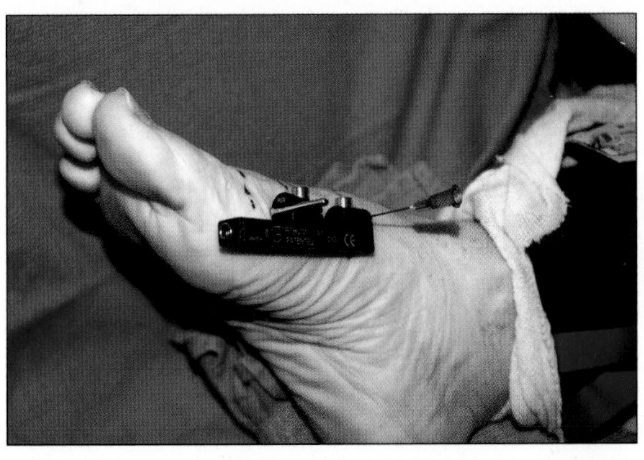
A

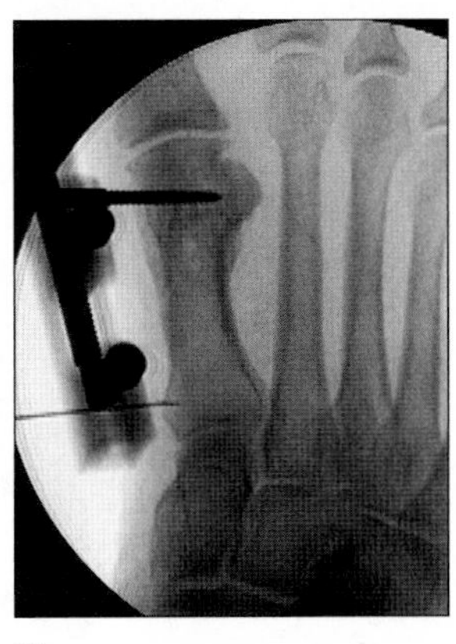
B

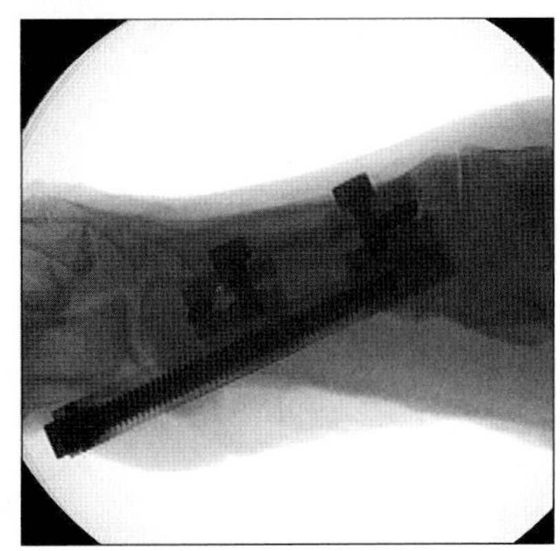
C

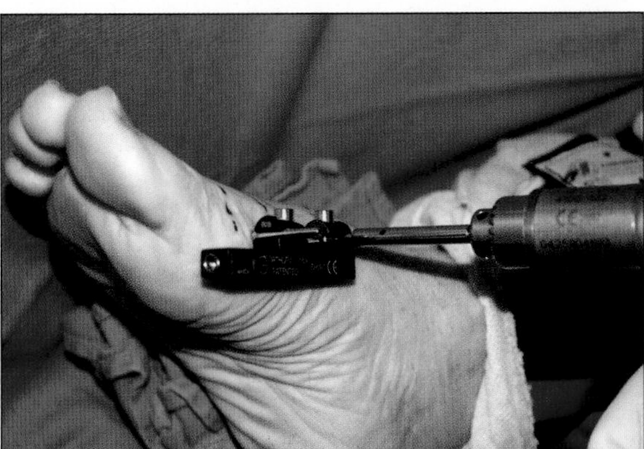
D

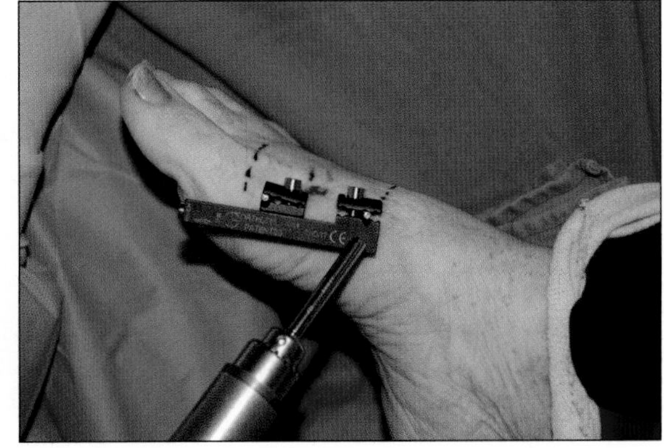
E

FIGURE 9

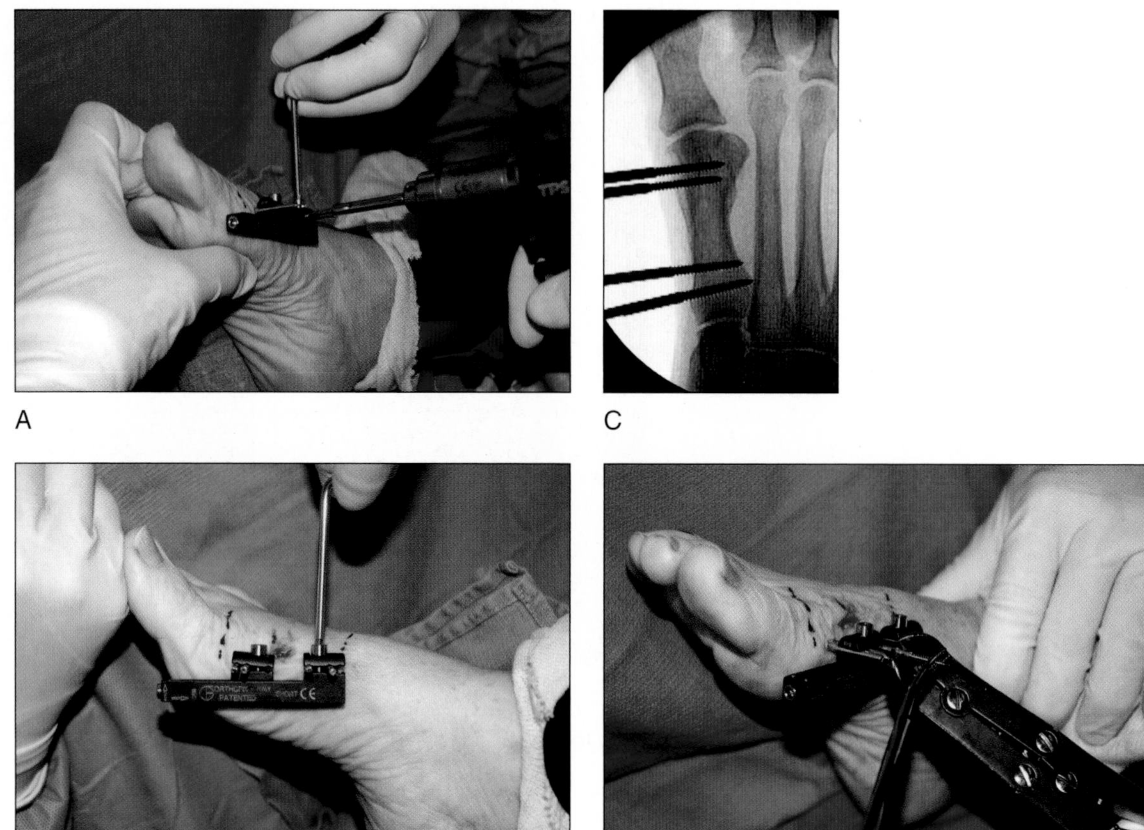

A B C D

FIGURE 10

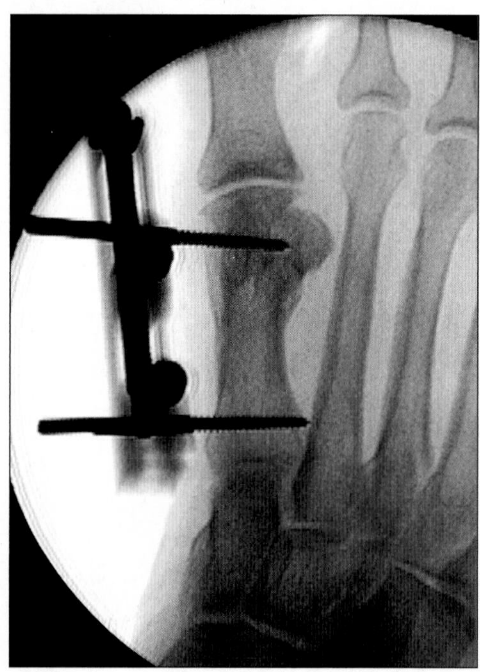

FIGURE 11

Pearls

- *The external fixator must be preset to ensure slight compression is still possible after the corticotomy (i.e., do not have the external fixator completely compressed when the corticotomy is performed because one needs to account for the saw blade thickness).*

Step 3: Corticotomy

- Attempt to make the corticotomy with the external fixator in place (otherwise you may lose control of the two metatarsal fragments).
- While the external fixator can be removed to facilitate access to the corticotomy site, repositioning the external fixator, despite best efforts, may lead to slight malalignment of the corticotomy.
- Corticotomy for the 1MT
  - Determine proper location for corticotomy (Fig. 12A).
  - Confirm proper corticotomy location on AP (Fig. 12B) and lateral (Fig. 12C) fluoroscopic views.

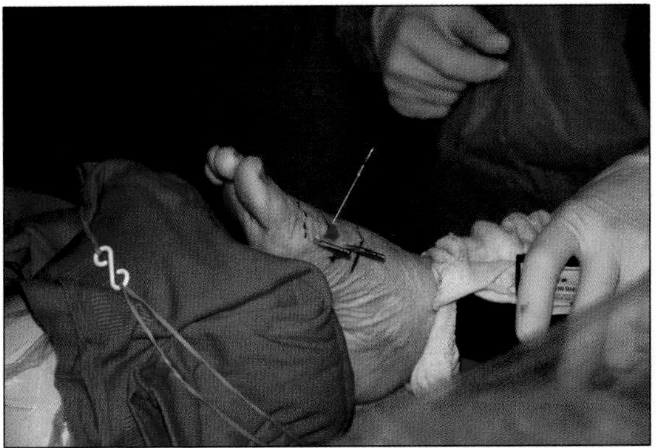

A

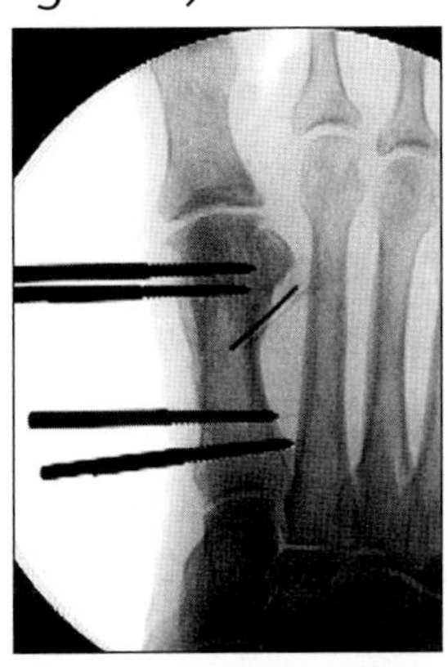

B

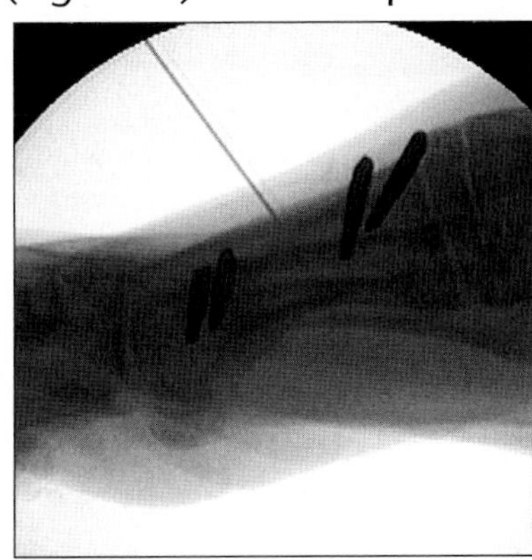

C

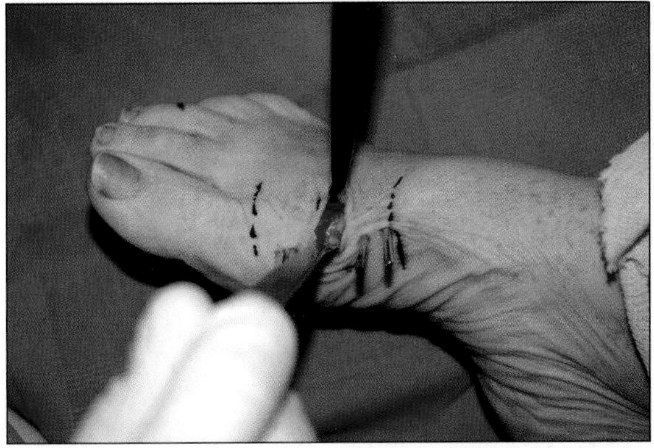

D

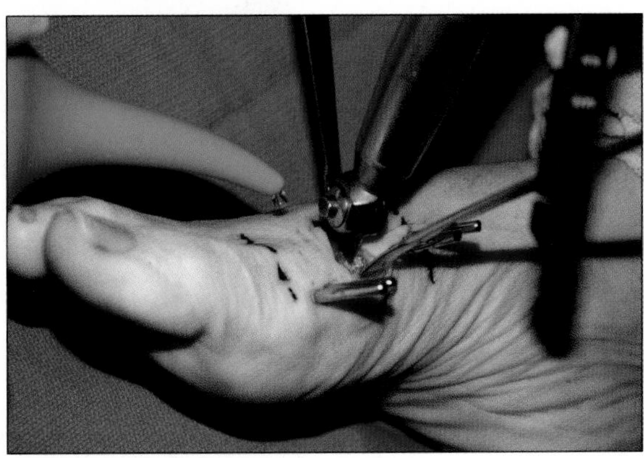

E

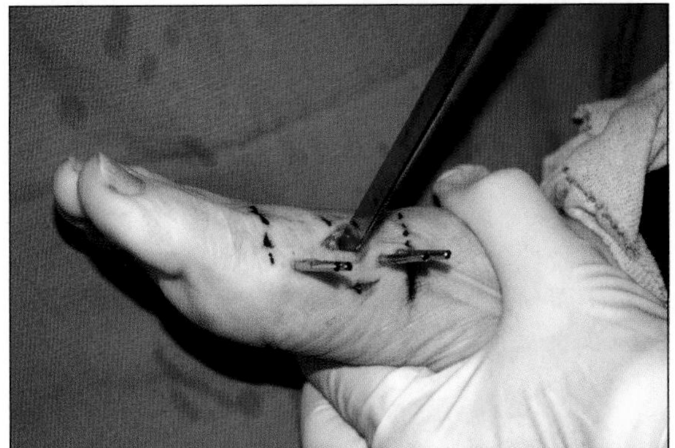

F

FIGURE 12

Pitfalls

- *Removing the external fixator to perform the corticotomy may lead to an inability to reposition the corticotomy anatomically.*

Instrumentation/ Implantation

- Micro-sagittal saw or Gigli saw, depending on surgeon preference
- Sterile cold saline/water irrigation to cool the saw blade while the corticotomy is being created
- Proper wrenches to adjust the external fixator

  - The corticotomy may be performed with a micro-sagittal saw while cold sterile water or saline is irrigated onto the saw blade (Fig. 12D). Alternatively, a Gigli saw may be used.
  - Regardless of technique, no periosteal stripping is required and this should be avoided. Figure 12E shows the minimal exposure and minimal periosteal stripping for corticotomy.
  - The corticotomy is made with adequate bone bridges to the adjacent intermediate pins (ideally at least 2–3 mm).
  - Figure 12F shows the corticotomy being completed and mobilized with an osteotome.
- Gently distract the external fixator to confirm that the corticotomy is complete, both clinically (Fig. 13A) and fluoroscopically (Fig. 13B).
- Then compress the corticotomy fully (Fig. 14A and 14B), check that the first metatarsal external fixator is in place without skin impingement (Fig. 15A), and perform wound closure (Fig. 15B).

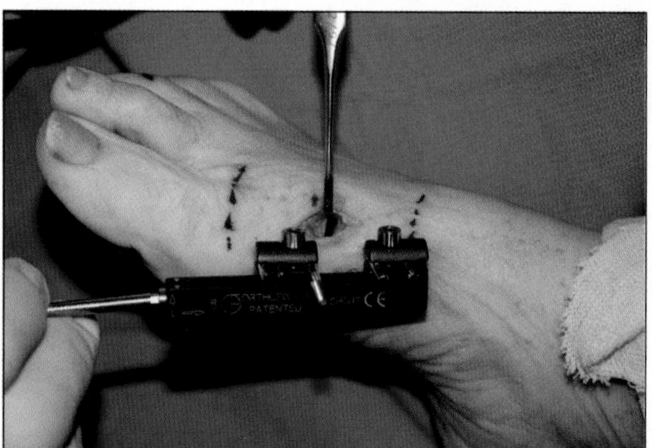

A

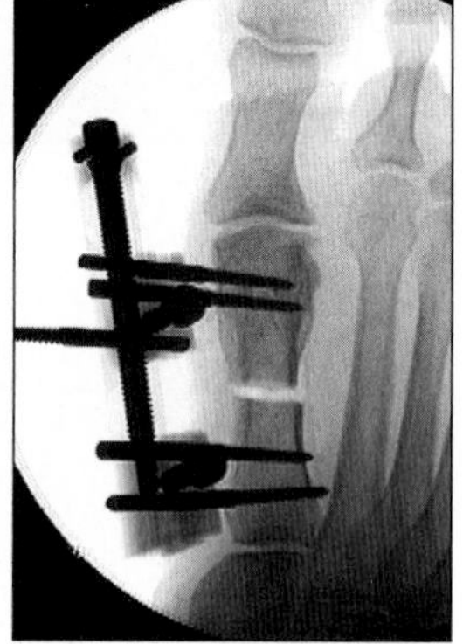

B

FIGURE 13

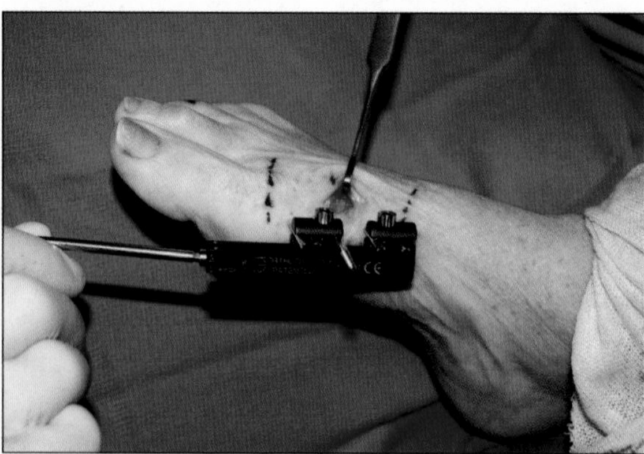

A

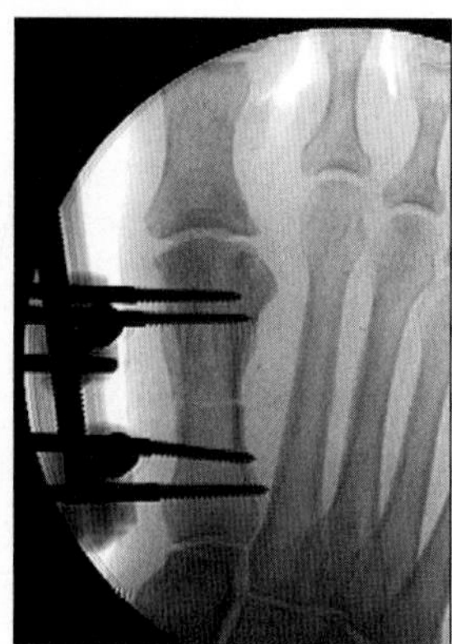

B

FIGURE 14

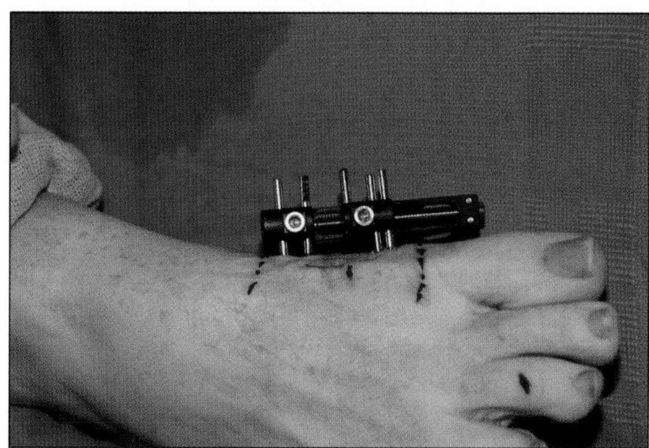

A

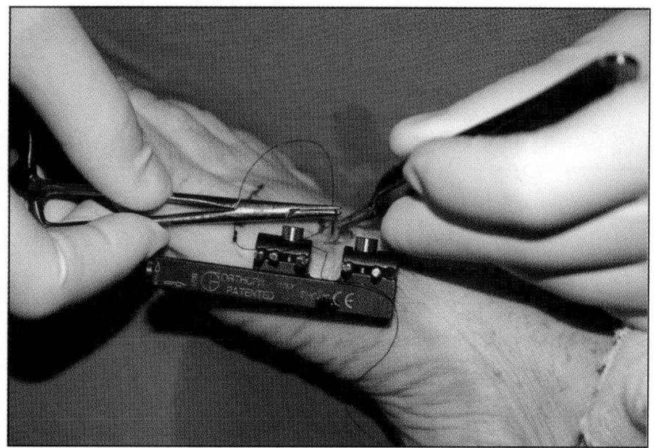

B

FIGURE 15

- 4MT corticotomy
  - Figure 16A shows the clinical view of a 4MT corticotomy. Note that the pins closest to the osteotomy are in the surgical approach since the 4MT is particularly short in this patient.
  - Slightly distract the corticotomy to confirm it is complete using fluoroscopy (Fig. 16B).
  - Fully compress the corticotomy (Fig. 16C).

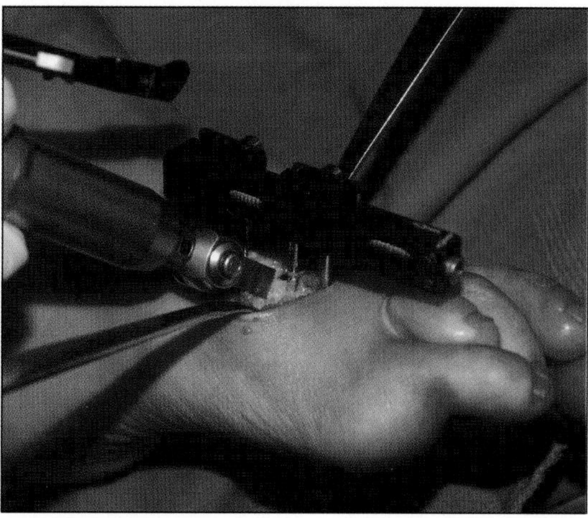

A

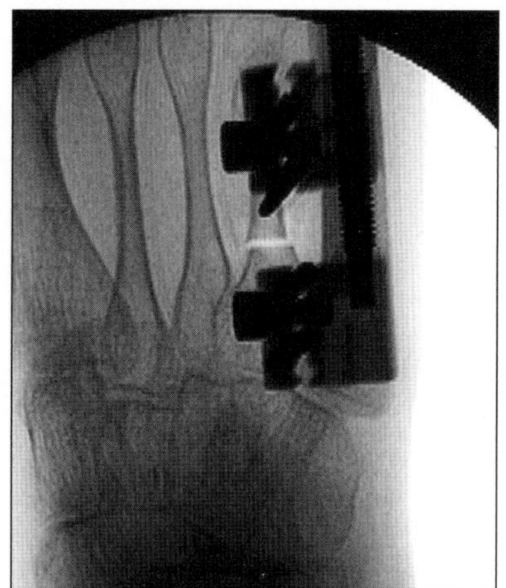

FIGURE 16 B C

PEARLS

- *Reinforced patient instruction and review with a family member often avoids inadvertent inappropriate distraction technique.*
- *Close initial follow-up is important to identify potential problems.*

PITFALLS

- *Miscommunication leads to undesirable accelerated distraction (risking failure of regenerate formation and nonunion), distraction that is too slow (early undesirable consolidation), or inadvertent compression.*

Postoperative Care and Expected Outcomes

- The patient is placed on non–weight-bearing status until adequate healing and external fixator removal.
- Maintain compression for approximately 10 days.
- Begin incremental distraction on postoperative day 10.
  - Distract 0.50–0.75 mm/day, in 0.25-mm increments.
  - This typically corresponds to ¼ turn 2 or 3 times daily.
- Clear instructions and patient compliance are mandatory.
- Close follow-up (at least weekly) in the first several weeks is necessary to ensure that distraction is occurring at proper rate.
- Daily pin care is mandatory.
- The external fixator is distracted until desired metatarsal length is achieved.
  - Figure 17 shows a 4MT external fixator at 4 weeks' follow-up without skin impingement.
  - Figure 18 shows serial AP radiographs for a 4MT lengthening in the patient shown in Figure 1.
    - Radiograph after 10 days of compression and 7 days of distraction (Fig. 18A).
    - Radiograph after 3 weeks of distraction (Fig. 18B).
    - Radiograph after 7 weeks of distraction (Fig. 18C).
    - Radiograph after external fixator removal at 10 weeks (Fig. 18D).

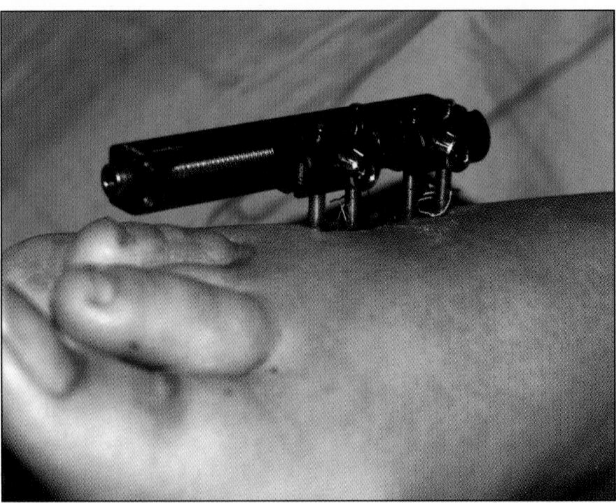

FIGURE 17

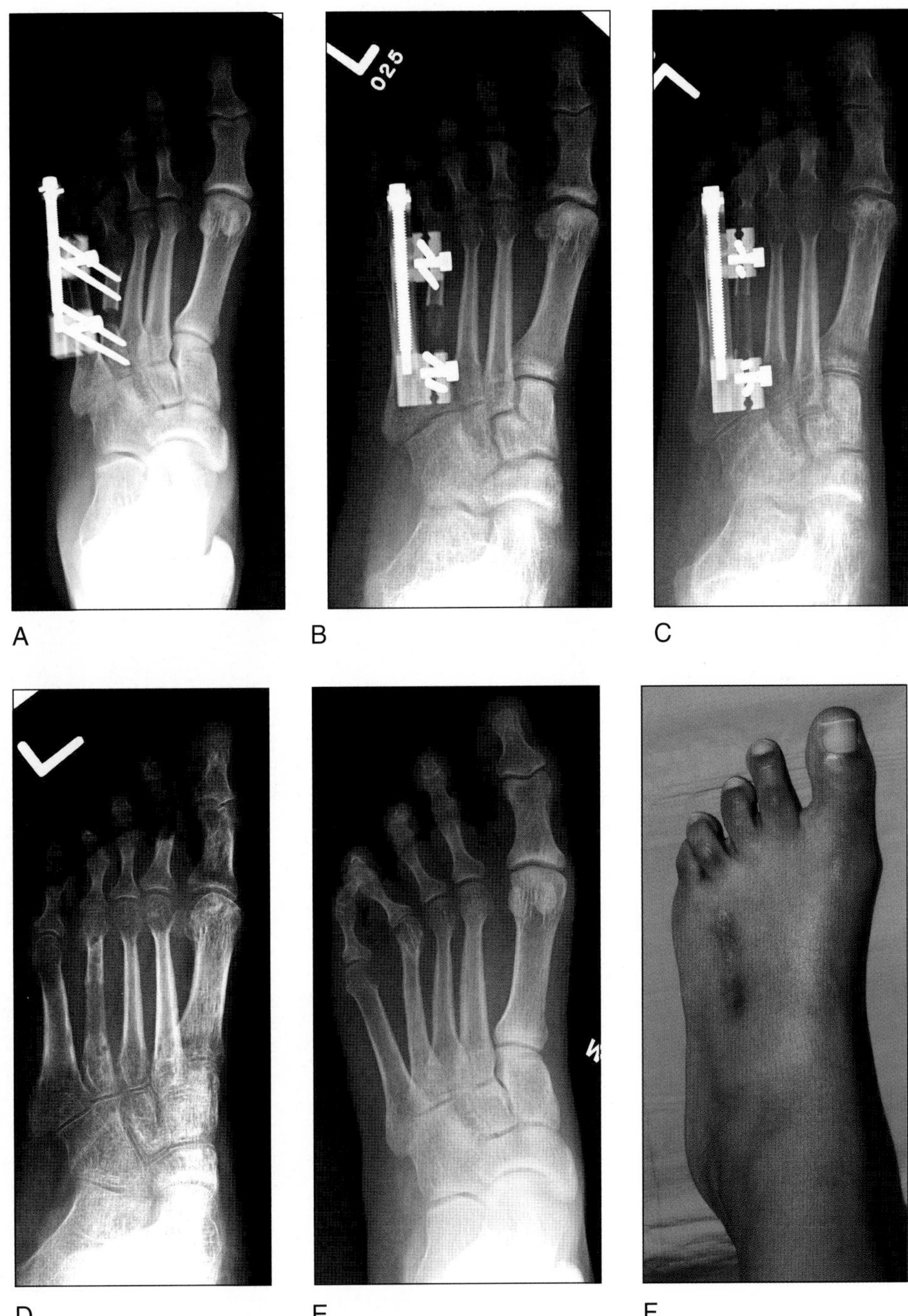

FIGURE 18

- Final follow-up at 2 years (Fig. 18E). Note that there is no correction of the fourth toe deformity.
- Clinical view of final follow-up with slight lateral deviation of the fourth toe (Fig. 18F).

- The external fixator is maintained until an adequate callus forms to allow fixator and pin removal.
- A cam walker or casting may be considered for 2–3 more weeks while the pin sites heal, followed by advancement to full weight bearing on the forefoot.

- Serial follow-up of 1MT lengthening of example patient in this chapter
  - Preoperative radiograph (Fig. 19A).
  - After 10 days of compression and 14 days of distraction (Fig. 19B).
  - After 8 weeks of distraction (Fig. 19C); note comparison to contralateral foot to determine ideal length restoration.
  - Final follow-up (Fig. 19D).

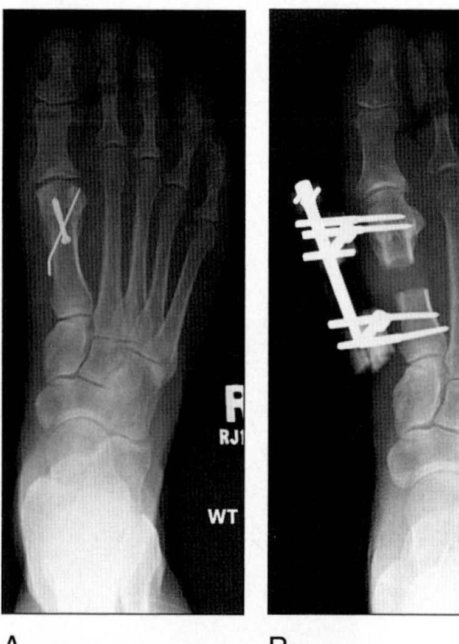

A B

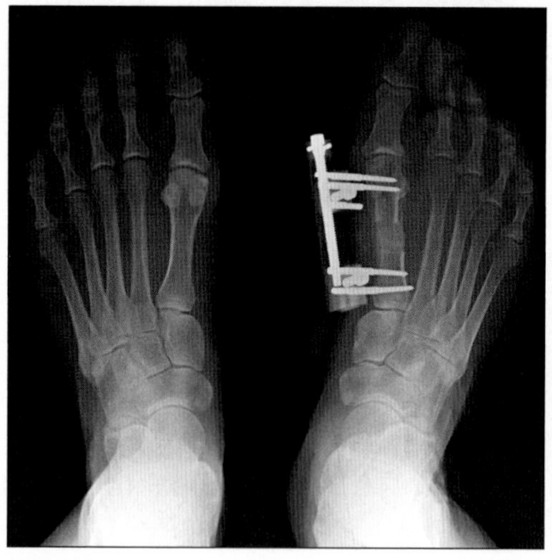

C

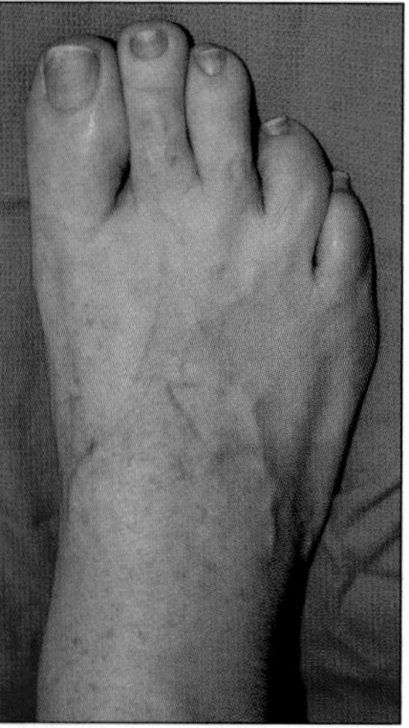

D

FIGURE 19

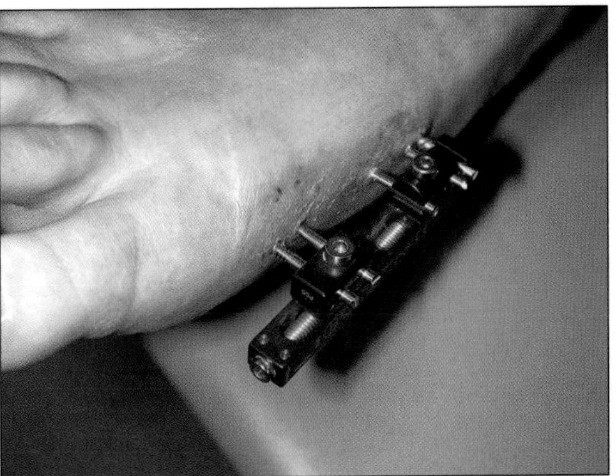

A

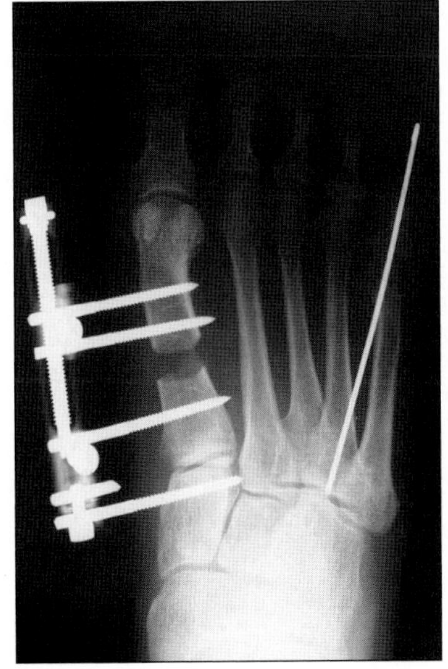

B

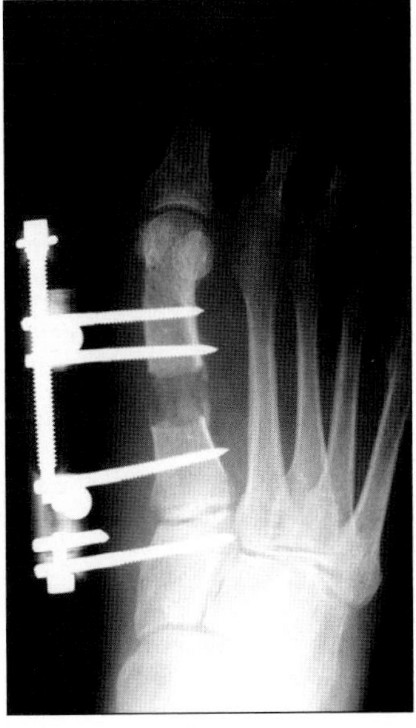

C

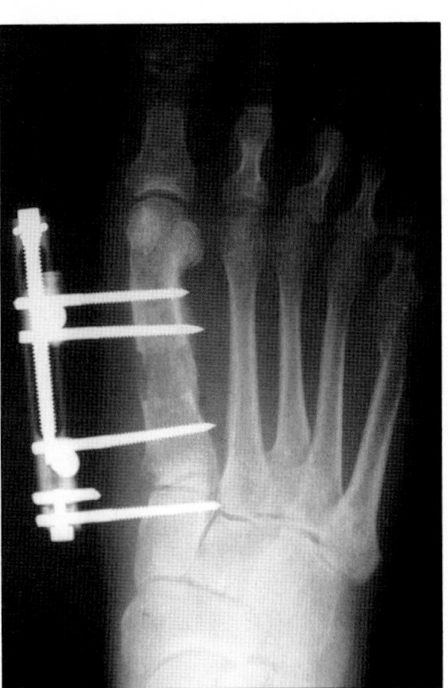

D

FIGURE 20

- Serial follow-up of another patient with 1MT lengthening (see preoperative evaluation in Fig. 2A).
  - Clinical picture of external fixator in place (Fig. 20A).
  - After 10 days of compression and 3 weeks of distraction (Fig. 20B).
  - After 6 weeks of distraction (Fig. 20C).
  - After 11 weeks of distraction (Fig. 20D).

Evidence

Given multiple Level IV series with relatively consistent successful outcomes of distraction osteogenesis for metatarsal lengthening, a grade B recommendation for metatarsal lengthening may be provided.

Baek GH, Chung MS. The treatment of congenital brachymetatarsia by one-stage lengthening. J Bone Joint Surg [Br]. 1998;80:1040-4.
Choi IH, Chung MS, Baek GH, Cho TJ, Chung CY. Metatarsal lengthening in congenital brachymetatarsia: one-stage lengthening versus lengthening by callotasis. J Pediatr Orthop. 1999;19:660-4.
Hurst JM, Nunley JA 2nd. Distraction osteogenesis for the shortened metatarsal after hallux valgus surgery. Foot Ankle Int. 2007;28:194-8.
Kim HT, Lee SH, Yoo CI, Kang JH, Suh JT. The management of brachymetatarsia. J Bone Joint Surg [Br]. 2003;85:683-90.
Kim JS, Baek GH, Chung MS, Yoon PW. Multiple congenital brachymetatarsia: a one-stage combined shortening and lengthening procedure without iliac bone graft. J Bone Joint Surg [Br]. 2004;86:1013-5.
Kucukkaya M, Kabukcuoglu Y, Tezer M, Kuzgun U. Correcting and lengthening of metatarsal deformity with circular fixator by distraction osteotomy: a case of longitudinal epiphyseal bracket. Foot Ankle Int. 2002;23:427-32.
Masada K, Fujita S, Fuji T, Ohno H. Complications following metatarsal lengthening by callus distraction for brachymetatarsia. J Pediatr Orthop. 1999;19:394-7.
Oh CW, Satish BR, Lee ST, Song HR. Complications of distraction osteogenesis in short first metatarsals. J Pediatr Orthop. 2004;24:711-5.
Oh CW, Sharma R, Song HR, Koo KH, Kyung HS, Park BC. Complications of distraction osteogenesis in short fourth metatarsals. J Pediatr Orthop. 2003;23:484-7.
Oznur A, Alpaslan AM. Lengthening of short great toe and correction of all lesser toe deformities by distraction-lengthening. Foot Ankle Int. 2003;24:345-8.
Robinson JF, Ouzounian TJ. Brachymetatarsia: congenitally short third and fourth metatarsals treated by distraction lengthening—a case report and literature summary. Foot Ankle Int. 1998;19:713-8.
Song HR, Oh CW, Kyung HS, Kim SJ, Guille JT, Lee SM, Kim PT. Fourth brachymetatarsia treated with distraction osteogenesis. Foot Ankle Int. 2003;24:706-11.
Wada A, Bensahel H, Takamura K, Fujii T, Yanagida H, Nakamura T. Metatarsal lengthening by callus distraction for brachymetatarsia. J Pediatr Orthop B. 2004;13:206-10.

PROCEDURE 16

Internal Fixation of the Sesamoid Bone of the Hallux

Geert I. Pagenstert, Victor Valderrabano, and Beat Hintermann

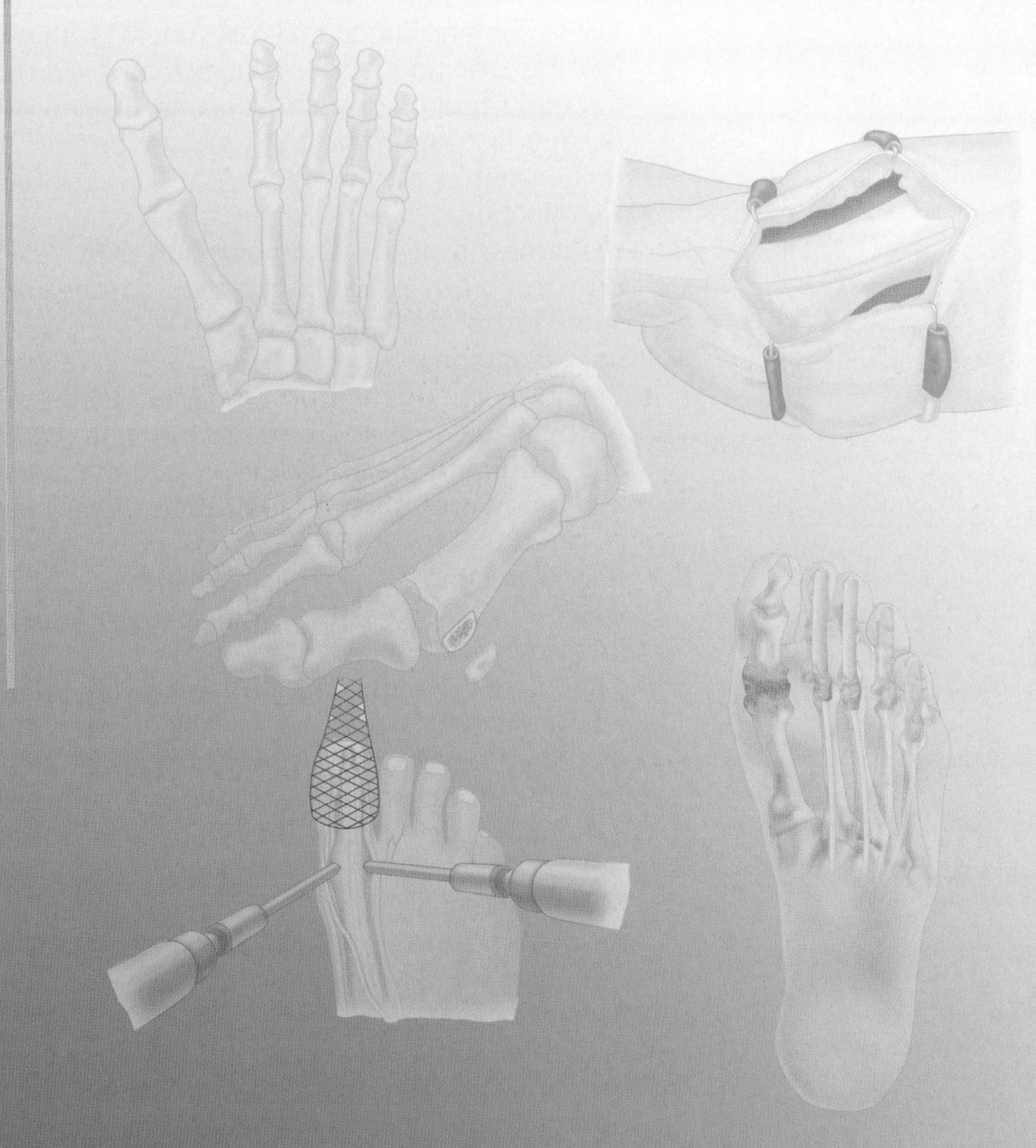

PITFALLS

- *Fracture fragments smaller than 3 mm may be too small for screw fixation and may be excised (Biedert and Hintermann, 2003; Rodeo et al., 1993).*
- *Almost all painful sesamoid fragmentations into two parts occur transverse to the long axis (fracture, nonunion, congenital bipartite sesamoid) (Inge and Ferguson, 1933). If such is the case, longitudinal or multiple sesamoid fragmentations may be unsuitable for screw fixation.*

Controversies

- Distinguishing between symptomatic congenital bipartite sesamoid and old fracture nonunion may be difficult. Both have blunt edges on radiographs and computed tomography (CT) scans and increased uptake on bone scans. However, differentiation will not change treatment strategy and is unnecessary (Blundell et al., 2002).

Indications

- Symptomatic sesamoid bone fracture, fracture nonunion, or congenital bipartite sesamoid bone after at least 6 weeks' failure of nonsurgical treatment
- Acute displaced sesamoid bone fracture or congenital bipartite sesamoid of more than 5 mm

Examination/Imaging

- Clinical evaluation
  - Inspection and functional assessment of the whole foot for structural abnormalities that stress the fractured sesamoid, such as plantar flexion, short or long first ray, or hallux valgus deformity (Pagenstert et al., 2006)
  - Examination of the hallux-sesamoid complex for tenderness over the sesamoids and pain provocation by exacerbation with dorsiflexion stress test of the hallux (Fig. 1)
- Plain radiographs
  - Weight-bearing anteroposterior and lateral views of the whole foot and ankle to evaluate osseous architecture for hallux valgus, flexed metatarsus, and amount of fracture-dislocation (Pagenstert et al., 2006)
  - Special sesamoid tangential (skyline) and oblique views (Fig. 2A) to assess arthritis and number of fragments
- Longitudinal CT scans (Fig. 2B) are most helpful to assess vitality of the fracture site. Blunt fracture edges or fractured bipartite sesamoids may need débridement of a necrotic and avital fracture zone.
- We do not regularly utilize magnetic resonance imaging (MRI).
  - MRI may give additional information about surrounding ligaments and tendons in cases of traumatic trans-sesamoidal fracture-dislocation of the hallux (turf toe).
  - In chronic sesamoid conditions, MRI may help in assessing cartilage destruction, inflammation, osteomyelitis, or bone edema (Karasick and Schweitzer, 1998).
- We do not regularly utilize bone scans. They may be used to rule out sesamoid pathology (negative predictive value). However, increased uptake is present in 25% of the sedentary and active population without sesamoid symptoms (Chisin et al., 1995).

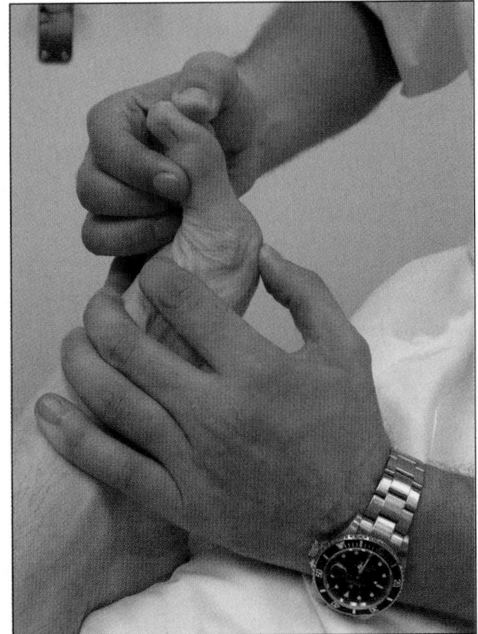

FIGURE 1

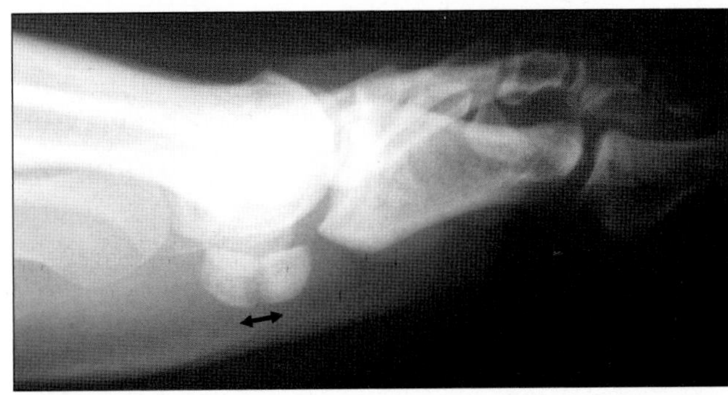

A

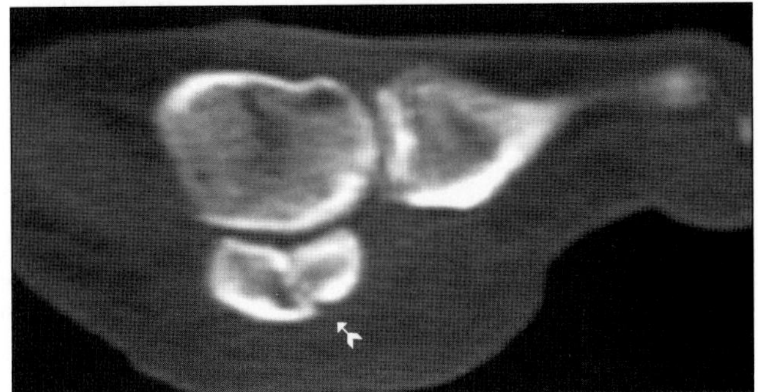

B

FIGURE 2

Treatment Options

- In acute sesamoid fractures with less than 5 mm of fragment displacement, nonoperative treatment with a solid sole for 6–8 weeks is usually successful.
- In chronic sesamoid conditions with less than 3 mm of fragment displacement, débridement and bone packing of the fracture site with autologous bone from the first metatarsal head may be used. Stability is inherent in the intact flexor hallucis brevis tendon sheath, which closes about the sesamoid bone (Anderson and McBryde, 1997).
- Total sesamoid excision results in reasonable pain management and return to activity (Brodsky et al., 2000; Saxena and Kristdakumtorn, 2003). The flexor hallucis brevis and plantar plate have to be repaired meticulously. However, hallux valgus, hallux varus, and cock-up deformities will occur in 10–20% of cases. In addition, transfer metatarsalgia (lack of great toe pushoff) may occur (Aper et al., 1994).

Surgical Anatomy

- Hallux sesamoid bones are 13.5 ± 3 mm long. In males, the sesamoid bones are larger than in females and the medial sesamoid is more elliptically shaped and bigger compared to the more circular-shaped lateral one (Pretterklieber, 1990).
- Failure of the sesamoid to ossify completely during childhood results in a multipart sesamoid bone.
  - Bipartite sesamoids are much more common than tripartite or multiple parts.
  - Despite incomplete ossification, the sesamoid parts are firmly connected with fibrocartilaginous tissue to act as one bone. Spontaneous fusion can occur later in life (Inge and Ferguson, 1933).
  - Fractures usually run through the fibrocartilaginous zone (Rodeo et al., 1993).
- The sesamoids of the hallux act as a complex. Reconstruction with internal sesamoid fixation has to incorporate intraoperative evaluation and eventually the repair of the following contributory anatomic structures (Fig. 3):
  - Each hallux sesamoid is surrounded by the corresponding tendon sheath of the flexor hallucis brevis, which is firmly attached to the base of the proximal phalanx and plantar plate. The intersesamoid ligament connects both sesamoids to form a solid pedestal to elevate the first ray and absorb stress during gait (Aper et al., 1994).

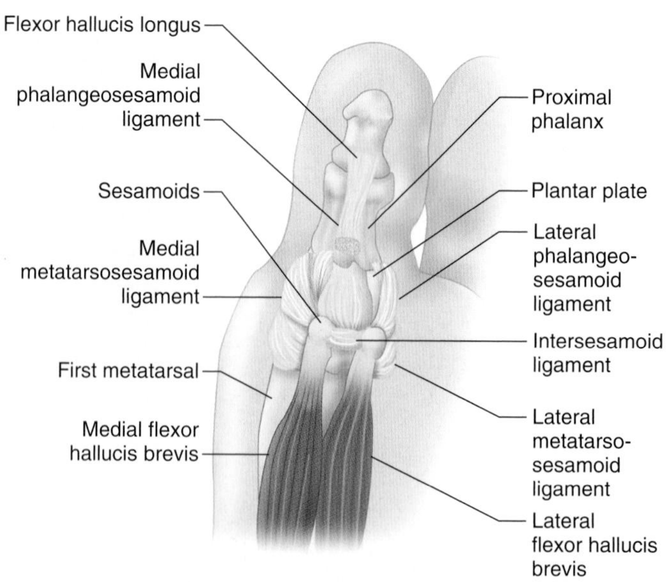

FIGURE 3

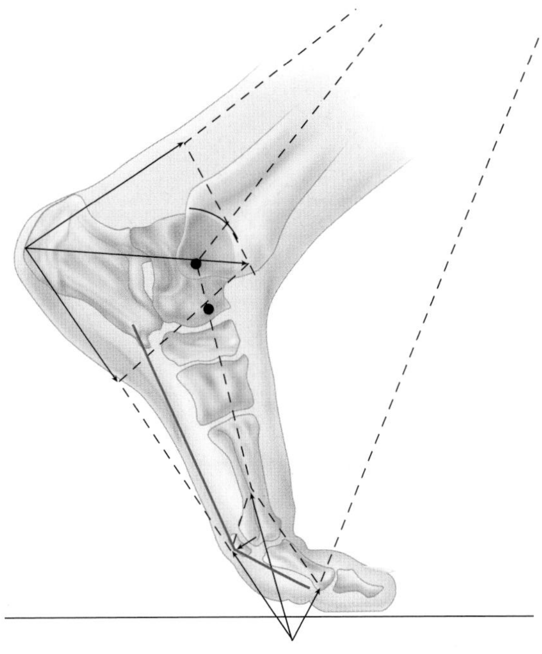

FIGURE 4

Pearls

- *Keep the leg free to allow moving the foot into desired positions for fluoroscopy during surgery.*

Pitfalls

- *Fixation of the leg on the operating table will not allow proper fluoroscopy.*

Equipment

- Fluoroscan with draping for sterile use

- The sesamoid complex act as fulcrum to the flexor hallucis brevis and longus tendons, increasing their lever arms and great toe push-off power, similar to the relationship of the patella and the quadriceps tendon (Fig. 4) (Aper et al., 1994, 1996).

Positioning

- Supine position of the patient is fine for isolated sesamoid bone fixation and combined deformity corrections.
- A tourniquet is needed except during percutaneous fixation.
- Drape the patient to the midshank.

Pearls

- *Correction of hallux valgus is described in detail in Procedures 1–3.*
- *Correction of a plantar-flexed first ray is described in detail in Procedure 00.*
- *Repair of hallucal dislocations (turf toe) is described in detail in Procedure 9.*

Portals/Exposures

- The surgical approach to internal sesamoid fixation is dependent on the concomitant morbidities.
- Acute, largely displaced sesamoid fractures (>5 mm)
  - These are defined as trans-sesamoidal fracture-dislocations of the hallux (turf toe) with significant soft tissue disruption (Rodeo et al., 1993).
  - An open approach is used via a medial internervous skin incision over the first metatarsophalangeal (MTP) joint for isolated medial sesamoid fracture-dislocation, with expansion to an L-shaped incision for bilateral sesamoid fracture-dislocation (Fig. 5).
  - Fracture-dislocation of the hallux through the lateral sesamoid bone without injury to the medial sesamoidal attachment does not occur; therefore, an isolated approach to the lateral sesamoid is not needed.
  - The first and second distal digital nerves run close to the outer side of the medial and lateral sesamoid bones and have to be visualized for ligamento-capsular repair (for more detail, see Procedure 9).
- Chronic medial sesamoid fracture combined with hallux valgus (Pagenstert et al., 2006)
  - A standard medial internervous skin incision over the first MTP joint is done. Capsulotomy and bony corrections are made as needed for hallux valgus repair (see Procedure 1).
  - The medial sesamoid fracture is reached from inside the joint capsule, avoiding the distal digital nerve (Fig. 6).
- Chronic lateral or medial sesamoid stress fracture with metatarsus primus flexus
  - The flexed metatarsus is usually treated by a proximal osteotomy of the first ray using a separate skin incision at the dorsomedial foot. Therefore, the sesamoid fracture is handled separately as described below.
- Chronic lateral or medial sesamoid fractures without comorbidities
  - A stab incision distal to the sesamoid bone is made, followed by blunt separation of soft tissues down to the sesamoid bone (Fig. 7).

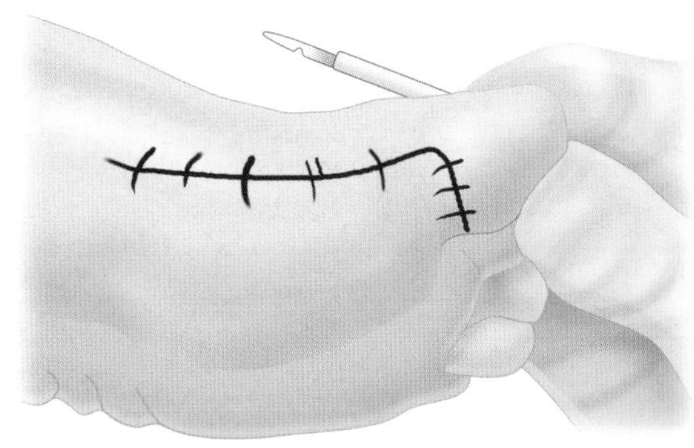

FIGURE 5

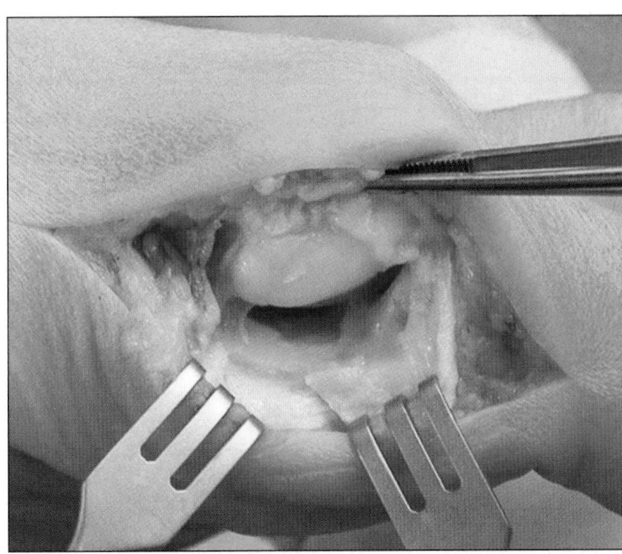

FIGURE 6

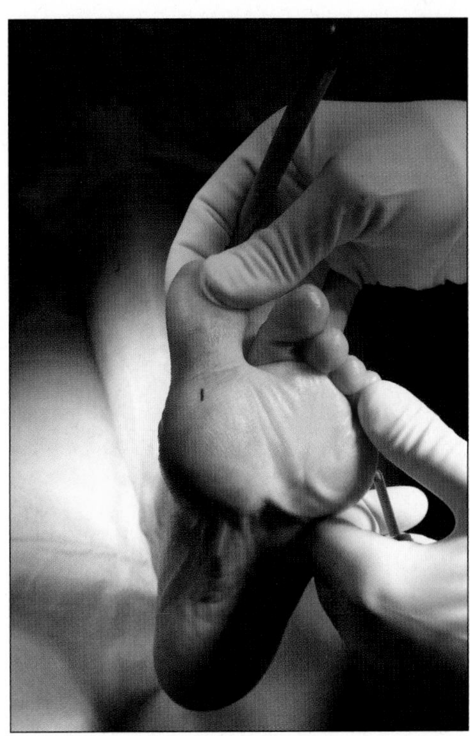

FIGURE 7

Pearls

- *Alternatively, the screw can be inserted over a Kirschner wire through arthrotomy (Fig. 9).*

Procedure

Step 1

- In closed internal sesamoid fixation, the hallux is dorsiflexed and the fractured sesamoid bone is pressed against the metatarsal head to stabilize the fracture fragments (Fig. 8).
- The stab incision is made in the skin distal to the weight-bearing area of the sesamoid bone, and the soft tissues are divided bluntly by a clamp.

Step 2

- A guidewire is inserted under fluroscopic control from the distal pole, perpendicular to the fracture line and subchondral to the sesamoid joint line.
- The length of the screw is measured as the difference between the inserted guidewire and a second guidewire that is held next to the first and is advanced to the sesamoid cortex. The usual range is between 12 and 16 mm.

Step 3

- Insert an appropriate self-drilling/tapping headless cannulated compression screw (Bold screws; Newdeal, Lyon, France). The screw should engage the proximal and distal cortex to enhance stability (Fig. 10).
- Close the stab incision with a Steri-Strip. Apply a compression dressing in neutral hallux position.

Controversies

- In one patient, the screw had to be removed because of intermittent pain with exercise 1 year after surgery. Since then, we have used suture cerclage in open approaches, but continue to use percutaneous screw fixation in the absence of large fracture-displacement or hallux valgus deformity.

Postoperative Care and Expected Outcomes

- Postoperative care for isolated percutaneous screw fixation
  - Weight bearing over the heel is permitted immediately after surgery, using a shoe with a stiff and convex sole to prevent dorsiflexion of the first MTP joint until wound healing is accomplished (usually 2 weeks); thereafter, free walking over the forefoot is allowed.
  - Normal shoes may be worn after 6 weeks.
  - Return to full athletic activity is not recommended before 8–12 weeks after surgery.
  - No suture removal or wound care is needed with percutaneous sesamoid fixation since the stab incision has been closed by a sterile strip.
- Postoperative care for screw fixation in combination with deformity correction

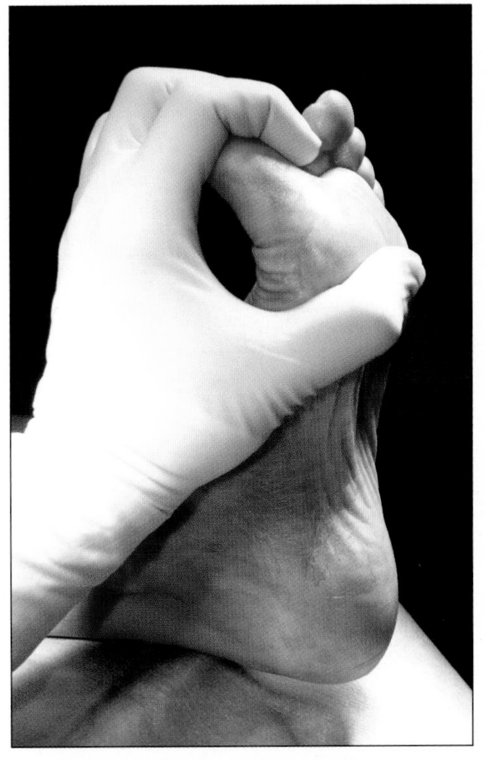
FIGURE 8

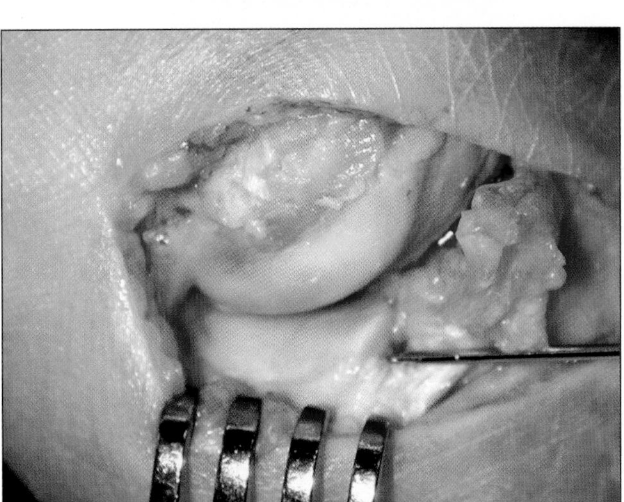
FIGURE 9

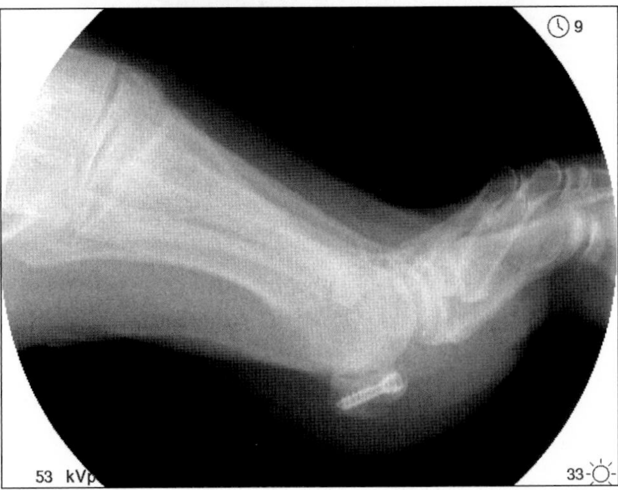

FIGURE 10

- Specifics of postoperative care are dictated by the deformity correction procedure.
- Protection of the great toe against passive dorsiflexion is needed as for isolated screw fixation of the sesamoid.

■ Persistent sesamoid pain may be caused by (1) unrecognized foot deformity and continuous stress to the hallux sesamoids; (2) development of arthritis, avascular necrosis; or (3) screw irritation.
- Focused therapy (deformity correction, screw removal) may prevent total excision as definite treatment of persistent sesamoid pain.

■ Blundell and colleagues (2002) fixed nine sesamoid fractures in athletes with percutaneous cannulated screws and revealed excellent results.
- All athletes went back to their previous level of activity. No complication was reported.
- The authors concluded that percutaneous screw fixation is a safe and fast procedure. They questioned the importance of diagnosing the etiology of painful sesamoid bipartition since treatment is the same anyway.

■ We performed screw fixation in eight athletes and suture fixation with grafting in two nonathletes and had excellent results with full recovery.
- All athletic patients were endurance athletes (running, dancing): six females and two males. Two lateral and eight medial sesamoid bone nonunions have been treated.
- In one patient, an accompanying forefoot-driven pes cavovarus was corrected with extension osteotomy of the first metatarsus. In four patients,

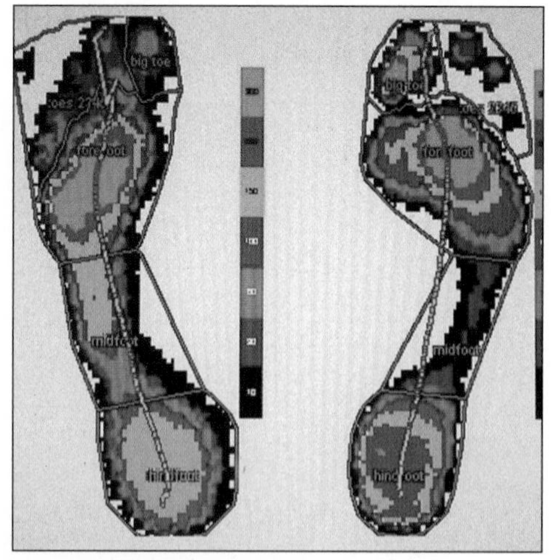

A

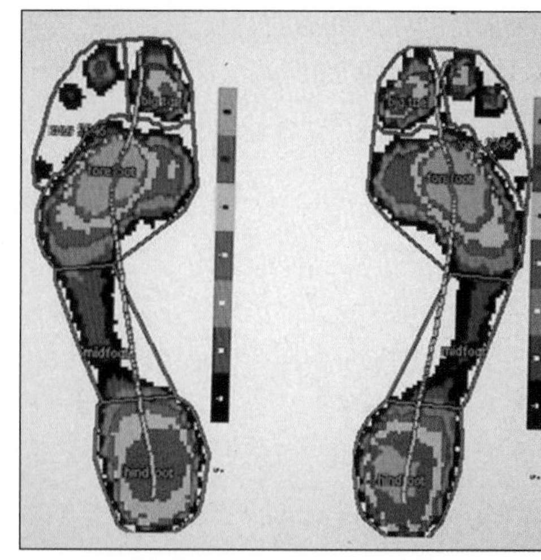

B

FIGURE 11

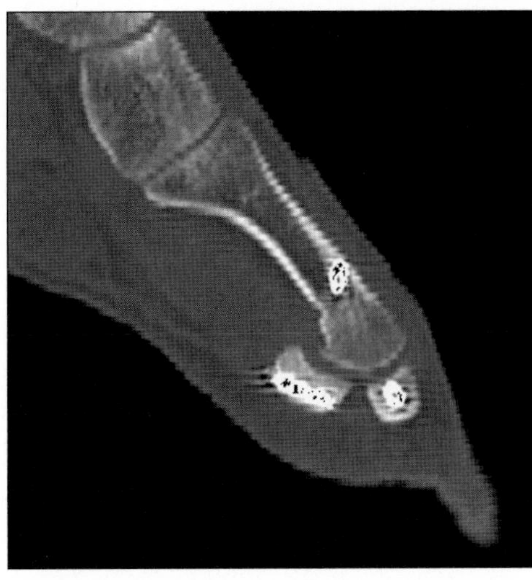

FIGURE 12

concomitant hallux valgus deformity was corrected in combined open surgery. In two of these patients, screws, and in the other two, sutures, were used to stabilize the sesamoid bone during the open approch. All others were treated by percutaneous screw fixation. Local anesthesia was sufficient in one of these cases.

- All patients went back to their preinjury athletic or occupational activity level within 12 weeks after surgery. Clinical healing was documented with pedobarography (Fig. 11A and 11B). Osseous healing of the fractures was proved by CT scan in three cases (Fig. 12). No sesamoid had to be excised. No hallux deformity occurred.

Evidence

Anderson RB, McBryde AM. Autogenous bone grafting of hallux sesamoid nonunions. Foot Ankle Int. 1997;18:293-6.

This study describes the authors' technique to repair painful sesamoid fracture nonunions without the use of internal fixation material. It includes the results of 21 athletes with an average of 4.6 years' follow-up. In two cases, union was not achieved because of hypermobility at the fracture site. These sesamoids were excised. All athletes went back to activity. (Level IV evidence [case series])

Aper RL, Saltzman CL, Brown TD. The effect of hallux sesamoid excision on the flexor hallucis longus moment arm. Clin Orthop Relat Res. 1996;(325):209-17.

This is a biomechanical cadaver study including 12 feet. Decreased moment arm of the flexor hallucis longus was noted with excision of one or both sesamoid bones.

Aper RL, Saltzman CL, Brown TD. The effect of hallux sesamoid resection on the effective moment of the flexor hallucis brevis. Foot Ankle Int. 1994;15:462-70.

This is a biomechanical cadaver study including nine feet. Decreased moment arm of the flexor hallucis brevis was noted with excision of both sesamoid bones.

Biedert R, Hintermann B. Stress fractures of the medial great toe sesamoids in athletes. Foot Ankle Int. 2003;24:137-41.

This study presents the authors' technique of proximal sesamoid pole excision in painful sesamoid nonunions. It includes the results of six patients with an average follow-up of 4.2 years. Five athletes returned to previous activity. (Level IV evidence [case series])

Blundell CM, Nicholson P, Blackney MW. Percutaneous screw fixation for fractures of the sesamoid bones of the hallux. J Bone Joint Surg [Br]. 2002;84:1138-41.

This study describes the authors' technique to repair painful bipartite sesamoid conditions (fractures, nonunions) with the use of a self-tapping cannulated compression screw. It includes the results of nine athletes. All athletes went back to previous activity. (Level IV evidence [case series])

Brodsky JW, Robinson AHN, Krause JO, Watkins D. Excision and flexor hallucis brevis reconstruction for the painful sesamoid fractures and non-unions: surgical technique, clinical results and histo-pathological findings. J Bone Joint Surg [Br]. 2000;82:217.

This abstract describes the authors' results in 20 athletes with an average of 6.5 years' follow-up. Despite flexor repair, 20% hallux valgus formation was noted. All athletes went back to activity. (Level IV evidence [case series])

Chisin R, Peyser A, Milgrom C. Bone scintigraphy in the assessment of the hallucal sesamoids. Foot Ankle Int. 1995;16:291-4.

This scintigraphic study included 86 asymptomatic infantry recruits and 27 asymptomatic sedentary adults. Twenty-nine percent of the recruits and 26% of the adults had pathologically increased scintigraphic uptake in at least one sesamoid bone of the hallux. (Level II evidence [prognostic study])

Inge GAL, Ferguson AB. Surgery of sesamoid bones of the great toe. Arch Surg. 1933;27:466-89.

This is a retrospective radigraphic study including 1025 radiographs of consecutive feet. Incidence, anatomy, epidemiology, and development of bi- and multipartite sesamoid bones of the hallux were studied. (Level II evidence [prognostic study])

Karasick D, Schweitzer ME. Disorders of the hallux sesamoid complex: MR features. Skeletal Radiol. 1998;27:411-8.

This study is a description of MRI findings in normal and various pathologic conditions of the hallux-sesamoid complex.

Pagenstert GI, Valderrabano V, Hintermann B. Medial sesamoid nonunion combined with hallux valgus in athletes. Foot Ankle Int. 2006;27:135-40.

This study reports the authors' technique of combined surgical treatment of hallux valgus and chronic sesamoid fracture in professional athletes. It includes the results of two athletes. Full athletic activity was reported after 10 and 12 weeks. (Level IV evidence [case series])

Pretterklieber ML. Dimensions and arterial vascular supply of the sesamoid bones of the human hallux. Acta Anat. 1990;139:86-90.

This is a descriptive anatomic study including 21 cadaver feet.

Rodeo SA, Warren RF, O'Brien SJ, et al. Diastasis of bipartite sesamoids of the first metatarsophalangeal joint. Foot Ankle Int. 1993;14:425-34.

This study reports the authors' technique of distal sesamoid pole resection and plantar plate repair. It includes the results of four athletes with traumatic fracture of the fibrocartilaginous junction of a bipartite sesamoid bone. All patients went back to previous level of activity. (Level IV evidence [case series])

Saxena A, Krisdakumtorn T. Return to activity after sesamoidectomy in athletically active individuals. Foot Ankle Int. 2003;24:415-9.

This study describes the authors' technique of total sesamoid excision and flexor brevis and plantar plate repair. It includes the results of 26 cases with an average follow-up of 4.2 years. All patients returned to previous activity; 10% hallux varus and valgus deformity was reported.

SECTION II

MIDFOOT

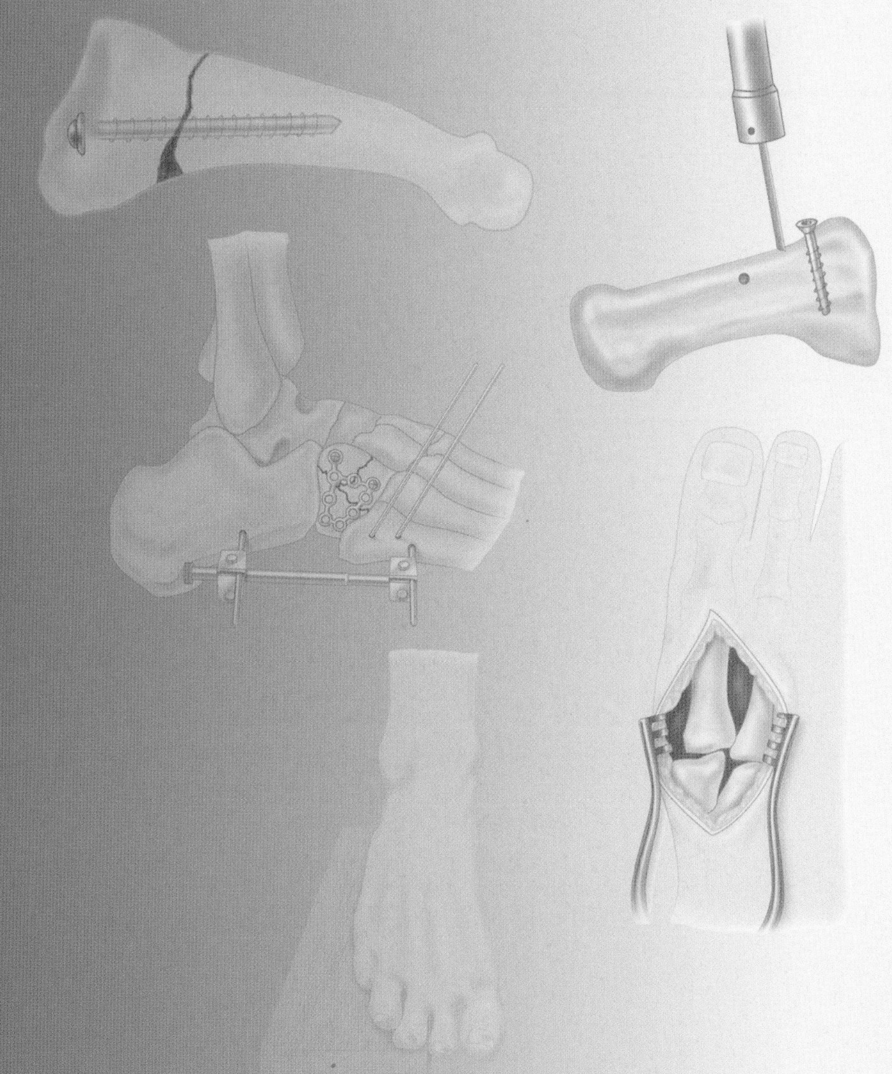

PROCEDURE 17

Cavovarus Correction in Charcot-Marie-Tooth Disease

Glenn B. Pfeffer

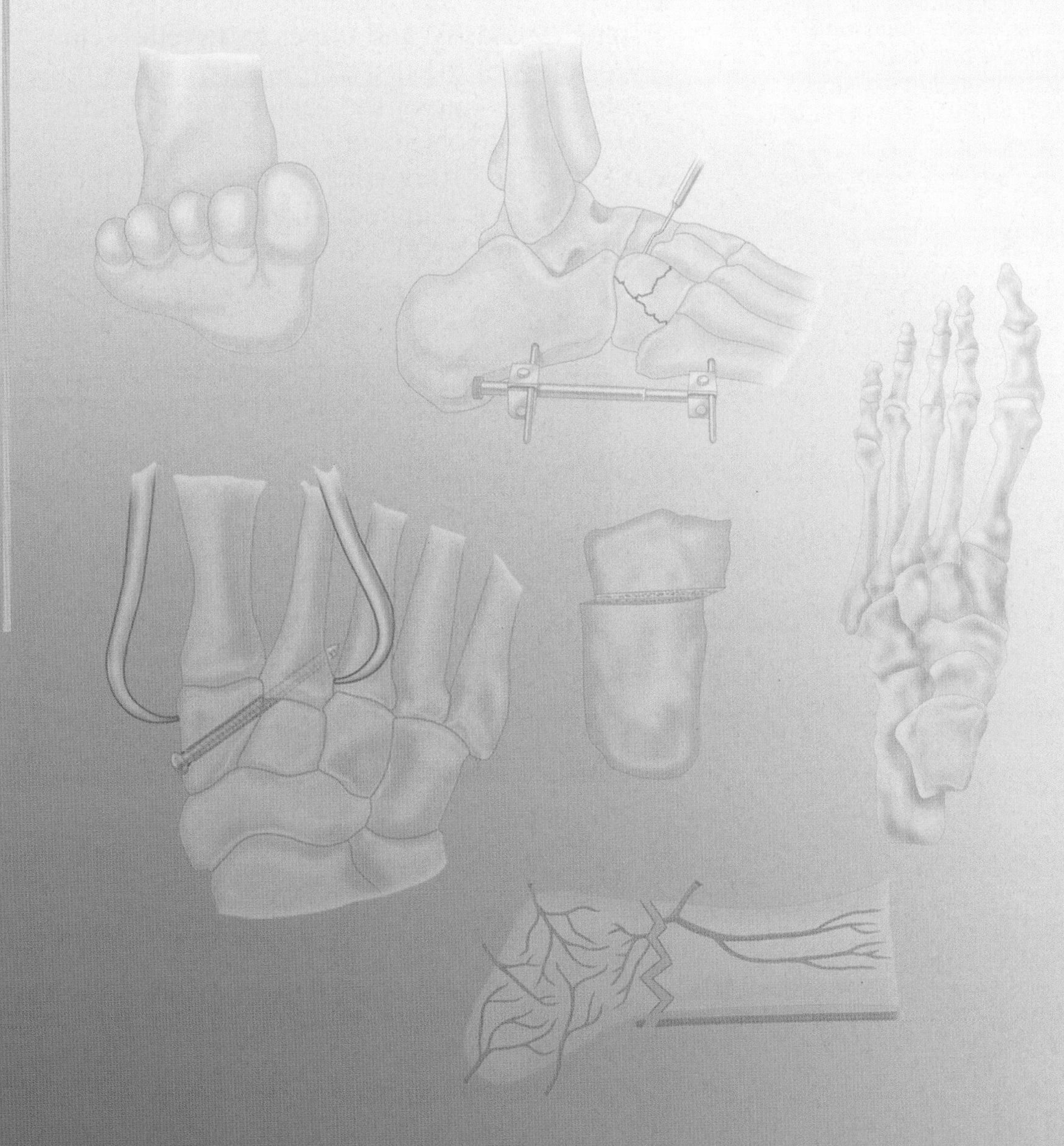

PITFALLS

- *Charcot-Marie-Tooth (CMT) disease includes a wide spectrum of hereditary motor and sensory neuropathies. These diseases are often progressive, which can compromise the long-term results of a surgical reconstruction.*
- *The feet of older adolescents and adults usually require simultaneous osteotomies, tendon transfers, and soft tissue balancing. Young adolescents and children may benefit from soft tissue procedures alone, especially in the early stages of the disease.*

Indications

- Chronic pain or deformity that interferes with activities of daily living
- Failure of conservative measures, including bracing, shoe modification, and physical therapy
- A relatively flexible deformity without arthritic changes in the involved joints

Examination/Imaging

Physical Examination

- CMT disease can also affect the hips (dysplasia), spine (scoliosis), and upper extremities (Fig. 1). Weakness of the first dorsal interosseous muscle in the hand is one of the earliest signs of upper extremity involvement.
- A complete orthopedic examination of the lower extremities is required. There is often atrophy of the anterior and lateral compartments of the leg.

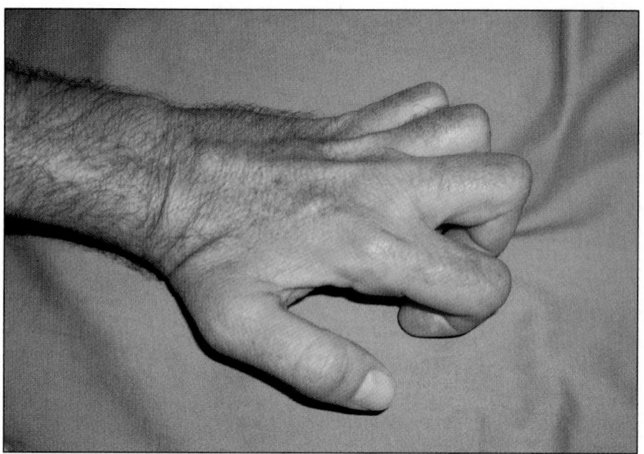

FIGURE 1

- Examine the foot from all sides while the patient is standing (Fig. 2A and 2B).
  - Closely examine the lateral foot to evaluate the apex of the sagittal deformity (Fig. 3).
  - Document the calluses on the plantar aspect of the foot (Fig. 4).

Controversies

- Early surgical intervention may prevent the progression of deformity and minimize impairment. There are no established guidelines, however, that address the appropriate age for surgery. Each case should be dealt with on an individual basis.
- In children younger than 14, it is often preferable to take an incremental approach to surgery, rather than correcting all deformities at once. This chapter examines the surgical options most appropriate for the older adolescent and adult with CMT disease.
- Patients with mild to moderate involvement can often be treated successfully with nonoperative care. Cushioned shoes for shock absorption, soft inserts for metatarsalgia, high-topped shoes and lace-up ankle braces for ankle instability, and bracing for footdrop can help avoid surgery. Physical therapy for range of motion, strength, and proprioception can also be helpful.
- The overarching goals of surgery are preservation of joint motion, creation of a plantigrade foot, and balance of muscle forces.

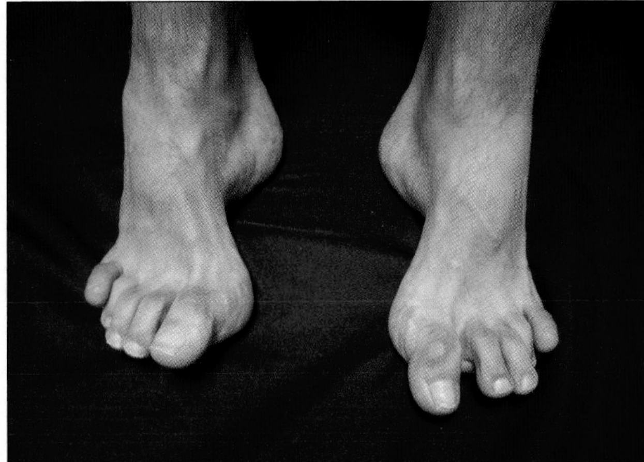

A

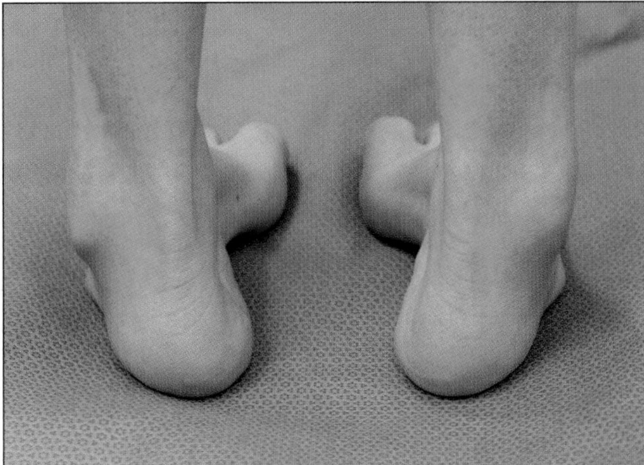

B

FIGURE 2

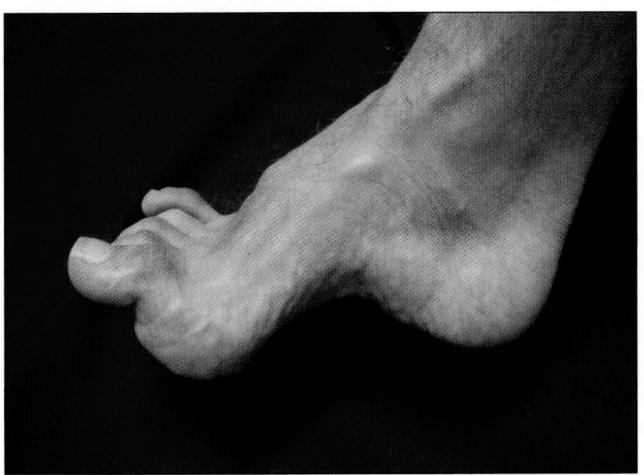

FIGURE 3

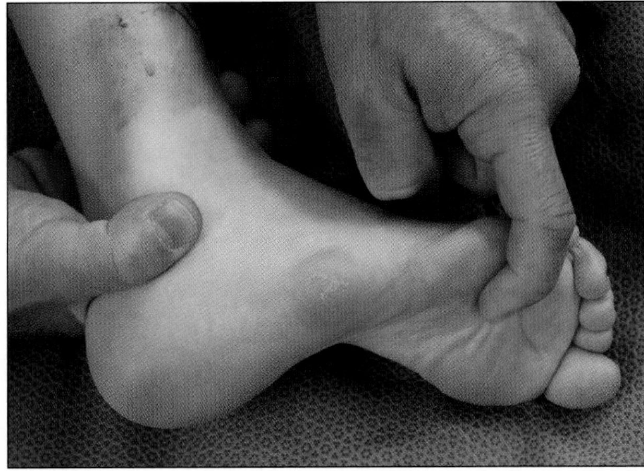

FIGURE 4

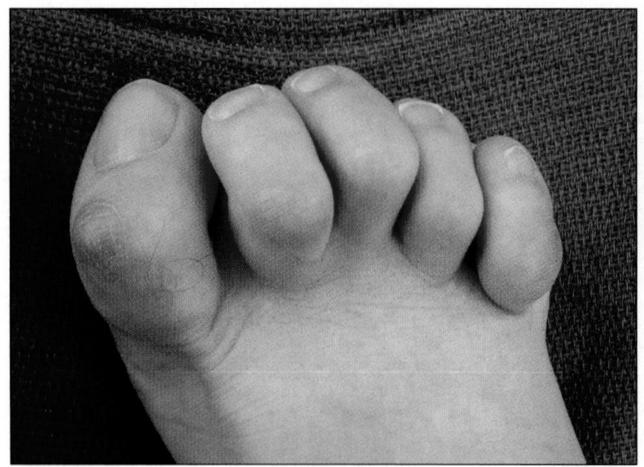
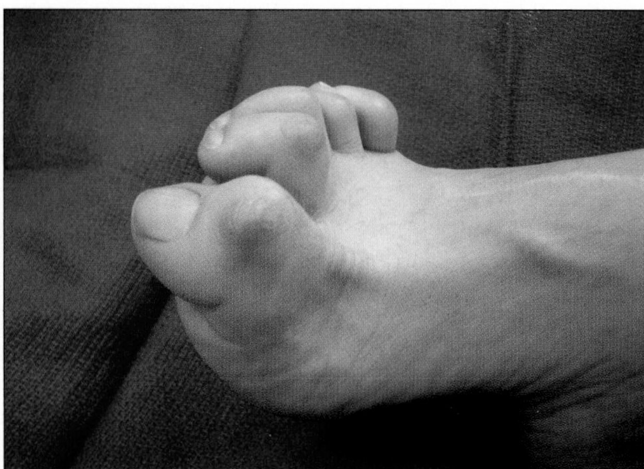

A B
FIGURE 5

- Determine if claw toes are passively correctable (Fig. 5A and 5B).

■ A Coleman block test (Paulos et al., 1980) can be helpful in sorting out forefoot-driven heel varus.
  - When the patient stands with a block beneath the lateral border of the foot, the medial column is unsupported and the first metatarsal head drops off the side of the block (Fig. 6A).
  - If the subtalar joint is flexible and there is no fixed varus deformity of the heel, the hindfoot will no longer be in varus when viewed from behind (Fig. 6B).

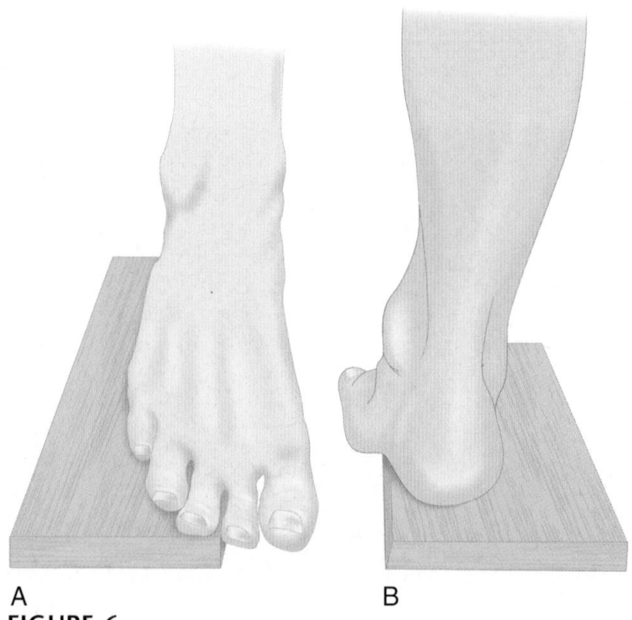

A B
FIGURE 6

- Document motor strength, including knee flexion and extension. Measure sensibility.
  - Typically the peroneus longus, long toe extensors and posterior compartment muscles will maintain strength long after the foot intrinisics, peroneus brevis, and tibialis anterior become weak.
  - Evaluate the imbalance between muscle agonists and antagonists (i.e., peroneus longus and tibialis anterior; posterior tibial and peroneus brevis; toe intrinsic flexors and extrinsic extensors).
- Observe the patient's gait. A footdrop is often effectively treated with an ankle-foot orthosis. The addition of an anterior tibial shelf often provides better balance to the patient. Surgery may still be required if a nonplantigrade foot deformity precludes effective bracing.
- A dynamic electromyogram may be particularly helpful when evaluating potential tendon transfers preoperatively.
- Multiple incisions are frequently required, which can create problems with skin healing. In patients with previous surgery, make sure that both the dorsalis pedis and posterior tibial pulses are present. If not palpable, a Doppler evaluation is indicated.
- Spasticity, asymmetric reflexes, or marked hyperreflexia is not typical of CMT disease. If these symptoms are noted, magnetic resonance imaging of the spine should be obtained.
- A neurologic consultation with electromyography/ nerve conduction study and genetic testing (Athena Diagnostics, Worcester, MA) is often appropriate. What is often considered idiopathic cavovarus is probably a form of CMT disease.
- Document ankle laxity. Although patients often complain of instability during gait, objective ankle laxity is not often present. Extreme varus laxity can masquerade as normal subtalar motion.
- Is the foot flexible? During the non–weight-bearing examination, the subtalar, transverse tarsal, and tarsal-metatarsal joints should be reasonably flexible. A fixed deformity will most commonly require a triple arthrodesis, which is not appropriate in a foot that has some preservation of motion in the hindfoot.
- Evaluate gastrocnemius and soleus tightness. Typically both the gastrocnemius and the soleus will have to be surgically lengthened at the level of the Achilles tendon.

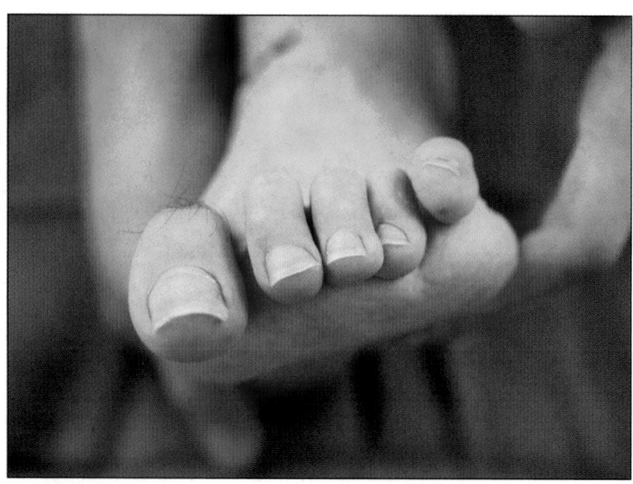

FIGURE 7

Treatment Options

- Many surgical options are used to address the wide array of deformity and motor imbalance that occurs. This chapter presents one of the most common operative approaches, which includes Achilles lengthening, triplane calcaneal osteotomy, Steindler release of the plantar fascia, peroneus longus–to–peroneus brevis transfer, closing wedge metatarsal or midfoot (Cole) osteotomy, correction of claw toes, interphalangeal fusion of the great toe, and extensor tendon transfers to the metatarsal necks. While often performed at the same time, forefoot reconstruction can be performed during a separate operative procedure.

- With the hindfoot held in neutral, evaluate forefoot cavus (valgus) caused by flexion of the medial metatarsals from over-pull of the peroneus longus (Fig. 7). Commonly only the first metatarsal is involved, although the second and third may be as well. Involvement of the fourth and fifth metatarsals that requires operative correction is rare. If a plantar-flexed metatarsal is not corrected, the surgical outcome will be poor.

Imaging

- Standing anteroposterior (AP) (Fig. 8A) and lateral (Fig. 8B) radiographs of the foot and ankle should be carefully examined to evaluate arthritic changes and determine the need for corrective osteotomies. Standing AP and lateral images of the foot should be repeated using a Coleman block, which presents a more accurate view of the foot and its true deformity.
- The calcaneal pitch angle (normal < 30°) and the talus–first metatarsal angle (Meary's line; normal = 0°), are particularly useful in preoperative planning. If the calcaneal pitch corrects with the Coleman block in place, a corrective osteotomy of the heel may not be needed.
- On the lateral standing radiograph, determine if the apex of the cavus is at the metatarsal-cuneiform joint or the midfoot. The deformity should be surgically corrected through its apex.
- A three-dimensional computed tomography reconstruction can be helpful in the assessment of complex deformities and revision surgery (Fig. 9).

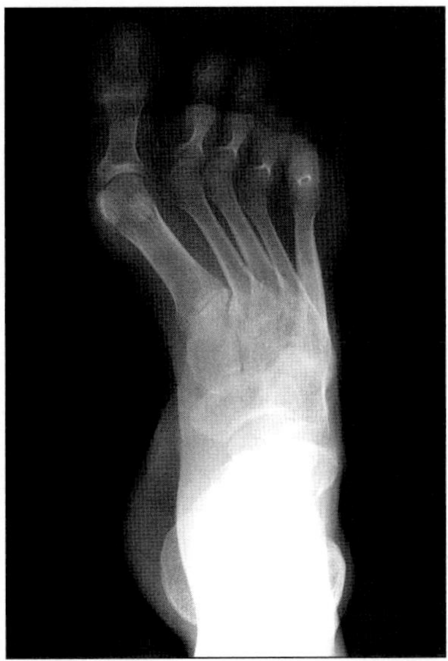

A

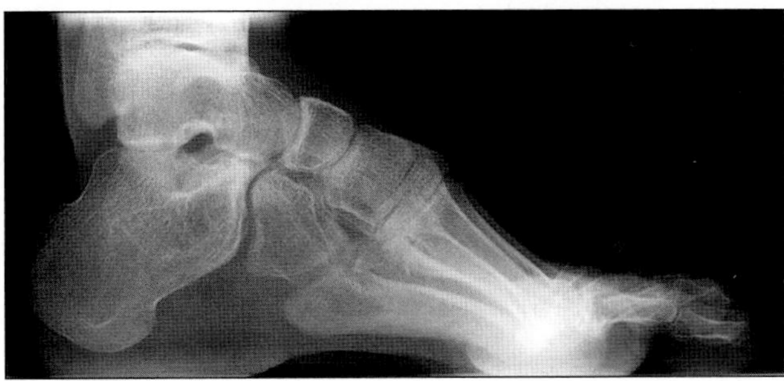

B

FIGURE 8

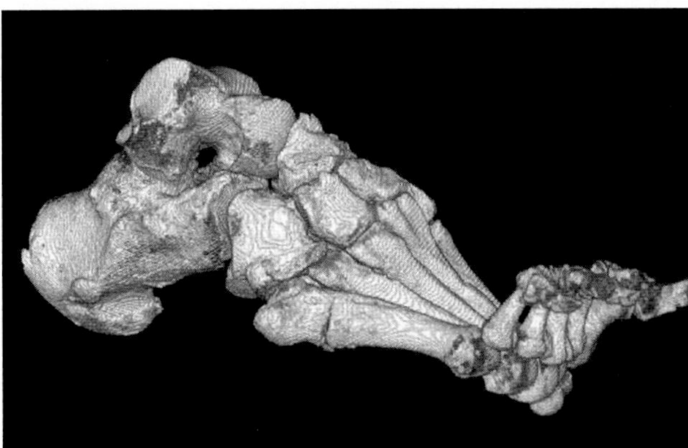

FIGURE 9

Surgical Anatomy

- Varus heel (Fig. 10A)
- Valgus forefoot (Fig. 10B)
- High calcaneal pitch angle (Fig. 11A)
- Meary's line (Fig. 11B)

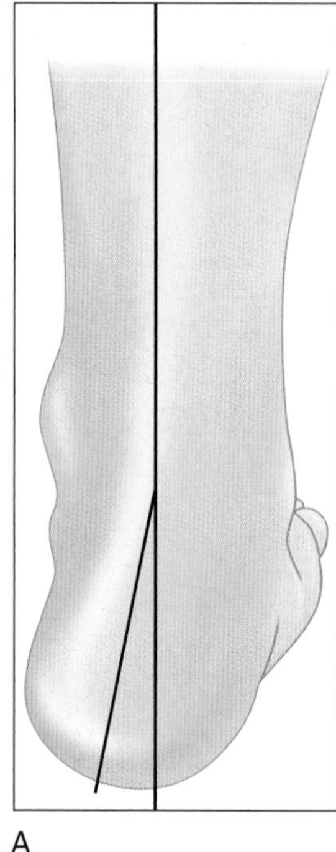
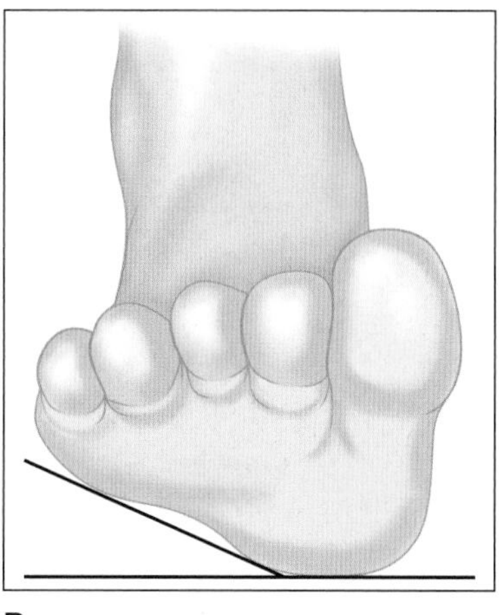

A B

FIGURE 10

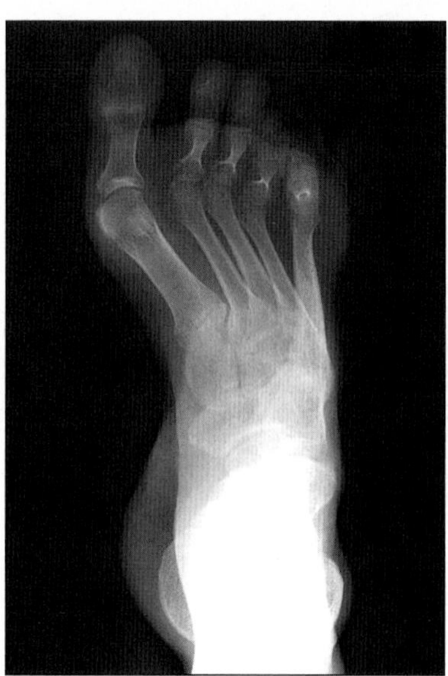
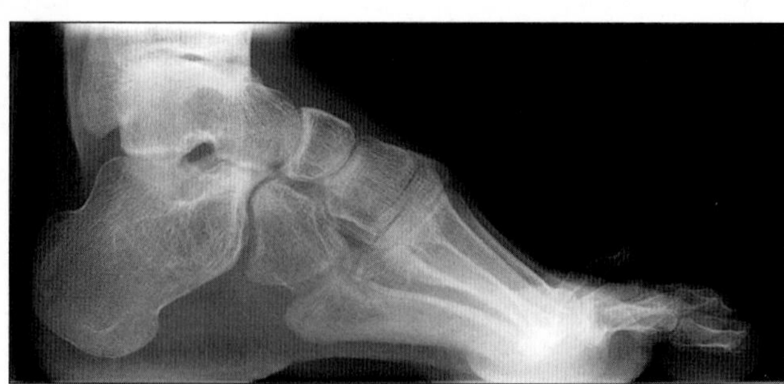

A B

FIGURE 11

PEARLS

- *The patient should be very well padded because of potential susceptibility to pressure palsies.*

PEARLS

- *Once the patient is under anesthesia, perform a fluoroscopic examination of the ankle for laxity. The surgical approach can be modified depending on the results of this examination.*
- *If ankle laxity has to be corrected, two incisions are preferable: one for the ligament reconstruction and tendon transfer, and the other for the calcaneal osteotomy. With one incision, too large a flap has to be dissected to expose both the calcaneal tuberosity and the anterior ankle. It is unusual, however, to find pathologic ankle laxity in these patients, and one incision can almost always be used to expose the heel and the peroneal tendons.*

Positioning

- Place the patient in a partial lateral decubitus position to gain easy exposure to the lateral side of the foot. A deflated beanbag is placed behind the ipsilateral hip to help support the patient in this position. The beanbag can easily be removed during the surgery, allowing the patient to drop down into a supine position.
- Use a thigh tourniquet.
- A femoral-sciatic or popliteal block will help with postoperative pain control (Fig. 12). CMT disease is not a contraindication to a regional block.

Portals/Exposures

- If indicated, perform a triple-cut lengthening of the Achilles tendon using a #11 blade, leaving the lateral insertion intact (Fig. 13). It is usually not sufficient to perform a Strayer procedure to lengthen the gastrocnemius alone.
- Begin the incision with a #15 blade just proximal to the tip of the fibula.
- Extend it distally over the calcaneal tuberosity, along the posterior border of the peroneal sheath. The incision should have a straight component over the portion of the calcaneus that will be osteotomized.

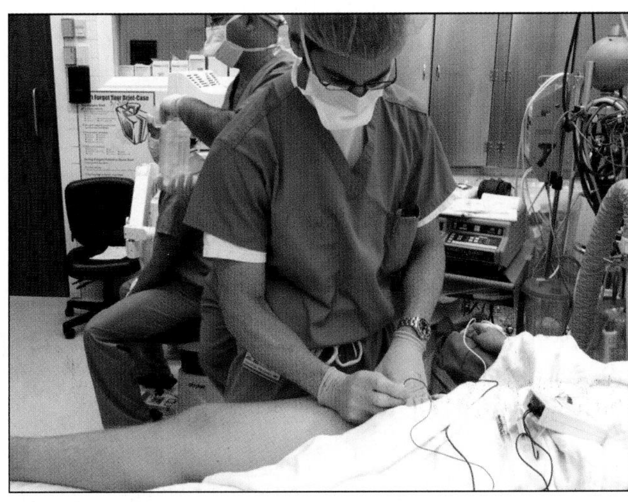

FIGURE 12

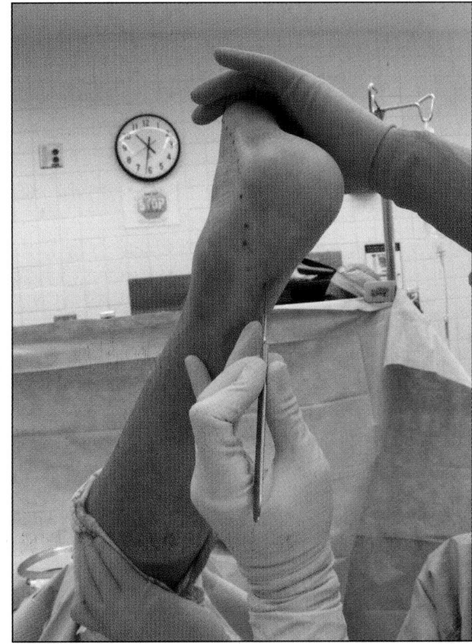

FIGURE 13

- Extend the incision distally over the peroneals, ending at the insertion of the peroneus brevis (Fig. 14). If a midfoot osteotomy is required, the incision can be extended distally over the lateral axis of the cuboid.
- Identify and protect the sural nerve (Fig. 15).

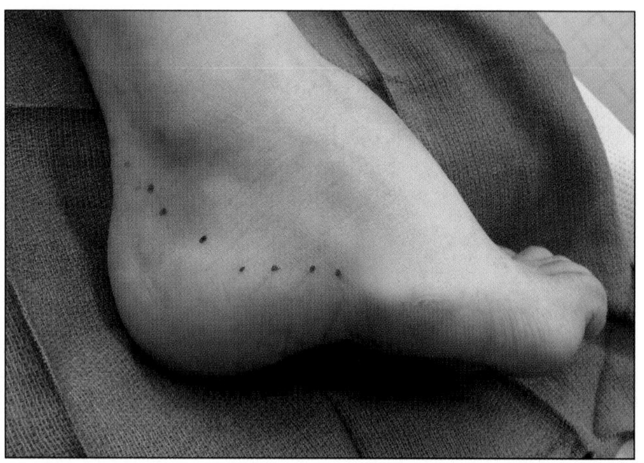
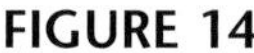

FIGURE 14

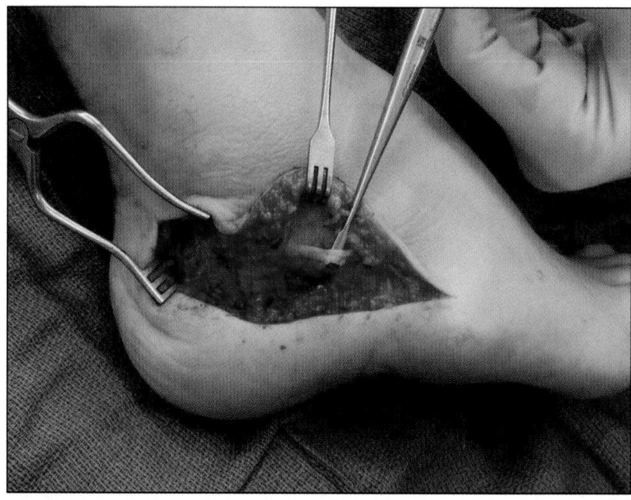

FIGURE 15

> **PEARLS**
>
> - *The calcaneal osteotomy is performed as anteriorly as possible in the tuberosity, to allow for maximal correction of the heel deformity. The osteotomy is usually located at the posterior border of the peroneal sheath.*
> - *A centimeter of bone is the most that can usually be removed from the calcaneus without shortening the heel unduly. Superior displacement of the tuberosity adds some length to the calcaneus, because of the obliquity of the cut.*
> - *When the calcaneus is displaced superiorly, the Achilles tendon is effectively lengthened, and an additional triple-cut lengthening may not be required.*

Procedure

Step 1

- Expose the lateral wall of the calcaneus. Under fluoroscopic guidance, determine the appropriate position of the osteotomy. This is usually just posterior to the peroneal sheath.
  - Under cool water lavage, use a micro-sagittal saw to cut perpendicular to the axis of the tuberosity (Fig. 16A). Superiorly, it should exit 1 cm posterior to the subtalar joint.
  - The osteotomy should be angled obliquely (Fig. 16B and 16C), from superior-proximal to inferior-distal, to allow rotation of the heel out of varus (as opposed to a medial displacement osteotomy used in the correction of pes planus, which is oriented closer to the axis of the tibia). Avoid the subtalar joint superiorly.
- If a simple closing wedge is all that is needed, leave the medial cortex intact; compress the osteotomy, and place three or four 16-mm × 25-mm staples using a 3M Power Stapalizer (Fig. 17). Excellent rigid fixation will be obtained without the need for compression screws.

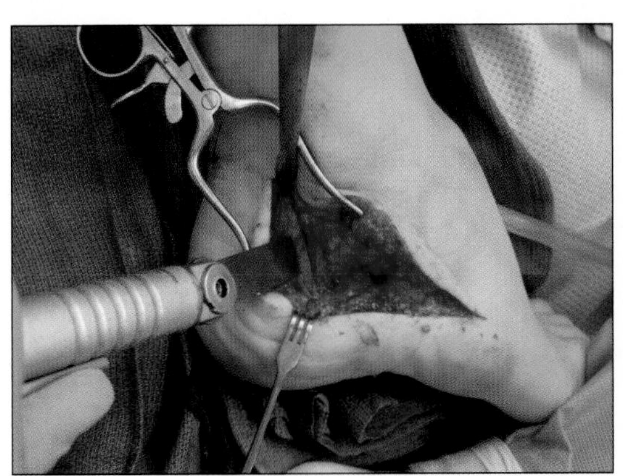

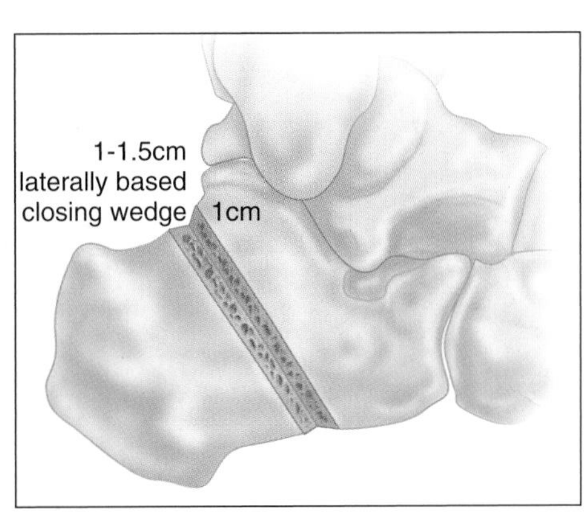

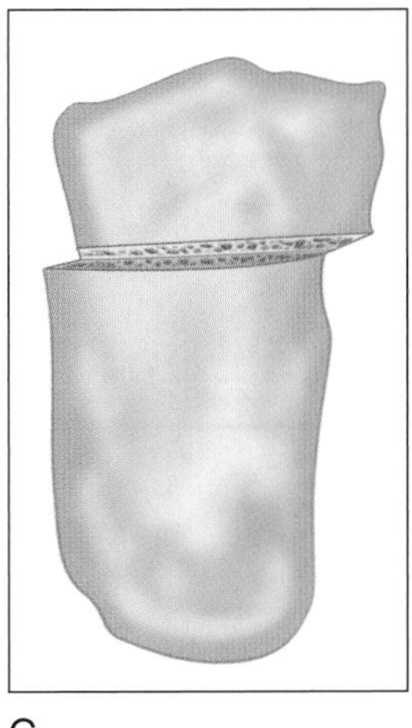

A B C

FIGURE 16

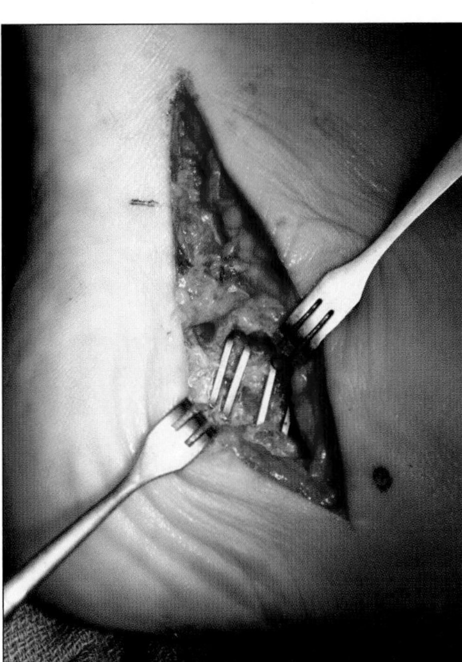

FIGURE 17

PITFALLS

- *A simple lateral displacement osteotomy of the tuberosity is rarely sufficient. Either a Dwyer or a triplane osteotomy is almost always needed in patients with CMT deformity.*

- Many patients require correction of both heel varus and a high calcaneal pitch angle (hindfoot cavus) by a triplane osteotomy. In such a case, continue the cut through the medial cortex, being very careful not to damage the neurovascular bundle.
  - Carefully make the distal cut of the osteotomy first, as there are several structures at risk anteriorly (peroneal tendons, neurovascular bundle, and subtalar joint). The second cut is made posterior and parallel to the first, removing the appropriate amount of bone (usually 7–10 mm).

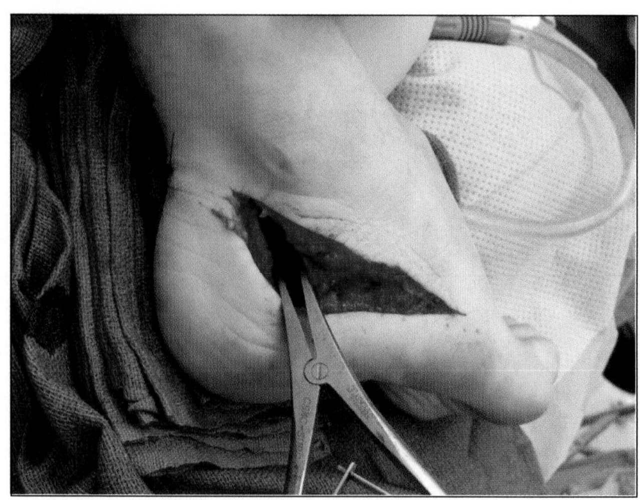
FIGURE 18

- Gently widen the osteotomy with a lamina spreader to facilitate displacement of the tuberosity (Fig. 18). The medial nerves will not be stretched by this maneuver.
- Displace the osteotomy approximately 1 cm superiorly and 1 cm laterally, to centralize the weight-bearing axis of the heel.
- Close the osteotomy laterally and hold it with one or two fluoroscopically placed 6.5- to 7.3-mm cannulated screws (Fig. 19A). One screw may be sufficient if good bone purchase is obtained (Fig. 19B).

- Use a reciprocating power rasp to smooth down the lateral wall of the calcaneus (Fig. 20).

Step 2

- If a peroneal tendon transfer is planned, extend the incision over the peroneals, as noted above (Fig. 21). Use the skin marker to note the resting length of both tendons, which will help place the longus at the appropriate resting length. Protect the sural nerve that crosses obliquely.
- Divide the peroneus longus as it passes beneath the cuboid. Use a Pulvertaft weave to transfer the longus into the distal most aspect of the brevis. Three weaves of the tendon create a very strong transfer. Use 3-0 Ethibond suture to secure the transfer (Fig. 22). The fibrous tunnel of the distal peroneal sheath may have to be removed, and the trochlear process smoothed down, to facilitate unobstructed motion of the transfer.
- If a midfoot osteotomy is not required, the wound is irrigated and closed in layers, using an absorbable subcutaneous suture and alternating horizontal mattress and simple 3-0 nylon sutures in the skin.

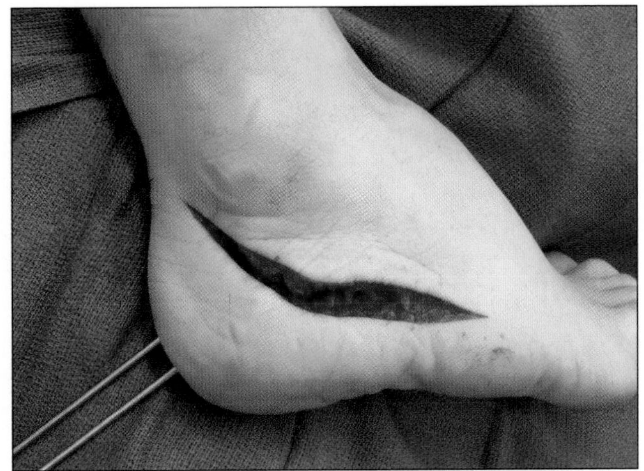

A

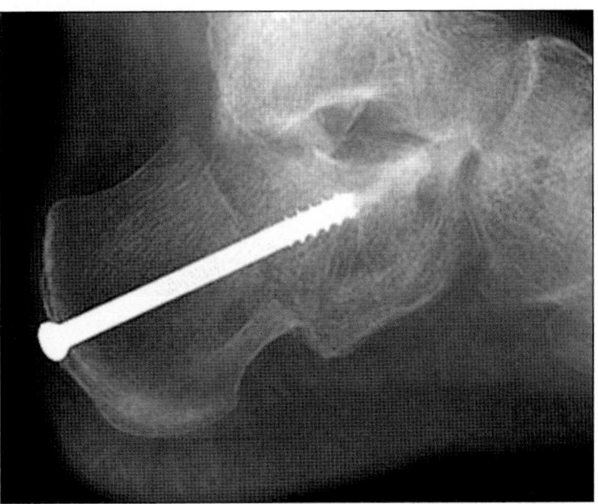

B

FIGURE 19

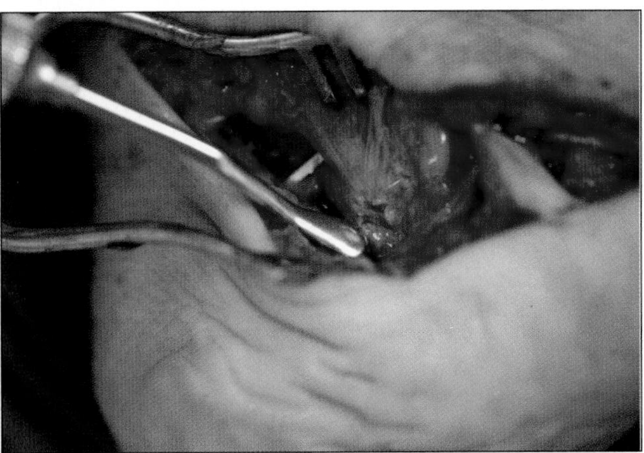

FIGURE 20

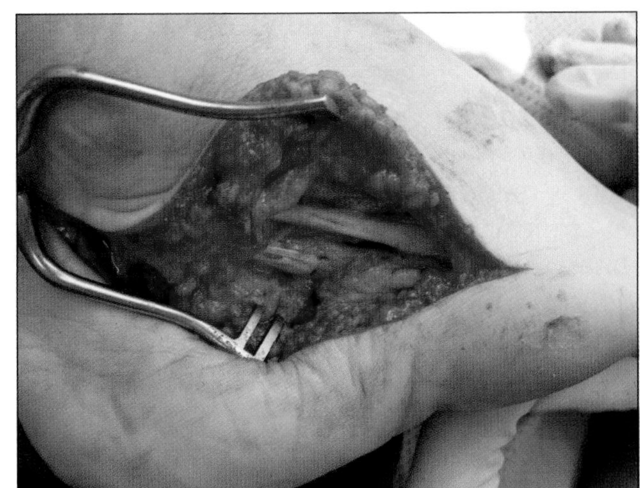

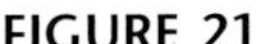

FIGURE 21

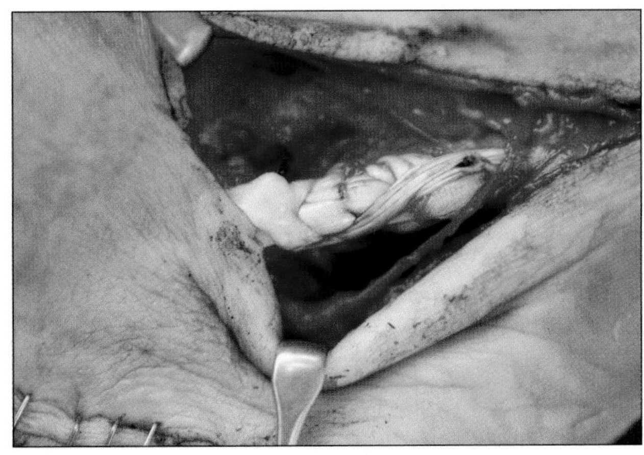

FIGURE 22

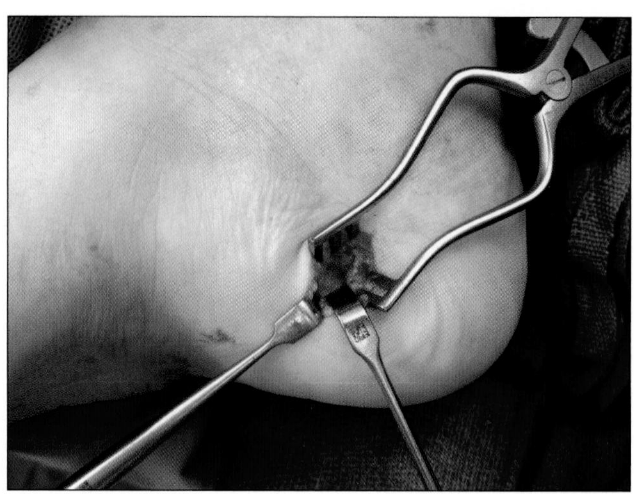

FIGURE 23

PITFALLS

- *Stay close to the calcaneus to avoid inadvertent injury to the lateral plantar nerve.*

STEP 3

- Remove the beanbag and place the patient into a supine position with the foot slightly externally rotated.
- Make a 3-cm oblique incision over the medial heel where the plantar fascia attaches. This incision will avoid the medial calcaneal nerve branch, which is easily injured with a longitudinal incision.
- Divide the superficial abductor fascia and strip the abductor muscle and its deep fascia from their attachments on the medial calcaneus (Fig. 23). Avoid injury to the first branch of the lateral plantar nerve, which runs deep to the abductor.
- Locate the medial edge of the plantar fascia and divide the fascia with a small tenotomy scissors, pushing from medial to lateral. Use a small key elevator to strip the calcaneal attachments of the plantar intrinsic muscles.
- Irrigate and close the skin with simple nylon sutures.

PEARLS

- *Occasionally, an osteotomy of the second metatarsal will be required (approximately 25% of cases). If two osteotomies are anticipated, base the initial incision more laterally, between the metatarsals. If more than two basilar osteotomies are needed, a better correction will be obtained with a midfoot osteotomy (see below). A midfoot osteotomy will also facilitate the correction of an adduction deformity.*

STEP 4

- Most frequently, the forefoot cavus (valgus) can be corrected with a closing wedge osteotomy at the base of the first metatarsal.
  - Make a 4-cm incision based over the base of the first metatarsal (Fig. 24). Identify the extensor hallucis longus and retract it laterally.
  - Identify the first metatarsal–cuneiform joint and, with a micro-sagittal saw, make a cut in the metatarsal 1.5 cm distal and parallel to the joint (Fig. 25A and 25B). Irrigate with cool water lavage when using the power saw. During the cut, place slight plantar pressure on the distal metatarsal, which will start to hinge open the osteotomy prior

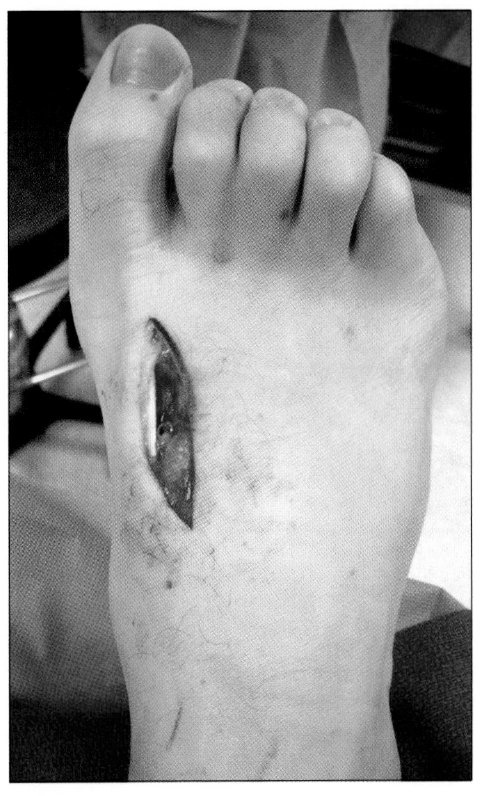

FIGURE 24

to completion of the cut. It is essential to leave the plantar cortex intact.

- Make a second oblique cut several millimeters distal to the first cut (see Fig. 25B). Only a small amount of bone (3–5 mm) must be removed because of the bone loss that occurs from the saw blade.

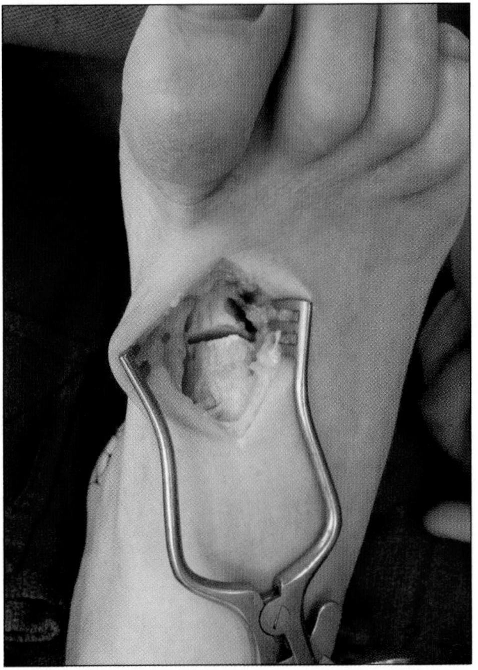

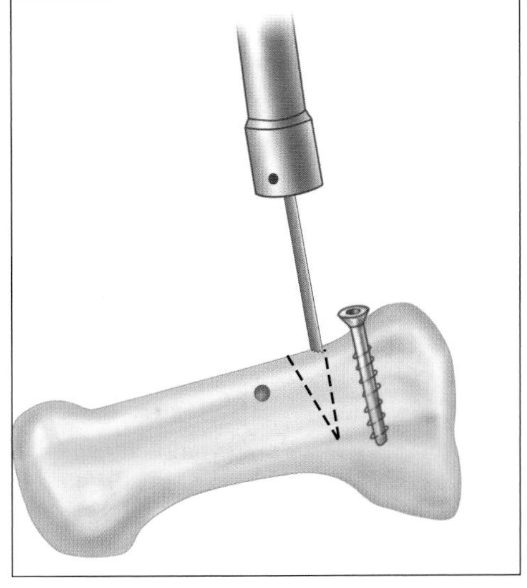

FIGURE 25 A B

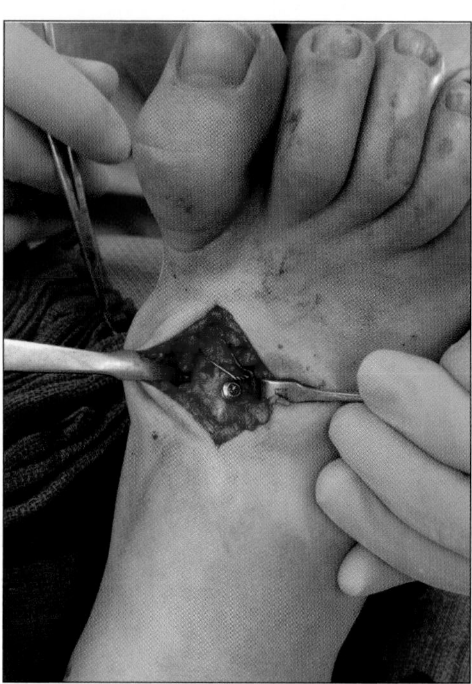

FIGURE 26

- Place a 4.0 partially threaded screw into the proximal fragment (see Fig. 25B). Do not seat it completely.
- Use a 0.062-inch Kirschner wire (K-wire) or comparable drill to make a transverse hole 1 cm distal to the osteotomy, just dorsal to the longitudinal axis of the metatarsal (see Fig. 25B). Pass a 22-gauge wire through the hole from medial to lateral. Use a small hemostat to grab the wire in the first metatarsal space. Place the wire in a figure-of-8 configuration around the screw head. Using a partially threaded screw allows the wire to seat securely beneath the screw head.
- Carefully close the osteotomy, tighten the wire, and advance the screw (Fig. 26). Do not overtighten the screw, which can cause the wire to break. Carefully examine the transverse alignment of the metatarsal heads. Repeat a similar osteotomy on additional metatarsals, as needed.

Step 5

- If the apex of the sagittal foot deformity is in the midfoot, the best correction is with a Cole osteotomy through the navicular-cuneiform joints medially and the cuboid laterally.
    - This truncated closing wedge osteotomy provides excellent multiplanar correction of the deformity. It also places the incisions on either side of the foot, away from the multiple dorsal incisions that may be needed to correct claw toes.

Pearls

- *If only the medial ray is involved, a closing wedge osteotomy of the medial cuneiform may be sufficient.*
- *Small plates can also be used to secure the Cole midfoot osteotomy, although they tend to be bulkier and are more likely to require removal in the future.*

Controversies

- Some surgeons are concerned about the rate of nonunion from this osteotomy. The broad cancellous surfaces, however, have little trouble healing.
- Others are concerned about potential arthritis of the adjacent joints because of inadvertent injury during the osteotomy cuts. Careful placement of the K-wires under fluoroscopic guidance completely avoids this potential complication. The decrease of motion that results from fusion of the navicular-cuneiform joints is insignificant.

  - This osteotomy should be used if more than two metatarsals require an osteotomy, or an adduction of the midfoot needs correction.
- The lateral incision should be extended over the longitudinal axis of the cuboid. Medially, an incision is made over the navicular-cuneiform joint, in the plane between the tibialis posterior and tibialis anterior tendons. Protect both of these tendons, particularly the tibialis anterior, which is vulnerable during the saw cuts.
- Under fluoroscopic guidance, place two 0.062-inch K-wires approximately 1.5 cm apart, from medial to lateral (Fig. 27A).
  - The pin placement is oblique, as the cuboid is inferior to the medial navicular-cuneiform joint.
  - The more distal pin passes through the medial cuneiform and exits through the distal cuboid; the more proximal pin passes medially across the navicular and exits through the proximal cuboid (Fig. 27B and 27C).
  - Avoid penetration of the fourth and fifth metatarsal–cuboid joints.
- Using blunt dissection and a small key elevator, completely dissect the soft tissue envelope around the bone of the midfoot. Protect the neurovascular structures dorsally and plantarly with small Hohmann retractors.

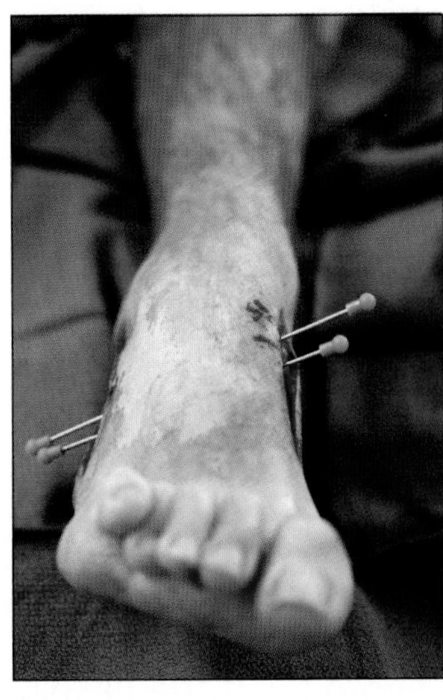

A

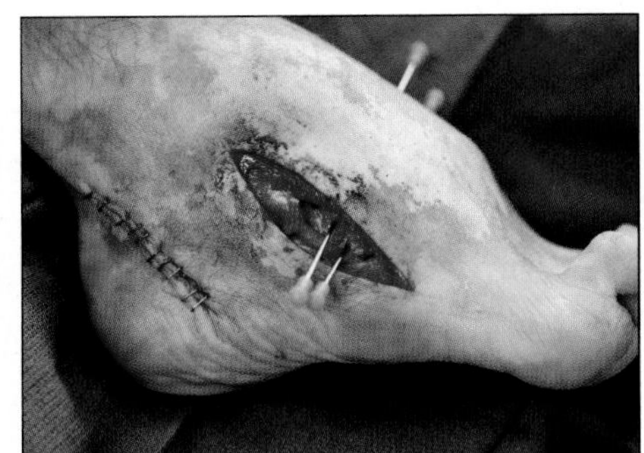

B

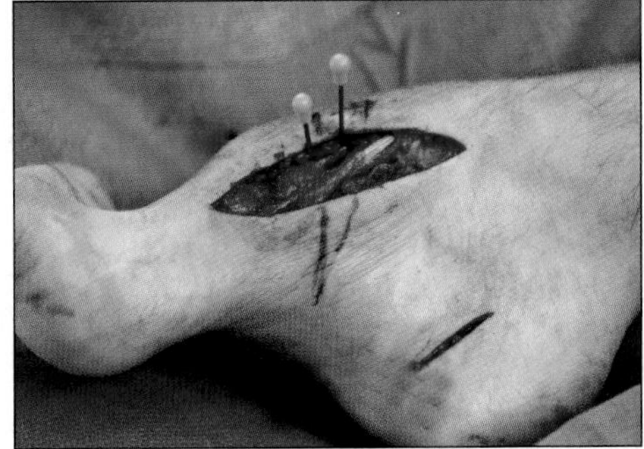

C

FIGURE 27

- Cut along the inside of each pin, removing a trapezoidal wedge of bone that includes the navicular-cuneiform joints (Fig. 28). Irrigate with cool saline lavage.
  - Make every effort to create flat cuts, without redirecting the saw blade. Imagine that the apex of the wedge is at the plantar fascia, which enables a trapezoidal piece of bone to be resected.
  - Adduction of the midfoot can be corrected with appropriately placed bone cuts.
  - Remove the K-wires.
- The forefoot can now be dorsiflexed and rotated into the correct position. Make sure that the transverse metatarsal arch is well aligned and that the forefoot valgus is corrected.
- Place the two K-wires temporarily across the osteotomy and place three 16-mm × 20-mm 3M power staples across the osteotomy sites both medially and laterally. Excellent fixation can be obtained in this manner (Fig. 29).
- Deflate the tourniquet. Obtain hemostasis and close the wounds in two layers, with alternating 3-0 nylon horizontal mattress and simple sutures in the skin.

Step 6

- Claw toes should be corrected using standard techniques that involve resection of the distal aspect of the proximal phalanx (see Procedure 7). The extensor digitorum longus tendon of each toe is transferred to the distal metatarsal using a deep periosteal stitch (Fig. 30). A small drill hole in the bone can be used, but is time consuming and probably unnecessary, given that the foot will be immobilized for at least 6 weeks in neutral position.
- If clawing of the great toe is present, the interphalangeal joint should be fused through a transverse incision. The extensor hallucis longus is transferred into the distal metatarsal through a transverse drill hole.
- Correction of the forefoot deformity, by either metatarsal or midfoot osteotomy, can create extrinsic flexor tightness, especially in the lesser toes. Even after the clawing is corrected, hyperflexion of the toe may persist. A closed or open tenotomy of the flexor digitorum longus to the toe will correct this problem (Fig. 31).

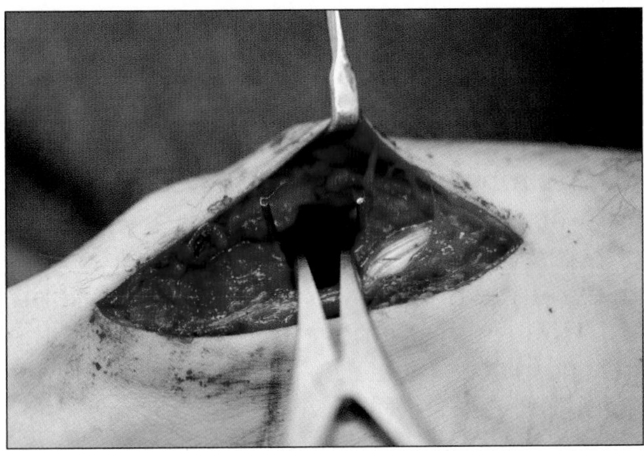

FIGURE 28

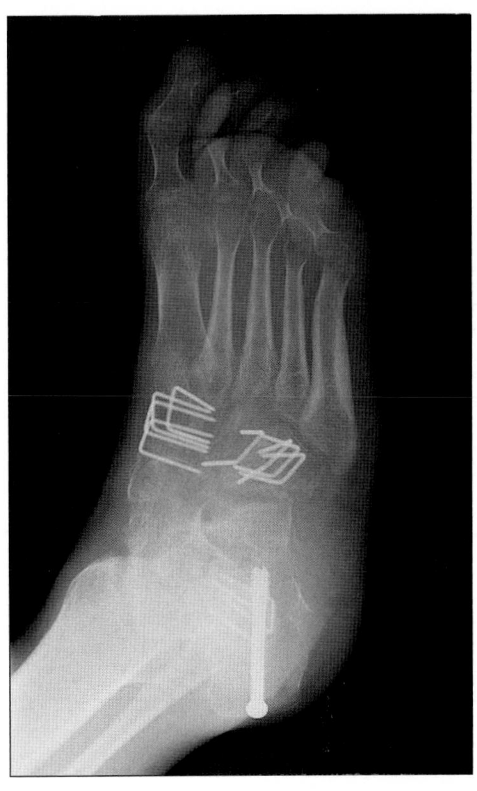

FIGURE 29

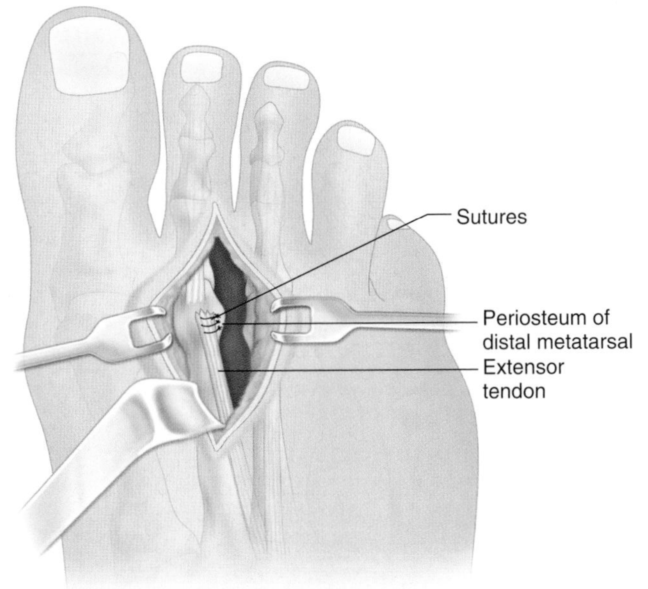

FIGURE 30

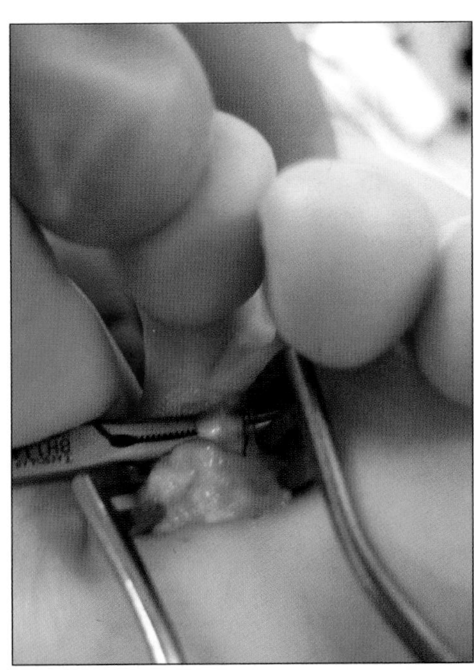

FIGURE 31

Postoperative Care and Expected Outcomes

- A bulky dressing and a three-sided splint are applied in the operating room after all of the osteotomies are checked for a final time by fluoroscan.
- The patent returns to the office 10–12 days after surgery for the placement of a short-leg non–weight-bearing cast. Sutures are removed at this point, if the wounds are completely healed. Anteroposterior (Fig. 32A) and lateral (Fig. 32B) radiographs are taken in the cast.
- Six weeks after surgery, the cast is removed and radiographs are taken. An additional short-leg, nonremovable cast is applied. The patient can start weight bearing as tolerated. This second cast is removed at 10 weeks postoperatively. Physical therapy should be started at this point, along with appropriate shoewear.

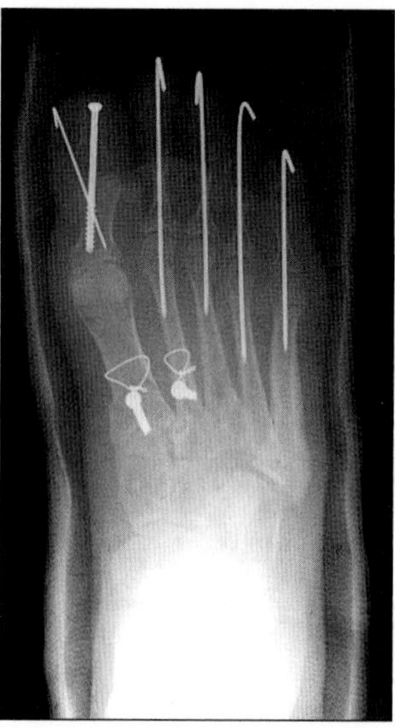

A

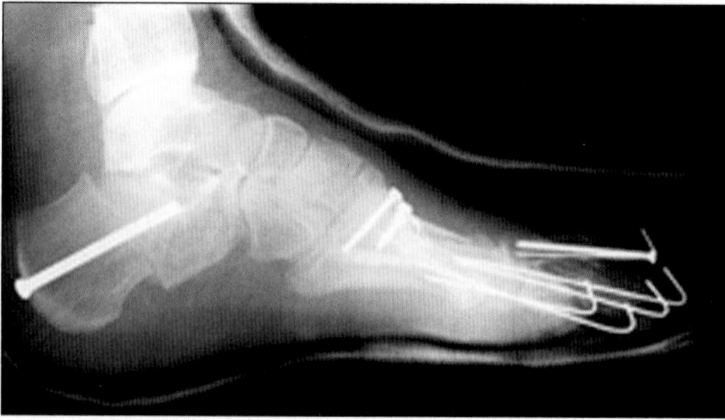

B

FIGURE 32

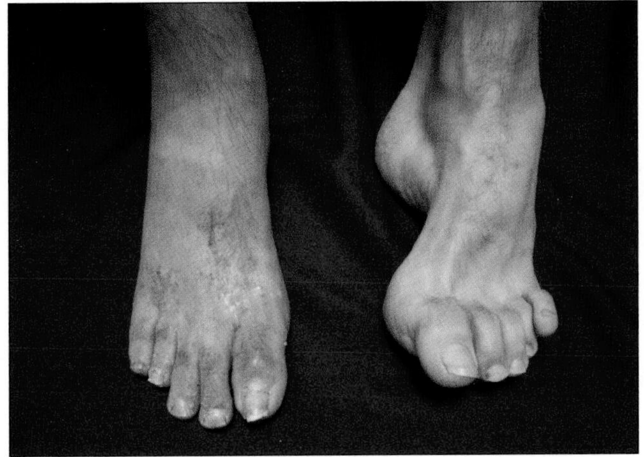
A

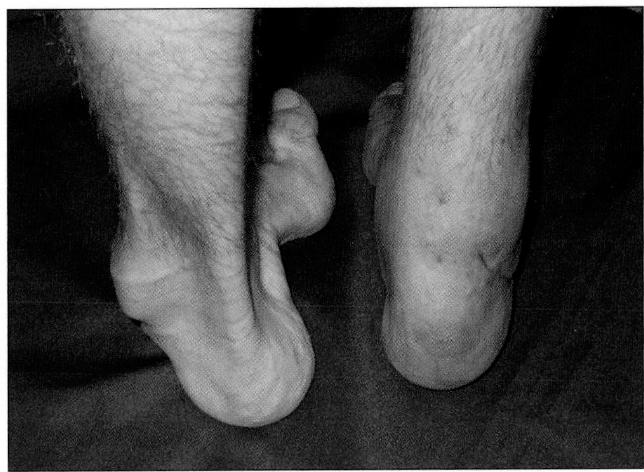
B

FIGURE 33

- An excellent and enduring correction of the deformity can be expected (Fig. 33A and 33B). The right foot has had surgery.

Evidence

Cole WH. The treatment of claw-foot. J Bone Joint Surg [Am]. 1940;22:895-905.

Original description of the Cole osteotomy for midfoot cavus. (Level V evidence)

Guyton GP. Current concepts review: orthopaedic aspects of Charcot-Marie-Tooth disease. Foot Ankle Int. 2006;27:1003-10.

An excellent review of the topic and the literature.

Mann RA, Missirian J. Pathophysiology of Charcot-Marie-Tooth disease. Clin Orthop Relat Res. 1988;(234):221-8.

This paper examines CMT deformity and the contribution of muscle imbalance. (Level V evidence)

Nagel MK, Chan G, Guille JT. Prevalence of Charcot-Marie Tooth disease in patients who have bilateral cavovarus feet. J Pediatr Orthop. 2006;26:438-43.

Seventy-eight percent of children with "idiopathic" cavovarus feet were diagnosed with CMT disease by neurophysiologic and genetic testing. (Level IV evidence)

Paulos L, Colemann SS, Samuelson KM. Pes cavovarus: review of surgical approach using selective soft-tissue procedures. J Bone Joint Surg [Am]. 1980;62:942-53.

Review of 39 feet in children with cavovarus deformity. The use of the Coleman block test to distinguish forefoot-driven heel varus is described. (Level IV evidence)

PROCEDURE 18

Charcot Neuroarthropathy of the Midfoot/Hindfoot

Lew C. Schon and Su-Young Bae

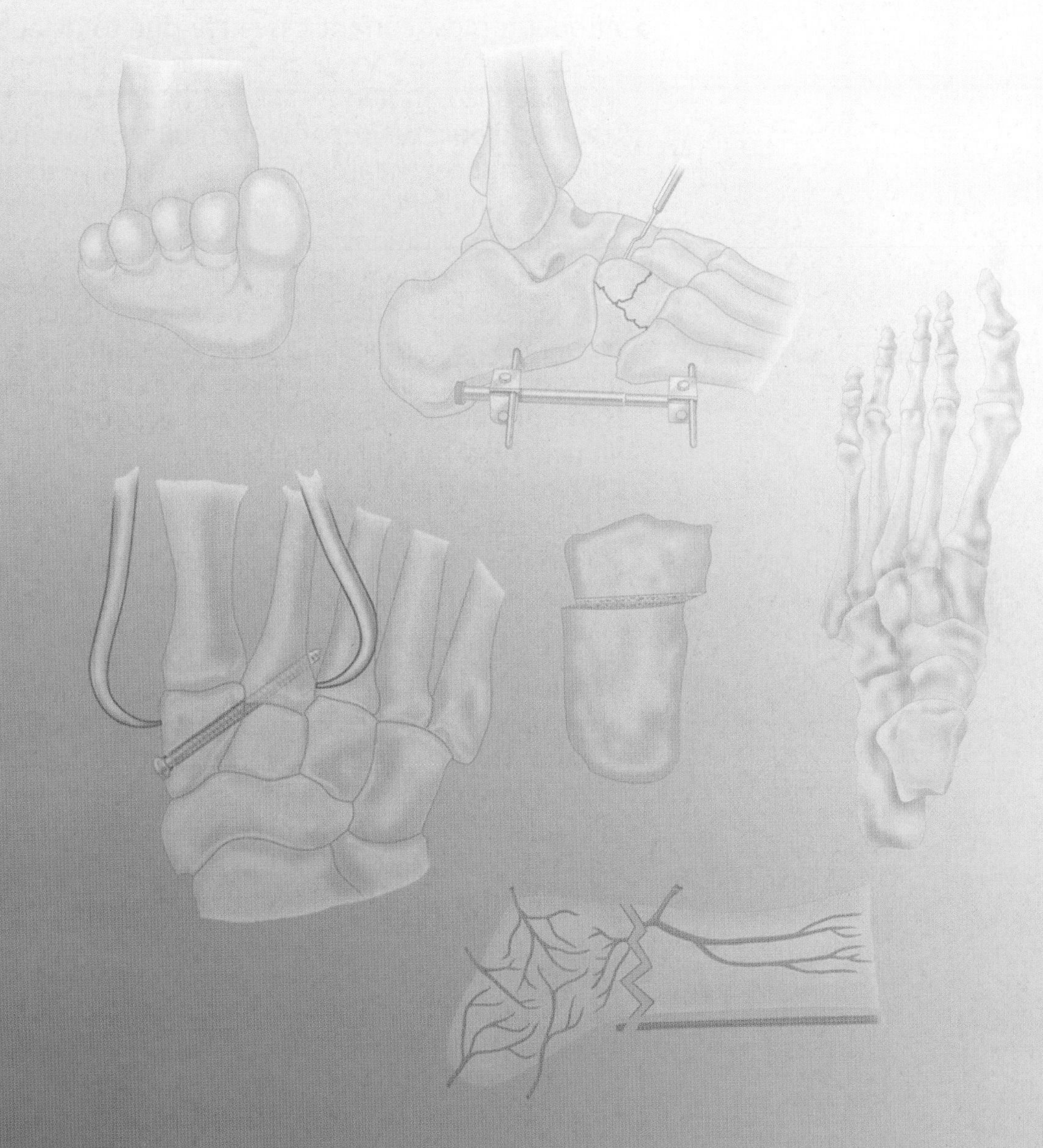

Midfoot Osteotomy and Arthrodesis Using Internal Fixation and External Fixation

Charcot Neuroarthropathy

Definition

- Charcot described neuroarthropathic arthropathy typically due to syphilis in the late 1880s.
- Although most current cases are due to diabetes, 20–30% of cases occur as a result of other neuropathic conditions: alcohol neuropathy, rheumatologic neuropathy, hereditary neuropathy, steroid-induced neuropathy, spinal injury, spinal tumor, spina bifida (syringomyelia), and many coexisting conditions.
- Refers to aggressive destruction of the bones and joints as a result of repetitive microtrauma, recognized or unrecognized acute trauma, arthritis or avascular necrosis. Often there is an inciting event that goes unrecognized, and the destructive process is magnified by repetitive trauma.
- Charcot neuroarthropathy:
  - May present in an acute or chronic fashion.
  - Can involve any portion of the foot and ankle.
  - Can lead to severe deformities with risk for ulcers and infection and possibly osteomyelitis.

Pathogenesis

- Neuropathic patients have either acute trauma (fracture, ligament injury, tendon disruption or dislocation) or repetitive microtrauma or spontaneous avascular necrosis of either the navicular or the talus. Arthritis may also be a precursor by triggering inflammation or destruction that may also lead to Charcot collapse.
- The situation that begins as above is compounded by the patient's activity coupled with lack of awareness that the foot is swelling, deforming, and the like.
- Often obesity will aggravate the situation by increasing the stresses to these vulnerable bones and joints.

Natural History

- Without mechanical relief for the foot and ankle, the bones and joints progressively become destroyed.
- The foot becomes deformed and unstable. The midfoot can develop a rocker-bottom deformity. There may be abduction or adduction of the forefoot or midfoot. The hindfoot may assume a varus or valgus deformity.
- Bony prominences occur at the apex of the deformities, and over fragmented, dislocated, or displaced bones.
- The hindfoot and midfoot joints collapse, leading to equinus of the talus in the ankle joint and relative dorsiflexion of the metatarsals or cuneiforms on the more proximal mid- or transverse tarsus.
- Progressive Achilles tendon contracture occurs.
- The foot contacts the shoe or ground with vulnerable bony prominences.
- These pressure areas become ulcerated.
- The ulcers lead to superficial and deep infection.
- Osteomyelitis and septic joints may develop.
- Uncontrolled infection leads to limb loss.

Indications

- Recurrent ulcer
- Deep infection
- Instability
- Severe malalignment
- Unbraceable deformity
- Inability to wear shoes

Examination/Imaging

Physical Findings

- Acute
  - Swollen, warm, erythematous foot and ankle are seen.
  - Gross foot deformities include rocker-bottom foot, severe abduction and pronation, or less often adduction and supination.
  - Deformity can be flexible and unstable.
  - Equinus contracture may occur.
  - Bony prominences occur at the apex of deformities.
  - Ulcers manifest over the prominences.

- Chronic
  - Deformities include rocker-bottom foot (Fig. 1A) and severe abduction, adduction, supination, and/or pronation (Fig. 1B).
  - Deformities are not reducible.
  - If destruction occurs through fracture, the deformity can be stiff and stable.
  - If the deformity is through a dislocation, the deformity can be unstable.
  - Additional findings include:
    - Mild swelling
    - Mild warmth
    - Mild to no erythema
  - The foot tends to be thicker due to soft tissue and bony changes.

Physical Examination

- General
  - Evaluate the patient for systemic infection.
  - Peripheral vascular status should be assessed; check pulses.
  - Cardiac/renal/pulmonary function may be impaired.
- Local
  - Charcot type: location—which joints are involved
  - Charcot stage: clinical severity of deformity
  - Charcot phase (Eichenholtz): acute, subacute, chronic
  - Neuropathy: decrease in two-point discrimination; decrease in sensitivity to light touch, vibration, and temperature
  - Ischemia
    - Dorsalis pedis and posterior tibialis pulses may be decreased. Perform a side-to-side comparison.
    - Additional signs and symptoms include: cool foot, painful ulcer, gray base, eschars, odor, weak or absent pulses
  - Depth of ulcer and infection
  - Rule out
    - Deep venous thrombosis
    - Osteomyelitis (probe to bone)

Radiographs

- Acute Charcot neuroarthropathy
  - Subluxation, dislocation, and/or fracture of any part of the midfoot and hindfoot may not be distinguishable from normal acute trauma.
- Chronic Charcot neuroarthropathy
  - Deformity: resulting from fracture and/or dislocation

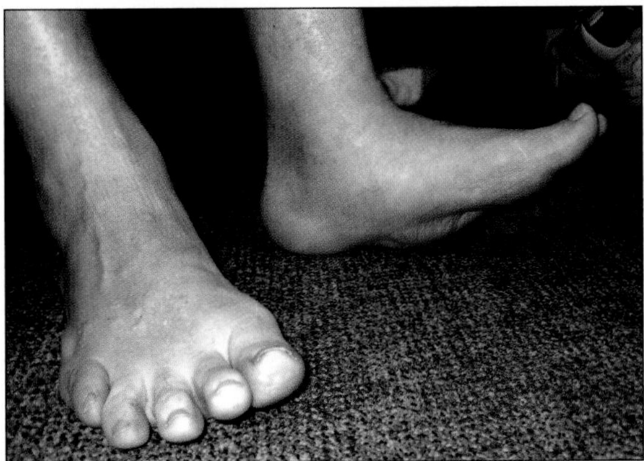
A

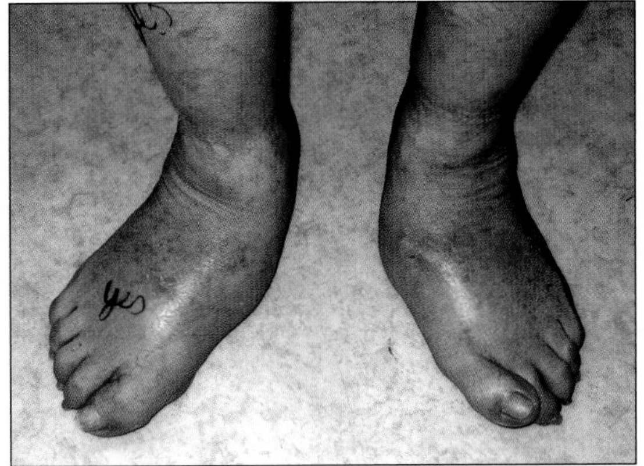
B

FIGURE 1

- Hypertrophic arthritis
- Avascular changes to bone with sclerosis and fragmentation, deformity (loss of normal shape)
- Consolidation of bone fragmentation
- Zones of radiodensity with bone remodeling
- Joint subluxation/dislocation
- Bone fractures with hypertrophic malunions and nonunions

Location of Charcot Process

- Forefoot: metatarsal heads, toes
- Midtarsus
  - Common location; involves complex pattern types described in midfoot classification below.
  - Figure 2A and 2B illustrate a type I deformity with abduction and collapse of the arch occurring at the metatarsal-cuneiform joints medially and the fourth and fifth metatarsal-cuboid joints laterally.
- Peritalar region: avascular necrosis of talus, subtalar destruction results in varus/valgus of hindfoot

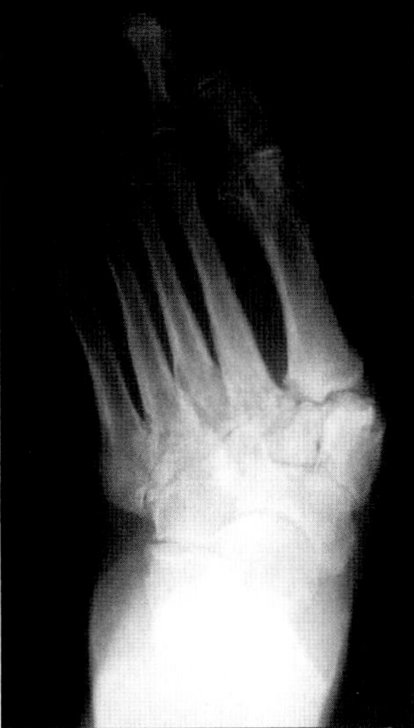
A

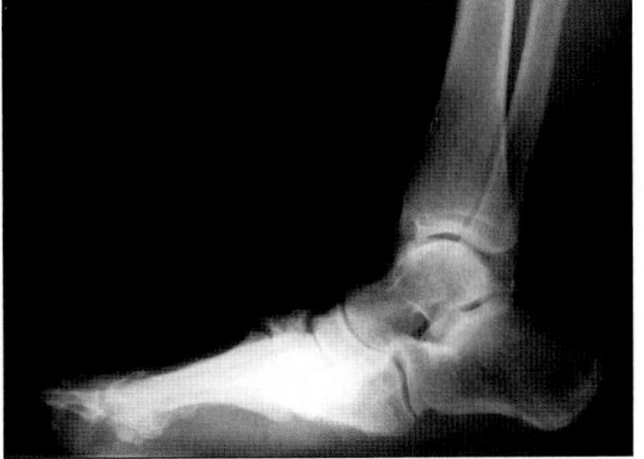
B

FIGURE 2

- Calcaneus: avulsion fracture of posterior tuberosity
- Ankle: fracture, destructive arthritis, avascular necrosis of distal tibia
- Tibia

Pitfalls

- *A swollen, warm Charcot foot in a patient with glucose control problems warrants further evaluation to rule out an occult foot infection. If there is a callus, ulcer, or eschar, débride it to potentially unroof an abscess. If there are no skin lesions, an abscess can be hidden in the deep fascial spaces in the arch or along tendons. In this situation, MRI or needle aspiration can reveal an abscess.*

Treatment Options

- Postoperative shoe for toe ulcers or forefoot plantar ulcers (add unloading orthotic device)
- Ankle-foot orthosis (AFO) for stability and to accommodate deformity
- Débridement of ulcer
- Casting for nonhealing ulcer, acute or subacute phase of Charcot neuroarthropathy, unbraceable or unshoeable deformity
- Treatment of underlying Charcot neuroarthropathy
  - Immobilization
  - Crutches, walkers, and wheelchairs to off-load foot and ankle
- Maintenance of stable, ulcer-free foot
  - Shoewear adaptations
  - Accommodative insoles
  - Custom-molded AFO or Charcot rocker orthotic walker
  - Double metal upright AFO with shoe with steel shank and rocker sole; consider Steven Craig modification for added strength (additional L-shaped bracket supports metal upright–to–shoe caliper connection)

Differential Diagnosis: Infection Versus Charcot Neuroarthropathy

- Assess the ulcer.
  - Neuropathic ulceration: result of repetitive pressure
    - Pink-based ulcer
    - Warm foot with pulses
    - Not typically painful
  - Vascular ulcer (result of ischemia)
    - Gray, yellow-based ulcer or eschar
    - Cool foot with decreased pulse
    - Can be painful
- Probe the wound: osteomyelitis is diagnosed if bone is felt at the base of the ulcer.
- Palpate for deep abscess; if uncertain, aspirate the area, avoiding if possible a cellulitic or grossly infected entry point.
- Look for signs of spreading infection.
  - Cellulites: warm, red, swollen with tenderness and streaking
  - Systemic: fever, chills, malaise, nausea, vomiting, confusion, elevated blood glucose, white blood cell count with shift, erythrocyte sedimentation rate, C-reactive protein
- Elevation test: when the foot is elevated, the erythema in a Charcot neuroarthropathy will decrease, which does not occur with infection.
- Mechanical test: as with elevation, off-loading, resting, bracing, or casting will decrease the swelling, redness, and warmth associated with a Charcot neuroarthropathy, but not with infection.
- Radiologic clues of infection include more osteolysis (large ovoid shape), bone erosions, fluffy periosteal changes, and gas in soft tissues.
- Bone scan: when in doubt, get a scan.
  - Uptake on technetium-99m and indium-111 scans in osteomyelitis.
  - Technetium-99m sulfur colloid scan shows uptake on white blood cell count with none on marrow test in osteomyelitis.
  - Technetium-99m–HMPAO (Ceretec) may be useful.
- Magnetic resonance imaging (MRI): marrow changes and bony destruction with infection are the same as with Charcot neuroarthropathy; particularly useful to look for soft tissue abscess.

Surgical Anatomy

- Bony anatomy
  - Metatarsal-cuneiform joints make up the arch of the foot and are vulnerable to destruction in Charcot neuroarthropathy.
  - The second metatarsal-cuneiform joint is recessed relative to the first and the third metatarsocuneiform joint.
  - The fourth and fifth metatarsal-cuboid joints have more mobility than the first, second, and third metatarsal-cuneiform joints.
  - The three cuneiforms are wedge-shaped bones between the navicular and the medial three metatarsals.
  - The talonavicular and calcaneocuboid joints are responsible for inversion and eversion of the foot in conjunction with the subtalar joint and also are often involved in the Charcot process.
- Soft tissue anatomy
  - The anterior tibialis tendon inserts on the medial cuneiform.
  - The peroneus brevis inserts on the fifth metatarsal tuberosity.
  - The abductor hallucis takes origin along the navicular, medial cuneiform, and first metatarsal medially.
  - The posterior tibialis tendon inserts on the navicular medially.
  - The dorsalis pedis artery is dorsal to the second metatarsal-cuneiform joint.
  - The medial and lateral plantar nerves run under the mid-tarsus. When the bones have dislocated or deformed, these nerves are compromised by being compressed between the plantar prominence and the floor during standing or walking.
  - The deep peroneal nerve and the superficial peroneal nerve run dorsal to the medial and middle cuneiforms.

Classification of Midfoot Charcot Neuroarthropathy (Fig. 3A and 3B)*

- Deformity types
  - Type I: deformity at the metatarsal-cuneiform joints medially and the fourth and fifth metatarsal-cuboid joints laterally.
  - Type II: deformity at the navicular-cuneiform joint medially and the fourth and fifth metatarsal-cuboid joints laterally.
  - Type III: major deformity in the perinavicular region, with prominence plantar centrally or plantar laterally.
  - Type IV: deformity at the transverse tarsal joints with variable prominences.
- The type I foot typically has abduction and plantar prominence under the medial cuneiform.
- The type II foot typically has a plantar lateral prominence under the cuboid.
- The type III foot typically has a prominence under the cuboid or fifth metatarsal and may be supinated and adducted.
- The type IV foot will often have pronation and plantar prominence under the naviculum and the distal plantar calcaneus.

*Figure 3A and 3B are modified with permission from Schon LC, Weinfeld SB, Horton GA, Resch S. Radiographic and clinical classification of acquired midtarsus deformities. Foot Ankle Int. 1998;19:394-404. Copyright © 2008 by the American Orthopaedic Foot and Ankle Society, Inc.

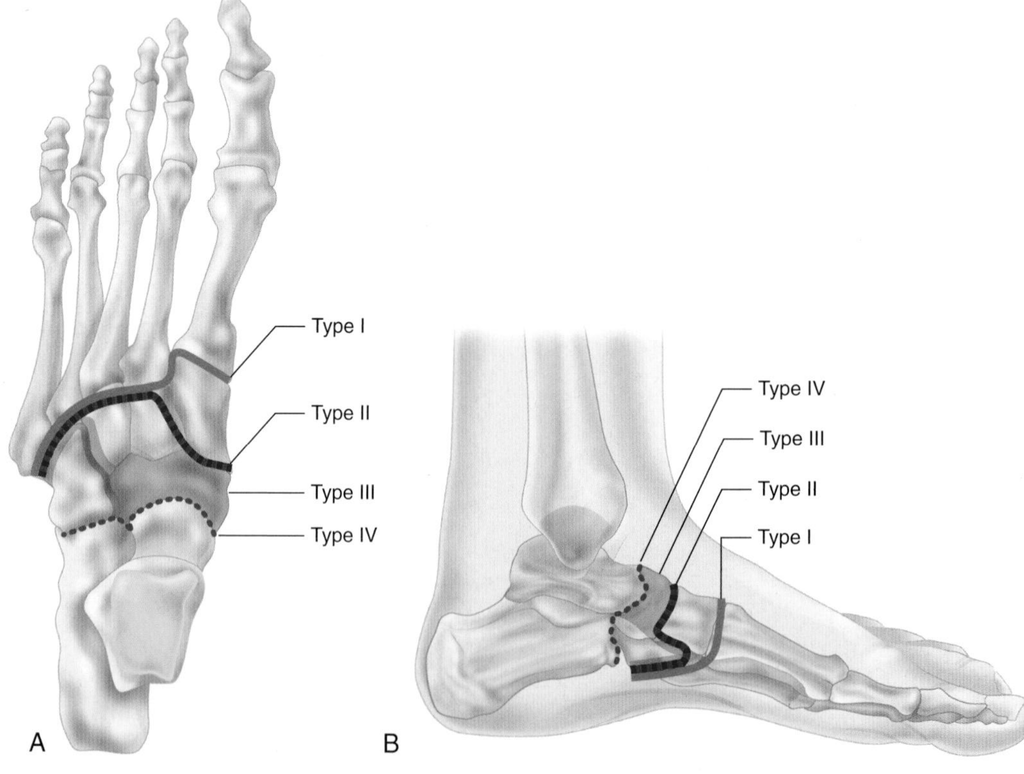

FIGURE 3

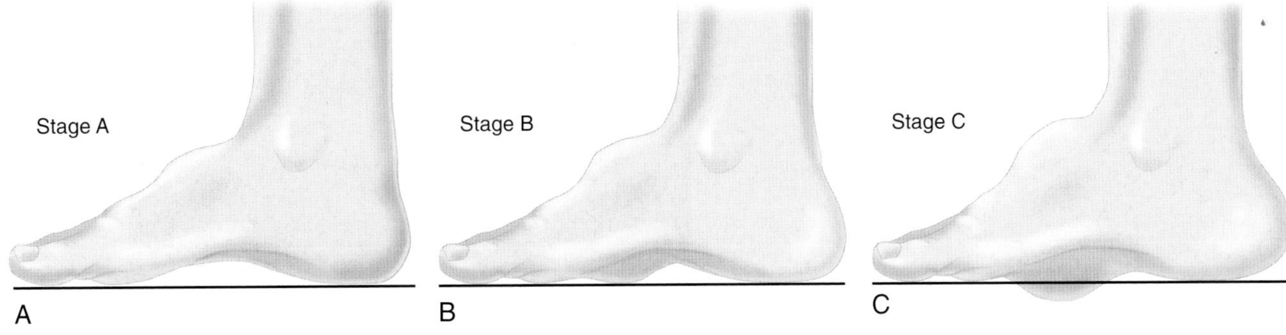

FIGURE 4

PEARLS

- *Stage A feet have a high success rate with nonoperative treatment, whereas Stage C feet have a very high incidence of ulcers, infections, and osteomyelitis and difficulty with modified shoes and braces. Therefore, Stage C feet often require surgical reconstruction.*
- *Stage B feet are a challenge, but with great effort and compliance can have successful nonoperative treatment.*

Clinical Staging Based on Severity of the Deformity

- The clinical severity of the rocker-bottom deformity can be assessed to help determine prognosis (Fig. 4).
  - Stage A: midtarsus is above the metatarsal-calcaneal plane.
  - Stage B: midtarsus is co-planar with the metatarsal-calcaneal plane (mild to moderate rocker bottom).
  - Stage C: midtarsus is below the metatarsal-calcaneal plane (severe rocker bottom).

Portals/Exposures

- A curvilinear incision is made along the plantar margin of the medial bony prominence of the midfoot Charcot deformity (Fig. 5). Full-thickness skin flaps are preserved, and the deep dissection proceeds to the fascia of the abductor hallucis muscle.
- The muscle is retracted plantarly to identify the first metatarsal, medial cuneiform, and navicular or talus as needed (Fig. 6).

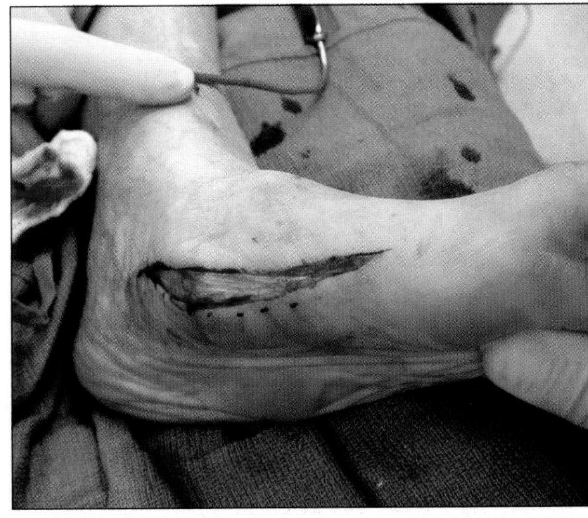

FIGURE 5

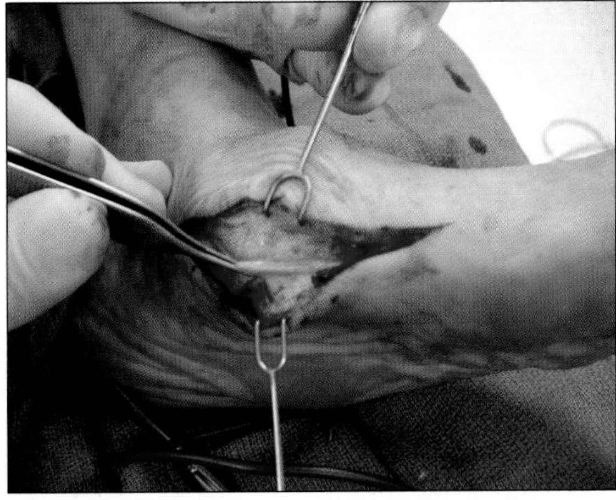

FIGURE 6

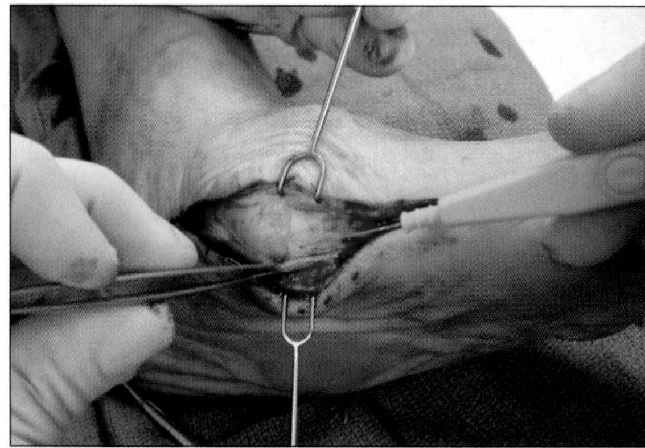

FIGURE 7

- The periosteum is incised and elevated longitudinally at the junction of the medial and plantar aspects of the medial ray using an electrocautery blade, and the plantar soft tissues are then dissected from the bone using a periosteal elevator across the midfoot (Fig. 7).
- The insertion of the anterior and posterior tibial tendons may be identified and preserved as part of the thick soft tissue sleeve, but complete detachment should be avoided.
- Sometimes a lateral incision may be used to expose the lateral rays, especially in the case of a dislocation of the fourth and fifth metatarsal-cuboid joints.
  - A lateral incision is made over the dorsal aspect of the fourth and fifth metatarsal-cuboid joints (Fig. 8; the metatarsal bases are on the left and the cuboid is seen proximally).
  - Through the dorsolateral exposure, the periosteal elevator is inserted into the fourth and fifth metatarsal-cuboid joints.

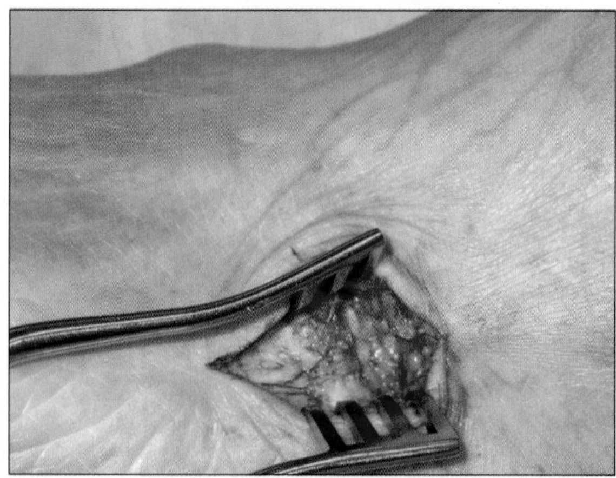

FIGURE 8

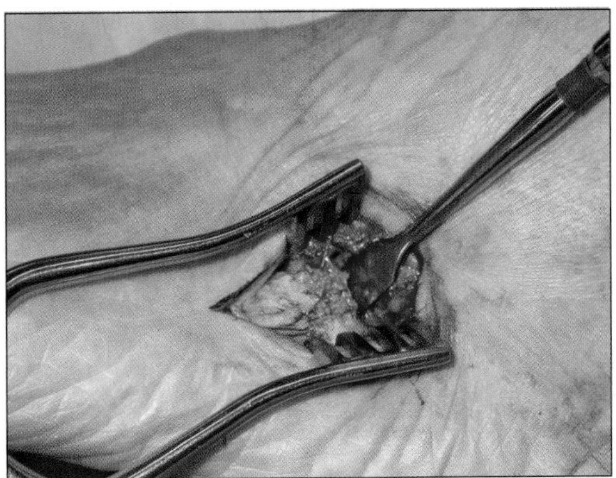

FIGURE 9

- The elevator is angled to go under the subluxed bases of the fourth and fifth metatarsals (Fig. 9; the metatarsal bases are on the left). Then the distal articular surface of the cuboid can be released and levered dorsally to reduce it from its plantar position.

Procedure

Preoperative Planning and Principles

- Consider Achilles lengthening.
- Identify the plane of the deformity.
- Use techniques including anatomic arthrodesis, derotational osteotomies, and closing wedge arthrodesis.
- Apply rigid fixation (screws, plates, external frames).

General Principles of Correction of the Midfoot Charcot Deformity

- Mild to moderate deformity: correction through anatomic midfoot fusion, resection of joint surfaces without wedge
  - No infection, no ulcer: internal fixation with plantar plate
  - Noninfected superficial ulcer or marginal infection (history of infection or suspicious infection): minimal internal fixation with screws and added external ring fixator as a neutralization frame
  - Active infection or deep ulcer: external frame only
- Severe deformity: correction though transpedal wedge resection
  - No infection, no ulcer: internal fixation with plantar plate ± screws

- Noninfected superficial ulcer or marginal infection: minimal internal fixation with screws and added external ring fixator as a neutralization frame
- Active infection or deep ulcer: external frame only

Step 1: Transpedal Wedge Resection

- The soft tissue envelope is protected during removal of the wedge of midtarsal bones and joints through the medial approach.
- The transpedal wedge is planned by using Kirschner wires (K-wires) across the apex of the deformity and checking the placement using the mini C-arm.
  - In Figure 10, the K-wires are seen at the bases of the metatarsals and the distal aspect of the cuneiforms and cuboid. This is the plane of the deformity in this type I foot.
  - The saw blade penetrates the bones within the boundary of the deformity to remove a medially based wedge.
  - In the sagittal plane, the wedge is trapezoidal with a wider plantar base to address the rocker-bottom deformity.
  - It is critical to save as much bone stock as possible at the bases of the metatarsals.
- The wedge of bone removed should be designed to correct the rocker-bottom and the abduction deformities.
  - If both are corrected, a plantar-based and medially based wedge of bone is removed.

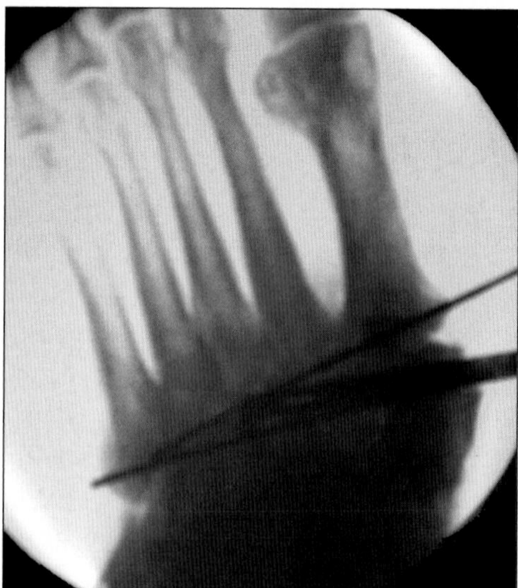

FIGURE 10

- If only a rocker-bottom deformity is corrected, a plantar-based wedge is removed.
- If there is an adduction deformity, then a laterally based wedge is planned.

- Figures 11–14 illustrate the transpedal wedge resection.
  - In this foot (also shown in Fig. 2) with a type I deformity, the saw is seen cutting the proximal aspect of the wedge with the blade positioned perpendicular to the hindfoot (Fig. 11).
  - The wedge is defined with a chisel in the proximal osteotomy and the saw blade detached from the handle in the distal cut (Fig. 12). The distal cut is made perpendicular to the axis of the forefoot. A trapezoidal wedge is removed to address the abduction and the rocker-bottom deformity.

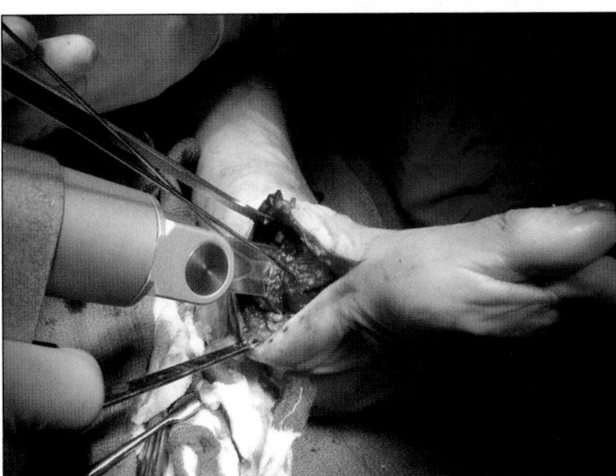

FIGURE 11

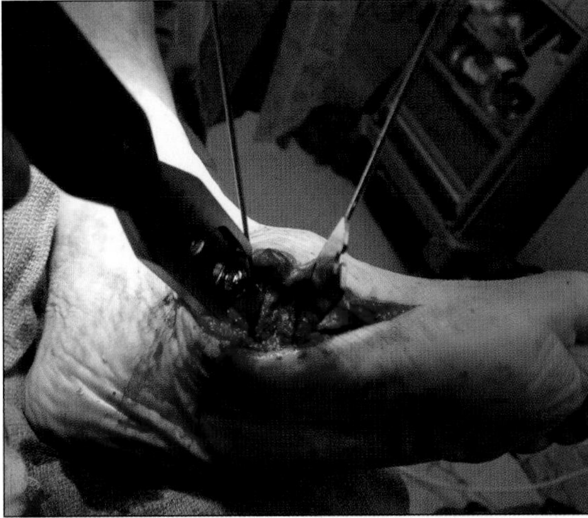

FIGURE 12

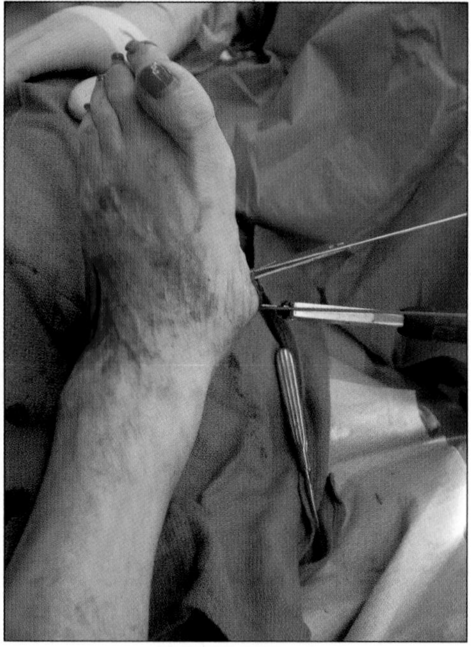

FIGURE 13

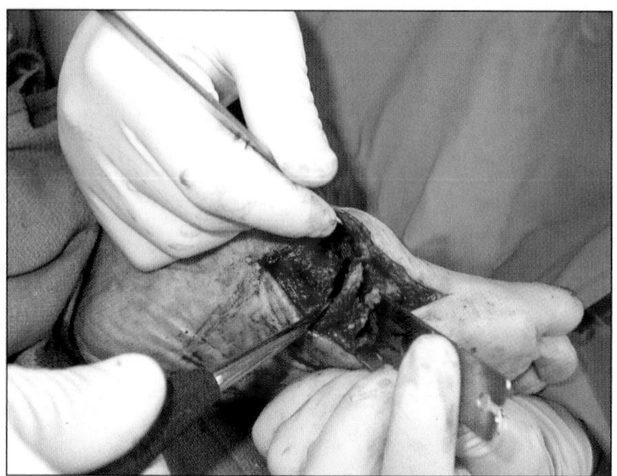

FIGURE 14

Pearls

- *Cannulated screws (6.5–8.0 mm) can be placed from the posterolateral aspect of the talus into the naviculum or cuneiforms when dealing with a type III or IV deformity. The guidewire is placed 2–4 cm dorsal to the dorsal aspect of the calcaneus, just lateral to the Achilles tendon, spreading the soft tissue to avoid the sural nerve. As long as the placement stays lateral to the midline, the risk to the tibial nerve is very low. Mini-fluoroscopic guidance is necessary.*
- *If a prior hallux amputation was performed, the 6.5- to 8.0-mm cannulated screws can be placed from the first metatarsal head into the medial cuneiform. If needed, these screws can run all the way to the talus.*

- In Figure 13, the wedge is seen from the dorsal perspective. Note the dorsolateral incision. The saw blade can be watched as it cuts the distal end of the cuboid, or the micro-sagittal saw can be used through the dorsal approach to complete the transpedal wedge.
- The wedge of bone, which includes the damaged articular surfaces, is removed (Fig. 14).

Step 2: Screw Insertion

- Each joint fused should be stabilized by one to two 4.0- to 5.0-mm cannulated or solid screws. Whenever possible, the screws should be nearly perpendicular to the surfaces.
- Medially, one screw is placed from the dorsomedial cortex of the first metatarsal shaft to the medial cuneiform or even into the navicular.
- We usually add the second screw plantar to the first screw but directed toward the second cuneiform.
- A third screw is inserted from the medial cuneiform or navicular toward the second metatarsal base; it may go further into the third metatarsal base.
- An additional screw may be used to fix the third metatarsal to the lateral cuneiform.

- The lateral two screws are inserted from the plantar lateral cortex of the fifth metatarsal toward the cuboid. The more distal of the two screws may start on the fifth metatarsal and go through the fourth metatarsal into the cuboid (Fig. 15).
- If the calcaneocuboid joint is to be fused, one or two 6.5-mm axial screw(s) from the calcaneal tuberosity to the cuboid and into the fourth metatarsal can be placed (Fig. 16A and 16B).

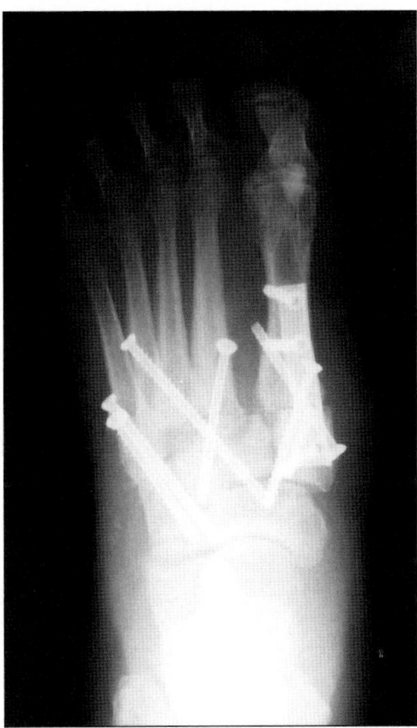

FIGURE 15

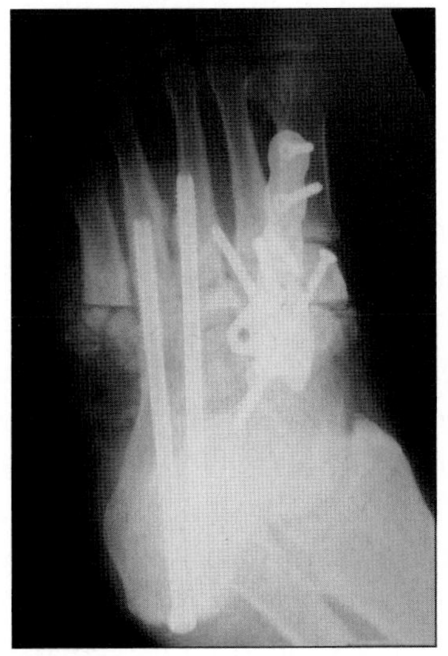

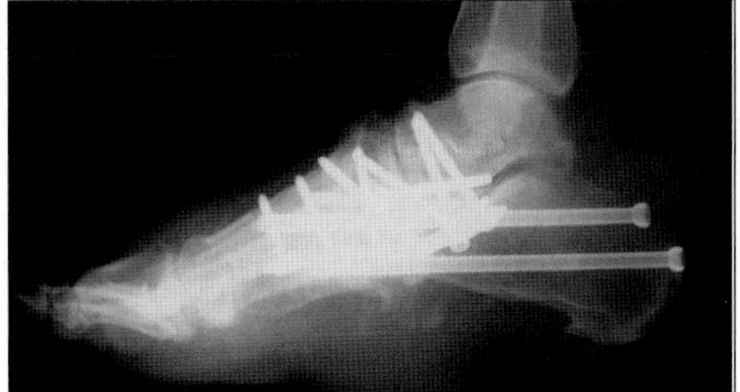

A B

FIGURE 16

Pearls

- *Although the semitubular plate is commonly used plantarly, if fixation is needed under the navicular and/or the talus, a plate that has a wider area for screw placement can be used. The Depuy humerus plate (nonlocking) is well suited for this application (see Fig. 16A and 16B).*

Step 3: Plate Application

- A plantar medial column plate can be applied under the joints to be fused. This plate is on the tension side of the construct, making it a very rigid means of fixation.
  - Typically in a type I deformity, the plate is placed under the medial cuneiform and under the first metatarsal. A four-hole small-fragment plate is used with two screws into the medial cuneiform and the other two into the first metatarsal (see Fig. 15).
  - In a type II deformity, the plate is placed under the medial cuneiform and medal pole of the naviculum.
  - In a type III deformity, the plate is placed under the head of the talus and under the remaining naviculum, ending under the medial cuneiform.
  - In a type IV deformity, the plate can be placed under the talus and navicular.
- At times it is necessary to span all the medial joints for stability (see Fig. 16A and 16B).
- Although the senior author has applied lateral plantar plates to the underside of the cuboid and fourth and/or fifth metatarsals, he has used a dorsal plate for the last 10 years. This plate does not provide the same rigidity as the plantar plate, which is on the tension side of the construct. In general, this dorsolateral plate is used for additional stability when the screws are insufficient.

Pearls

- *Avoid placing the wires in a parallel fashion. Convergence or divergence of the wires creates better construct stability.*

Step 4: External Fixation

- A fine wire frame can be applied for fixation in the face of an active ulcer or osteomyelitis (Fig. 17). Also, it can be useful when there is poor bone stock for screw fixation.
  - When used in active infection, no internal screws should be used.
  - If used with a resected chronic osteomyelitis or resected ulcer, supplementary screws may be used as determined by the surgeon.
- Begin with an olive wire from the medial aspect of the head of the first metatarsal, aiming at the head of the fifth metatarsal laterally. The surgeon should hold the metatarsals in alignment to facilitate the wire's passage through as many metatarsal heads as possible. The ring frame is now attached above the wire and held in place with wire holders. It is very

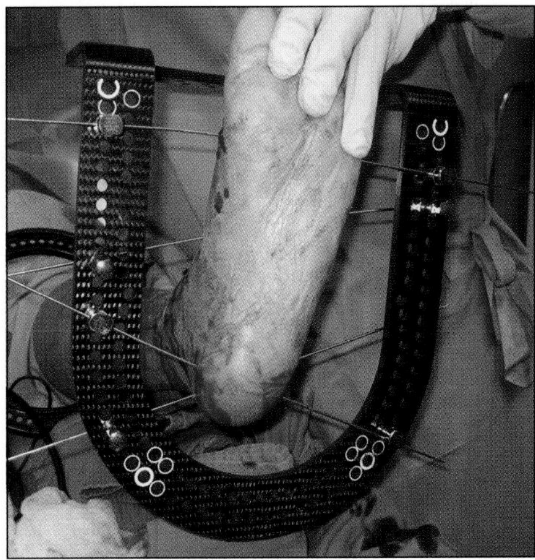

FIGURE 17

important to make sure that the frame is equidistant from the foot on each side and that the sole and frame are in the same plane.

- Again using an olive wire, go from the lateral posterior calcaneus (distal to the peroneal tendons), aiming medial to just posterior to the neurovascular bundle. The pin holder attached to the ring should be used to help guide the placement of the wire.
- The third wire (without olive) is started on the medial aspect, above the ring from the first cuneiform aiming toward the fifth metatarsal base or toward the head, depending on bone quality or technical issues. The wire should be placed through the pin holder so it is parallel to the ring.
- The fourth wire is started posteromedially, just posterior to the tibial neurovascular bundle. This wire is directed posterolaterally. The wire should be on the opposite side of the ring from the second wire.
- To tension the wires, always tighten the pin holders in one side, and then tension on the other side. The wires should be left short in one side of the frame (where they are tightened first), and long in the other (where the tensioning maneuver is done).
- If an osteotomy was done and there is a need for additional compression of the site, advance the pin holders one hole closer to the site of the osteotomy prior to tensioning. A compressive force will be exerted across the osteotomy when the fixator is tensioned.

Complications

- Inadequate correction
- Broken hardware
- Loss of fixation
- Extension of Charcot neuroarthropathy into adjacent joints
- Osteonecrosis of talus
- Pin site infection
- Deep infection
- Incomplete or delayed union

Postoperative Care and Expected Outcomes

- Postoperative care
  - Protect the foot with non–weight bearing for 3 months.
  - When a frame is used, it is typically removed at 3 months.
  - Cast or brace for an additional 3–12 months.
  - Use of crutches, walker, or canes is helpful until full healing is achieved.
- Outcomes
  - Favorable results with surgical correction are based on appropriate indication, planning, and applying appropriate fixation.
  - In our study, outcomes included improved footwear, no amputation at 5- to 8-year follow-up, and easier foot maintenance in 60 transpedal arthrodesis cases.
  - Review of 250 (including those 60 cases) of our Charcot midfoot and hindfoot cases performed over the last 18 years revealed few failures. Most patients have improved foot function, better shoewear, and fewer ulcers or hospital visits for foot problems.
  - Approximately 10% of cases will develop a proximal or distal Charcot neuroarthropathy in the same limb within 10 years.

Evidence

Kann JN, Parks BG, Schon LC. Biomechanical evaluation of two different screw positions for fusion of the calcaneocuboid joint. Foot Ankle Int. 1999;20:33-6.

Biomechanical study demonstrating the superiority of an axially placed calcaneocuboid screw from posterior to anterior versus an obliquely placed screw. (Controlled biomechanical study)

Marks RM, Parks BG, Schon LC. Midfoot fusion technique for neuroarthropathic feet: biomechanical analysis and rationale. Foot Ankle Int. 1998;19:507-10.

Study demonstrating the superiority of a plantar plate versus multiple oblique screws for midfoot fixation. (Controlled biomechanical study)

Pinzur MS. Neutral ring fixation for high risk non-plantargrade Charcot midfoot deformity. Foot Ankle Int. 2007;28:961-6.

Using a prospective algorithm, 26 patients had correction of Charcot midfeet with stabilization with a three-ring external fixator. At a minimum 1-year follow-up, 24 were able to ambulate with shoes with custom insoles. There was one unrelated death, one amputation, four patients with recurrent ulcerations, and two stress fractures related to the wires. (Level IV evidence [uncontrolled case series])

Schon LC, Easley ME, Cohen I, Lam PW, Badekas A, Anderson CD. The acquired midtarsus deformity classification system—interobserver reliability and intraobserver reproducibility. Foot Ankle Int. 2002;23:30-6.

The authors presented a classification scheme for midtarsal deformities based on clinical and radiographic assessment of Charcot cases. They demonstrated intraobserver reproducibility (97%) and interobserver reliability (81%) based on testing 75 American Orthopaedic Foot and Ankle Society members supplied with a teaching booklet and two examination booklets.

Schon LC, Easley ME, Weinfeld SB. Charcot neuroarthropathy of the foot and ankle. Clin Orthop Relat Res. 1998;(349):116-31.

The authors characterized 50 ankles, 22 hindfeet, 131 midfeet, and 18 forefeet and made recommendations for treatment of Charcot neuroarthropathy in these areas. (Retrospective review)

Schon LC, Weinfeld SB, Horton GA, Resch S. Radiographic and clinical classification of acquired midtarsus deformities. Foot Ankle Int. 1998;19:394-404.

A total of 131 radiographs of feet were analyzed and clinical records reviewed to determine a classification for assessing these deformities. Radiographic types I through IV were identified and clinical stages A through C were defined.

Simon SR, Tejwani SG, Wilson DL, Santner TJ, Denniston NL. Arthrodesis as an early alternative to nonoperative management of Charcot arthropathy of the diabetic foot. J Bone Joint Surg [Am]. 2000;82:939-50.

A total of 14 patients with stage I Eichenholtz Charcot feet without ulceration underwent successful fusion with return to independent ambulation. (Level IV evidence [uncontrolled prospective study])

PROCEDURE 19

Midfoot Arthrodesis in Charcot Foot Deformity with "Charcot Screws"

Roman Lusser and Beat Hintermann

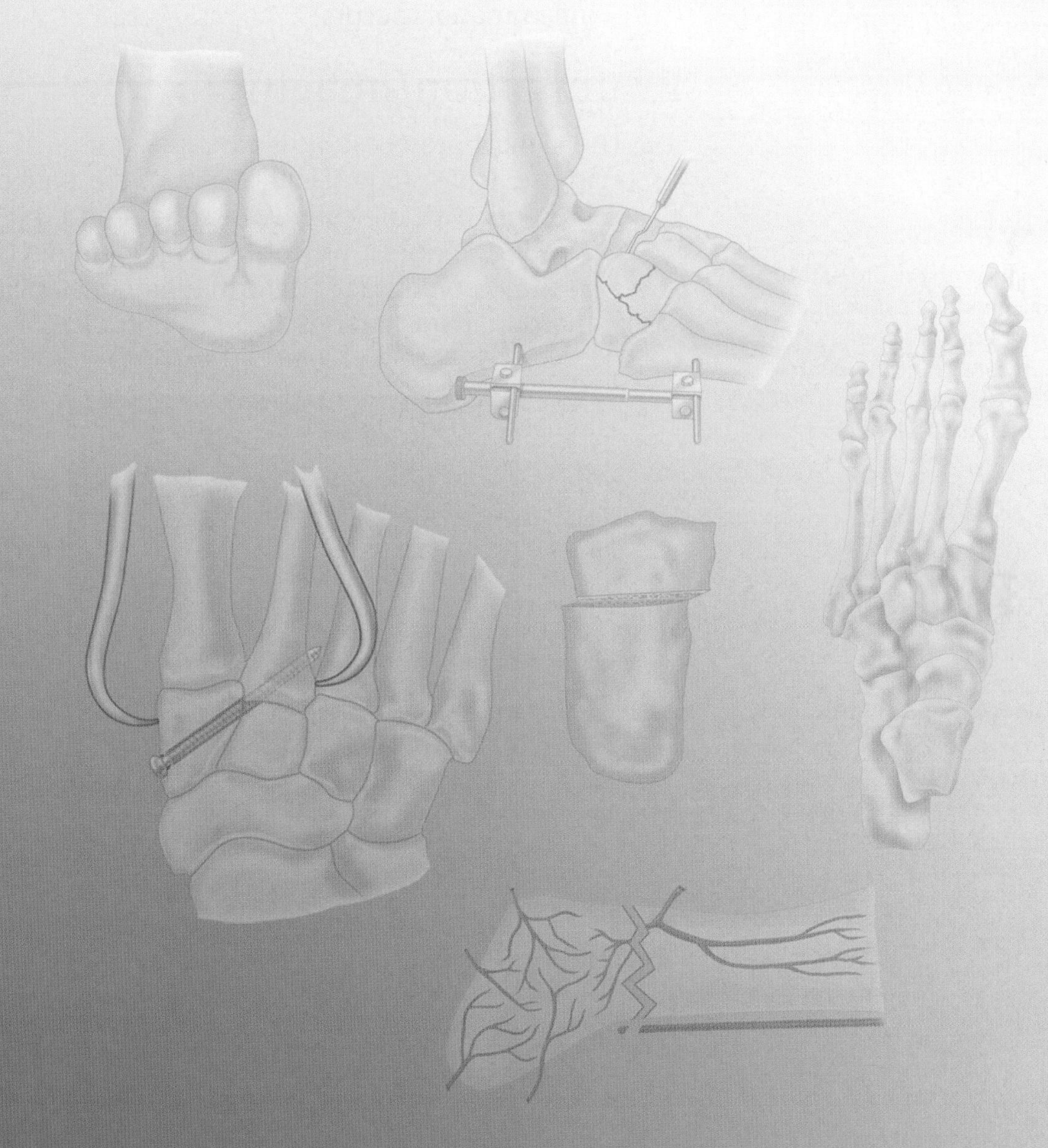

PITFALLS

- *Contraindications:*
  - *Infection of the soft tissue or bone.*
  - *Relative: pre-existing ulcers should be closed before operative treatment (full-contact cast).*
- *Acute stage (Eichenholtz stage I) of a Charcot joint needs conservative treatment (immobilization, full-contact cast, bisphosphonates).*

Controversies

- Operation in the acute early stage (Eichenholtz I) in cases with moderate inflammatory reaction (Simon et al., 2000).
- Operation in cases with a fresh fracture before the inflammation occurs.

Treatment Options

- Exostosectomy only
- Arthrodesis:
  - Screws and plate on the plantar aspect of the medial column
  - Compression blade-plates
  - Custom intramedullary rods/nails
- External fixation
- Amputation

Indications

- Patients with a Charcot arthropathy, Eichenholtz stage II or III and Brodsky classification type I and II with
  - Severe deformity
  - Marked instability
  - Chronic recurrent ulceration
  - Joint instability
  - Persistent pain without response to nonoperative treatment
  - Acute fractures in a very early stage (before inflammation occurs)

Examination/Imaging

- The clinical presentation is essential.
  - In the acute stage (Eichenholtz I), the patient presents with difficulty with shoe-fitting, painless swelling, redness, warmth, and hyperemia (Fig. 1).
  - In the chronic stage, deformity and instability are the dominant findings (Fig. 2A and 2B).

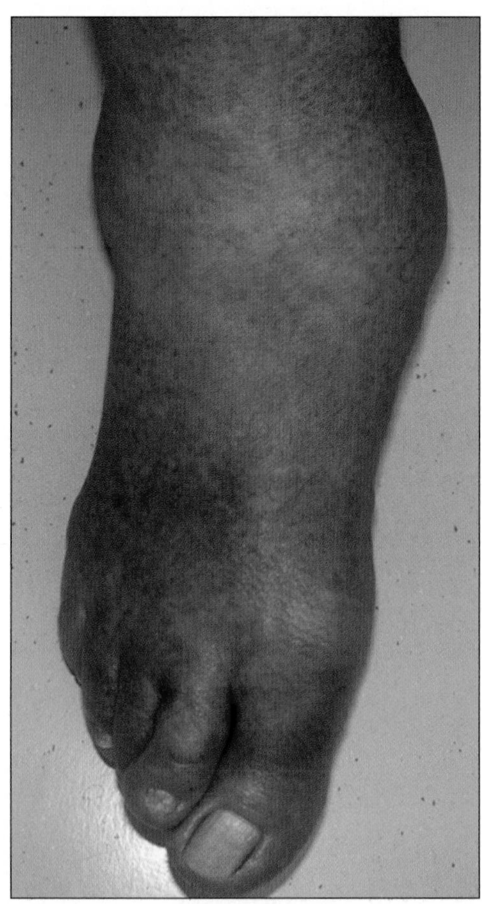

FIGURE 1

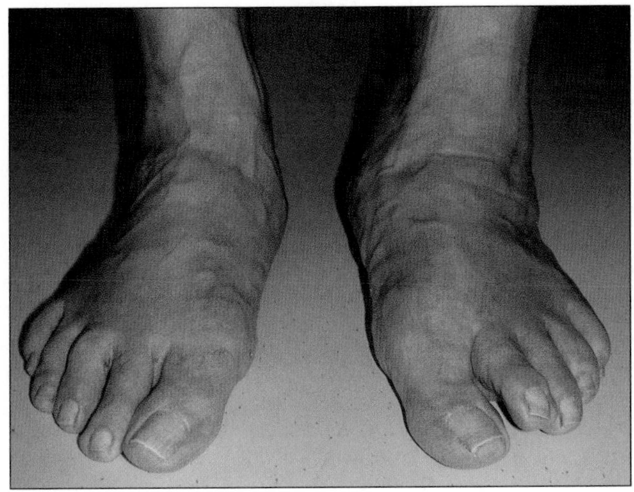
A

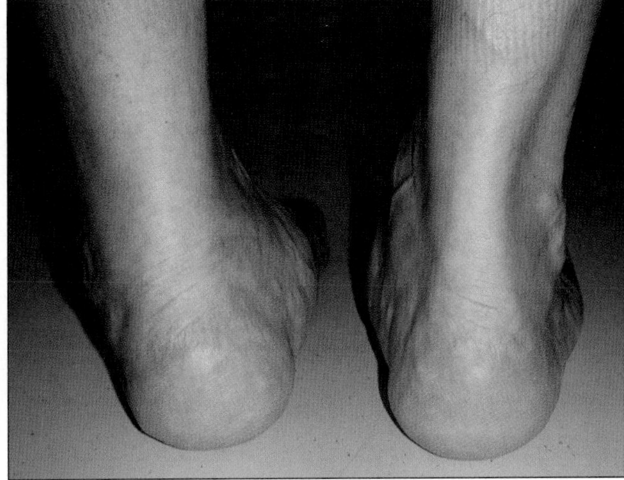
B

FIGURE 2

- Laboratory parameters: normal to slight increase in C-reactive protein levels, normal white cell count, and mild increase in erythrocyte sedimentation rate (exclusion of infection).
- Vascular and neurologic (e.g., degree of sensory neuropathy with Semmes-Weinstein monofilaments) status should be checked preoperatively.
- Plain radiographs: anteroposterior and lateral views of bilateral foot and ankle. Weight-bearing radiographs are required to analyze the degree of deformity (Fig. 3A–C).

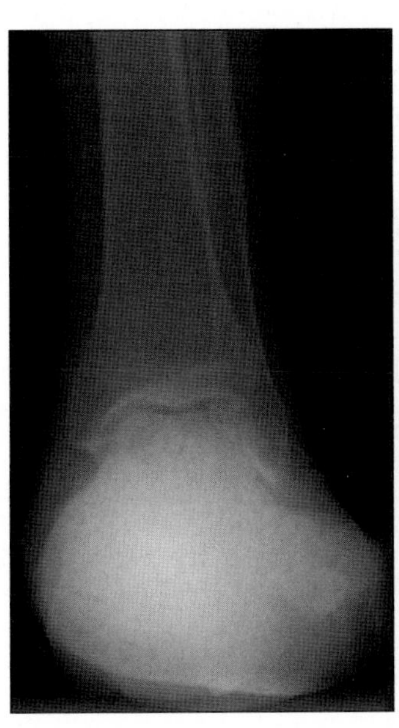
A

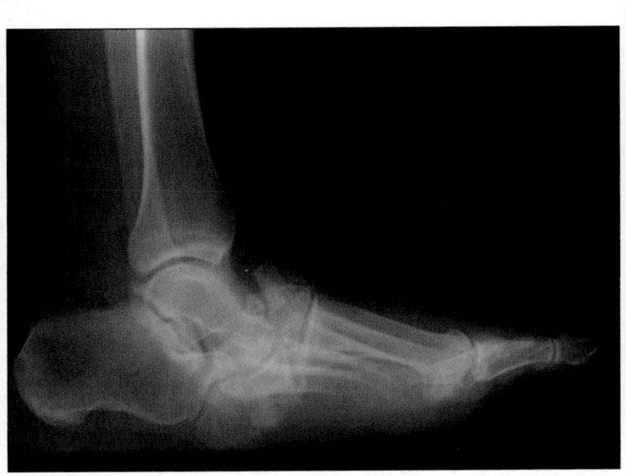
B

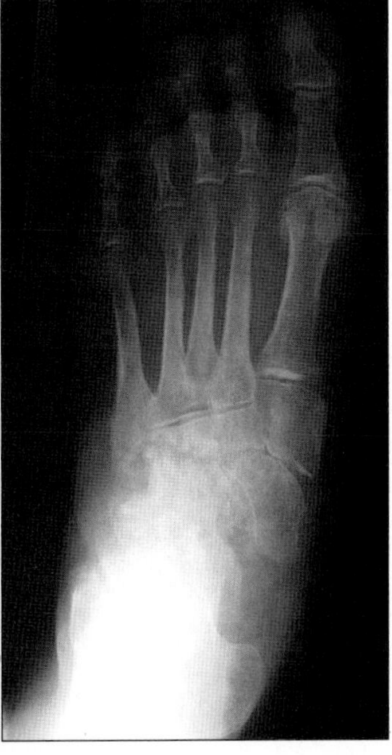
C

FIGURE 3

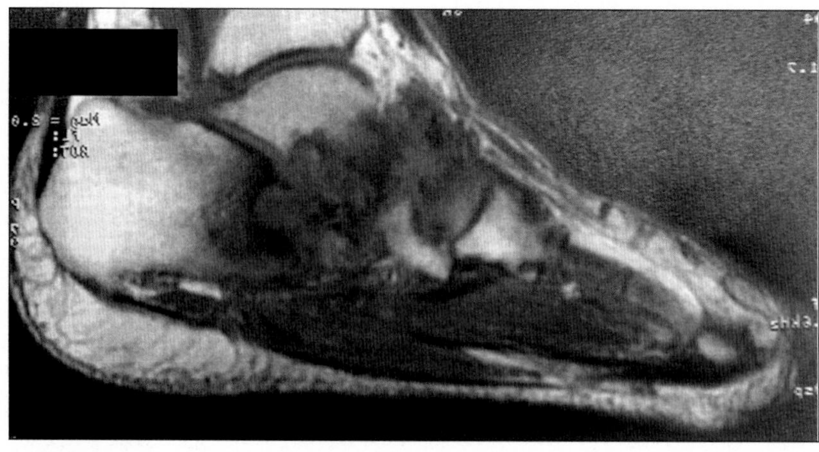

FIGURE 4

- Computed tomography scan in cases of difficult-to-interpret plain films to delineate the pattern and extent of joint involvement.
- Magnetic resonance imaging to rule out the presence of an abscess if the distinction from an acute infection cannot be made by the clinical assessment (Fig. 4).
- ^{111}In-labeled monoclonal antigranulocyte scintigraphy: differentiation between osteomyelitis and Charcot arthropathy (cannot be made by ^{99m}Tc scintigraphy).
- Bone biopsy: differentiation between osteomyelitis and Charcot arthropathy.

Surgical Anatomy

- Depending on type and activity of Charcot neuroarthropathy, the foot will be destabilized and deformed.

Positioning

- Position the patient in supine on a radiolucent operating table.
- A tourniquet at the thigh may be used; however, in the case of any vasculopathy, it is not recommended to use a tourniquet.

Portals/Exposures

- A dorsomedial incision is made directly to the bone.
- Expose the unstable area at the original talonavicular joint.
- A spreader and Hohmann retractor may be used to reduce the Chopart joint (Fig. 5).

PEARLS

- *The opposite pelvis could be underlayed by cushions to produce a slight external rotation of the leg.*

PEARLS

- *The subtalar joint can also be exposed through the same approach.*

PITFALLS

- *Damage to the anterior tibial tendon may result in loss of dorsiflexion power.*

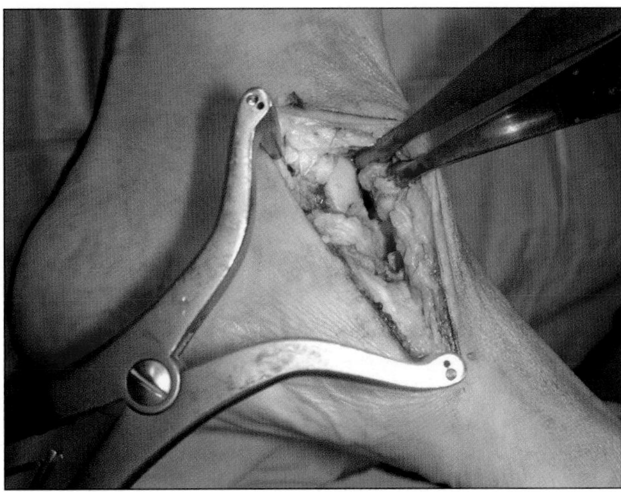

FIGURE 5

Instrumentation

- Distractor or spreader

Controversies

- An additional lateral approach has been proposed; however, in our experience, a single medial approach allows for enough access to the dislocated Chopart joint.

Pearls

- *Using demineralized bone matrix and autologous growth factors from a platelet-rich plasma concentration system enhances bone healing and makes use of iliac crest spongiosa often unnecessary.*

Procedure

Step 1: Preparation for the Midfoot Arthrodesis

- Resect all cartilage of the subtalar, talonavicular, navicular-cuneiform, and tarsometatarsal joints using chisel and curettes.
- Preserve all bony fragments for grafting.
- Harvest bone graft from the iliac crest.

Step 2: Reduction of the Midfoot

- Reduce the midfoot by using a distractor and Hohmann retractor (see Fig. 5); adduction and plantar flexion of the foot may additionally help to get an appropriate reduction with restoration of the arch.
- Insert a Kirschner wire (K-wire) percutaneously lateral to the Achilles tendon to the posterior aspect of talus and then brought through the talar head and navicular into the first cuneiform and metatarsal shaft.
  - Alternatively, the guiding K-wire can be inserted from *distally* into the first metatarsal head through the first cuneiform, navicular, and talus to exit just lateral to the Achilles tendon.
- Enlarge the skin incision to insert the drill bit.
- Drill a 4.5-mm hole for a 6-mm screw; drill a 6.5-mm hole for an 8-mm screw.
- Enlarge the hole proximally for the screw head with a 5.5-mm and 7.5-mm drill bit, respectively.
- Measure the required screw length.

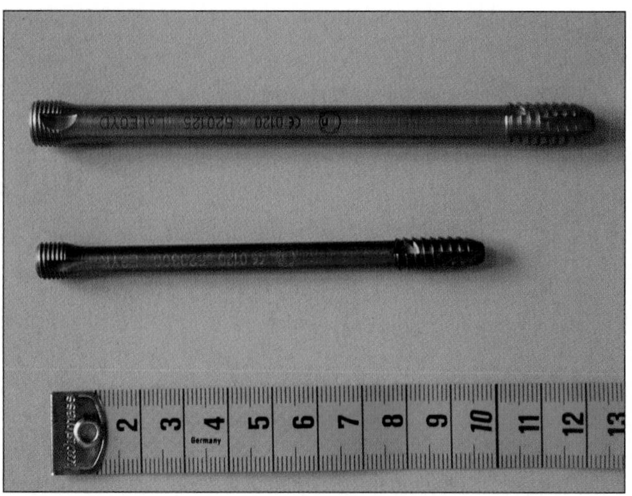

FIGURE 6

- Insert the cannulated screw (Newdeal/Integra; Fig. 6), which is driven until it enters into the first metatarsal head.
  - An additional screw can be inserted analogously from the talus into the base of the second and/or third metatarsal.
  - Alternatively, a screw can be inserted through the calcaneus into the base of the third metatarsal.
  - Additional screws can be inserted to stabilize the subtalar joint.
- Fluoroscopy or radiography is used to check appropriate reduction and position of screws (Fig. 7A and 7B)

Pearls

- *If, after correction and stabilization, there is still a bony prominence beneath the cuboid bone, exosectomy is done through a lateral incision.*
- *The use of strong screws (see Fig. 6) is necessary to avoid implant failure due to prolonged bone healing.*
- *The use of a guiding device may facilitate proper positioning of the K-wire (Fig. 8A and 8B).*

Pitfalls

- *Inappropriate correction and persisting plantar bony prominence may cause recurrent ulceration.*

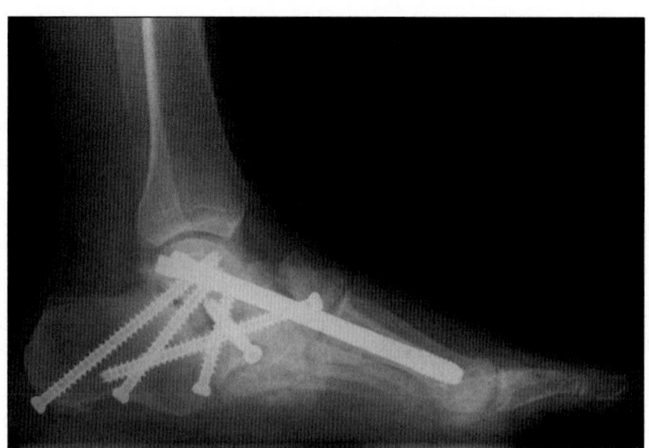

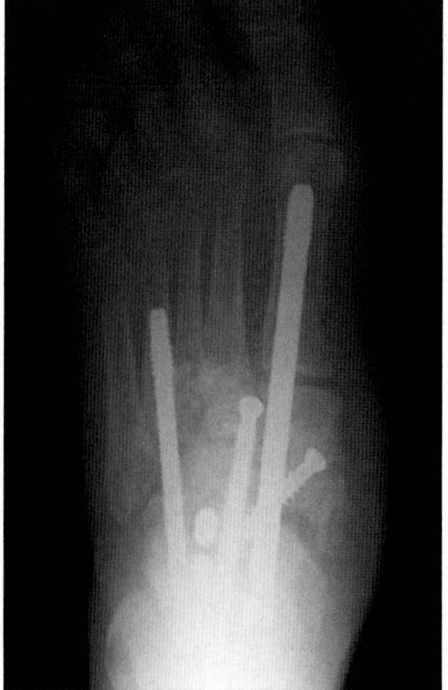

FIGURE 7 A B

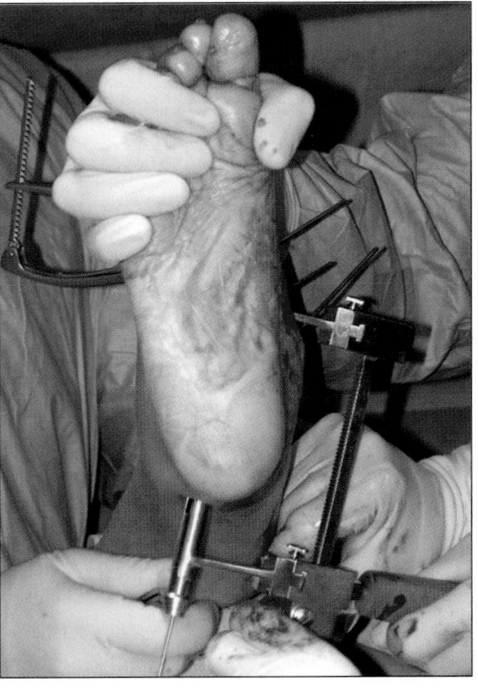

A

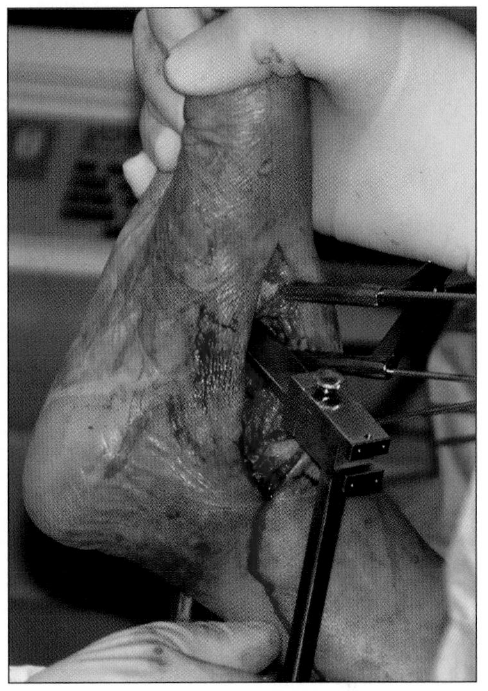

B

FIGURE 8

- Harvested bone is impacted at the arthrodesis site.
- If the foot cannot be brought to minimally 10° of dorsiflexion, heel cord lengthening is done.

Step 3: Wound Closure

- Irrigate the medial wound.
- Close the incision with skin sutures using interrupted stitches.
- Apply a sterile, compressive cotton-wool dressing and below-the-knee splint.

Controversies

- There is controversy as to whether the heel cord should always be lengthened.

Pitfalls

- *Weight bearing too early can cause collapse of the arch.*
- *There is danger of deep venous thrombosis.*

Postoperative Care and Expected Outcomes

- The patient is kept on bed rest for 48 hours.
- Perform the first change of dressings after 48 hours with application of a removable split soft cast. No more than 15 kg of partial weight bearing is allowed in the soft cast.
- After satisfactory wound healing and removal of the stitches, a full-contact cast is administered.
- Full weight bearing is allowed in the full-contact cast. This cast is replaced every 4 weeks for at least 6–12 months.
- Clinical and radiologic follow-up is done after 8 and 16 weeks, then every 4–6 months.
- Low-molecular-weight heparin or an oral anticoagulant is prescribed as long as the cast is on.

Evidence

Anderson JJ, Woelffer KE, Holtzman JJ, Jacobs AM. Bisphosphonates for the treatment of Charcot neuroarthropathy. J Foot Ankle Surg. 2004;43:285-9.

This prospective study including 13 patients evaluated the effects of the bisphosphonate pamidronate on associated signs of Charcot. (Level IV evidence)

Brodsky JW, Rouse AM. Exostectomy for symptomatic bony prominences in diabetic Charcot feet. Clin Orthop Relat Res. 1993;(296):21-6.

This clinical study describes the appearance of symptomatic bony prominences in Type I Charcot feet. (Level IV evidence)

Chantelau E. The perils of procrastination: effects of early vs. delayed detection and treatment of incipient Charcot fracture. Diabet Med. 2005;22:1707-12.

This prospective case-control study demonstrates that the early detection of incipient Charcot foot is facilitated by imaging techniques other than plain X-rays. (Level III evidence)

Jeffcoate W, Lima J, Nobrega L. The Charcot foot. Diabet Med. 2000;17:253-8.

An impressive review of the clinical manifestations of the Charcot foot in diabetes mellitus, with particular reference to theories concerning aetiology. (Level V evidence)

Johnson JE. Surgical treatment for neuropathic arthropathy of the foot and ankle. Instr Course Lect. 1999;48:269-77.

A practical review about the surgical possibilities in Charcot feet. (Level V evidence)

Lipman BT, Collier BD, Carrera GF, Timins ME, Erickson SJ, Johnson JE, Mitchell JR, Hoffmann RG, Finger WA, Krasnow AZ, Hellman RS. Detection of osteomyelitis in the neuropathic foot: nuclear medicine, MRI and conventional radiography. Clin Nucl Med. 1998;23:77-82.

A clinical study comparing the diagnostic efficacy of (1) combined three-phase bone scintigraphy and In-111 labeled WBC scintigraphy (Bone/WBC), (2) MRI, and (3) conventional radiography in detecting osteomyelitis of the neuropathic foot. (Level III evidence)

Pinzur M. Surgical versus accommodative treatment for Charcot arthropathy of the midfoot. Foot Ankle Int. 2004;25:545-9.

Using a simple treatment protocol with the desired endpoint being long-term management with commercially available, therapeutic footwear and custom foot orthoses, more than half of the patients with Charcot arthropathy at the midfoot level can be successfully managed without surgery. (Level III evidence)

Pinzur MS, Lio T, Posner M. Treatment of Eichenholtz stage I Charcot foot arthropathy with a weightbearing total contact cast. Foot Ankle Int. 2006;27:324-9.

This preliminary study supports the use of total contact cast therapy and weightbearing in the treatment of acute Charcot foot arthropathy. When the total contact cast was changed every 14 days, all subjects were able to use commercially available depth-inlay shoes and custom orthoses. (Level IV evidence)

Pitocco D, Ruotolo V, Caputo S, Mancini L, Collina CM, Manto A, Caradonna P, Ghirlanda G. Six-month treatment with alendronate in acute Charcot neuroarthropathy: a randomized controlled trial. Diabetes Care. 2005;28:1214-5.

This randomized clinical study addresses the reliability of long-term alendronate therapy in Charcot feet. (Level I evidence)

Sammarco GJ, Conti SF. Surgical treatment of neuroarthropathic foot deformity. Foot Ankle Int. 1998;19:102-9.

The authors of this study could show that surgical reconstruction of midfoot, hindfoot, and ankle neuroarthropathic deformity is a viable alternative to amputation for patients who fail nonoperative care. Proper preoperative evaluation and assessment will result in a rate of complications comparable to foot surgery in nondiabetic patients. (Level IV evidence)

Simon SR, Tejwani SG, Wilson DL, Santner TJ, Denniston NL. Arthrodesis as an early alternative to nonoperative management of Charcot arthropathy of the diabetic foot. J Bone Joint Surg [Am]. 2000;82:939-50.

This is the first clinical study which demonstrates the potential for early operative treatment to restore anatomical alignment and improve function of diabetic patients with stage-I Charcot arthropathy. (Level IV evidence)

PROCEDURE 20

Open Reduction and Internal Fixation of Lisfranc/Tarsometatarsal Injuries

Andrew K. Sands

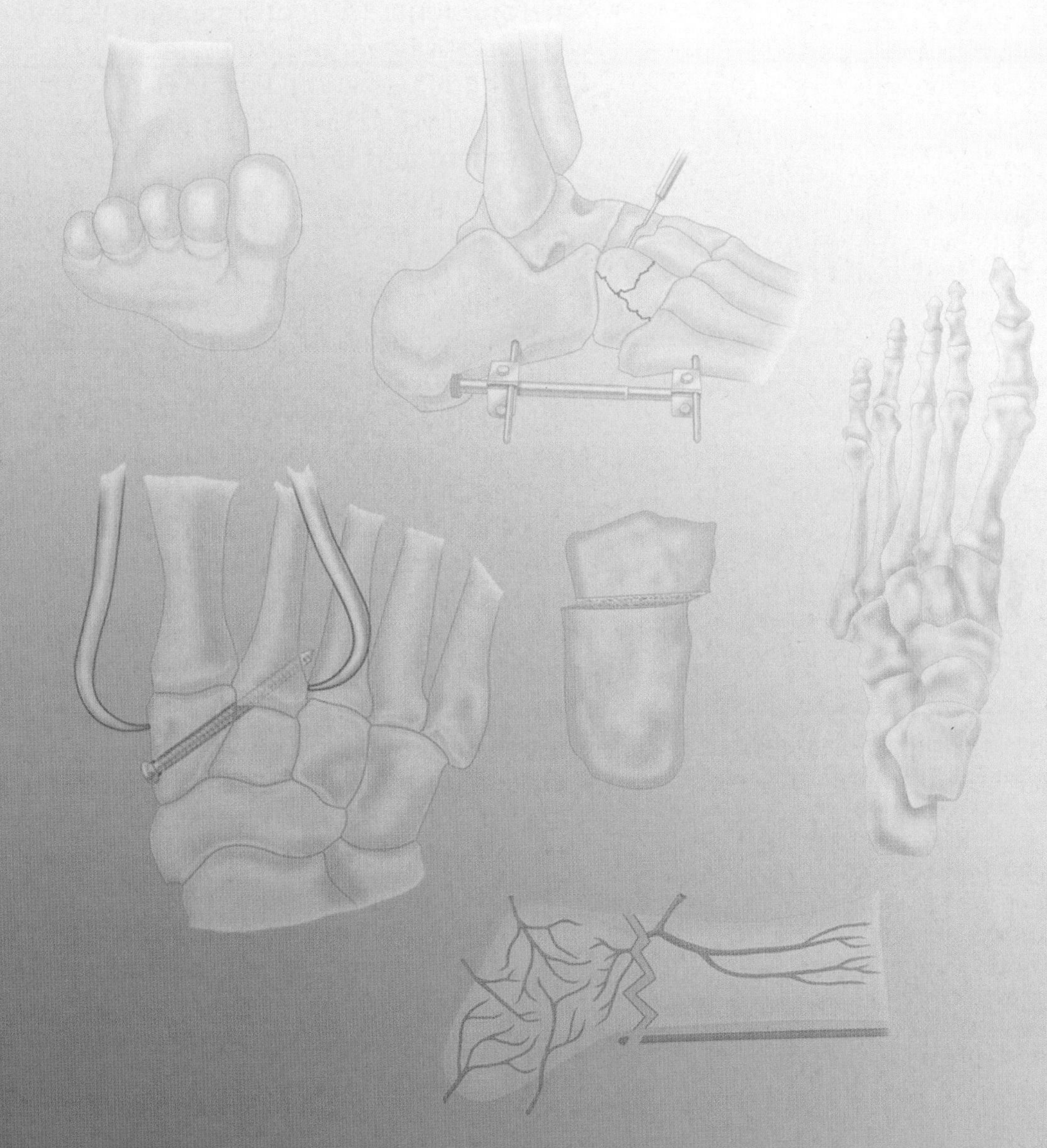

Andrew K. Sands would like to acknowledge the assistance of Edmund Choi, MD with this chapter.

PITFALLS

- *Displaced injuries lead to midfoot arthritis and often require later reconstruction with midfoot fusion.*

Controversies

- Open reduction and internal fixation (ORIF) versus immediate fusion: In the cervical spine, if one is treating a purely ligamentous C1-2 injury, immediate fusion would be advocated. Similarly, purely ligamentous injuries to the midfoot are being treated with immediate fusion. Conversely, fractures/avulsions will heal better when treated with ORIF.

Treatment Options

- There is often an associated equinus contracture with this injury pattern requiring a calf lengthening at the time of ORIF. It is thought that performing a calf lengthening at this time helps prevent degeneration in the midfoot.
- Newer ideas on treatment include immediate fusion in the case of pure ligamentous injuries. The technique, approach, choice of implant and screw pattern, and technique are the same. The joint surfaces are prepared for fusion instead of pure ORIF.
- In the case of a nondisplaced injury, closed cast or cam walker treatment (strict non–weight bearing) can be tried as long as the patient is warned that future fusion may be more likely.

Indications

- Lisfranc/tarsometatarsal (TMT) injuries with instability and displacement

Examination/Imaging

- On examination, the patient will report severe pain, worse than for a typical twisting injury. There will be midfoot swelling and ecchymosis (often with a plantar medial pattern).
- Plain radiographs
  - Anteroposterior (AP), oblique, and lateral views with weight bearing as tolerated
    - On the AP view, the first TMT (1TMT) and second TMT (2TMT) joints are assessed for alignment and displacement. There is often a gap between the bases of the first metatarsal (1MT) and second metatarsal (2MT) bases (Fig. 1).
    - The third TMT (3TMT) can be best viewed on the oblique view. It should line up with the lateral cuneiform (Fig. 2). The fourth metatarsal (4MT) and fifth metatarsal (5MT) bases are also viewed. The 4MT should line up with the cuboid border in this view.
    - On the lateral view, dorsal displacement at the TMT can be seen, indicating a higher energy pattern (Fig. 3).
  - Intertarsal injuries and displacement should also be looked for. If they exist, they should be addressed first.
  - Stress view
    - Obtaining this view is painful and should be done under an ankle block or in the operating room before ORIF.
    - The heel can be grasped with the contralateral hand and the forefoot with the ipsilateral hand. A gentle valgus stress can be applied (Fig. 4).
    - In a typical homolateral pattern, the midfoot will displace (under radiograph views for documentation).
- Computed tomography
  - Can be helpful in assessing other associated tarsal injuries
  - Good bony resolution
- Magnetic resonance imaging is not needed because there is no bony resolution.

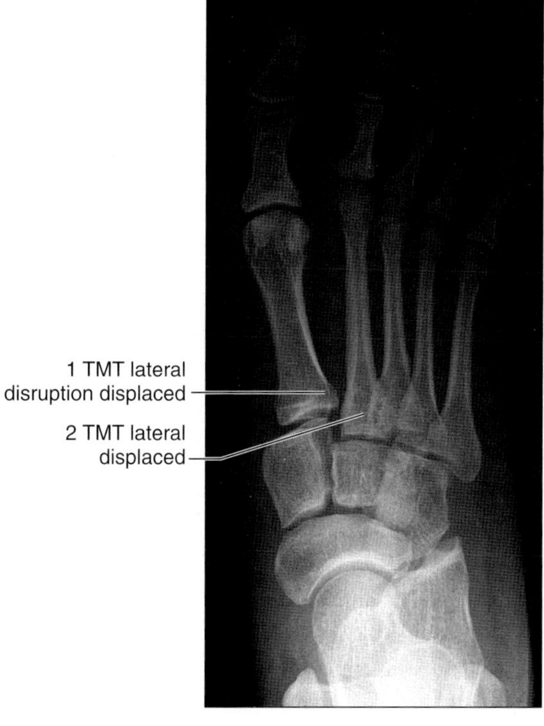

FIGURE 1

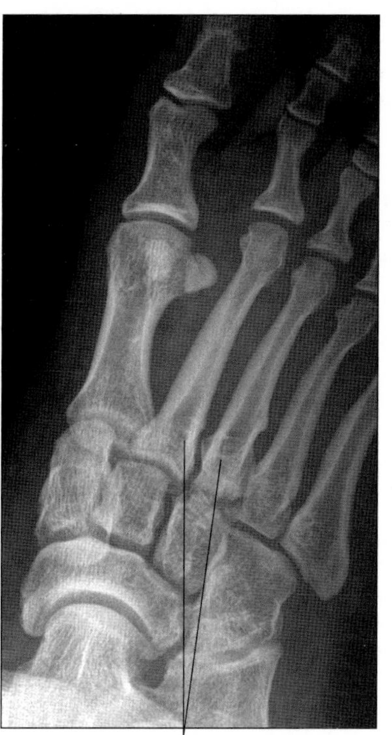

FIGURE 2

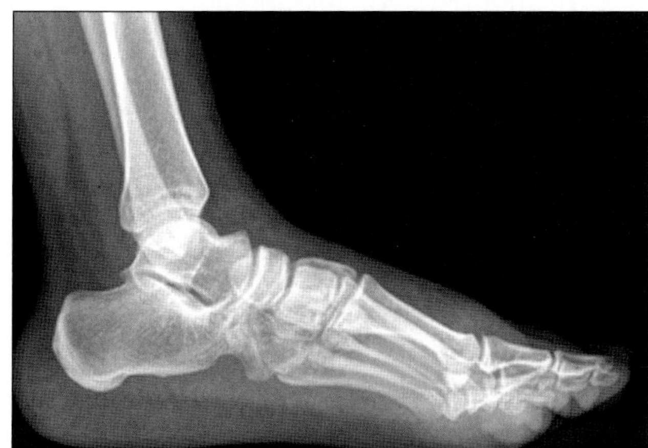

FIGURE 3

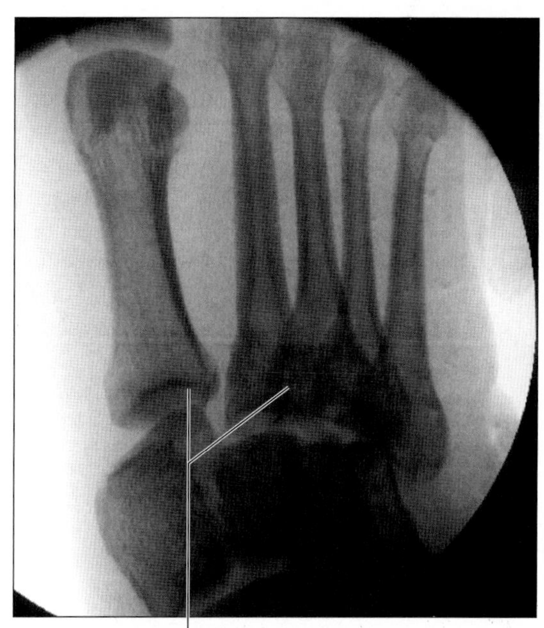

FIGURE 4

Controversies

- Associated fracture of the plantar base of the 2MT
- Before the midfoot is reduced, some advocate ORIF of the 2MT base. Others believe that the bony injury will be adequately reduced and will allow bony healing without specific ORIF.

Surgical Anatomy

- The main stabilizer of the midfoot is the plantar ligament, which goes from the plantar base of the medial cuneiform to the plantar medial base of the 2MT. The amount of force required to disrupt this ligament is considerable. However, the dorsal ligaments are not as strong and can be disrupted more easily. If ORIF is performed, it is often possible to repair these dorsal ligaments at the time of closure for added stability.
- Since there is essentially no soft tissue on the dorsum of the foot, care must be taken with the approach. Double dorsal incisions allow access to every area needed. Healing is without problem unless the area between the incisions is violated. The dorsal flap between the incisions is protected by the dorsalis pedis artery.

Positioning

- Supine with ipsilateral bump
- Allows access to the dorsal and medial foot as well as the medial calf if calf lengthening is to be performed

Portals/Exposures

- Dorsomedial
  - This incision is placed over the 1MT and centered over the TMT area (Fig. 5). The incision is deepened between the extensor hallucis longus and extensor hallucis brevis tendons.
  - The capsule over the 1TMT as well as the periosteum is incised and reflected, although it is frequently disrupted by the injury. Closure of this layer later can help with healing.
  - The subperiosteal dissection is carried medially and laterally, taking care to avoid the communicating branch of the dorsalis pedis artery as it goes plantar between the 1MT and 2MT.
  - This allows access to the 1TMT and the medial half of the 2TMT (Fig. 6A and 6B).

Pearls

- *Take care to protect the dorsalis pedis artery in the central area between the incisions. If it is disrupted, the entire dorsal flap of the foot can become necrotic.*

Controversies

- A common approach used in Europe that is not as popular in North America is the straight incision from the base of the second toe, straight up the foot, across the ankle and up the anterolateral leg, if needed. This approach is especially useful in limb-sparing procedures for injuries resulting from massive trauma. The soft tissue on the top of the foot can be shifted medially and laterally to allow access to the entire midfoot.

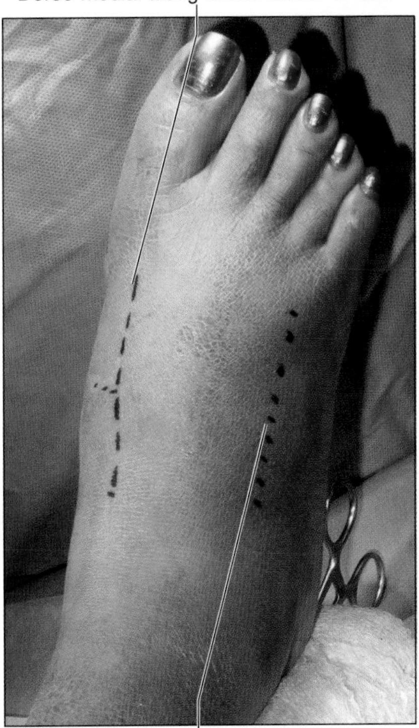

FIGURE 5

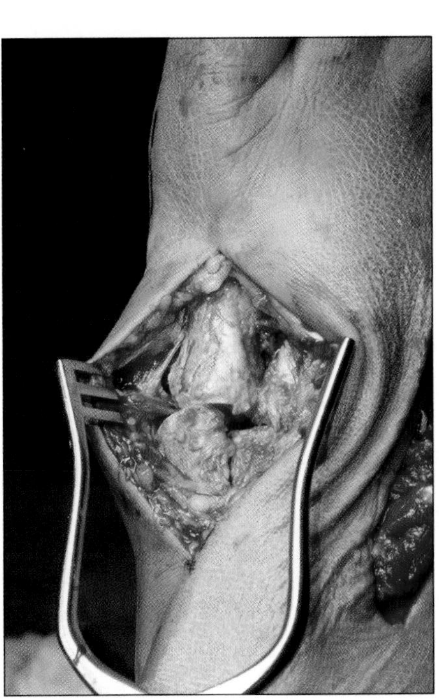
A

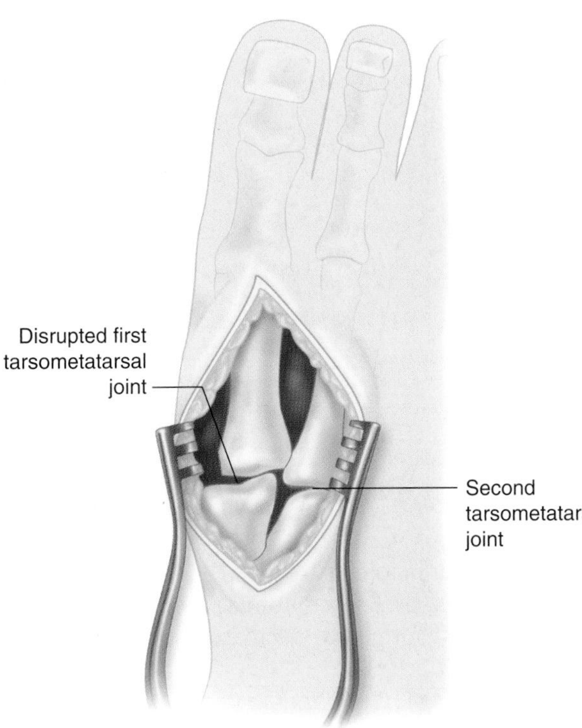

B

FIGURE 6

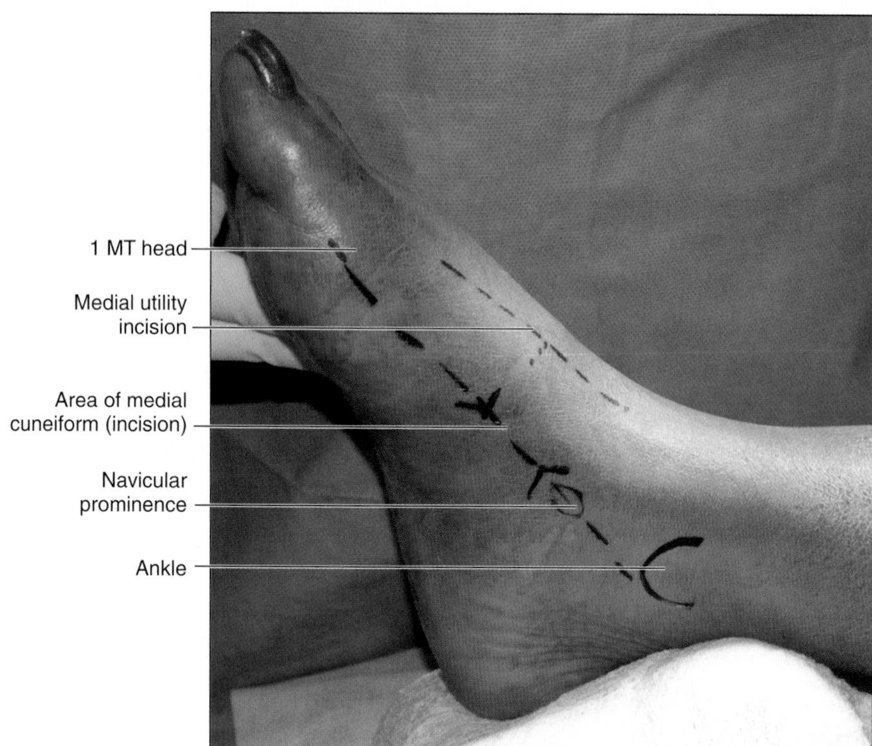

FIGURE 7

- Dorsolateral
  - This incision is placed over the 4MT, also centered over the TMT area. Attempts should be made to maintain as wide a bridge as possible between the two incisions (see Fig. 5).
  - The incision is deepened through the extensor digitorum brevis, and the extensor digitorum communis tendons are retracted. The lateral half of the 2TMT, as well as the 3TMT and 4TMT, are now visible.
- Medial
  - A small incision is made to allow screw placement from the medial incision to the base of the 2MT (Fig. 7).

Controversies

- Percutaneous versus ORIF: Since the main principle in treating this injury is perfect anatomic reduction (thought to decrease subsequent arthritic degeneration), it is imperative that ORIF with direct visualization be done. Percutaneous cannulated screws are not adequate to make sure this is achieved.

Procedure: Dual Dorsal Approach

Step 1: Reduction of Base of 2TMT Fracture

- After the approach is made, work back and forth to clear out the joints. Remove any flakes or pieces impeding perfect anatomic reduction.
- Address any intertarsal instability by reduction and Kirschner wires (K-wires). Screws can be placed transversely but should be aimed over the transverse arch so as not to injure the neurovascular structures.

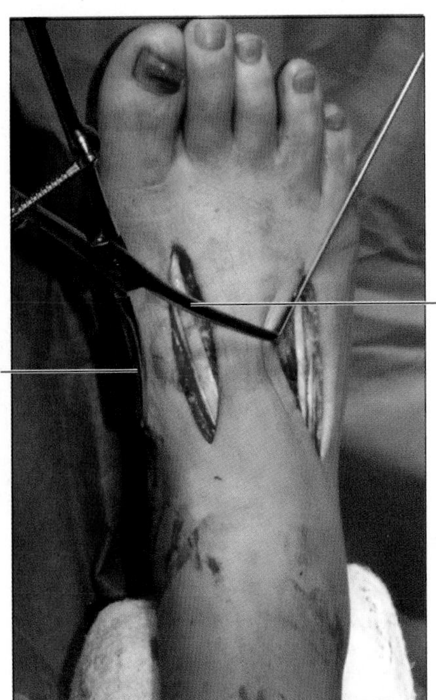

FIGURE 8

> **PEARLS**
>
> - *Despite many techniques, there is one constant: perfect anatomic reduction. This gives the best result and helps prevent future arthritis.*

- Reduce the base of the 2TMT into the keystone at the lateral TMT area.
  - Hold the reduction with a Weber clamp placed from the lateral base of the 2MT to the medial surface of the medial cuneiform (Figs. 8 and 9). Gently apply reduction pressure to bring the keystone into correct reduction.

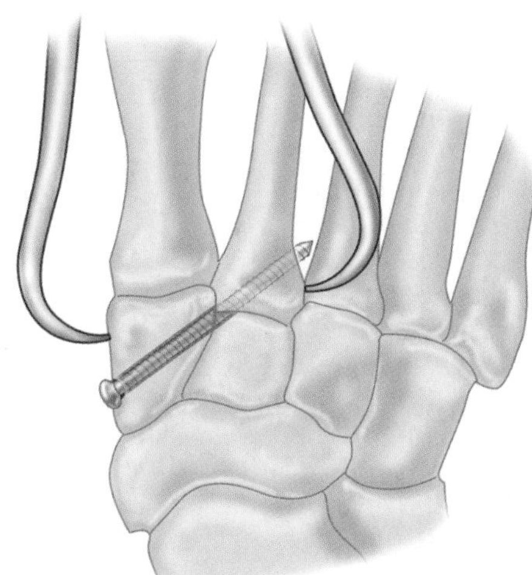

FIGURE 9

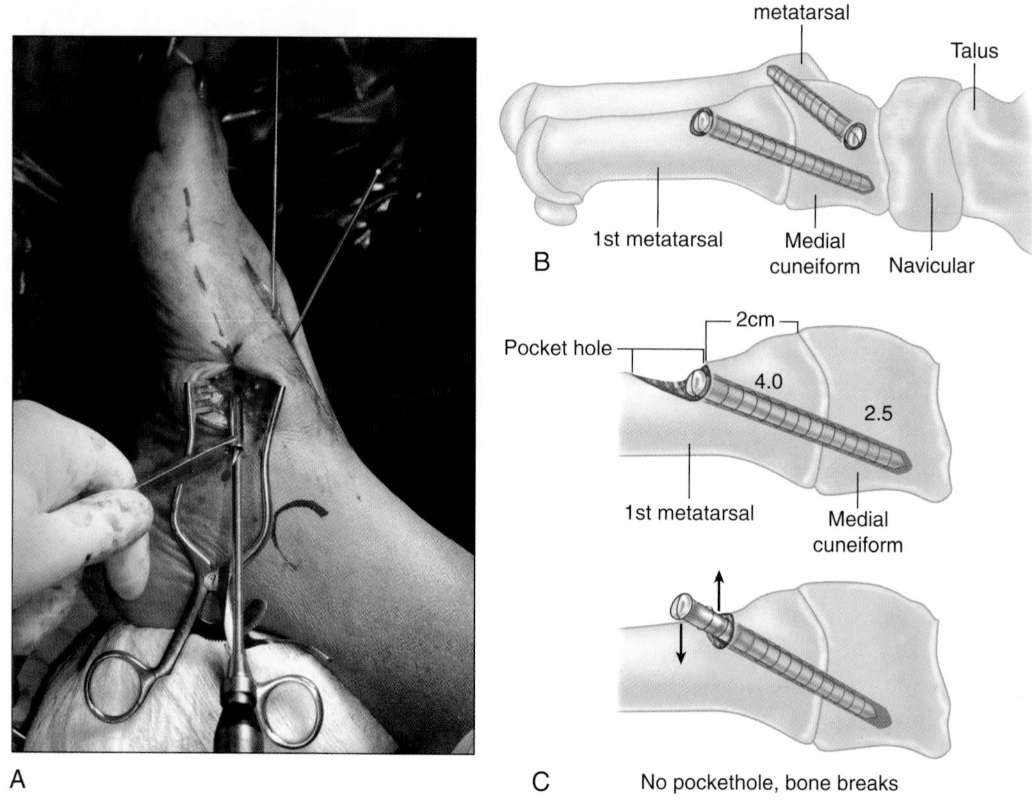

FIGURE 10

- Place a 4.0 solid cortical fully threaded screw from the medial cuneiform to the base of the 2MT by drilling in 4.0 cm through the 1MT and then 2.5 cm into the medial cuneiform (Fig. 10A–C). Use the ACL aiming guide if assistance is needed in aiming the screw direction. Gently tighten the lag screw, reducing the base of the 2MT.
- Place a second lag screw from the medial cuneiform into the base of the 2MT.

PEARLS

- *Pocket hole—why and how to make it: Just as in building a bookcase, if one is butt-joining two surfaces, the pocket hole is used to prevent breakout at the joint. If there is no pocket hole, the screw head would engage the bottom and a dorsal torque would cause breakout and loss of fixation. Use the 6-mm round burr to make a "ramp" for the screw head to come down as it engages the base of the metatarsal (see Fig. 10B and 10C).*

Step 2: Reduction of 1TMT with Internal Fixation

- Reduce the 1TMT and place two K-wires from the base of the 1MT into the medial cuneiform. Place the wires wide enough so as not to interfere with the screw.
- Use the 6-mm round burr to make a pocket hole 2 cm from the base of the 1MT (Fig. 11). Drill 4.0 cm, then 2.5 cm, and then place a lag screw from the base of the 1MT into the plantar medial aspect of the medial cuneiform (Fig. 12).
- If more stability is needed, a lag screw can also be placed from the dorsal medial cuneiform to the plantar base of the 1MT.

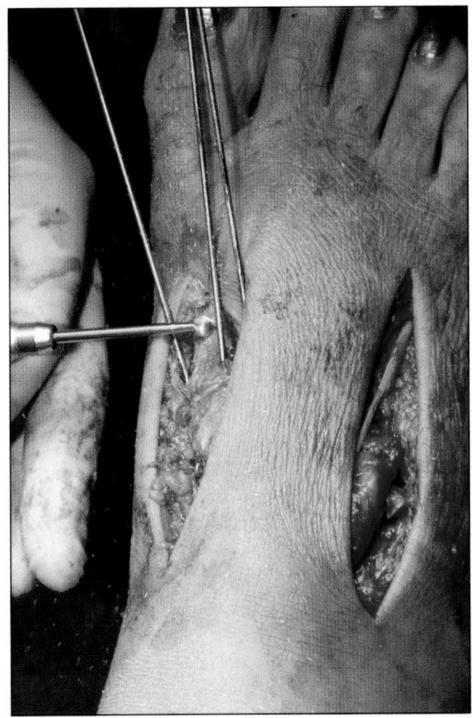

FIGURE 11

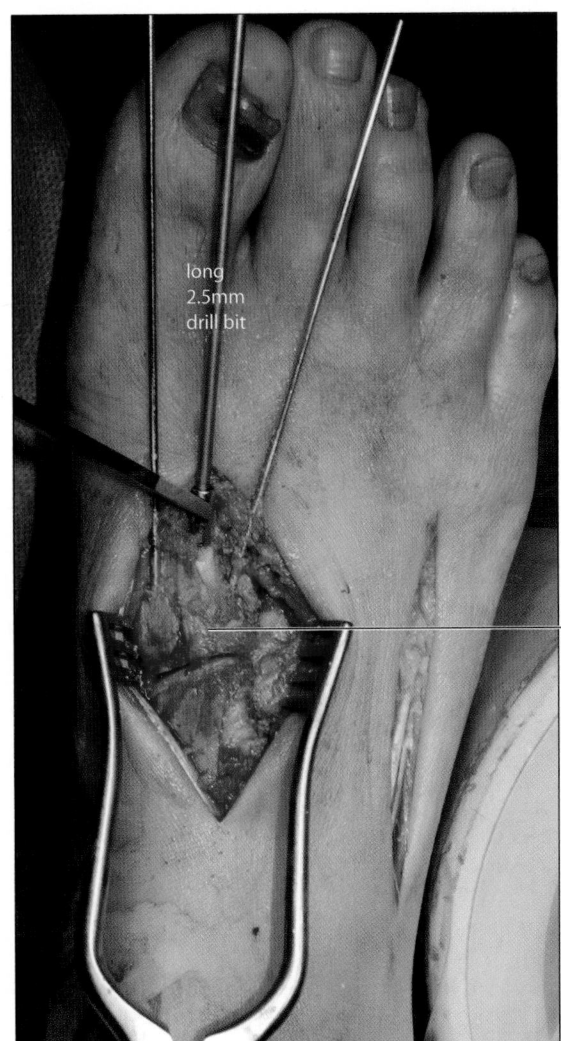

FIGURE 12

Controversies

- Starting point—1TMT versus 2MT base: While not as important as a perfect reduction, some think that the starting point is not the base of the 2MT being pulled into the keystone but rather the 1TMT injury being reduced. This leads to a reduced and stabilized medial column from which the reduction of the other joints can be based around.

Step 3: Reduction of 3TMT, 4TMT, and 5TMT

- Now working through the lateral incision, reduce the 3TMT and insert a K-wire. Drill 4.0/2.5 cm and place a lag screw from the base of the third metatarsal (3MT) into the midfoot (either the middle or lateral cuneiform) (Fig. 13).

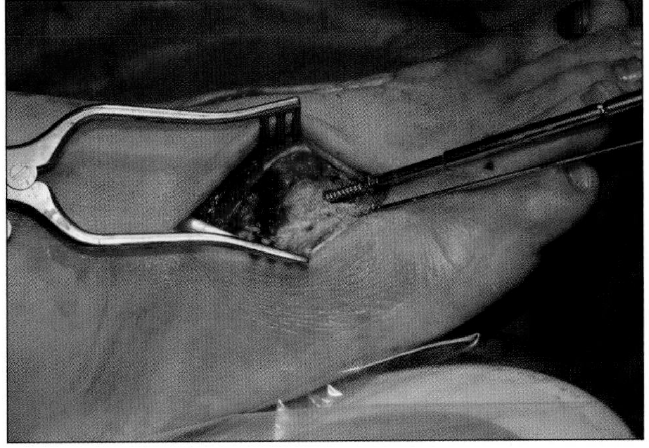

FIGURE 13

Controversies

- ORIF of the 4MT and 5MT
- Percutaneous K-wire is adequate for stabilization of the 4TMT and 5TMT, and it makes for easier removal. Another option (used more in Europe) is screw fixation of the 4TMT and 5TMT.

Pearls

- *Why long drill bits? Since the angle of the drilling is very flat (so the screw goes into the cuneiforms and does not miss by being too plantar), the bit must be long. If a short bit is used, the chuck will grind into the toes. The long bit allows the chuck to be distal to the toes.*

Instrumentation/Implantation

- Dental instrument
- Pointed reduction (Weber) clamps: big and small
- Aiming guide (ACL)
- Long drill bits
- 6-mm round burr
- K-wires

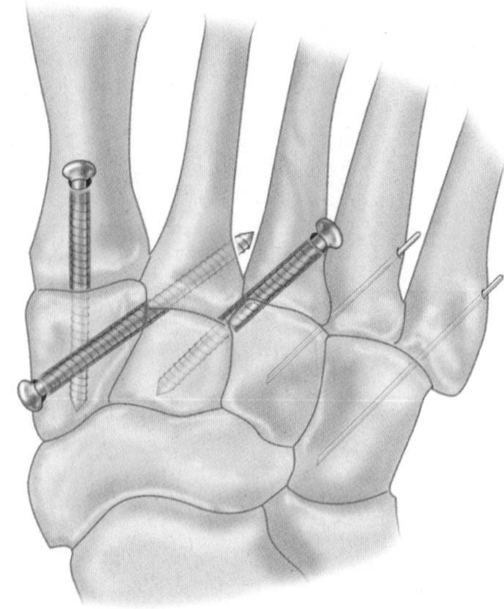

FIGURE 14

- The 4MT and 5MT usually come medial with the 3MT. If not, reduce them using the dental tool. Fixation can be accomplished with K-wires, one or two as needed (Fig. 14).

Step 4: Closure and Technique Summary

- Close the periosteum and joint capsule layer if they are present and not too badly shredded by the injury. It helps healing.
- Since there is no subcutaneous layer in the foot, extensive closure can lead to nerve injury. A few 2-0 simple stitches are placed to draw the skin edges together and reduce tension. The skin should then be closed using an absorbable suture in a running, everting, tension-relieving mattress stitch.
- Technique summary
  - Starting point: 2MT into keystone
  - Screw and technique: solid 4.0 fully threaded large-core/small-head (cortical) screw and lag technique

Controversies

- Lag screws versus non–lag screw technique: Lag screws compress across the joint. This could damage the articular surface and perhaps cause fusion. The non–lag screw technique can have a distracting effect if not done properly, leaving the joints malpositioned. Since these are (for the most part) non-mobile joints, and since any motion is atavistic, loss of motion is not a negative and may yield more stability to the reconstruction.
- Solid versus cannulated screws: The thought is that cannulated screws are easier to place. While this may be true initially, if one takes a bit of time to practice placing screws in this area, one finds the proper placement of screws is not difficult. Then, the use of cannulated screws is not needed. This is an advantage as cannulated screws are far weaker (especially in resisting bending forces) and more expensive than solid screws.

Controversies

- Removal of hardware—what and when? When 3.5-mm screws were used, there was much more incidence of screw breakage if they were left in place. Since the advent of 4.0 solid screws, with the associated increased resistance to bending failure, the incidence of screw failure in areas such as the midfoot in particular has markedly decreased. In light of this, 1TMT, 2TMT, and 3TMT screws can be left in place and never routinely removed. The K-wire across the 4TMT and 5TMT should be removed at 8 weeks, as some motion at this area is desirable. In cases in which screws are placed across the 4TMT and 5TMT, these screws are removed at 8 weeks. Sometimes Europeans also remove all the TMT screws at 8 weeks. However this can lead to loss of fixation and re-displacement.

Postoperative Care and Expected Outcomes

- For 2 weeks, the patient is kept non–weight bearing in a three-sided splint with the ankle at neutral, especially if calf lengthening has been performed.
- Then for 4–6 weeks, a cam walker boot with a nighttime ankle L-shaped splint at 90° is used still with strict non–weight bearing. Also, the patient should begin range-of-motion exercises (hyperflexion range of motion and biomechanical ankle platform system, ankle range of motion, complex range of motion).
- After 6–8 weeks, if follow-up radiographs are satisfactory, the K-wires are pulled. The patient then may begin weight bearing in a cam walker with cane-assistance outside the home and barefoot weight bearing inside the home. The patient is also fitted for a visco-cushioned insert with medial support and visco-cushioned sole "running sneakers."
- After 8–10 weeks, if radiographs are still satisfactory, the patient may begin full weight bearing in sneakers and orthotics and progress to formal physical therapy.

Evidence

Alberta FG, Aronow MS, Barrero M, Diaz-Doran V, Sullivan RJ, Adams DJ. Ligamentous Lisfranc joint injuries: a biomechanical comparison of dorsal plate and transarticular screw fixation. Foot Ankle Int. 2005;26:462-73.

This study evaluates 10 matched pairs of cadaveric lower limbs to assess the biomechanical comparison of dorsal plate versus transarticular screw fixation. Measurements were made in the loaded and unloaded condition. (Level V evidence [cadaveric study])

Coetzee JC, Ly TV. Treatment of primarily ligamentous Lisfranc joint injuries: primary arthrodesis compared with open reduction and internal fixation. A prospective, randomized study. J Bone Joint Surg [Am]. 2006;88:514-20.

This prospective study evaluates 41 patients randomized to either ORIF of Lisfranc injuries or primary arthrodesis. Follow-up averaged 42.5 months. Outcome was determined by American Orthopaedic Foot and Ankle Society (AOFAS) scores, visual analog pain scale, and a clinical questionnaire. (Level I evidence [randomized controlled trial])

Kuo RS, Tejwani NC, Digiovanni CW, Holt SK, Benirschke SK, Hansen ST, Sangeorzan BJ. Outcome after open reduction and internal fixation of Lisfanc joint injuries. J Bone Joint Surg [Am]. 2000;82:1609-18.

This study is a retrospective review of 48 patients treated with open reduction and screw fixation. Follow-up averaged 52 months. Outcome was determined by AOFAS and Musculoskeletal Functional Assessment scores. (Level IV evidence [case series])

Lee C, Birkedal JP, Dickerson EA, Vieta P, Web LX, Teasdall RD. Stabilization of Lisfranc joint injuries: a biomechanical study. Foot Ankle Int. 2004;25:365-70.

This study examined 10 matched-pair cadaveric limbs to assess the average stiffness of cortical screw fixation versus Kirschner wire fixation. (Level V evidence [cadaveric study])

Mulier T, Reynders P, Dereymaeker G, Broos P. Severe Lisfranc injuries: primary arthrodesis or ORIF? Foot Ankle Int. 2002;23:902-5.

This study is a retrospective review of 28 patients treated with ORIF or with complete arthrodesis. Follow-up averaged 30.1 months. Outcome was determined by the Baltimore Painful Foot Score. (Level III evidence [case cohort])

Richter M, Wippermann B, Krettek C, Schratt HE, Hufner T, Thermann H. Fractures and fracture dislocations of the midfoot: occurrence, causes and long-term results. Foot Ankle Int. 2001;22:392-8.

This study is a retrospective review of 155 patients with midfoot fractures treated either nonoperatively or with open reduction. Follow-up averaged 9 years for 97 patients. Outcome was determined by AOFAS, AOFAS-Midfoot, Hannover Scoring system, and Hannover Questionnaire scores. (Level III evidence [retrospective cohort])

Teng AL, Pinzur MS, Lomasney L, Mahoney L, Havey R. Functional outcome following anatomic restoration of tarsal-metatarsal fracture dislocation. Foot Ankle Int. 2002;23:922-6.

This study is a retrospective review of 11 patients treated operatively. Follow-up averaged 41.2 months. Outcome was determined by AOFAS score, clinical alignment, and radiographic analysis. (Level IV evidence [case series])

PROCEDURE 21

Painful Accessory Navicular: Augmented Kidner Procedure with Flexor Digitorum Longus Transfer

Andrew K. Sands

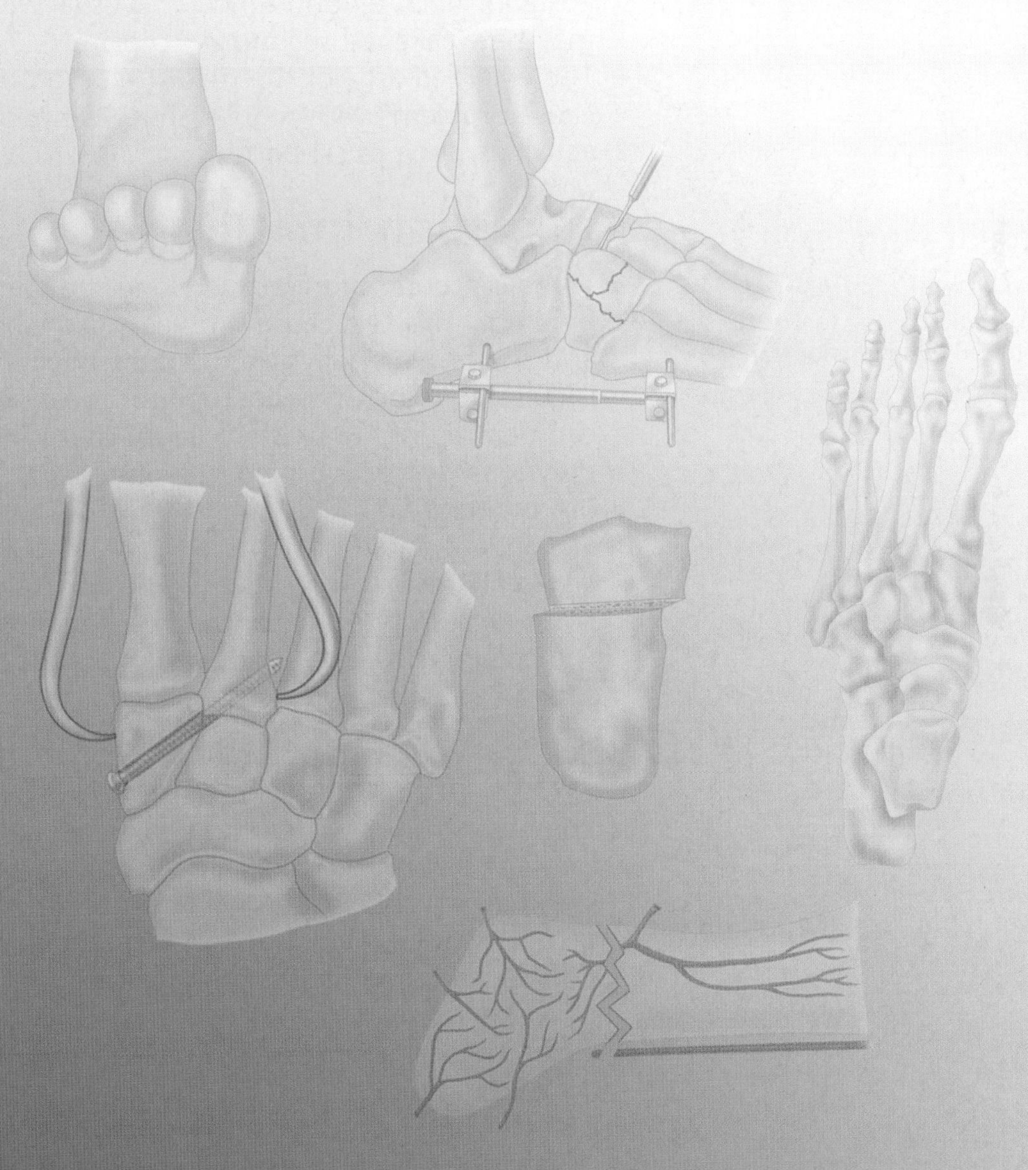

Andrew K. Sands would like to acknowledge the assistance of Edmund Choi, MD with this chapter.

Augmented Kidner Procedure with Flexor Digitorum Longus Transfer

Indications

- Presence of a painful accessory navicular with or without flatfoot.
- Often associated with equinus contracture as well. Posterior tibial tendon function is usually intact but may be weakened secondary to pain.
- The enlarged area of the medial hindfoot may also cause problems with regular shoewear and for sports activities, such as ski boots.

Treatment Options

- Initial treatment can consist of immobilization of the foot and ankle to see if bony union can be achieved.

Examination/Imaging

- There is a bony prominence along the medial hindfoot. This can cause problems with shoe fitting and sports, especially when a tight boot is worn, such as in skiing/snowboarding or roller skating. Pain can be present if a twisting injury causes motion at a previously securely-bound bony interface.
- Plain radiographs
  - Standing anteroposterior (Fig. 1A) and lateral (Fig. 1B) views will show the deformity.
  - The accessory navicular may be attached to the medial navicular by bone or fibrous tissue, or may be unattached within the posterior tibialis tendon.

Surgical Anatomy

- The posterior tibialis tendon comes distally into the foot just behind the medial malleolus.
  - It makes a sharp bend when it goes from vertical to horizontal (Fig. 2A). This can also be a zone of circulatory compromise that can lead to tendinopathy.
  - The tendon then travels distally to the medial navicular area, continues under the foot, and fans out to form a medial support for the foot. It inserts onto the navicular and the cuneiforms, the cuboid, and the bases of the middle metatarsals (Fig. 2B).
  - It is thought that, when the accessory navicular is present, this distal extension is weaker and less extensive.

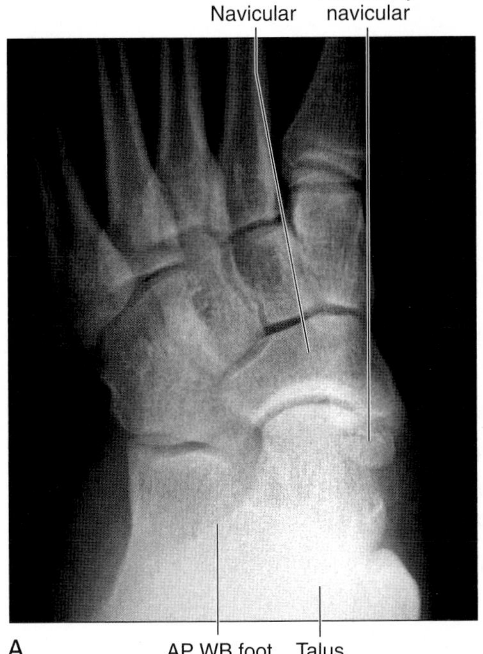

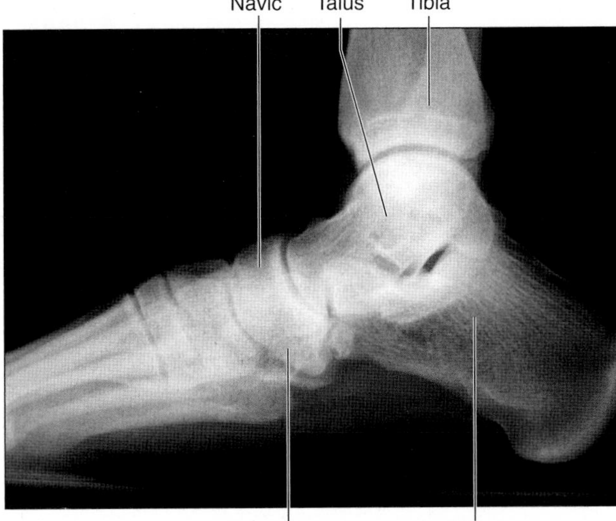

FIGURE 1 A B

- Care must be taken to maintain a shell of bone in the posterior tibialis tendon when performing a repair. The bony shell can be re-approximated to the medial navicular with a screw and washer. Attempting to attach the stripped posterior tibialis tendon to the bone does not result in good healing and bonding.
- A medial utility incision can give good exposure of the posterior tibialis and flexor digitorum longus (FDL) tendons as well as the bony structures.

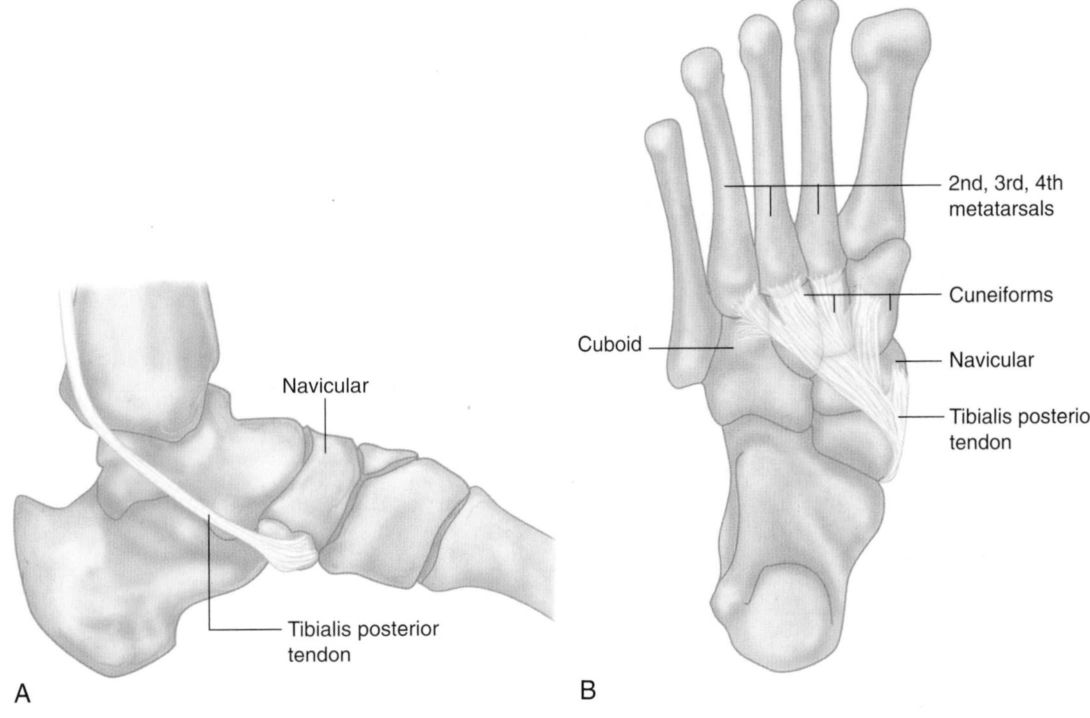

FIGURE 2 A B

Positioning

- The patient is placed supine with a contralateral bump under the pelvis.
- This "super"-supine position allows excellent exposure to the medial foot for the medial utility incision.

Portals/Exposures

- A medial utility incision allows excellent access to the surgical field. The medial prominence of the navicular is marked. A point 1 cm below the medial malleolar tip is marked. The center of the first metatarsal head is marked. A straight line can then be drawn connecting these three points, approximately along the medial border of the plantar skin pattern. The proximal half of the marked line can be used for this procedure.
- The incision is carried down through the subcutaneous tissue (Fig. 3A and 3B). The vertical veins along the medial aspect of the foot are cauterized.
- The FDL is found just posterior and inferior to the posterior tibialis tendon. A small clamp can be placed behind it. Confirmation can be obtained by moving the lesser toes—the correct tendon will be seen gliding over the clamp.
- Once the FDL is found, it is followed distally to the master knot of Henry (Fig. 4A and 4B). There are often large veins along the deep medial border, and care must be taken to cauterize them as the dissection is carried toward the master knot of Henry.

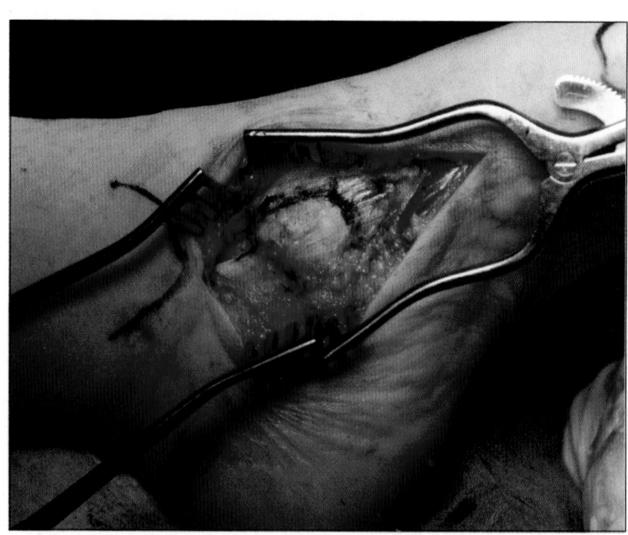

A

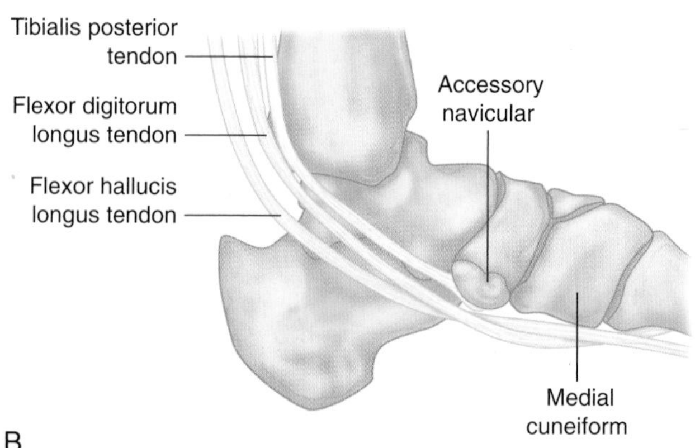

B

FIGURE 3

- Once the master knot is found, the FDL is again confirmed and transected (Fig. 5). The paratenon is stripped and is used for the augmented tendon transfer once the bony procedure is completed.

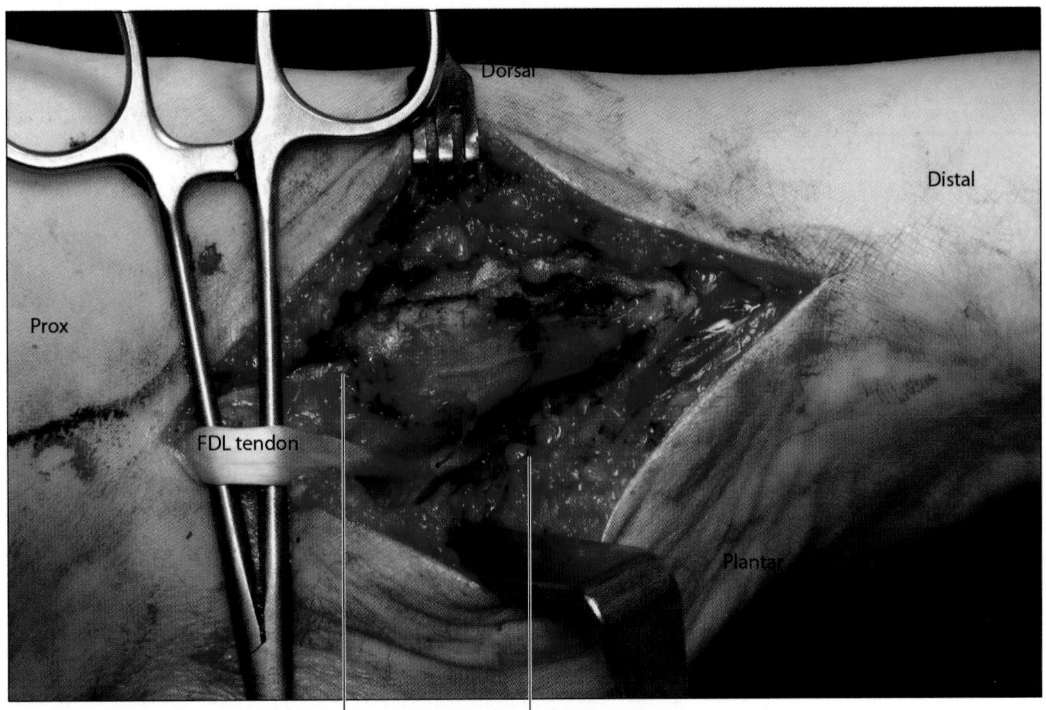

A

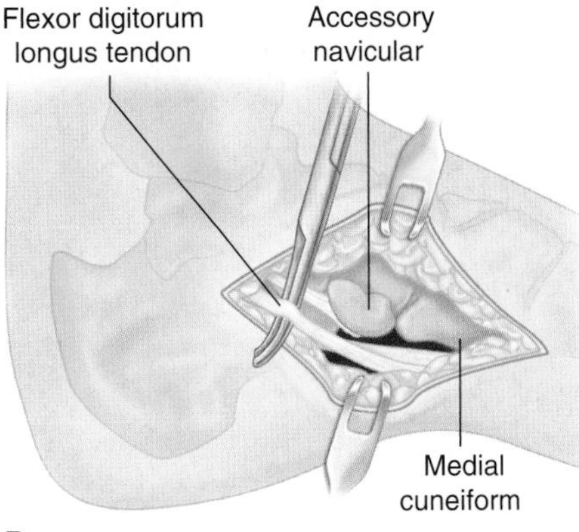

B

FIGURE 4

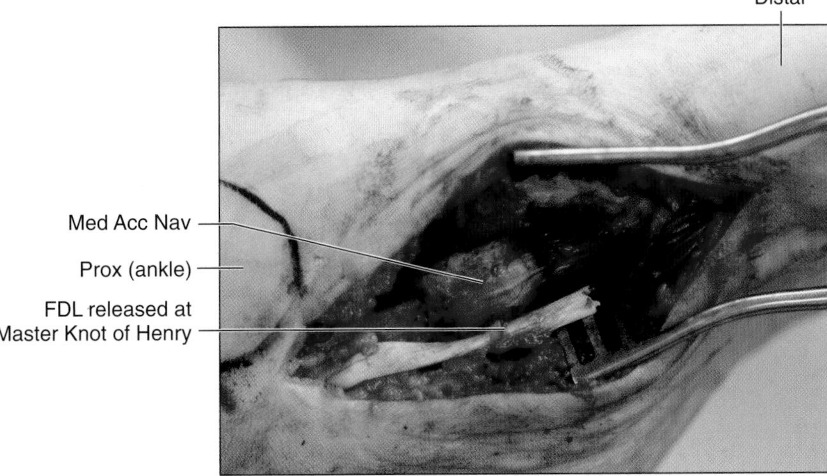

FIGURE 5

Procedure

Step 1: Exposure of the Posterior Tibial Tendon Sheath

- Carry the incision deep through the subcutaneous tissue to the tendon sheath.
- Enter the sheath, but take care to avoid injury to the posterior tibialis tendon. Follow it distally to the accessory navicular.
- Using a sharp chisel or osteotome, cut down into the gap between the bones (or, if fused, make a plane along the medial border of the cuneiform) and flip the posterior tibialis and attached accessory navicular outward, taking care to keep it attached along the plantar aspect if possible (Fig. 6A and 6B).

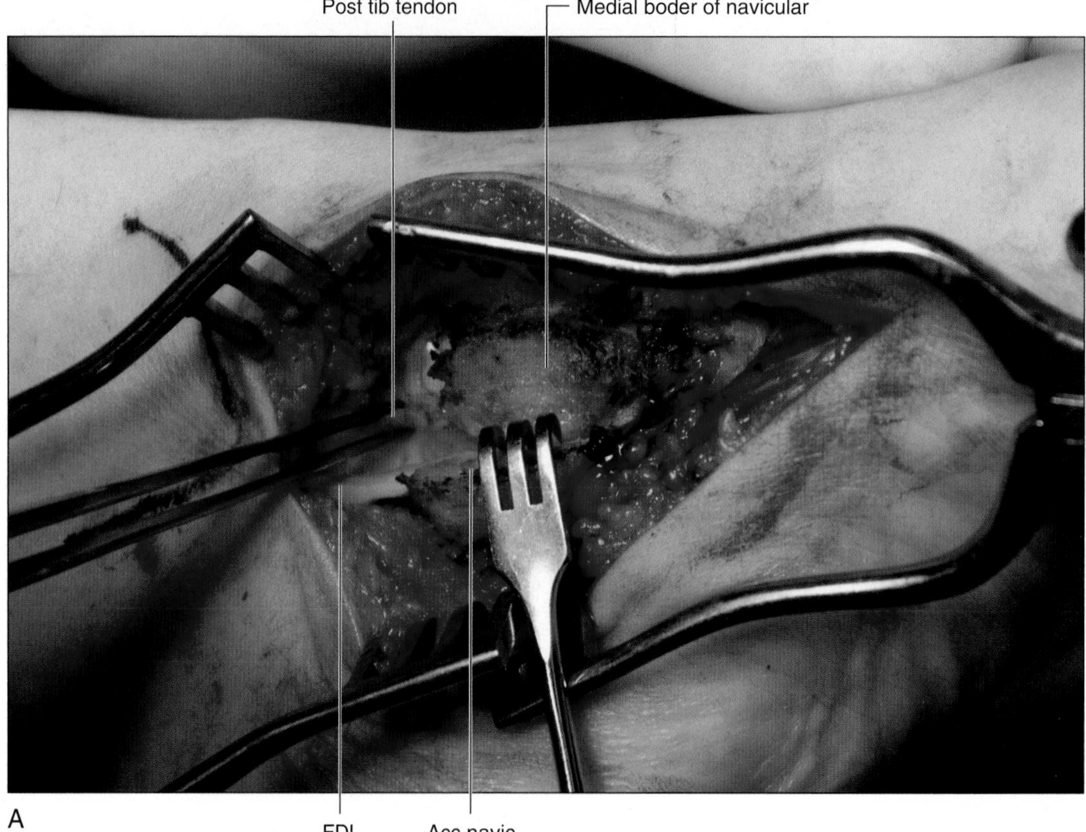

A

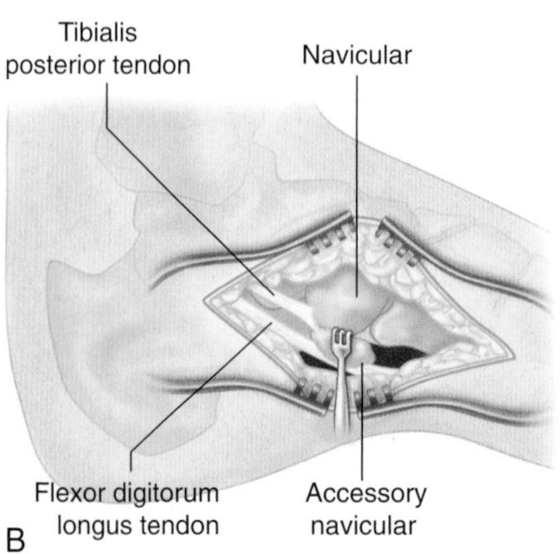

B

FIGURE 6

Step 2: Excision of Accessory Navicular and Augmentation of Posterior Tibial Tendon Insertion

- The bony prominence is removed with a rongeur, taking care to maintain the bony shell of cortical bone along the tendon (Fig. 7).
- The medial navicular can also be shaved down to just below the medial border of the cuneiform. This allows the resulting medial border of the foot to be flush once the repair is completed.
- The shell of bone is pre-drilled in the middle portion of the bony shell. The navicular is also pre-drilled, taking care so as not to enter the talonavicular joint (Fig. 8).

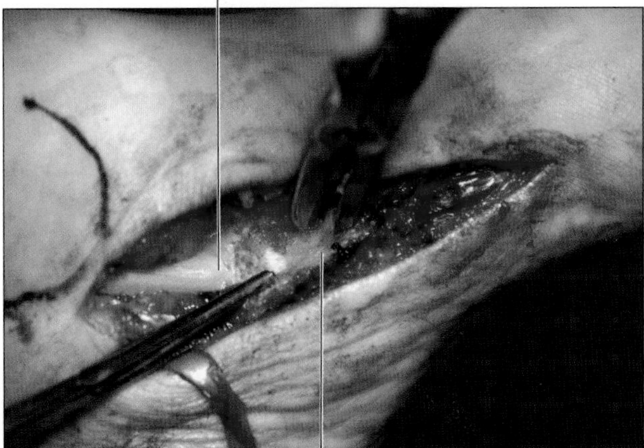

FIGURE 7

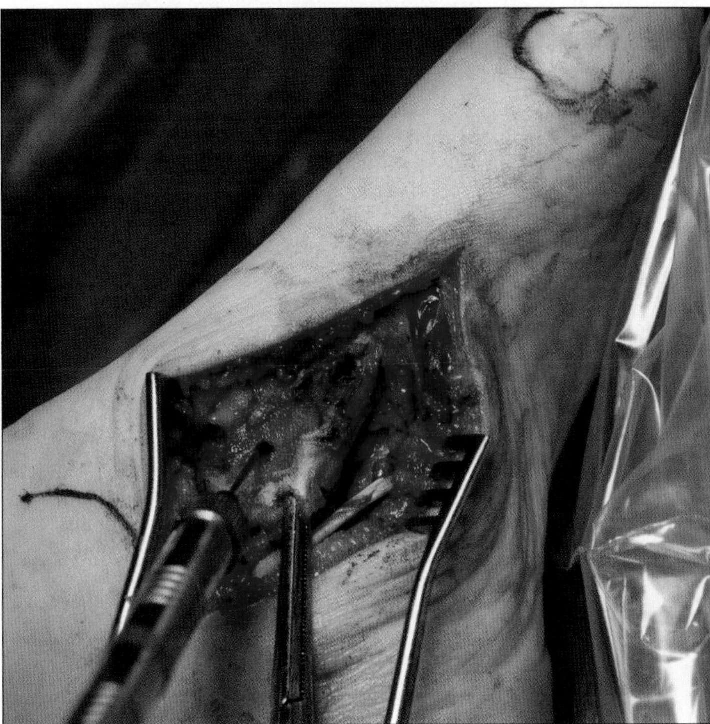

FIGURE 8

PEARLS

- *When drilling the pilot hole into the navicular, take care to aim distally. The talonavicular joint is spherical and, if one drills straight across from the medial navicular border, the joint will be entered and damaged. This can also be done under fluoroscopic control. The trajectory and depth of the drill can be aimed using the mini-fluoroscopy machine (Fig. 11A and 11B).*

Controversies

- Trough with suture versus drill hole with interference screw
  - The tendon either can be attached to the underside of the navicular-cuneiform joint in a bony trough with suture only through the bone, or can be brought through a drill hole into the bone and fixed with an interference screw. The author's preference is to use a trough with a suture, with no experience of the problem of pullout. A similar notion is presented by Levy et al. (2000) for biceps repair. The biceps repair is tacked to the paratenon, where the tendon stays and adheres.
  - A large pull-through tunnel with an interference screw may also be unnecessarily expensive.

- The screw with washer is inserted through the shell of bone and into the navicular body until the bony shell is in contact with the medial navicular (Fig. 9). The tendon profile should be even with the medial cuneiform.
- The FDL can then be transferred into a bony trough on the underside of the navicular-cuneiform joint, further augmenting the posterior tibialis tendon (Fig. 10).
  - The bony trough can be made on the underside medial ridge of the navicular-cuneiform joint with a rongeur. A 2.5-cm drill hole can be made from dorsal to plantar through the body of the cuneiform.
  - A suture (0 monofilament absorbable on a large needle) is fed backward down through the drill hole. The suture is then whip-stitched from distal to proximal for approximately 2 cm.
  - Another drill hole is made through the body of the navicular into the trough. The same suture is then passed upward and is tied by dorsally pulling the FDL up into the bony trough.
  - Supplemental sutures can be added along the side to further secure the transfer.

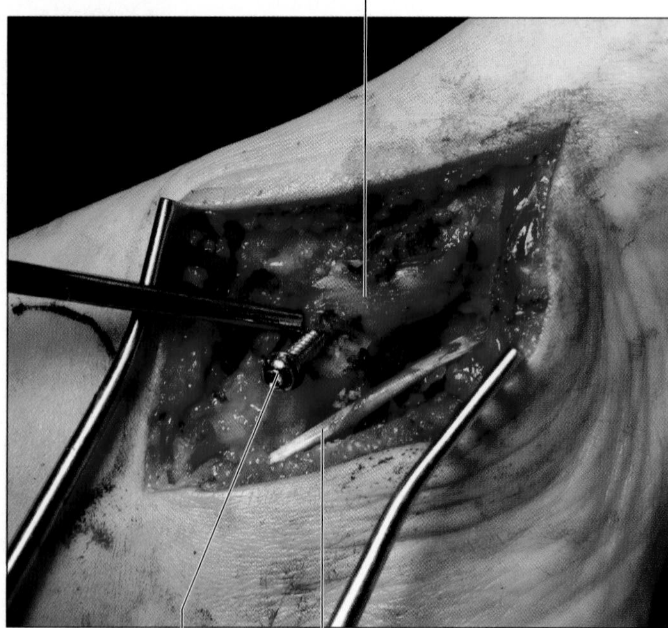

FIGURE 9

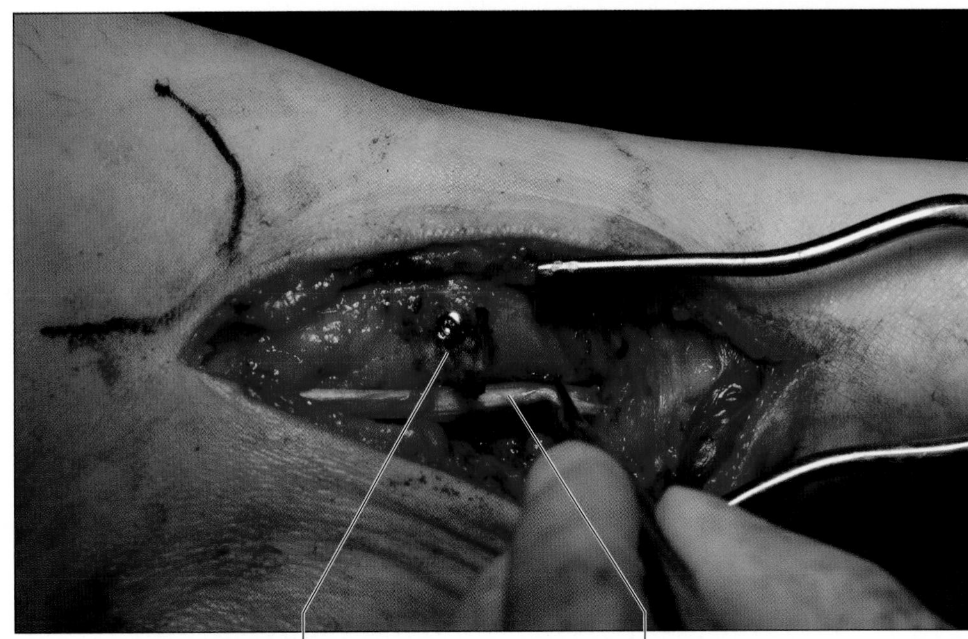

FIGURE 10

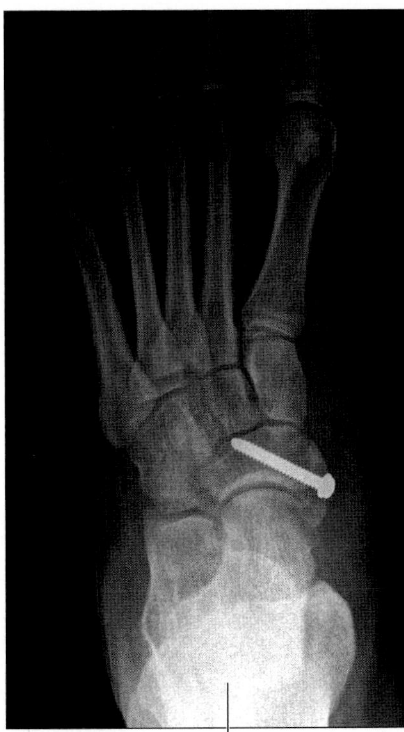

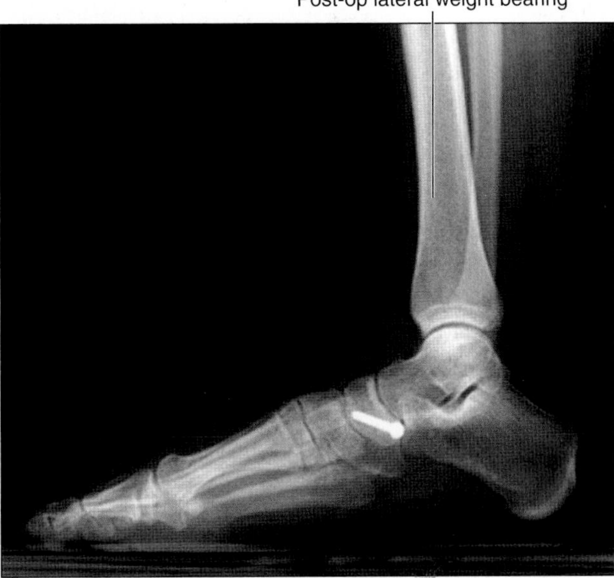

A B

FIGURE 11

Postoperative Care and Expected Outcomes

- The patient is placed into a three-sided plaster splint with the ankle and hindfoot in neutral.
- At the first postoperative visit another cast or a cam walker can be applied. The patient should be non–weight bearing but can be allowed to place the foot down gently during activities such as tooth brushing as long as the foot and ankle are protected in the splint or the cam walker boot.
- After 6 weeks gentle range of motion begins. Weight bearing is progressed to full. More aggressive physical therapy is begun at 12 weeks if needed.

Evidence

Bennett GL, Weiner DS, Leighley B. Surgical treatment of symptomatic accessory tarsal navicular. J Pediatr Orthop. 1990;10:445-9.

This study is a retrospective review of surgical treatment of 50 consecutive patients with symptomatic accessory tarsal naviculars that failed conservative treatment. Outcome was determined by clinical and subjective assessment. (Level IV evidence [case series])

Kopp FJ, Marcus RE. Clinical outcome of surgical treatment of the symptomatic accessory navicular. Foot Ankle Int. 2004;25:27-30.

This study is a retrospective review of surgical treatment of 13 consecutive patients for symptomatic accessory navicular. Follow-up averaged 103.4 months, and outcome was judged by clinical results utilizing American Orthopaedic Foot and Ankle Society (AOFAS)-Midfoot scores. (Level IV evidence [case series])

Levy HJ, Mashoof AA, Morgan D. Repair of chronic ruptures of the distal biceps tendon using flexor carpi radialis tendon graft. Am J Sports Med. 2000;28:538-40.

This study is a case series of five patients with chronic distal biceps tendon ruptures treated with flexor carpi radialis tendon graft through suture anchors. Follow-up was a minimum of 2 years, and outcome was determined by clinical assessment. (Level IV evidence [case series])

Macnicol MF, Voutsinas S. Surgical treatment of the symptomatic accessory navicular. J Bone Joint Surg [Br]. 1984;66:218-26.

This study is a retrospective series of the treatment of 47 patients with the Kidner operation. (Level IV evidence [case series])

Prichasuk S, Sinphurmsukskul O. Kidner procedure for symptomatic accessory navicular and its relation to pes planus. Foot Ankle Int. 1995;16:500-3.

This study is a case series of surgical treatment of symptomatic accessory navicular in relation to pes planus in 28 patients. Follow-up averaged 3.2 years, and outcome was determined by radiographic and clinical assessment. (Level IV evidence [case series])

Ray S, Goldberg VM. Surgical treatment of accessory navicular. Clin Orthop Related Res. 1983;(177):61-6.

This study is a retrospective review of surgical management of the accessory navicular using the Kidner procedure in 29 feet. Follow-up averaged 4.5 years, and outcome was judged by subjective assessment. (Level IV evidence [case series])

PROCEDURE 22

Painful Accessory Navicular Treated with Fusion

Glenn B. Pfeffer

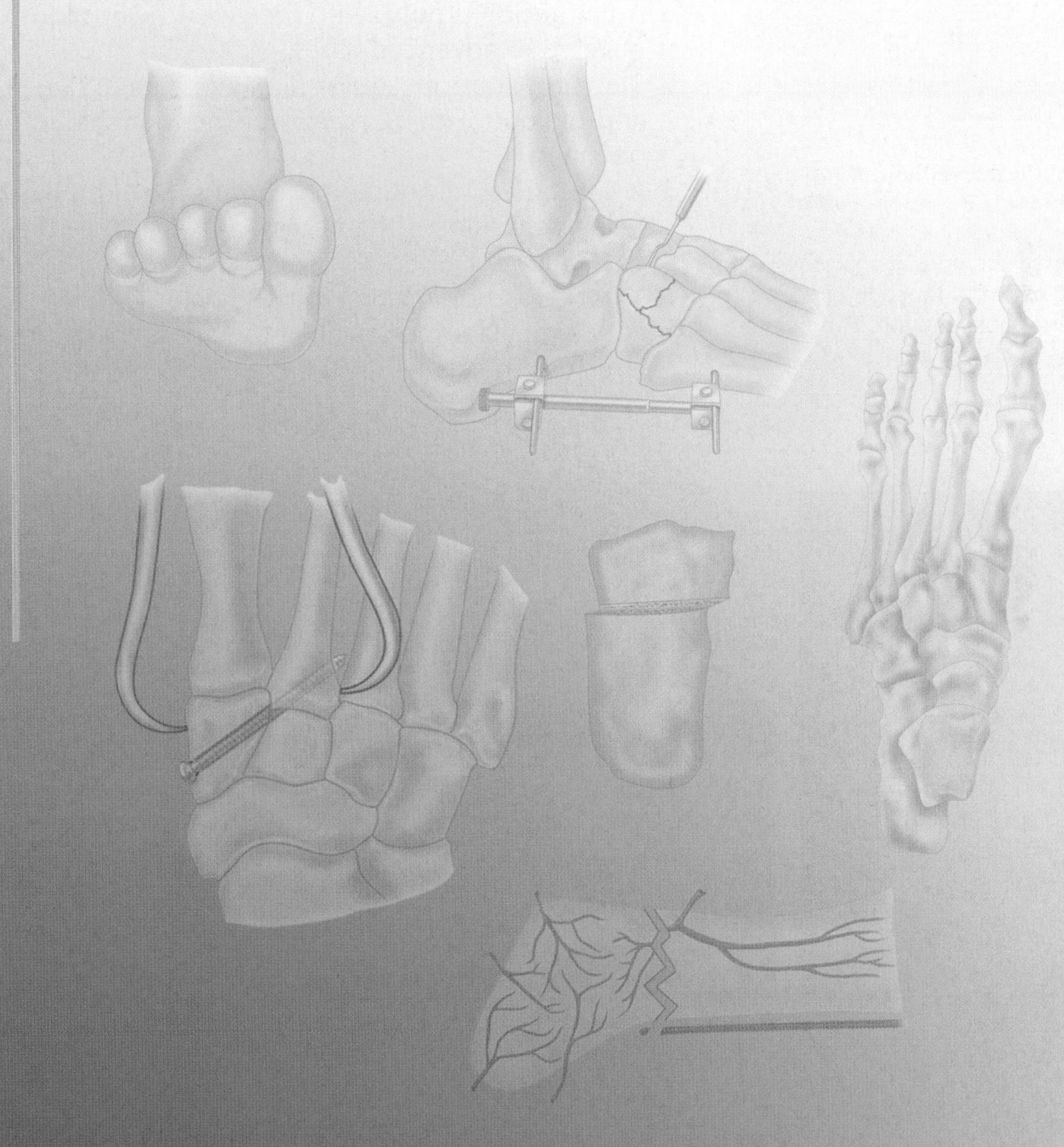

Pitfalls

- *The accessory navicular has to be of sufficient size to accept a screw without fragmentation. If increased heel valgus has developed on the symptomatic side, a calcaneal osteotomy should be added to the procedure.*

Controversies

- There is a high failure rate of simple excision of a large type II accessory navicular, with or without advancement of the posterior tibial tendon. Fusion of the painful synchondrosis preserves the normal anatomy of the foot and function of the posterior tibial tendon, without the need for additional procedures.

Indications

- Painful type II accessory navicular
- Failure of conservative care

Examination/Imaging

- The hallmark of the examination is focal pain over the accessory navicular.
- Posterior tibial tendon function may be compromised by pain at the accessory navicular, although unassisted toe rise is still possible.
- A flatfoot deformity, with increased heel valgus, may develop in advanced cases.
- Standing anteroposterior (Fig. 1A), lateral (Fig. 1B), and oblique (Fig. 1C) views of the foot should be obtained.
- A computed tomography scan through the navicular helps determine if the accessory piece is of sufficient size to accept a screw.
- Magnetic resonance imaging is helpful if concomitant posterior tibial tendinopathy is present, which is unusual.

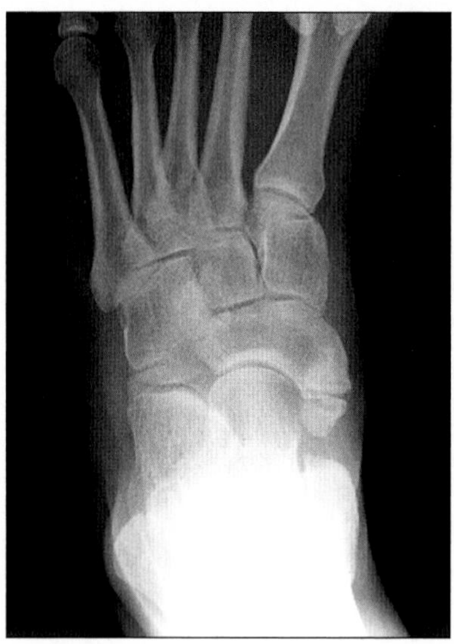

A

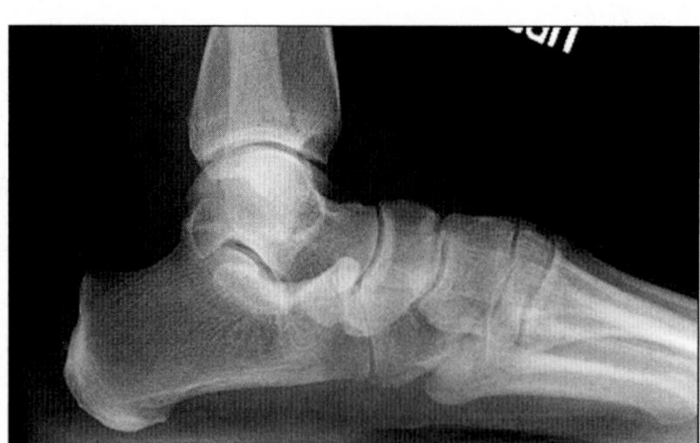

B

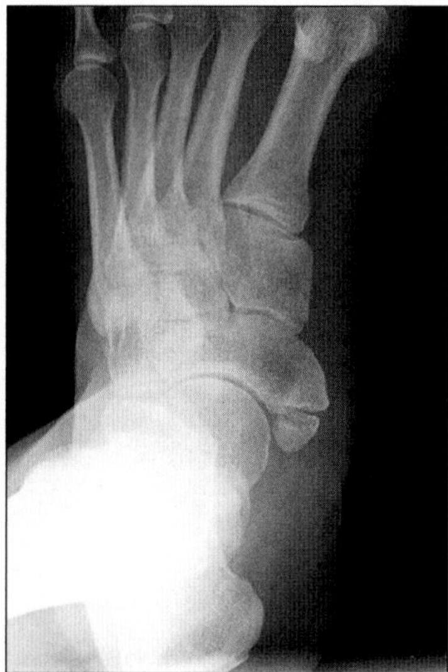
C

FIGURE 1

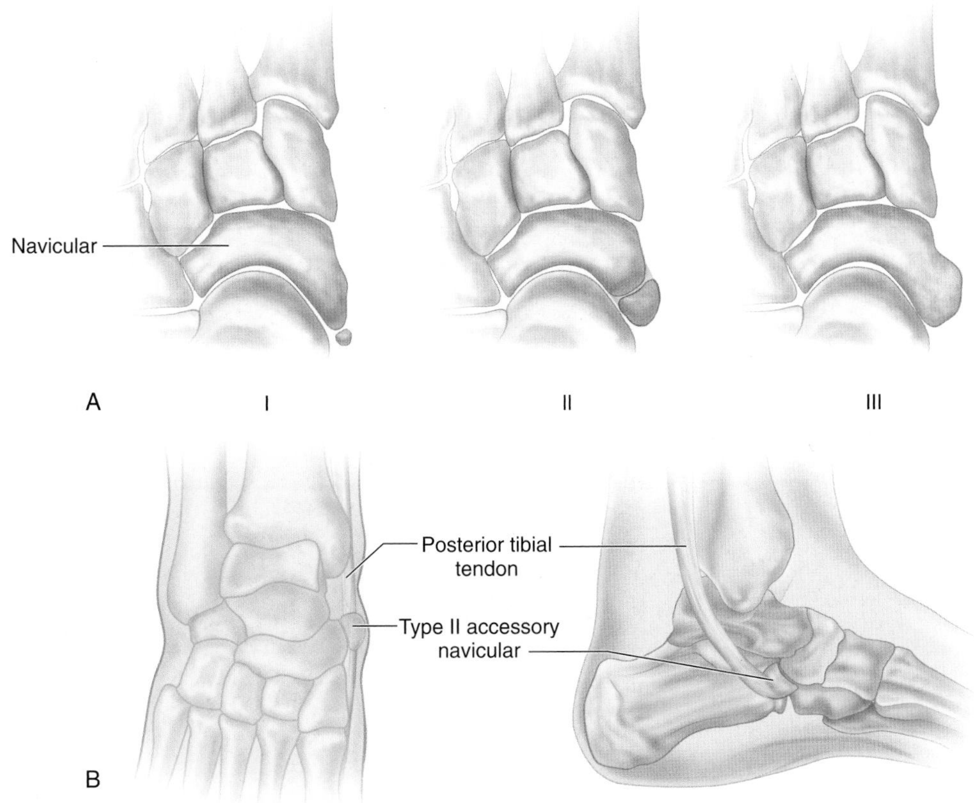

FIGURE 2

Treatment Options

- Orthotics may be helpful for mild symptoms.
- A walking cast for 4–6 weeks should be tried prior to operative intervention.
- Physical therapy may be beneficial in select cases.

Surgical Anatomy

- There are three types of accessory navicular (Fig. 2A).
- This procedure is used for type II accessory navicular (Fig. 2B).

Positioning

- The patient is placed supine.
- A bump under the contralateral hip will help externally rotate the leg.
- An ankle tourniquet may be used, but a thigh tourniquet is preferable as it places no tension on the posterior tibial muscle or tendon during the repair.

PEARLS

- *The incision should not be curved along the course of the posterior tibial tendon. A longitudinal incision facilitates placement of the pin and cannulated screw.*

PITFALLS

- *Loupe magnification will be helpful.*

Portals/Exposures

- The longitudinal incision starts 1.5 cm distal to the anterior edge of the medial malleolus and extends 2 cm distal to the accessory navicular (Fig. 3).

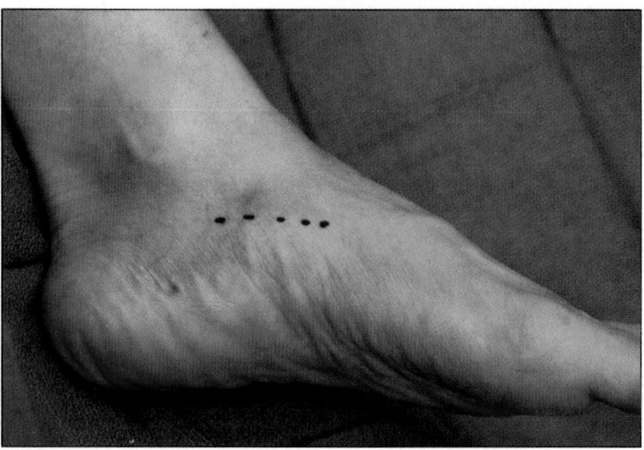

FIGURE 3

Procedure

STEP 1

- Open the posterior tibial tendon sheath along its superior border (Fig. 4).
- A mild synovitis may be present, which should be débrided.

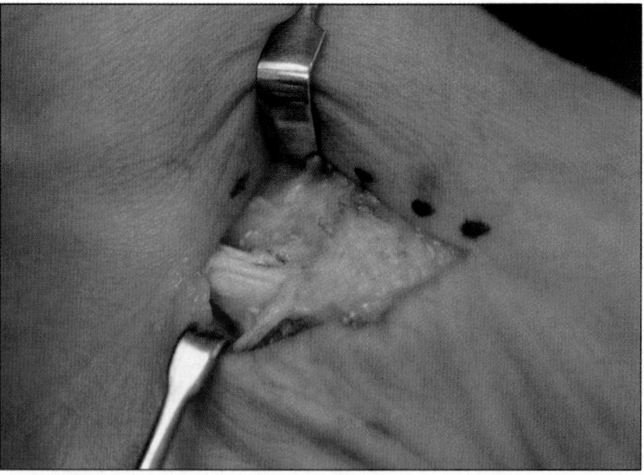

FIGURE 4

Pearls

- *It is essential to evaluate the oblique angle of the synchondrosis from the preoperative radiographs. Otherwise, a false plane may be created as the accessory navicular is detached from the navicular.*
- *The attachment of the posterior tibial tendon must be kept intact. Care is taken not to damage the spring ligament.*

Pearls

- *The underlying approach to this procedure is similar to that of a scaphoid nonunion in the wrist, including removal of fibrous tissue and sclerotic bone, bone graft to fill the defect, and application of internal rigid fixation.*

Step 2

- Locate the synchondrosis of the navicular.
- Walk along the bone with a round-tipped beaver blade to identify the junction between the body of the navicular and the accessory piece (Fig. 5).

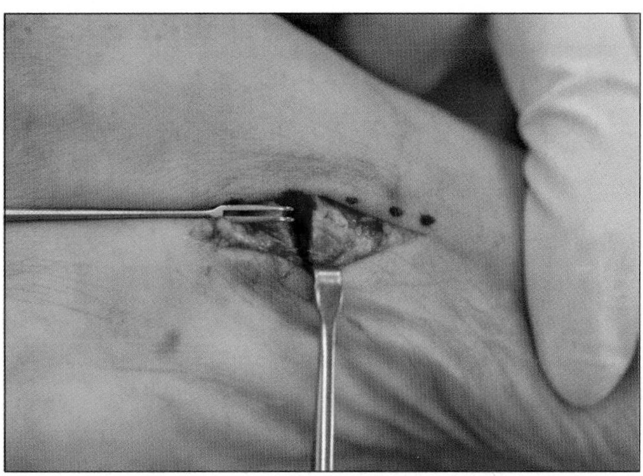

FIGURE 5

Step 3

- Remove the fibrocartilaginous tissue from each bony piece.
- Sclerotic bone often caps the bone ends and should be lightly débrided with a 3-mm burr while irrigating with cool saline (Fig. 6).

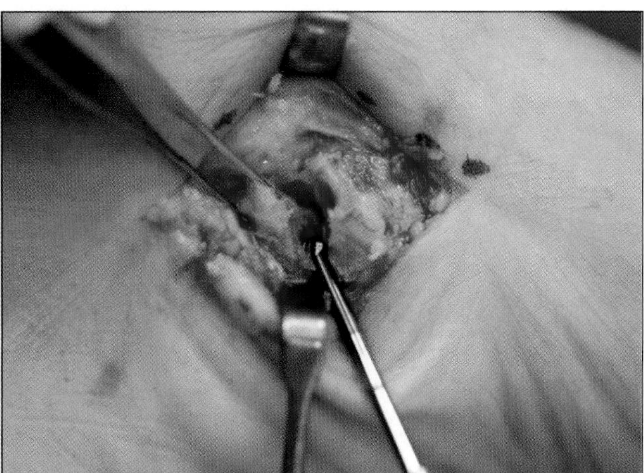

FIGURE 6

Step 4

- Use a 2- to 3-mm curette to débride the bone pieces back to healthy cancellous bone (Fig. 7).
- Care must be taken to keep the cortical shell of the accessory navicular intact.
- Adequate cancellous bone must be preserved in the tip of the accessory navicular to hold the proximal portion of the cannulated headless screw (Fig. 8).

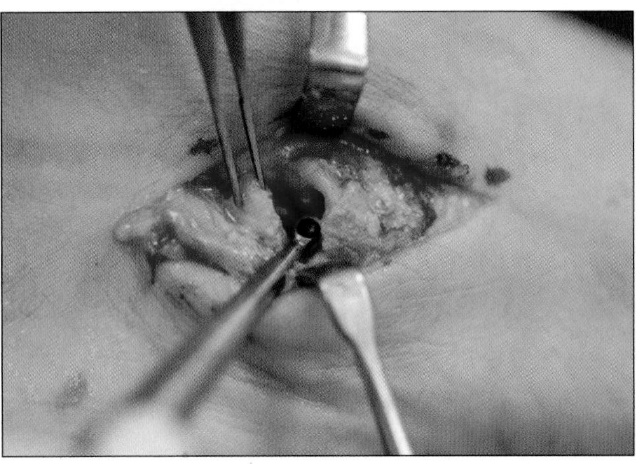

FIGURE 7

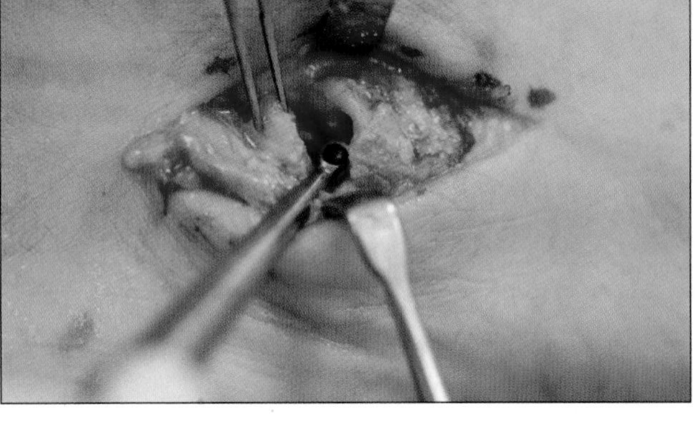

FIGURE 8

Step 5

- Cancellous bone is morcellized and placed into the concave defects in each piece.
- The graft should be easily compressible so that it can contour to the space (Fig. 9).
- Either the lateral calcaneus or proximal tibial are excellent harvest sites.

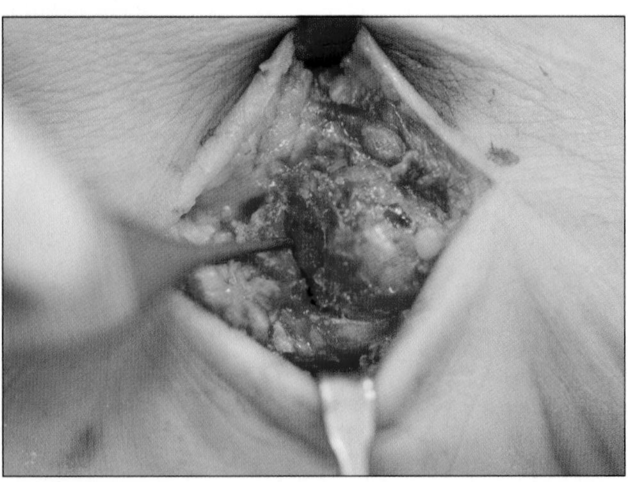

FIGURE 9

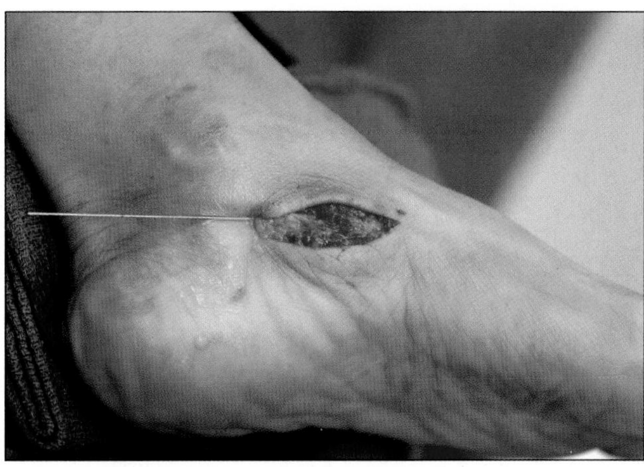

FIGURE 10

Step 6

- Using a mini-driver, position a 0.045-inch guidewire (Acutrak 2, titanium alloy mini-cannulated screw set) across the reduced pieces (Fig. 10). Confirm the placement by fluoroscan.
- Determine the appropriate screw length. The screw does not have to engage the far cortex as it will have excellent compression in the dense cancellous bone of the navicular.

Step 7

- Compress the pieces with a towel clip, and drill as needed. Often just the cortical bone of the accessory navicular piece requires drilling.

Pearls

- *A small incision in the posterior tibial tendon provides the best access for the screw, without removing any of the posterior tibial tendon attachment into the accessory navicular (Fig. 11).*

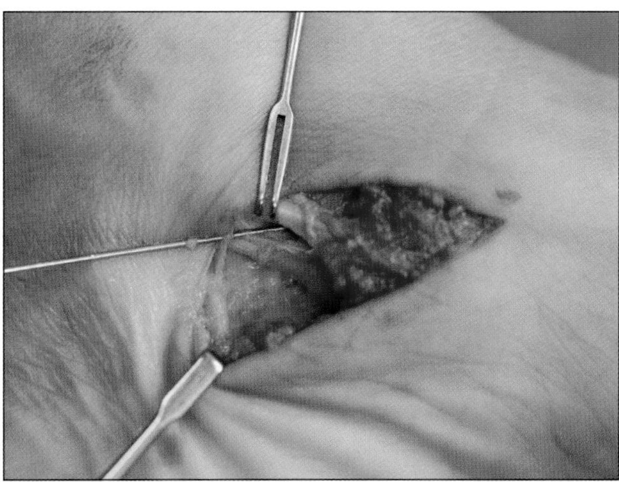

FIGURE 11

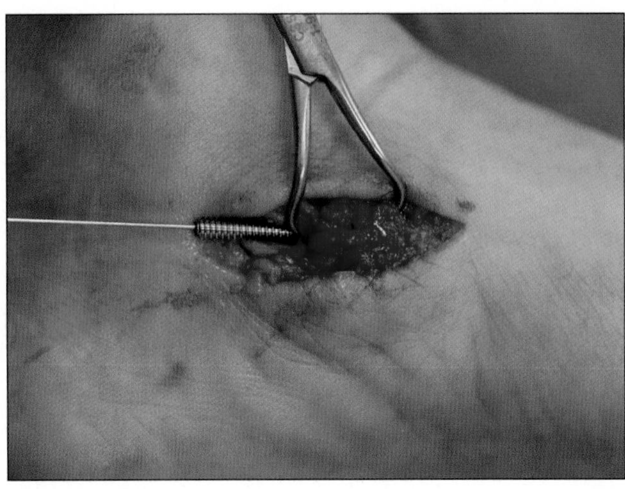

A

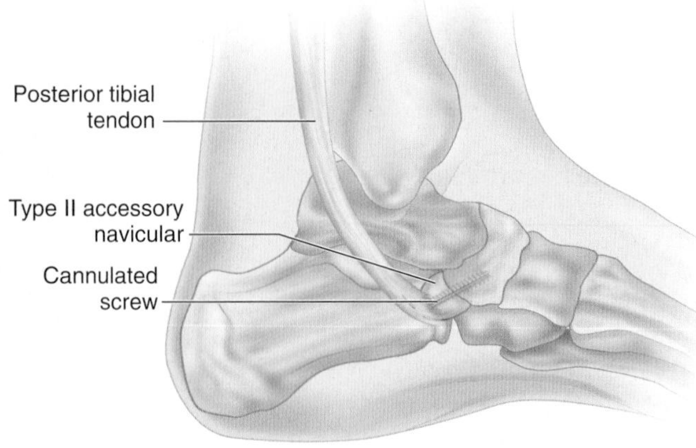

B

FIGURE 12

- Carefully place the Acutrak 2 miniscrew and confirm final position by fluoroscopy.
  - Compression of the pieces will be evident as the screw enters (Fig. 12A and 12B).
  - Place the ankle in plantar flexion and the foot in supination during screw placement to relax the posterior tibial tendon and diminish pull on the accessory piece.
- The tendon can be repaired with two 3-0 Ethibond sutures, burying the knots within the tendon. Repair the tendon sheath using similar suture.
- Deflate the tourniquet, obtain hemostasis, and close the skin with simple nylon sutures.
- Place a bulky splint with the foot in supination and the ankle in slight plantar flexion.

Postoperative Care and Expected Outcomes

- The patient is seen 10–12 days postoperatively and the sutures are removed. Apply a non–weight-bearing cast with the foot in supination and the ankle in neutral.
- Change the cast at 1 month after surgery and bring the foot into a neutral position. The patient is kept non–weight bearing for 6 weeks postoperatively. At 6 weeks, the cast is removed and weight bearing is allowed in a cast boot, if healing is evident clinically and by radiography (Fig. 13A and 13B). Physical therapy may be beneficial to restore range of motion and strength.

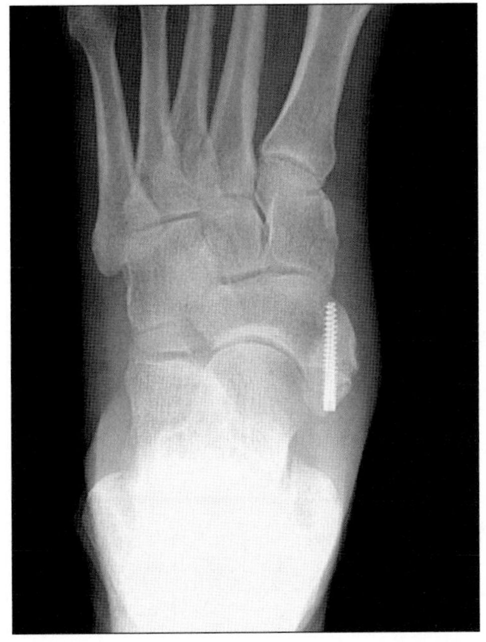
A

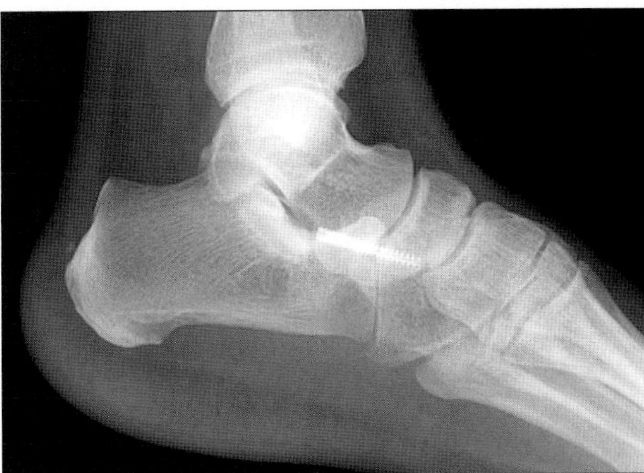
B

FIGURE 13

- All patients can be expected to do well and be symptom free, unless there is a nonunion of the attempted fusion.

Evidence

Kidner FC. The pre hallux (accessory scaphoid) in its relation to flat foot. J Bone Joint Surg. 1929;11:831.

The first description of a surgical procedure to treat a painful accessory navicular. (Level IV evidence)

Knupp M, Hintermann B. Reconstruction in posttraumatic combined avulsion of an accessory navicular and the posterior tibial tendon. Tech Foot Ankle Surg. 2005;4:113-8.

This technique article reviews a modification of the Kidner procedure first published by Malicky et al. in 1999 (see below). The technique involves fusion of the accessory navicular piece to the body of the navicular, with more bone resection than the method described in this procedure. (Level IV evidence)

Kopp FJ, Marcus RE. Clinical outcomes of surgical treatment of the symptomatic accessory navicular. Foot Ankle Int. 2004;25:27-30.

This study reviews 14 feet that underwent surgical treatment for symptomatic accessory navicular with excision of the piece and advancement of the posterior tibial tendon (Kidner procedure). The clinical status of each patient improved significantly. The authors use the American Orthopaedic Foot and Ankle Society Midfoot scale to evaluate the results in the study. (Level IV evidence)

Malicky ES, Levine DS, Sangeorzan BJ. Modification of the Kidner procedure with fusion of the primary accessory navicular bones. Foot Ankle Int. 1999;20:53-4.

The authors fused the accessory navicular to the body in an effort to avoid the complications associated with excision of the piece. (Level V evidence)

PROCEDURE 23

Open Reduction and Internal Fixation of Proximal Fifth Metatarsal (Jones' or Stress) Fracture

Mark E. Easley and James A. Nunley II

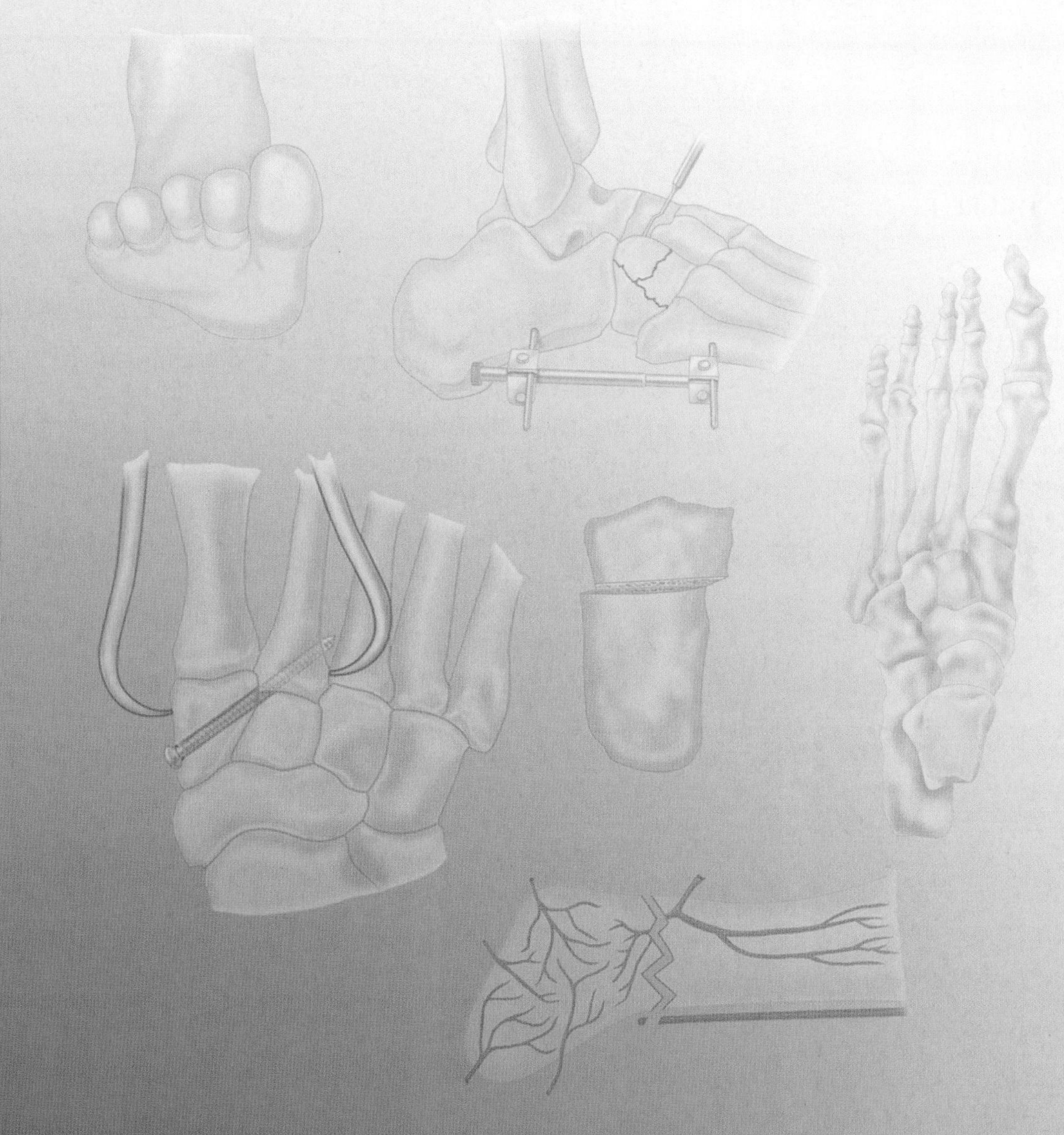

Indications

- Fracture in zone II or III of the proximal fifth metatarsal (5MT) (Fig. 1)
- Acute fracture in an athlete
- Delayed union

> **PITFALLS**
>
> - *Varus hindfoot alignment maintaining a continued risk to 5MT overload*

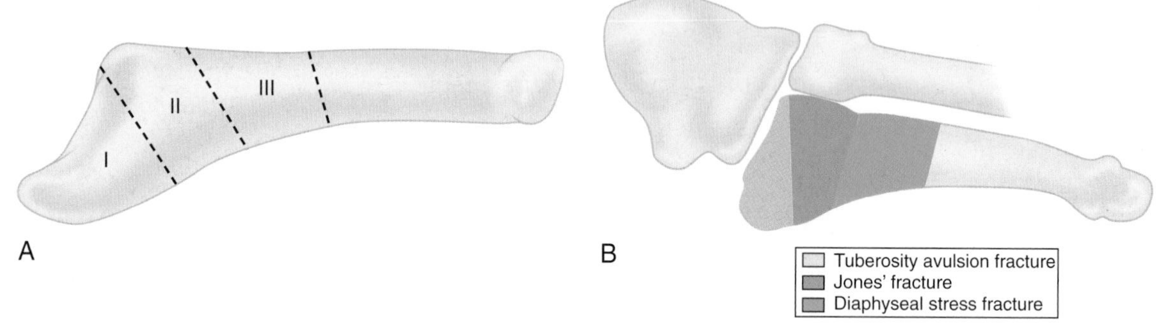

FIGURE 1

Examination/Imaging

- Tenderness at the base of the 5MT
- Hindfoot alignment
- Radiographs demonstrating fracture in zone II of the 5MT
  - Fracture in base of the 5MT extending into articulation of fourth metatarsal and 5MT bases on anteroposterior (Fig. 2A), oblique (Fig. 2B), and lateral (Fig. 2C) views.

> ## Treatment Options
>
> - Nonoperative treatment with casting, protected weight bearing
> - Intramedullary screw fixation
> - External bone stimulation
> - Tension band technique/plating

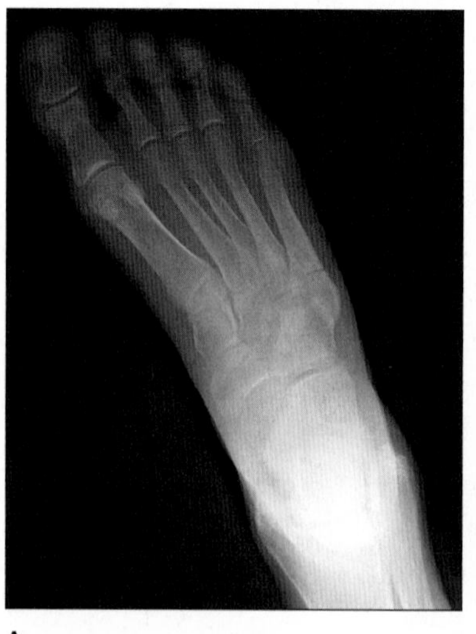
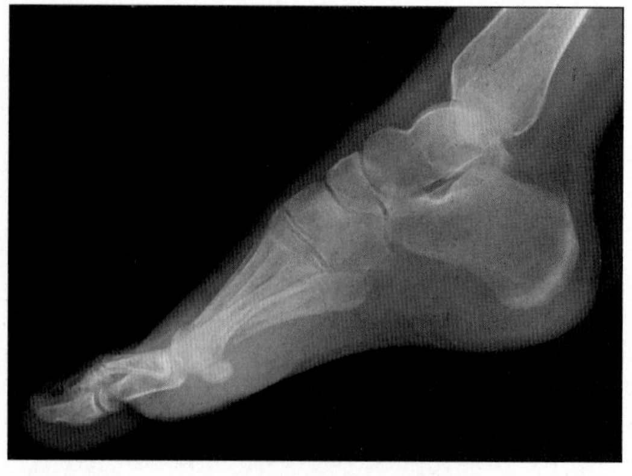

A B C

FIGURE 2

PEARLS

- *Bump under ipsilateral hip to improve access to lateral foot*
- *Patient's operated foot on edge of table to facilitate passing instruments/implants and to allow shifting foot over edge of table for easy fluoroscopic access*
- *Bump under operated foot to improve ability to pass instruments/implants*

Surgical Anatomy

- There is a watershed area of relatively less perfusion in zone II of the 5MT base (Fig. 3A).
- The 5MT is a curved bone (relevant to fixation with a straight implant [screw]) (Fig. 3B).
- At-risk structures include the peroneus brevis and longus and the sural nerve (Fig. 3C).

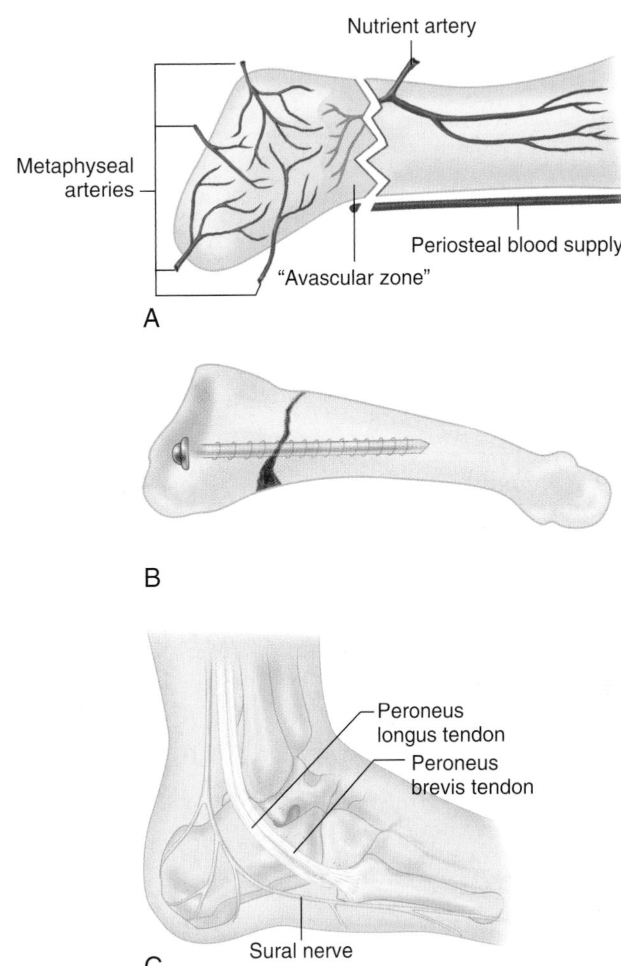

FIGURE 3

Positioning

- Supine in a modified lateral position with the foot on the edge of the operating table to allow easy access to the lateral foot
- Bump/bolster under ipsilateral hip
- Bump/bolster under operated foot

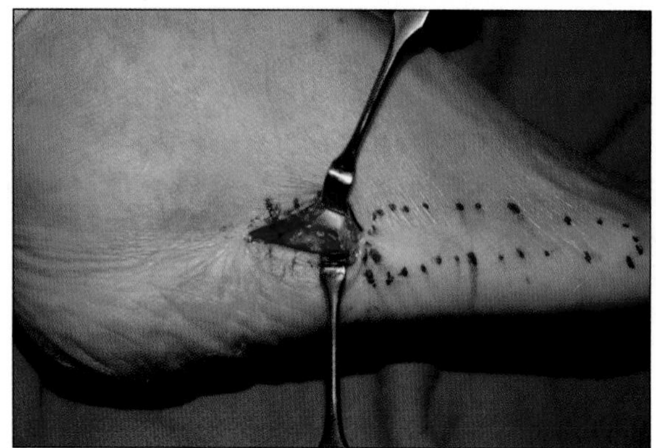
A

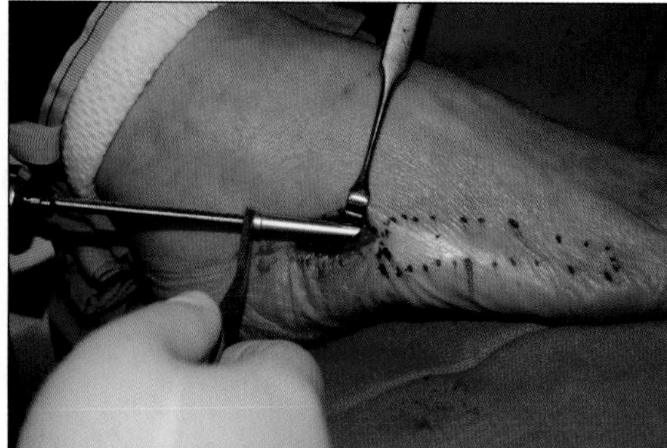
B

FIGURE 4

Portals/Exposures

- The approach is 2–4 cm proximal to the 5MT base, in line with the 5MT on the lateral foot (Fig. 4A). This approach allows optimal positioning of drill guide (Fig. 4B).
- Establish protection of structures at risk.
  - Identify sural nerve and carefully retract dorsally/superiorly.
  - Identify peroneus brevis tendon and retract dorsally/superiorly.
  - Identify peroneus longus tendon and retract plantarward/inferiorly.

Pearls

- *The surgeon may wish to mark the 5MT based on palpation to optimize the incision.*
- *Exposure must be adequate to place the drill and drill guide at the superior and medial aspect of the 5MT base.*

Pitfalls

- *Be sure to identify the sural nerve and peroneal tendons to ensure they are protected from the drill and implant.*

Instrumentation

- Standard blunt retractors

Procedure

Step 1

- Optimal guide pin placement is high and inside on the proximal 5MT, without soft tissue obstruction (Fig. 5A).
- Guide pin placement requires verification in the 5MT intramedullary canal in anteroposterior (Fig. 5B), oblique (Fig. 5C), and lateral (Fig. 5D) intraoperative fluoroscopic views.

Pearls

- *Use a high and inside (superior and medial) starting point on the 5MT base.*
- *There is no need to pass the guide pin the full length of the 5MT; it can be passed just enough to get the threads of the screw across the fracture site.*

Step 2

- Determine ideal screw diameter by successively drilling and tapping with increasingly greater drills and corresponding taps.
  - The drill should pass over the guide pin (Fig. 6A and 6B).
  - The tap is introduced into the metatarsal (Fig. 7A and 7B).

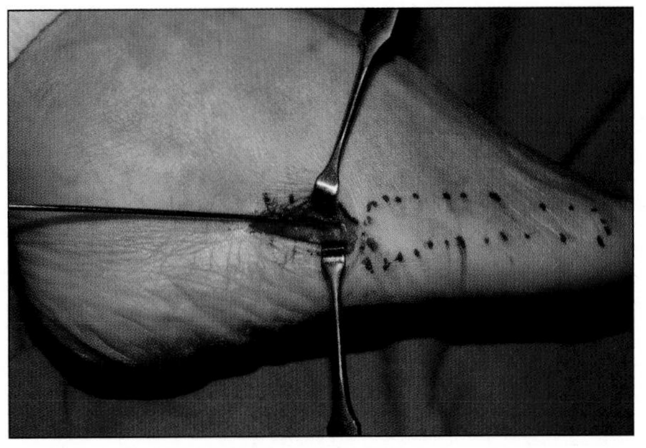

A

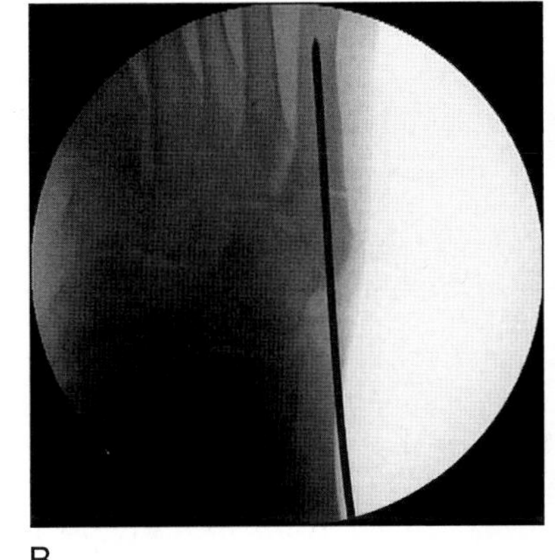

B

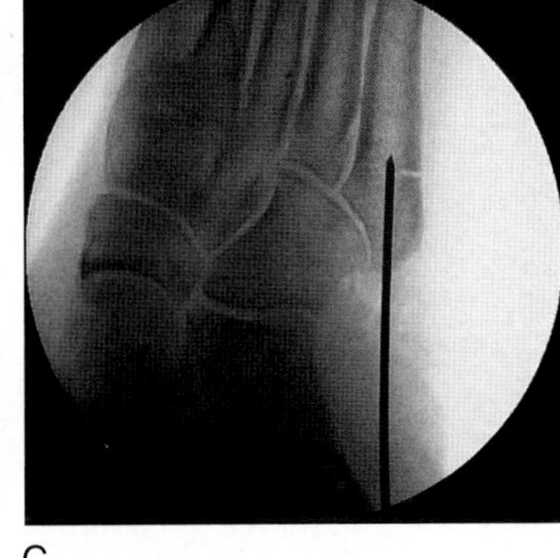

C

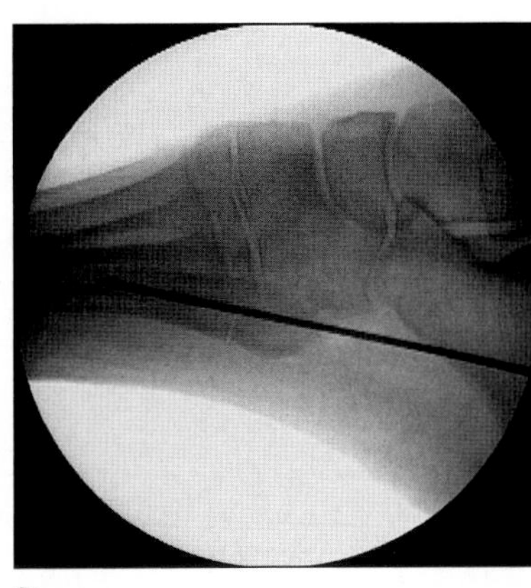

D

FIGURE 5

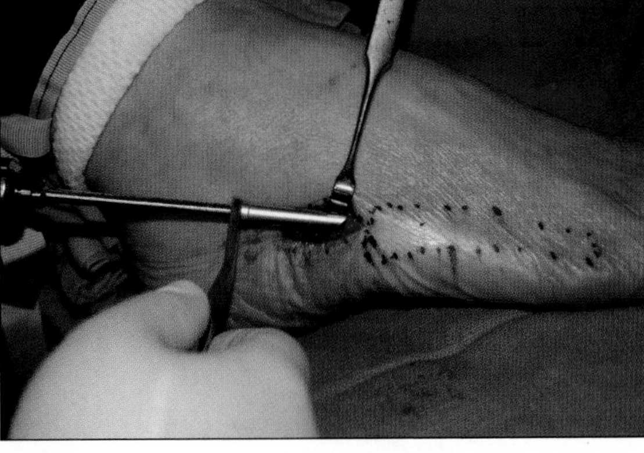

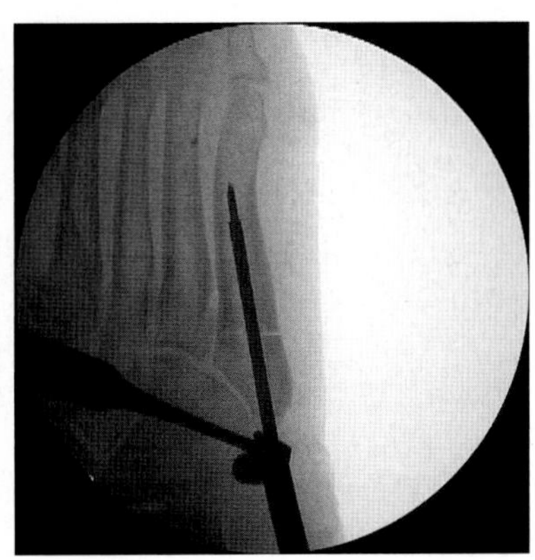

FIGURE 6 A B

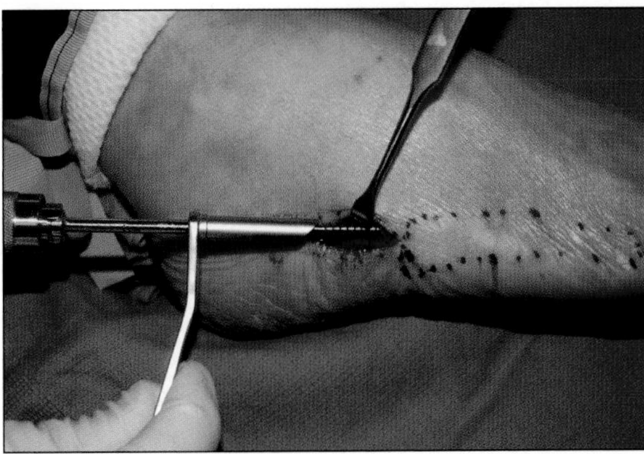

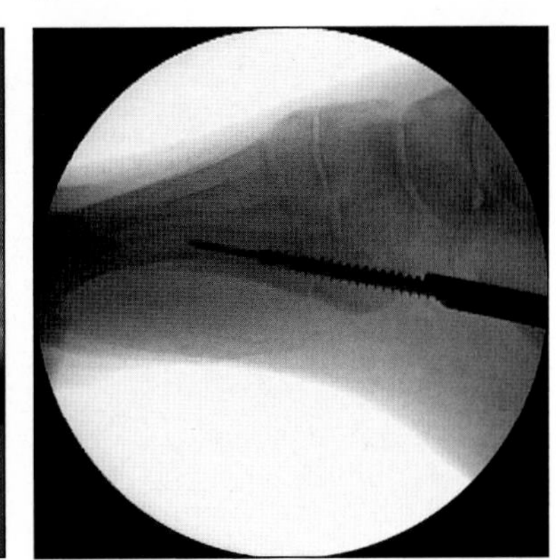

FIGURE 7 A B

Pitfalls

- *ALL THREE fluoroscopic views/ angles must be obtained to confirm that the guide pin is contained in the 5MT.*
- *The sural nerve and peroneal tendon must be protected every time an instrument or implant is passed.*

Instrumentation/ Implantation

- Satisfactory fluoroscopy unit
- Soft tissue protector for guide pin

Pearls

- *The threads of the tap/screw only need to cross the fracture site; there is no need to place the screw the entire length of the metatarsal.*
- *Hold the distal fragment as the tap is advanced; once the distal fragment begins to torque with each turn, proper screw diameter is determined.*

- Overdrill guide pin with smaller diameter cannulated drill.
- The ideal tap size provides proper intramedullary interference to allow adequate screw purchase (Fig. 8A and 8B).
  - If a 4.5-mm diameter tap has purchase in the distal fragment, then that is the ideal screw; if not, go to the next greater diameter.
  - Most 5MTs will accommodate 5.5-mm taps, and many will require 6.5-mm taps for adequate purchase.
- A calibrated tap may aid in determining ideal screw length.

Pitfalls

- *Advancing the screw too far and unnecessarily into the 5MT risks gapping at the fracture site as a straight implant is advanced into the curved bone.*
- *The starting point must be ideal or the distal fragment's medial cortex may be violated, creating a stress riser.*
- *Follow the guide pin with the drill to avoid shearing the pin within the 5MT (difficult to retrieve).*

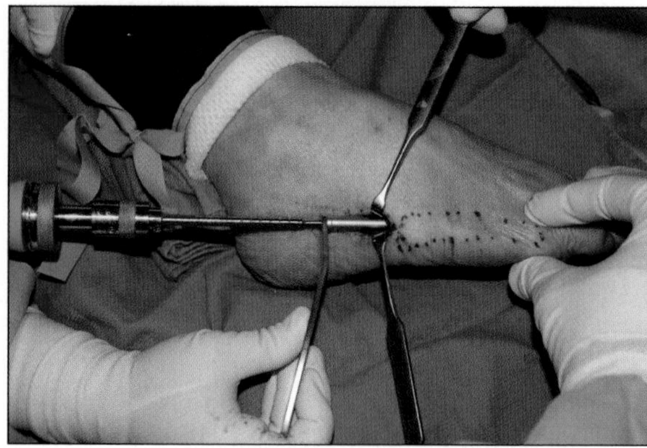

A

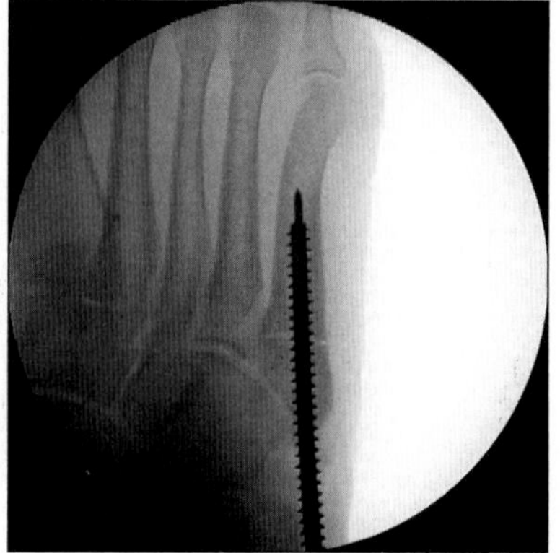

FIGURE 8 B

Step 3

- Based on ideal tap diameter, the screw diameter is selected.
- Screw length is determined by a calibrated tap and confirmed with a cannulated or noncannulated depth gauge.
- The guide pin is removed.
- Before implanting the selected screw, it may be held immediately adjacent to the bone to roughly determine if it appears appropriate, that all threads will cross the fracture site, and that the screw will not need to pass excessively into the metatarsal to be fully seated (Fig. 9).
- A soft tissue protector is placed.
- Screw insertion is done while holding the distal fragment (Fig. 10A and 10B).

Instrumentation/Implantation

- Soft tissue protector that accommodates all drill and tap sizes
- Multiple cannulated drill bits and taps that correlate with 4.5-, 5.5-, and 6.5-mm screws
- Consider a comprehensive 5MT fracture kit

Instrumentation/Implantation

- Solid or cannulated screws
- Average thread length: 16 mm (thus the screw does not need to be long to advance the threads completely across the fracture site)

Controversies

- Cannulated screws may be used; we recommend solid screws.

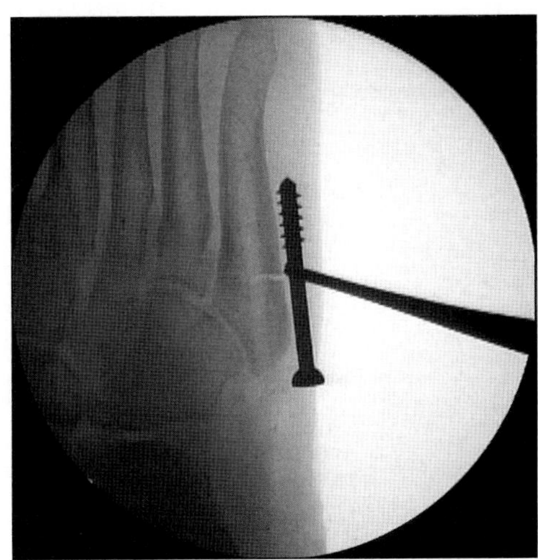

FIGURE 9

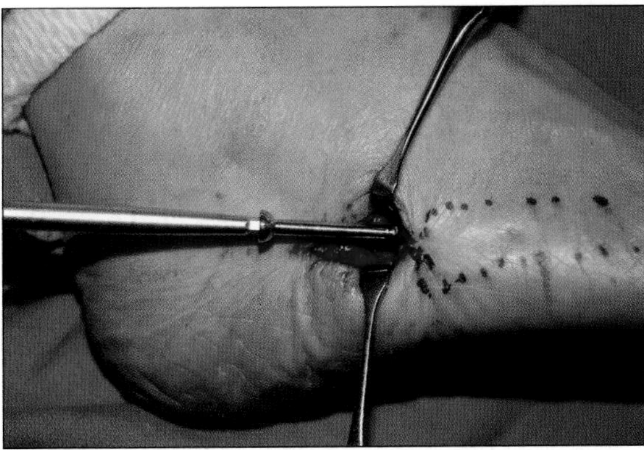

A

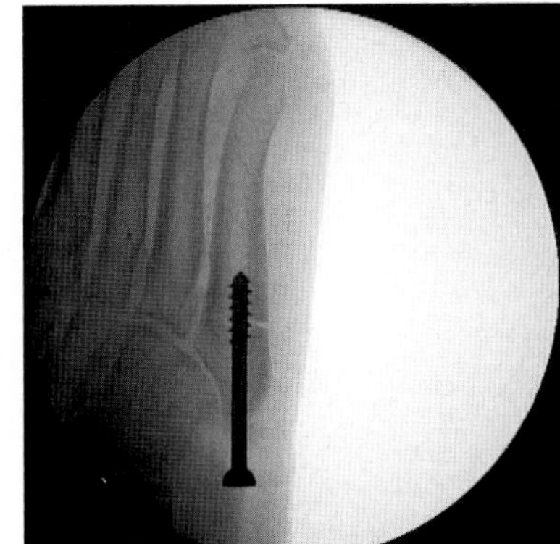

B

FIGURE 10

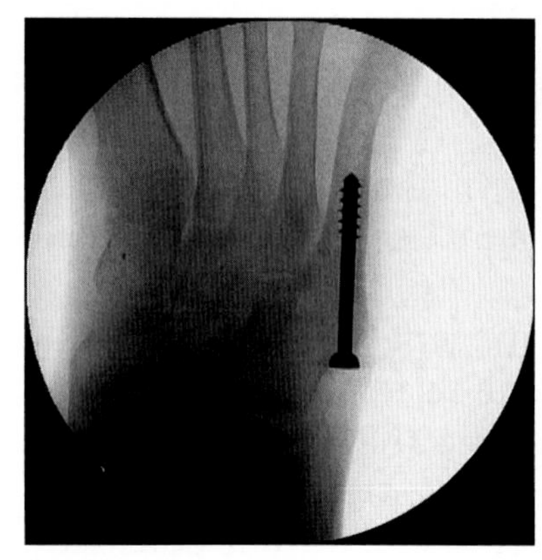
A

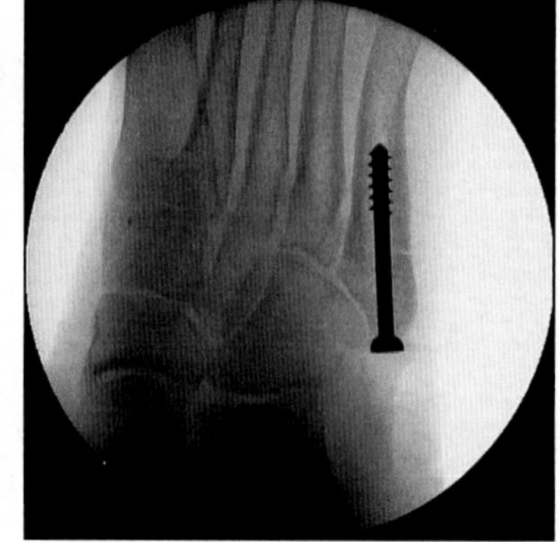
B

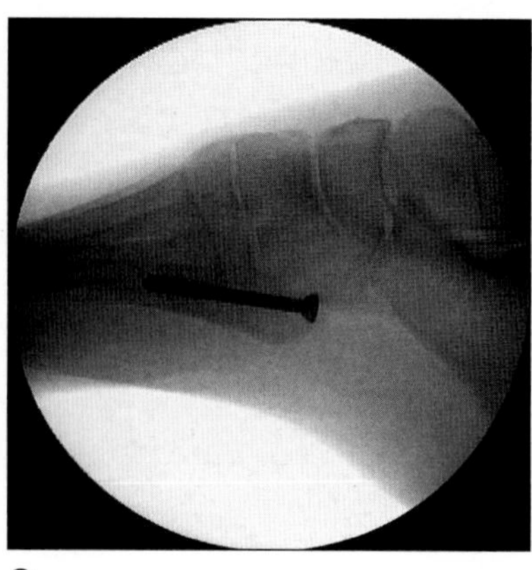
C

FIGURE 11

- When the same interference noted with the tap is achieved, fluoroscopic confirmation of proper screw fixation is made (Fig. 11A–C). The screw head should be in full contact with the 5MT base and all threads should be crossing the fracture site.

Step 4

- If heel varus is present, consideration should be given to correction of cavus/varus foot alignment to prevent 5MT overload.
  - Possible lateralizing/valgus-imparting calcaneal osteotomy.
  - Possible dorsiflexion first metatarsal osteotomy for a forefoot-driven hindfoot varus.

Pearls

- *The screw should only be long enough to allow the threads to cross the fracture site.*
- *The screw should torque the distal fragment as it is fully inserted to confirm proper interference fit.*

Pitfalls

- *A screw that is too long will potentially begin gapping the lateral fracture site (straight implant in a curved bone) and may create a distal fragment stress fracture.*

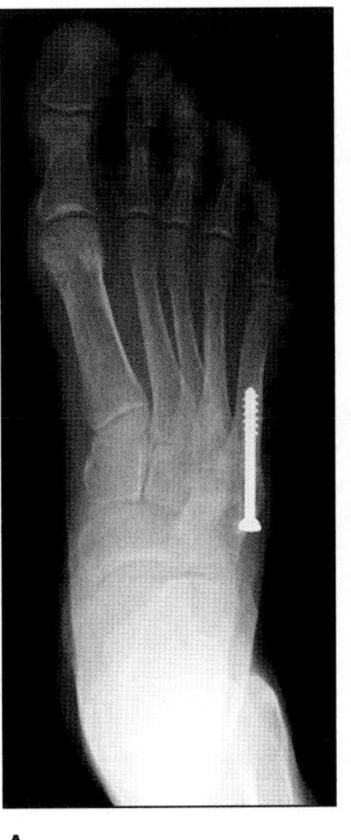
A

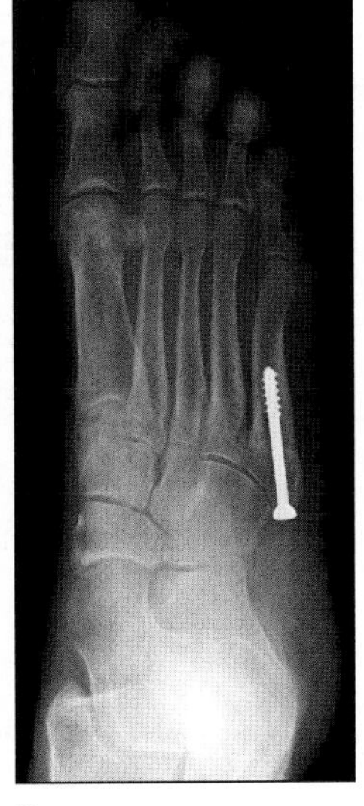
B

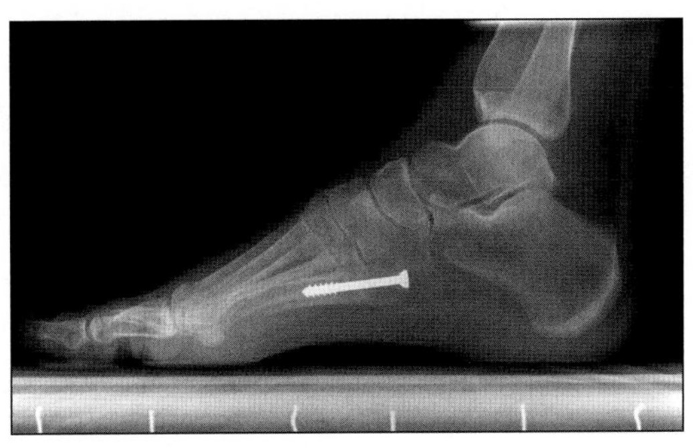
C

FIGURE 12

PEARLS

- *Support above the ankle (cam boot or cast) for at least 6 weeks is recommended to limit the pull of the peroneal tendons and stress of the lateral plantar fascia on the base of the 5MT.*

PITFALLS

- *Do not advance weight bearing or recommend return to activity until there is radiographic evidence for healing.*

Postoperative Care and Expected Outcomes

- The patient is restricted to protected weight bearing in a cam walker, splint, or cast for approximately 4 weeks.
- Begin progressive advancement of weight bearing in a cam walker for an additional 3–4 weeks.
- If there is radiographic evidence for 5MT base healing, the patient may advance to full weight bearing in a regular shoe.
- If there is a delay in healing, consider external bone stimulation.
- The patient is restricted from sports participation until the fracture site is nontender and radiographic healing is evident (approximately 10–12 weeks).
- Figure 12 shows the anteroposterior (Fig. 12A), oblique (Fig. 12B), and lateral (Fig. 12C) radiographs of a healed 5MT fracture at 4 months' follow-up.

Evidence

Chuckpaiwong B, Queen RM, Easley ME, Nunley JA. Distinguishing Jones and proximal diaphyseal fractures of the fifth metatarsal. Clin Orthop Relat Res. 2008;466:1966–70.

Nunley JA. Fractures of the base of the fifth metatarsal: the Jones fracture. Orthop Clin North Am. 2001;32:171–80.

Porter DA, Rund AM, Dobslaw R, Duncan M. Comparison of 4.5- and 5.5-mm cannulated stainless steel screws for fifth metatarsal Jones fracture fixation. Foot Ankle Int. 2009;30:27–33.

Portland G, Kelikian A, Kodros S. Acute surgical management of Jones' fractures. Foot Ankle Int. 2003;24:829–33.

Sides SD, Fetter NL, Glisson R, Nunley JA. Bending stiffness and pull-out strength of tapered, variable pitch screws, and 6.5-mm cancellous screws in acute Jones fractures. Foot Ankle Int. 2006;27:821–5.

(Grade I recommendation) (Level IV/V evidence)

PROCEDURE 24

Open Reduction and Internal Fixation of the Cuboid Fracture/Nutcracker Injury

Andrew K. Sands

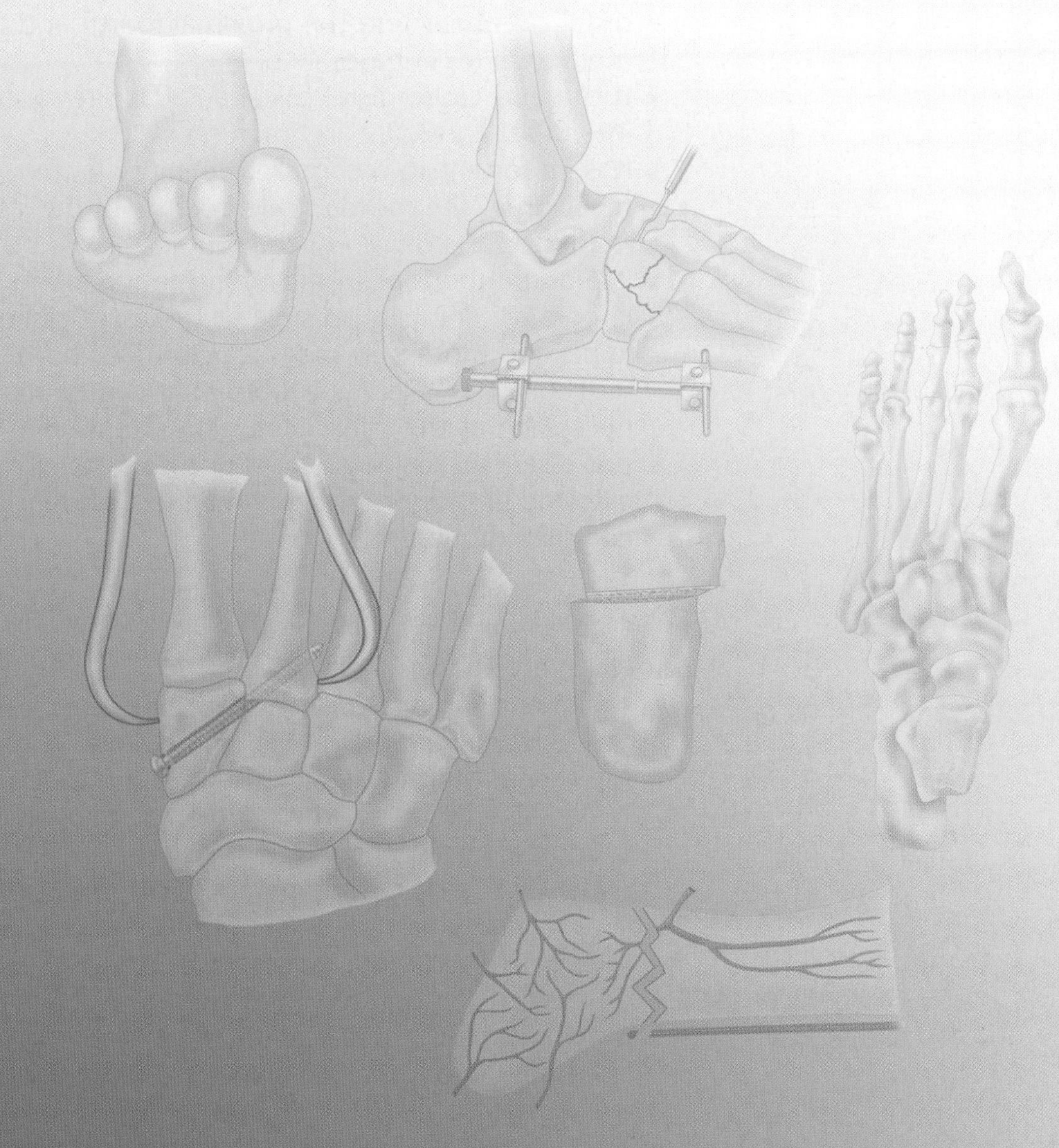

Andrew K. Sands would like to acknowledge the assistance of Edmund Choi, MD with this chapter.

Nutcracker Injury

Indications

- Injuries about Chopart joints (talonavicular and calcaneocuboid) can cause forced abduction around the talonavicular joint with subsequent compression and injury of the lateral column.
- This "nutcracker" injury can lead to avulsion fractures medially about the navicular and compression fractures of the cuboid as it is crushed between the distal calcaneus and the proximal fourth and fifth metatarsal (MT) bases.
- It can also cause distal calcaneus fractures and intertarsal and MT base fractures.
- It is important to recognize the injury pattern and to reconstruct the mechanical structure of the lateral (and medial) column of the foot.
- It is also important to maintain motion along the cuboid/MT joints if possible as these are essential joints and motion in them is helpful for normal foot function. The calcaneocuboid joint can be fused if necessary, as this is an expansion sliding joint and not essential. As long as it is not fused at either extreme of motion, there is no effect on hindfoot complex motion.

Examination/Imaging

- Plain radiographs
  - Obtain three views of the foot: anteroposterior (Fig. 1A), lateral (Fig. 1B), and oblique (Fig. 1C).
  - Observe the overall alignment of the foot and any associated injuries. There are areas of overlap and double density, however.
  - Get good-quality preoperative films and note the proximal migration of the fifth MT and lateral column shortening if present (see Fig. 1).
- Computed tomography reconstructions of the foot show a three-dimensional picture of the injury and associated injuries in the areas of double-density overlap (Fig. 2).
- Magnetic resonance imaging is not as useful as plain radiographs; however it may show bony injuries not appreciated on plain radiographs.

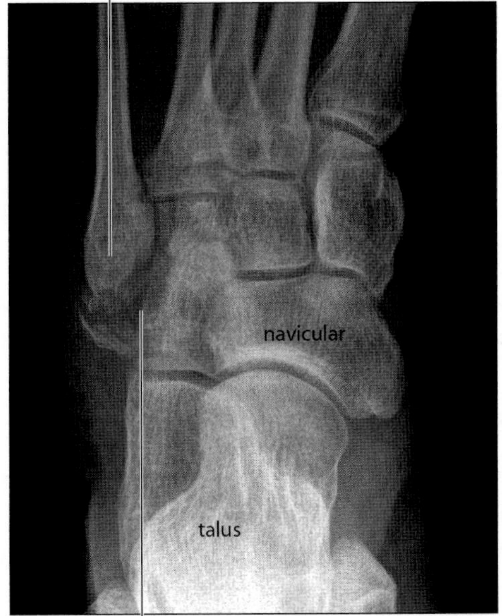

A

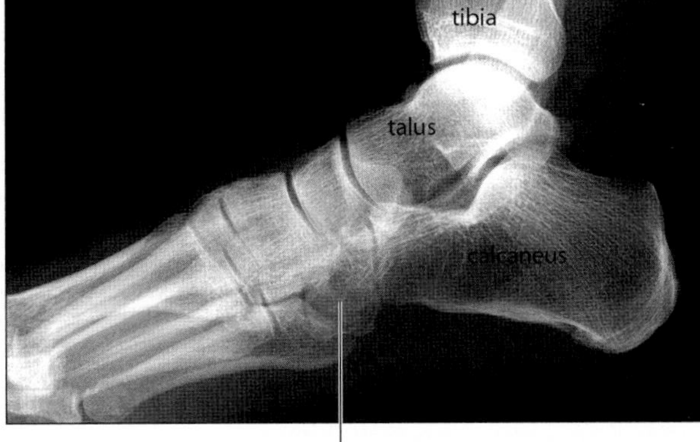

B

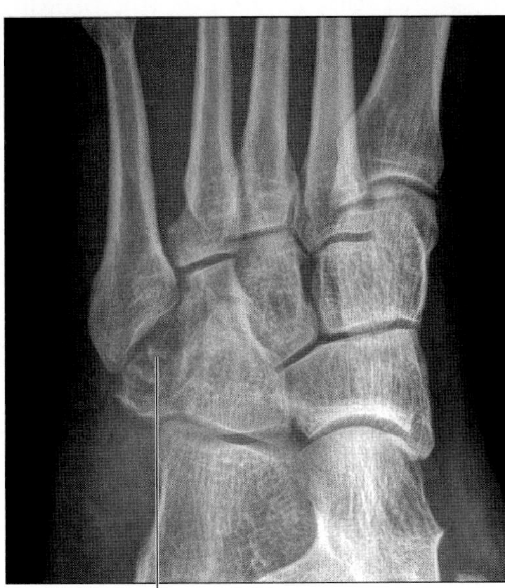

C

FIGURE 1

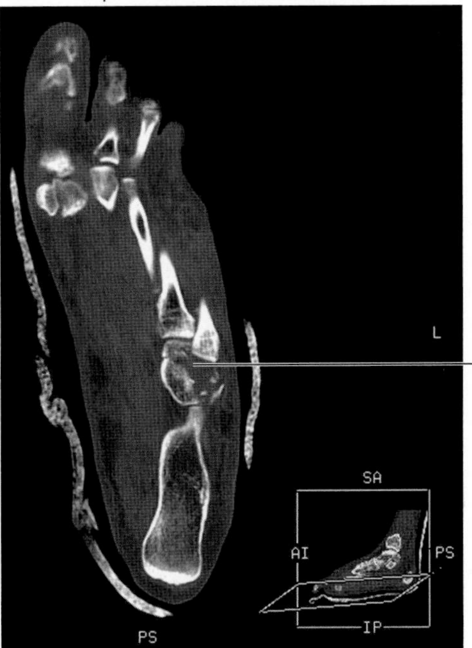

FIGURE 2

Surgical Anatomy

- The tarsal cuboid bone articulates distally with the fourth and fifth MTs, forming the fourth and fifth tarsometatarsal (TMT) joints.
- Proximally, the cuboid articulates with the calcaneus, forming the calcaneocuboid joint (Fig. 3A).
- The medial surface articulates with the lateral cuneiform and navicular (Fig. 3B).
- The plantar surface has a peroneal sulcus, through which passes the peroneus longus tendon (Fig. 3C).

Positioning

- If the cuboid injury is purely lateral in nature, then a lateral position can be used.
- The total hip positioner is helpful, along with the foam tunnel (i.e., open reduction and internal fixation of the calcaneus fracture). This allows access to the lateral foot as well as the proximal lateral tibia if autologous bone grafting is needed.
- If the patient's hips are stiff and lack sufficient external rotation to address a combined injury with a medial component, then a more "sloppy" lateral position can be used with a beanbag or a large ipsilateral bump.
- If there is good external rotation at the hip, then the leg can be rotated to allow access to any part of the foot.

Portals/Exposures

- Repair of a nutcracker injury is done through a lateral approach.
- The extensor digitorum brevis (EDB) muscle belly is dorsolateral on the foot and should be retracted medially in this approach.
- The peroneal tendons are lateral and plantar, and care should be taken to not injure them in the approach or reconstruction. The peroneus longus runs under the groove in the cuboid as it traverses the plantar aspect of the foot before inserting on the plantar base of the first MT. It is especially susceptible to injury.
- A straight lateral approach between the EDB belly and the peroneals allows access to the sinus tarsi and distal calcaneus, distally along the cuboid and more distally into the lateral TMT joints and MT bases and intertarsal area. The dissection can then be carried subperiosteally from lateral to medial to expose the cuboid.

Pearls

- *The cuboid crush is often a severe impaction injury. It is often not possible to achieve perfect reduction as in other fractures. An attempt should be made to reconstruct the joint surfaces, then to reconstruct the anatomy of the bone, and finally to stabilize the construct and bone-graft the defect. Even if eventually one or both joints become arthritic, it is important to preserve the alignment and relative length of the lateral column.*

Pitfalls

- *The lateral approach can lead to injury to the sural nerve, and the patient should be forewarned.*
- *If the sural nerve is accidentally cut in the lower foot, trace the nerve higher up and posterior to the lateral malleolus in order to cut it higher up to avoid lower Tinel's sign and neuroma. If the nerve is divided higher up, there is less incidence of bothersome neuroma.*

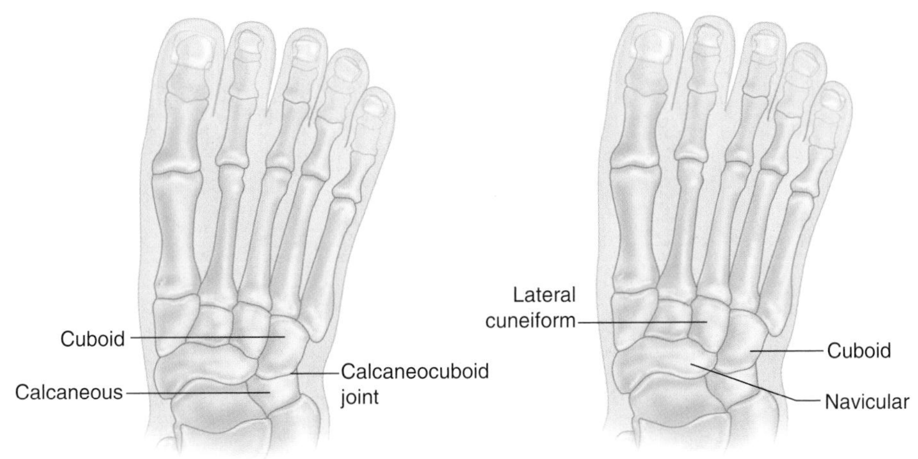

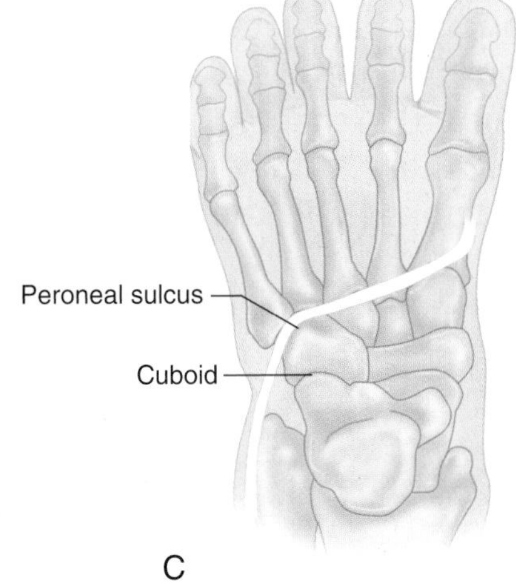

FIGURE 3

Procedure

Step 1

- The cuboid fracture site is prepared using the lateral incision between the EDB and peroneals, entering the sinus tarsi and exposing the calcaneocuboid, lateral (and superior) cuboid, and lateral TMT joints (Fig. 4A and 4B).
- Take care to expose enough to achieve reduction, but do not strip the soft tissue off of the fragments.
- Using a Freer elevator, the cuboid and surrounding joints can be examined.

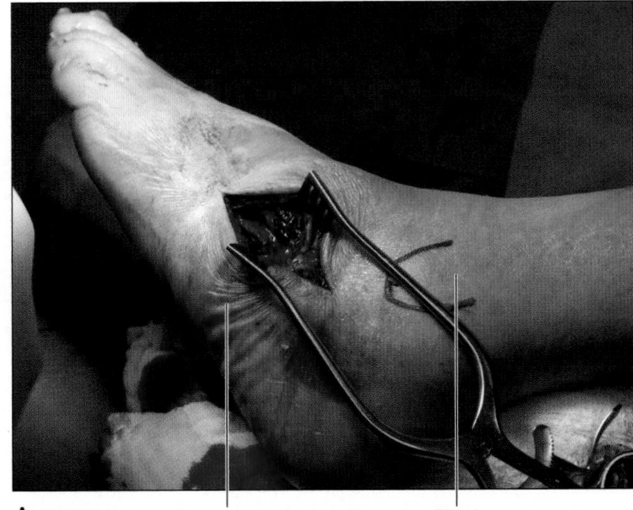

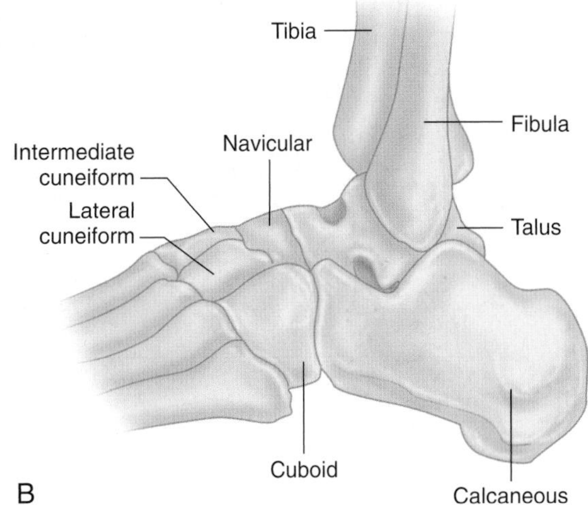

FIGURE 4

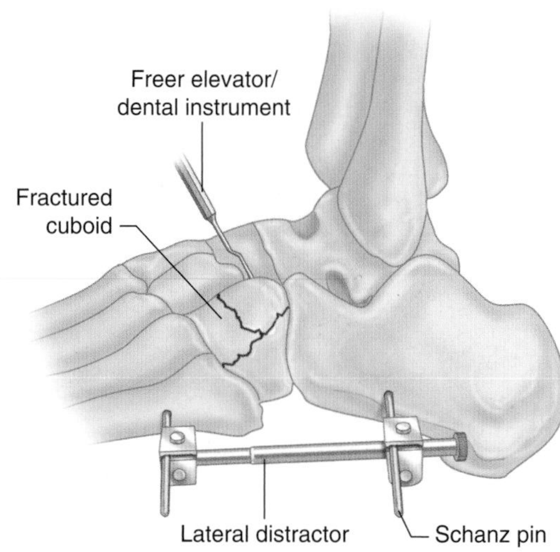

FIGURE 5

Step 2

- Usually it is necessary to apply a lateral distractor to bring the lateral column out to length and to open up the areas to be fixed (Fig. 5). Schanz pins are placed in the calcaneus and more distally into the MTs. The bar can then be applied and the lateral column distracted.
- Care should be taken to preserve any osteochondral fragments. Sometimes these small periarticular fragments can only be held with small Kirschner wires.

Step 3

- The joint surfaces are then extracted from the central crushed portion and buttressed out against the adjacent joint surfaces. The lateral cortex, which is often blown outward, can then be fitted back into place (Fig. 6A and 6B).

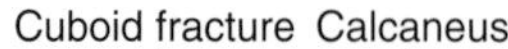

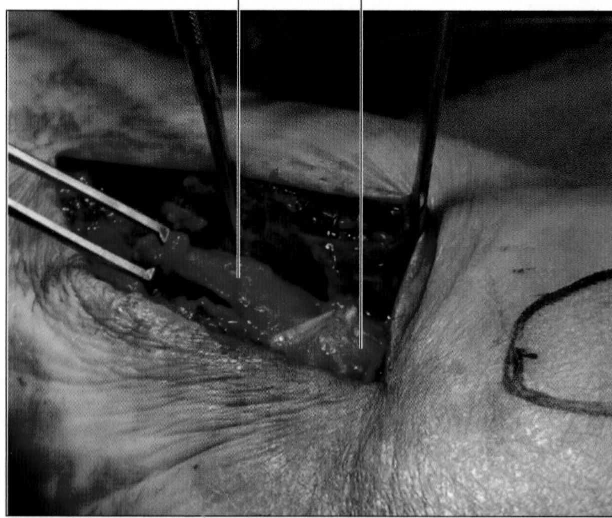

A

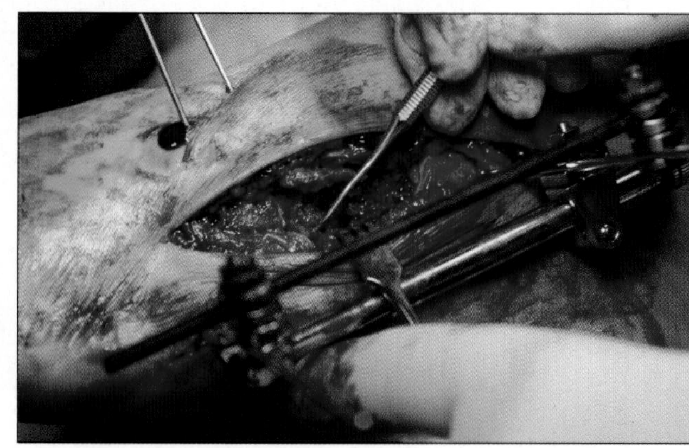

B

FIGURE 6

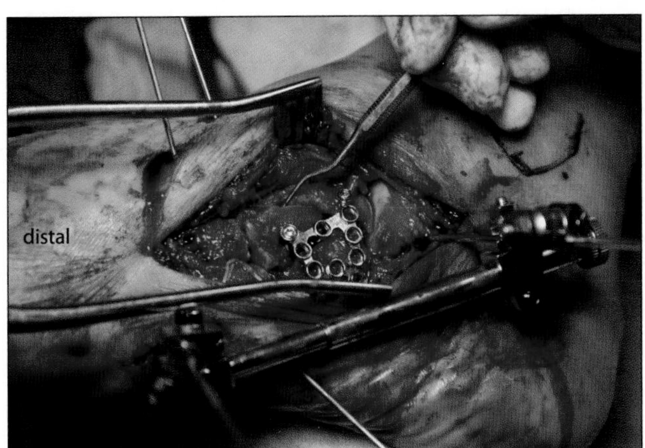

A

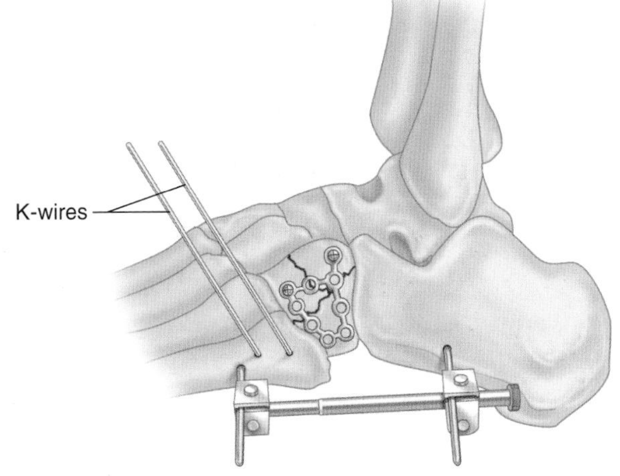

B

FIGURE 7

- Once the fit has been checked and the length and geometry corrected, the cortex can again be flipped up. The empty central core can then be filled with autologous cancellous bone graft and/or allograft of bone morphogenic protein putty/cancellous bits.
- The cuboid plate can then be positioned and secured with screws (Fig. 7A and 7B) placed under fluoroscopic control (Fig. 8). Any small unstable areas that had been provisionally fixed with small wires can remain in place as part of the construct (Fig. 9A–C).
- The subcutaneous layers are loosely tacked back together. The skin is closed with tension-relieving running everting stitches.

PEARLS

- *If there is no retained external fixator, then the plate is being asked to hold a crushed bone without much structural support.*
- *If necessary, a cervical spine–type distractor can be used to gently and carefully distract the lateral column out to length (see Fig. 9A–C, with the distractor over the pins along with the carbon rod).*

FIGURE 8

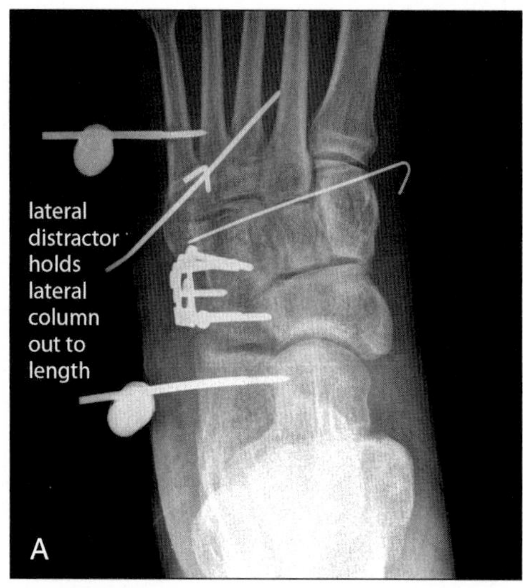

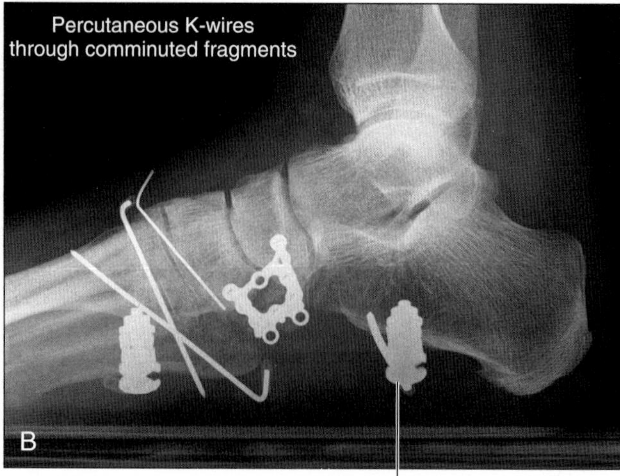

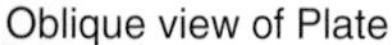

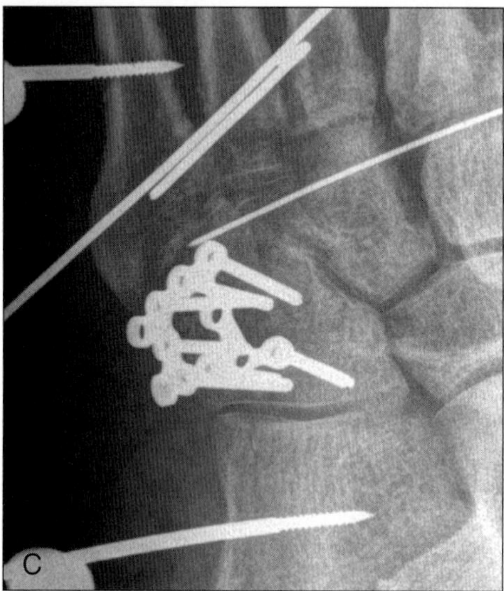

FIGURE 9

Postoperative Care and Expected Outcomes

- An external fixator that has been used and left on obviates the need for more rigid casting.
- Some sort of protective device can be used, but early range of motion can begin.
- Strict non–weight bearing should be maintained for 3 months with the external fixator left in place at least 8 weeks.
- After 3 months the construct should be stable enough to begin progressive weight bearing in a cushioned "running sneaker" with a visco-cushioned orthotic. Formal physical therapy can then begin with emphasis on complex hindfoot range of motion with the biomechanical ankle platform system (BAPS).

Evidence

Ebraheim NA, Haman SP, Lu J, Padanilam TG. Radiographic evaluation of the calcaneocuboid joint: a cadaver study. Foot Ankle Int. 1999;20:178-81.

This study evaluates 18 cadaver feet to assess the radiographic evaluation of the articular cuboid surface. In six specimens, fractures and 1-mm stepoff of the cuboid fractures were simulated. (Level V evidence [cadaveric study])

Hsu JC, Chang JH, Wang SJ, Wu SS. Nutcracker fracture of the cuboid in children: a case report. Foot Ankle Int. 2004;25:423-5.

This case report is of a 9-year-old girl treated with open reduction of a cuboid fracture. Follow-up was 2 years. Outcome was determined by radiographic and clinical examination, and patient subjective assessment. (Level V evidence [case report])

Sangeorzn BJ, Swiontkowski MF. Displaced fractures of the cuboid. J Bone Joint Surg [Br]. 1990;72:376-8.

This study is a series of four patients with cuboid fractures treated operatively. (Level IV evidence [case series])

Weber M, Locher S. Reconstruction of the cuboid in compression fractures: short to midterm results in 12 patients. Foot Ankle Int. 2002;23:1008-13.

This study is a retrospective review of 12 patients with cuboid fractures treated operatively either with plate fixation or screw fixation alone. Follow-up ranged from 12 to 47 months. Outcome was determined by radiographic and clinical examination, and patient subjective assessment. (Level IV evidence [case series])

SECTION III

Hindfoot/Ankle

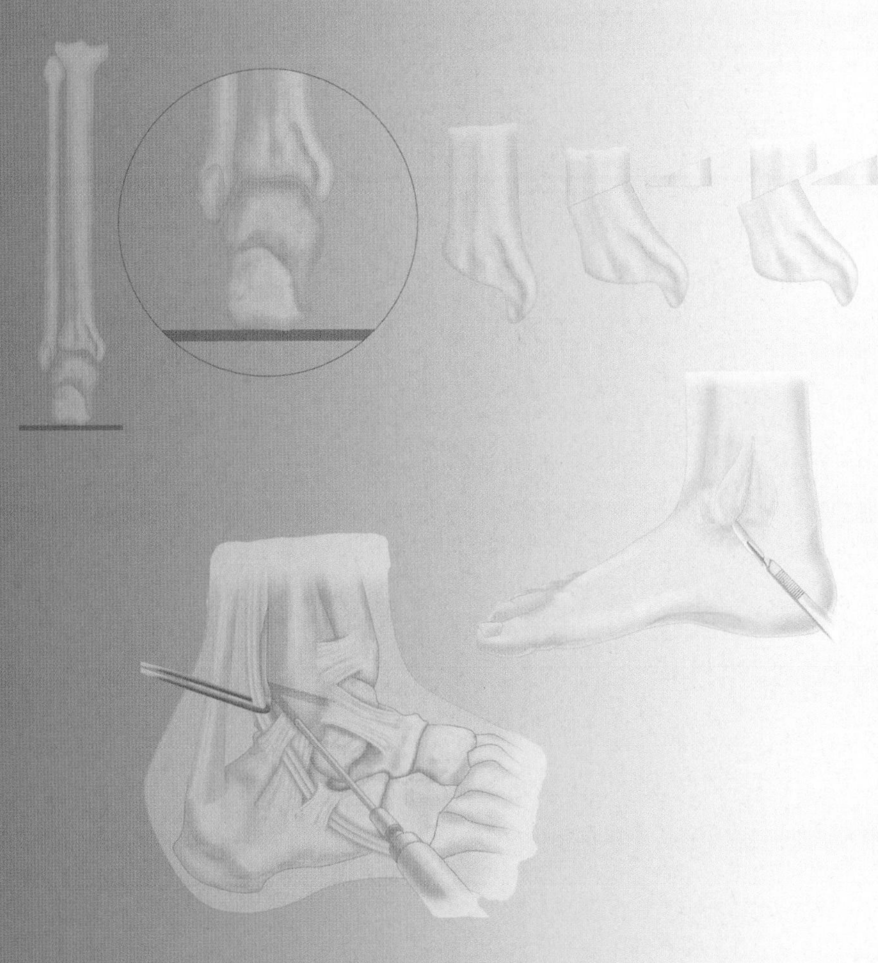

PROCEDURE 25

Total Ankle Arthroplasty with a Current Three-Component Design (HINTEGRA Prosthesis)

Beat Hintermann

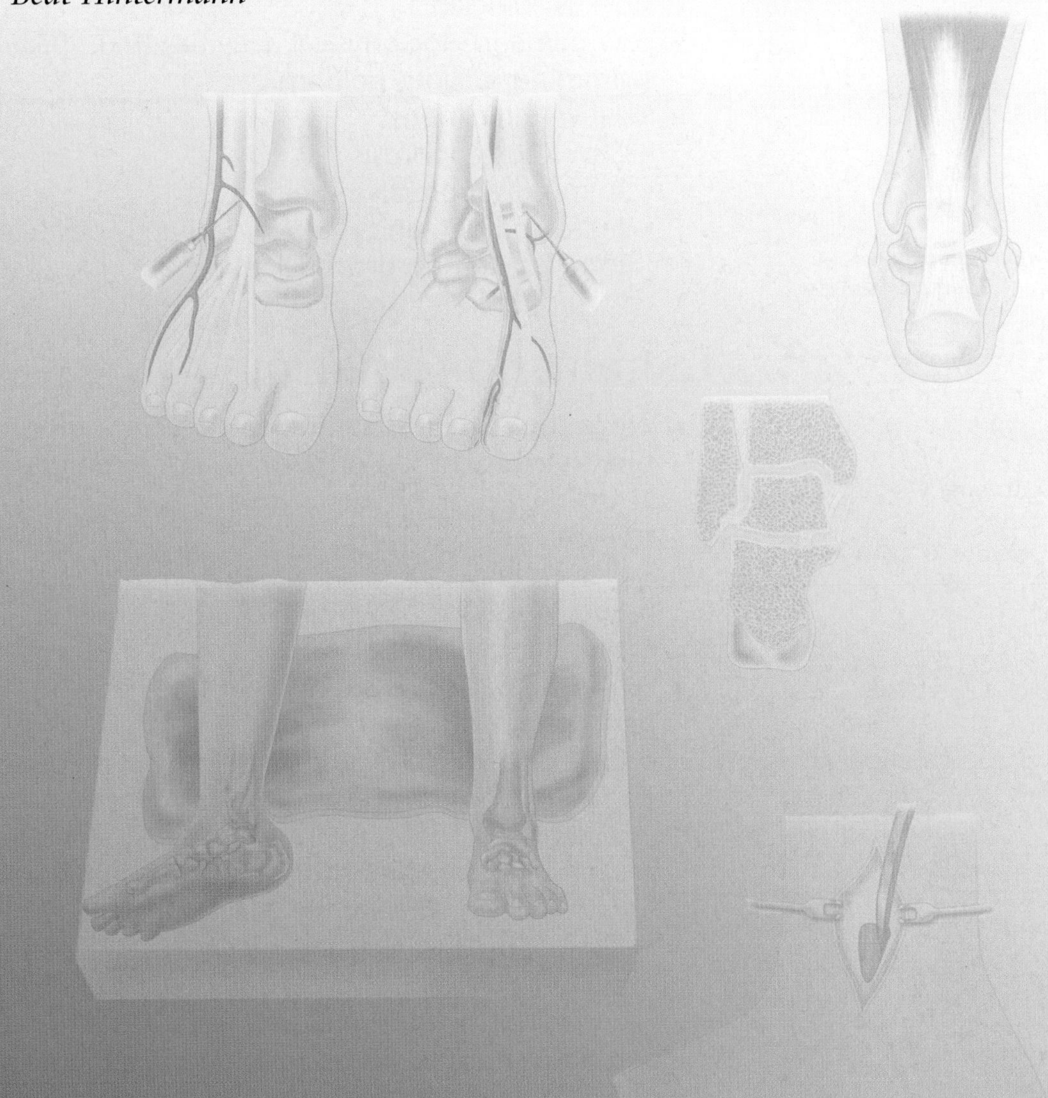

Pitfalls

- *Infection*
- *Avascular necrosis of more than one third of talus*
- *Nonmanageable instability*
- *Nonmanageable malalignment*
- *Neuromuscular disorder*
- *Neuroarthropathy (Charcot arthropathy)*
- *Diabetic syndrome*
- *Suspected or documented metal allergy or intolerance*
- *Highest demands for physical activities (e.g., contact sports, jumping)*

Controversies

- Diabetic syndrome without polyneuropathy
- Avascular necrosis of talus

Treatment Options

- Medication
- Local therapy
- Shoe modifications and orthoses

Indications

- Primary osteoarthritis (e.g., degenerative disease)
- Systemic arthritis (e.g., rheumatoid arthritis)
- Posttraumatic osteoarthritis (if instability and malalignment are manageable)
- Secondary osteoarthritis (e.g., infection, avascular necrosis) (if minimally two thirds of the talar surface is preserved)
- Salvage for failed total ankle replacement or for nonunion and malunion of ankle fusion (if bone stock is sufficient)
- Low demands for physical activities (e.g., hiking, swimming, biking, golfing)
- Relative indications:
  - Severe osteoporosis
  - Immunosuppressive therapy
  - Increased demands for physical activities (e.g., jogging, tennis, downhill skiing)

Examination/Imaging

- While the patient is standing, perform a thorough clinical investigation of both lower extremities to assess:
  - Alignment
  - Deformities
  - Foot position
  - Muscular atrophy
- While the patient is sitting with free-hanging feet, perform an assessment of:
  - Extent to which a present deformity is correctable
  - Preserved joint motion at the ankle and subtalar joints
  - Ligament stability of the ankle and subtalar joints with anterior drawer and tilt tests
  - Supination and eversion power (e.g., function of posterior tibial and peroneus brevis muscles)
- Plain weight-bearing radiographs, including anteroposterior views of ankle (Fig. 1A) and foot (Fig. 1B), and lateral view of the foot (Fig. 1C), to determine/rule out
  - Extent of destruction of tibiotalar joint (e.g., tibia, talus, fibula)
  - Status of neighboring joints (e.g., associated degenerative disease)
  - Deformities of the foot and ankle complex (e.g., heel alignment, foot arch, talonavicular alignment)

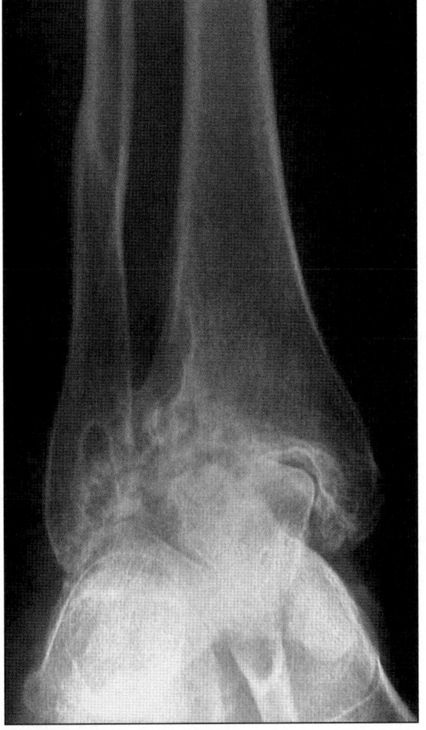

A

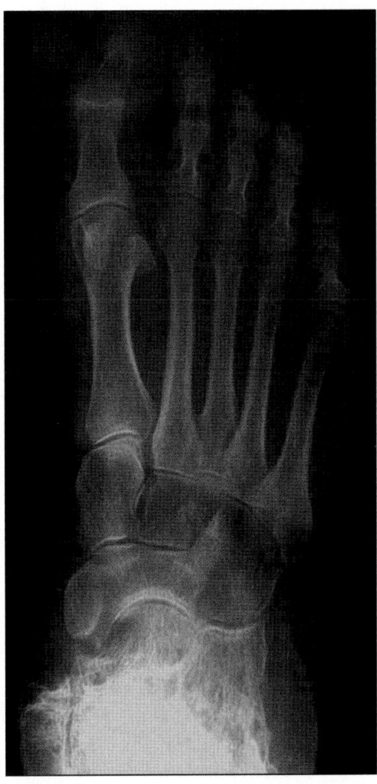

B

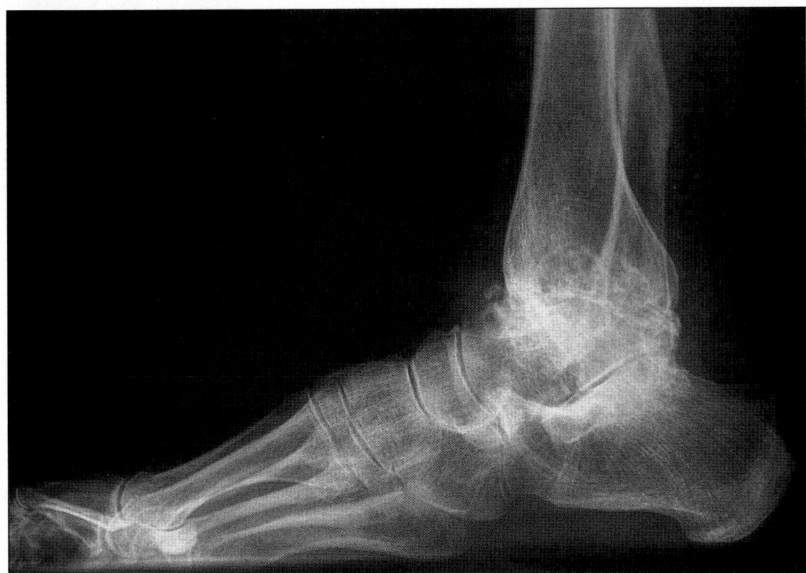

C

FIGURE 1

- Tibiotalar malalignment (e.g., varus, valgus, recurvatum, antecurvatum)
- Bony condition (e.g., avascular necrosis, bony defects)

- Computed tomography scan may be obtained for assessment of
  - Destruction of joint surfaces and incongruency
  - Bony defects
  - Avascular necrosis
- Single-photon emission computed tomography with superimposed bone scan (Fig. 2A and 2B) may be used to visualize
  - Morphologic pathologies and associated activity process
  - Biologic bone pathologies and associated activity process
- Magnetic resonance imaging may be used to identify
  - Injuries to ligament structures
  - Morphologic changes of tendons
  - Avascular necrosis of bones (e.g., talar body, tibial plafond)

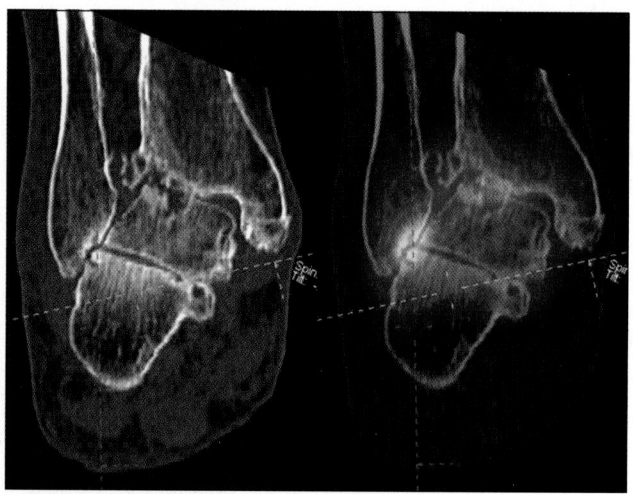

A

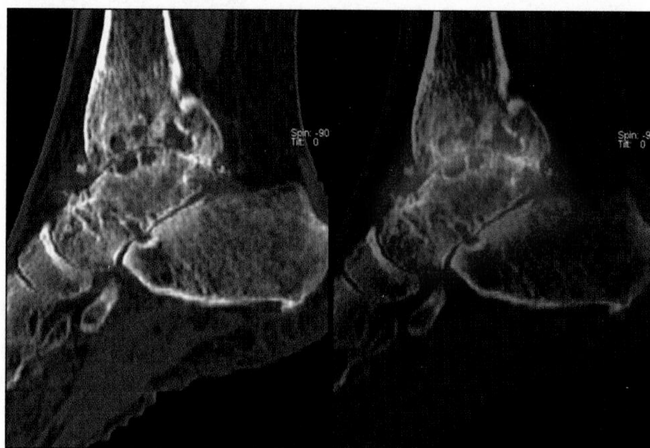

B

FIGURE 2

Surgical Anatomy

- The superior extensor retinaculum is a thickening of the deep fascia above the ankle, running from the tibia to the fibula (Fig. 3). It includes, from medially to laterally, the tendons of the tibialis anterior, extensor hallucis longus, and extersor digitorum longus.
- The anterior neurovascular bundle lies roughly halfway between the malleoli (Fig. 4A); it can be found consistently between the extensor hallucis longus and extensor digitorum longus tendons.
- The neurovascular bundle contains the tibialis anterior and the deep peroneal nerve. The nerve supplies the extensor digitorum brevis and extensor hallucis brevis and a sensory space (interdigital I–II).
- On the height of the talonavicular joint, the medial branches of the superficial peroneal nerve cross from lateral to medial (Fig. 4B). This nerve supplies the skin of the dorsum of the foot.
- On the posterior aspect of the ankle, the medial neurovascular bundle is located behind its posteromedial corner, and the flexor hallucis longus tendon on its posterior aspect (Fig. 4C).

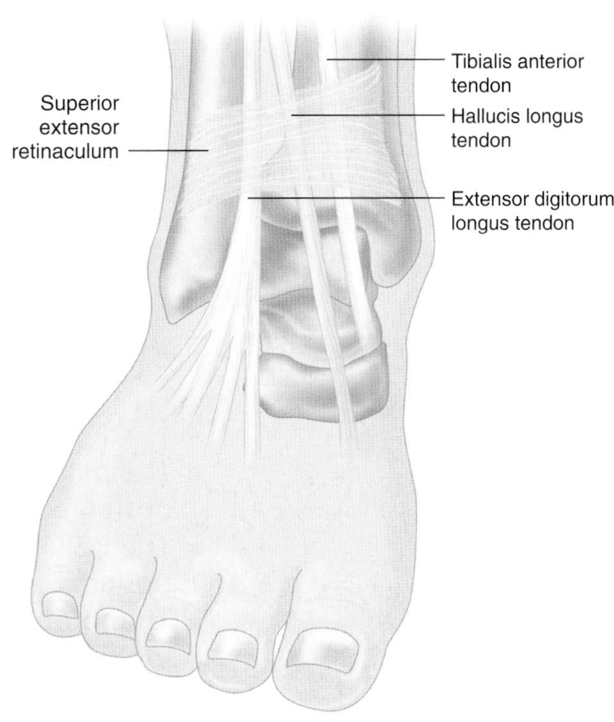

FIGURE 3

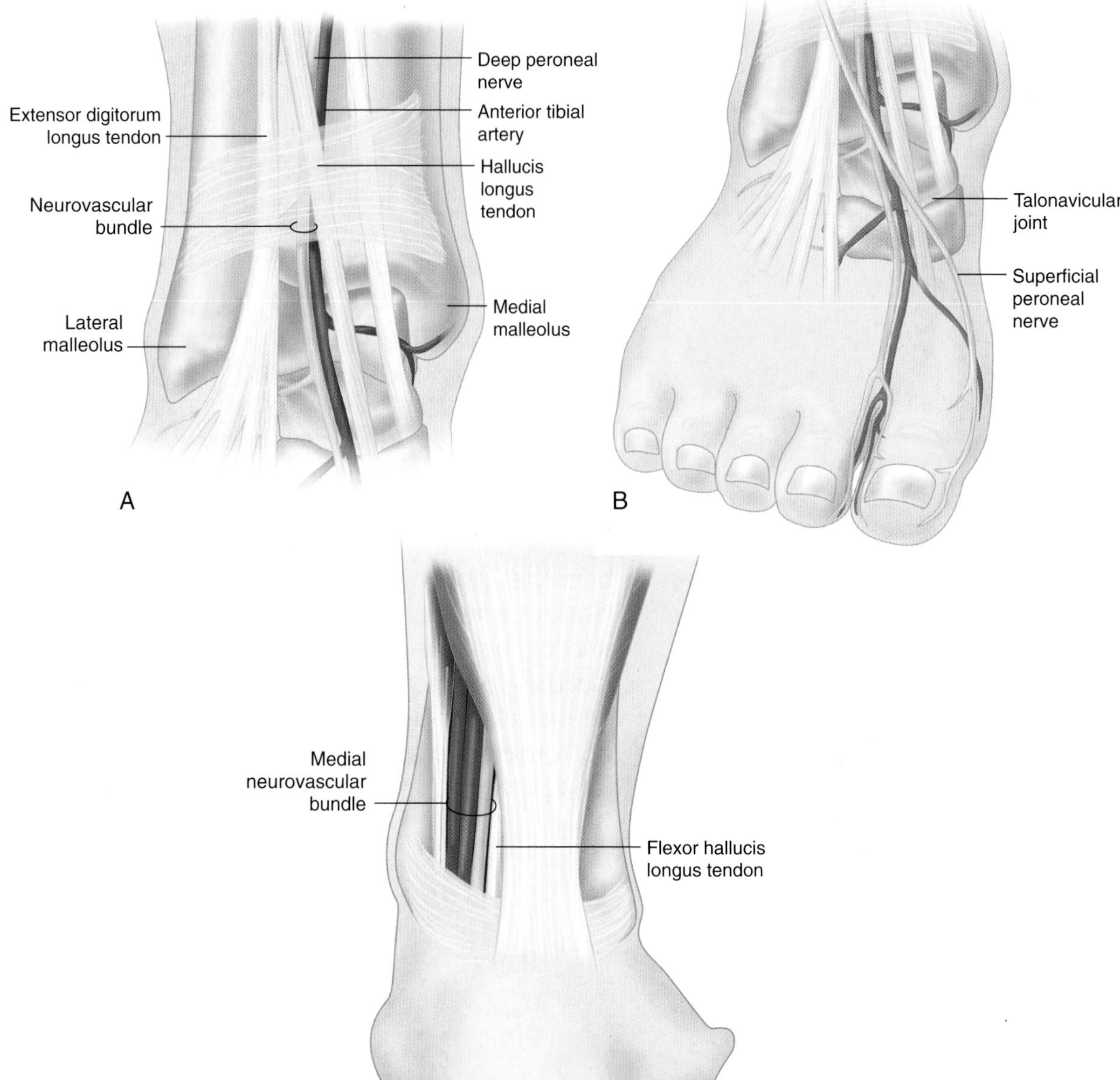

FIGURE 4

> **Pearls**
>
> - *The affected foot is supported with a block to facilitate fluoroscopy during surgery.*
> - *The contralateral nonaffected leg is also draped if there is significant deformity to be corrected.*

Positioning

- The patient is positioned with the feet on the edge of the table.
- The ipsilateral back is lifted until a strictly upward position of the foot is obtained.
- The tourniquet is mounted at the ipsilateral thigh.

Portals/Exposures

- An anterior longitudinal incision of 10–12 cm in length is made to expose the retinaculum (Fig. 5A and 5B).

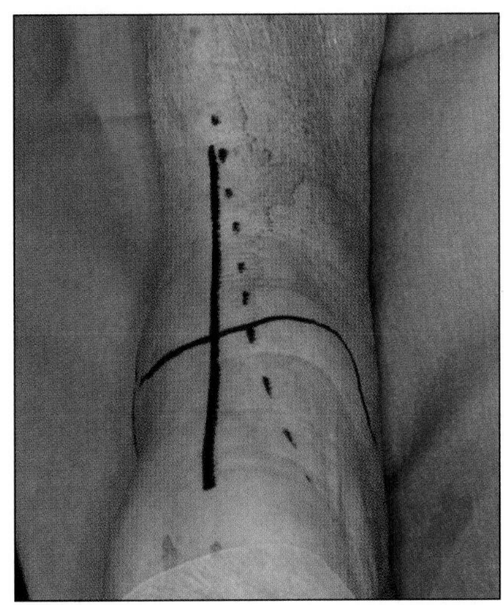

A

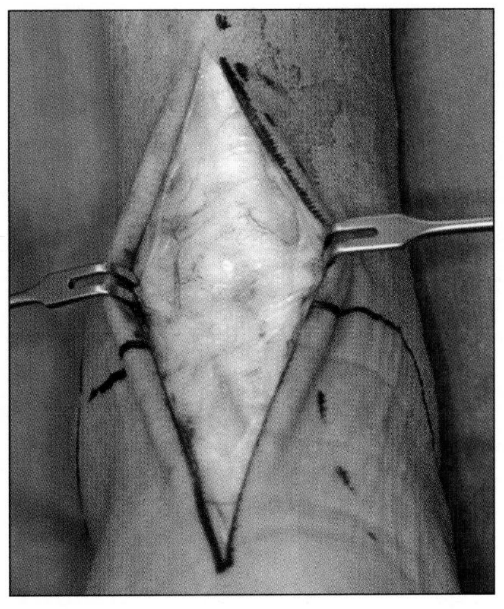

B

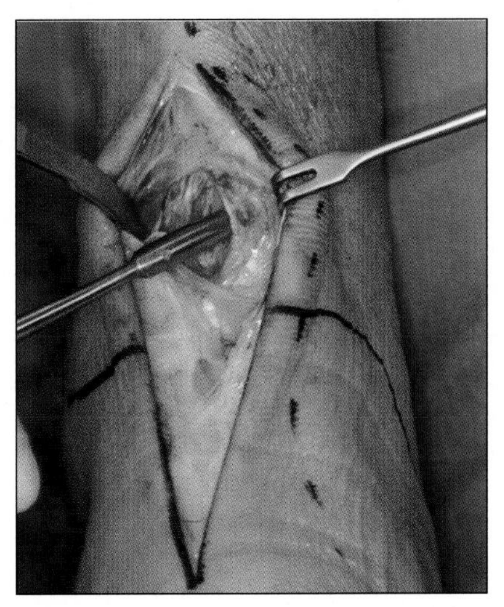

C

FIGURE 5

Pearls

- *The soft tissue beneath the anterior tibial tendon is always free from the neurovascular bundle and thus is called the "safe spot" while approaching the anterior ankle joint.*

Pitfalls

- *If old scars from previous surgeries or injuries are not respected, breakdown of critical areas may occur.*

Instrumentation

- A self-retaining distractor may be helpful; care must be taken, however, that no tension is applied to the skin.

- The retinaculum is dissected along the lateral border of the anterior tibial tendon, and the anterior aspect of the distal tibia is exposed.
- While the soft tissue mantle is dissected with the periosteum from the bone (Fig. 5C), attention is paid to the neurovascular bundle that lies behind the long extensor hallucis tendon.
- A capsulotomy (Fig. 6A) and a capsulectomy are made, and a self-retaining retractor is inserted to carefully keep the soft tissue mantle away (Fig. 6B).
- Osteophytes on the tibia are removed, particularly on the anterolateral aspect.
- Osteophytes on the talar neck and anterior aspect of the medial malleolus are also removed.
- The fibula usually cannot be fully visualized at this stage.

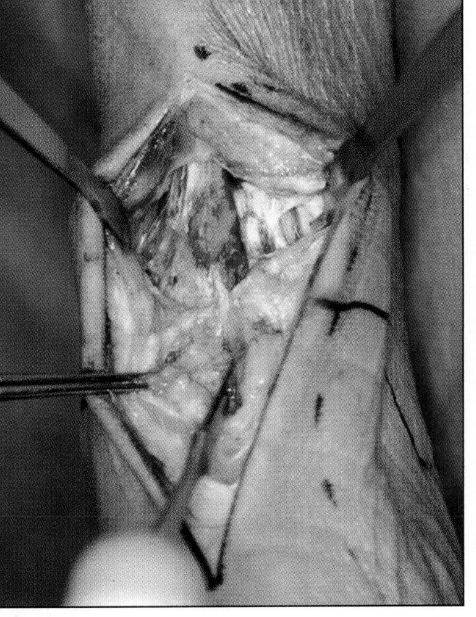

A

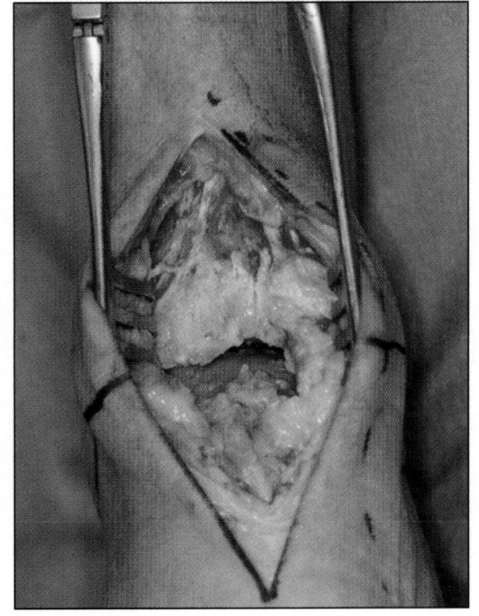

B

FIGURE 6

Procedure

Step 1: Tibial Resection

- The tibial cutting block with its alignment rod is positioned using the tibial tuberosity as the proximal reference (Fig. 7A), and the anterolateral border of the ankle as the distal reference (e.g., the medial corner of the resection block is supposed to merge the anterolateral corner of the tibiotalar joint; see Fig. 7A).
- The final adjustment is made as follows:
  - *Sagittal plane:* The rod is moved until a position parallel to the anterior border of the tibia has been achieved (see Fig. 7A).
  - *Frontal (coronal) plane:* After preliminary fixation of the block with a long pin, the tibial resection block is rotated until proper varus/valgus alignment and ligament tension have been achieved.
  - *Vertical adjustment:* The tibial resection block is moved proximally until the desired resection height is achieved (Fig. 7B). Usually resection of approximately 2 mm on the apex of the tibial plafond is desired.
  - *Rotational adjustment:* The tibial resection block is rotated to get a parallel position of its medial surface to the medial surface of the talus (to avoid damaging the malleoli with the saw blade during resection).

Instrumentation/ Implantation

- The Hintermann distractor, mounted with one pin to the anteromedial aspect of the distal tibia and one pin to the anteromedial talar neck, serves to provide a better view into the tibiotalar joint while the collateral ligaments are tightened.

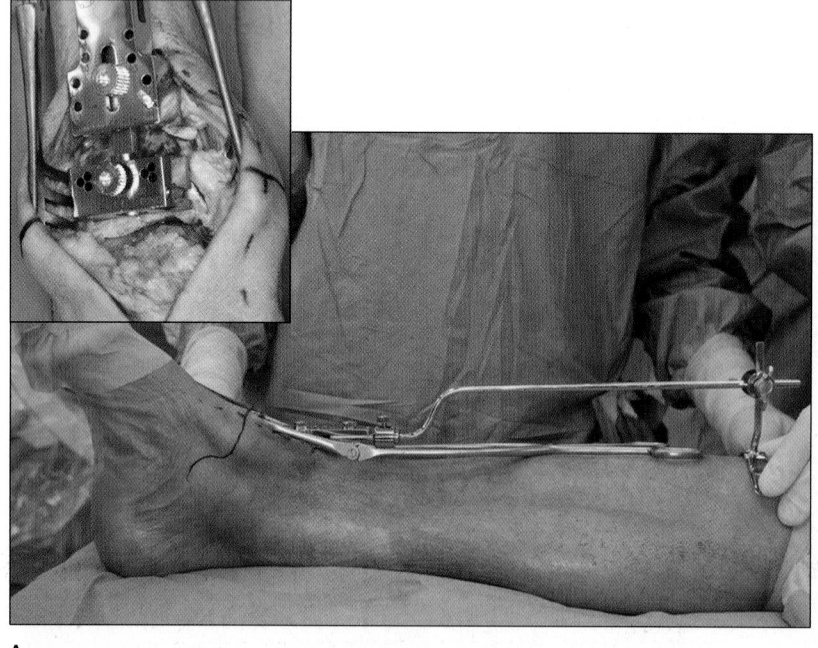

A

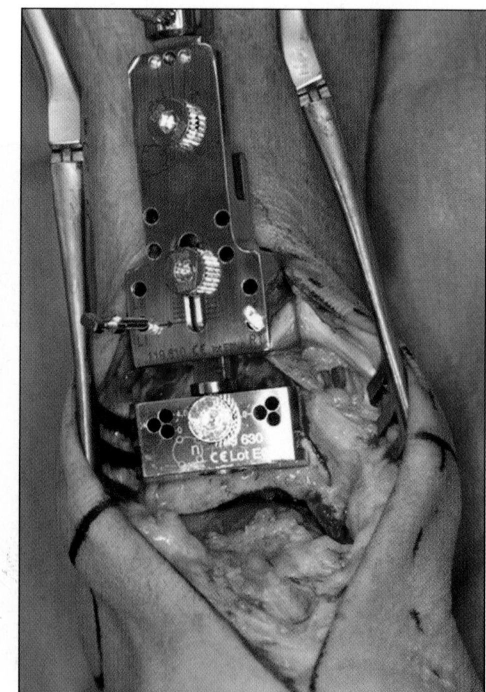

B

FIGURE 7

- The tibial cutting guide is slid into the cutting block, creating a slot in which the saw blade will be guided (Fig. 8A). The width of the slot limits the excursion of the saw blade, thereby protecting the malleoli from being hit and fractured.

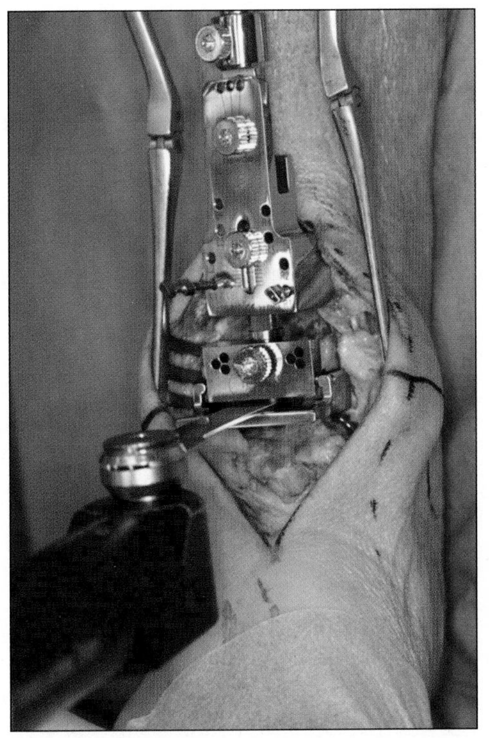
A

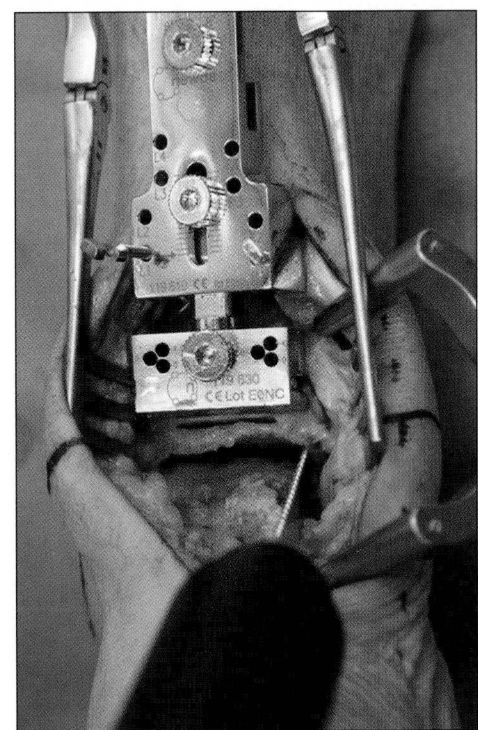
B

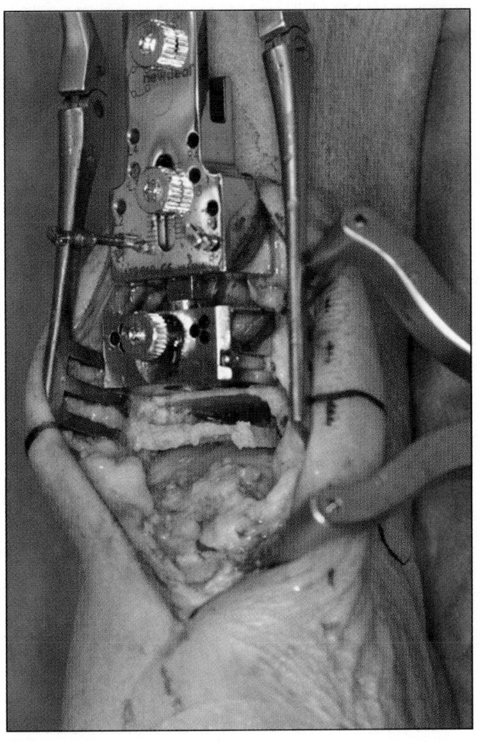
C

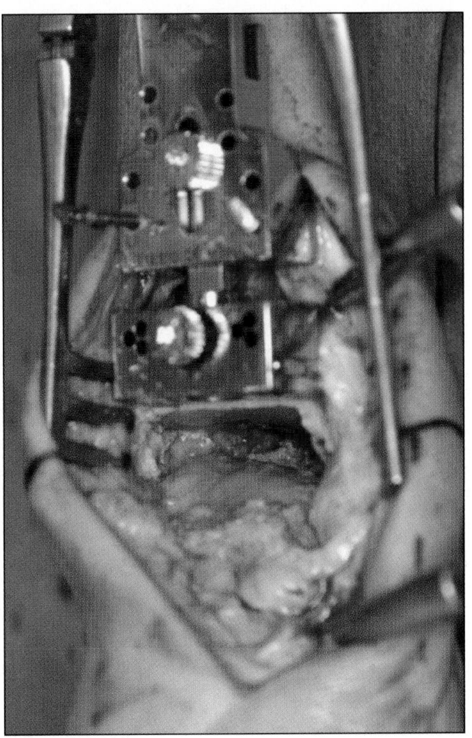
D

FIGURE 8

Controversies

- Some bone and capsular tissue on posterior aspect of the joint might be left in place at this stage of surgery (it is much easier to be removed once the talar cuts are performed), as long as it may not hinder insertion of the talar cutting block.

- Once the tibial cut is made, a reciprocating saw may be used to finalize the cuts, particularly for the vertical cut on medial side (Fig. 8B).
- Remaining bone, including the posterior capsule, is removed with a rongeur (Fig. 8C and 8D).

Pearls

- *Proper frontal (coronal) plane alignment may best be achieved while pulling the talus distally with a rasp (placed in the center of the tibiotalar joint), thereby tightening the medial and lateral ligaments. The tibial resection block is adjusted to get a position parallel to the upper surface of the talus. A second pin is used for fixation.*
- *In varus ankles there is usually need of more tibial resection, whereas in valgus ankles, and/or in the presence of high joint laxity, less bone resection is advised.*
- *If in doubt (e.g., if the anterior border of the tibia is projected onto the gauge between two markers), the bigger size might be selected.*

Pitfalls

- *Attention should be paid so as not to insert the saw blade too deeply into the joint as the tibial nerve might be at risk.*

Step 2: Talar Resection

- The talar resection block is inserted into the tibial cutting block (Fig. 9A).
- The resection block is moved distally as much as possible to properly tension the collateral ligaments (Fig. 9B).
- All distractors and spreaders must be removed before the foot is moved into neutral position (e.g., with respect to dorsi-/plantar flexion, and pronation/supination) (Fig. 9C).
- Once the foot is in neutral position, the resection block is fixed by two pins (medially and laterally, respectively).
- The tibial resection block is removed, and the distractor (HINTERMANN spreader) is again mounted to distract the joint; proper fit of the resection bloc to the talus is checked.

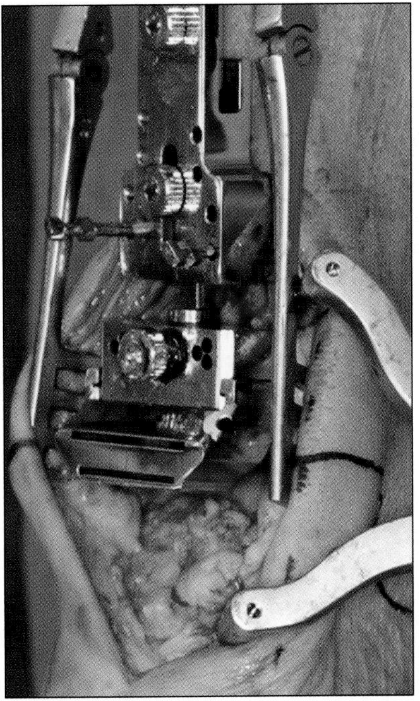

A

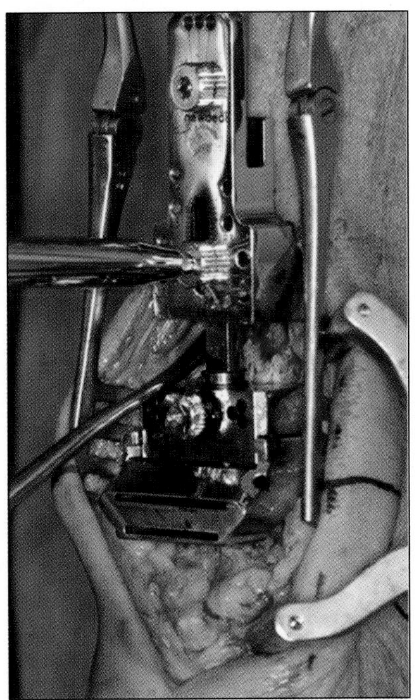

B

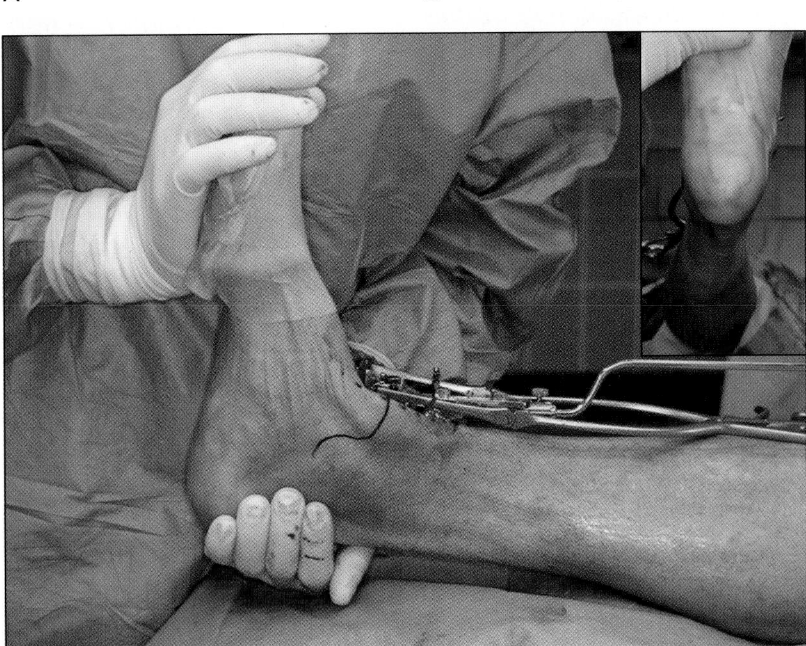

C

FIGURE 9

Pearls

- *In the case of major extrusion of the talus out of the mortise, as is often the case in posttraumatic deformities, the talar resection block can be removed and the anterior vertical cut is made freehand such that just a minimal step of 2–3 mm in the anterior talus is created.*
- *The posterior capsule should be removed completely until fat tissue and tendon structures are visible to get full dorsiflexion.*

Pitfalls

- *Positioning of the resection block too posterior will lead to insufficient bony support of the talar component, thus creating sagittal plane instability.*

- The resection of the talar dome is made with the oscillating saw through the upper slot of the talar cutting block (Fig. 10A and 10B).
- A second limited cut is made through the inferior slot of the talar cutting block, and the vertical cut is done with the talar osteotome (Fig. 10C and 10D).
- The 12-mm-thick spacer, representing the thickness of the tibial and talar components and the thinnest 5-mm inlay, is inserted into the created joint space. While the foot is held in neutral flexion position, the surgeon should check:
  - If an appropriate amount of bone has been resected
  - If the achieved alignment is appropriate
  - If the medial and lateral stability are appropriate
- *If the spacer cannot be properly inserted into the joint space, and if there is no obvious contracture of the remaining posterior capsular present, additional bony resection might be considered. In most instances, such additional resection should be done on tibial side. The tibial cutting block is repositioned using the same fixation holes for the pins. The distal resection block is moved proximally as desired, and a new cut is performed with the saw blade.*
- *If the alignment is not appropriate, and if an associated deformity of the foot itself (e.g., varus, valgus heel) can be excluded, a corrective cut should be considered. In most instances, the resection should be done on the tibial side. The desired angular correction on the tibial resection block is made, and the tibial cutting block is repositioned using other fixation holes for the pins. The distal resection block is moved proximally or distally to achieve the height of the original cut such that an angular bony resection will result.*
- *If the ankle is not stable on both sides, the use of a thicker inlay might be advised. If the ankle is not stable on one side, a release of the contralateral ligaments, and/or ligament reconstruction on the affected side, should be considered. Ligament reconstruction is better done once the definitive implants have been inserted, and if there is still an obvious instability.*
- The spacer is removed and the distractor (HINTERMANN spreader) mounted using the same pins.

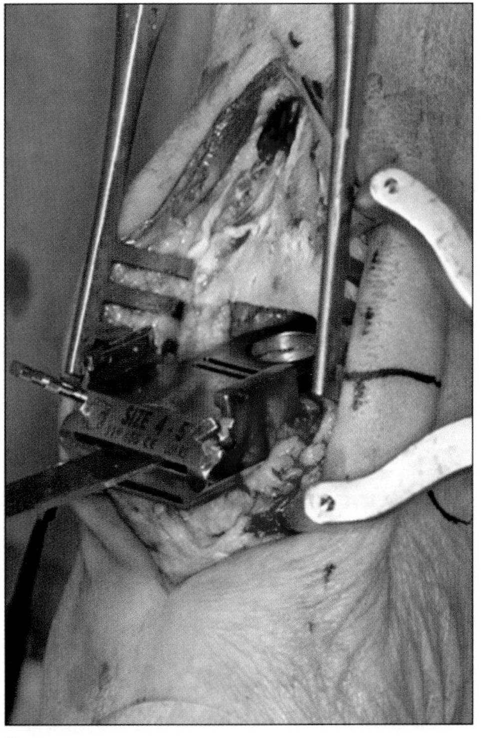

A

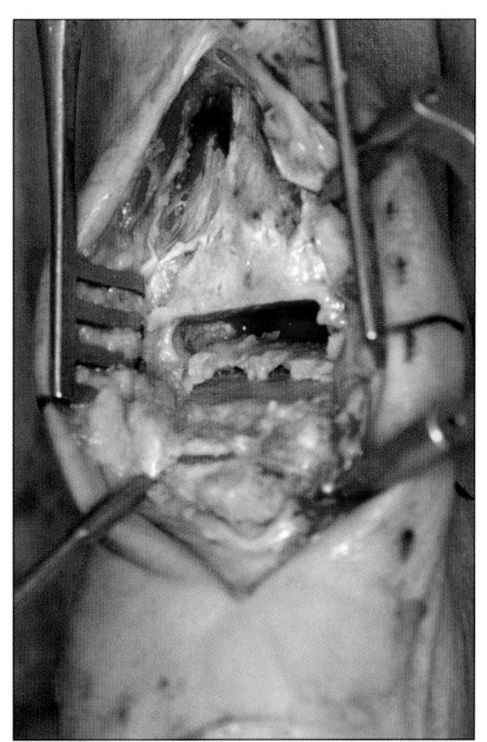
B

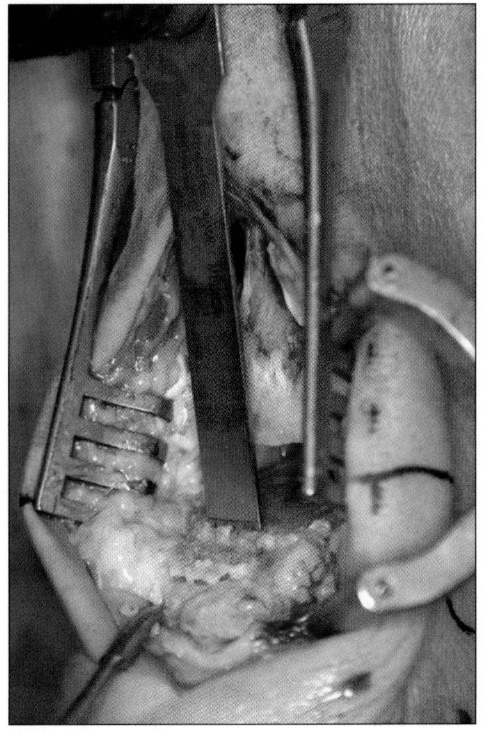
C

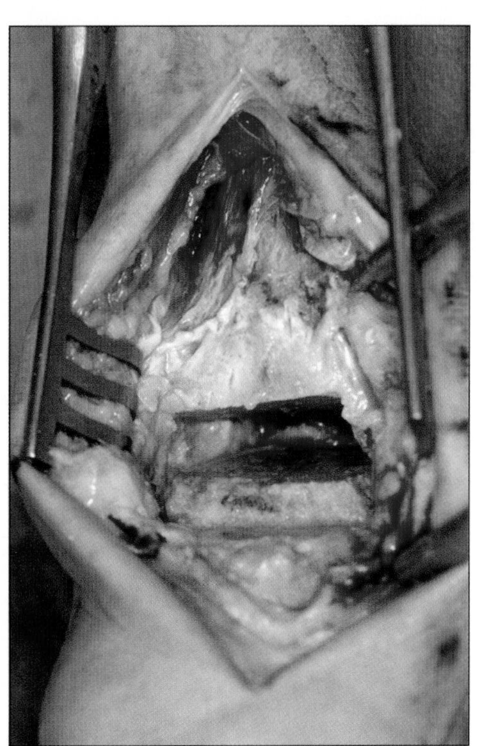
D

FIGURE 10

- The size of the resected talar block is determined as follows:
  - The medial side of the talus is taken as the reference; the resection block should be positioned along the medial border of the talus such that 1–2 mm of bone will be removed from the medial side of talus (Fig. 11A).
  - On the lateral side, the resection block is supposed to remove as little bone as possible on its posterior aspect; usually, there will be more bone to be removed on the lateral aspect of the talus as there are osteophytes (see Fig. 11A).
  - On the posterior side, the resection block is supposed to remove 2–3 mm of bone additionally to remaining cartilage (Fig. 11B).
  - The talar size should not oversize the previously determined tibial component by more than one size; if so, a smaller talar size must be selected.
- Once the appropriate size of talar cutting block is selected, it is fixed by two to three short pins.
- Medial and lateral resections of the talus are made with the reciprocating saw that is guided along the talar cutting block. The cuts should be made as follows:
  - Medial side: 6 mm deep, as the reference is the upper surface of the talus
  - Lateral side: 8 mm deep, as the reference is the upper surface of the talus
- On the posterior aspect of the talus, 2–3 mm of bone should be removed (see Fig. 11B).
- On the medial and lateral sides, the cuts are finalized by using a chisel to make an almost horizontal cut along the base of the existing cuts, thereby avoiding extensive loss of bone stock and potentially damaging the vascular supply of the talus.
- The medial and lateral gutters are cleaned using a rongeur.
- The remaining bone and capsule of the posterior compartment is removed (Fig. 11C).

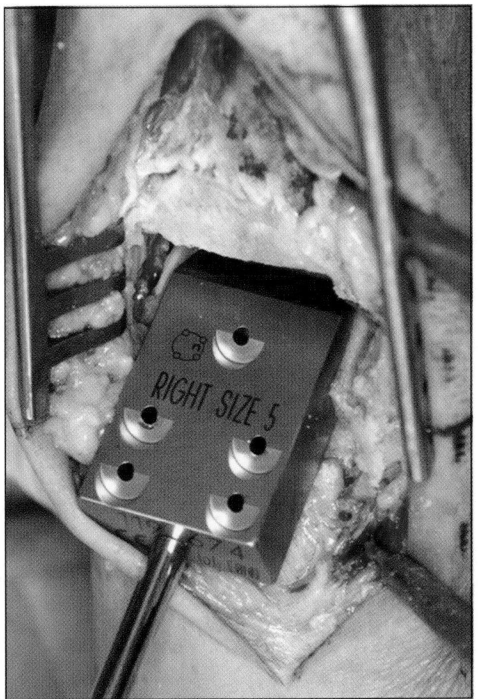

A

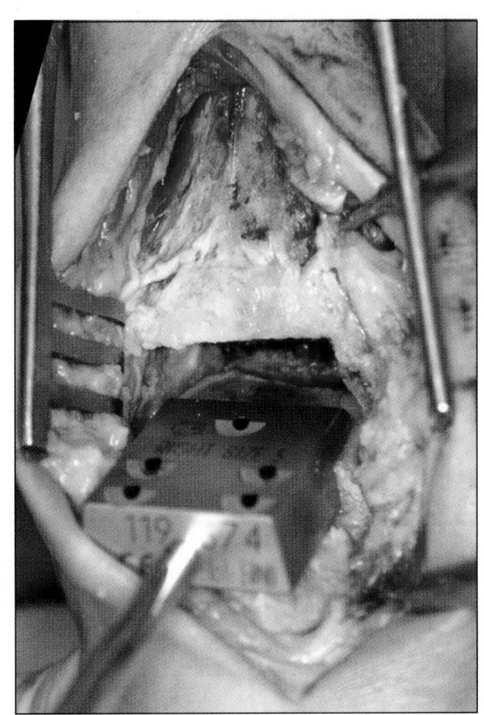

B

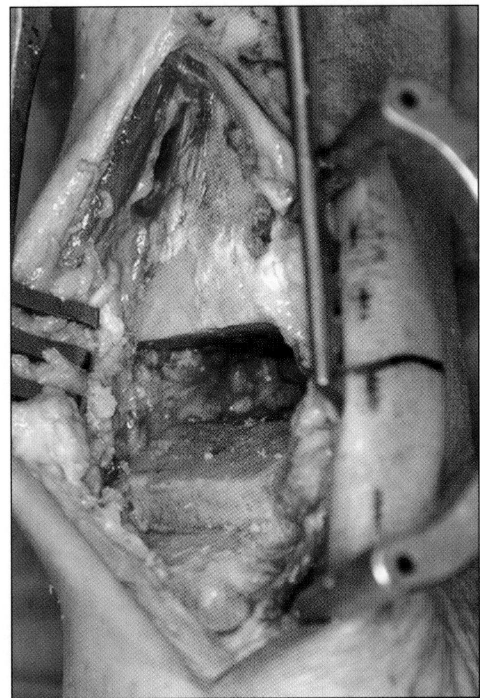

C

FIGURE 11

Step 3: Insertion of Trial Implants and Finalizing of Cuts

- Talar trial
  - The first talar trial is inserted using the small impactor (Fig. 12A).

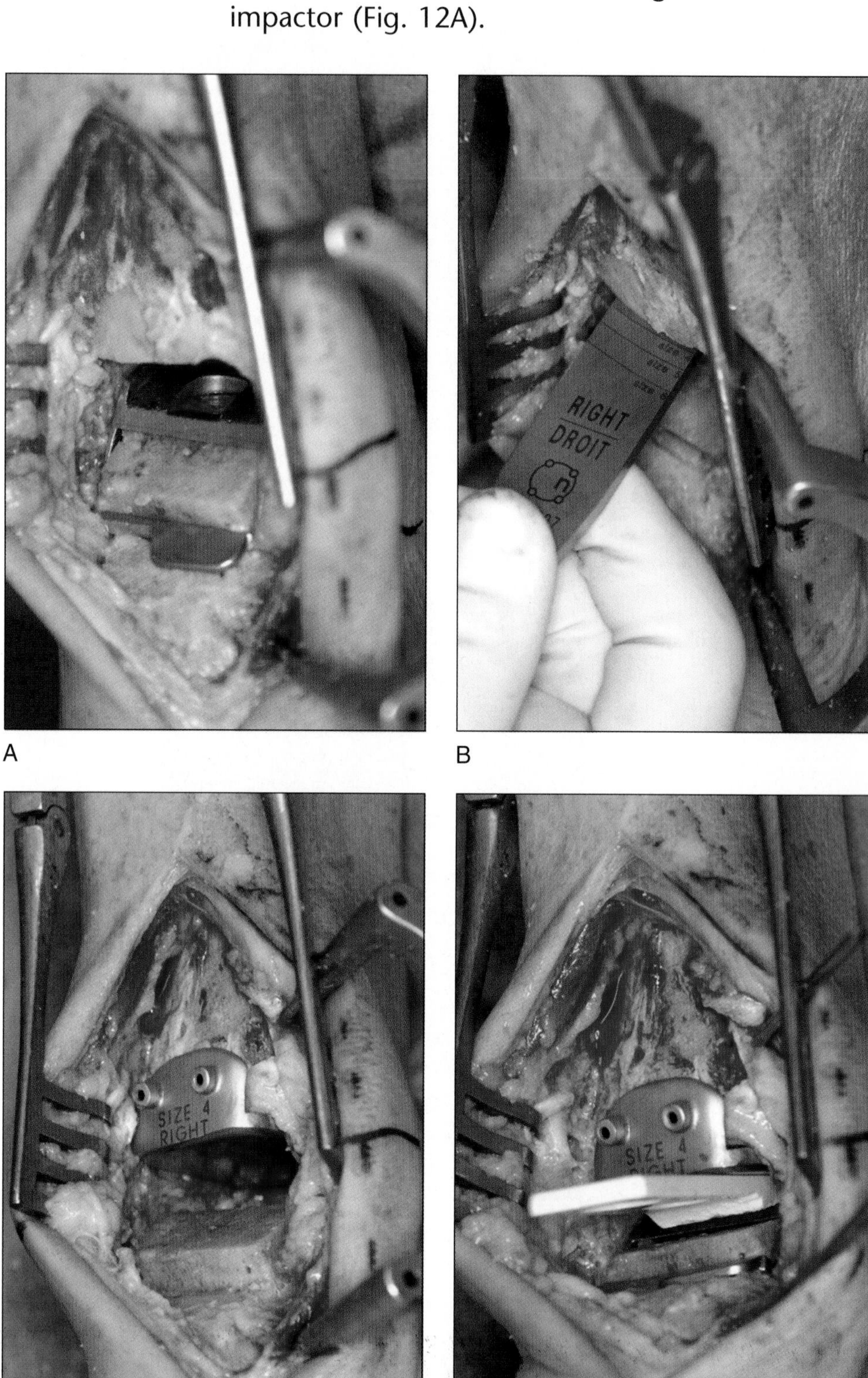

A B C D

FIGURE 12

PEARLS

- *The contact point should be between 40% and 45% of the tibial component when the anterior border is taken as 0% and the posterior border as 100%, respectively. If the point of contact is too posterior, ligament balance will not be able to be achieved.*

  - The window on the posterior aspect of the trial allows checking its proper fit to the posterior resection surface of the talus.
- Tibial trial
  - The tibial depth gauge is used to determine the size of tibial implant to be selected (Fig. 12B). It is inserted with the appropriate side (right/left) against the tibial surface, and the posterior edge is hooked in on the posterior border of the tibia. The size to be selected can be taken from the scale on the depth gauge.
  - The tibial trial is inserted (Fig. 12C). Attention should be paid to get the tibial component in close contact with the medial malleolus.
- Trial inlay
  - The 5-mm inlay trial is inserted (Fig. 12D) and the distractor (HINTERMANN spreader) is removed; if not enough soft tissue tension can be achieved, the 7-mm or 9-mm trial is inserted.
- It is highly recommended to use fluoroscopy to check the position of implants while the foot is held in neutral position (Fig. 13A), particularly checking for the following (Fig. 13B):
  - Appropriate length of the tibial component (its posterior border should be in line with the posterior aspect of the tibia, thereby fully covering the tibial surface)

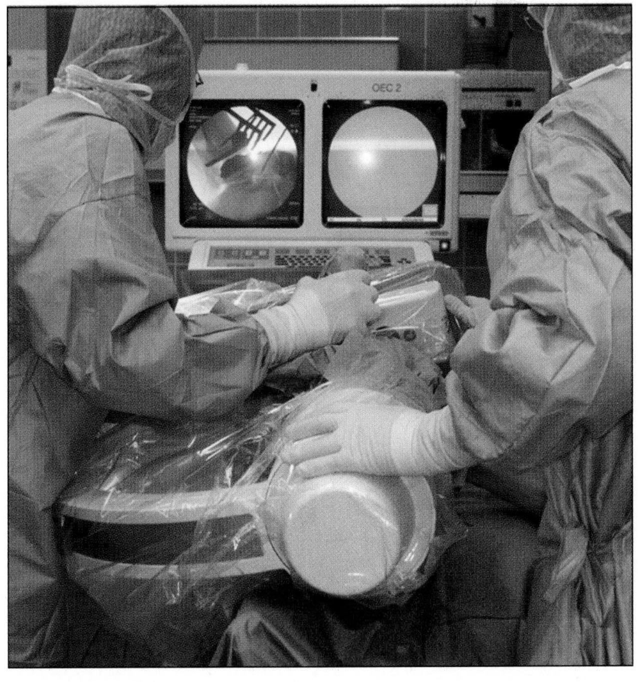

A

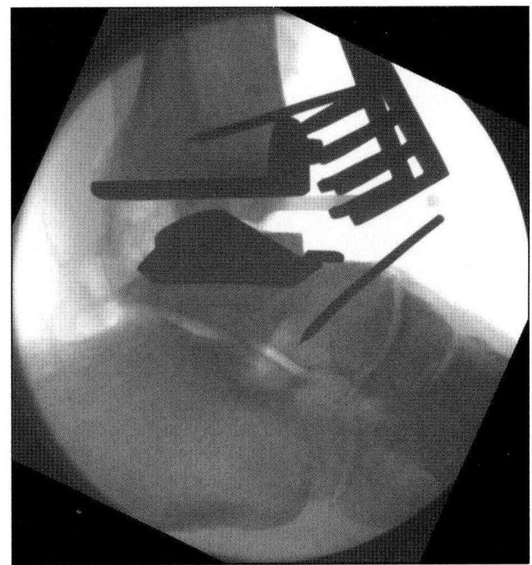

B

FIGURE 13

  - Proper fit of the tibial component to the tibial surface
  - Proper fit of the posterior edge of the talar component to the posterior surface of the talus
  - Point of contact of the talar component with the tibial component
- If proper position of the talus has been achieved, resection of the anterior surface of the talus is made using a rongeur and/or the oscillating saw (Fig. 14A).
- The second talar trial (same size as the first talar trial) is positioned on the talus using the small impactor to get proper fit against all resection surfaces (Fig. 14B).
- Two drill holes are made with the provided 4.5-mm drill, and the trial is removed (Fig. 14C).
- The bony surfaces are carefully checked. If there are cysts, they are removed with a curette (Fig. 14D); filling with cancellous bone taken from the removed bony material is recommended. If there is sclerotic bone left on the surface, drilling with a 2.0-mm drill is recommended.

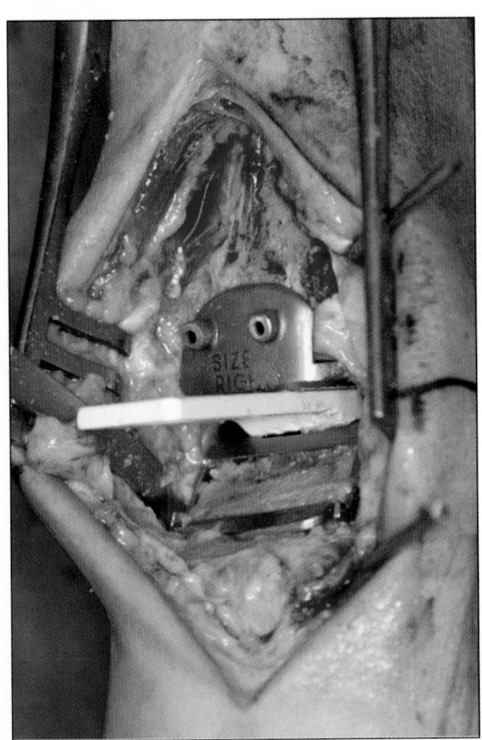

A

FIGURE 14

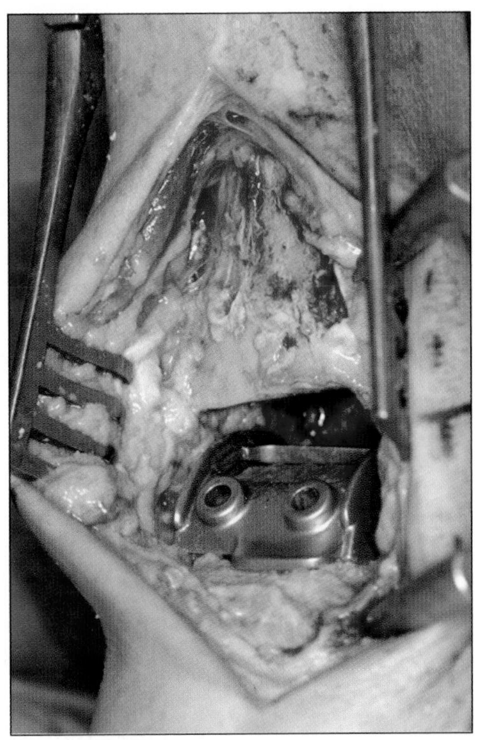

B

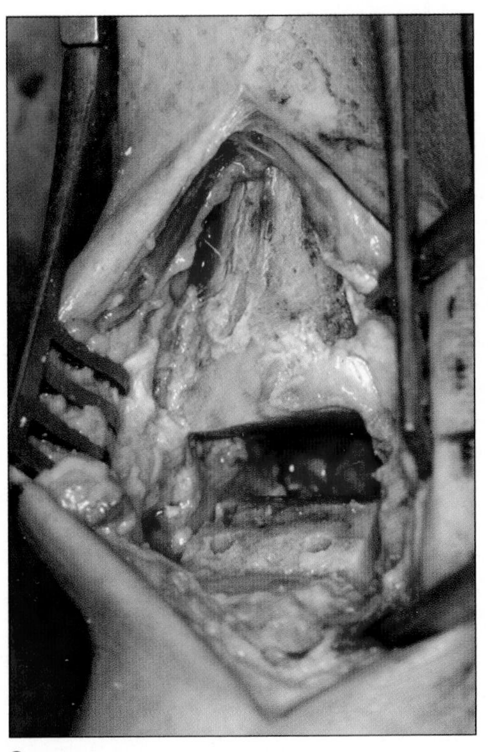

C

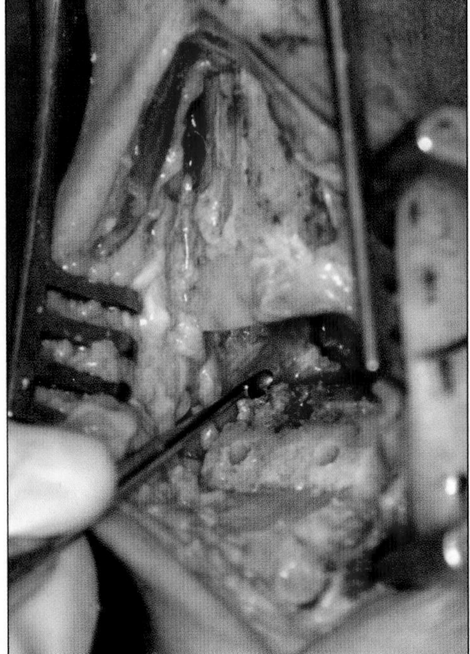

D

FIGURE 14, cont'd

Pearls

- *If the foot is moved in dorsiflexion with the surgeon's maximal power, settling of the implant may be improved, and remaining soft tissue contracture on the posterior aspect of the ankle may be released.*
- *Fluoroscopy allows detecting any remaining bony fragments or osteophytes that could be a potential source of pain or motion restriction.*

Step 4: Insertion of Implants

- The final implants, as selected before, are inserted as follows:
  - The talar component is filled with bone matrix (TBX) to get the cysts filled (Fig. 15A) and then inserted such that the pegs can glide into the two drilled holes (Fig. 15B). A hammer and impactor are used to get a proper fit of the component to the bone (see Fig. 15B).
  - The tibial component is inserted along the medial malleolus until proper fit to the anterior border of the tibia is achieved (Fig. 15C). A hammer and impactor may be used for appropriate fit to bone (Fig. 15D).
  - The inlay (same size as the talar component!) is inserted (Fig. 15E).
- The distractor (HINTERMANN spreader) is removed, and achieved stability and motion are checked clinically.
- Screw fixation of the tibial component is needed to achieve stability against rotational and translational forces during the osteointegration process (Fig. 15F).

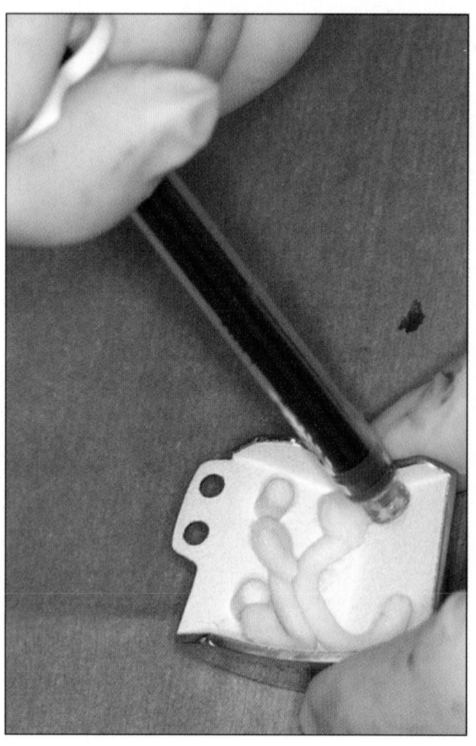

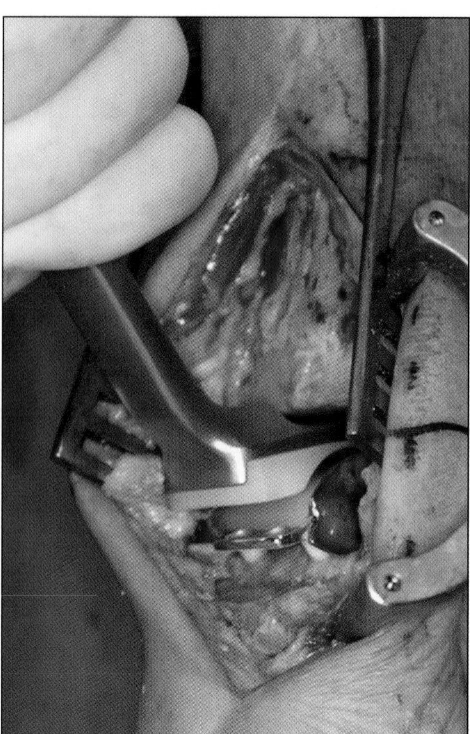

A B

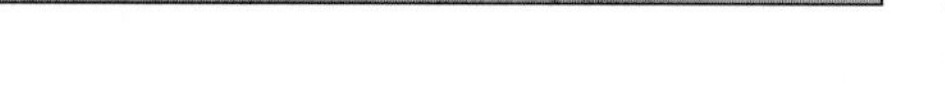

FIGURE 15

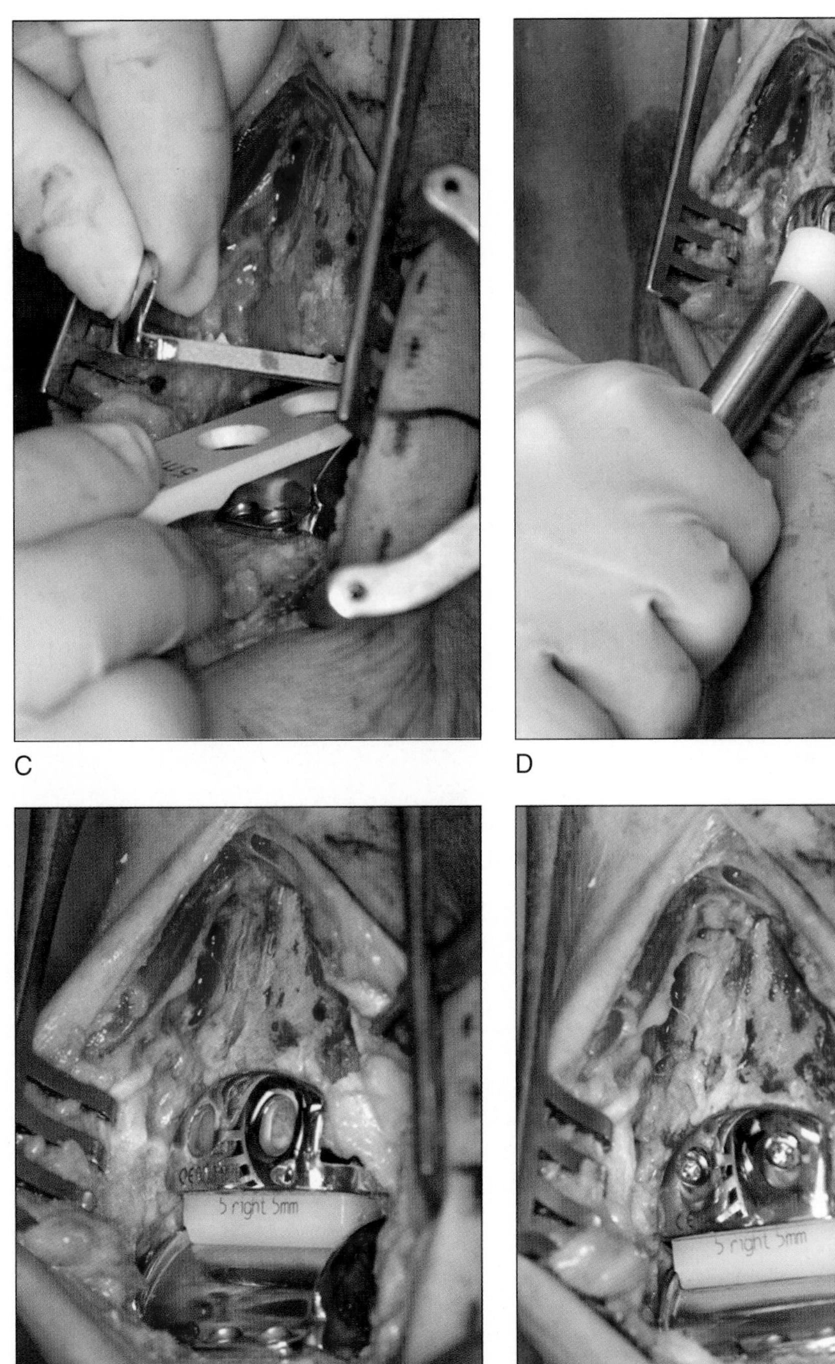

C D E F

FIGURE 15, cont'd

Pearls

- *Active motion and lymphatic drainage may support recovery of soft tissues during the first 6 weeks.*
- *In the case of additional osteotomies of the calcaneus, ligament reconstruction, and/or tendon transfer, cast immobilization for 6 weeks is advised.*
- *In the case of additional fusion of adjacent joints, cast immobilization for 8 weeks is advised.*
- *In the case of additional supramalleolar osteotomy, non–weight bearing for 8–10 weeks is advised.*

- It is also highly recommended to check the position of the implants by fluoroscopy, as described for the trial implants (Fig. 16A–C).

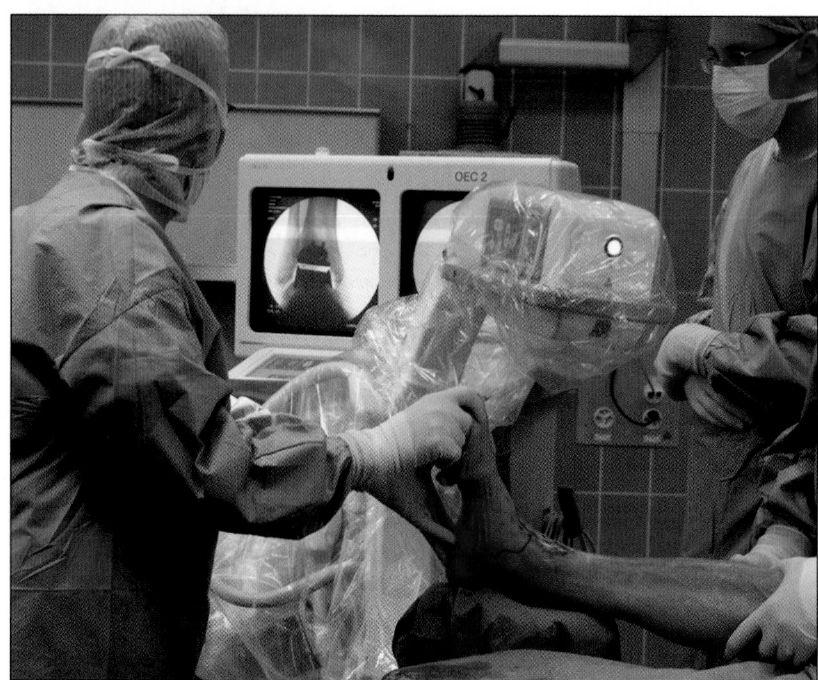

A

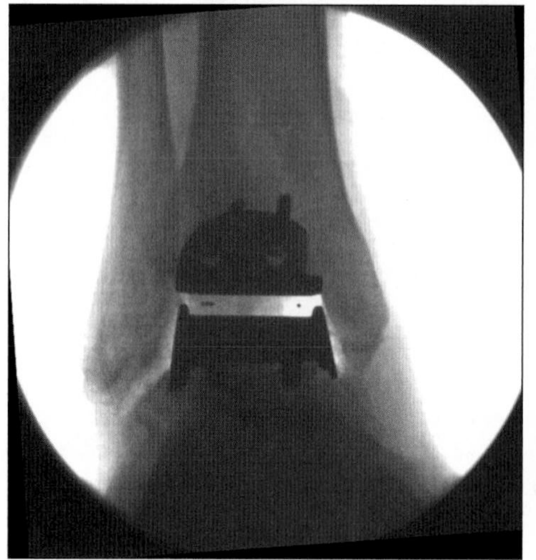

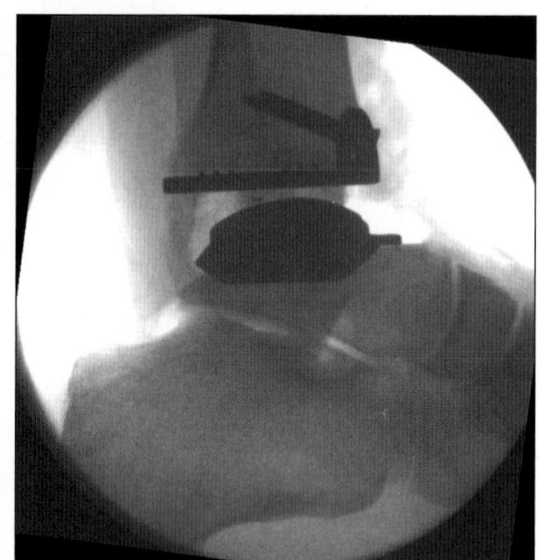

FIGURE 16 B C

Step 5: Wound Closure

- Wound closure is obtained by suture of the tendon sheath and retinaculum (Fig. 17A) and of the skin (Fig. 17B).
- A careful dressing is made to avoid any pressure to the skin (Fig. 17C and 17D).
- A splint is used to keep the foot in neutral position (Fig. 17E).

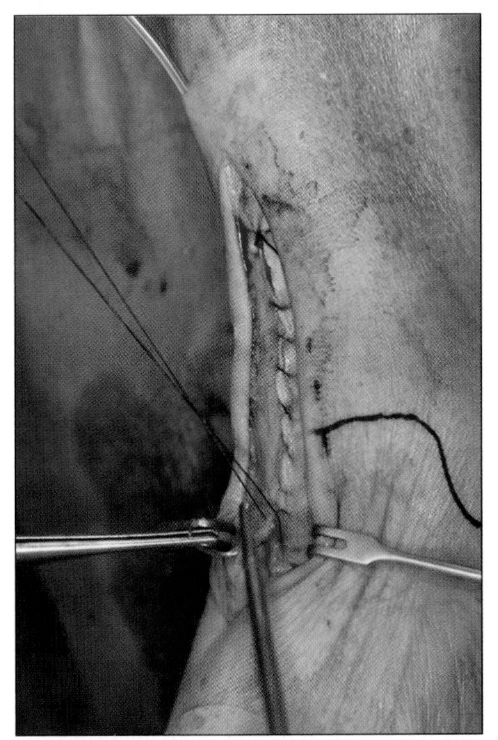

A

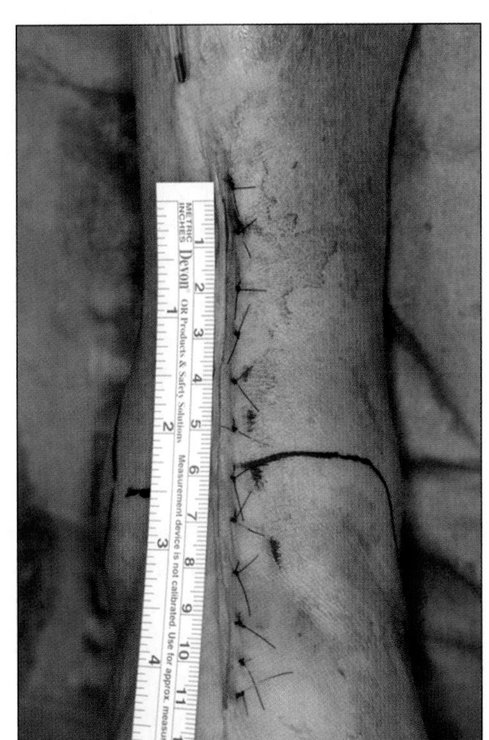

B

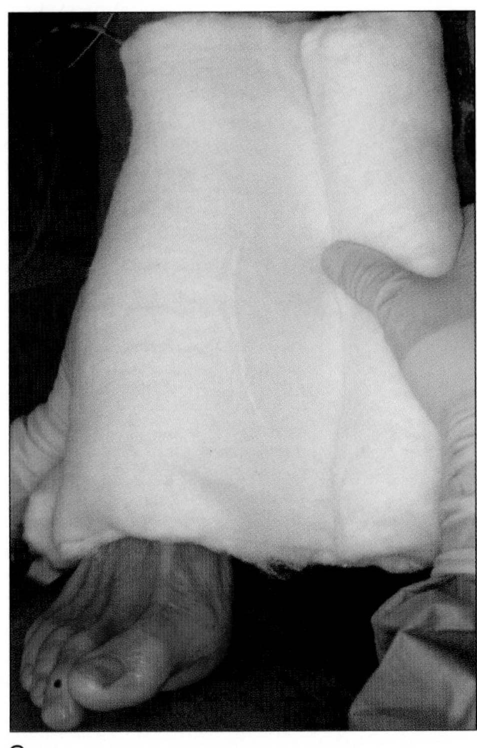

C

D

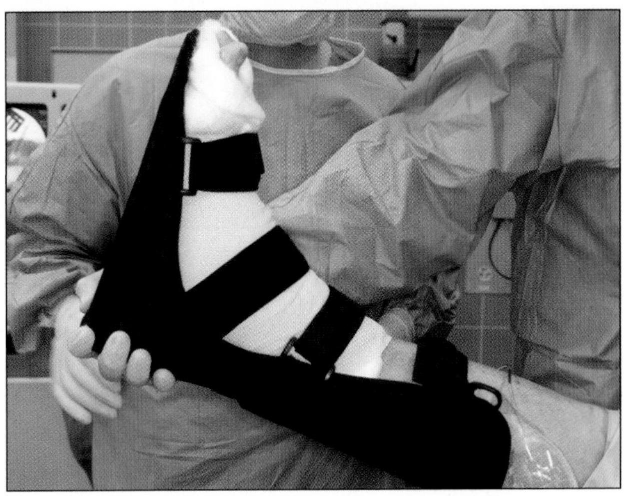

E

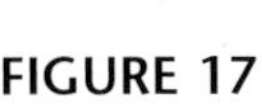

FIGURE 17

PITFALLS

- *Too-aggressive motion during the first postoperative days may lead to breakdown of soft tissues.*

Postoperative Care and Expected Outcomes

- The dressing and splint are removed and changed after 2 days.
- When the wound condition is dry and proper, typically 2–4 days after surgery, the foot is placed in a stabilizing cast or walker that protect the ankle against eversion, inversion, and plantar flexion movements for 6 weeks.
- Weight bearing is allowed as tolerated. Usually, full weight bearing is achieved after 1 week.
- A rehabilitation program should be started for the foot and ankle after cast or walker removal, including stretching and strengthening of the triceps surae.
- The first clinical and radiologic follow-up is made at 6 weeks, to check wound situs and osteointegration and position of the implants (Fig. 18A and 18B).
- The patient should be advised to wear a compression stocking to avoid swelling for a further 4–6 months.

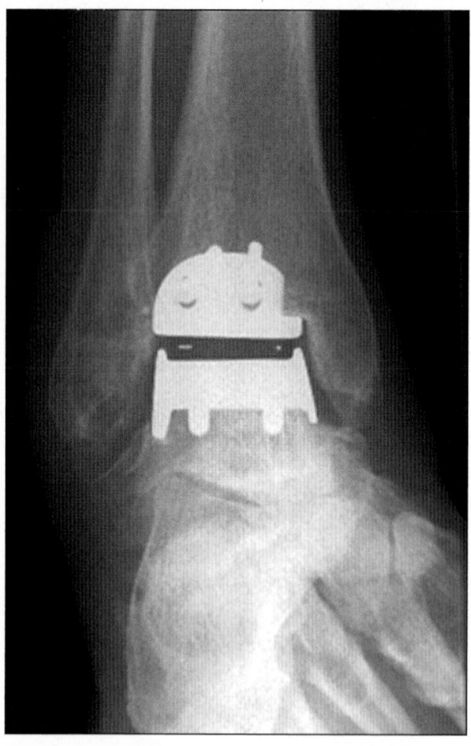

A

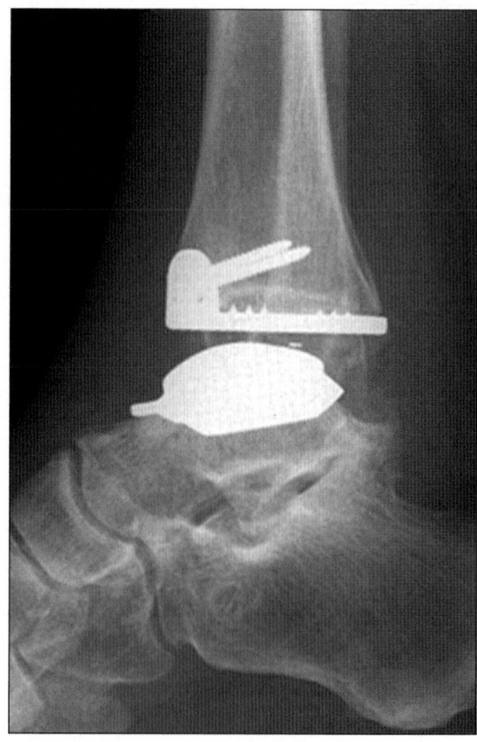

B

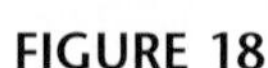

FIGURE 18

Evidence

Hintermann B. Total Ankle Arthroplasty: Historical Overview, Current Concepts and Future Perspectives. Berlin: Springer, 2004.

A recent comprehensive work reporting existing experience with total ankle arthroplasty.

Hintermann B, Valderrabano V, Dereymaeker G, Dick W. The HINTEGRA ankle: rationale and short-term results of 122 consecutive ankles. Clin Orthop Relat Res. 2004;(424):57-68.

This clinical study highlights the clinical and functional outcome of patients undergoing the implantation of a HINTEGRA ankle prosthesis. (Level IV evidence)

Valderrabano V, Nigg BM, von Tscharner V, Stefanyshyn DJ, Goepfert B, Hintermann B. Gait analysis in ankle osteoarthritis and total ankle replacement. Clin Biomech. 2007;22:894-904.

This study provides data for the clinical-biomechanical understanding of the normal, arthritic, and total ankle replacement. (Level III evidence)

Valderrabano V, Pagenstert G, Horisberger M, Knupp M, Hintermann B. Sports and recreation activity of ankle arthritis patients before and after total ankle replacement. Am J Sports Med. 2006;34:993-9.

A clinical study addressing the sports level in patients after total ankle replacement. (Level IV evidence)

PROCEDURE 26

Salvage of Failed Total Ankle Arthroplasty

Beat Hintermann

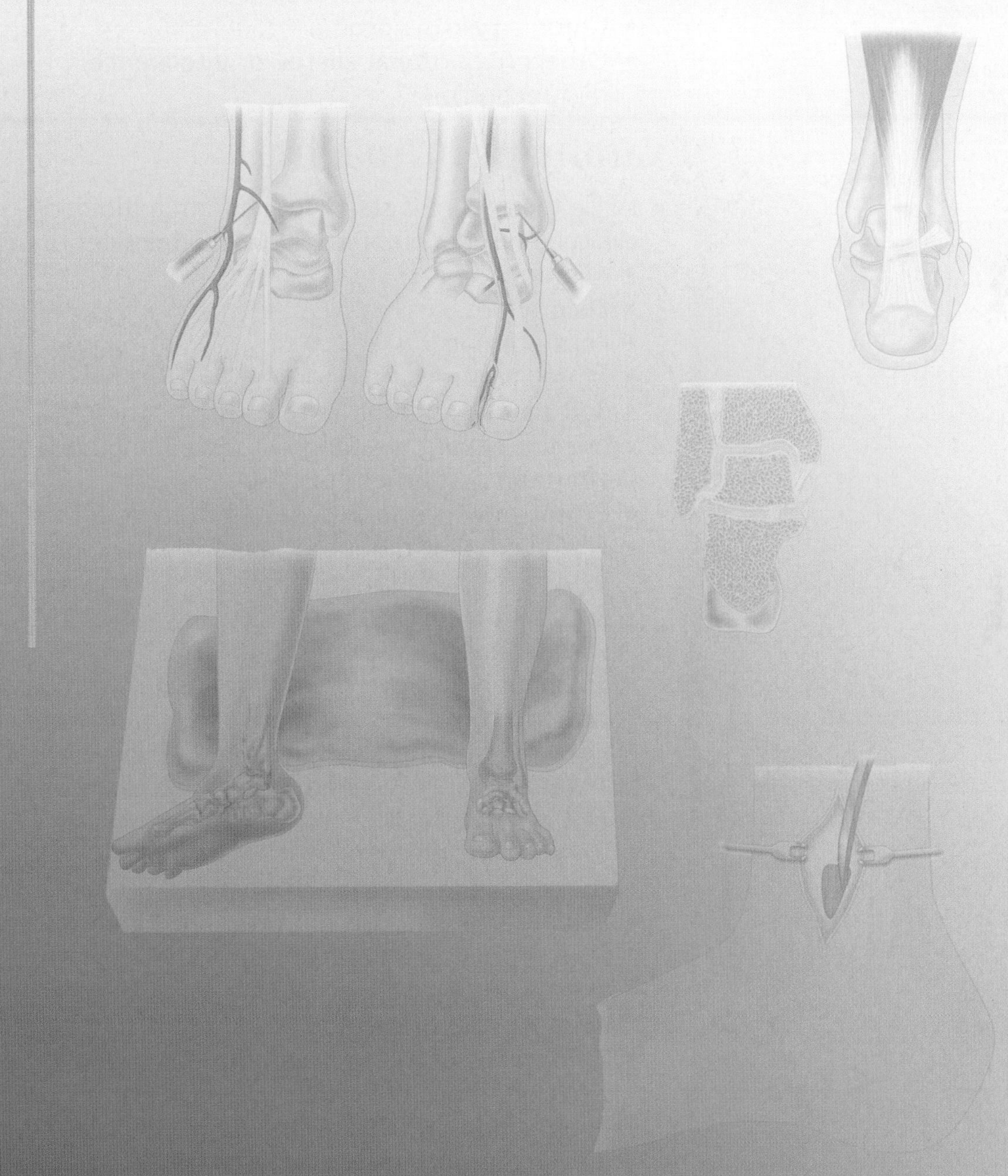

PITFALLS

- *Active infection*
- *Neuroarthropathy (Charcot arthropathy)*

Controversies

- Controversy about appropriate salvage procedure
  - Revision arthroplasty
  - Tibiotalar arthrodesis
  - Tibiocalcaneal arthrodesis

Treatment Options

- Revision arthroplasty
- Tibiotalar arthrodesis
- Tibiocalcaneal arthrodesis

Indications

- Failed arthroplasty of the ankle due to
  - Primary loosening of component
  - Late loosening of component
  - Progressive nonmanageable malalignment
  - Nonmanageable instability
  - Avascular necrosis of bone underlying bone
  - Deep infection
  - Periprosthetic fracture
  - Breakdown of soft tissues
  - Chronic pain syndrome
  - Others (e.g., metal allergy or intolerance, dysfunction)

Examination/Imaging

- While the patient is standing, perform a thorough clinical investigation of both lower extremities to assess:
  - Alignment
  - Deformities
  - Foot position
  - Muscular atrophy
  - Soft tissue condition (e.g., existing scars)
- While the patient is sitting with free-hanging feet, perform an assessment of:
  - Extent to which a present deformity is correctable
  - Preserved joint motion of the ankle and subtalar joints
  - Ligament stability of the ankle and subtalar joints with anterior drawer and tilt tests
  - Supination and eversion power (e.g., function of posterior tibial and peroneus brevis muscles)
- Plain weight-bearing radiographs, including anteroposterior (AP) views of foot and ankle and lateral view of the foot, to determine/rule out
  - Component position
  - Lucency zone beneath component
  - Extent of destruction of underlying bone stock (e.g., tibia, talus, fibula)
  - Status of neighboring joints (e.g., associated degenerative disease)
  - Deformities of the foot and ankle complex (e.g., heel alignment, foot arch, talonavicular alignment)
  - Bony condition (e.g., avascular necrosis, bony defects, osteoporosis)
  - Figure 1 shows a 67-year-old male patient, 5.8 years after primary arthroplasty, evidencing cyst formation on AP (Fig. 1A) and lateral (Fig. 1B) plain radiographs.

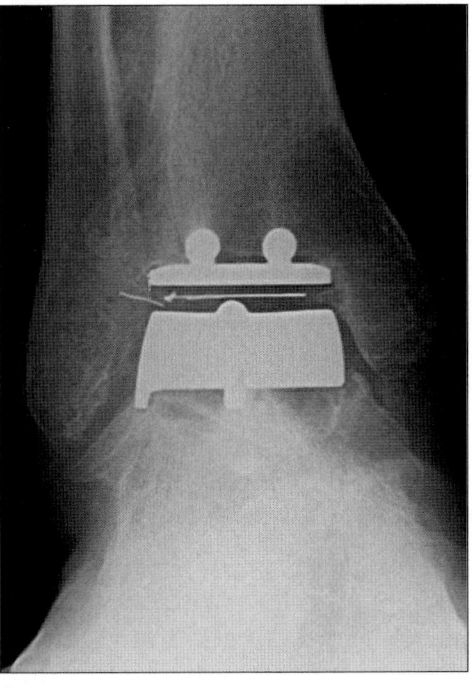
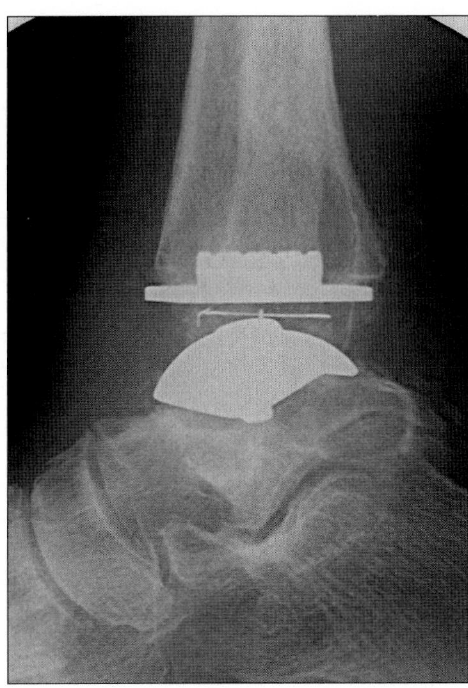

FIGURE 1 A B

- Computed tomography scan may be obtained for assessment of
  - Bone-implant interface
  - Bony defects
  - Cyst formation
  - Avascular necrosis
  - Figure 2 shows coronal (Fig. 2A) and sagittal (Fig. 2B) views of the same patient as in Figure 1.

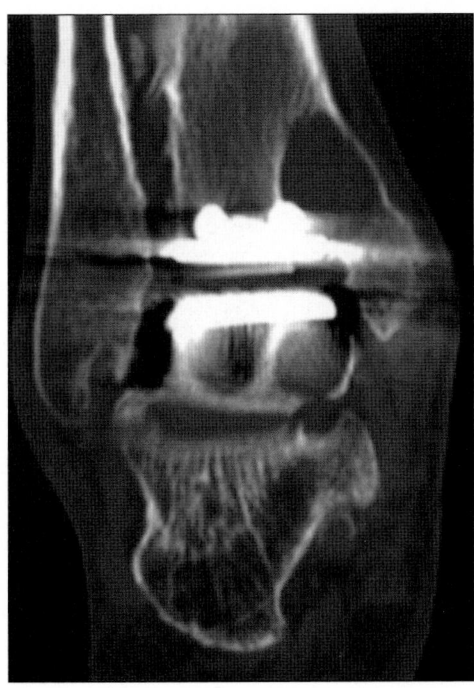
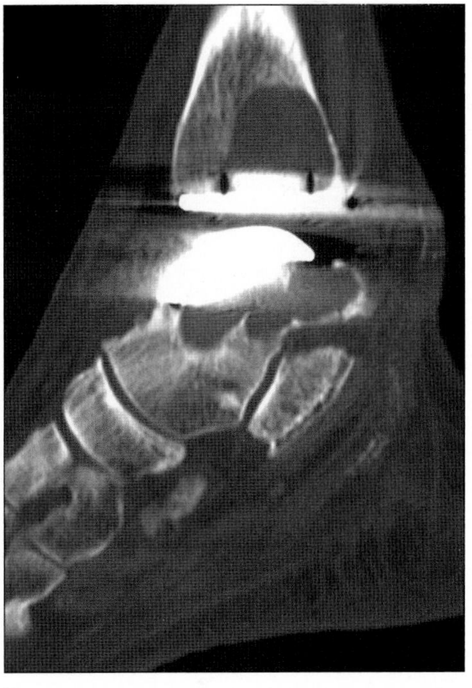

FIGURE 2 A B

- Single-photon emission computed tomography with superimposed bone scan may be used to visualize
  - Bone-implant interface
  - Stress reaction (e.g., medial malleolus, fibula)
  - Bony impingement
  - Morphologic pathologies and associated activity process

Surgical Anatomy

- The superior extensor retinaculum is a thickening of the deep fascia above the ankle, running from the tibia to the fibula (Fig. 3). It includes, from medially to laterally, the tendons of the tibialis anterior, extensor hallucis longus, and extensor digitorum longus.
- The anterior neurovascular bundle lies roughly halfway between the malleoli (Fig. 4A); it can be found consistently between the extensor hallucis longus and extensor digitorum longus tendons.
- The neurovascular bundle contains the tibialis anterior and the deep peroneal nerve. The nerve supplies the extensor digitorum brevis and extensor hallucis brevis and a sensory space (interdigital I–II).
- On the height of the talonavicular joint, the medial branches of the superficial peroneal nerve cross from

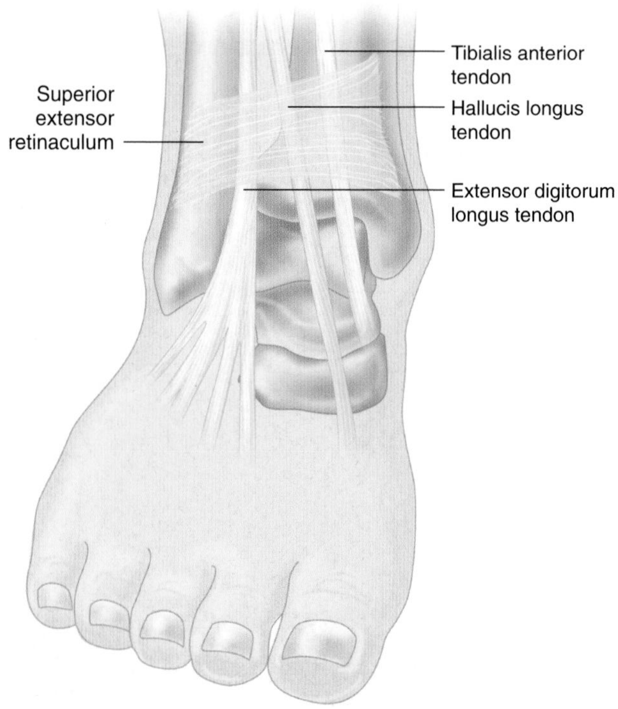

FIGURE 3

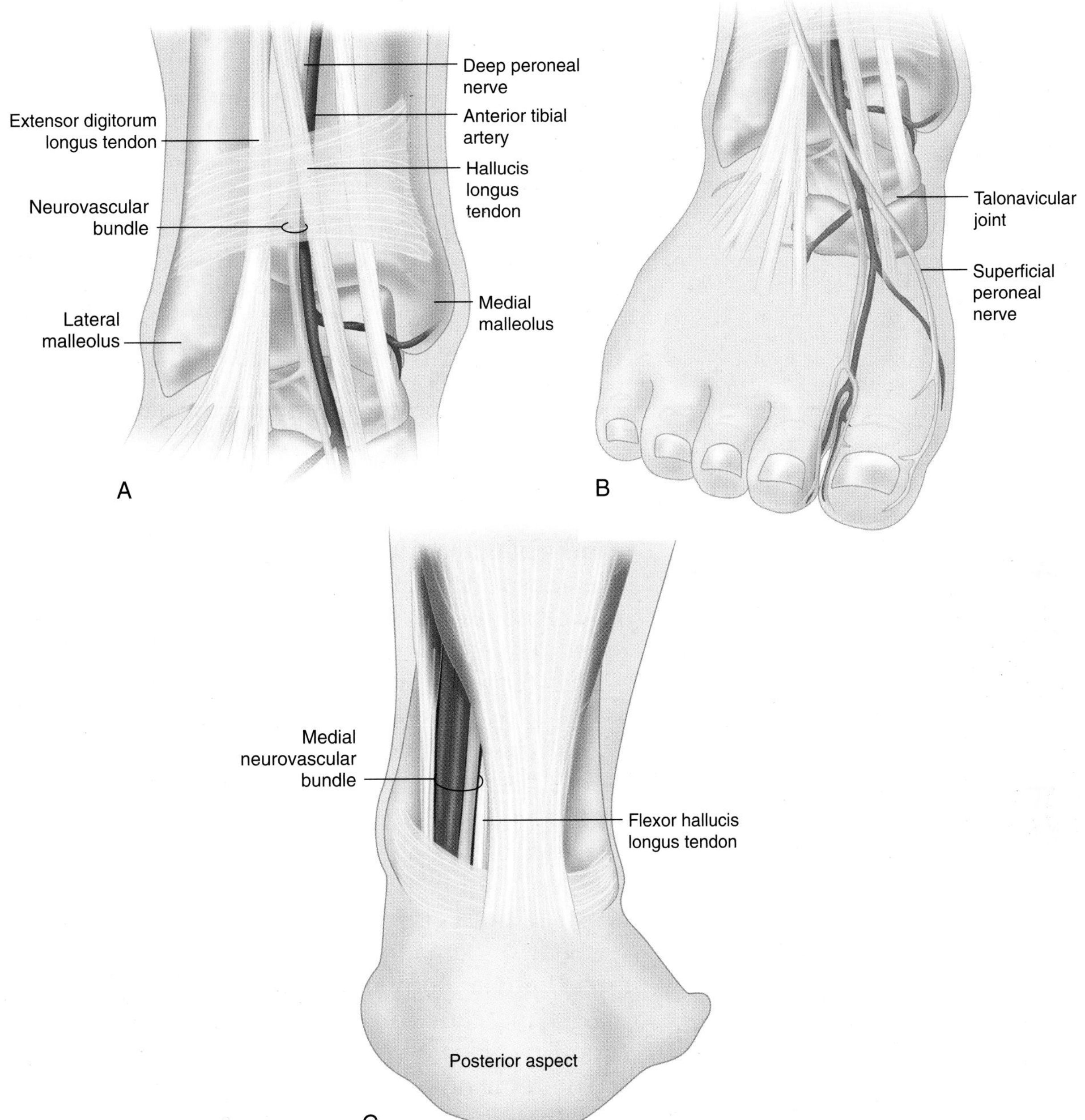

FIGURE 4

lateral to medial (Fig. 4B). This nerve supplies the skin of the dorsum of the foot.

- On the posterior aspect of the ankle, the medial neurovascular bundle is located behind its posteromedial corner, and the flexor hallucis longus tendon on its posterior aspect (Fig. 4C).

PEARLS

- *The affected foot is underlet with a block to facilitate fluoroscopy during surgery.*

PEARLS

- *To remove a tibial component with stem fixation, a window at the anterior tibial cortex may be created.*
- *To remove a talar component, a small impactor may be inserted percutaneously from the lateral foot sole to gain access to the anterolateral corner of the implant (Fig. 6).*

PITFALLS

- *If old scars from previous surgeries or injuries are not respected, breakdown of critical areas may occur.*

Instrumentation

- A self-retaining distractor may be helpful; care must be taken, however, that no tension is applied to the skin.

Positioning

- The patient is positioned with the feet on the edge of the table.
- The ipsilateral back is lifted until a strictly upward position of the foot is obtained.
- The tourniquet is mounted at the ipsilateral thigh.

Portals/Exposures

- Usually, the scar from the previous incision is used.
- The scarred extensor retinaculum is exposed through a 10- to 12-cm incision.
- The retinaculum is dissected along the lateral border of the anterior tibial tendon, and the anterior aspect of the distal tibia is exposed.
- While the soft tissue mantle is dissected with the periosteum from the bone, attention is paid to the neurovascular bundle that lies behind the long extensor hallucis tendon.
- A capsulotomy and capsulectomy are made, and a self-retaining retractor is inserted to carefully keep the soft tissue mantle away.
- The prosthesis is exposed and explored with regard to instability, dysfunction, loosening, bony impingement, and wear. The components are then removed.
  - In most instances, the polyethylene insert is removed first.
  - The tibial component is removed next, taking care not to damage the bone stock (Fig. 5A).
  - The talar component is then removed, again taking care not to damage the bone stock (Fig. 5B).
- The remaining bone surfaces are carefully débrided from any soft tissue formation and avascular bone. Figure 5C shows the talar surface after débridement and Figure 5D shows excised cyst material from the same patient as in Figure 1.
- The medial and lateral compartments are débrided as well.
- While the foot is held in neutral position, the overall defect is measured.

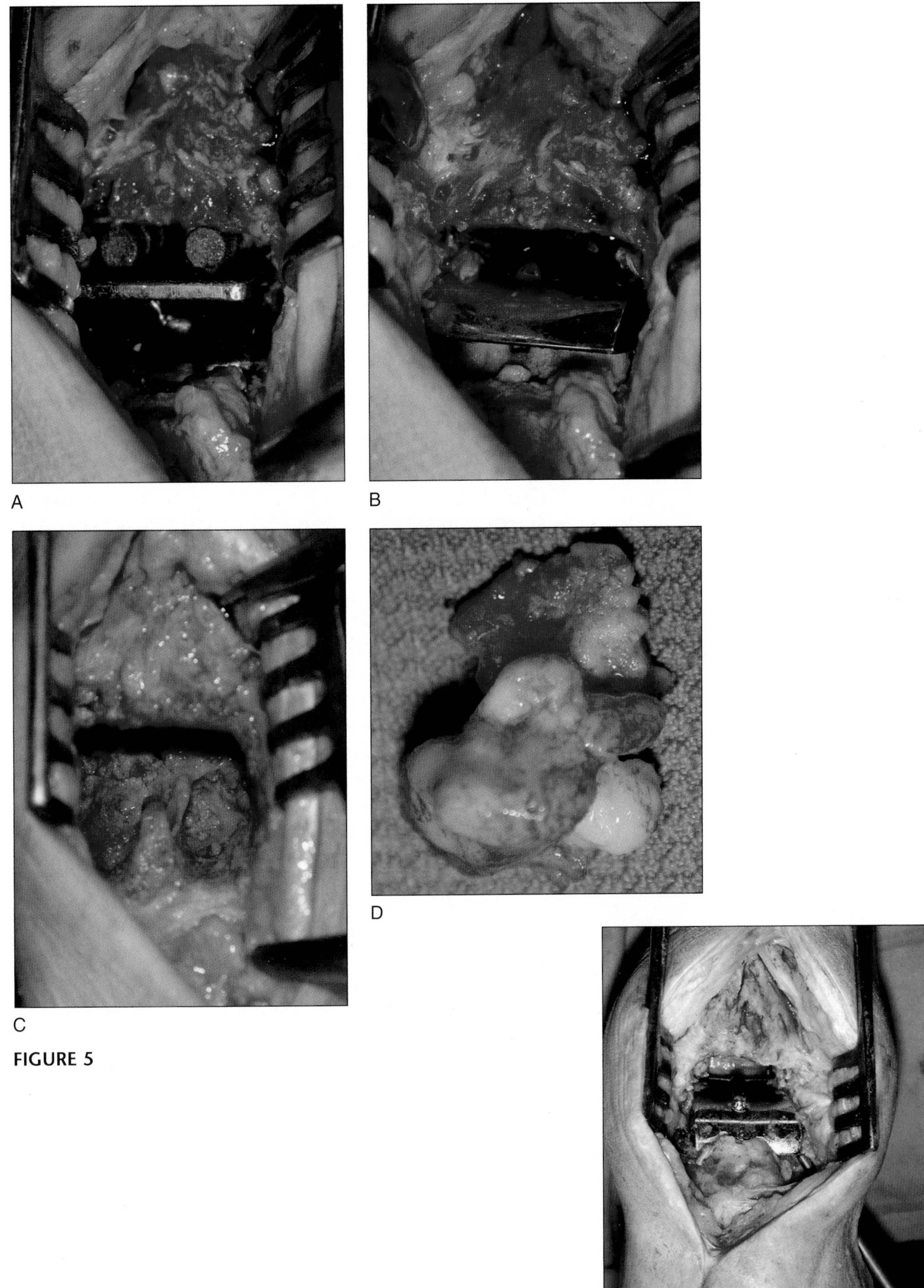

FIGURE 5

FIGURE 6

Procedure: Revision Arthroplasty

- Revision arthroplasty is considered if
  - Bone stock on the talar side is sufficient to get proper anchorage of the implant (see Fig. 1).
  - The condition of the bone stock allows for appropriate component fixation and osteointegration (see Fig. 2).
  - Associated problems are manageable (e.g., stability of the ankle, alignment of hindfoot).

Step 1

- Posterior scars and capsular structures are carefully removed.
- A tibial resection block is fixed to the tibia.
- Minimal bone is resected at the bony cortex (Fig. 7A).
- A trial implant is inserted and its stability is tested.

Step 2

- A flat cut is made on the talar side, taking care to remove as little bone as possible to retain enough to support the flat revision talar component (Fig. 7B).
- A talar resection block is mounted, and medial and lateral cuts are done.
- The medial and lateral gutters are débrided.
- A trial implant is fixed to the talus, and its position is checked by fluoroscopy (Fig. 8A and 8B).
- If appropriate position (particularly in the AP plane) is achieved, drill holes for the pegs are made.

Step 3

- The resection surfaces of the tibia and talus are carefully débrided, and drill holes may be made to break down osteosclerotic areas.
- Remaining defects in the center of the tibial metaphysis are filled with bone matrix and/or cancellous bone from iliac crest.
- The tibial component is inserted and impacted; two screws are inserted to increase primary stability against rotational and translational forces.
- Remaining defects in the talar body are filled with bone matrix and/or cancellous bone from iliac crest.
- The talar revision component is inserted and impacted.
- A polyethylene insert of appropriate thickness is inserted.
- Overall stability and range of motion are carefully tested.
- Position of the implants is checked by fluoroscopy.

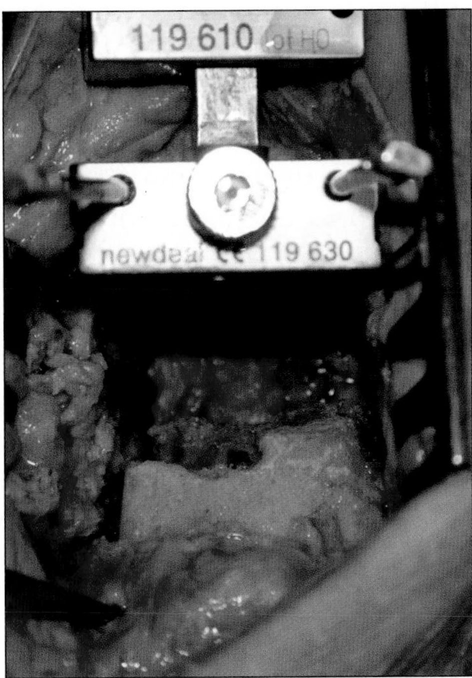

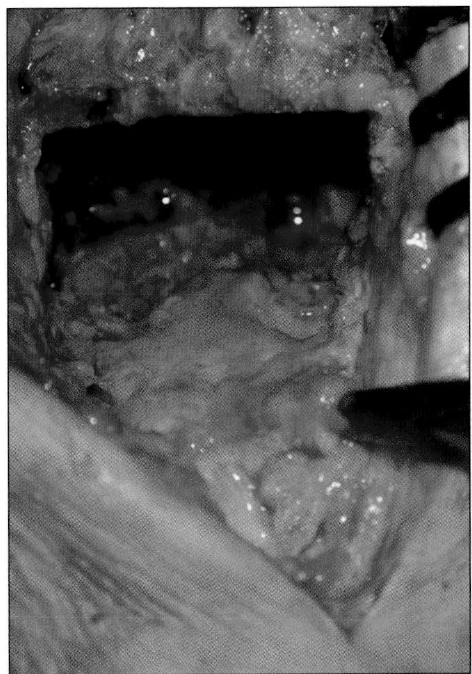

FIGURE 7 A B

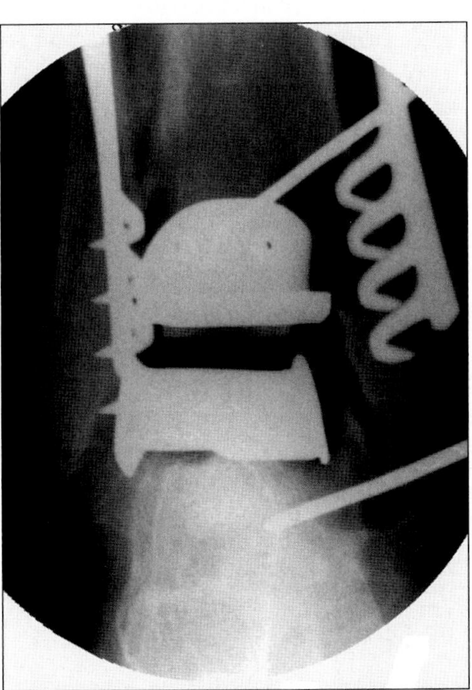

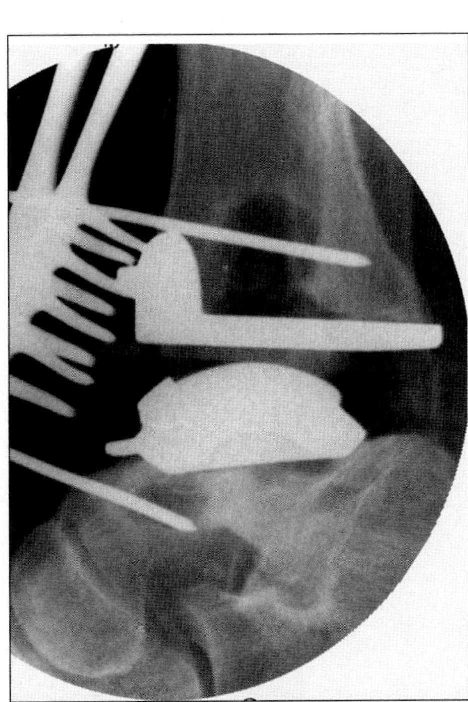

FIGURE 8 A B

Step 4

- Wound closure is obtained by suture of the tendon sheath and retinaculum, and the skin.
- A careful dressing is made to avoid any pressure to the skin.
- A splint is used to keep the foot in neutral position.

Pearls

- *Firm, tripodal bony support of the components may be sufficient to achieve stable osteointegration.*
- *In the case of lateral instability, reconstruction of lateral ligaments is done.*
- *In the case of peroneus brevis dysfunction, peroneus longus–to–peroneus brevis transfer is done.*

Pitfalls

- *Inappropriate balancing or bad quality of soft tissues may result in increased movement of the polyethylene insert during dorsiflexion–plantar flexion of the foot.*

Procedure: Tibiotalar Arthrodesis

- Tibiotalar arthrodesis is considered if
  - Bone stock on the talar side is sufficient to get proper anchorage of screws. Figure 9 shows AP (Fig. 9A) and lateral (Fig. 9B) radiographs of a 52-year-old male patient 27 months after revision arthroplasty (removal of MOBILITY prosthesis and insertion of HINTEGRA prosthesis) following primary loosening, as evidenced by chronic pain.
  - The condition of the bone stock does not allow for appropriate component fixation.
  - Revision arthroplasty is not advised (e.g., nonmanageable instability and/or malalignment, bad soft tissue condition, chronic pain syndrome).

Step 1

- The foot is held in neutral position (for dorsiflexion–plantar flexion, eversion-inversion) and slight external rotation (approximately 10° of abduction).
- A bone graft from the iliac crest (autograft) or the femoral head (allograft) is shaped to fit exactly into the defect (Fig. 10A and 10B).
- An anterolateral plate is fixed by three locking screws to the talar neck.

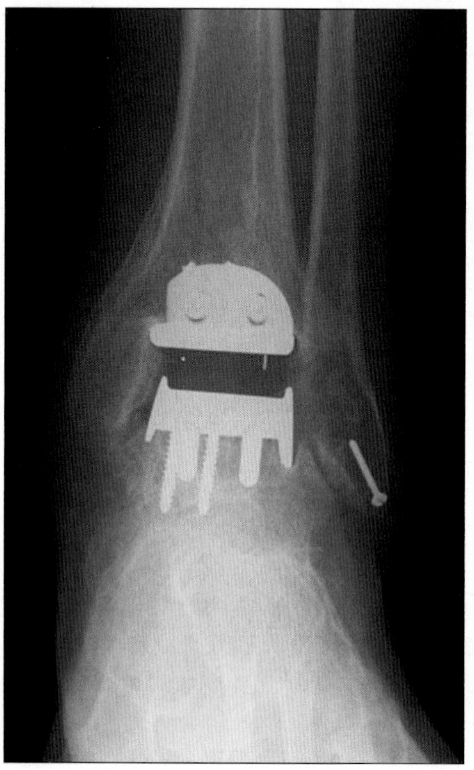

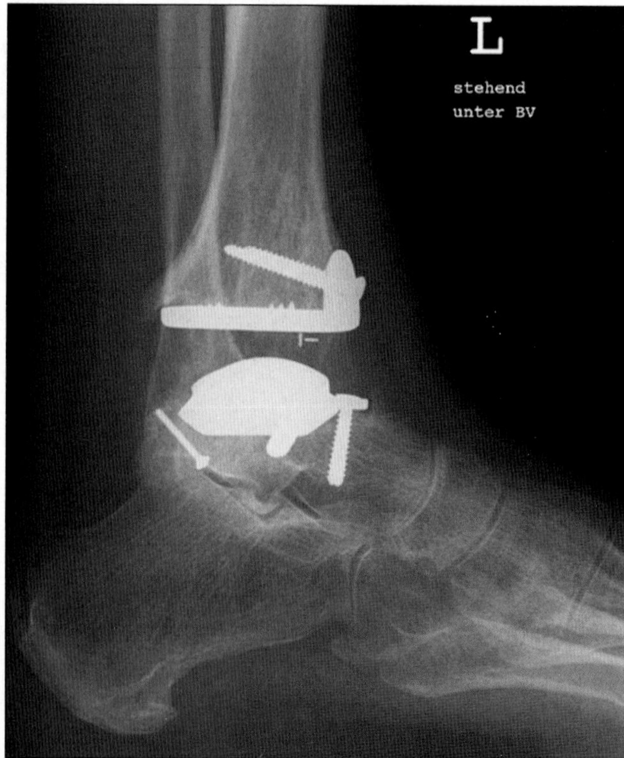

FIGURE 9 A B

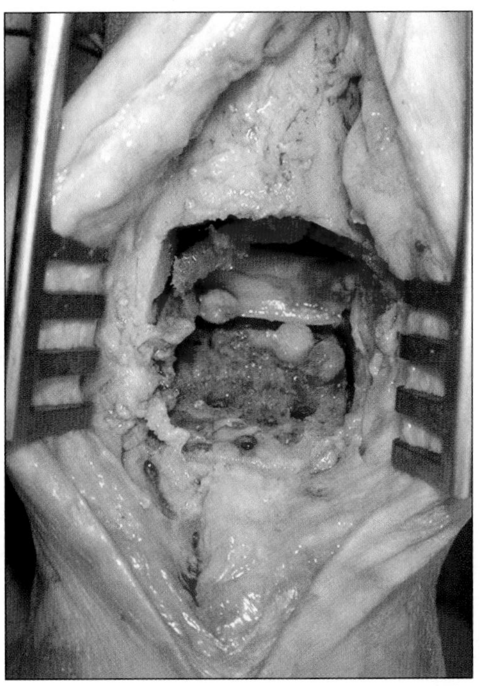

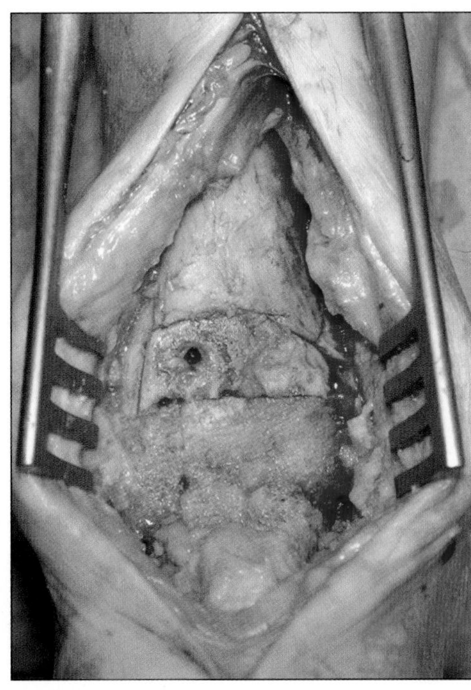

FIGURE 10 A B

- A compression device (fixed to the plate and tibia) is used to apply maximal axial compression.
- The plate is fixed to the tibia.

Step 2

- A second anteromedial plate is fixed analogously to the talar neck and tibia.
- An oblique screw is inserted through both the medial and lateral plates to get anchorage into the posterior aspect of the talar body (Fig. 11).
- Step-by-step wound closure is performed.

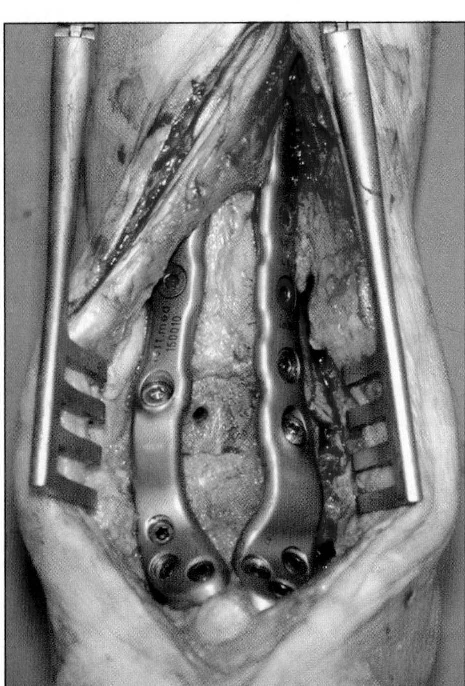

FIGURE 11

PEARLS

- *The posterior scarred capsule may be left in place, which increases the primary stability of the graft.*
- *Fluoroscopy is used to check appropriate screw and plate position (Fig. 12).*
- *The use of bone matrix and blood platelet concentrate may support bone healing.*

PITFALLS

- *Screws that are too long may damage the subtalar joint.*

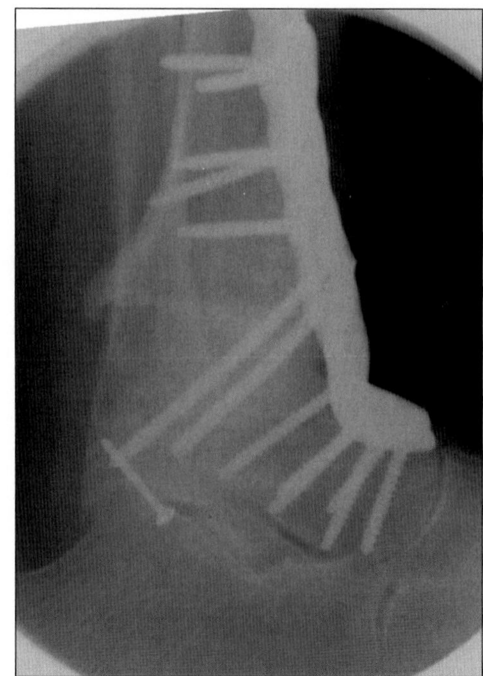

FIGURE 12

Procedure: Tibiocalcaneal Arthrodesis

- Tibiocalcaneal arthrodesis is considered if
  - Bone stock on the talar side is not sufficient to get proper anchorage of screws. Figure 13 shows AP and lateral radiographs of a 39-year-old male patient with painful total ankle arthroplasty after 22 months, as evidenced by loosening and subsidence of both components, instability, and varus malalignment.
  - The condition of the bone stock does not allow for appropriate component fixation.
  - Revision arthroplasty is not advised (e.g., nonmanageable instability and/or malalignment, bad soft tissue condition, chronic pain syndrome).
  - There is extensive avascular necrosis of the talar body.

PEARLS

- *The posterior scarred capsule may be left in place, which increases primary stability of the graft.*
- *Fluoroscopy is used to check appropriate nail and screw position.*
- *The use of bone matrix and blood platelet concentrate may support bone healing.*
- *Compression applied between the calcaneus and tibia may increase the stability of the overall fixation and thus increase bone healing.*

STEP 1

- The subtalar joint is approached through a small lateral incision at the sinus tarsi.
- The subtalar joint is débrided.
- The foot is held in neutral position (for dorsiflexion–plantar flexion, eversion-inversion) and slight external rotation (approximately 10° of abduction).
- A bone graft from the iliac crest (autograft) or the femoral head (allograft) is shaped to fit exactly into the defect.

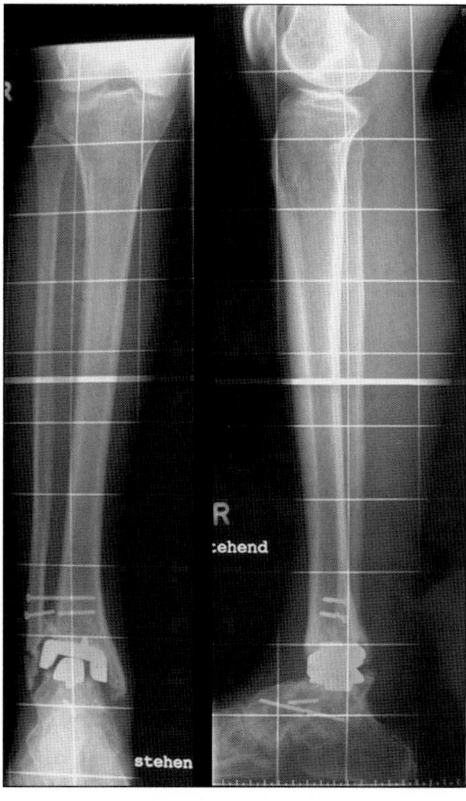

FIGURE 13

STEP 2

- A 2- to 3-cm incision is made at the plantar aspect of the foot.
- A guidewire is inserted through the calcaneus and talus into the tibial metaphysis.
- Drills of increasing size are used to get a 10- to 12-mm drill hole.
- A retrograde nail is inserted and fixed by screws according to the specifications of the manufacturer.
- Step-by-step wound closure is performed.

Postoperative Care and Expected Outcomes

- The dressing and splint are removed and changed after 2 days.
- When the wound condition is dry and proper, typically 2–4 days after surgery, the foot is placed in a stabilizing cast that protects the ankle against eversion, inversion, and dorsiflexion–plantar flexion movements for 6–8 weeks.

PITFALLS

- *Too-aggressive motion during the first postoperative days may lead to breakdown of soft tissues.*

- In the case of tibiotalar or tibiocalcaneal fusion, weight bearing of 15–20 kg is allowed until the first radiologic follow-up at 8 weeks. Full weight bearing is allowed if bone healing has occurred, usually after 8–12 weeks.
- In the case of revision arthroplasty, full weight bearing is allowed after 2 weeks.
- A rehabilitation program should be started for the foot and ankle after cast removal, including stretching and strengthening of the triceps surae.
- Clinical and radiologic follow-up is done at 2, 4, 6, and 12 months, checking for osteointegration and position of the implants.
  - Figure 14 shows stable osteointegration of components at 1-year follow-up in AP (Fig. 14A) and lateral (Fig. 14B) views (same patient as Fig. 1).
  - Figure 15 shows bone healing of a tibiotalar arthrodesis at 4 months in AP (Fig. 15A) and lateral (Fig. 15B) views of the ankle and an AP view of the foot (Fig. 15C) (same patient as Fig. 9).
  - Figure 16 shows bone healing of a tibiocalcaneal arthrodesis at 6 months in AP (Fig. 16A) and lateral (Fig. 16B) views (same patient as Fig. 13).
- The patient should be advised to wear a compression stocking to avoid swelling for a further 4–6 months.

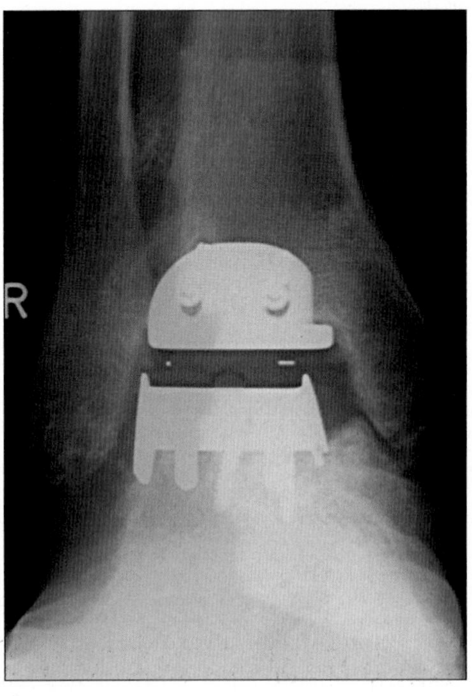

A

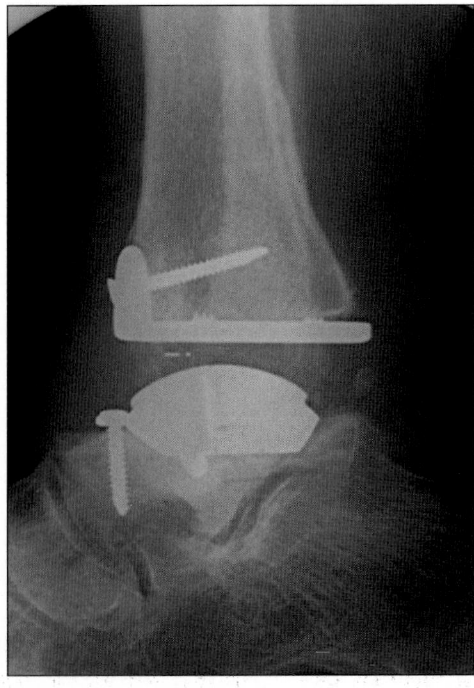

B

FIGURE 14

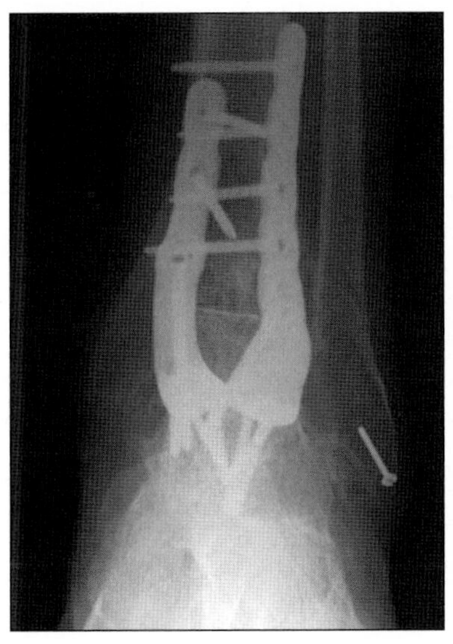
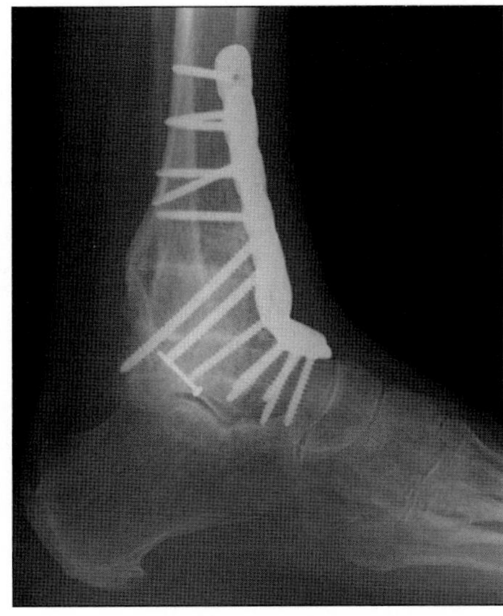
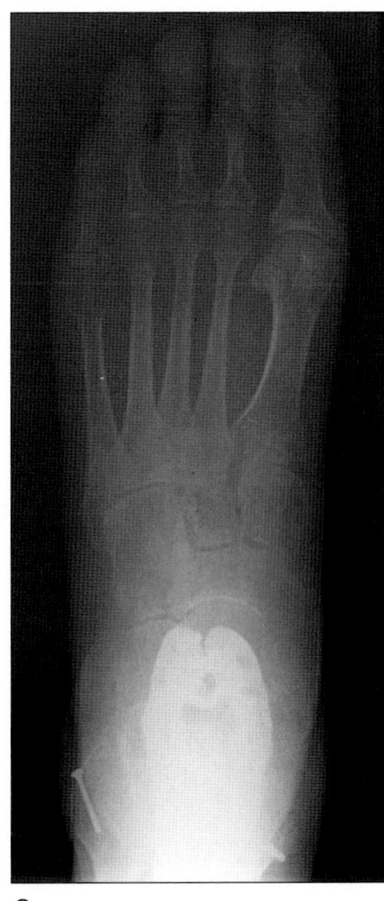

A B C

FIGURE 15

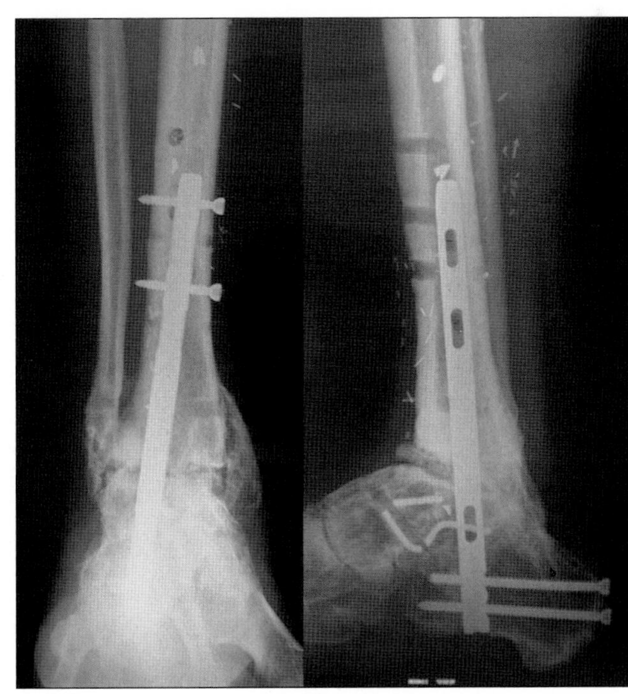

A B

FIGURE 16

Evidence

Hintermann B, Knupp M, Barg A. Revision arthroplasty for failed total ankle replacements. J Bone Joint Surg [Am]. 2009 (submitted).

A prospective clinical study analyzing outcomes in a patient group consisting of 62 patients undergoing revision arthroplasty. (Level IV evidence)

Hintermann B, Valderrabano V, Dereymaeker G, Dick W. The HINTEGRA ankle: rationale and short-term results of 122 consecutive ankles. Clin Orthop Relat Res. 2004;(424):57-68.

This clinical study highlights the clinical and functional outcome of patients undergoing the implantation of a HINTEGRA ankle prosthesis. (Level IV evidence)

Plaass C, Knupp M, Barg A, Hintermann B. Anterior double plating for rigid fixation of isolated tibiotalar arthrodesis. Foot Ankle Int. 2009 (submitted)

A prospective clinical study addressing the reliability of the anterior double plating system for isolated tibiotalar arthrodesis. The patient cohort of 29 patients includes nine ankles that failed total ankle replacement. (Level IV evidence)

PROCEDURE 27

Ankle Arthrodesis for Salvage of the Failed Total Ankle Arthroplasty

Donald R. Bohay

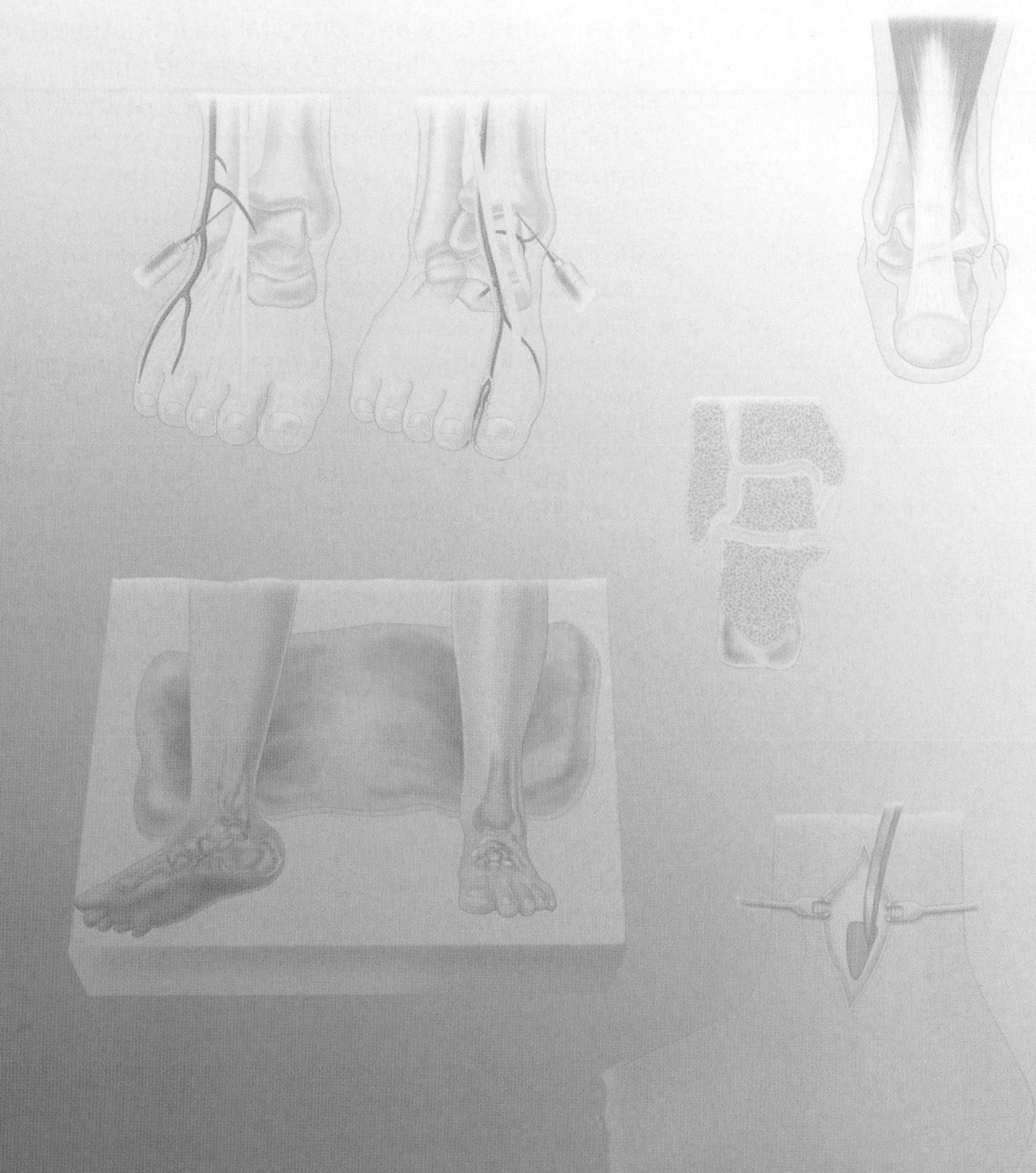

Indications

- Failed total ankle arthroplasty (TAA) where the option for revision of the implants is contraindicated or not selected, including
  - Aseptic loosening of any one or all of the components
  - Pain without radiographic evidence of loosening
  - Infection

Examination/Imaging

- A careful history and physical examination remain critical for the clinician to begin planning intervention in this situation. Any history of trauma, infection, or pattern of discomfort can give important clues as to the nature of the TAA failure. There are situations wherein the history will reveal definitive circumstances that cause pain and that can reduce the discomfort for the patient.
- The clinical examination includes careful evaluation of ankle position, skin condition, previous incisions, swelling, range of motion, and specific areas of tenderness. In addition, clinical evaluation of the ipsilateral foot, particularly as it pertains to deformity and whether it is supple or fixed, is recommended. Attention to contracture of the Achilles tendon and/or gastrocnemius should be standard.
- The radiographic evaluation includes standing anteroposterior, lateral, and mortise views of both ankles in the standing position as well as standing radiographs of the feet. The weight-bearing position is critical in this assessment, as are the foot radiographs, to help establish an accurate assessment of the lower extremity. Particular attention should be paid to the component position, osteolysis and cyst formation, fractures, bone loss, and the condition of the ipsilateral subtalar joint and foot.
- Computed tomography (CT) is another useful diagnostic tool. This study allows for the planning of the arthrodesis as it pertains to bone loss/defects and the status of the subtalar joint. Although scatter from the metal implants can make complete visualization of the bone directly associated with the TAA difficult, CT remains very useful.

Surgical Anatomy

- The revision nature of this procedure makes the surgical anatomy unpredictable at times and, as is the case for revision surgery in general, more hazardous.
- The incision should follow the original surgical incision and lead to an interval between the tibialis anterior and the extensor hallucis longus. The superficial peroneal nerve has a branch that becomes the dorsal cutaneous nerve to the hallux that is generally found at the distal extent of the incision (Fig. 1).
- The capsule below will be very scarred and contracted. Once it is entered, the TAA implants will become visible.

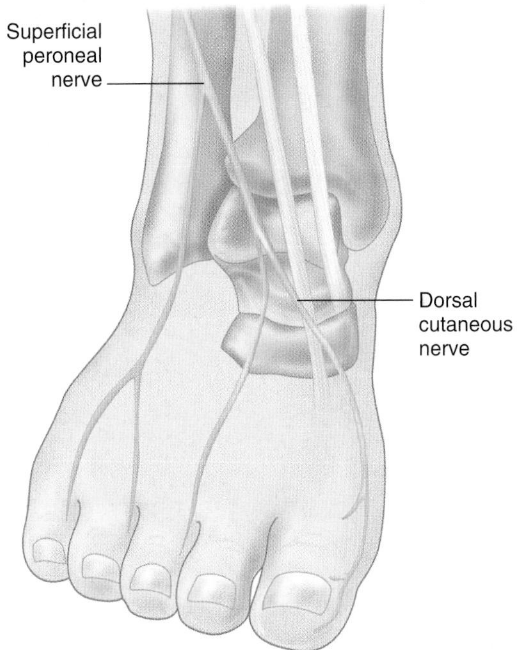

FIGURE 1

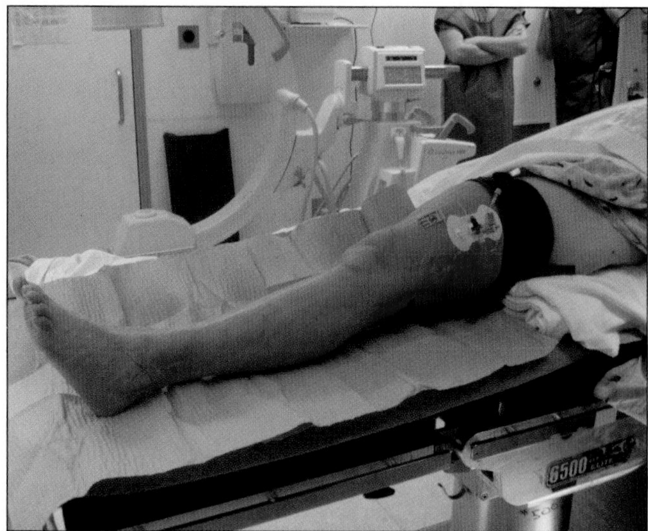

A

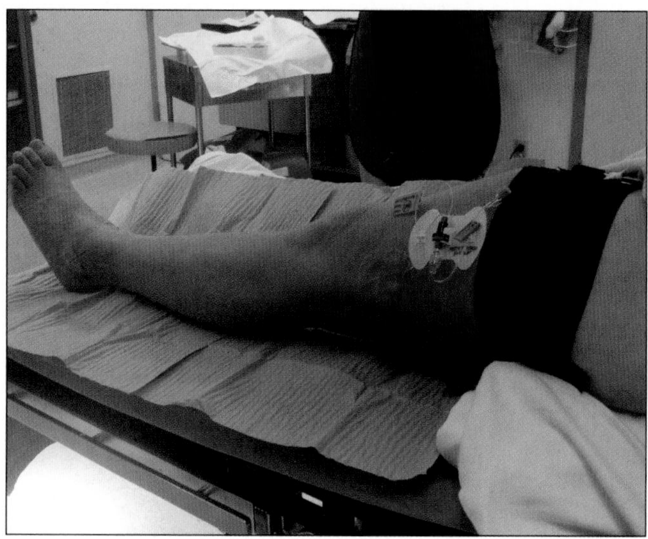

B

FIGURE 2

Positioning

- Supine position with a thigh tourniquet is standard.
- An ipsilateral bump under the hip should allow neutral positioning of the limb.
- All pressure points should be well padded and the table appropriately positioned to allow fluoroscopic imaging (Fig. 2A and 2B).

Pearls

- *The first assistant should be very gentle in retraction of the skin, and only blunt-ended retractors should be used.*

Portals/Exposures

- After appropriate preoperative antibiotic is administered, the limb is elevated and exsanguinated and the tourniquet inflated.

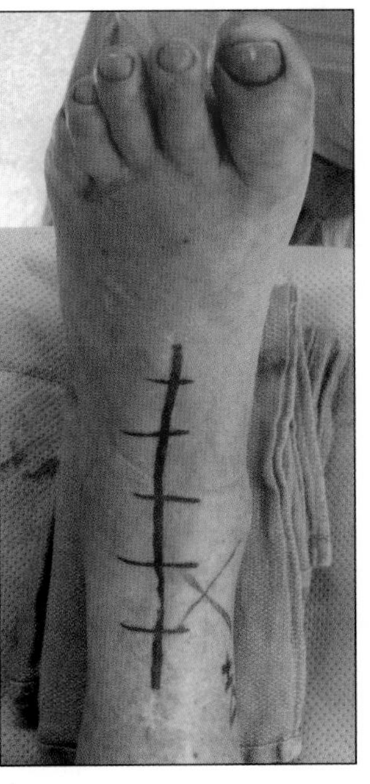

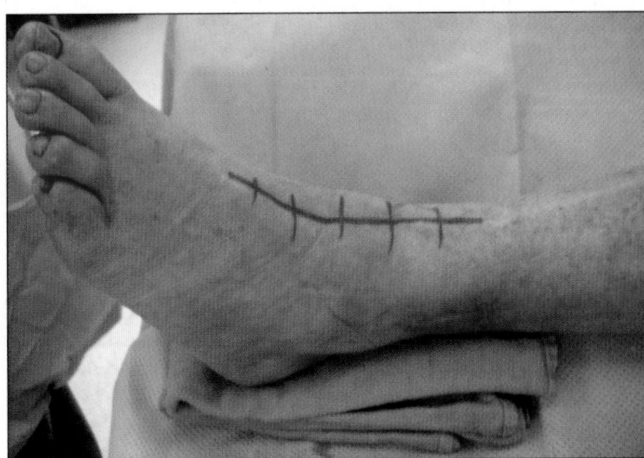

A B

FIGURE 3

- The standard approach to TAA will allow exposure of the ankle capsule deep to the interval between the tibialis anterior and extensor hallucis longus (Fig. 3A and 3B and Fig. 4). Care should be taken to avoid the medial branch of the superficial peroneal nerve as it crosses at the distal extent of the incision to become the dorsal cutaneous nerve (Fig. 5).

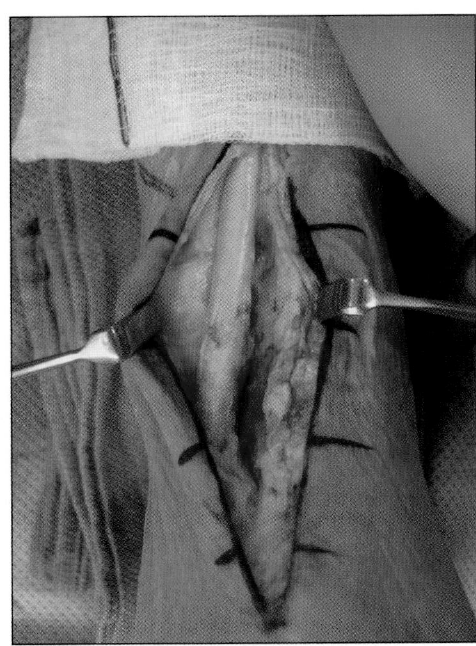

FIGURE 4

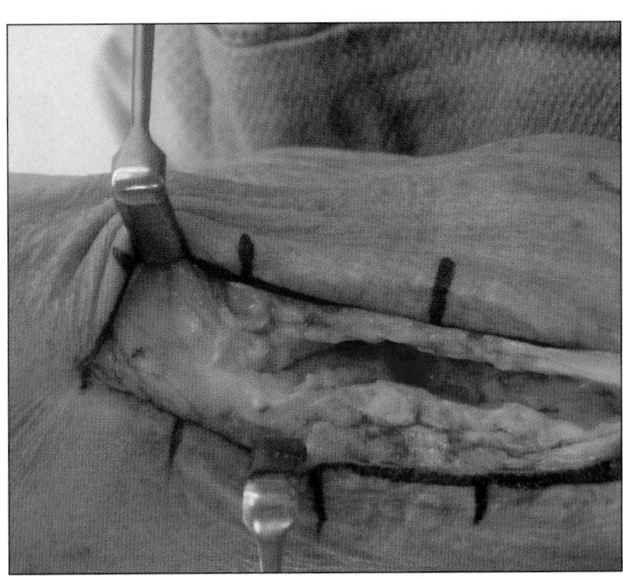

FIGURE 5

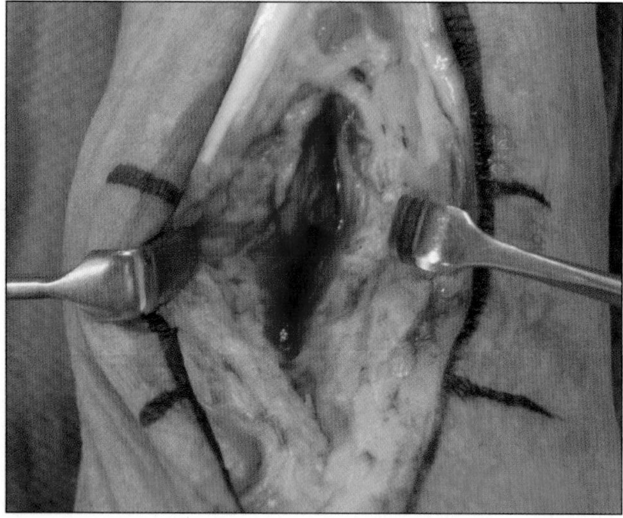
A

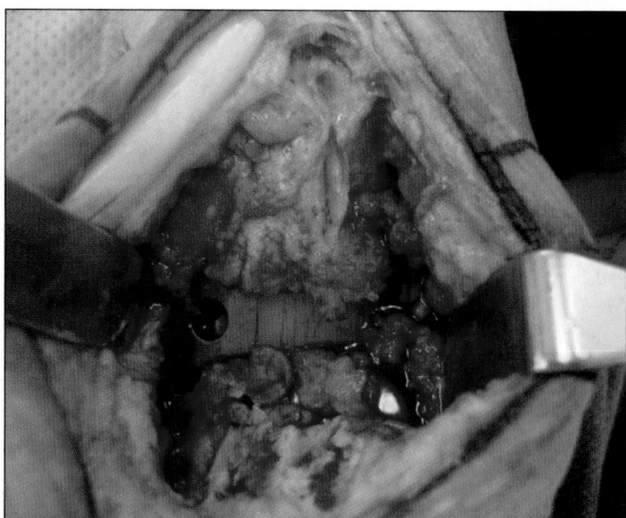
B

FIGURE 6

- Once the capsule is exposed (Fig. 6A), it may be removed by sharp dissection to expose the total ankle prosthesis (Fig. 6B).
- As the capsule is removed, the components will become visible and are often encased in this capsular scar.
  - Once exposed, the implants may be removed and placed on the back table (Fig. 7).
  - If there is a fibrous bond from the implant to the host bone, it should be carefully removed with a combination of sharp and blunt dissection and the use of small flexible osteotomes if needed.

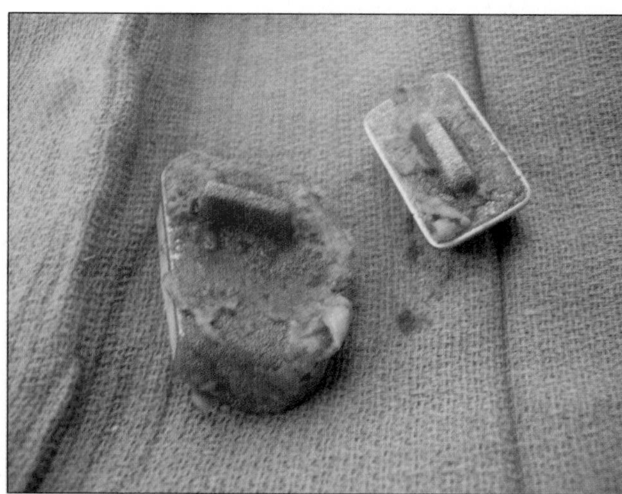

FIGURE 7

PEARLS

- *If the provisional K-wires are in the way during this phase of the procedure, they can be removed and either repositioned out of the void if possible or replaced after the graft is impacted.*

Procedure

STEP 1

- The void left following removal of the implants is prepared by removing any further fibrous tissue, and the subchondral bone is drilled using a 2.0-mm drill (Fig. 8A–C).
- The ankle is then positioned appropriately with attention to the need for Achilles tendon lengthening if needed.
- Once the position is satisfactory clinically and radiographically, provisional fixation is placed using 0.062-inch Kirschner wires (K-wires).

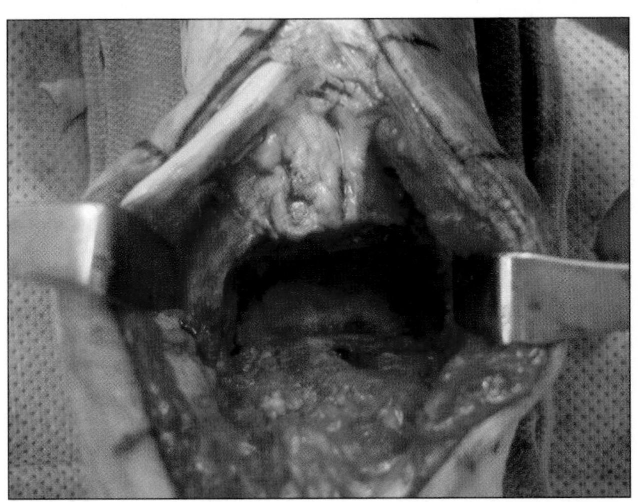
A

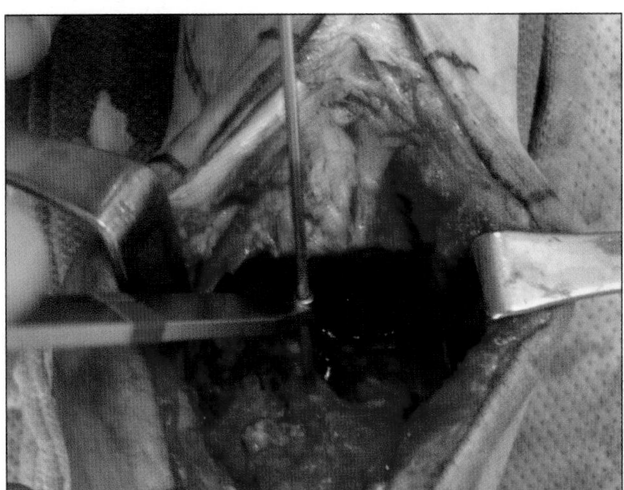
B

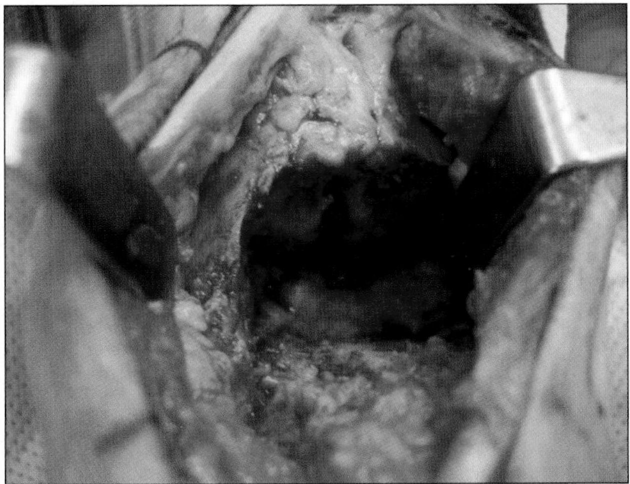
C

FIGURE 8

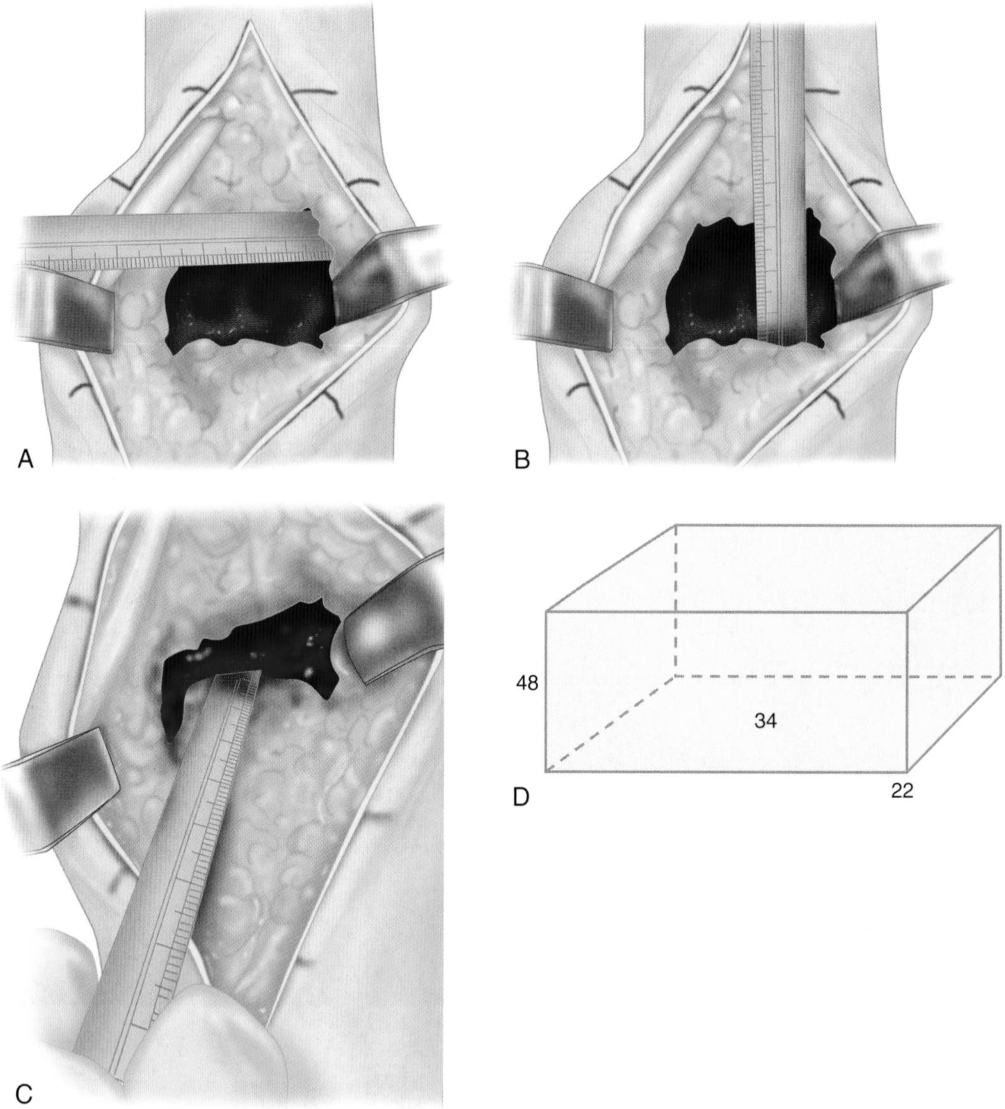

FIGURE 9

- The defect is measured in the *x*, *y*, and *z* axes (Fig. 9A–C), and the allograft size and shape are determined (Fig. 9D).

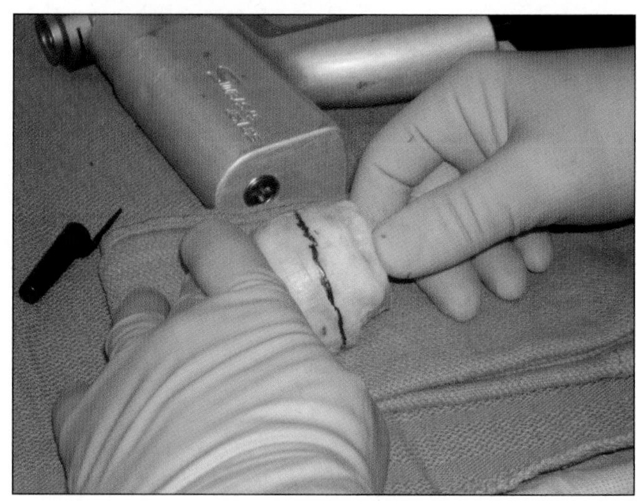

FIGURE 10

- A large femoral head allograft is secured for cutting (Fig. 10). Care should be taken while utilizing a large oscillating saw to shape the allograft (Fig. 11A–C).
- The graft is then impacted into the void (Fig. 12). Typically, the graft will need to be removed and refashioned to satisfy the architecture of the void.

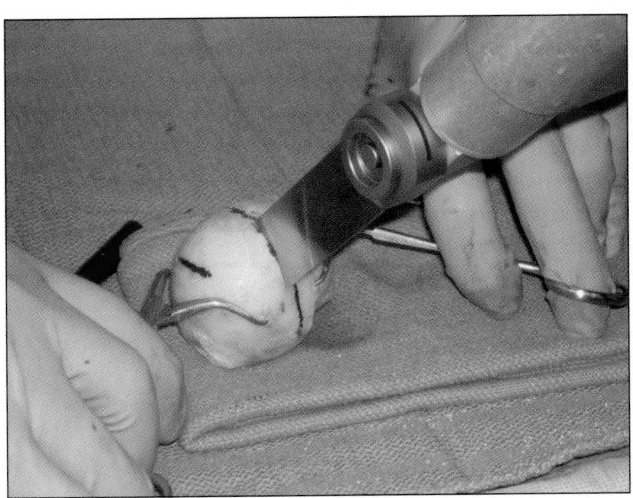

A

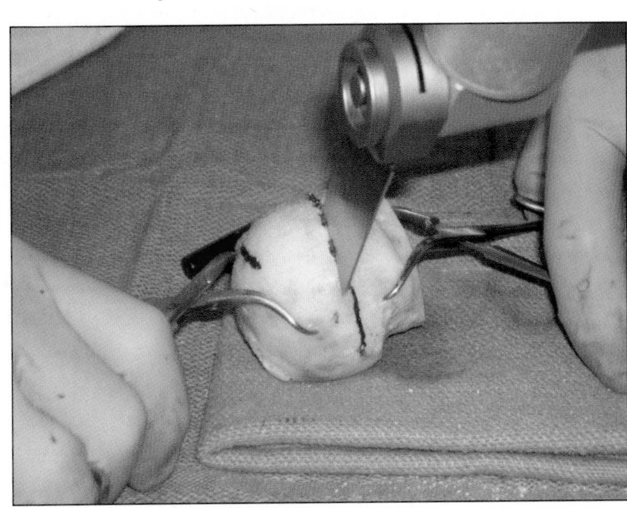

B

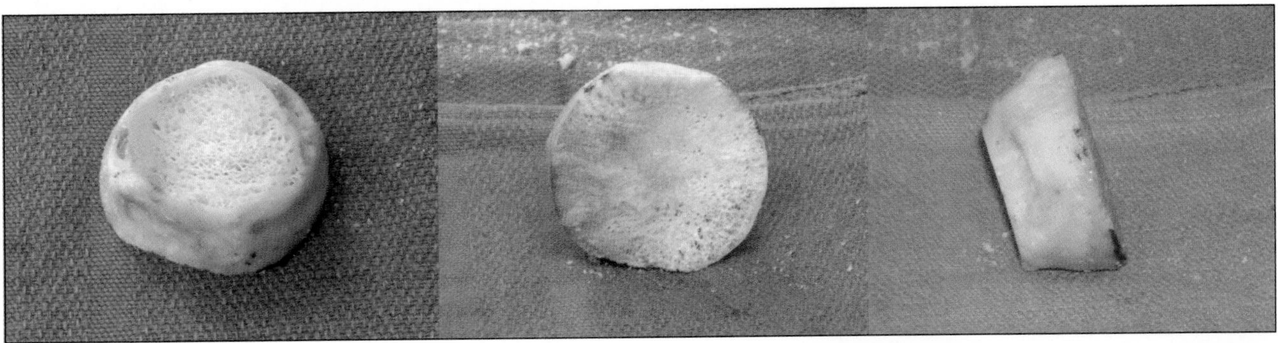

C

FIGURE 11

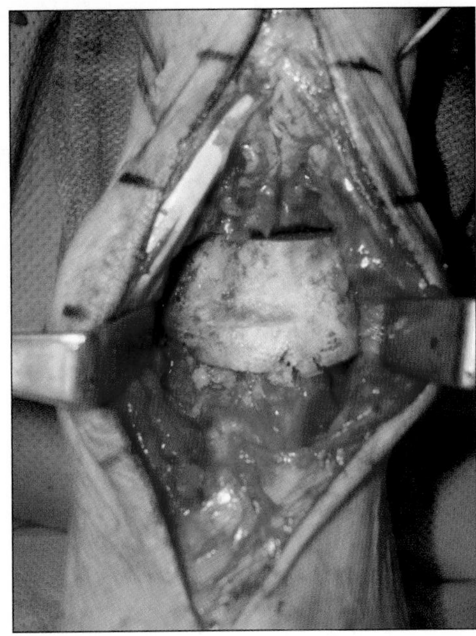

FIGURE 12

Pearls

- *Technically, the third screw is most demanding and could be considered optional, but additional screws should be utilized to provide rigid fixation.*

Step 2

- Once the graft is positioned and secured provisionally, the clinical and radiographic postion is verified (Fig. 13A and 13B). The procedure then turns to the internal fixation of the arthrodesis.
- Large 6.5-mm screws with a 16-mm thread length are utilized.
  - The goal is to place one screw from the anterolateral tibia into the remaining talar body through the allograft and a second from the anteromedial tibia into the opposite talar body and graft.
  - A third screw from the back of the tibia into the talar head is then placed.
- The first screw begins with a small defect made in the corner of the anterolateral tibia with a pineapple-shaped burr. This divot will allow for the screw to enter at an oblique angle and maintain the bone bridge (Fig. 14).
  - A short 4.5-mm drill is used to create a pilot hole, followed by a long 3.5-mm drill into the talar body across the allograft (Fig. 15). Appropriate length is determined by depth gauge and a 6.5-mm screw (16-mm thread length) placed.
  - Care must be taken to avoid fracture of the bone bridge and avoiding screw thread penetration into the subtalar joint.
  - Screw placement is checked by fluoroscopy (Fig. 16A and 16B).

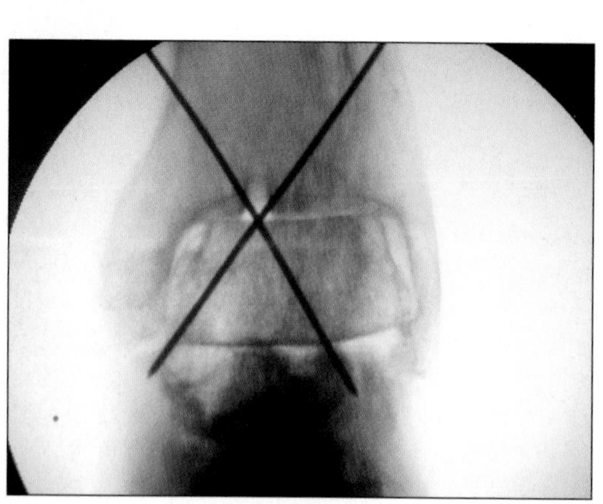
A

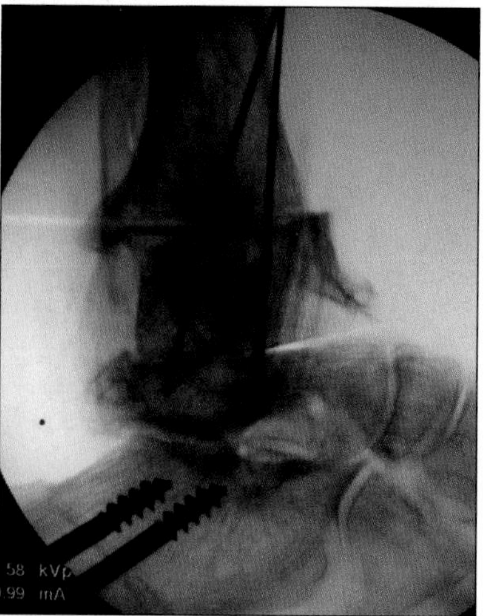

B

FIGURE 13

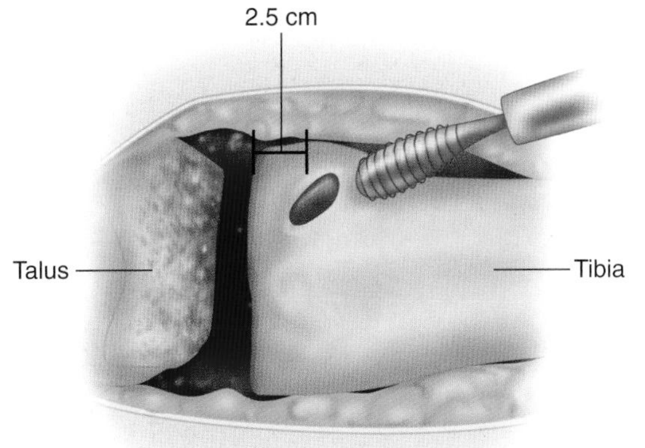

FIGURE 14

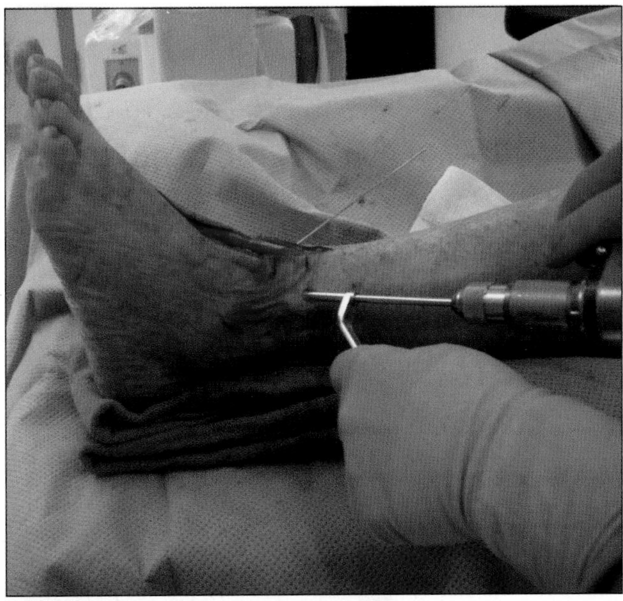

FIGURE 15

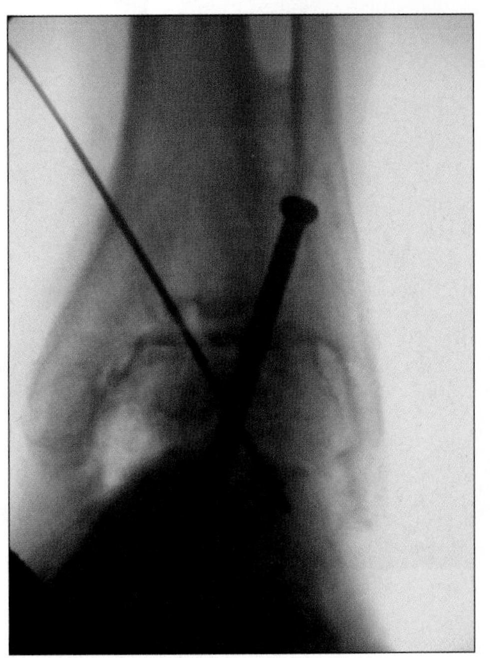

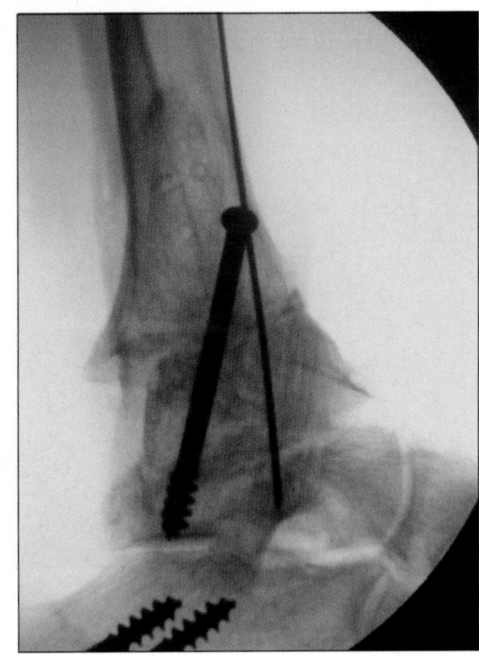

FIGURE 16 A B

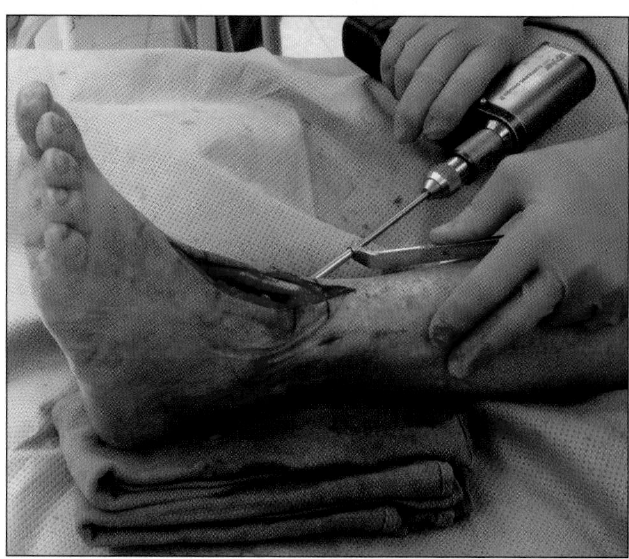

FIGURE 17

- The second screw is placed from the anteromedial tibia following the same preparatory stages as for the first screw (Fig. 17).
- Once the second screw is placed and confirmed by fluoroscopy, a third screw can be addressed (Fig. 18A and 18B).
    - The limb is elevated by the surgical assistant at the foot of the table (Fig. 19). The fluoroscopy unit is positioned for a cross-table lateral view, and an incision is made posterolateral to the Achilles tendon.

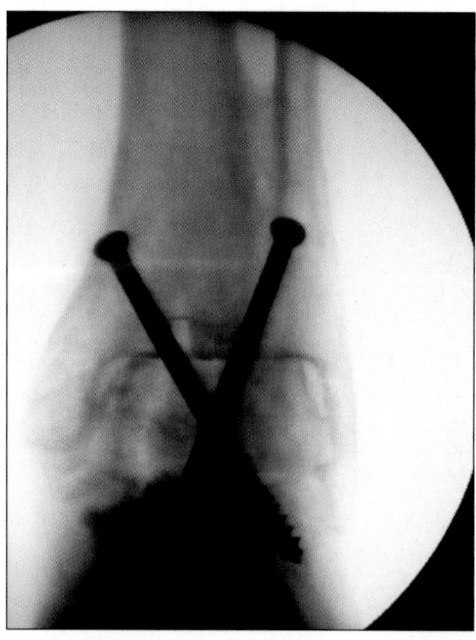

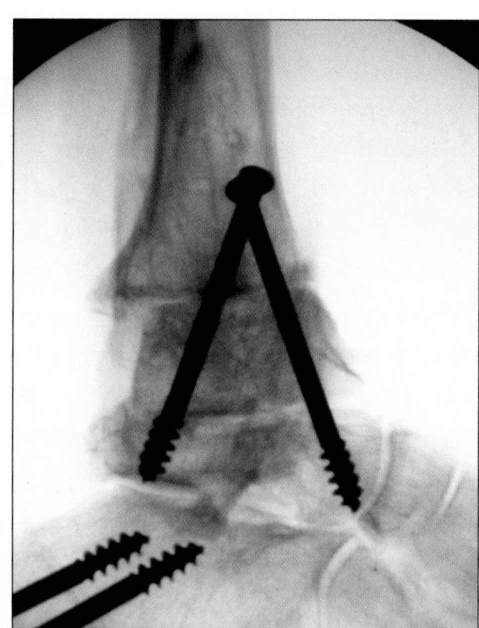

A B

FIGURE 18

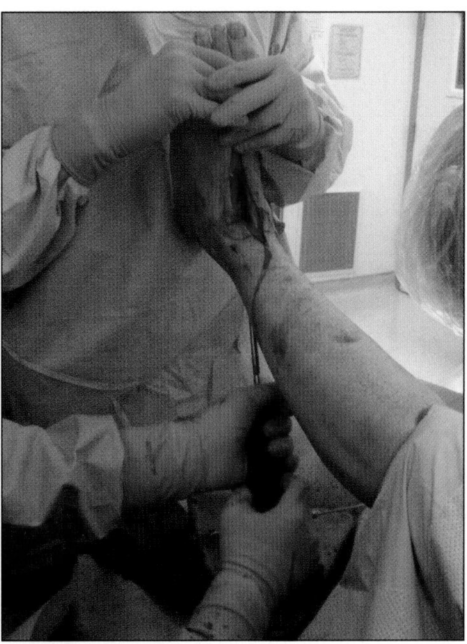

FIGURE 19

- The 4.5-mm drill is placed posteriorly at the midline or slightly lateral, aiming for the neck of the talus (the second toe is a reasonable target). The 3.5-mm drill is placed through the gliding hole and disconnected from the drill.
- With care, an anteroposterior image of the foot is made to confirm the placement of the drill in the talar head (Fig. 20). Once confirmed, the drill is removed and the screw length measured.
- The standard 6.5-mm, 16-mm thread length screw is placed, completing the primary screw placement.

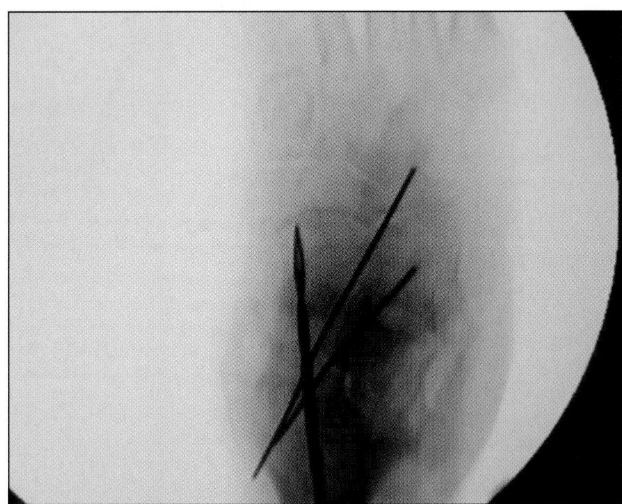

FIGURE 20

- Additional screws can be placed from the medial malleolus through the graft and then from the distal tibia through the graft. Identical technique is utilized with the same set of drills and screws, with fluoroscopic confirmation of screw placement (Fig. 21A–C).

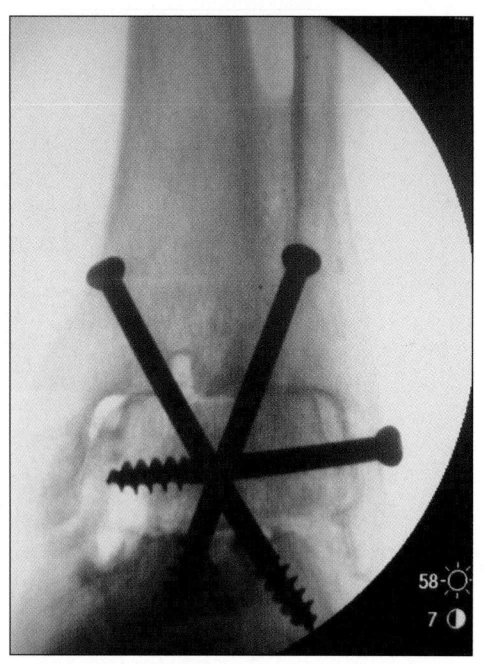

A

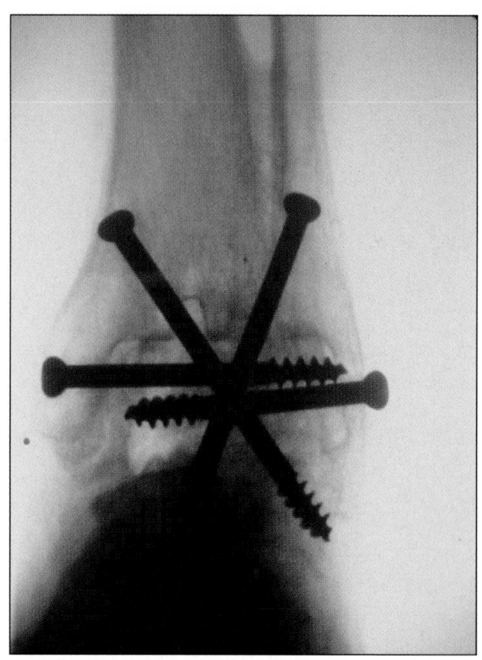
B

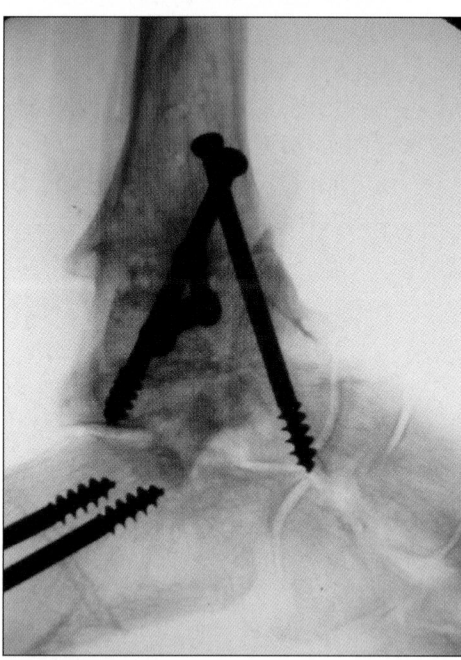
C

FIGURE 21

Step 3

- Supplemental bone grafting to fill any intercalary defects can be accomplished utilizing the remaining femoral head allograft. The use of bone substitutes or internal/external bone stimulation can be used at the discretion of the surgeon.
- Wound closure generally proceeds in a routine manner.
  - Closure is done in layers with 3-0 monocryl in the subcutaneous layer and 3-0 nylon or staples for the skin (Fig. 22A and 22B).
  - A bulky Jones dressing with a posterior splint is applied (Fig. 23).

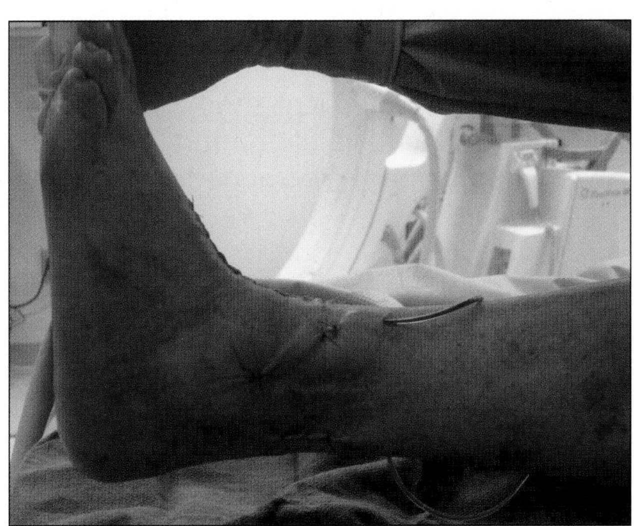

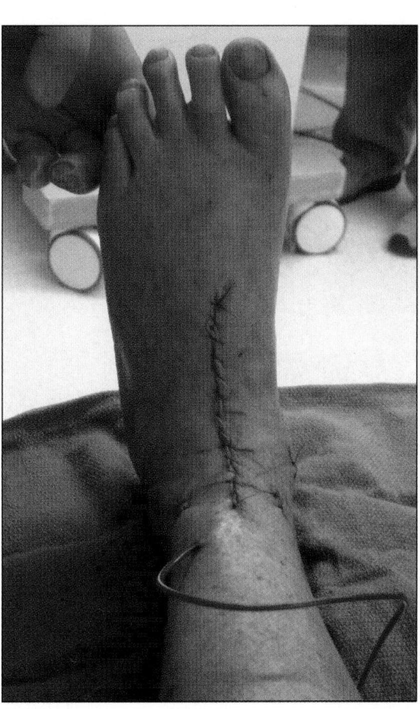

FIGURE 22 A B

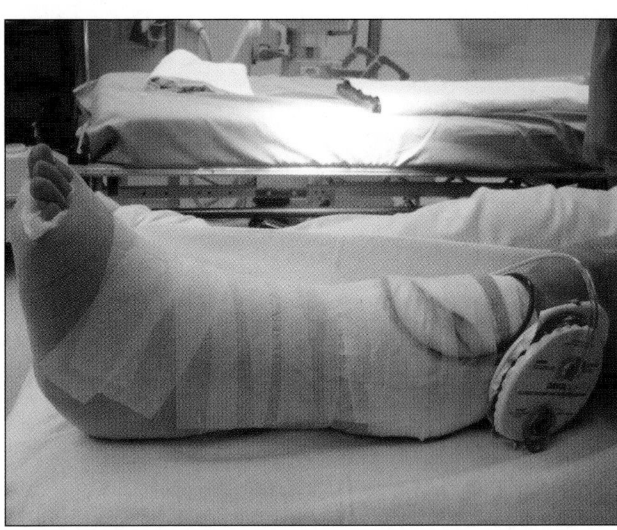

FIGURE 23

Postoperative Care and Expected Outcomes

- The patient is kept non–weight bearing in the postoperative splint and is followed up in the office 2 weeks after surgery. The dressing is removed, sutures taken out, and a non–weight-bearing fiberglass cast applied. Routine radiographs of the ankle are taken.
- The patient is then seen 4 weeks later for radiographs and examination. Generally, protected weight bearing in a fracture brace does not start until approximately 8–10 weeks postoperatively, depending on the nature of the surgery and the maturation of the fusion radiographically.
- Once the patient has progressed to full weight bearing in the fracture boot, shoewear can be addressed. The use of a rocker-bottom adaptation to the shoe may be a benefit for some but not all patients.
- Swelling can linger easily for 1 year and, once abated, the patient should have significant resolution of preoperative discomfort. The time to maximal improvement can range from 1 to 2 years.

Evidence

Carlsson AS, Montgomery F, Besjakov J. Arthrodesis of the ankle secondary to replacement. Foot Ankle Int. 1998;19:240-5.

Study of 21 failed TAAs in which external fixation was the primary technique. All had fused at final follow-up. (Level III evidence [Retrospective review])

Culpan P, LeStrat V, Piriou P, Judet T. Arthrodesis after failed total ankle replacement. J Bone Joint Surg [Br]. 2007;89:1178-83.

Study of 16 failed TAAs converted to fusion using autograft and internal fixation; 15 of 16 arthrodeses were successful. (Level III evidence [Retrospective review])

Groth HE, Fitch HF. Salvage procedures for complications of total ankle arthroplasty. Clin Orthop Relat Res. 1997;(224):244-50.

Review of techniques addressing treatment of the complications of TAA, including arthrodesis. (Level IV evidence)

Hopgood P, Kumar R, Wood PL. Ankle arthrodesis for failed total ankle replacement. J Bone Joint Surg [Br]. 2006;88:1032-8.

Study of 23 failed total ankle replacements treated with three different fixation techniques. Seventeen had fused, and the review suggested that, if tibiotalocalcaneal fusion is needed, the best results may be with an intramedullary nail. (Level III evidence [Retrospective review])

Johl C, Kircher J, Pohlmann K, Jansson V. Management of the failed total ankle replacement with a retrograde short femoral nail: a case report. J Orthop Trauma. 2006;20:60-5.

Report of tibiotalocalcaneal fusion with an intramedullary nail and bone graft for a failed total ankle replacement. (Level IV evidence [Case report])

Kitaoka HB, Romness DW. Arthrodesis for failed ankle arthroplasty. J Arthroplasty. 1992;7:277-84.

Study of 38 failed total ankle replacements treated with arthrodesis using external fixation. Reported union rate of 89%. (Level III evidence [Retrospective review])

Kotnis R, Pasapula C, Anwar F, Cooke PH, Sharp RJ. The management of failed ankle replacement. J Bone Joint Surg [Br]. 2006;88:1039-47.

Study of 16 failed total ankle replacements of which 2 were the result of infection. Five patients had revision total ankle replacement. Discussing the technique for fusion with both infected and noninfected failures, the authors concluded that hindfoot fusion appears to be preferable to revision total ankle replacement. (Level III evidence [Retrospective review])

Pelton K, Hofer JK, Thordarson DB. Tibiotalocalcaneal arthrodesis using a dynamically locked retrograde intramedullary nail. Foot Ankle Int. 2006;27:759-63.

Study of 33 patients treated with tibiotalocalcaneal arthrodesis using an intramedullary nail. One patient had a failed TAA treated the same way; no independent report on this single patient was provided. (Level III evidence [Retrospective review])

Ritter M, Nickisch F, DiGiovanni C. Technique tip: posterior blade plate for salvage of failed total ankle arthroplasty. Foot Ankle Int. 2006;27:303-4.

Technique of staged tibiotalocalcaneal fusion with antibiotic spacer and débridement followed 6–8 weeks later by arthrodesis using a blade plate and posterior approach. (Level IV evidence)

PROCEDURE 28

Ankle Arthrodesis Using Ring/Multiplanar External Fixation

Mark E. Easley and Stefan G. Hofstaetter

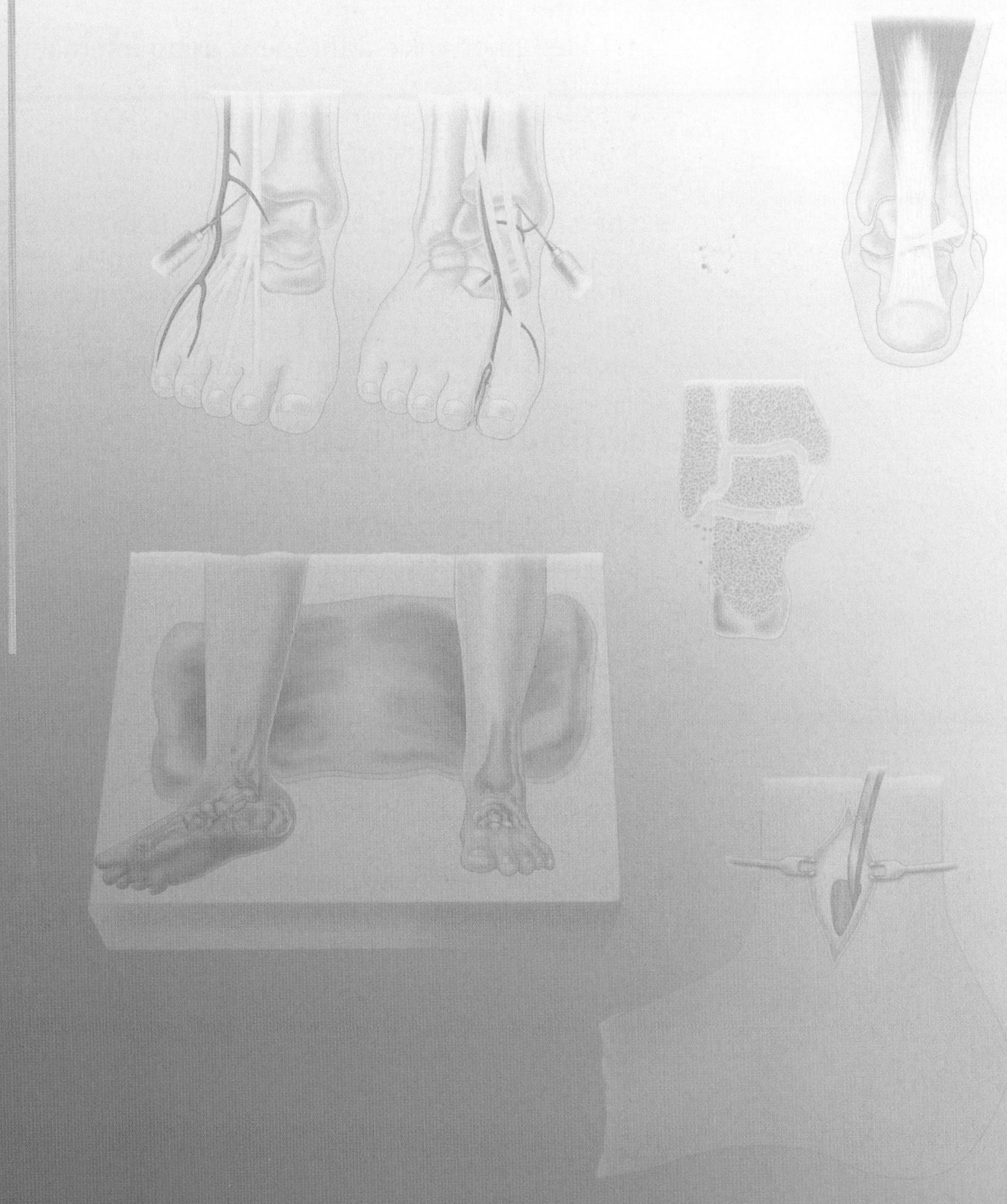

Figures from Easley M, Looney C, Wellman S, Wilson J. Ankle arthrodesis using ring external fixation. Tech Foot Ankle Surg. 2006,5:1–14.

Pitfalls

- *Patient with prior total joint arthroplasty (pin tract infection may seed joint implant)*
- *Anticipated noncompliance with pin care*

Indications

- Ankle arthrodesis
  - Symptomatic end-stage ankle arthritis (posttraumatic, inflammatory, primary)
  - Failed nonoperative management
- External fixation
  - History of sepsis/osteomyelitis at the arthrodesis site (Fig. 1A and 1B)
  - Compromised soft tissue envelope
  - Inadequate bone stock to support internal fixation at the arthrodesis site
  - Failed prior ankle arthrodesis using internal fixation (Fig. 1C)
  - Failed total ankle arthroplasty (Fig. 1D)
  - Anticipated noncompliance with non–weight-bearing status
- The case illustrating this procedure is that of a patient with posttraumatic end-stage ankle arthritis, an inability to comply with a non–weight-bearing status (for other medical reasons), and adequate support at home to maintain adequate pin care.

Examination/Imaging

Physical Examination

- Range of motion (ROM)
  - Typically limited, painful ankle ROM
  - Preferably asymptomatic, full hindfoot ROM (following ankle fusion, greater stress will be experienced on the hindfoot articulations)
- Alignment (clinical)
  - Must be assessed with the patient weight bearing
  - Assess deformity that will need to be corrected to re-establish a plantigrade foot (equinus, varus/valgus)
- Soft tissue envelope (previous incisions) often less important with external fixation compared to internal fixation since limited exposure typically suffices to prepare the tibiotalar joint for arthrodesis
- Vascular examination to confirm that adequate perfusion is present to allow healing

Imaging

- Obtain weight-bearing radiographs of the foot and ankle.
  - Confirm end-stage tibiotalar arthritis
  - Assess malalignment
  - Assess associated deformity and compensatory alignment in the foot

Treatment Options

- Ankle arthrodesis using internal fixation
- Distraction arthroplasty
- Ankle fresh/fresh frozen allograft (ankle replacement with allograft ankle)
- Total ankle arthroplasty

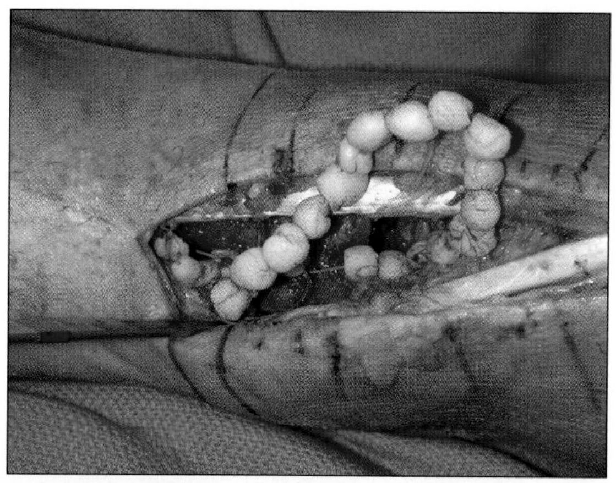
A

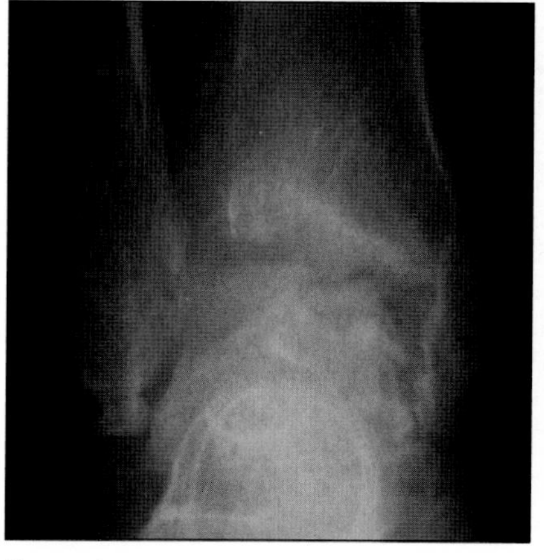
B

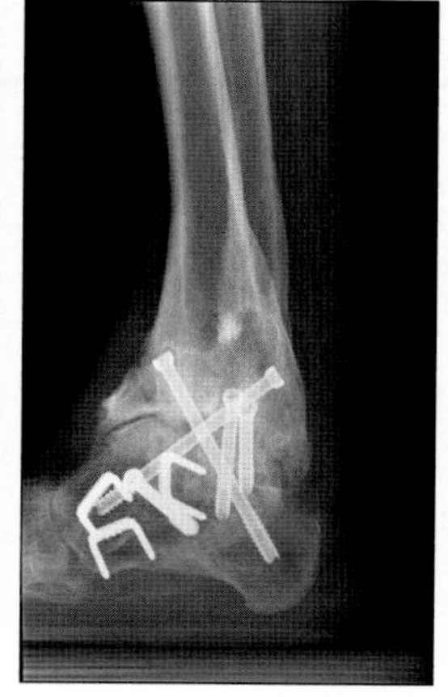
C

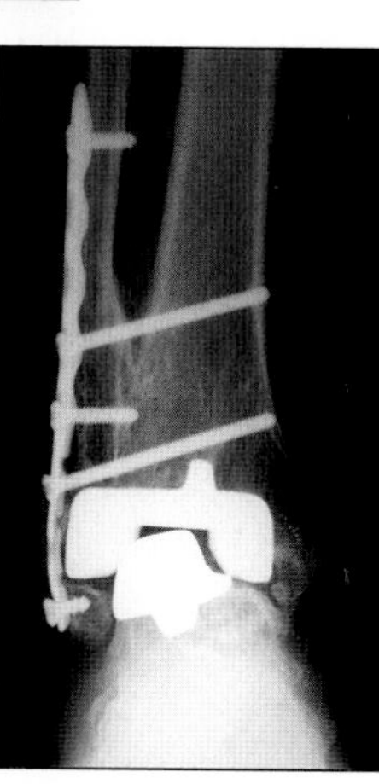
D

FIGURE 1

- If avascular necrosis (AVN) of the talus is suspected, consider magnetic resonance imaging to predetermine how much bone will need to be resected to achieve viable tibiotalar surfaces for healing (usefulness may be limited by previously placed hardware).

Surgical Anatomy

- Neurovascular structures must be respected with the surgical approach (ankle) and half-pin and thin wire placement (lower leg, ankle, and foot).
  - Anteriorly: superficial peroneal nerve, deep peroneal nerve, and anterior tibial/dorsalis pedis artery
  - Posteromedially: posterior tibial artery, tibial nerve and its branches
  - Laterally: sural nerve
- Ideally, despite external fixation, the muscles and respective tendons should remain mobile, particularly the ones responsible for toe movement (flexor and extensor digitorum longus, flexor and extensor

Pearls

- *Positioning the foot and lower leg with the toes directed to the ceiling facilitates placing the external fixator congruently on the foot and ankle.*

Pitfalls

- *Be sure to allow enough space for the calf. A bump to support the calf may distort soft tissues of the lower leg. When the bump under the calf is removed, the proximal ring should not impinge on the skin of the lower leg (be sure to leave adequate space between the external fixator and the calf).*

hallucis longus, and intrinsics). Thus, half-pin and thin wire placement must respect these structures as well.

- Ideally, thin wires should be extra-articular, since potential pin tract infections could lead to septic arthritis.
- "Safe" zones have been established for thin wire placement (Fig. 2A–C).

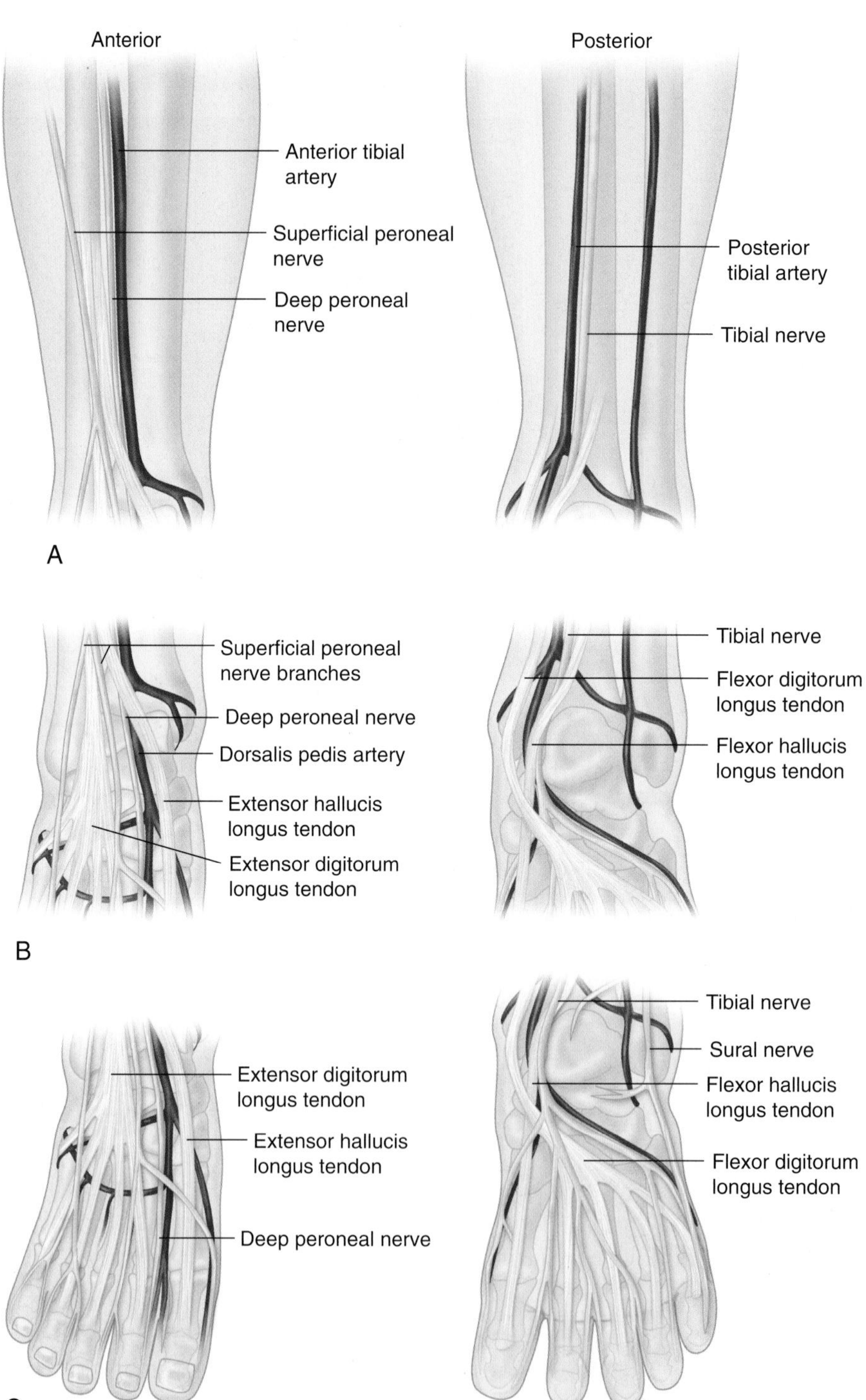

FIGURE 2

Positioning

- Supine with foot (toes) directed toward ceiling (Fig. 3)
- Bump/bolster under ipsilateral hip to maintain position
- Bump/bolster under ipsilateral calf to suspend foot and ankle and facilitate external fixator frame placement

Equipment

- Radiolucent operating table
- Bump/bolsters

Portals/Exposures

- The surgical approach is the same as for ankle arthrodesis using internal fixation.
  - Open anterior, mini-arthrotomy, arthroscopic, and open transfibular approaches are all options, and are often dictated based on prior surgical approaches.
  - In this chapter, we highlight an anterior approach (see video) and a mini-arthrotomy technique (illustrated here).
- Dual arthrotomy technique (Fig. 4)
  - While distracting the joint with a lamina spreader through one arthrotomy, the joint surfaces are prepared though the other.
  - The lamina spreader is moved to the other arthrotomy to complete joint preparation. Periosteal stripping is kept to a minimum.
  - In this case, a second spreader is used to further facilitate exposure.

Pitfalls

- *While minimally invasive techniques have advantages, the surgical approach should not be limited to the point that the joint surfaces are inadequately prepared.*

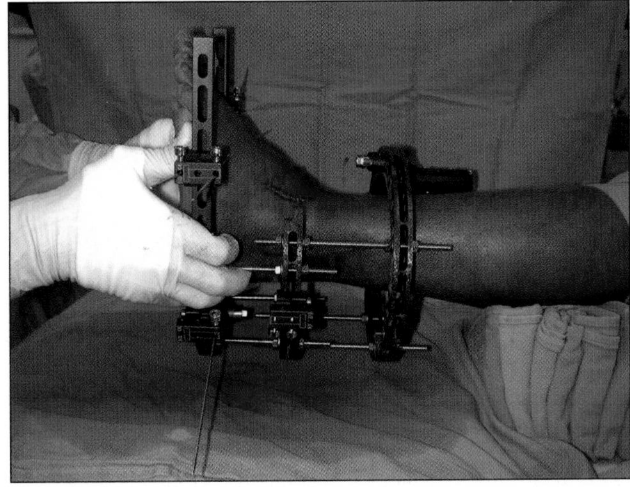

FIGURE 3

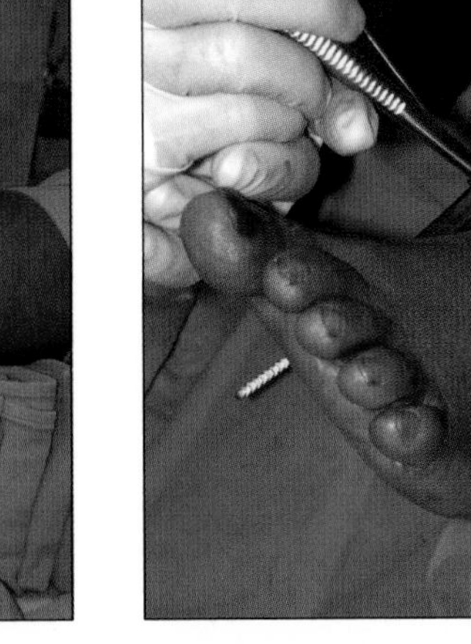

FIGURE 4

- During the procedure:
  - Protect the superficial peroneal nerve, deep neurovascular bundle, and extensor tendons.
  - Maintain careful soft tissue handling; avoid direct tension on wound margins.
  - Minimize periosteal stripping at the tibiotalar joint to maintain optimal blood supply at the arthrodesis site.

Pearls

- *The tibial and talar surfaces must be vascular; neither external fixation nor any other method of fixation can promote fusion without adequate vascularity at the arthrodesis site.*

Pitfalls

- *Alignment is essential, particularly if a prebuilt or traditional ring external fixator is used.*
- *Err into valgus, not varus; err into external rotation, not internal rotation.*

Procedure

Step 1: Preparation and Provisional Pinning

- Ring external fixation is not a substitute for proper joint preparation in ankle arthrodesis.
- Remove all residual cartilage using an elevator (Fig. 5). Following this, a drill and/or chisel are introduced to penetrate the subchondral bone.
- Remove any bone suspicious for AVN.
- Penetrate subchondral bone to facilitate mesenchymal stem cell migration to the arthrodesis site.
- Maintain the architecture of the tibiotalar joint subchondral surfaces.
  - Improves stability of arthrodesis
  - May increase surface area for fusion
- The surgeon may need to consider a posterior capsular release or tendo-Achilles lengthening if a plantigrade foot position cannot be achieved.
- Bone grafting
  - Use cancellous allograft chips mixed with a platelet-rich product (Fig. 6).
  - Choice is based on surgeon preference.

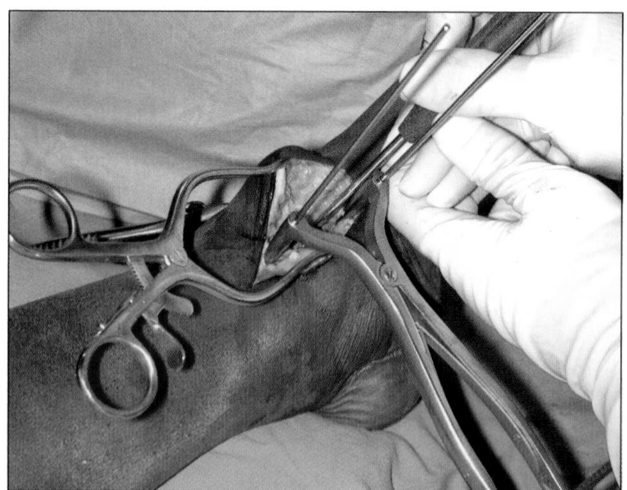

FIGURE 5

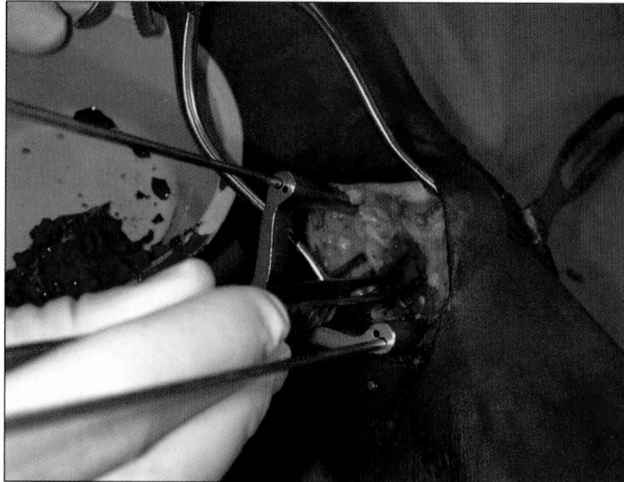

FIGURE 6

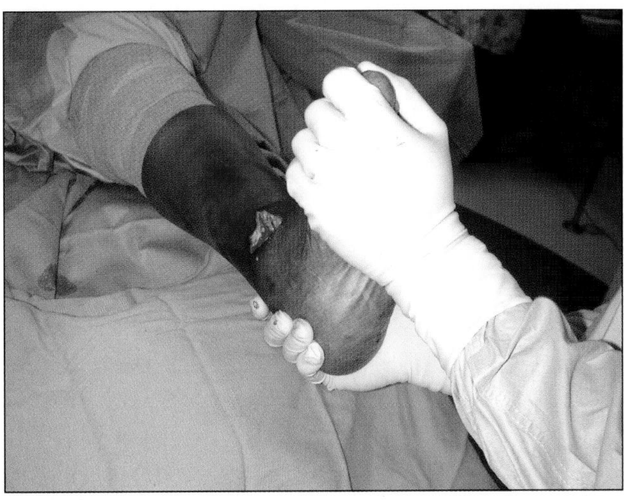

FIGURE 7

Instrumentation/ Implantation

- Chisel or drill to prepare the articular surface for fusion
- Steinmann pin to stabilize ankle arthrodesis while external fixator is being assembled about the foot and ankle
- Fluoroscopy unit to confirm satisfactory alignment and bony apposition at the arthrodesis site

- Provisionally pin the tibiotalar joint in anatomic alignment with appropriate apposition of tibial and talar fusion surfaces: neutral dorsiflexion/plantar flexion; slight hindfoot valgus; second metatarsal aligned with the tibial crest (Fig. 7).
  - Sagittal plane
    - Neutral plantar flexion/dorsiflexion (for ankle and foot)
    - Talar dome centered under tibial plafond
  - Coronal plane
    - Neutral at the ankle
    - Slight (5°) hindfoot valgus
  - Rotation: second metatarsal aligned with the tibial crest
- Figure 8 shows fluoroscopic images of the ankle provisionally pinned in ideal alignment in anteroposterior (Fig. 8A) and lateral (Fig. 8B) views.

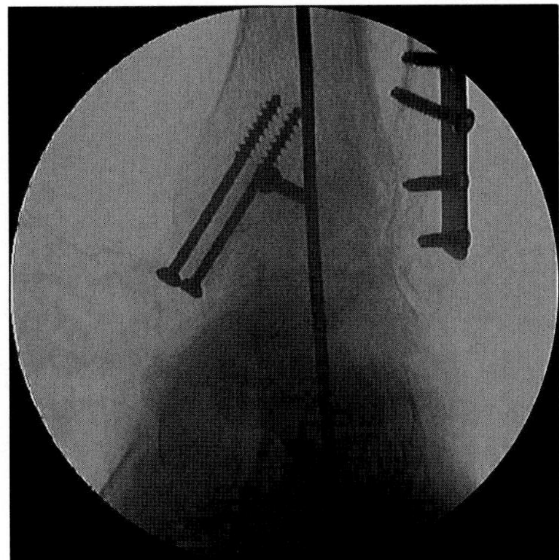

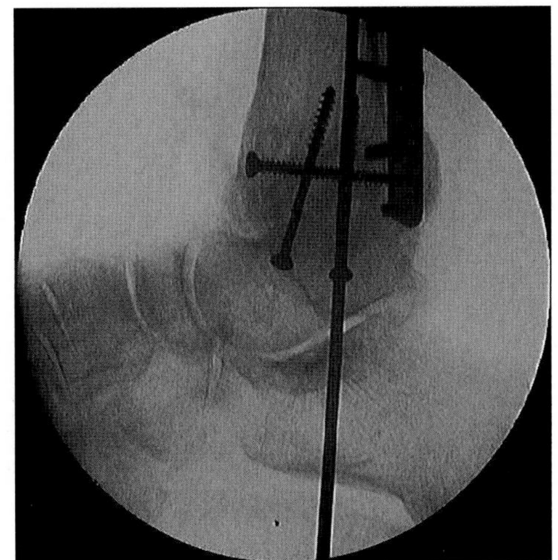

FIGURE 8 A B

Pearls

- *In order to limit heat generation and potential skin/bone necrosis and resultant pin infection and/or loosening, thin wires and half-pins should be inserted while cold saline is irrigated on them or while they are held with a sponge moistened with cold saline.*
- *To optimize frame construct stability, place pins in a straight axis and directly on the frame.*

Pitfalls

- *Adequate space must be left for the calf and the posterior aspect of the calcaneus.*
- *If the calcaneal wires are tensioned first in an open ring construct, then subsequent tensioning of the forefoot or more distal wires will lead to loss of tension in the calcaneal wires.*
- *All wires and half-pins should achieve bicortical fixation. Unicortical drilling and pin placement leads to excessive heat generation and potential pin infection/loosening.*

Step 2: External Fixator Assembly/Attachment to Lower Leg and Foot

- The surgeon will need to be familiar with the particular frame system he or she employs; be sure to meet with the frame system's representative to become familiar with the intended frame and the recommended tensioning for the thin wires.
- In this example case, a prebuilt frame assembled on a back table is used (Fig. 9A). The frame is positioned congruently about the lower leg and foot (here with thin wires already positioned in foot) (Fig. 9B), while the calf is supported by a bolster and the leg is perpendicular to the operating room table to facilitate frame placement.

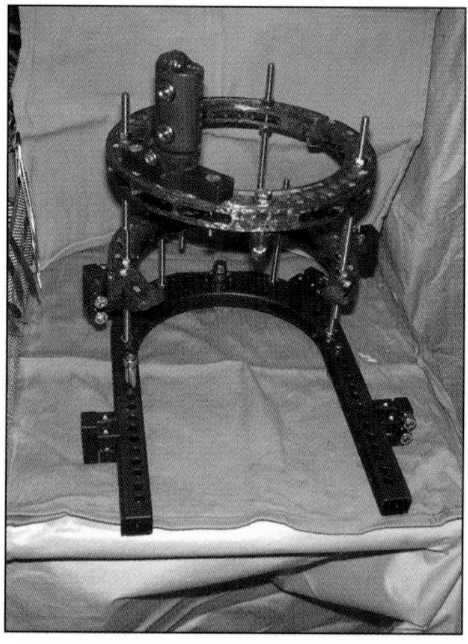

A

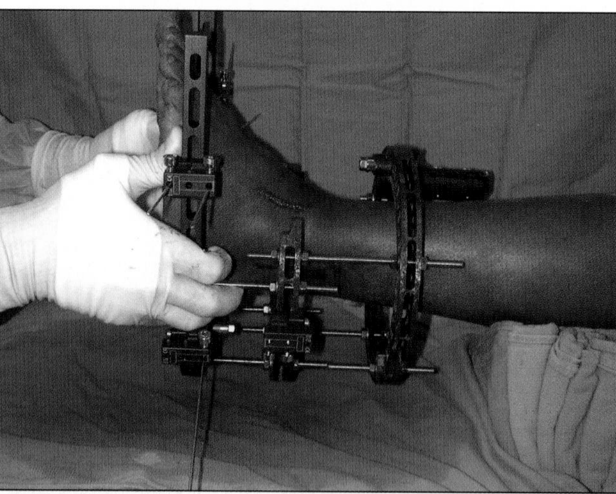

B

FIGURE 9

- The frame should allow adequate space for the calf and posterior heel. The bolster under the calf may give a false sense of adequate space; be sure to check to see if adequate space is available for the calf with bolster removed. At least 1 cm should separate the foot portion of the frame from the posterior heel (Fig. 10A).
- Securing the foot:
  - The plantar aspect of the foot should be inferior to the foot portion of the frame. This will facilitate placing the thin wires in the foot in ideal position, and facilitate postoperative weight bearing even without a supplemental foot tread added to the construct.
  - A thin wire is placed in the forefoot to "suspend" the frame from the foot (Fig. 10B), and the foot is centered in the foot portion of the frame, but not yet tensioned. The wire need only capture.

Instrumentation/ Implantation

- External fixator system with corresponding wrenches and tensioning device

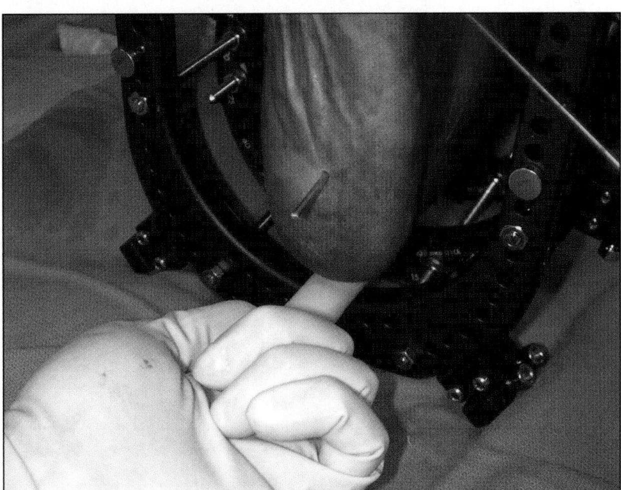

A

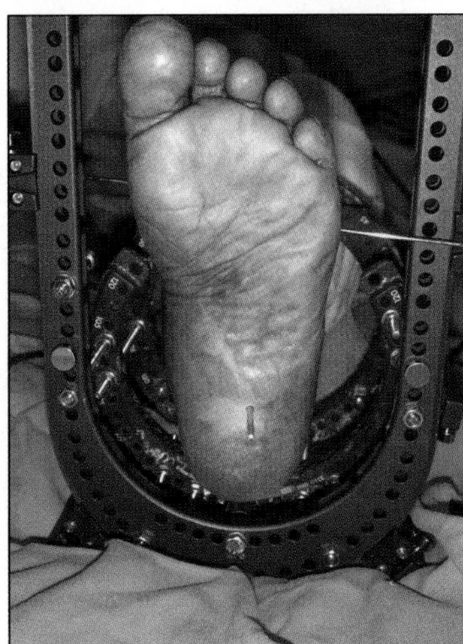

B

FIGURE 10

- Two calcaneal wires are placed 60–80° to one another, but not yet tensioned (Fig. 11A and 11B).
- A midfoot/supplemental forefoot wire is placed, typically supported by at least one post attached to the frame, but not yet tensioned.
- The foot portion of the ring may be closed anteriorly to avoid frame distortion during thin wire tensioning.
- After placing the midfoot wire, all wires are tensioned (the final calcaneal wire is tensioned at this point) (Fig. 11C). If the surgeon chooses to leave the anterior foot portion of the ring open, then tensioning should begin with the forefoot wires that will serve to complete the anterior portion of the ring and permit successful calcaneal wire tensioning.

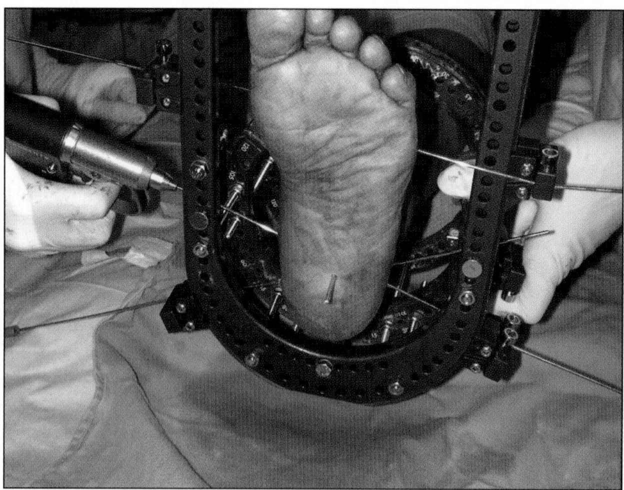

A

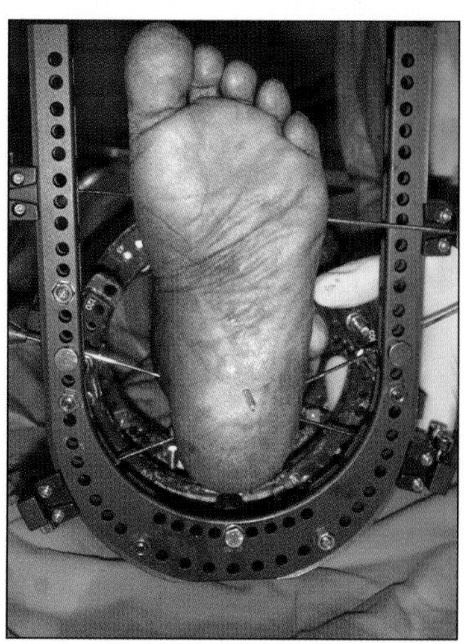

B

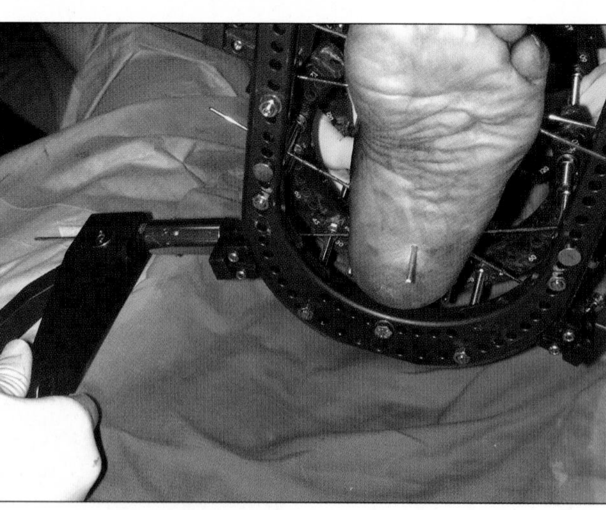

C

FIGURE 11

- Securing the proximal ring or proximal ring block to the lower leg
  - One or more thin wires may be placed across the proximal rings and tensioned. Alternatively, these thin wires may be secured to the proximal ring without tensioning while ideal ring position on the lower leg is established.
    - Again, a prebuilt, traditional ring external fixator construct should be properly positioned before any of the wires in the foot or lower leg are placed, since further adjustments are limited. However, subtle adjustments can be made to the ankle, hindfoot, and proximal ring block position at this stage, despite the provisional pin placed across the ankle.
    - While maintaining respect for vital structures, the thin wires should be placed as close to 90° to one another as possible.
  - As the surgeon holds the external fixator by the foot portion with the proximal ring block centered in ideal position over the lower leg, an assistant places one or more thin wires, one or more half-pins, or a combination of half-pins and thin wires to secure the proximal ring block (Fig. 12A).
    - Typically, the entire frame construct is secure once one half-pin is simultaneously anchored to the tibia and proximal ring block.
    - Ideally, two half-pins are placed in the medial tibia and a third in the anterior tibia, directed slightly medially to achieve bicortical purchase.
    - The proximal ring should be well centered on the lower leg (Fig. 12B).

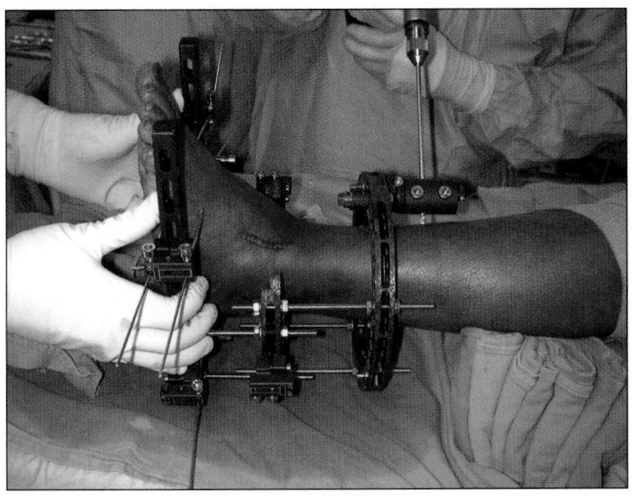

A

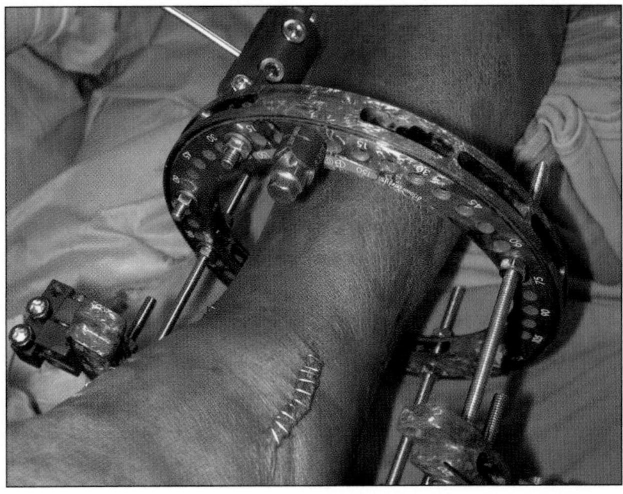

B

FIGURE 12

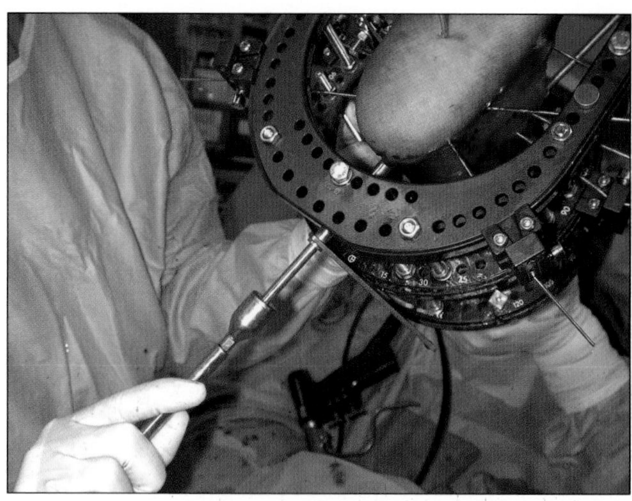

FIGURE 13

- To augment fixation in the foot, a supplemental half-pin may be placed axially, from posterior to anterior in the calcaneus, and attached to the foot portion of the frame after the proximal ring block is secured (Fig. 13).

Step 3: Talar Wires and Tibiotalar Compression

- Talar wire placement
  - Once the foot portion of the frame and proximal ring block are secured, one or two talar wires are added and secured only to the foot portion of the frame, not the proximal ring block.
  - An intermediate partial ring, attached to the foot portion of the frame, serves to support the talar wires. Often, the talar wires need to be suspended from the intermediate partial ring with posts.
  - Figure 14A shows the frame with talar wires in place from the perspective of the lateral foot and ankle. A close-up view (Fig. 14B) demonstrates one talar wire attached directly to the intermediate ring and the second suspended from a post.
  - The talar wires need to be tensioned like the other thin wires.
- Tibiotalar joint compression
  - With all wires and half-pins secured, the distal ring block (foot and intermediate portions) is advanced toward the proximal ring block using the threaded rods connecting the proximal and distal portions of the frame. With appropriate compression, this should become increasingly more difficult.
  - Figure 15A shows the frame construct completed. In Figure 15B, compression is being applied (advancing threaded rods secured to the distal frame construct toward the proximal ring).

Pearls

- *Talar wires must be placed and secured to the foot portion of the frame to avoid subtalar joint compression.*
- *With appropriate compression, the talar wires may bend (noted on fluoroscopic images).*

Pitfalls

- *Talar wires maintain the subtalar joint during compression; if they are not placed, then compression of the foot portion of the frame to the proximal ring block will produce not only desired tibiotalar compression but also undesired subtalar compression.*
- *Placing the talar wires through the malleoli will restrict tibiotalar compression; they should only penetrate the talus.*

Instrumentation/ Implantation

- External fixator system with corresponding wrenches and tensioning device

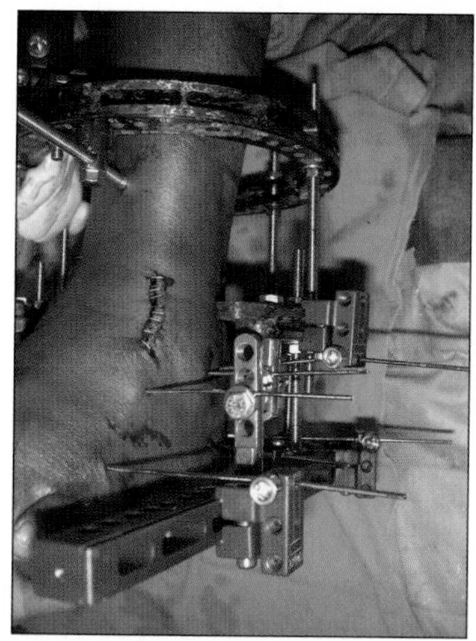

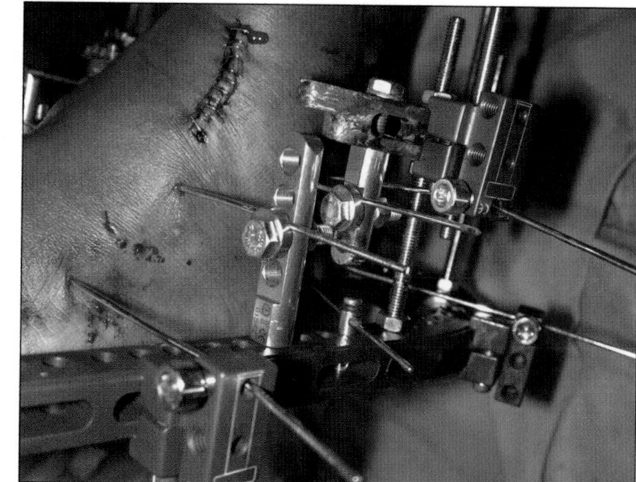

FIGURE 14 A B

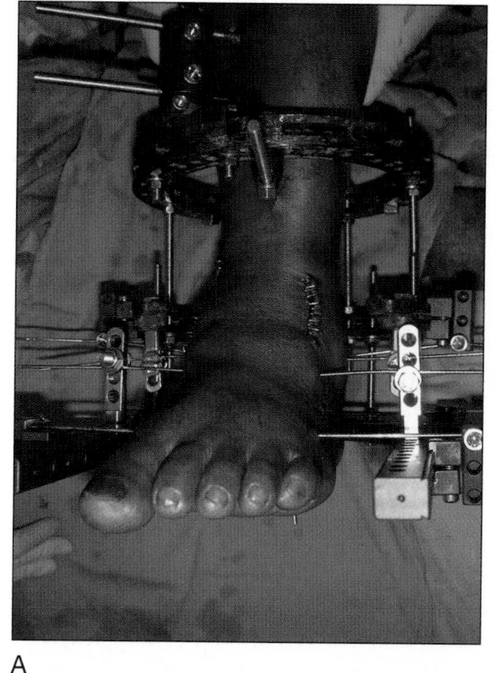

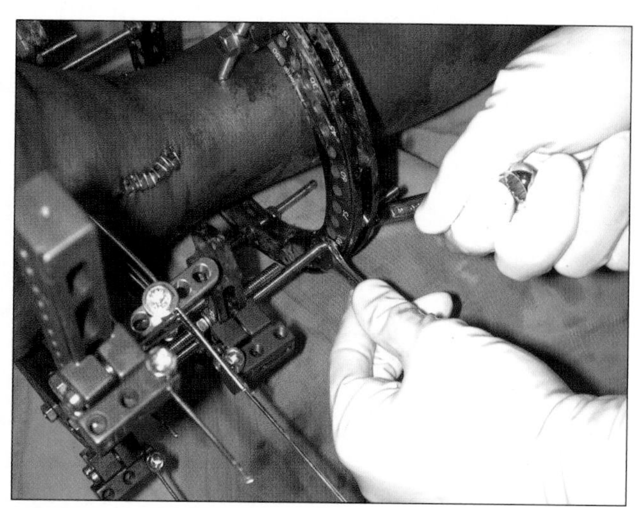

A B

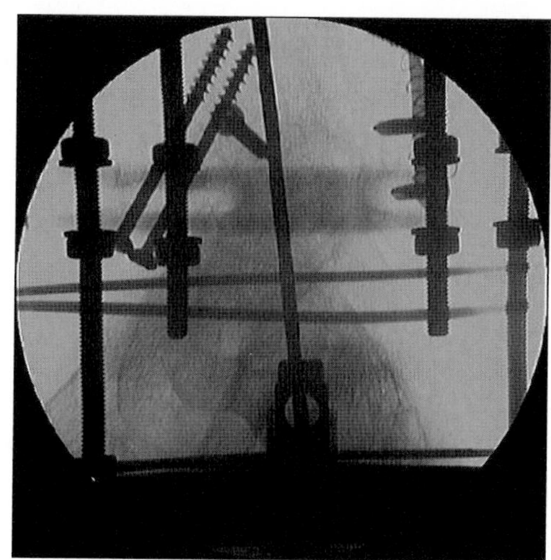

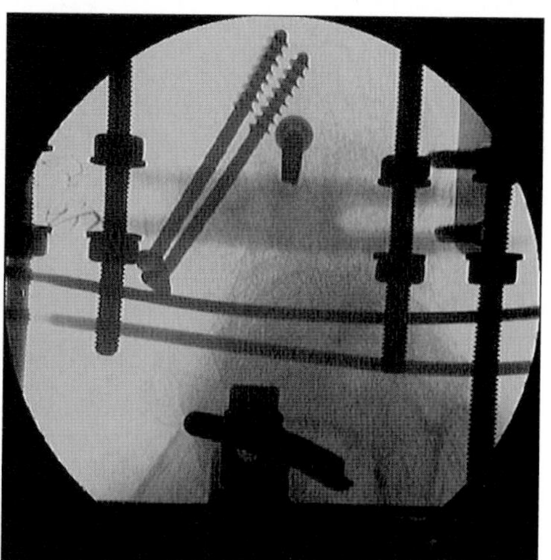

FIGURE 15 C D

Controversies

- Some surgeons consider subtalar joint distraction desirable during tibiotalar compression; we only add this when we identify mild, early arthritic changes in the subtalar joint.

PEARLS

- *Typically pins remain clean when the skin immediately surrounding the pin is stable, thereby reducing the skin irritation.*
- *Unlike ankle arthrodesis performed with internal fixation, further tibiotalar compression can be applied at follow-up visits and early weight bearing to tolerance is permitted.*

PITFALLS

- *A persistent pin tract infection, particularly with a lucency about the pin on postoperative radiographs, should prompt pin removal and placement of another pin in a different location.*

- Intraoperative fluoroscopy confirms that appropriate tibiotalar apposition has been achieved (Fig. 15C and 15D).
- The provisional pin may be left in place during compression to act as an "internal rail" to guide compression, but is not necessary and may be removed even prior to applying compression.

Postoperative Care and Expected Outcomes

- External fixation is maintained until there is radiographic evidence for healing.
- Occasionally, bridging trabeculation across the tibiotalar joint is obscured by the external fixator; in this case, a computed tomography scan may be useful to confirm fusion.
- Typically, healing in uncomplicated ankle arthrodeses takes 10–14 weeks.
- An advantage of external fixation over internal fixation for ankle arthrodesis is that greater compression may be applied at the arthrodesis site postoperatively. We routinely apply further compression at each postoperative visit in the first 6 weeks, particularly when postoperative radiographs suggest any gapping at the arthrodesis site.
- Once the surgical approach site is healed, weight bearing to tolerance is permitted. A tread attached to the foot portion of the frame may facilitate weight bearing and protect the foot.
- Once-daily pin care is recommended, with a gauze moistened with a 50:50 mixture of saline and hydrogen peroxide to remove any tissue debris that collects at the pin-skin interface.
- Skin irritated at a pin site should be carefully cleaned and then stabilized with dressings that apply slight pressure on the skin to limit its movement about the pin.
- A short course of an oral antibiotic and a topical antibiotic at the pin site usually treats minor pin tract infections adequately when combined with dressings that limit irritated skin motion about the pin.

Evidence

A Grade B recommendation can be made for ankle arthrodesis using external fixation given several Level IV studies that demonstrate satisfactory outcomes using this technique.

Easley ME, Montijo HE, Wilson JB, Fitch RD, Nunley JA 2nd. Revision tibiotalar arthrodesis. J Bone Joint Surg Am. 2008;90:1212–23.

Katsenis D, Bhave A, Paley D, Herzenberg JE. Treatment of malunion and nonunion at the side of an ankle fusion with the Ilizarov apparatus. J Bone Joint Surg Am. 2005;87:302–9.

Ogut T, Gilsson RR, Chuckpalwong B, Le IL, Easley ME. External ring fixation versus screw fixation for ankle arthrodesis: a biomechanical comparison. Foot Ankle Int. 2009;30:353–60.

Paley D, Lamm BM, Katsenis D, Bhave A, Herzenberg JE. Treatment of malunion and nonunion at the site of an ankle fusion with the Ilizarov apparatus. Surgical technique. J Bone Joint Surg Am. 2006;88(Suppl 1):119–34.

Salem KH, Kinzi L, Schmeiz A. Ankle arthrodesis using Ilizarov ring fixators: a review of 22 cases. Foot Ankle Int. 2006;27:764–70.

PROCEDURE 29

Arthroscopic Ankle Arthrodesis

Carol Frey

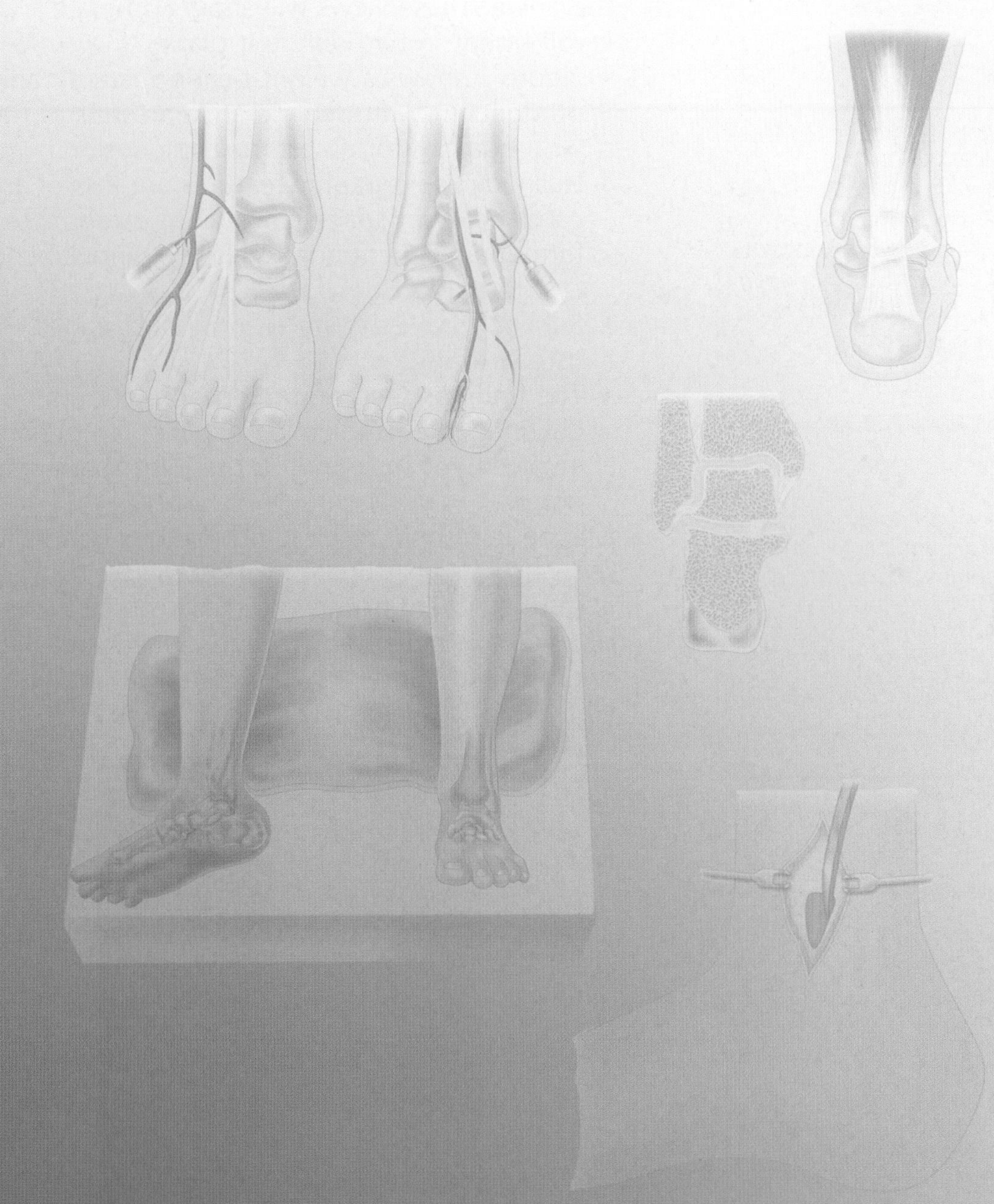

PITFALLS

- *You cannot correct gross deformity of the ankle with an arthroscopic fusion.*
- *Patients with significant varus or valgus tilt, marked anteroposterior translation, or significant bone loss are best treated by open arthrodesis.*

Controversies

- Avascular necrosis of the body of the talus.
- A patient with poor skin quality, extensive scar formation, vascular damage, or neuropathy is a poor candidate for an open procedure, but can still have an arthroscopic procedure.

PITFALLS

- *Weight-bearing radiographs are necessary to simulate loading the respective joints in an attempt to identify joint collapse and deformity. Without weight-bearing radiographs of the ankle, the amount of joint space involvement is often underestimated.*

Indications

- Degenerative joint disease of the ankle from any cause, including trauma, rheumatoid arthritis, hemophilic arthritis, and idiopathic degenerative joint disease
- Arthritis from infections

Examination/Imaging

- Weight-bearing anteroposterior and lateral views of the ankle. These views will show complete involvement in two different planes.
  - Figure 1 shows a weight-bearing lateral radiograph of a patient with degenerative arthritis of the ankle who qualifies for an arthroscopic fusion.
  - Hallmark radiographic features are loss of articular cartilage, joint space narrowing, osteophyte formation, subchondral sclerosis, and subchondral cyst formation.
  - Subchondral cysts are seen in later stages of osteoarthritis.
  - The findings seen on radiographs should be confined to the ankle joint space. No periarticular involvement surrounding the joint space should be noted.
- Magnetic resonance imaging (MRI) is generally not required in the evaluation of osteoarthritis; however, it can help identify early articular cartilage changes not seen on radiographs. With evidence of diffuse sclerosis and joint space collapse, MRI may be warranted to evaluate for osteonecrosis.

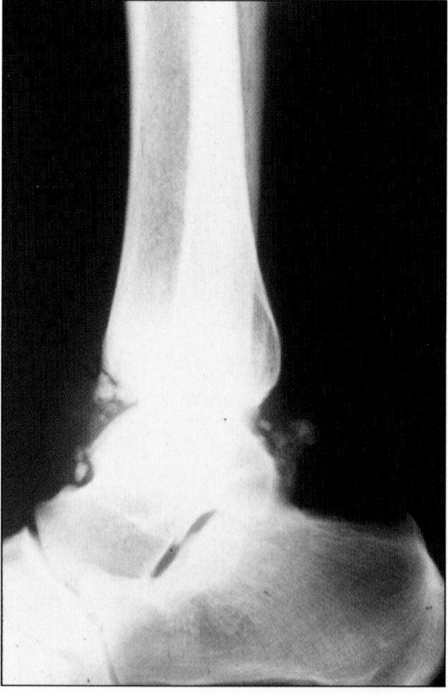

FIGURE 1

Treatment Options

- Anti-inflammatory medication
- Brace
- Injections of local anesthetic and cortisone
- Orthotic devices
- Shoe modifications

Surgical Anatomy

- The distal ends of the tibia and the fibula form an anatomic and functional unit with the talus (Fig. 2A and 2B).
- The inferior surface of the distal tibia is articular and corresponds to the dome of the talus.
  - It is concave in the anterior-posterior direction and slightly convex in the transverse direction.
  - It is divided into the wide lateral and the more narrow inner segment.
  - The lateral border is larger than the medial. The anterior border is longer than the posterior.
- With the talus in any position, the tibial plafond covers only two thirds of the surface of the talus.
- The posterior border of the inferior articular surface of the tibia is lower than the anterior.
- The talus is an intercalated bone between the tibia and fibula and the tarsal bones of the hindfoot.

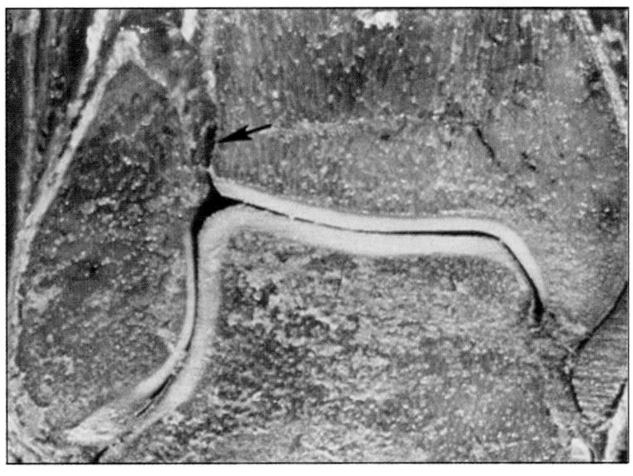

A

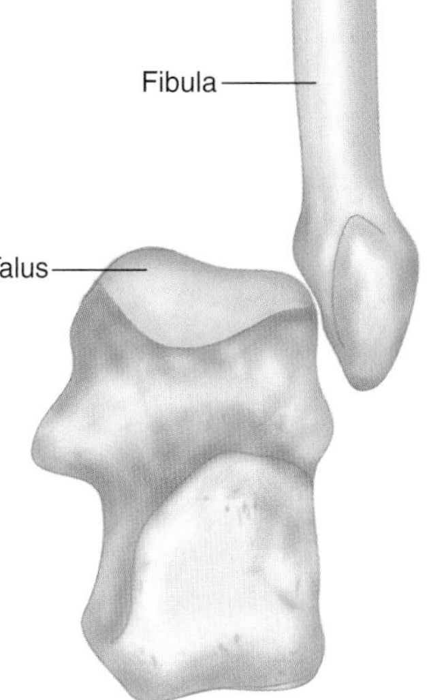

B

FIGURE 2

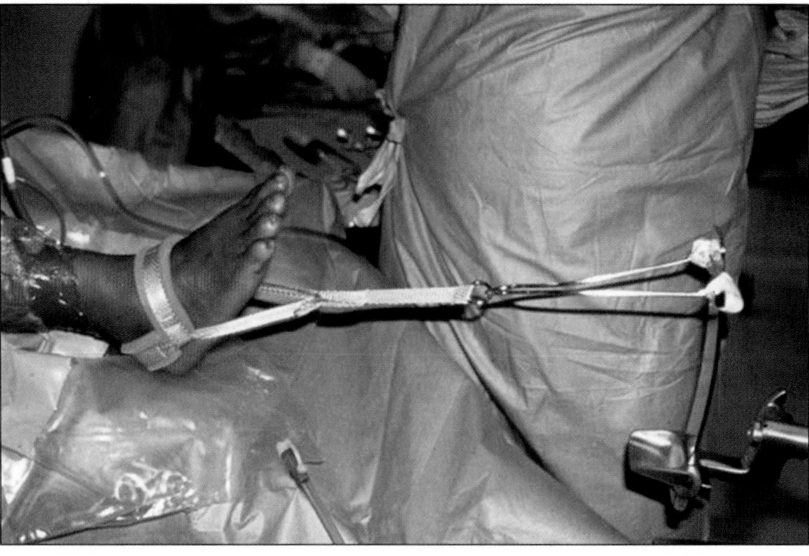

FIGURE 3

Pearls

- *Noninvasive joint distraction is recommended.*

Positioning

- Supine with or without a leg holder. A noninvasive distraction device is recommended (Fig. 3).

Portals/Exposures

- Standard ankle arthroscopic portals, including anteromedial, anterolateral, and posterolateral portals, can be used for an arthroscopic ankle fusion (Fig. 4).

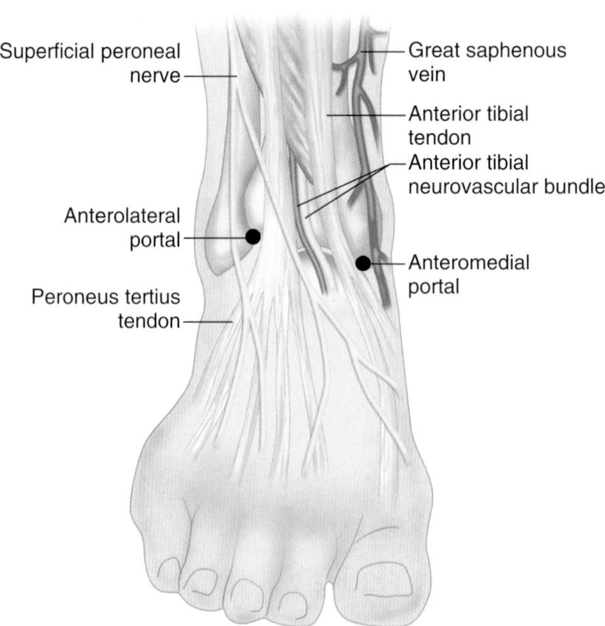

FIGURE 4

Procedure

Step 1

- Complete arthroscopic examination is undertaken.
- Anterior joint synovectomy is done as necessary to aid visualization.
- A combination of curettes, burrs, and shavers are needed to débride remaining cartilage on the talar dome, tibial plafond, and medial and lateral gutters.
  - Curved curettes are useful to reach over the most posterior aspect of the talar dome to débride remaining cartilage.
  - A motorized burr is then used to remove a thin layer of subchondral bone; around 2 mm of bone is enough (Fig. 5A).
  - Care must be taken to maintain the normal contour of the tibial plafond and talar dome so that there is good congruity of the bone surfaces at the conclusion of the procedure.
- Removal of anterior osteophytes of the tibial and talus will allow better visualization and positioning of the fusion (Fig. 5B).

Pearls

- *Failure to remove osteophytes can impair visualization and make it difficult to position the arthrodesis.*
- *Remove scar tissue impinging on the lateral and medial gutters to allow the talus to seat well into the tibial plafond at the conclusion of the case.*
- *Occasionally an Achilles tendon lengthening must be added to the procedure to obtain a neutral position.*

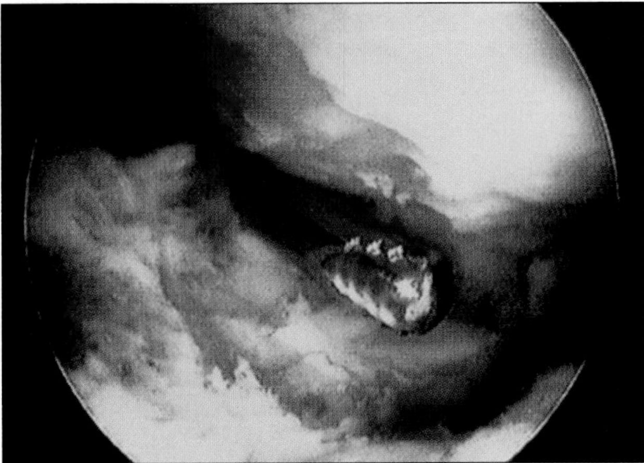

A

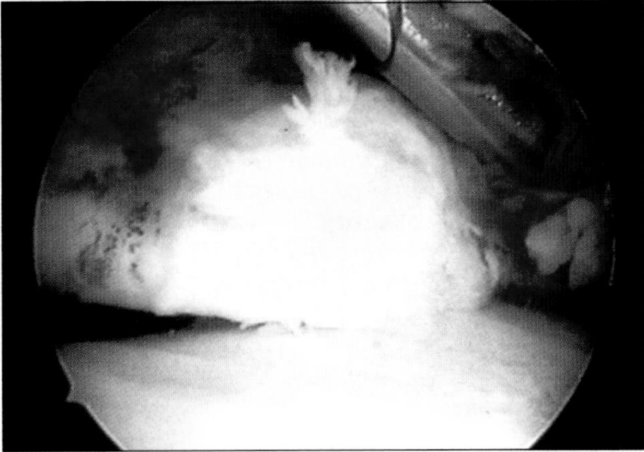

FIGURE 5 B

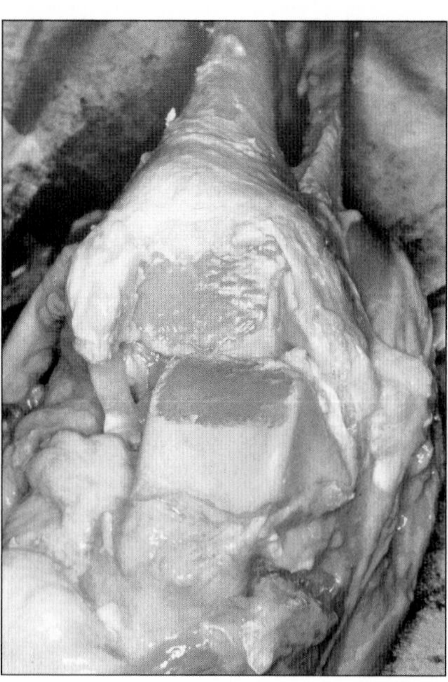

FIGURE 6

- With the use of a distraction device, most of the articular cartilage may be removed through the anteromedial and anterolateral portals. Figure 6 shows an ankle that has been sectioned after a débridement using just the anteromedial and anterolateral portals; 95% of the articular cartilage has been débrided.
- Motorized shavers and curettes may be introduced from the posterolateral portal to débride the most posterior aspect of the talus.

Step 2

- Guide pins for fixation (Fig. 7) are advanced under direct visualization from the medial malleolus and the posterior lateral tibia (just behind the fibula, if possible).
  - The general angle of the guide pins is 45° off vertical in the coronal plane and 45° off vertical in the sagittal plane.
  - Generally this directs the pins across the tibial plafond and down the neck of the talus.
- Care must be taken not to cross the subtalar joint.
- The pins are then backed out to just beneath the tibial surface.
- The arthroscope and noninvasive distractor are now removed.
- The fluoroscan can be used to confirm the position of the fusion and the guide pins.

Pearls

- *Occasionally a third screw is necessary for stability, which is placed lateral in the tibia and directed into the dome of the talus.*
- *Arthroscopic ankle arthrodesis should not be performed unless the surgeon is prepared to abandon the procedure and perform an open one if necessary.*

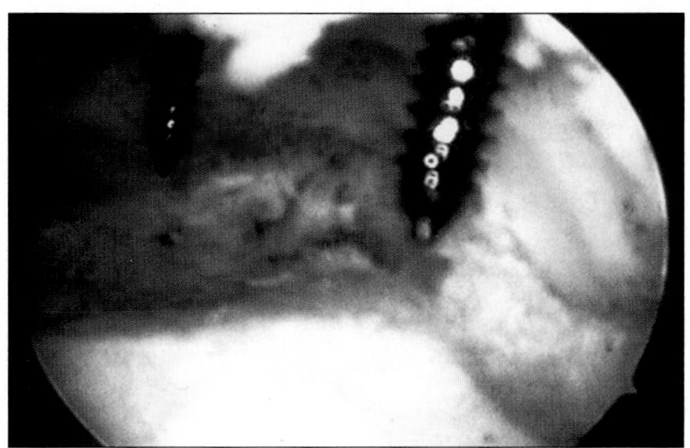

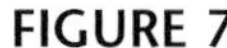

FIGURE 7

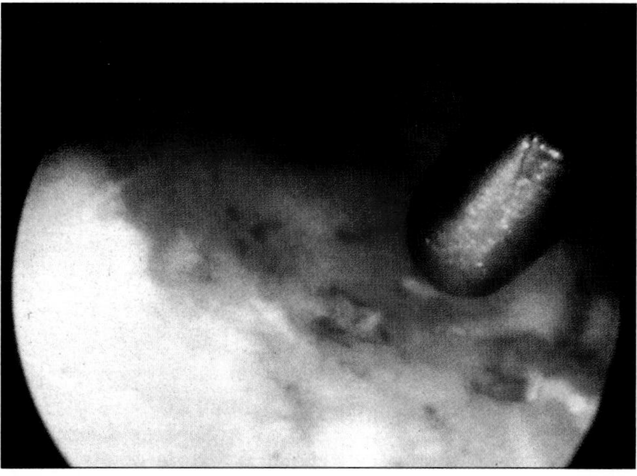

FIGURE 8

Instrumentation/ Implantation

- Arthroscopic curettes, including angled ones
- Fluoroscan
- Large-diameter cannulated cancellous screws (6.5–7.00 mm)
- Noninvasive distraction
- Arthroscopic pump
- 2.9-mm arthroscope
- Standard arthroscopic instrument tray

- Two 6.5-mm cannulated screws are then advanced and tightened (Fig. 8).
  - The lateral screw is advanced first.
  - Washers may be necessary if the bone is osteopenic.
- Position is confirmed on fluoroscan (Fig. 9A and 9B) and by direct visualization.
- Routine closure is undertaken.

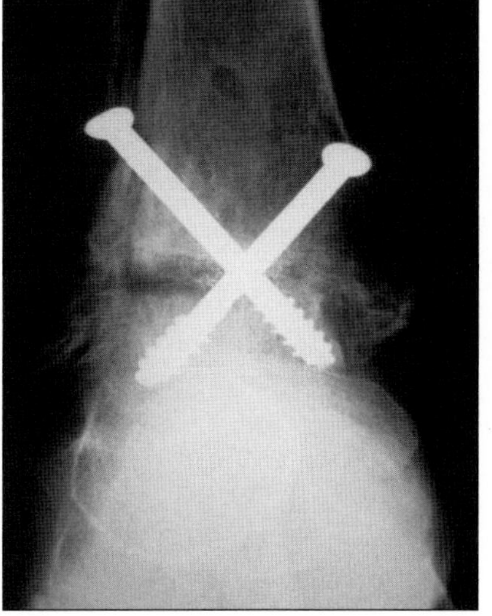

A

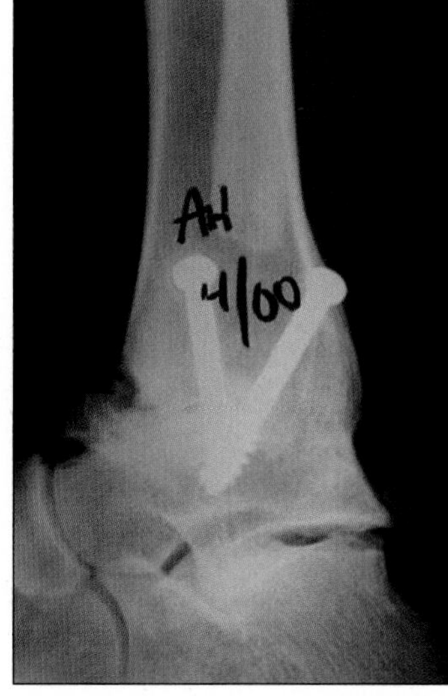

B

FIGURE 9

PEARLS

- *The average time to union after arthroscopic arthrodesis is 9 weeks.*

Postoperative Care and Expected Outcomes

- A compression dressing with a posterior splint is applied in the operating room with the foot and ankle in neutral position.
- The dressing is changed at 1 week, and a short-leg non–weight-bearing cast is applied that is utilized for 4 weeks.
- Sutures are removed at 2 weeks.
- Afterward, weight bearing as tolerated in a boot walker is recommended.
- The boot walker is used until there is radiographic evidence of fusion, at approximately 9–12 weeks postoperative.

Evidence

Glick JM, Morgan CD, Myerson MS. Ankle arthrodesis using an arthroscopic method: long-term follow-up of 34 cases. Arthroscopy. 1996;12:428-34.

This study reported high rates of fusion using arthroscopic techniques with few complications. Failure to remove the anterior osteophytes resulted in impaired visualization and inability to approximate the surfaces of the joint. (Level II evidence)

Morgan CD. Arthroscopic tibiotalar arthrodesis. In McGinty J (ed). Operative Arthroscopy. New York: Raven Press, 1991:695-701.

Morgan CD, Henke JA, Bailey RW, et al. Long-term results of tibiotalar arthrodesis. J Bone Joint Surg [Am]. 1985;67:546.

This study reported on a group of patients who underwent an open technique using in situ débridement with an anterior-lateral joint exposure but no fibular osteotomy. The fusion was fixed with a transmalleolar screw. There were high fusion rates, and this technique was duplicated when arthroscopic fusion of the ankle was undertaken. (Level I evidence)

Myerson MS, Allon SM. Arthroscopic ankle arthrodesis. Contemp Orthop. 1989;19: 21-7.

This study reported that the average time to union after arthroscopic arthrodesis is 9 weeks, with fewer complications than open techniques. The authors warned of a high learning curve. (Level II evidence)

Ogilvie-Harris DJ, Lieberman I, Fistulas D. Arthroscopically assisted arthrodesis for osteoarthritis ankles. J Bone Joint Surg [Am]. 1993;75:1167.

PROCEDURE 30

Rigid Fixation for Ankle Arthrodesis Using Double Plating

Christian Plaass and Beat Hintermann

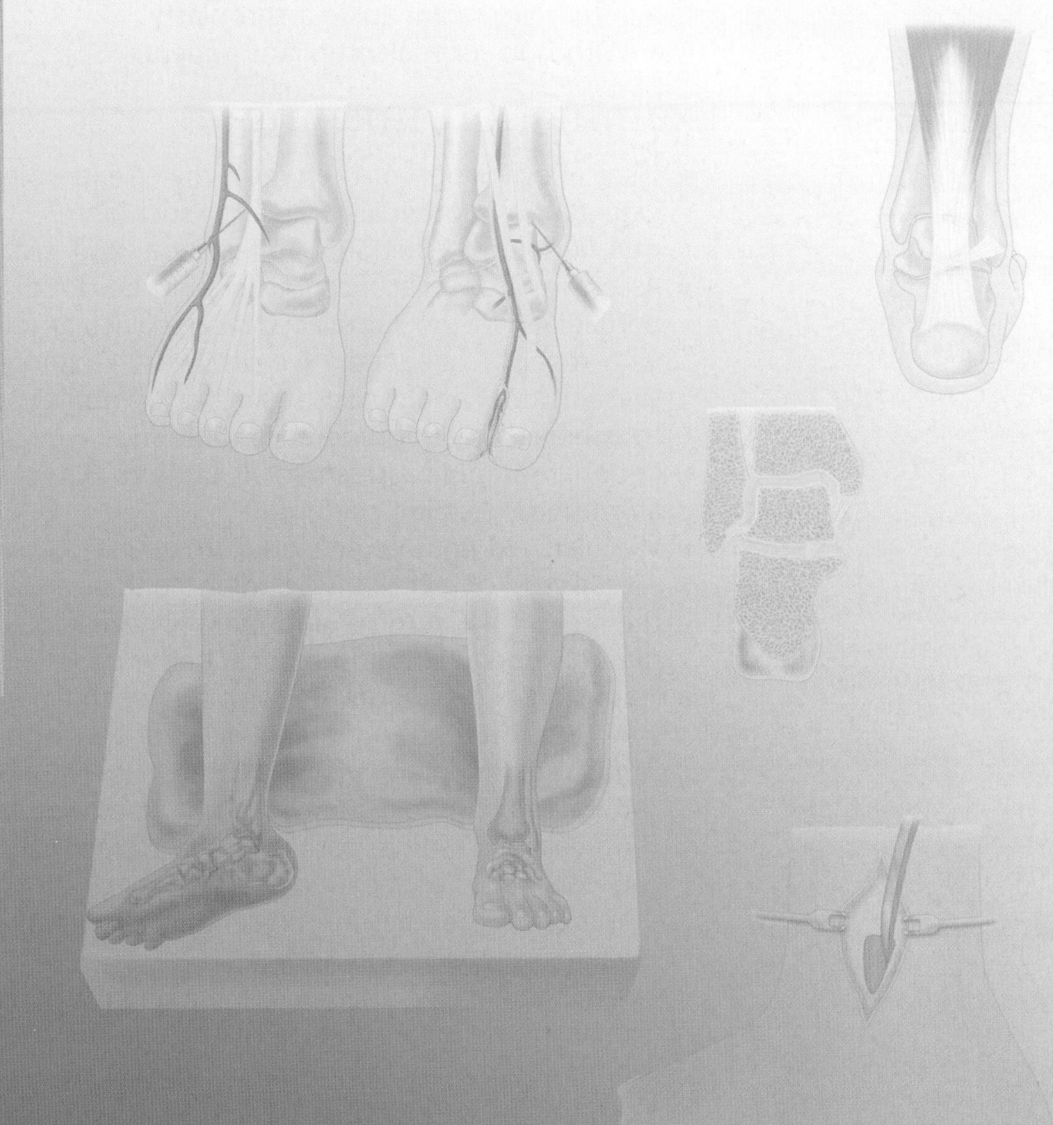

PITFALLS

- *Acute or chronic osteomyelitis has to be treated first, before internal fixation can be used.*
- *Chronic wounds and skin necrosis are relative contraindications.*

Controversies

- Peripheral arterial occlusive disease is a relative contraindication as delayed wound and bone healing may occur.
- Heavy smokers are at risk for bony fusion.

Treatment Options

- Conservative treatment with pain medication, shoe modifications, and orthoses may be undertaken.
- Total ankle replacement (TAR) has, in recent years, evolved to a viable alternative to ankle arthrodesis. Hence, the indication for ankle arthrodesis is more and more the existence of contraindications for TAR (neurologic disorders, gross ankle instability, severe deformity and bony defects) or failed ankle prostheses.
- In ankles with no deformity where TAR is not considered, a mini-open approach or mini-arthroscopic arthrodesis with a three- or four-screw technique may be a valuable alternative.
- Involvement of the subtalar joint may offer intramedullary tibiocalcaneal fixation using retrograde nailing.

Indications

- Isolated ankle arthrodesis in patients with painful posttraumatic or idiopathic ankle arthritis after failed conservative treatment, especially in cases
  - With severe deformity
  - With relevant comorbidities (diabetes, osteoporotic bone, rheumatoid arthritis, hemodialysis)
  - With neurologic disorders
  - With gross ankle instability
  - With bone defects (posttraumatic or after infection)
  - After failed total ankle arthroplasty
  - With non- or malcompliant patients

Examination/Imaging

- Clinical evaluation of the whole lower extremity is essential to address all problems, such as malalignment, functional impairment, and instability.
- Assessment of adjacent joints should be done, particularly of the subtalar and talonavicular joints, with regard to degenerative disease or dysfunction; if present, this should also be addressed during surgery to achieve a plantigrade and stable foot.
- Pedobarographic assessment is done to detect an asymmetric loading pattern.
- Vascular and neurologic status are assessed.
- Assessment of soft tissue condition and scarring in the area of the surgical approach is necessary, and a plastic surgeon should be consulted if necessary.
- Plain standard radiographs with full weight bearing
  - Anteroposterior and lateral views of the foot, and mortise and lateral views of the ankle, should be obtained. Figure 1A and 1B show radiographs of a 68-year-old female patient (on hemodialysis because of diabetic kidney insufficiency) 3 years after an ankle fracture, presenting as unstable valgus osteoarthritis.
  - A Saltzman view should be obtained in the case of malalignment to estimate the position of the hindfoot and the weight-bearing axes.
- A computed tomography (CT) scan should be done in cases with bone defects to further evaluate bone structures and define necessary surgical techniques and the use of allografts.
- A single-photon emission CT scan with superimposed bone scan may help to discern the status of adjacent joints of the ankle. It is particularly helpful in decision making as to whether arthrodesis of adjacent joints should be considered.

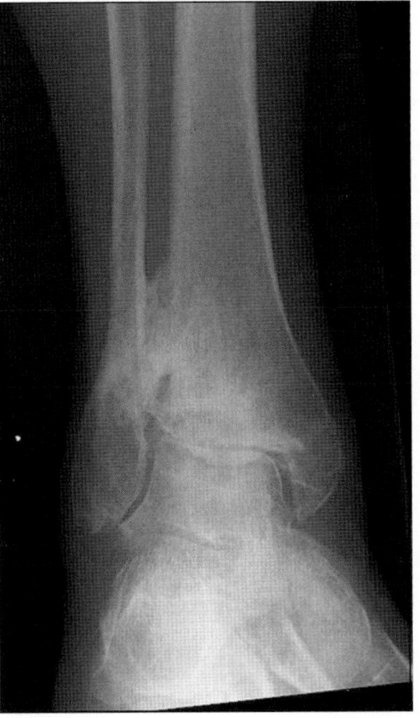

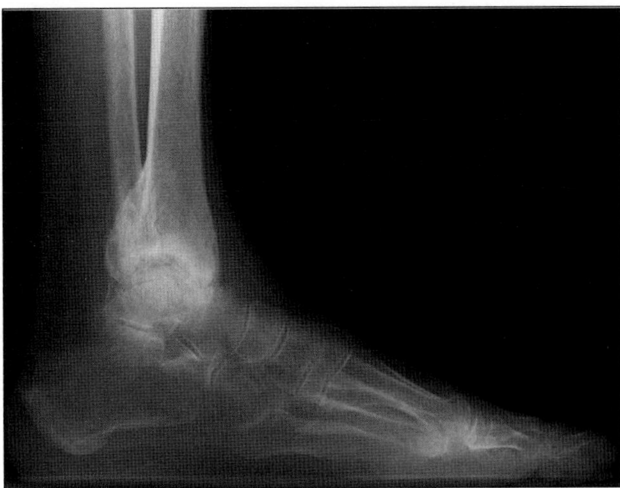

FIGURE 1 A B

Surgical Anatomy

- The superior extensor retinaculum is a thickening of the deep fascia above the ankle, running from the tibia to the fibula (Fig. 2). It includes, from medially to laterally, the tendons of the tibialis anterior, extensor hallucis longus, and extensor digitorum longus.

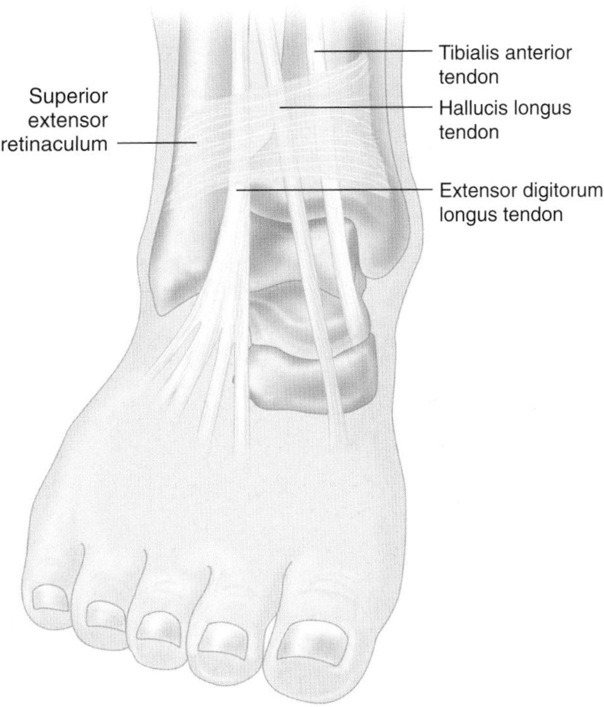

FIGURE 2

- The anterior neurovascular bundle lies roughly halfway between the malleoli (Fig. 3A); it can be found consistently between the extensor hallucis longus and extensor digitorum longus tendons.
- The neurovascular bundle contains the tibialis anterior and the deep peroneal nerve. The nerve supplies the extensor digitorum brevis and extensor hallucis brevis and a sensory space (interdigital I–II).
- The soft tissue beneath the anterior tibial tendon is always free from the neurovascular bundle and thus is referred to as the "safe spot" while approaching the anterior ankle joint.

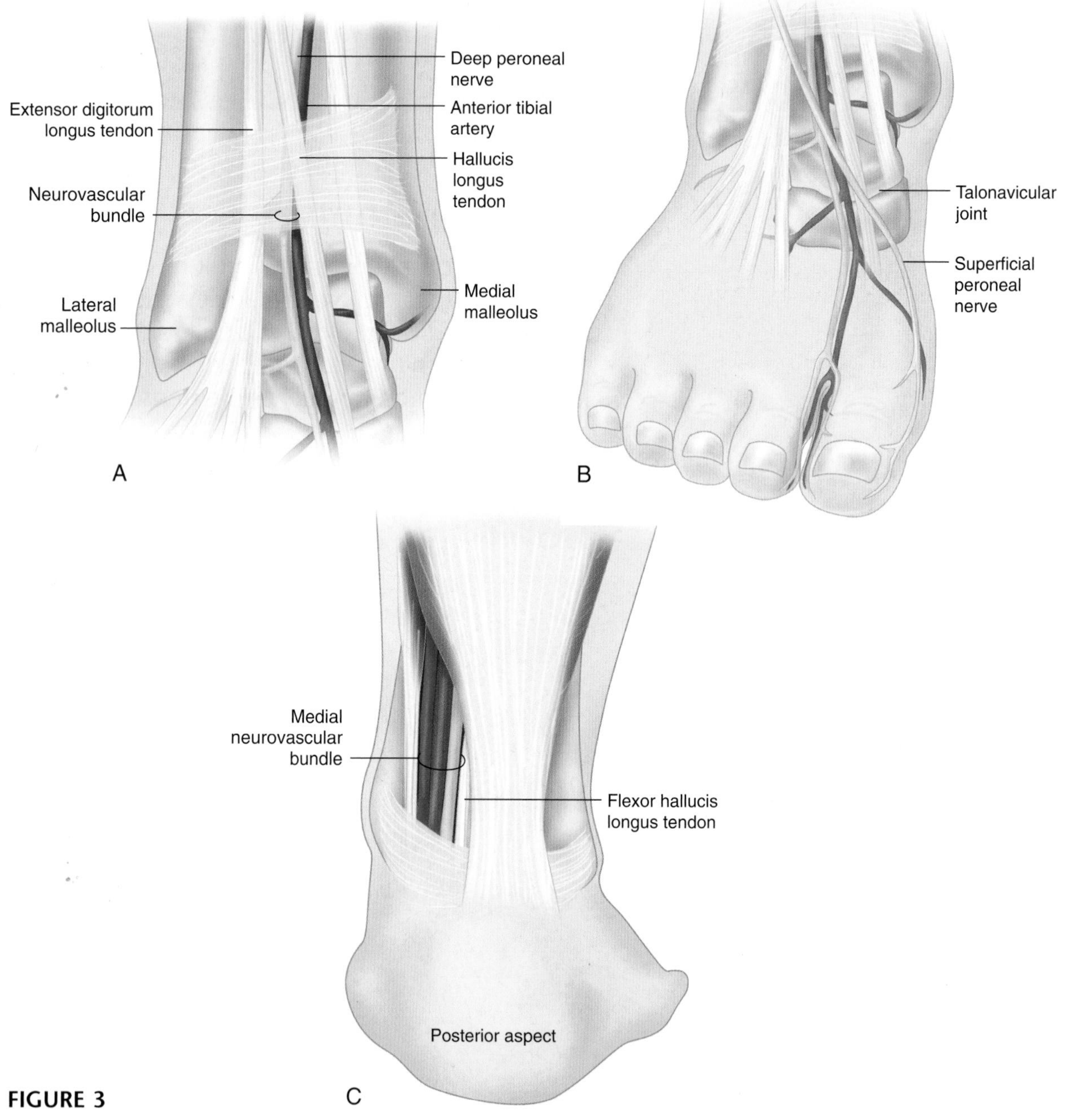

FIGURE 3

- On the height of the talonavicular joint, the medial branches of the superficial peroneal nerve cross from lateral to medial (Fig. 3B). This nerve supplies the skin of the dorsum of the foot.
- On the posterior aspect of the ankle, the medial neurovascular bundle is located behind its posteromedial corner, and the flexor hallucis longus tendon on its posterior aspect (Fig. 3C).

Pearls

- *Elevation of the operated leg with cushions or lowering of the opposite leg facilitates lateral radiography and achieves more space for the surgeon.*
- *Free draping of both legs may help to properly position the foot for fusion, particularly in the case of asymmetric deformity or malrotation of the affected leg.*

Pitfalls

- *Inappropriate draping can hinder appropriate reduction at the ankle for fusion.*

Positioning

- The patient is placed in the supine position on a radiolucent operating table.
- The ipsilateral pelvis should be supported by cushions to control external rotation of the leg, so that the patella is directed upward to allow easier operation.
- A tourniquet is placed at the thigh.
- Positioning of the distal shank on a cushion may help to properly reduce the ankle joint during surgery.
- The leg should be draped free to the knee joint to facilitate control of the position of the arthrodesis in all axes.

Portals/Exposures

- A 10- to 12-cm anterior longitudinal incision is directly lateral to the tibialis anterior tendon.
- The subcutaneous tissues are divided to the extensor retinaculum, paying attention to the medial branches of the superficial peroneal nerve and the veins.
- The extensor retinaculum is dissected longitudinally along the lateral border of the anterior tibial tendon.
- Exposure is obtained to the distal tibia beneath the anterior tibial tendon, which is held to medial by a small blunt retractor, and subperiosteal exposure of the distal tibia is obtained using two small Hohmann retractors.
- Arthrotomy of the ankle joint is performed, with removal of scarred capsule and loose bodies.
- The neck of the talus is exposed.
- A self-retaining retractor is positioned, taking care to not apply tension to the skin (Fig. 4).

Pearls

- *Strictly subperiosteal exposure of the distal tibia and talar neck may prevent any injury to the surrounding soft tissues, particularly the neurovascular structures.*
- *Using a distractor may help to expose the tibiotalar joint (Fig. 5).*

Pitfalls

- *Injury to the nerve structures (cutaneous dorsalis intermedius and medialis of the peroneus superficialis) that cross from lateral to medial*
- *Injury to the neurovascular bundle (dorsalis pedis artery, the corresponding vein and the peroneus profundus nerve) that is located laterally to the extensor digitorum tendon*

Controversies

- Several approaches to expose the ankle joint for arthrodesis have been proposed; if properly done, the described anterior approach is safe and allows preservation of the gross anatomy of the ankle joint. It is also beneficial in the case of bad scar tissue on the lateral or medial aspect of the ankle from previous injuries and surgeries.

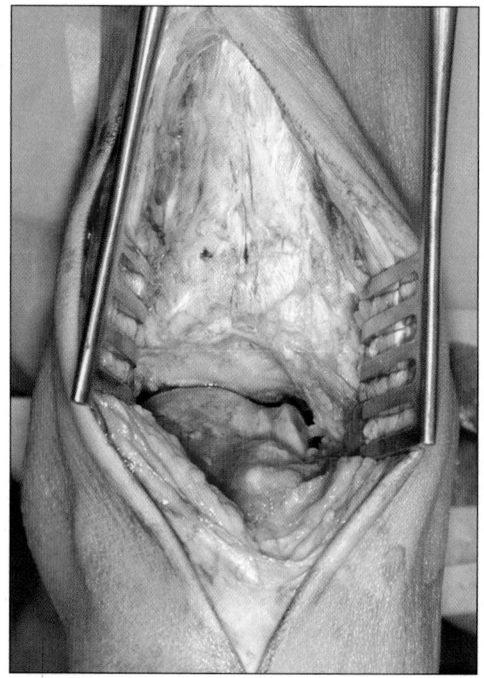

FIGURE 4

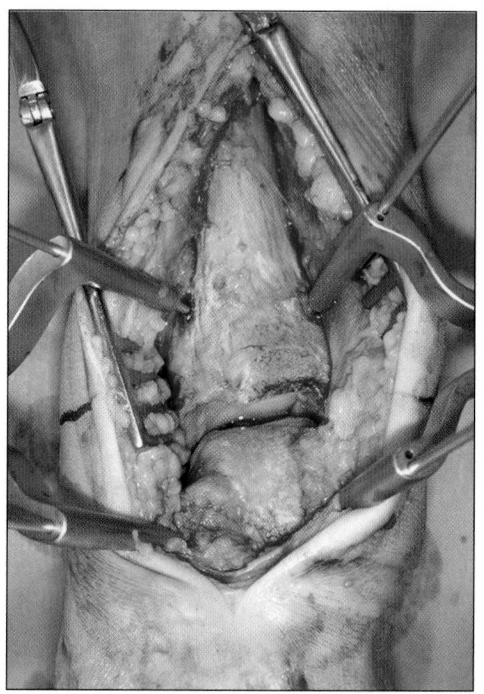

FIGURE 5

Procedure

Step 1

- Remaining cartilage is removed from the talar dome, the tibial plafond, and the medial gutter using chisel and curettes, paying attention to preserve the anatomic configuration of surfaces and the vascularity of remaining bone (Fig. 6).
- After denuding the subchondral bone, a 2.5-mm drill or a burr is used to break sclerotic bone areas.
- Cysts are cleaned and filled with cancellous bone graft or bone matrix.

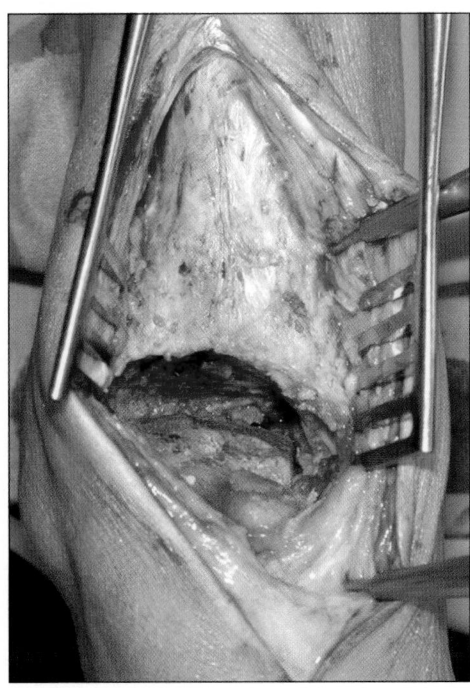

FIGURE 6

Pearls

- *Preservation of the convexity of the talar dome and concavity of the distal tibia may increase the stability obtained after internal fixation, particularly against rotational forces. In any case, the anterior and posterior rims of the distal tibia should be preserved to get high-contact stress at the anterior and posterior aspects during arthrodesis, which will increase the intrinsic stability of the arthrodesis.*
- *The lateral gutter does not need to be cleaned.*
- *In very sclerotic bone or cases of talus necrosis, opening the tourniquet during surgery may help in evaluating the vitality of the bone.*

Pitfalls

- *Incomplete removal of articular cartilage, or inadequate denuding of contact surfaces, may lead to delayed union or nonunion.*
- *Destroying the concavity of the distal tibia may lead to instability.*

Instrumentation/Implantation

- Using a sharp, curved chisel allows easier removal of the cartilage and preserves the anatomic shape of the bones.

Controversies

- Use of a burr may facilitate breakdown of sclerotic subchondral bone; however, its use may be associated with heat damage to the bony surface, which, in turn, may change the healing of fusion.

STEP 2

- Correct positioning in reduction before internal fixation is crucial for success of the surgery. Optimal position in all planes must be achieved.
- Once desired reduction is obtained, a 2.5-mm Kirschner wire may be inserted through the distal tibia into the talus. It is best placed in the center of the tibia and in the sagittal plane so as to not interfere with the plate position later on (Fig. 7A and 7B).
- The lateral plate is fixed by three interlocking screws to the lateral aspect of the talar neck (Fig. 8). Residual osteophytes hampering the plate placement have to be removed first.
- Compression of the talus against the tibia and the medial malleolus is achieved by a compression device and screw fixation to the tibia (Fig. 9).
- The medial plate is positioned accordingly and fixed with three interlocking screws to the talar neck and, thereafter, the tibia (Fig. 10).

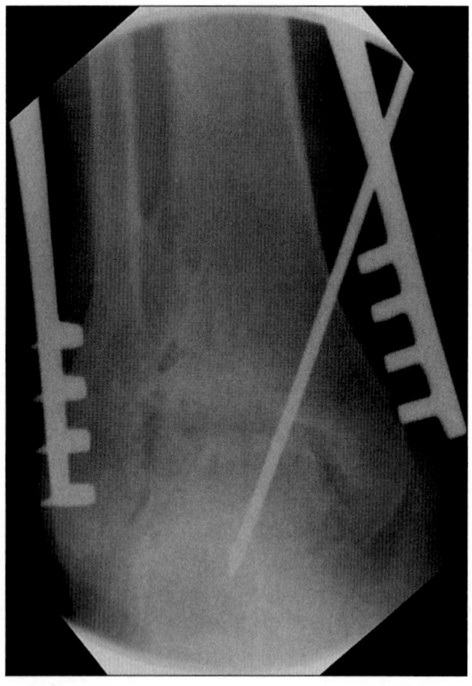

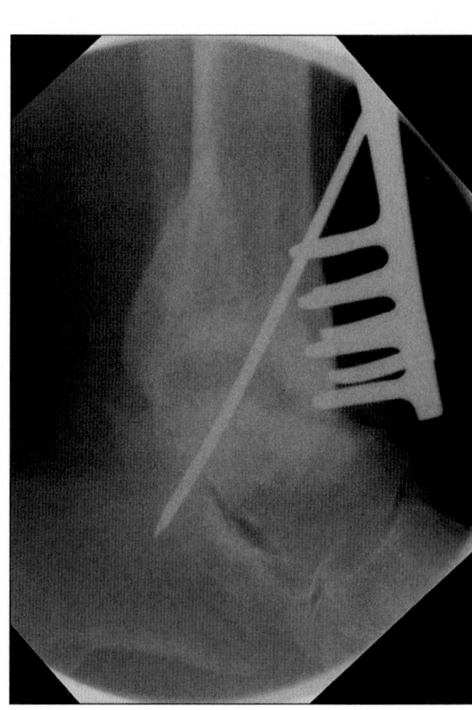

A B

FIGURE 7

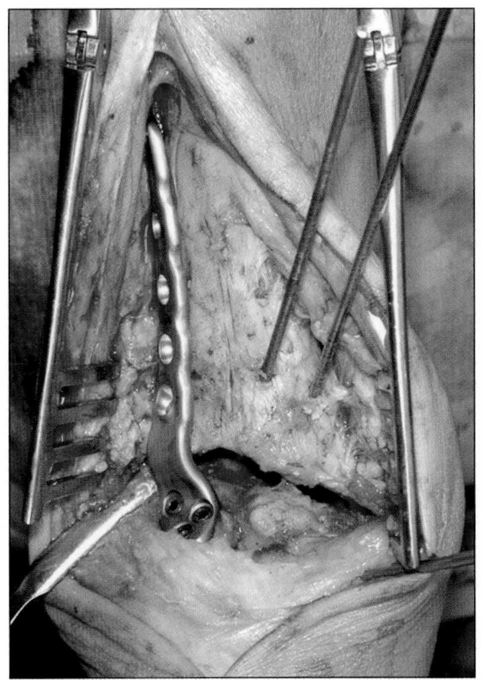

FIGURE 8

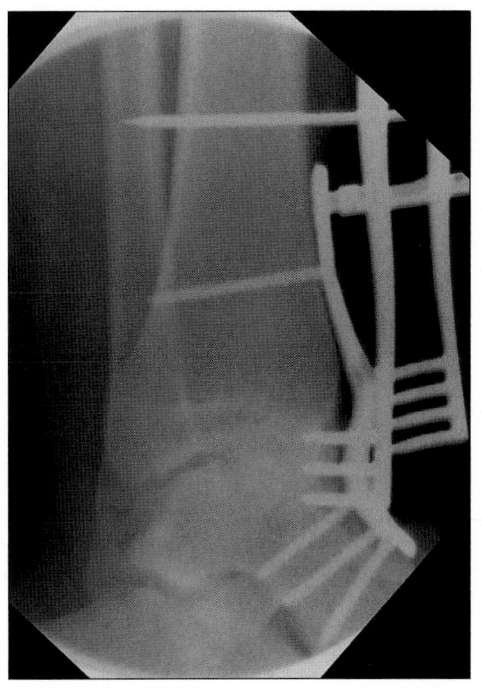

FIGURE 9

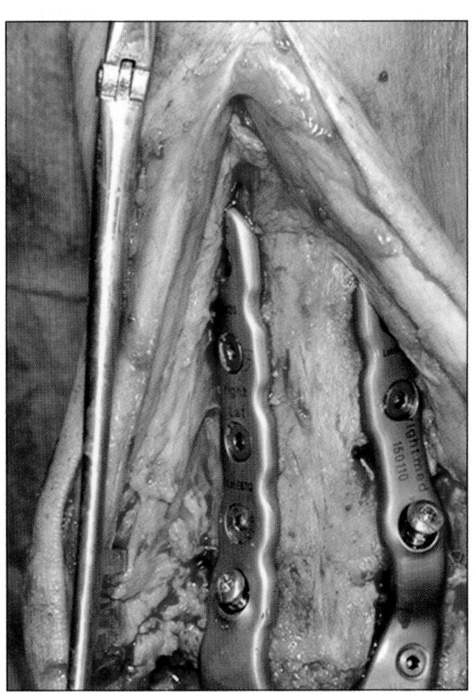

FIGURE 10

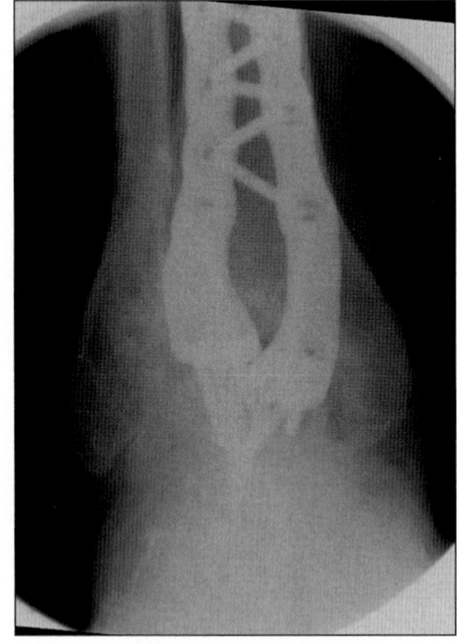

A

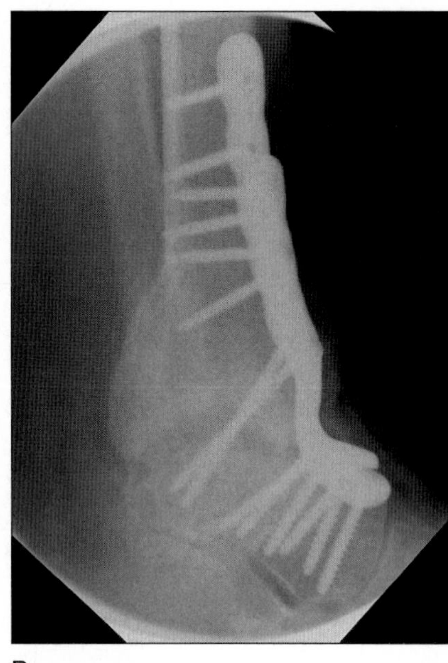

B

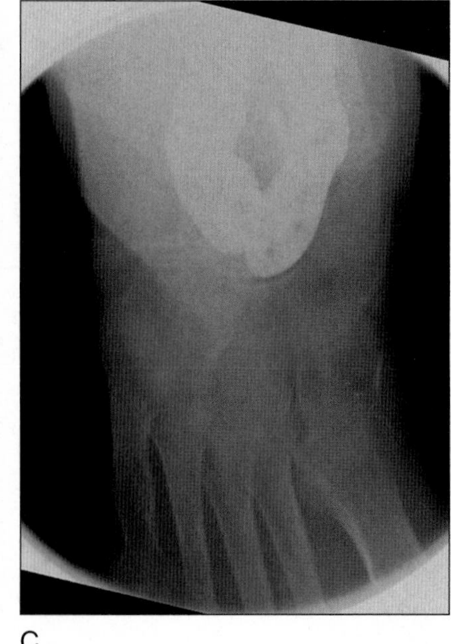

C

FIGURE 11

- Additional screws crossing and compressing the tibiotalar joint are placed in the dorsal part of the talus.
- A final check is performed by fluoroscopy (Fig. 11A–C).

Pearls

- *In cases of gross deformity or bone defects, reconstruction with an iliac crest allograft or an autograft may be necessary (Fig. 12).*
- *Demineralized bone matrix enhances bone healing and may be an alternative to autologous cancellous bone graft from the iliac crest. Platelet concentrate may be used to stimulate bone healing in critical conditions (e.g., smokers).*
- *Excessive length of the fibula causing lateral impingement may make shortening necessary. This can be easily done through the same anterior approach.*

Pitfalls

- *Fixation of the foot in any wrong position may cause functional impairment for walking and overuse of the adjacent joints, resulting in early degenerative disease.*

Instrumentation/Implantation

- The use of a fluoroscan or C-arm is highly recommended for proper positioning of the implants (e.g., so as not to damage the subtalar joint by improper screw positioning).

Controversies

- The use of isolated screw fixation is also possible; however, achieved stability is less and often additional fixation of the fibula is necessary.

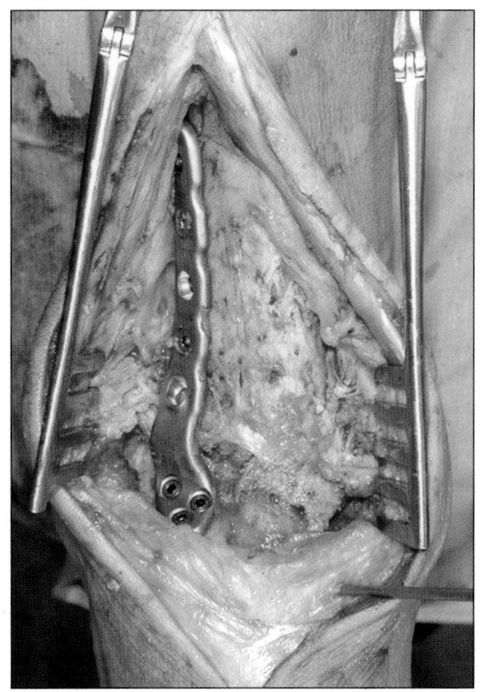

FIGURE 12

Pearls

- *A cotton-wool compression dressing allows reduction of postoperative hematoma and swelling.*

Pitfalls

- *In some instances, the extensor retinaculum cannot be fully closed due to the two plates; however, in our experience, no further problems were created by an incompletely closed retinaculum.*

Controversies

- A suction drain may evacuate blood out of the bone without preventing local hematoma formation; instead, a compressive dressing may be used to apply continuous pressure during the first 2 postoperative days.

Step 3

- The longitudinal incision of the extensor retinaculum is closed by continuous absorbable 0 suture.
- The skin is closed with interrupted nonabsorbable 3-0 sutures.
- A drain is not used routinely.
- A thick compressive dressing is applied, and the foot is placed in a reusable prefabricated splint.
- The tourniquet is deflated.

Postoperative Care and Expected Outcomes

- At the second postoperative day, the compressive dressings and prefabricated splint are replaced by a removable (synthetic) cast. This allows the use of an inflatable foot pump in case of substantial postoperative swelling.
- After subsidence of the swelling (mostly between days 6 and 14 postoperative), a below-knee walking cast is applied and left in place until the eighth postoperative week.
- Removal of the stitches should not be done before the 14th postoperative day.

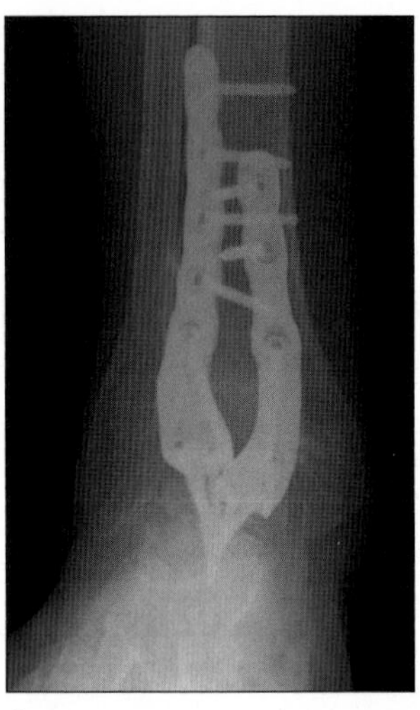
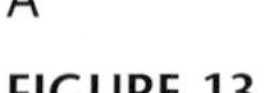
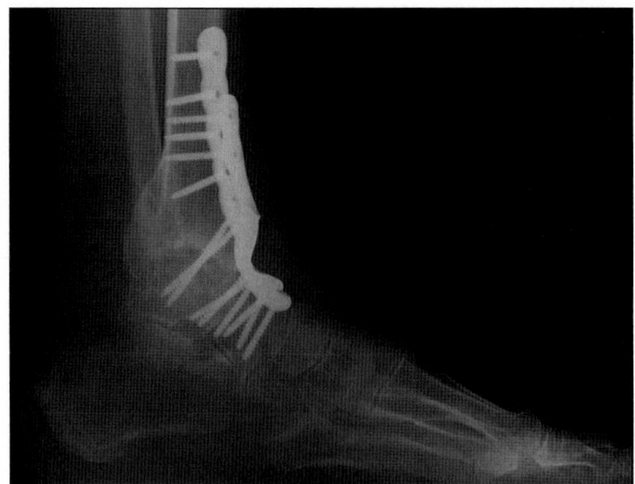

A B

FIGURE 13

Pearls

- *General measures such as the wearing of compressive stockings and strengthening exercises of the lower leg are encouraged.*
- *We recommend that patients stop smoking before surgery or reduce smoking as much as possible.*

Pitfalls

- *Potential complications include wound problems, infection (superficial or deep), malunion or nonunion of the fused joints, and late secondary arthritis of the adjacent joints.*

- Once the walking cast is applied properly, weight bearing is allowed as tolerated; usually full weight bearing is achieved after 10–14 days postoperative.
- At 8 weeks, the cast is removed and standard radiographs are taken (Fig. 13A and 13B). If bony fusion is considered not to be sufficient, a removable walking cast is applied for another 4–6 weeks. If the fusion is considered to be sufficient, the patient is permitted free ambulation in custom shoes.
- Low-molecular-weight heparin or an oral anticoagulant should be given, as long as the walking cast is in place or free full weight bearing is not permitted.

Controversies

- The recent literature on ankle arthrodesis procedures supports our personal experience that shoe modifications should be recommended for improving gait pattern.

Evidence

Alonso-Vázquez A, Lauge-Pedersen H, Lidgren L, Taylor M. The effect of bone quality on the stability of ankle arthrodesis: a finite element study. Foot Ankle Int. 2004;25:840-50.

This finite element study shows that bone quality has a marked effect on the initial stability of ankle arthrodeses at the arthrodesis site. To reduce the risk of bone failure, the stability provided should be increased. (Level V evidence)

Anderson T, Maxander P, Rydholm U, Besjakov J, Carlsson A. Ankle arthrodesis by compression screws in rheumatoid arthritis: primary nonunion in 9/35 patients. Acta Orthop. 2005;76:884-90.

The use of compression screws for fusion of the rheumatic ankle does not appear to give acceptable results regarding healing and function. (Level IV evidence [retrospective case series])

Buck P, Morrey BF, Chao EY. The optimum position of arthrodesis of the ankle: a gait study of the knee and ankle. J Bone Joint Surg [Am]. 1987;69:1052-62.

This study has shown the ideal position of fusion of the ankle to be neutral flexion, slight (0–5°) valgus angulation of the hind part of the foot, and 5–10° of external rotation. (Level IV evidence)

Cobb TK, Gabrielsen TA, Campbell DC, Wallrichs SL, Ilstrup DM. Cigarette smoking and nonunion after ankle arthrodesis. Foot Ankle Int. 1994;15:64-7.

The relative risk for nonunion increases 3.75-fold for active smokers in ankle arthrodesis. (Matched-pair analysis) (Level III evidence)

Collman DR, Kaas MH, Schuberth JM. Arthroscopic ankle arthrodesis: factors influencing union in 39 consecutive patients. Foot Ankle Int. 2006;27:1079-85.

Arthroscopic ankle arthrodesis led to nonunion in 12.8% of a group of patients who had no severe malalignment. A case with significant tibial plafond collapse was identified as not ideal for this technique. Ten patients experienced complications. Analysis showed that posttraumatic arthritis and obesity are significant risk factors for nonunion. Diabetes mellitus, polyneuropathy, and other comorbidities showed a tendency to increase the failure risk. (Level IV evidence [retrospective case series])

Cracchiolo A, Cimino WR, Lian G. Arthrodesis of the ankle in patients who have rheumatoid arthritis. J Bone Joint Surg [Am]. 1992;74:903-9.

Seven of 32 patients with rheumatoid arthritis showed nonunion after arthrodesis of the ankle, regardless of whether screw or external compression arthrodesis was used. (Level IV evidence [case series])

Frey C, Halikus NM, Vu-Rose T, Ebramzadeh E. A review of ankle arthrodesis: predisposing factors to nonunion. Foot Ankle Int. 1994;15:581-4.

This study retrospectively analyzed 78 ankle arthrodeses. Overall complications occurred in 56% of the patients, with 41% nonunions. Avascular necrosis, neurologic deficits, infections, major medical problems, and previous open fractures were identified as risk factors for nonunion. (Level IV evidence)

Helm R. The results of ankle arthrodesis. J Bone Joint Surg [Br]. 1990;72:141-3.

This study shows a high complication rate of ankle arthrodesis and the negative influence of varus/valgus malposition on function after ankle arthrodesis. (Level IV evidence [case series])

Hopgood P, Kumar R, Wood PL. Ankle arthrodesis for failed total ankle replacement. J Bone Joint Surg [Br]. 2006;88:1032-8.

After failed ankle replacement, bone loss in the body of the talus often makes isolated tibiotalar arthrodesis with screws difficult, making tibiotalacalcanear arthrodesis necessary. (Level IV evidence)

Kakarala G, Rajan DT. Comparative study of ankle arthrodesis using cross screw fixation versus anterior contoured plate plus cross screw fixation. Acta Orthop Belg. 2006;72:716-21.

In this study of 22 cases, patients with additional contoured plate arthrodesis showed faster and more secure healing than those with cross-screw fixation alone. Plate usage was also successful after failed cross-screw arthrodesis. (Level IV evidence [case study])

Morrey BF, Wiedeman GP. Complications and long-term results of ankle arthrodeses following trauma. J Bone Joint Surg [Am]. 1980;62:777-84.

This study shows a complication rate of 48% after ankle arthrodesis because of posttraumatic ankle arthritis, with infection in 23%, nonunion in 23%, malunion in 12%, loss of position in 15%, and delayed union in 7%. Varus and valgus angulation in the hindfoot led to a greater degree of symptoms in the subtalar area and the middle of the foot. Arthrodesis was recommended in neutral or slight dorsiflexion, as this is better tolerated than plantar flexion. (Level IV evidence)

PROCEDURE 31

Tibiotalocalcaneal Fusion with a Retrograde Intramedullary Nail

Alexej Barg, Beat Hintermann, and Markus Knupp

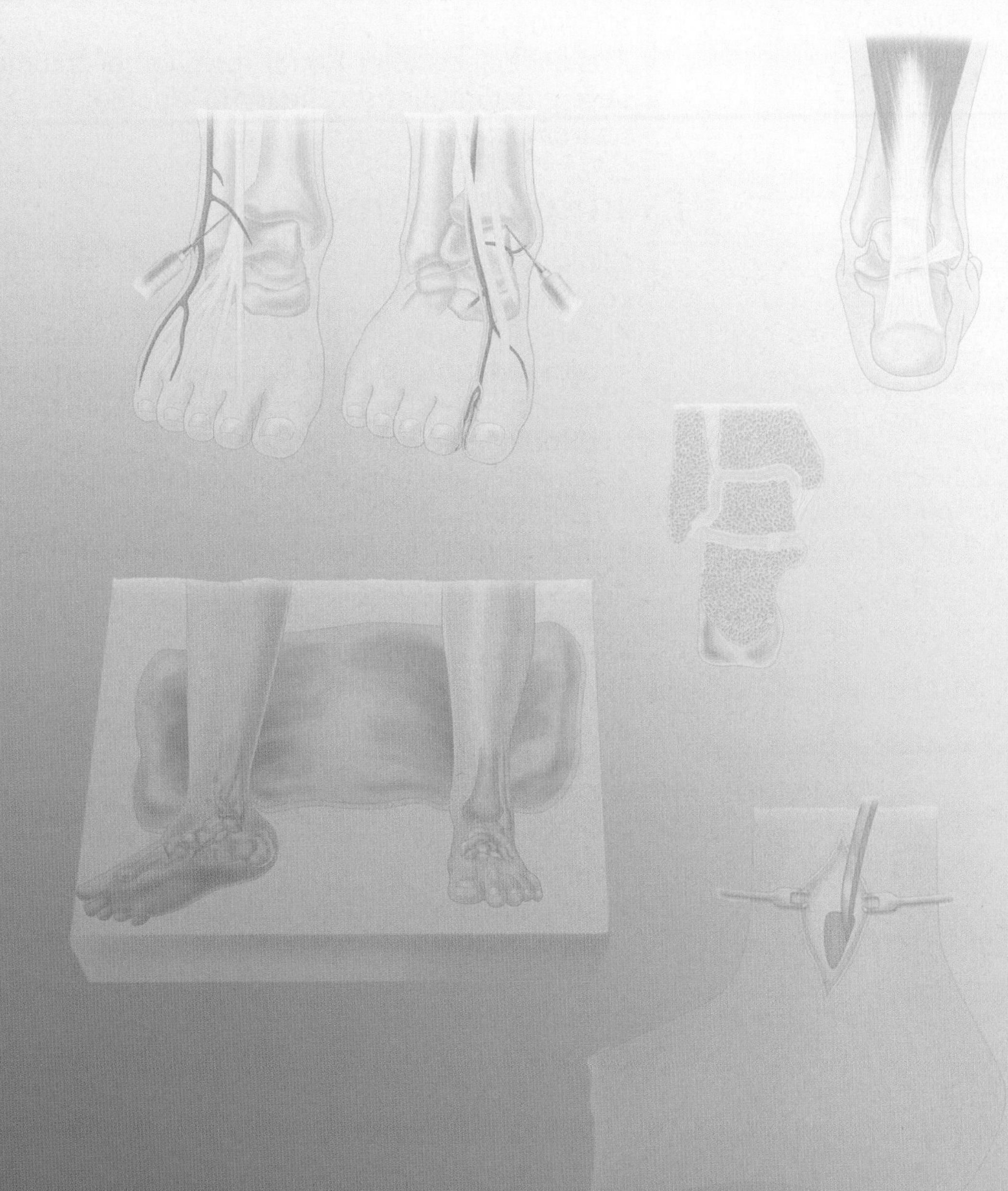

Pitfalls

- *Contraindications for this procedure (Mendicino et al., 2004):*
  - *Acute osteitis/osteomyelitis*
  - *Critical and poor skin or soft tissue condition*
  - *Severe deformity or blockage of medullary canal of tibia*
  - *Reflex sympathetic dystrophy of leg*
  - *Dysvascular extremity*

Treatment Options

- Medication, shoe correction, and orthoses
- Ankle arthrodesis using two ventral plates (Plaass et al., 2009)
- Tibiotalocalcaneal arthrodesis by using a blade-plate fixation (Chiodo et al., 2003)

Indications

- Posttraumatic/degenerative/inflammatory arthritis (Goebel et al., 2006)
- Rheumatoid arthritis (Anderson et al., 2005)
- Failed ankle arthrodesis (Eingartner et al., 2005)
- Failed ankle arthroplasty (Hopgood et al., 2006; Zwipp et al., 2005)
- End-stage talar osteonecrosis
- Diabetic patients with unstable Charcot neuroarthropathy (Caravaggi et al., 2006; Pinzur et al., 2005)
- Skeletal defects after tumor resection or trauma
- Severe deformities secondary to clubfoot or neuromuscular disease

Examination/Imaging

- Clinical examination, particularly to exclude all contraindications
  - Careful evaluation of medical history, particularly with regard to previous injuries and surgeries, metabolic and vascular problems, acute and chronic infection
  - Careful inspection of local wound and scar conditions
  - Checking for neurovascular status of affected leg
  - Assessment of hindfoot and foot alignment, instability, and remaining motion
  - Exclusion of all contraindications
- Plain radiographs under full weight bearing for assessment of malalignment, deformity, and instability
  - Foot: anteroposterior (AP) and lateral views; Figure 1 shows a lateral view of an ankle with severe osteoarthritis
  - Ankle: AP view; Figure 2 shows an AP view of an ankle with severe osteoarthritis
  - Hindfoot: Saltzman view for assessment of the hindfoot axis in relation to the tibial axis
  - In the case of lower extremity deformity: long film view of leg
- Computed tomography scan for assessment of bone status: triplane view of hindfoot complex, three-dimensional reconstruction
- Single-photon emission computed tomography for assessment of extent of degenerative changes in joints and proper evaluation of inflammatory activity
- Magnetic resonance imaging for assessment of bone vitality.

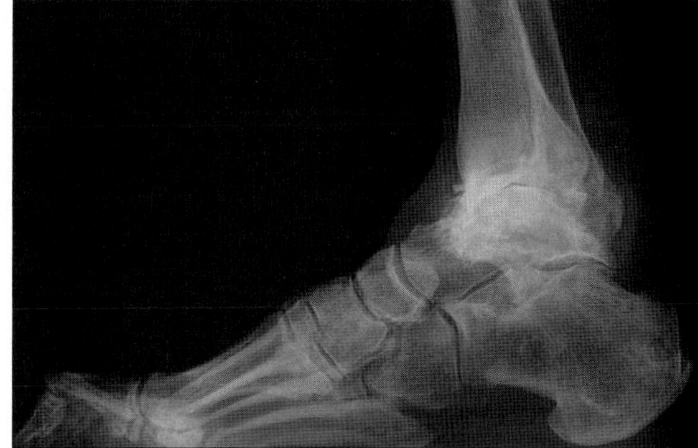

FIGURE 1

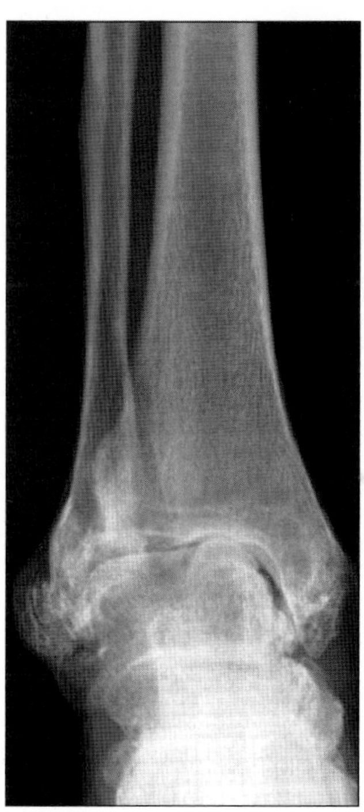

FIGURE 2

Surgical Anatomy

- Plantar approach to the calcaneus (Fig. 3)
  - Fat pad
  - Plantar fascia
  - Neurovascular structures (run medial to insertion area)
  - Figure 4 shows insertion area of nail (crosshairs) with plantar fat pad removed (Fig. 4A) and with plantar soft tissue removed (Fig. 4B)
- Anterior approach to the ankle (Fig. 5)
  - Extensor retinaculum
  - Anterior tibial and long extensor tendons
  - Neurovascular bundle
- Lateral approach to the subtalar joint (Fig. 6)
  - Peroneal tendons
  - Sinus tarsi

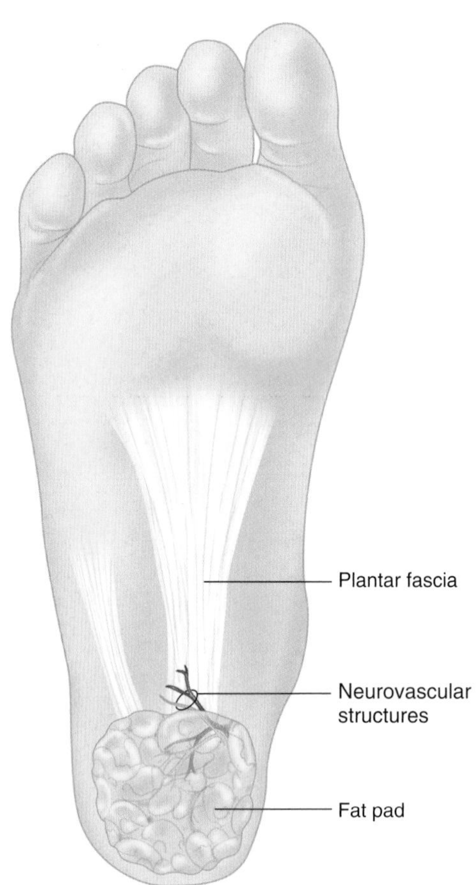

FIGURE 3

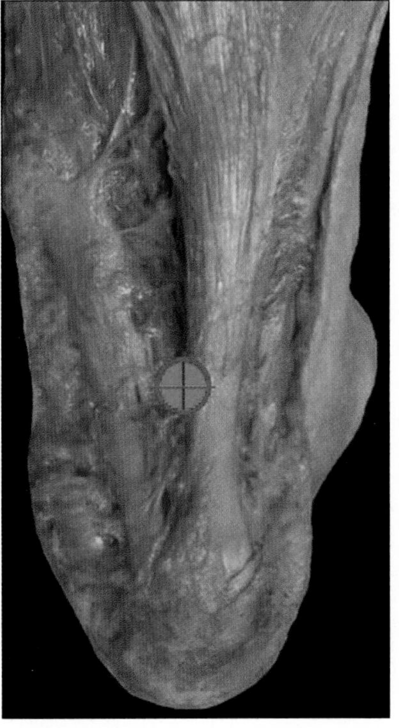
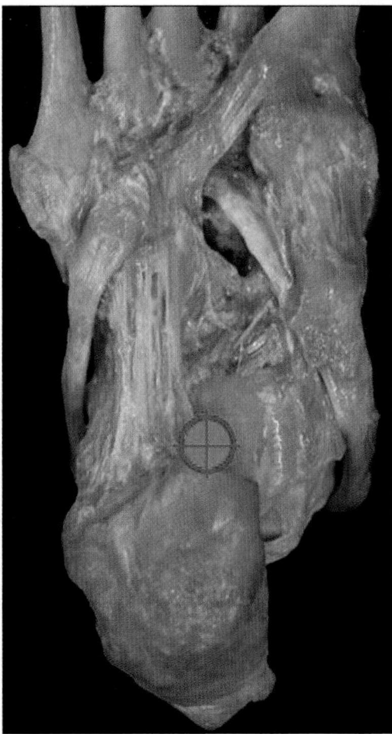

A B

FIGURE 4

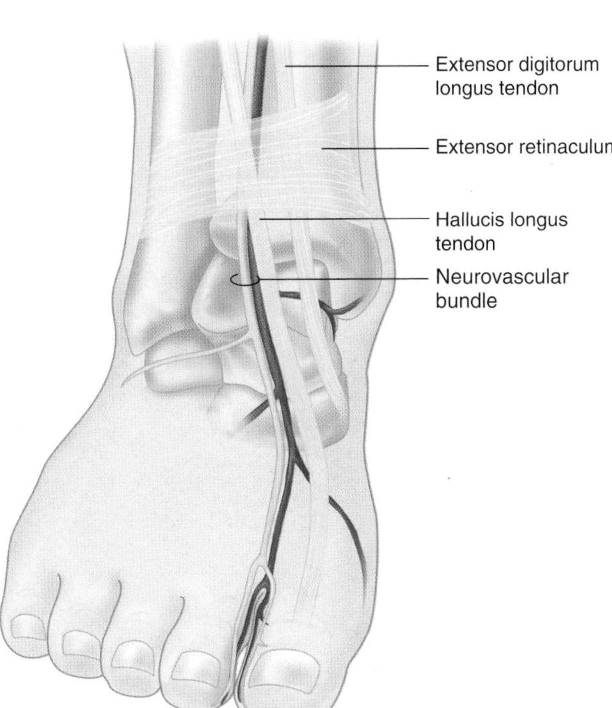

FIGURE 5

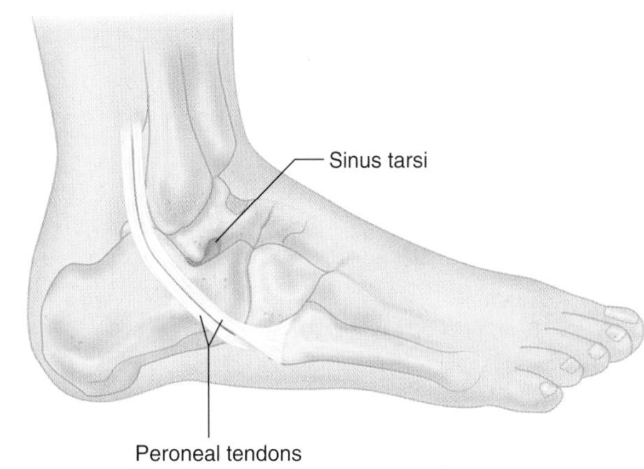

FIGURE 6

PEARLS

- *Positioning of heel at the edge of the operating table will facilitate surgery.*

Positioning

- Supine position
- Higher positioning of the operative lower leg on stable radiolucent cushion with the knee in approximately 40° of flexion.
- Tourniquet at the thigh
- C-arm, or better a fluoroscan, placed at the same side of the operated foot, to obtain easy fluoroscopic control during surgery
- Free draping of the whole limb

Portals/Exposures

ANTERIOR EXPOSURE OF ANKLE JOINT

- Landmarks
  - Palpate the lateral malleolus at the distal subcutaneous end of the fibula and the medial malleolus.
  - Identify the ankle joint line.
  - Identify the tendon of the musculus tibialis anterior.
- Skin incision
  - Make a 5- to 7-cm longitudinal incision in the middle over the distal tibia and ankle joint.
  - Identify the medial branch of the peroneal superficial nerve. Avoid any damage of it.
- Exposure (Fig. 7)
  - Incise the extensor retinaculum between the extensor hallucis longus and the tendon of musculus tibialis anterior.

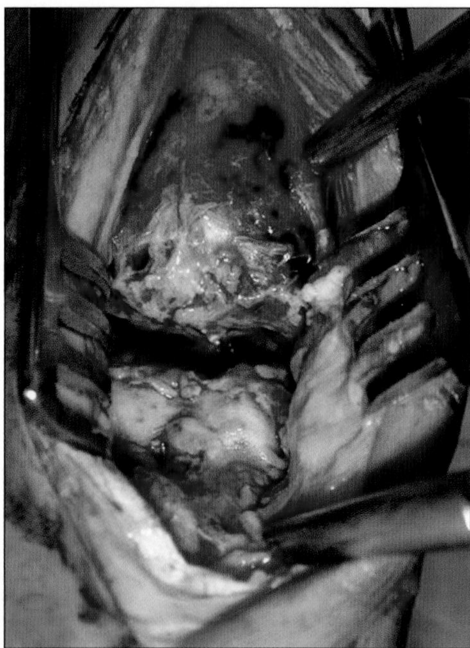

FIGURE 7

- Perform subperiosteal preparation of soft tissue with a rasp; take care to avoid vascular and neural structures.
- Perform arthrotomy.

LATERAL EXPOSURE OF SUBTALAR JOINT

- Landmarks
  - Palpate the lateral malleolus at the distal subcutaneous end of the fibula.
  - Identify the sinus tarsi by palpation.
  - Palpate the peroneal tendons.
- Skin incision
  - Make a short skin incision overlying the sinus tarsi anterior to the peroneal tendons.
  - Avoid any damage to peroneal tendons and sural nerve.
- Exposure (Fig. 8)
  - Perform sharp dissection of subcutaneous tissues until the sinus tarsi is visible.
  - The fatty tissues filling the sinus tarsi should be resected (or retracted anteriorly).
  - Perform arthrotomy and exposure of the subtalar joint.

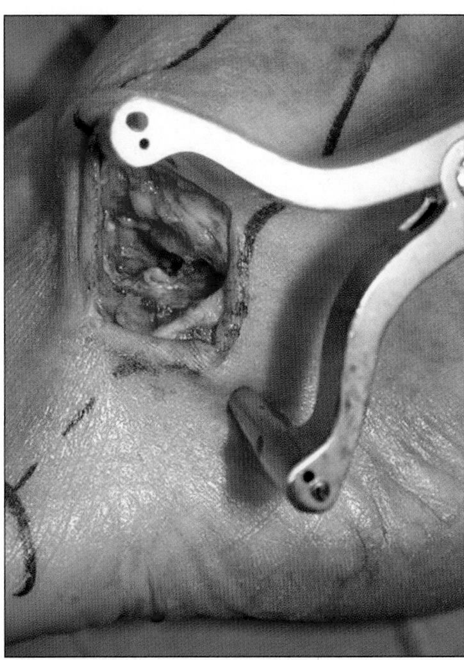

FIGURE 8

PEARLS

- *A distractor can be used to expose the ankle (see Fig. 5) and subtalar joints (see Fig. 6).*

PLANTAR APPROACH TO CALCANEUS

- Landmarks (Fig. 9)
  - Draw an imaginary line along the tibial shaft through the medial malleolus.
  - Draw an imaginary line through the center of the heel to the head of the second metatarsal.
- Skin incision
  - Make a 3-cm incision at the crossing point of the drawn lines.
- Exposure: prepare the entry point on the plantar site of the foot.
  - Make a sharp incision through the fat pad.
  - Make a longitudinal incision lateral to the medial part of the plantar fascia.
  - Perform blunt dissection of soft tissues to the plantar medial aspect of the calcaneus.

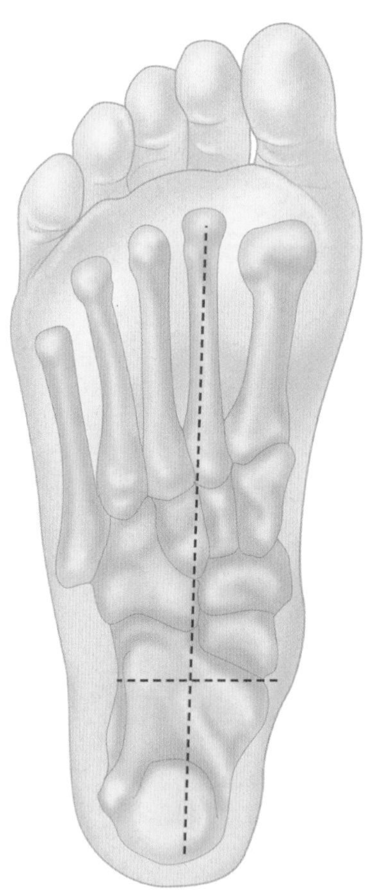

FIGURE 9

Procedure

Step 1: Débridement of Ankle and Subtalar Joints for Arthrodesis

- Complete removal of the articular cartilage, usually by using the curved chisel.
- If the subchondral bone appears sclerotic, multiple drill holes should be made in the joint surface.
- After removal of the joint spreader, the tibial, talar, and calcaneal bones should be mobile enough to fully correct the deformity.
- In the case of bone loss, a graft from the iliac crest or an allograft may be used.

Step 2: Insertion of Intramedullary Nail (Fig. 10)

- A guidewire is brought through the calcaneus and talus into the tibia under fluoroscopic control. The guidewire should be localized in the middle of the tibial intramedullary canal.
- Drill along the guidewire, and perform step-by-step enlargement of the drilling hole.
- Insert the nail with the support device manually into the medullary canal. Slight impaction may be used.
- Make a final check by fluoroscopy to ensure the correct positioning of the nail, especially the distal end, which should be located at the cortical side of the calcaneus.

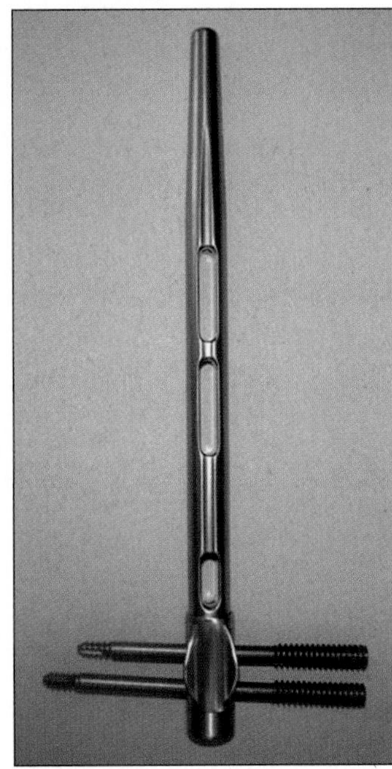

FIGURE 10

Step 3: Application of Compression and Fixation

- The calcaneal screw is percutaneously inserted, guided by the aiming devices.
- The compression frame is fixed by rods in the tibia.
- The desired tibiotalocalcaneal compression is applied.
- Tibial screws are placed in provided holes of the nail (Fig. 11).
- The compression frame is removed.
- A compression screw is inserted from plantar into the nail to get the calcaneal screws firmly fixed to the nail (Fig. 12).

Step 4

- Perform wound closure.
  - Interrupted absorbable 0 sutures for subcutaneous closure
  - Interrupted nonabsorbable 3-0 sutures for skin reapproximation
- Apply a dressing.
  - Compresses
  - Bandage
- Splint the foot.

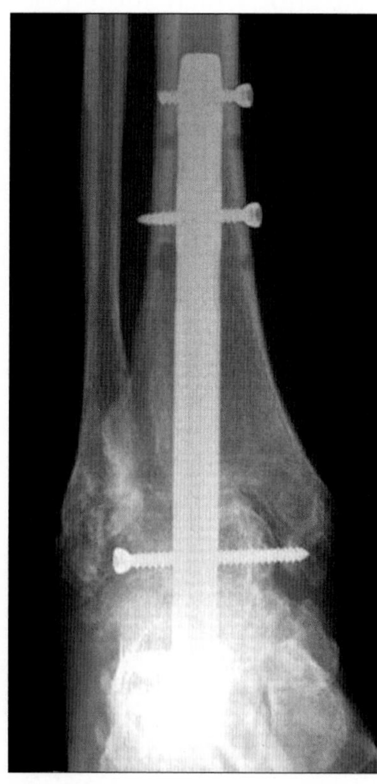

FIGURE 11

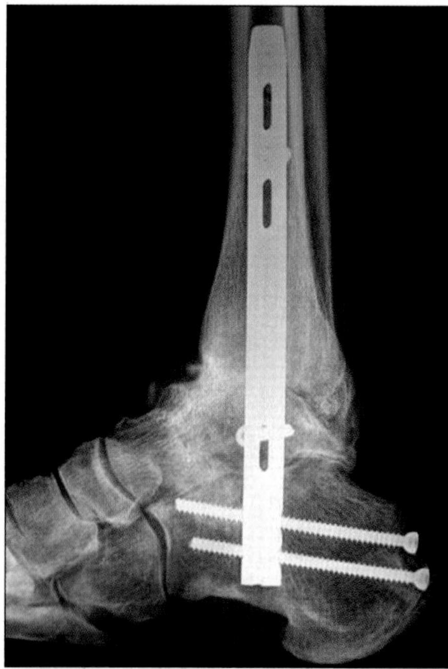

FIGURE 12

PEARLS

- *Antithrombotic socks are highly recommended to prevent swelling.*

Postoperative Care and Expected Outcomes

- Immobilize the foot in a splint until the wound is safely healed, usually for 2 weeks.
- Remove the skin suture 2–3 weeks after surgery.
- The patient should use a walking scotch cast or walker for another 8–16 weeks, until radiographically evident osseous consolidation has occurred.
- Weight bearing is allowed as tolerated, usually progressing to full weight bearing after 3 weeks.
- A rehabilitation program starts afterward, including drainage, gait training, and local measures.

Evidence

Anderson T, Linder L, Rydholm U, Montgomery F, Besjakov J, Carlsson A. Tibiotalocalcaneal arthrodesis as a primary procedure using a retrograde intramedullary nail: a retrospective study of 26 patients with rheumatoid arthritis. Acta Orthop. 2005;76:580-7.

This is a retrospective clinical study evaluating whether tibiotalocalcaneal arthrodesis is a suitable therapeutic option in patients with rheumatoid arthritis. Complications, functional outcome scores, and patient satisfaction were determined and radiographs were analyzed. (Level IV evidence)

Bennett GL, Cameron B, Njus G, Saunders M, Kay DB. Tibiotalocalcaneal arthrodesis: a biomechanical assessment of stability. Foot Ankle Int. 2005;26:530-6.

This controlled laboratory study includes biomechanical testing of four instrumentation techniques for tibiotalocalcaneal arthrodesis. (Level II evidence)

Caravaggi C, Cimmino M, Caruso S, Dalla Noce S. Intramedullary compressive nail fixation for the treatment of severe Charcot deformity of the ankle and rear foot. J Foot Ankle Surg. 2006;45:20-4.

Fourteen patients with diabetes and Charcot neuroarthropathy of the ankle were included in this clinical study. (Level III evidence)

Chiodo CP, Acevedo JI, Sammarco VJ, Parks BG, Boucher HR, Myerson MS, Schon LC. Intramedullary rod fixation compared with blade-plate-and-screw fixation for tibiotalocalcaneal arthrodesis: a biomechanical investigation. J Bone Joint Surg [Am]. 2003;85:2425-8.

This laboratory controlled study compared the two methods for fixation in tibiotalocalcaneal arthrodesis. (Level II evidence)

Eingartner C, Weise K. Revision of failed ankle arthrodesis. Oper Orthop Traumatol. 2005;17:481-501.

A retrospective clinical study including 16 patients with an average follow-up of 10.8 months. (Level IV evidence)

Goebel M, Gerdesmeyer L, Muckley T, Schmitt-Sody M, Diehl P, Stienstra J, Bühren V. Retrograde intramedullary nailing in tibiotalocalcaneal arthrodesis: a short-term, prospective study. J Foot Ankle Surg. 2006;45:98-106.

This prospective clinical study included 29 patients suffering from posttraumatic or postinflammatory arthrosis of both the subtalar and ankle joints. (Level IV evidence)

Hammett R, Hepple S, Forster B, Winson I. Tibiotalocalcaneal (hindfoot) arthrodesis by retrograde intramedullary nailing using a curved locking nail: the results of 52 procedures. Foot Ankle Int. 2005;26:810-5.

This is a retrospective clinical study including patients with combined ankle and subtalar arthritis or complex hindfoot deformities. All patients were controlled at follow-up averaging 34 months. (Level IV evidence)

Hopgood P, Kumar R, Wood PLR. Ankle arthrodesis for failed total ankle replacement. J Bone Joint Surg [Br]. 2006;88:1032-8.

In this clinical study, 23 patients with failed total ankle replacements were respectively reviewed. Ten patients were treated with a tibiotalocalcaneal nail. (Level IV evidence)

Mendicino RW, Catanzariti AR, Saltrick KR, Dombek MF, Tullis BL, Statler TK, Johnson BM. Tibiotalocalcaneal arthrodesis with retrograde intramedullary nailing. J Foot Ankle Surg. 2004;43:82-6.

This is a retrospective clinical study including 20 procedures. The average follow-up was 19.8 months. All postoperative complications were registered and analyzed. (Level IV evidence)

Niinimäki TT, Klemola TM, Leppilahti JI. Tibiotalocalcaneal arthrodesis with a compressive retrograde intramedullary nail: a report of 34 consecutive patients. Foot Ankle Int. 2007;28:431-4.

This is a retrospective clinical study including 34 patients with severe malalignment or arthrosis of the hindfoot. The mean follow-up was 24 months. (Level IV evidence)

Pelton K, Hofer JK, Thordarson DB. Tibiotalocalcaneal arthrodesis using a dynamically locked retrograde intramedullary nail. Foot Ankle Int. 2006;27:759-63.

A clinical study with 33 ankles reporting the dynamic retrograde intramedullary nailing as a good stabilization method. (Level IV evidence)

Pinzur MS, Noonan T. Ankle arthrodesis with a retrograde femoral nail for Charcot ankle arthropathy. Foot Ankle Int. 2005;26:545-9.

This clinical study including nine consecutive patients with type II diabetes and Charcot ankle arthropathy describes the midterm results after ankle arthrodesis.

Plaass C, Knupp M, Barg A, Hintermann B. Anterior double plating for rigid fixation of isolated tibiotalar arthrodesis. Foot Ankle Int. 2009 (submitted)

A prospective clinical study addressing the reliability of the anterior double plating system for isolated tibiotalar arthrodesis. The patient cohort of 29 patients includes nine ankles that failed total ankle replacement. (Level IV evidence)

Zwipp H, Grass R. Ankle arthrodesis after failed joint replacement. Oper Orthop Traumatol. 2005;17:518-33.

Four patients with loosened or infected total ankle replacement were treated with ankle fusion using tricortical bone grafts. (Level IV evidence)

PROCEDURE 32

Realignment Surgery for Valgus Ankle Osteoarthritis

Geert I. Pagenstert, Markus Knupp, Victor Valderrabano, and Beat Hintermann

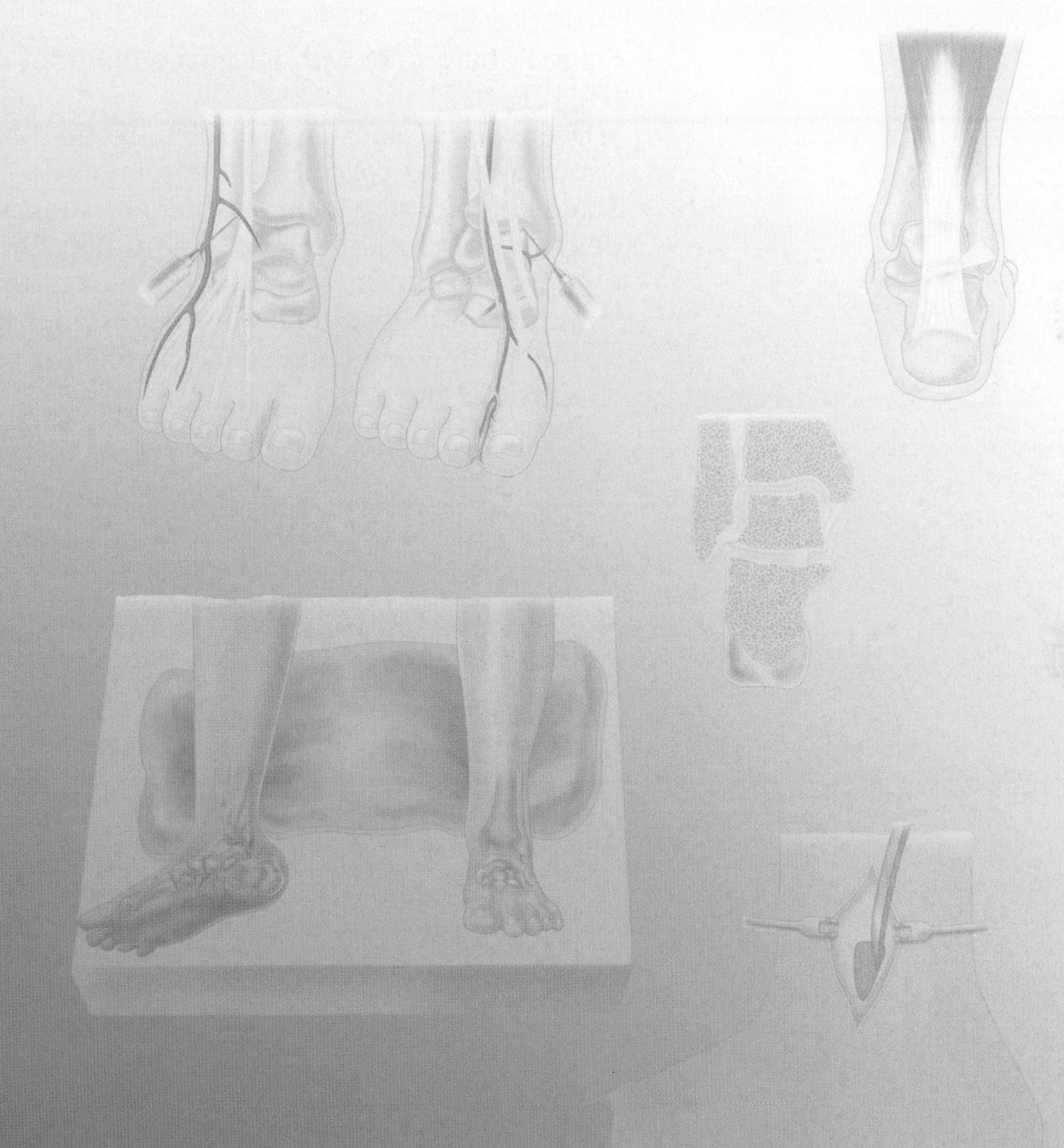

Indications

- Active patients with lateral ankle joint degeneration associated with valgus malalignment
- Lateral osteochondral lesion of the tibia or talus associated with valgus malalignment
- Depends on stage and extent of deformity
  - Stage I: deformity confined to the ankle (Fig. 1)
    - Lateral ankle joint collapse: medial closing wedge osteotomy of the distal tibia
    - Fibula malunion: derotation-lengthening osteotomy
  - Stage II: deformity with advanced hindfoot valgus (Fig. 2)
    - Heel still in valgus after tibial correction: added medial sliding calcaneus osteotomy
  - Stage III: deformity includes forefoot (supination deformity)–induced hindfoot valgus (Fig. 3)
    - Added flexion osteotomy/arthrodesis of the first ray, repair/augmentation of the posterior tibial tendon, and delta and spring ligaments; triceps release, as needed

Pitfalls

- *Loss of more than half of tibiotalar joint surface (plain radiographs, magnetic resonance imaging, arthroscopy) may be treated with ankle arthroplasty or fusion.*
- *Lack of compliance with the postoperative non–weight-bearing program caused by neurologic disease or poor health status may be treated by ankle arthrodesis.*
- *Insufficiency of the whole deltoid ligament complex may result in tibiotalar subluxation; such an unstable valgus ankle should be treated by ankle fusion.*

Controversies

- Although recovery of the joint surface from Outerbridge grade IV to I–II has been demonstrated by arthroscopy and biopsies (Takakura et al., 1999), further degeneration may occur over the years (Pagenstert et al., 2007).
- Inflammatory, systemic joint disease incorporating the ankle is usually treated with ankle arthroplasty.

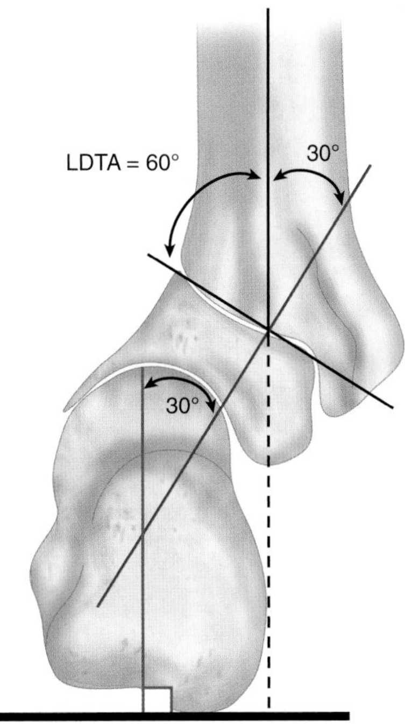

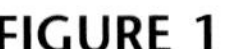

FIGURE 1

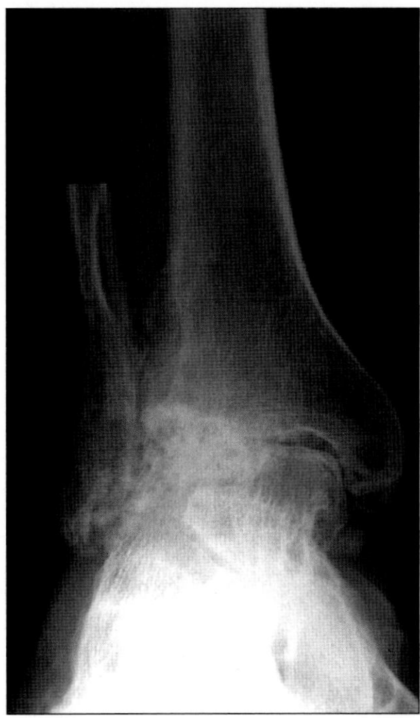

FIGURE 2

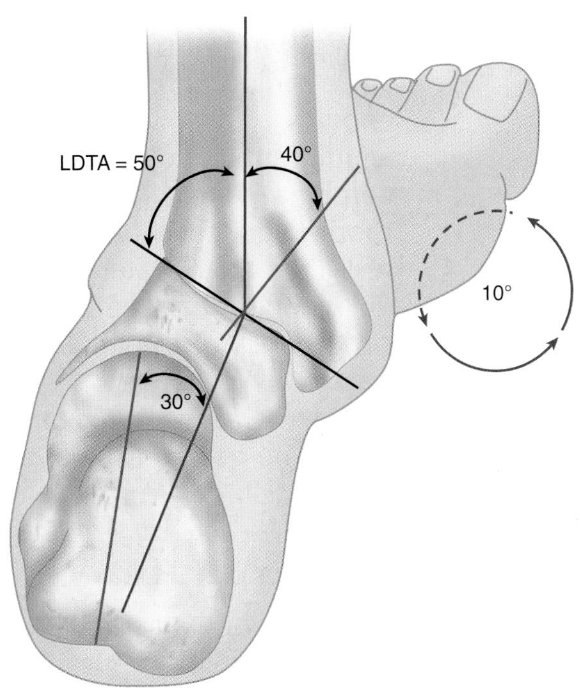

FIGURE 3

Treatment Options

- Resurfacing of destroyed articular surfaces by total ankle replacement (TAR) may allow for earlier weight bearing (Hintermann et al., 2004), but may not fully correct the deformity and instability (Wood and Deakin, 2003) and thus may fail. It may also limit sports activities in younger patients (Wood and Deakin, 2003; Valderrabano et al., 2006).
- Ankle fusion may enable high activity, but compensatory movements of adjacent foot joints will cause degenerative osteoarthritis in 44% of patients after 7 years (Takakura et al., 1999) and in 100% after 20 years (Fuchs et al., 2003).

Examination/Imaging

- While the patient is standing, perform a thorough clinical investigation of both lower extremities to assess:
  - Alignment
  - Deformities
  - Foot position
  - Muscular atrophy
  - Muscular function (particularly of posterior tibial muscle by heel rise tests)
- While the patient is sitting with free-hanging feet, perform an assessment of:
  - Extent to which a present deformity is correctable
  - Preserved joint motion of the ankle and subtalar joints
  - Ligament stability of the ankle and subtalar joints with anterior drawer and tilt tests
  - Supination and eversion power (e.g., function of posterior tibial and peroneus brevis muscles)
- Perform a radiographic evaluation of the deformity using standing weight-bearing plain radiographs centered on the ankle (anterior-posterior lower leg with mortise ankle (Fig. 4), dorsoplantar foot, lateral lower leg with whole foot and ankle)
- Obtain a hindfoot alignment view (Saltzman and El-Khoury, 1995) (Fig. 5).
- Radiographs of the whole leg are used for evaluation of alignment and preoperative planning. If no knee or hip symptoms or deformities are present, loaded ankle radiographs including the lower leg may be enough.
- Scintigraphy and computed tomography (CT) or the combination of both may be used to visualize morphologic and biologic bone pathologies restricted to the lateral ankle compartment (Fig. 6).
- CT scanning may be beneficial to assess the congruency of the fibula to the tibia after ankle fracture.
- Magnetic resonance imaging may help to further assess the posterior tibial tendon if its function remains clinically unclear.

Surgical Anatomy

- In white populations, the anterior tibial joint surface angle is in mild valgus (3° ± 3°) and perpendicular to the load axis, which runs down to the heel contact point with the ground (Isman and Inman, 1968; Paley, 2005; Fig. 7).

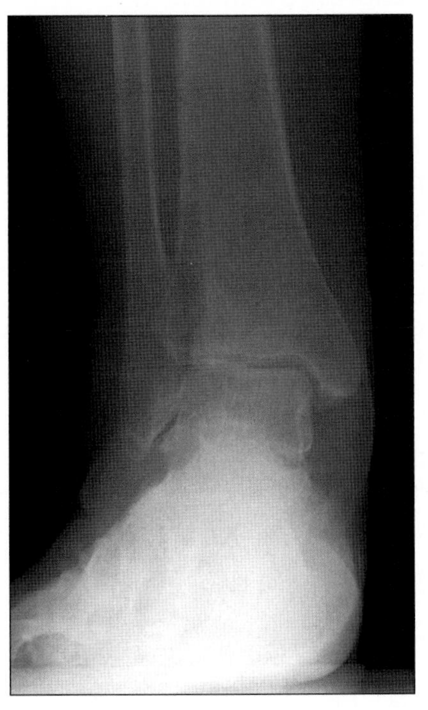

FIGURE 4

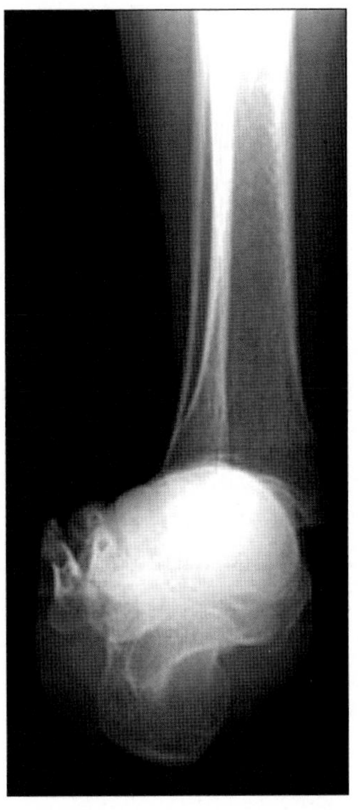

FIGURE 5

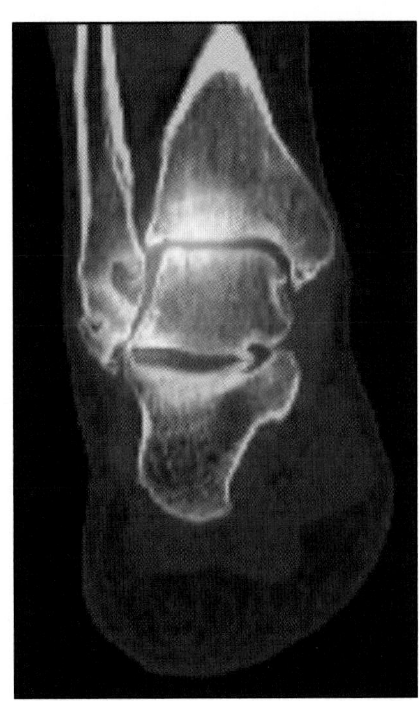

FIGURE 6

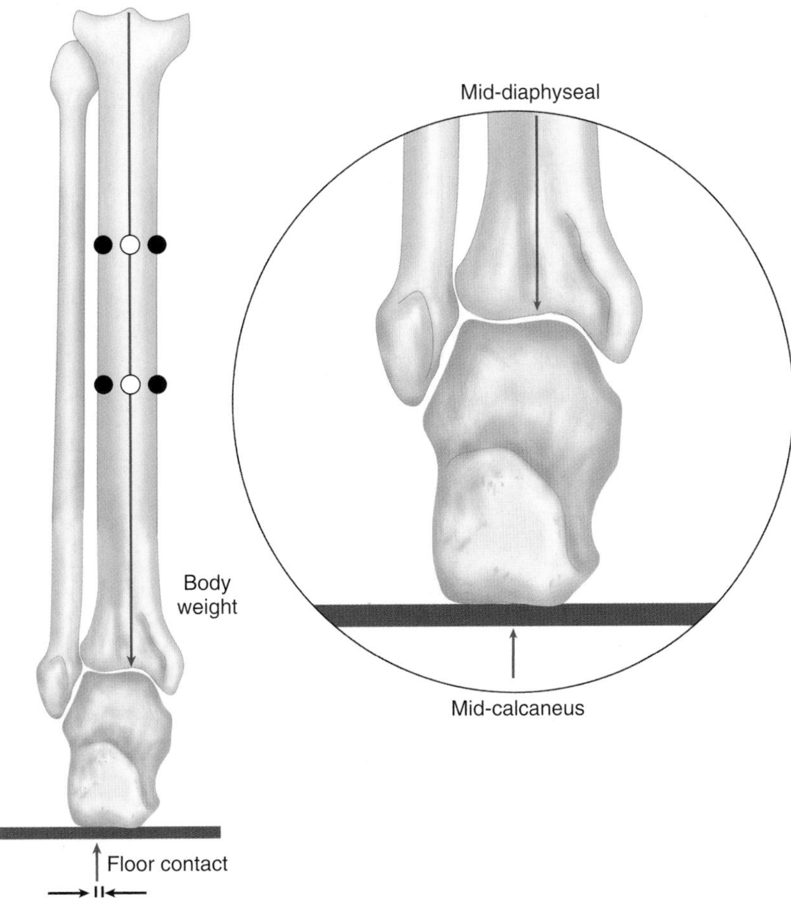

FIGURE 7

- The aim of surgical correction is to unload the osteoarthritic lateral tibiotalar and talofibular joints (Fig. 8A); an overcorrection to mild varus (max. 5°) is attempted.
- Shifting the heel contact point with the ground from the lateral to the medial site of the ankle will unload the collapsed tibiotalar joint (Takakura et al., 1995), thereby restoring congruency of the tibiotalar joint (Fig. 8B) (Pagenstert et al., 2007).
- The amount of distal tibia and heel deformity defines the sites of correction: deformity confined to the distal tibia can be corrected by tibia osteotomy alone (see Fig. 8B). With excessive heel valgus (Fig. 8C), additional calcaneus osteotomy is needed to shift the heel contact point medially to the mid-diaphyseal tibial axis (Fig. 8D).

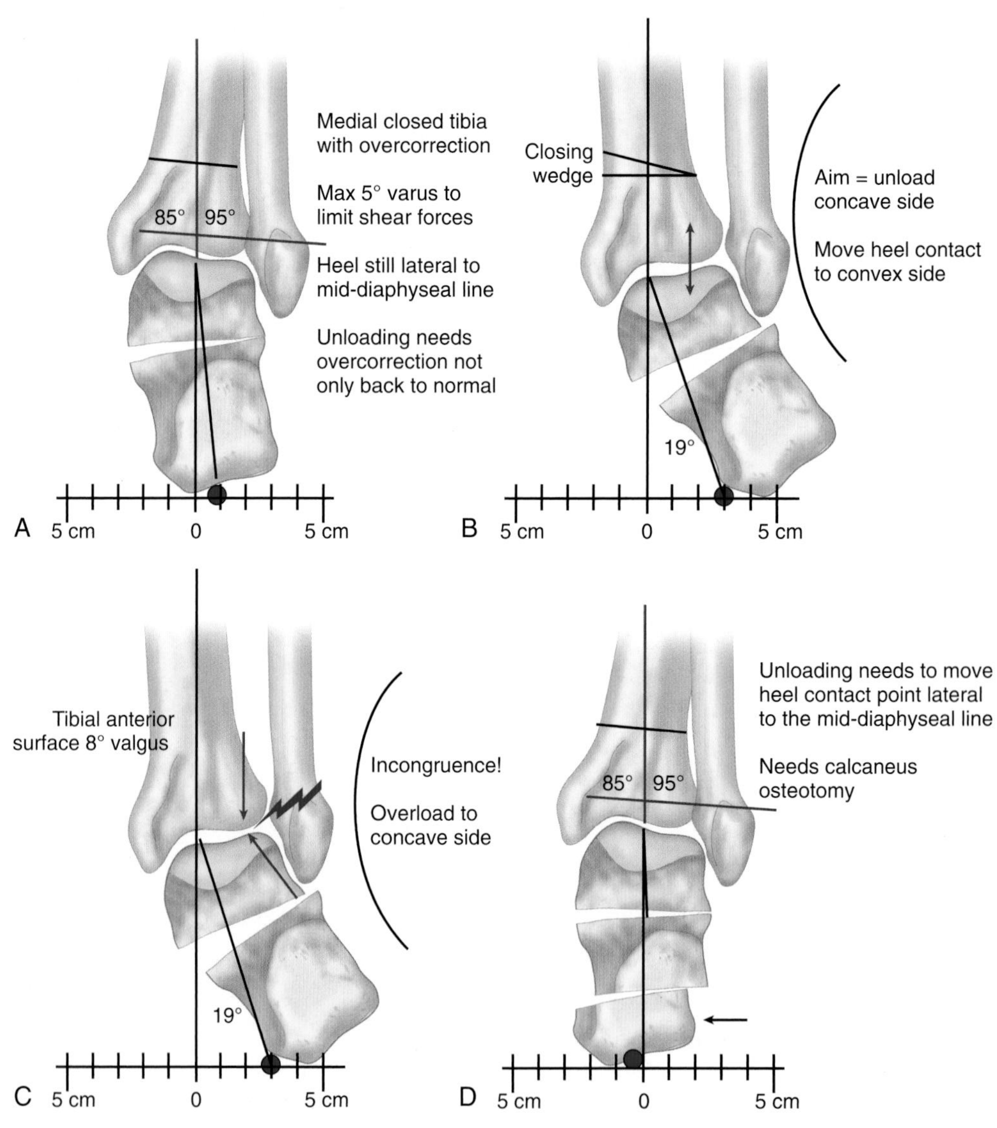

FIGURE 8

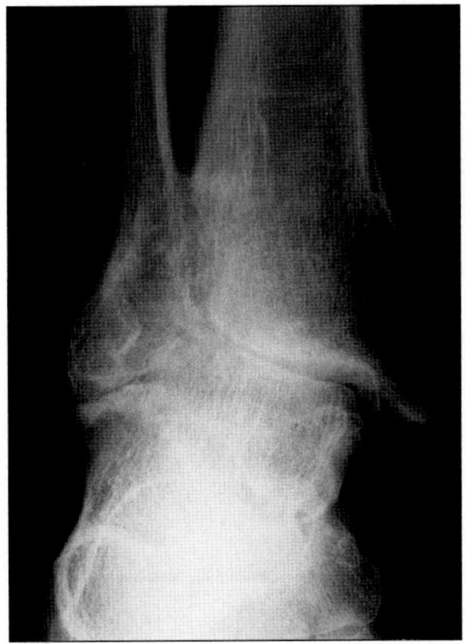

FIGURE 9

- After ankle fracture, malunion of fibula with shortening and external rotation may be the underlying cause of the valgus deformity (Pagenstert et al., 2007; Fig. 9).

Positioning

- Supine position (Fig. 10)
- Thigh tourniquet
- Pad under lower leg for elevation
- Heel flush with the operating table

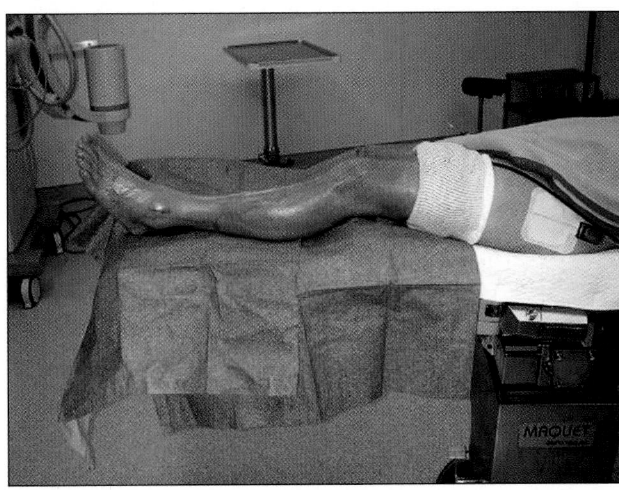

FIGURE 10

Pearls

- *Subperiosteal exposure at the osteotomy level helps to preserve soft tissues; in particular, Hohmann retractors will protect the flexor tendons during osteotomy.*
- *In a stage III osteoarthritic ankle in which TAR may become realistic in the near future, an alternative anterior approach is advised; TAR can then be used for future repair.*

Pitfalls

- *Damage to neurovascular structures and flexor tendons*

Portals/Exposures

- Arthroscopy is done using a slightly anteromedial central portal; an additional anterolateral or anteromedial portal is used to insert instruments.
- For tibial osteotomy, a medial skin incision is made directly over the distal tibial metaphysis (Fig. 11A–D).
  - The saphenous vein and nerve run posteromedial to the incision and usually do not hinder a direct bone approach.
  - Soft tissues are retracted en bloc with a retractor (Fig. 11E).
- For calcaneal osteotomy, a curved lateral skin incision is performed just posterior to the peroneal tendons (Fig. 12A–D).

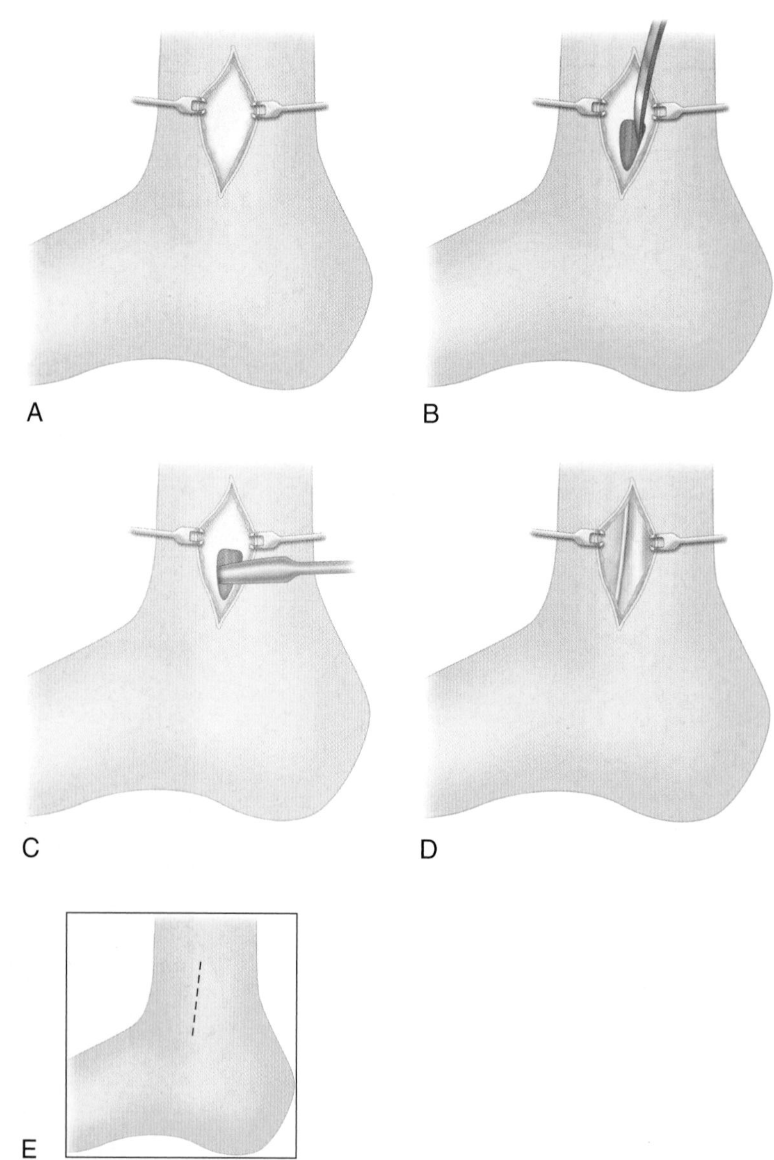

FIGURE 11

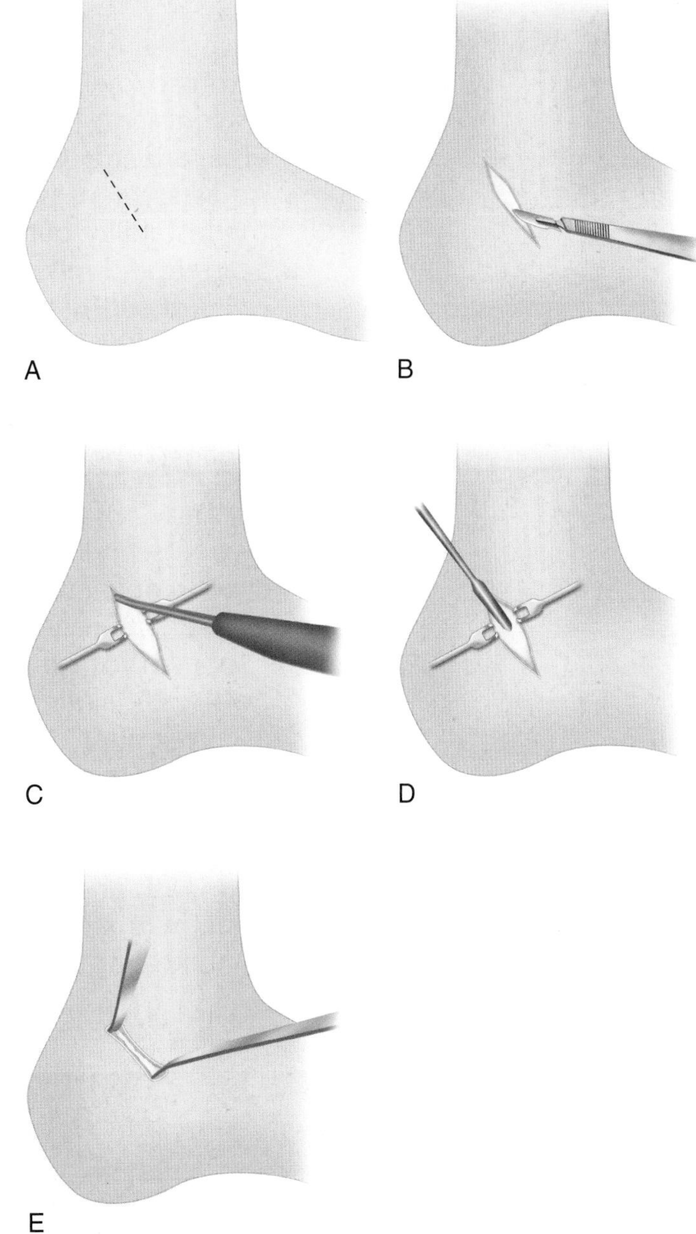

FIGURE 12

- The sural nerve is identified and retracted anteriorly.
- Dissection is continued straight to bone.
- Hohmann retractors are placed around the tuber to protect the soft tissues during saw osteotomy (Fig. 12E).

Procedure

Step 1: Ankle Arthroscopy

- Arthroscopy is done at the beginning of surgical realignment; Figure 13 shows an arthroscopic view of a cartilage lesion of the lateral ankle.
- An assessment is made of cartilage, ligaments, and the instability pattern.
- Scarred and inflammatory soft tissues are shaved in cases of soft tissue impingement.
- Osteophytes are débrided in cases of impingement or restricted range of motion.
- Microfracturing is done in cases of circumscribed confined chondral lesions.

Step 2: Tibial Osteotomy

- Two Kirschner wires (K-wires) are inserted under fluoroscopic control to guide the saw blade.
  - They are inserted perpendicular to the cortical bone, thus running typically slightly distally (Fig. 14A–C), aiming for direct contact of the medial cortex after closing the osteotomy.
  - A goniometer may be used.
- Osteotomy is done while following the K-wires with the saw blade (Fig. 15A); the wedge is mobilized (Fig. 15B) and removed (Fig. 15C).
- Bone matrix (e.g., TBX) may be used to improve bone healing (Fig. 15D).

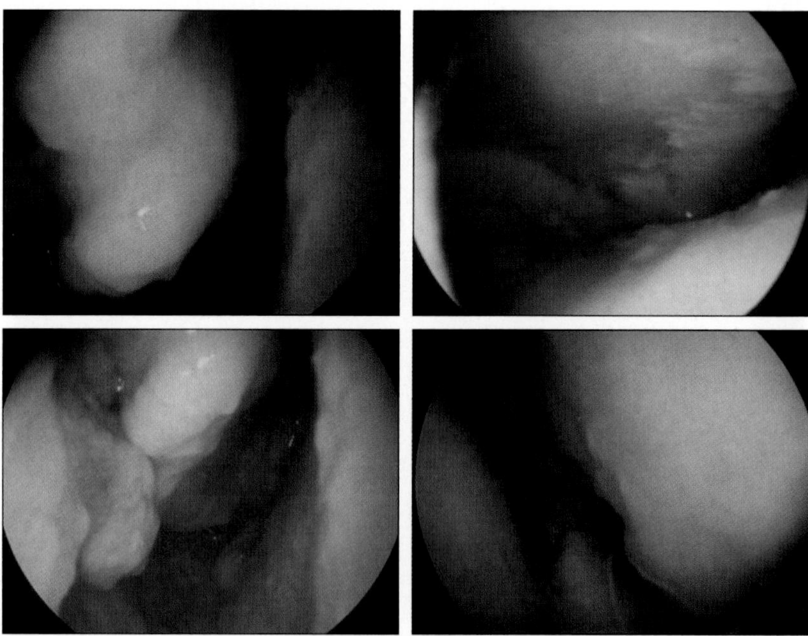

FIGURE 13

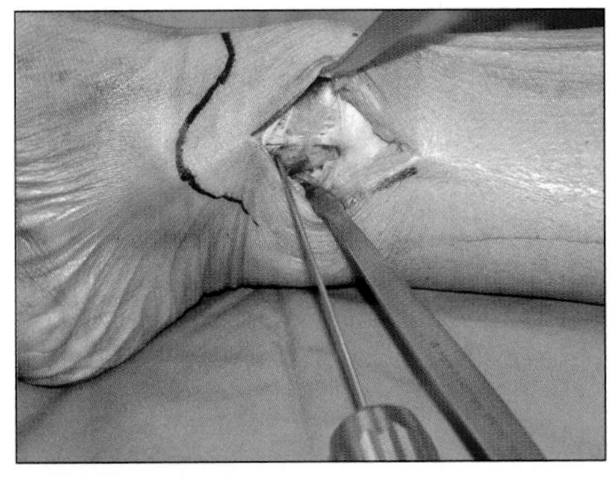
A

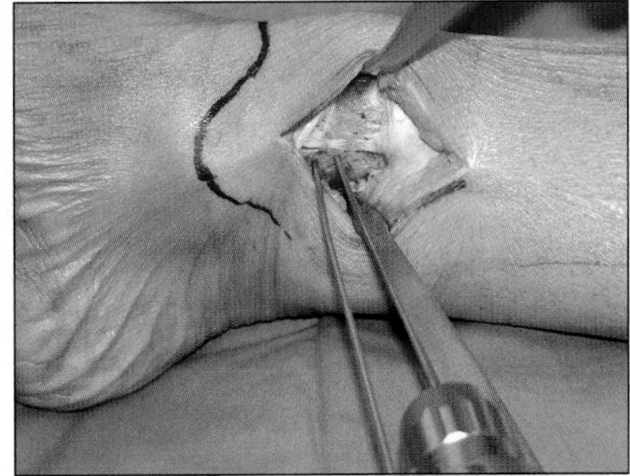
B

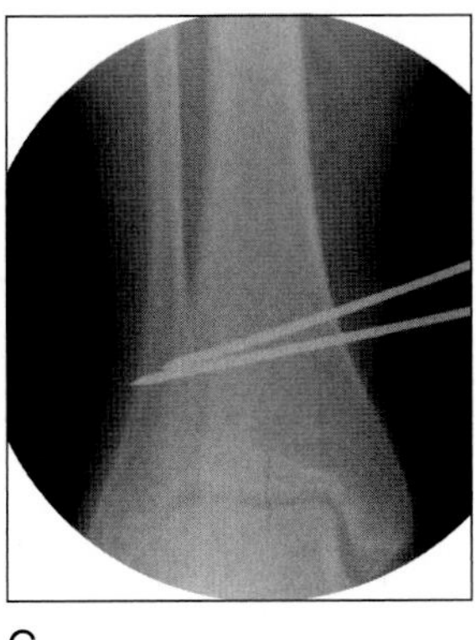
C

FIGURE 14

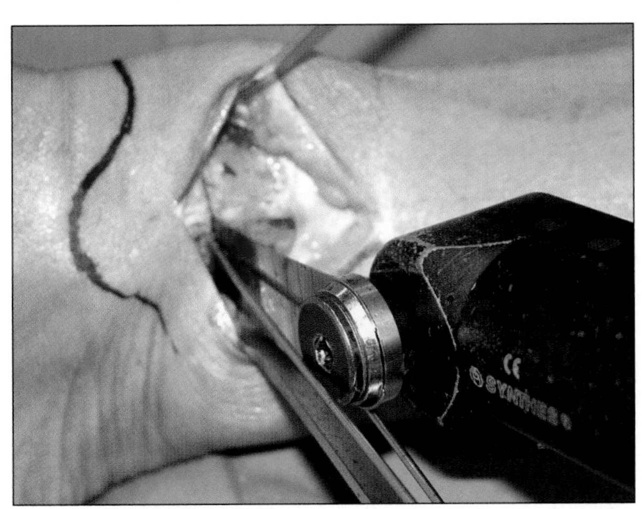

A

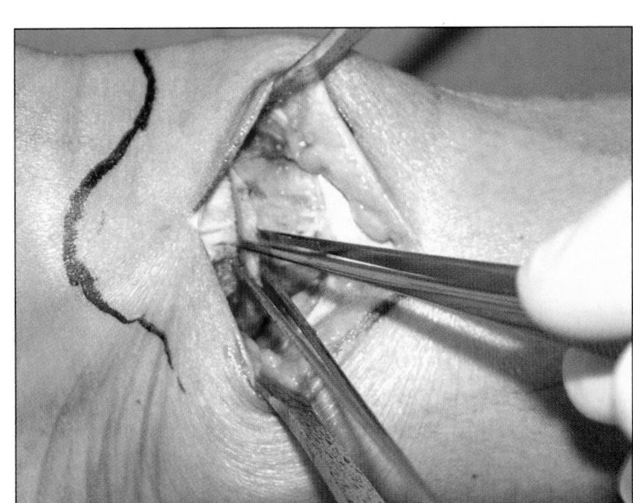
B

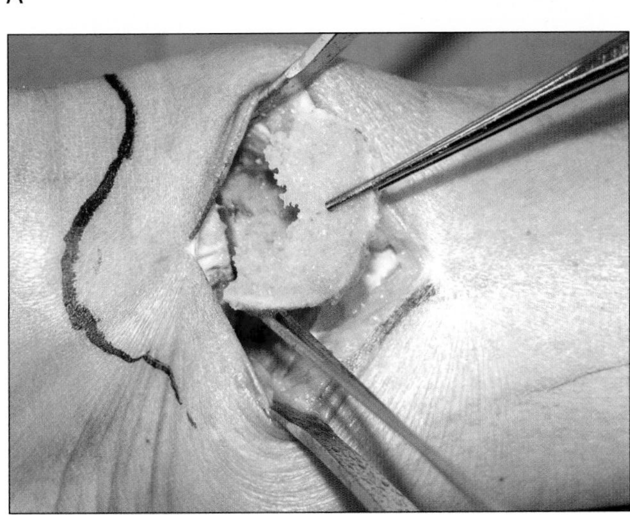
C

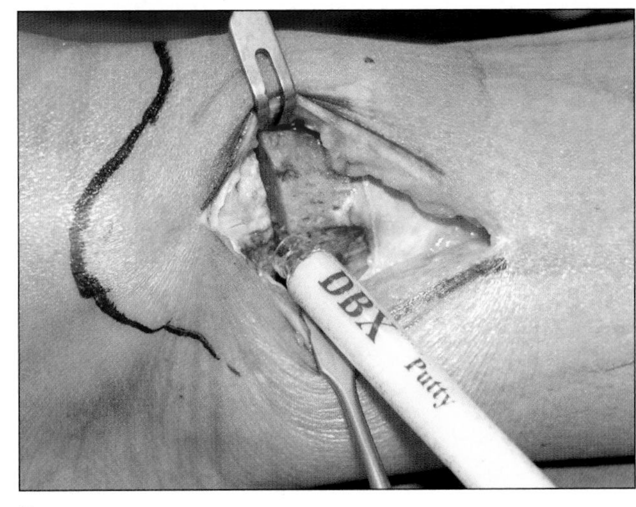

D

FIGURE 15

- The lateral cortex at the tip of the wedge is preserved to enhance stability of fixation and to use it as a hinge to translate the heel contact point to the convex side of the deformity. The osteotomy is slowly closed by manual compression.
- An anatomically shaped plate providing angular stability by locking screws is used (Fig. 16A).
  - First, the distal fragment is fixed (Fig. 16B and 16C).
  - Then, the osteotomy is closed by varus stress to the foot and/or ankle using a compression device on the distal plate, which is then fixed to the proximal fragment (Fig. 16D).
  - Oblique screw insertion may provide additional compression to the closed osteotomy.

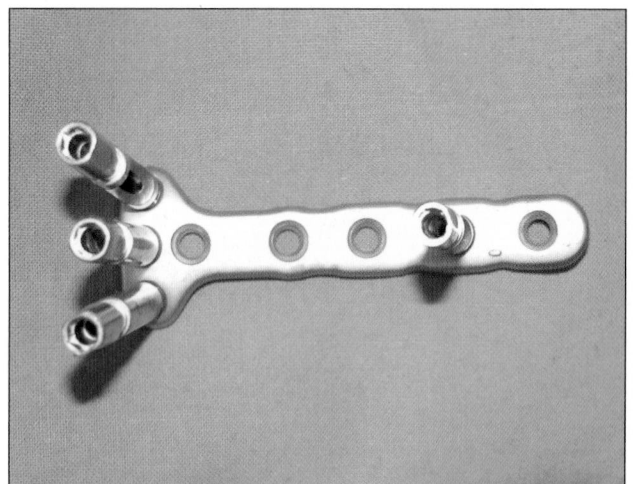

A

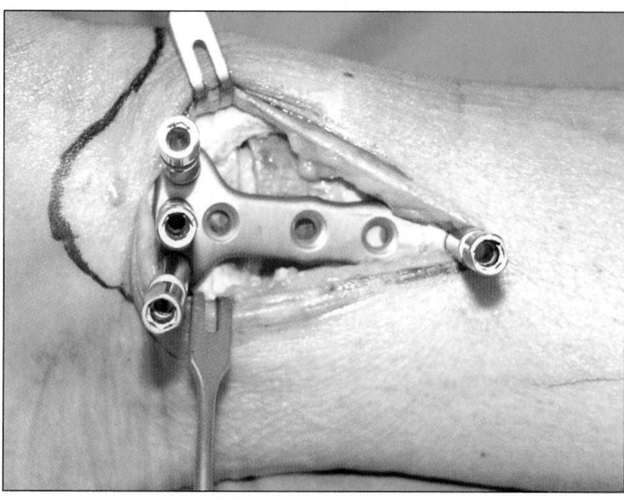

B

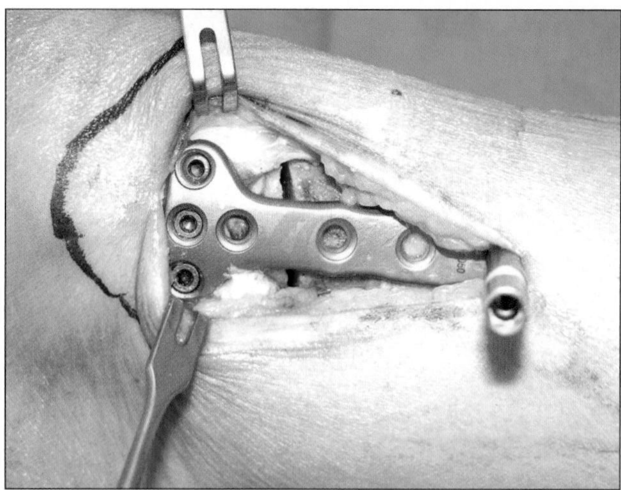

C

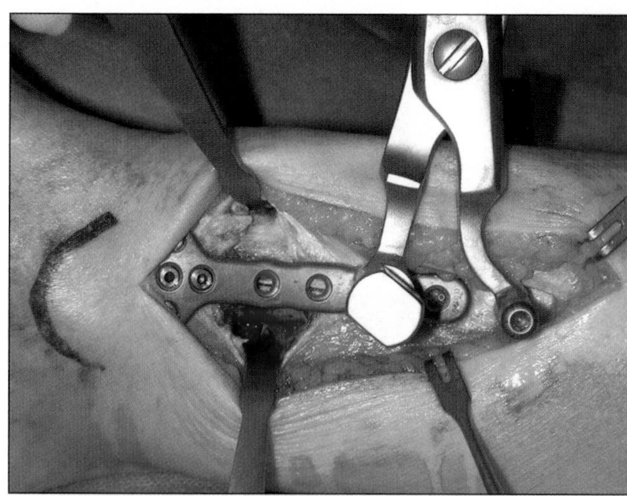

D

FIGURE 16

- Radiographs are then taken to confirm the overall position of the osteotomy and implant (Fig. 17).

- The internal fixation is finished (Fig. 18A–C), and the wound closed by interrupted sutures (Fig. 19).

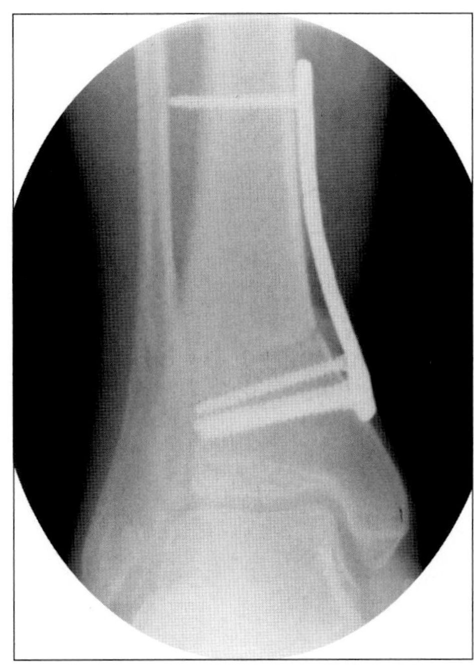

FIGURE 17

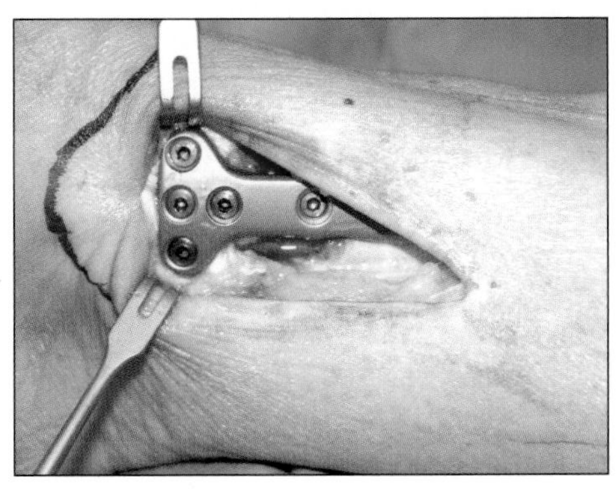

A

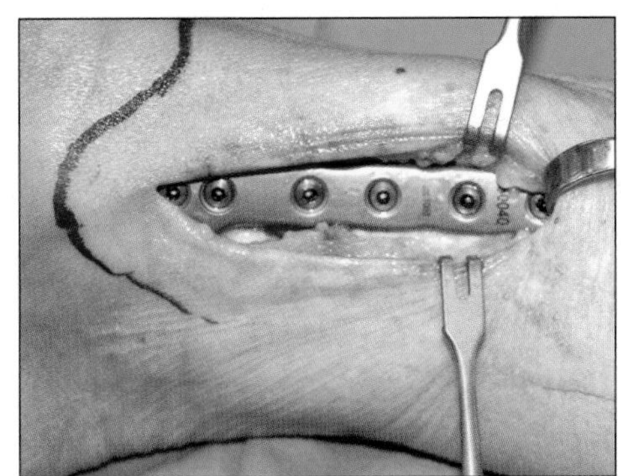

B

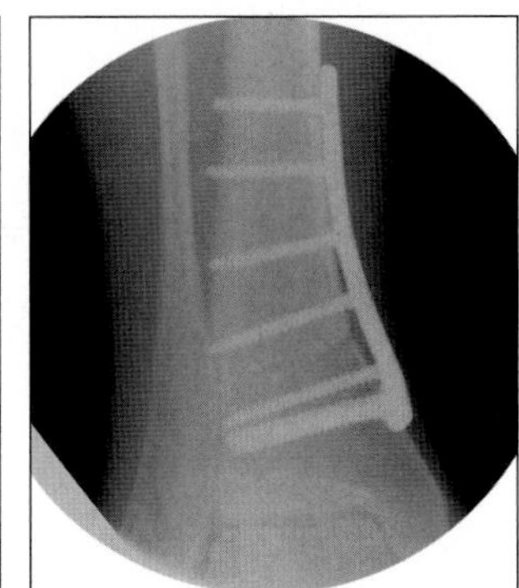

C

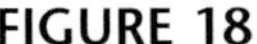

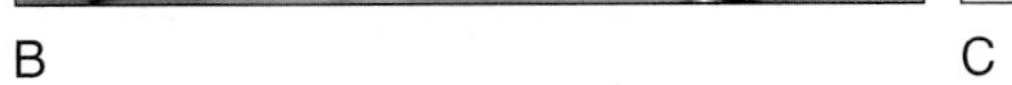

FIGURE 18

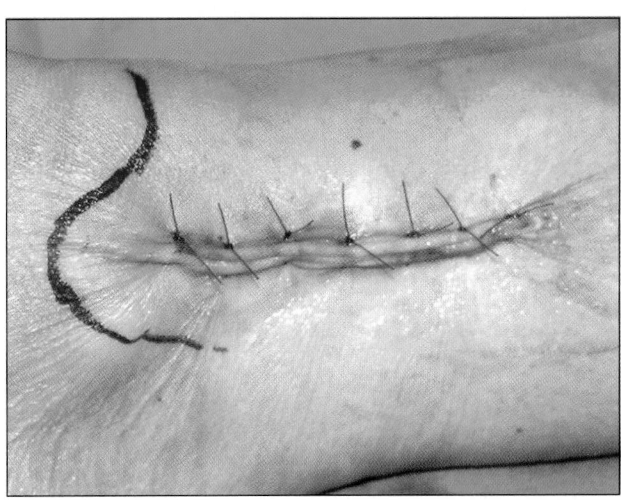

FIGURE 19

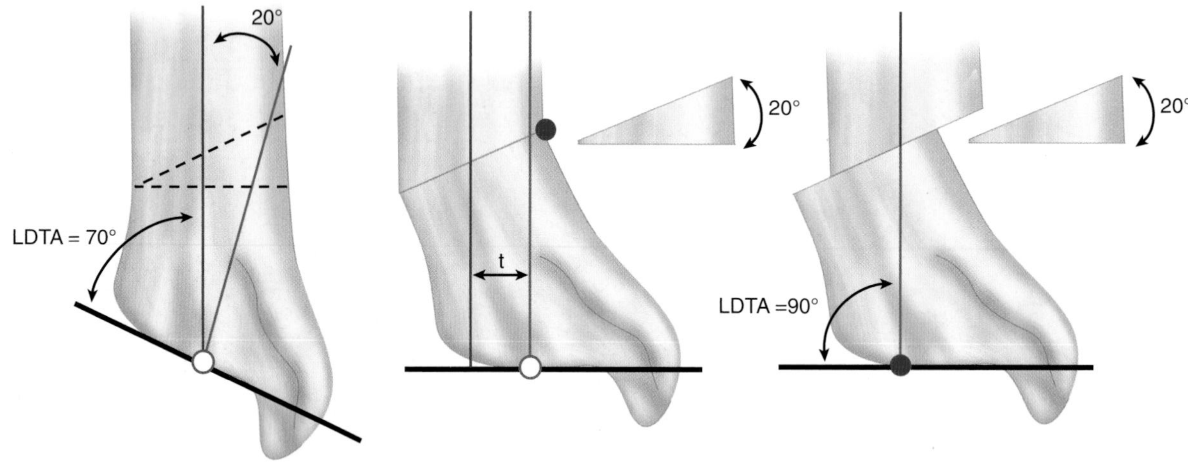

FIGURE 20

PEARLS

- *In tibia closing wedge osteotomy with a base of more than 10 mm thickness, closing of the osteotomy may cause relevant zigzag deformity of the distal tibia. In such cases, the lateral cortex is not preserved to allow adjustment by translation of the distal tibial fragment (Fig. 20). Usually translation is not necessary in wedges with smaller than a 10-mm base.*
- *The intact fibula does not hinder isolated tibial correction (Fig. 21A and 21B).*
- *A collapsed lateral malleolar gutter is usually decompressed by closing the medial tibial wedge (see Fig. 21B).*
- *Sagittal plane deformity of the distal tibial joint surface can be addressed by adding an anterior closing wedge osteotomy to correct the flexion deformity and a posterior closing wedge osteotomy to correct the extension deformity. The rotational center of the ankle in lateral view should be in line with the mid-diaphyseal axis of the tibia. Otherwise, translational adjustment has to be done.*

Controversies

- Mild shortening of the leg occurs with a tibia medial closing wedge osteotomy. However, usually this shortening is less than 1 cm and is not felt by the patient.
- Shortening of the medial tibia by the closing wedge osteotomy will theoretically decrease the tension of the posterior tibial tendon, which is often already impaired in valgus ankle arthritis. Re-evaluation of the heel, posterior tibial tendon, and forefoot with a heightened index of suspicion has to be done to indicate calcaneus and tendon dysfunction.

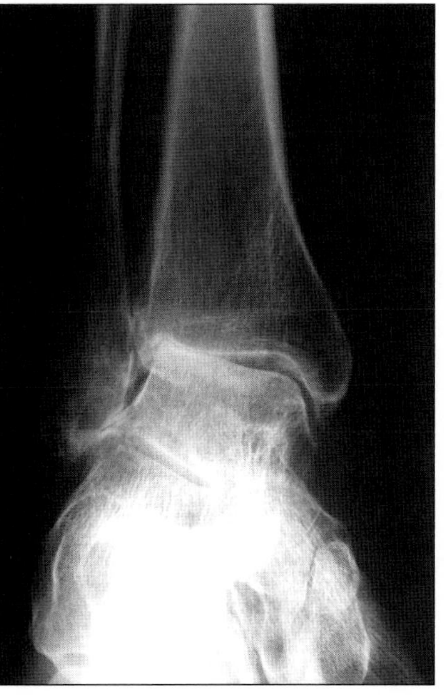
A

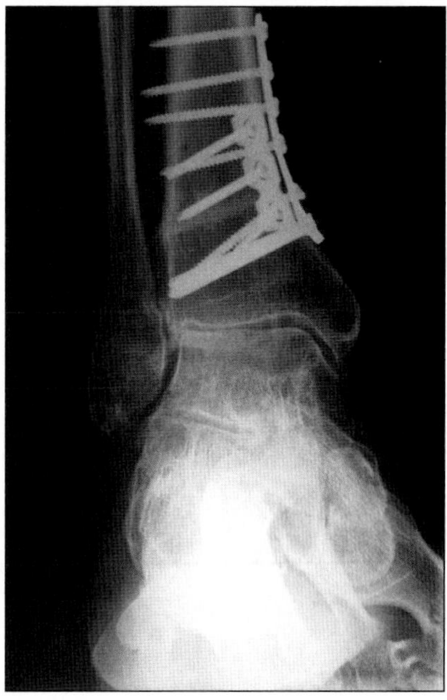
B

FIGURE 21

PEARLS

- *At times, scar tissue at the anterior syndesmosis has to be débrided or cut off the tibia to facilitate manipulation of the distal fibula fragment. A syndesmosis screw may be necessary.*
- *The correct rotation and length can be verified under fluoroscopy by leveling the small malleolar joint corner at the fibula with the tibia in mortise view.*

Step 3: Lateral Approach with Fibula Osteotomy

- In some instances, there is no talofibular impingement, as is typically the case after malunited ankle fractures. A lateral opening wedge osteotomy is thus preferred to preserve the ankle congruency, or to correct the position of the fibula (Fig. 22).
- The fibula is approached with a longitudinal lateral skin incision. Potential branches of the superficial peroneal nerve are retracted.
- The distal tibia is exposed by further preparation anteriorly to the fibula.

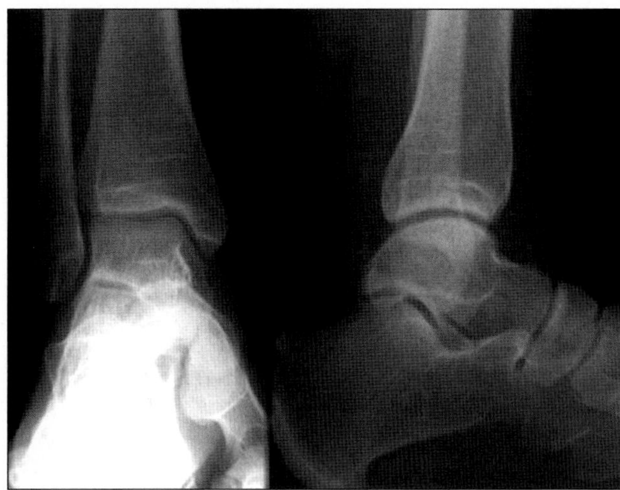

FIGURE 22

- To lengthen the fibula, two K-wires are inserted to mark the horizontal cuts of the Z-shaped osteotomy of the fibula.
  - Then, the distal horizontal cut is done anterior and the proximal horizontal cut is done posterior.
  - The vertical cut is usually 2 cm longer than the planned lengthening to assure a 2-cm overlap.
- To rotate the fibula, a oblique cut from dorsally-proximally to anteriorly-distally is done, which allows rotation, shortening, or lengthening of the distal fibula.
- For correction of the tibia, an incomplete cut is done by a saw and the osteotomy is opened as desired (Fig. 23A). A bone wedge is inserted, and stability is achieved by plate fixation (Fig. 23B).
- The fibula is fixed using one or two lag screws and an appropriate plate (see Fig. 23B).
- A postoperative radiograph is taken to confirm appropriate correction of fibula and tibia position (Fig. 24).

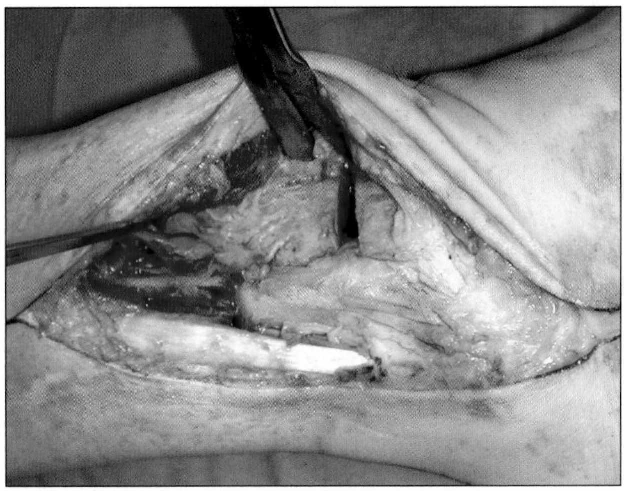
A

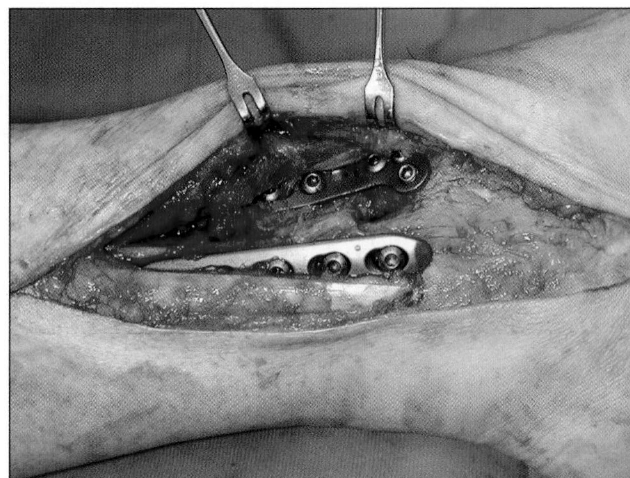
B

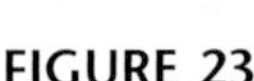
FIGURE 23

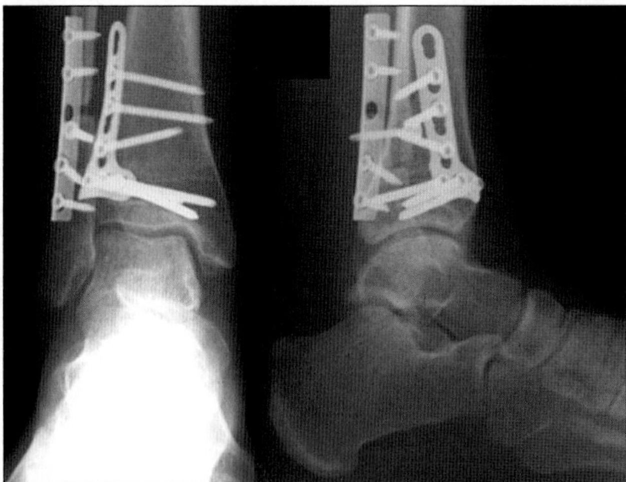
FIGURE 24

Pearls

- *Insert K-wires over step incisions proximal to the weight-bearing skin of the calcaneal tuber to prevent irritation and necrosis of the calcaneal fat pat.*
- *The first K-wire may be used as a joystick to manipulate the tuber until the second K-wire is fluoroscopically inserted for tuber fixation.*

Step 4: Calcaneal Osteotomy

- The calcaneus is exposed by a lateral oblique approach (see Fig. 12A–E).
- Osteotomy is performed with a saw blade (Fig. 25A).
- A laminar spreader is inserted (Fig. 25B) to open the osteotomy and stretch the tight soft tissues (Fig. 25C).
- The tuber fragment is displaced medially as much as desired (Fig. 25D).

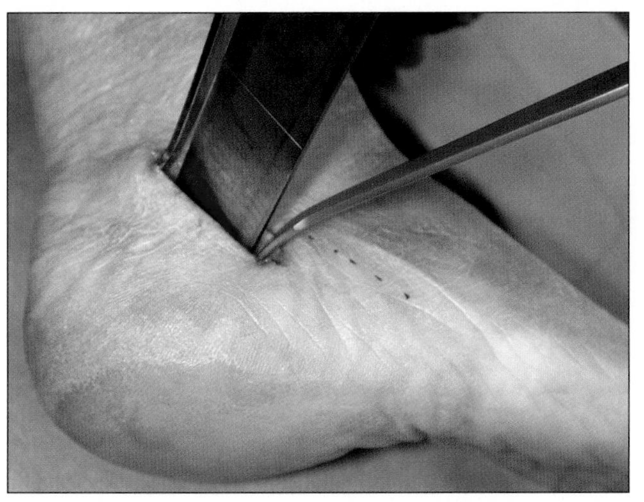

A

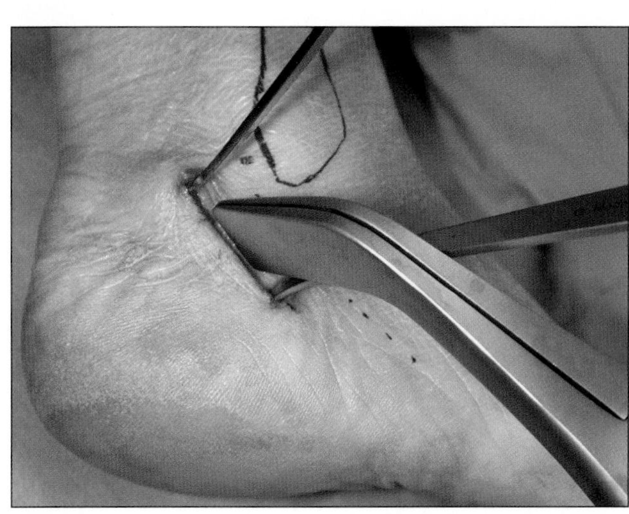

B

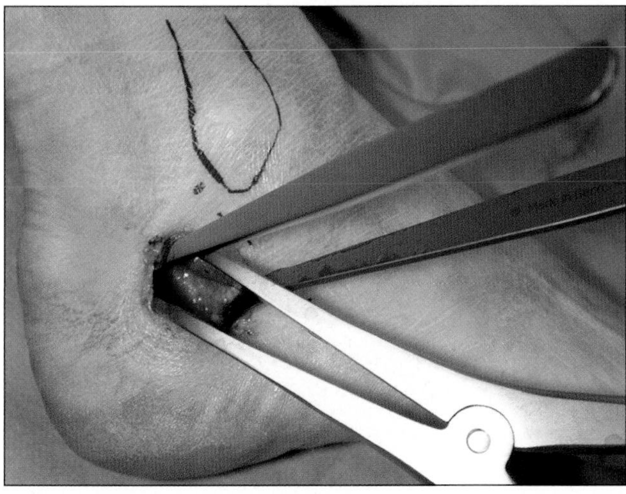

C

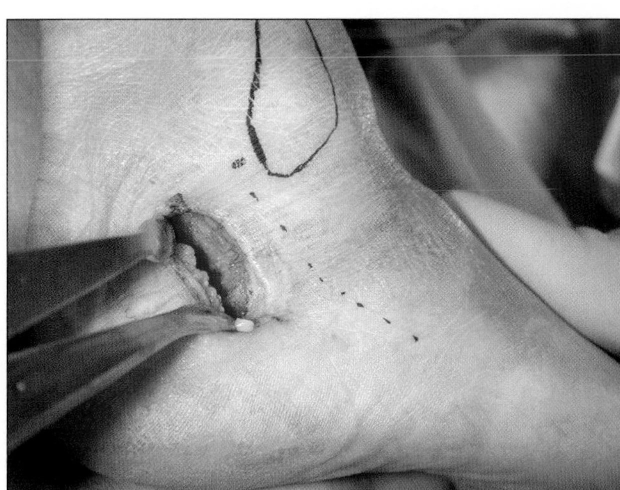

D

FIGURE 25

Controversies

- Usually one screw provides enough stability. However, rotational stability is increased by using two screws for calcaneal tuber fixation.

- Preliminary fixation is done with one or two K-wires under fluoroscopy (Fig. 26A) and achieved alignment is checked (Fig. 26B).
- The K-wires are subsequently used for guiding a cannulated compression screw (Fig. 27).
- The lateral bony stepoff is tamped.
- Postoperative radiographs are taken to confirm the postoperative position (Fig. 28A and 28B).
- Closure of the skin is accomplished by interrupted sutures (Fig. 29).

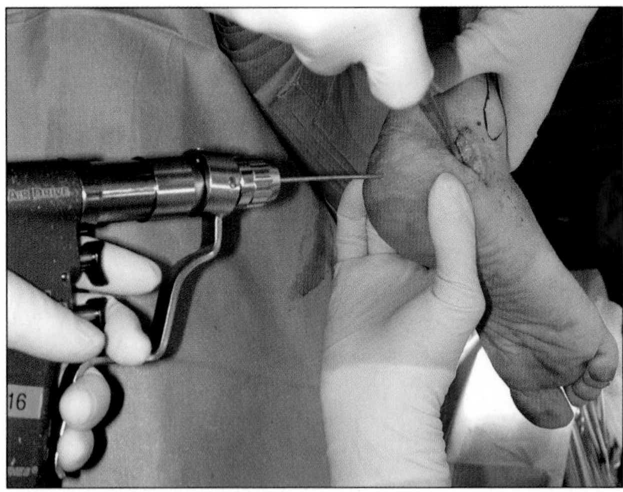

A

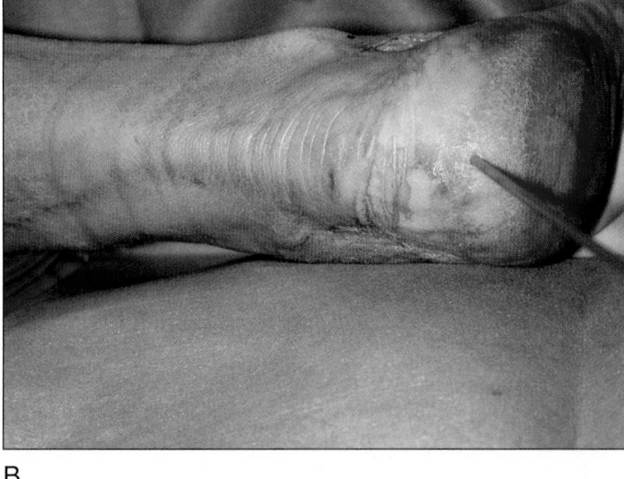

B

FIGURE 26

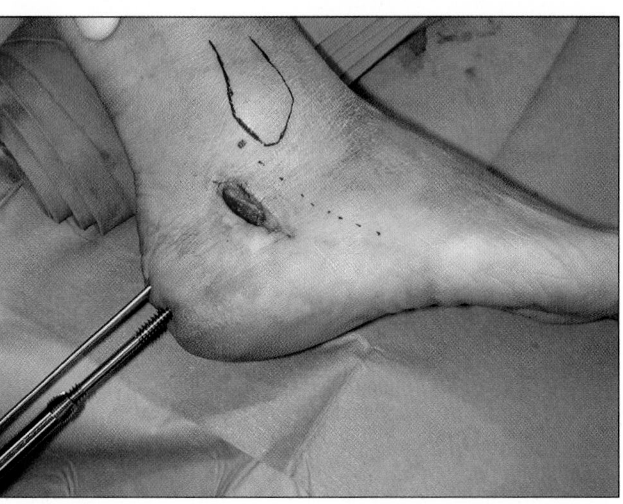

FIGURE 27

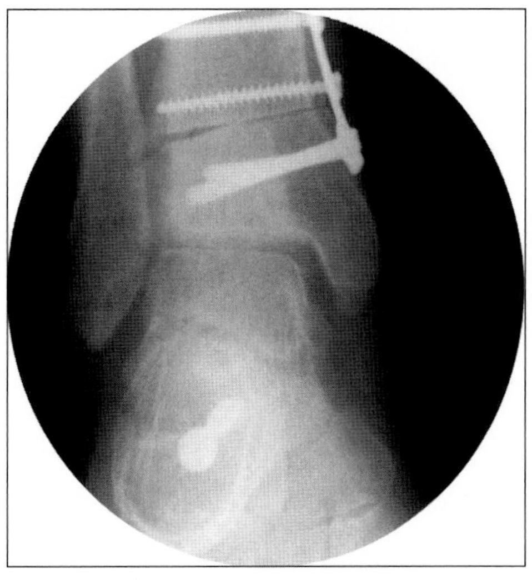
A

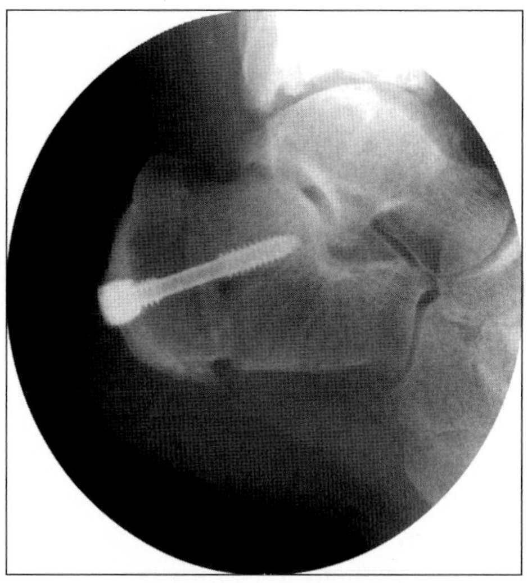
B

FIGURE 28

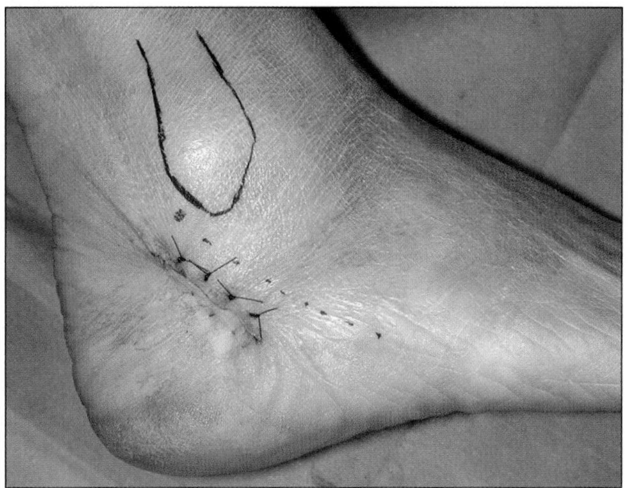

FIGURE 29

Step 5: Correction of Forefoot Supination

- If the deformity is flexible, soft tissue reconstruction can be used.
  - Repair and imbrication of the anterior delta and spring ligaments (Hintermann et al., 2006)
  - Repair of the posterior tibial tendon with or without augmentation with flexor digitorum tendon transfer (Hintermann et al., 1999)
- If the deformity is fixed:
  - For minimal correction, perform plantar-flexion osteotomy
    - At the first cuneiform
    - At the base of the first metatarsal
  - For major correction, perform plantar-flexing arthrodesis
    - At the navicular-cuneiform I joint
    - At the first tarsometatarsal joint

Pitfalls

- *Too-aggressive release of the heel cord may result in weakness at pushoff.*

Controversies

- There is no general agreement as to whether heel cord release is necessary; there is evidence that physical therapy may restore appropriate length of the heel cord in most instances.

Pitfalls

- *Removal of hardware is not recommended earlier than 8 months after surgery.*
- *Undercorrection of the valgus deformity is corrected by performing realignment surgery again. Overcorrection is unlikely.*
- *Progressive ankle arthritis may need further surgical treatment. However, total ankle arthroplasty and ankle fusion are facilitated in the well-aligned arthritic ankle.*

Step 6: Heel Cord Release

- Perform a Sinverskjöld test (assessment of dorsiflexion at the ankle with the knee in extension and flexion).
- If dorsiflexion of the ankle is decreased only with the knee in extension, a gastrocnemius release is performed until 10° of dorsiflexion with the knee in extension is achieved.
- If ankle dorsiflexion is decreased with the knee in extension and flexion, the Achilles tendon is released.

Postoperative Care and Expected Outcomes

Postoperative Care

- The foot is protected by a removable short-leg walking cast in neutral foot position for 6–8 weeks.
- Mobilization is permitted on crutches with partial weight bearing of 15–20 kg.
- A rehabilitation program starts immediately postoperatively, depending on achieved wound healing. It includes passive continuous motion and active motion without weight bearing.
- Once bone healing is achieved, usually after 8 weeks, free weight bearing as tolerated is allowed.
- Thereafter, a walker or stabilizing shoe may be recommended for another 4–8 weeks for walks on uneven ground, for high-risk sports activities, and for professional work outside.

Outcomes

- Athletes should anticipate return to sports in 8–12 months after their reconstruction.
- Between 1998 and 2003, the authors treated 22 patients with posttraumatic valgus ankle osteoarthritis of one ankle by realignment surgery. Average age at surgery was 47 years (range, 29–67 years). Fourteen patients had stage 1, three stage 2, and five stage 3 valgus ankle osteoarthritis.
  - All patients had a low tibial osteotomy and an average of two additional procedures (range, 0–6) per person.
    - Additional procedures in stage 1 included two fibula derotation-lengthening osteotomies and three collateral ligament repairs.
    - Additional procedures in stage 2 included three calcaneus osteotomies.
    - Additional procedures in stage 3 included three fibula corrections, four calcaneus osteotomies, one sinus tarsi screw, two flexion procedures at

the first ray, three repairs/augmentations of the posterior tibial tendon, five collateral ligament repairs, and one Achilles tendon lengthening.

- Chondral surgery was independent of stage and included microfracturing in three cases, cyst reaming in two, osteochondral bone transplant in one, and cheilectomy of talar and/or tibial osteophytes in eight cases.
- The surgical algorithm to correct varus and valgus ankle osteoarthritis with midterm results was published by the authors (Pagenstert et al., 2007).
- Average follow-up was 4.5 years (range, 3–6.5 years).
  - Eight patients (41%) were pain free. On average, the pain visual analog scale (minimum 1, maximum 10 points) decreased ($p < .0001$) from a preoperative mean of 6.6 ± 1.5 to 2.4 ± 1.6 at follow-up.
  - Tibiotalar arthritis and alignment as measured by the Takakura Score (1 = signs of arthritis, sclerosis, osteophytes, cysts but parallel tibiotalar joint space on loaded radiographs; 2 = signs of arthritis and tibiotalar joint tilt without subchondral bone contact; 3 = tibiotalar joint tilt and subchondral bone contact; 4 = total joint loss) decreased ($p < .0001$) from a preoperative mean of 2.4 ± 0.6 (range, 1–3) to 1.3 ± 0.4 (range, 1–3) at follow-up.
  - Function was evaluated by the ankle score of the American Orthopaedic Foot and Ankle Society (AOFAS score: minimum 0, maximum 100 points; 40 pain, 50 function, 10 alignment). AOFAS score increased ($p < .0001$) from 43 points preoperatively (range, 16–67) to 84 points (range, 63–100) at follow-up.
  - At follow-up, the Takakura Score correlated with improvement of pain ($r = .5$, $p = .004$) and function ($r = -.57$, $p < .001$).
- In two cases realignment surgery failed and progressive painful arthritis was treated by arthroplasty after 22 and 24 months. One fibula and one tibia nonunion needed revision fixation and grafting. One tibial undercorrection needed a second tibia medial closing wedge osteotomy.

Evidence

Fuchs S, Sandmann C, Skwara A, Chylarecki C. Quality of life 20 years after arthrodesis of the ankle: a study of adjacent joints. J Bone Joint Surg [Br]. 2003;85:994-8.

This retrospective study included 18 ankle arthrodeses. (Level IV evidence [case series])

Hintermann B, Knupp M, Pagenstert GI. Deltoid ligament injuries: diagnosis and management. Foot Ankle Clin. 2006;11:625-37.

This study reported the authors' technique of diagnosis and treatment of medial ankle instability. It included the results of 52 consecutive cases after an average follow-up of 4.4 years. (Level IV evidence [case series])

Hintermann B, Valderrabano V, Dereymaeker G, Dick W. The HINTEGRA ankle: rationale and short-term results of 122 consecutive ankles. Clin Orthop Relat Res. 2004;(424):57-68.

This prospective study reported the authors' technique of total ankle replacement. It included the results after an average follow-up of 19 months. (Level IV evidence [case series])

Hintermann B, Valderrabano V, Kundert HP. Lengthening of the lateral column and reconstruction of the medial soft tissue for treatment of acquired flatfoot deformity associated with insufficiency of the posterior tibial tendon. Foot Ankle Int. 1999;20:622-9.

This study reported the authors' technique to treat acquired flexible flatfoot deformity. It included 19 consecutive cases with an average follow-up of 2 years. (Level IV evidence [case series])

Isman RE, Inman VT. Anthropometric Studies of the Human Foot and Ankle (Technical Report 58). Berkeley, CA: Biomechanics Laboratory, University of California, Berkeley, 1968.

This cadaver study included 107 specimens.

Kofoed H, Stürup J. Comparison of ankle arthroplasty and arthrodesis: a prospective series with long term follow up. Foot. 1994;4:6-9.

This study reported the results of 14 Scandinavian total ankle replacements compared with 14 ankle fusions in patients matched for age, sex, and occupation. Mean follow-up was 7 years. (Level III evidence [comparative study])

Pagenstert GI, Hintermann B, Barg A, Leumann A, Valderrabano V. Realignment surgery as alternative treatment of varus and valgus ankle osteoarthritis. Clin Orthop Relat Res. 2007;(462):156-68.

This study reported the authors' technique to treat varus and valgus ankle osteoarthritis by off-loading realignment surgical procedures. It included the results of 35 cases with an average follow-up of 5 years. (Level IV evidence [case series])

Paley D. Foot and ankle considerations. In Paley D (ed). Principles of Deformity Correction. (Corrected 3rd Printing). Berlin: Springer, 2005.

This chapter describes the planning of correction of foot and ankle deformities without unloading of ankle arthritis.

Saltzman CL, el-Khoury GY. The hindfoot alignment view. Foot Ankle Int. 1995;16:572-6.

A modification of Cobey's method for radiographically imaging the coronal plane alignment of the hindfoot is described. The moment arm between the weight-bearing axis of the leg and the contact point of the heel is calculated on normative data of 57 asymptomatic adult subjects.

Takakura Y, Tanaka Y, Kumai T, Tamai S. Low tibial osteotomy for osteoarthritis of the ankle: results of a new operation in 18 patients. J Bone Joint Surg [Br]. 1995;77:50-4.

This study reported the authors' technique to treat varus ankle osteoarthritis by an off-loading supramalleolar osteotomy. It included the results with an average follow-up of 7 years. (Level IV evidence [case series])

Takakura Y, Tanaka Y, Sugimoto K, Akiyama K, Tamai S. Long-term results of arthrodesis for osteoarthritis of the ankle. Clin Orthop Relat Res. 1999;(361):178-85.

This study reported the authors' technique to treat end-stage ankle osteoarthritis by ankle fusion. It included the results of 43 cases with an average follow-up of 7.2 years. (Level IV evidence [case series])

Valderrabano V, Pagenstert G, Horisberger M, Knupp M, Hintermann B. Sports and recreation activity of ankle arthritis patients before and after total ankle replacement. Am J Sports Med. 2006;34:993-9.

This study reported the activity of 147 patients treated with 152 HINTEGRA total ankle replacements. It included the results with an average follow-up of 2.8 years. (Level IV evidence [case series])

Wood PL, Deakin S. Total ankle replacement: the results in 200 ankles. J Bone Joint Surg [Br]. 2003;85:334-41.

This study reported the authors' results of a consecutive patients series treated with Scandinavian total ankle replacements with an average follow-up of 4 years. (Level IV evidence [case series])

PROCEDURE 33

Osteochondral Lesion of the Ankle—OATS Procedure

Carol Frey

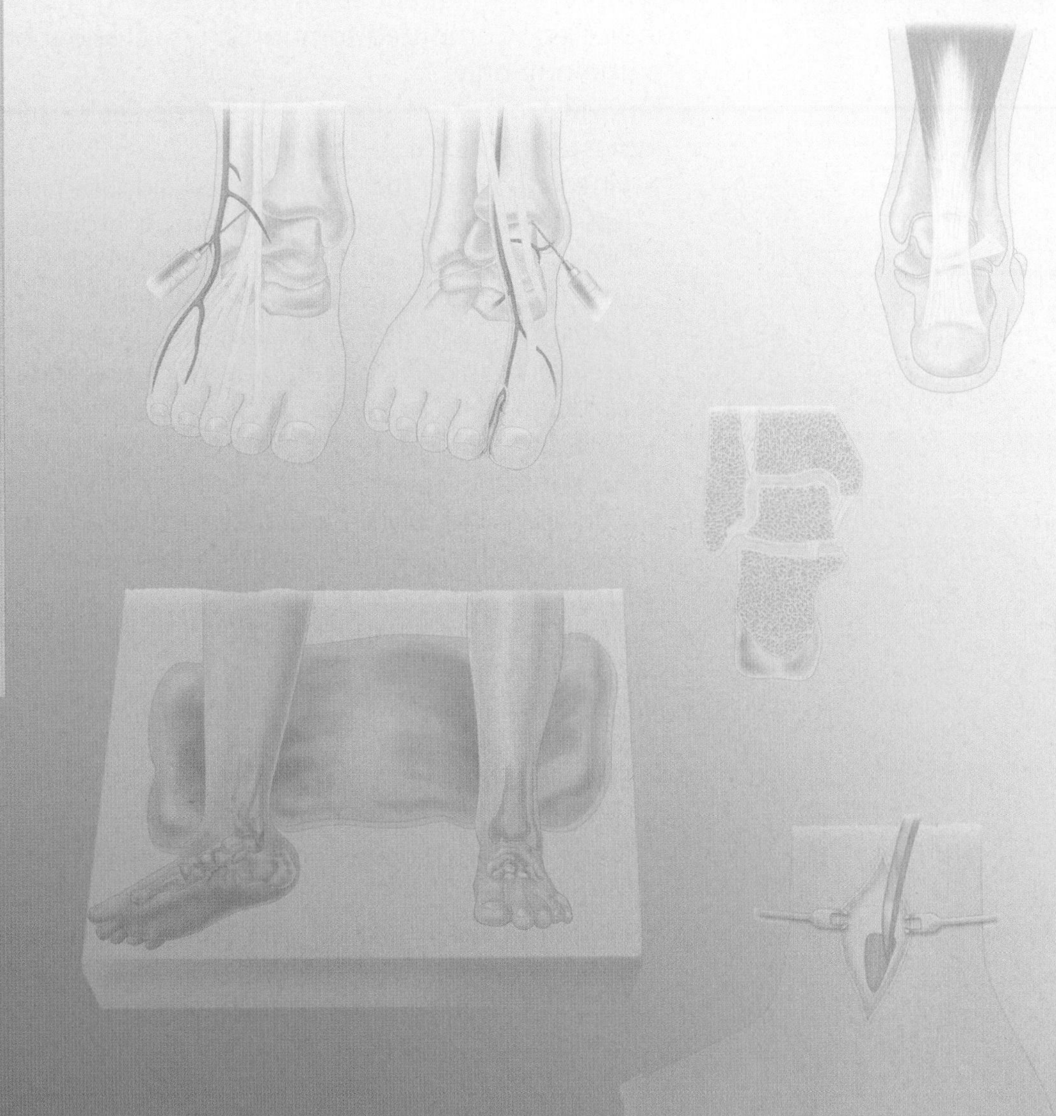

PITFALLS

- *More difficult to do surgery if the lesion is not focal, contained, and with a good shoulder of surrounding cartilage*

Controversies

- Primary treatment of cystic lesions, especially smaller than 15 mm

Treatment Options

- Drilling
- Microfracture
- Débridement
- Internal fixation
- Grafting techniques
- Excision of lesion
- Autologous chondrocyte implantation

Indications

- Cystic lesion of the talar dome 8–20 mm in diameter
- Precise definition of lesion
- Symptomatic lesion

Examination/Imaging

- Standard radiographs should be the first diagnostic study.
- If radiographs are normal but there are continued symptoms, magnetic resonance imaging (MRI) is indicated. Computed tomography will show bone pathology only.
- On MRI, increased signal in the articular cartilage indicates chondral softening.
  - Linear to ovoid foci of increased signal involving less than 50% of cartilage thickness indicate a superficial lesion of the cartilage extending down to less than 50% of the cartilage depth.
  - Linear to ovoid foci of increased signal involving greater than 50% of cartilage thickness indicate a cartilage defect extending down to greater than 50% of cartilage depth but not down to subchondral bone.
  - Complete loss of the articular cartilage or surface flap indicates loss of cartilage down to subchondral bone (Fig. 1).
- On MRI, five stages of osteochondral lesion (OCL) can be defined.
  - Stage I OCL shows subchondral trabecular compression and marrow edema.
  - Stage IIA OCL shows the formation of a subchondral cyst.
  - Stage IIB OCL shows incomplete separation of the fragment.
  - Stage III OCL shows an unattached, nondisplaced fragment with synovial fluid around the fragment.
  - Stage IV OCL shows a displaced fragment.
  - Stage V OCL shows a large cystic lesion (Fig. 2).

Surgical Anatomy

- Cartilage structure (Fig. 3)
  - Deep radial zone (40–60%): collagen oriented perpendicular to subchondral zone
  - Transitional zone (20–30%): more random collagen orientation
  - Superficial zone (<10%): parallel to surface

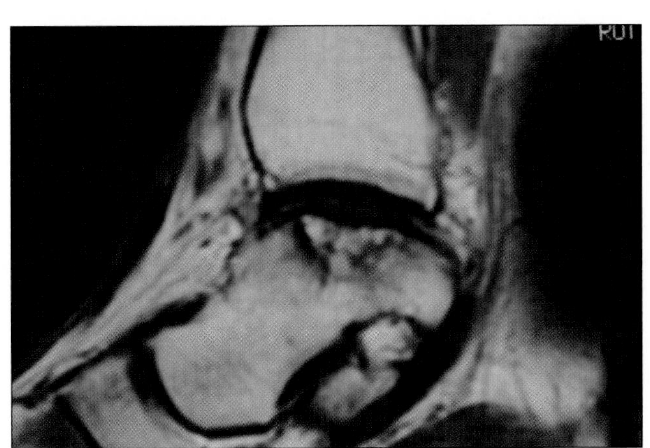

FIGURE 1

FIGURE 2

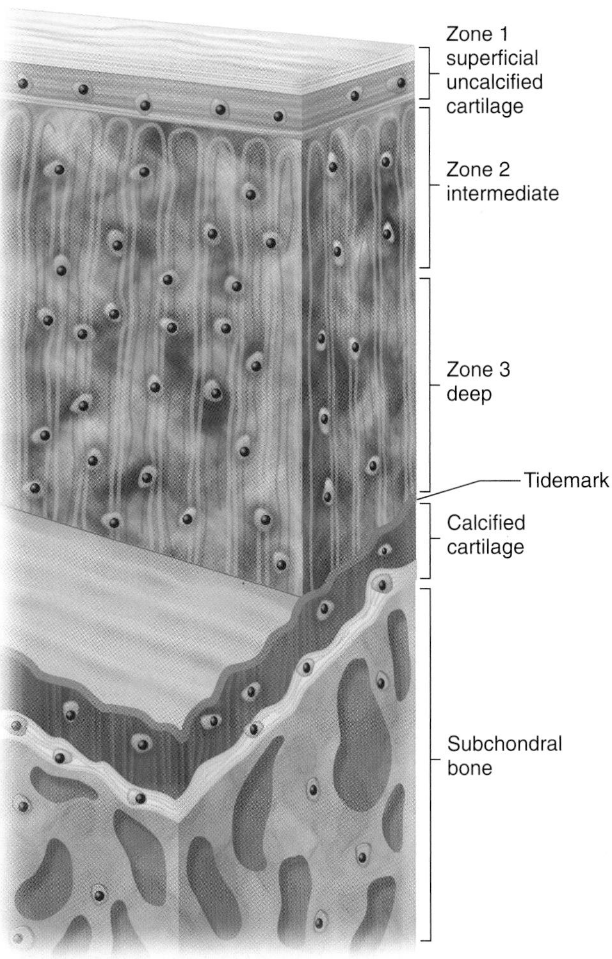

FIGURE 3

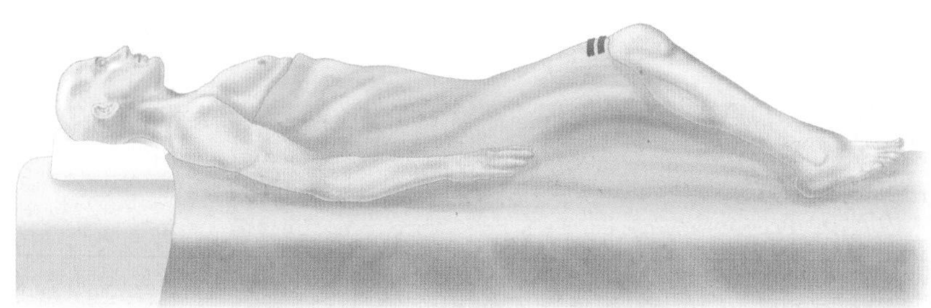

FIGURE 4

Positioning

- The patient is placed supine with the knee and ankle draped free (Fig. 4).
- An arthroscopic leg holder is not necessary.

Equipment

- Small Hohmann retractors

Portals/Exposures

- For posterior medial lesions, a curved longitudinal incision is made over the medial malleolus, adequate to expose the anteromedial and posteromedial ankle joint (Fig. 5).
- The saphenous vein, anteromedial and posteromedial nerves and vessels, and tendon structures are protected with small Hohmann retractors.

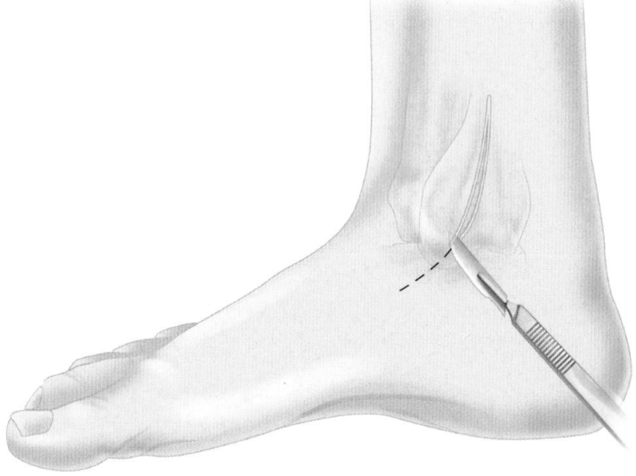

FIGURE 5

Instrumentation/ Implantation

- 4.0 arthroscope for knee
- Standard arthroscopic tray for ankle
- 2.9 arthroscope for ankle
- Arthroscopic curettes
- Noninvasive distractor for ankle
- Arthroscopic pump

Procedure

Step 1

- The ankle may be inspected with an arthroscope prior to the arthrotomy. Excess synovial tissue, loose bodies, and anterior tibial osteophytes may be removed at this time (Fig. 6A and 6B).
- The size of the lesion can be determined during the arthroscopy if there is good access to the lesion (Fig. 7).

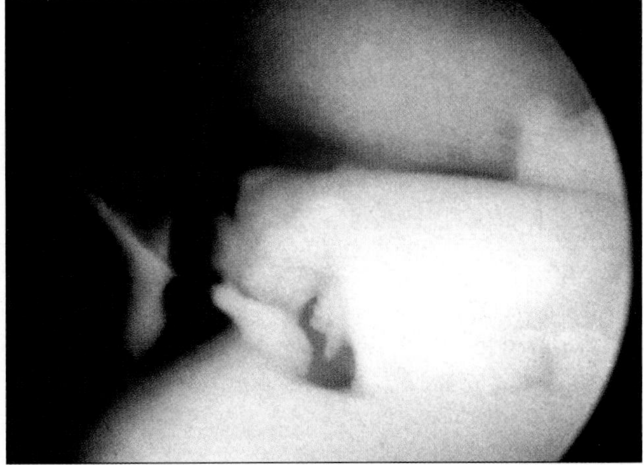

A

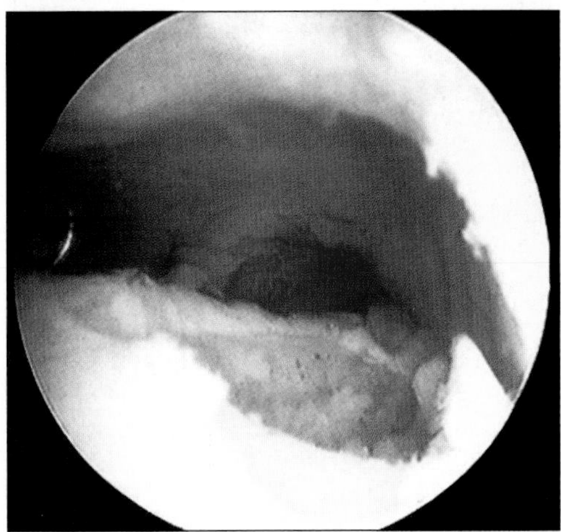

B

FIGURE 6

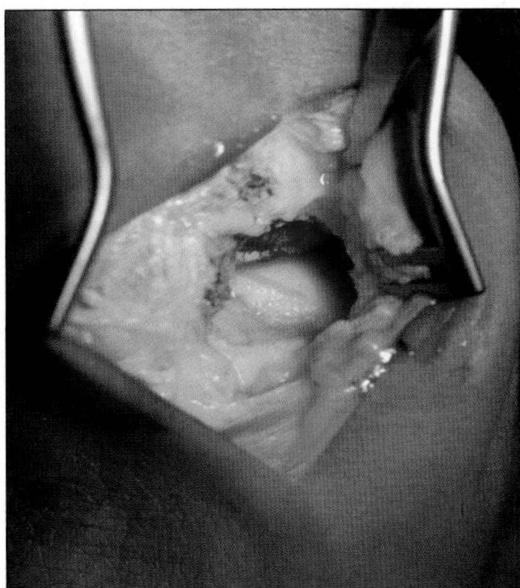

FIGURE 7

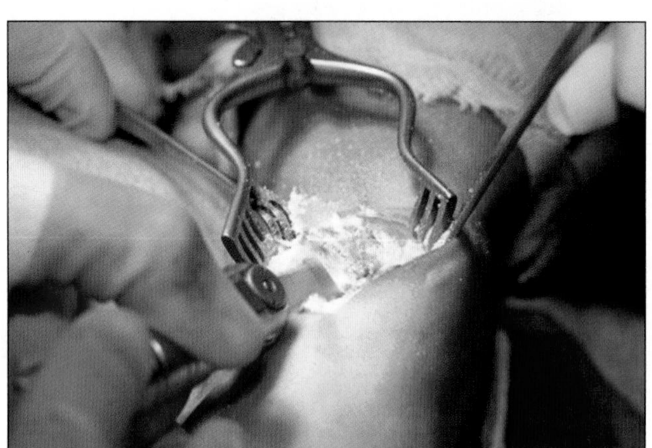

A

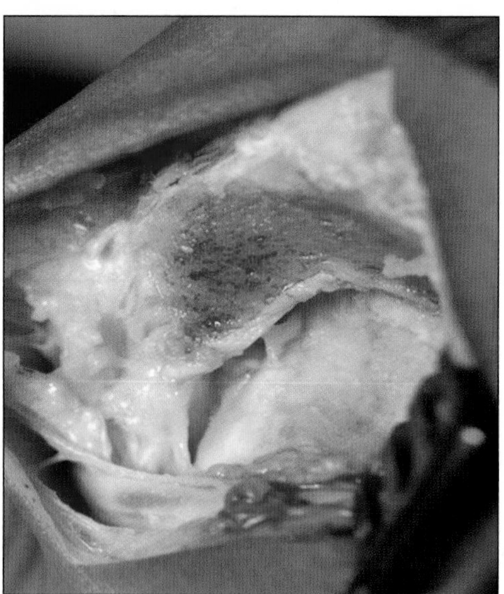

B

FIGURE 8

- If not, then a malleolar osteotomy is performed.
- An anteromedial arthrotomy is carried out.
  - The anterior joint is inspected.
  - Impingement spurs and loose bodies are removed.
- If there is overhang of bone from the distal anterior tibial plafond, it should be aggressively removed (Fig. 8A) for increased visualization (Fig. 8B).

Step 2

- If a medial malleolar osteotomy is necessary
  - The medial malleolus is predrilled with two 0.53-mm pins and then overdrilled with the AO Synthes 4.0-mm cannulated drill to a depth that crosses into the tibial plafond.
  - The two drill holes should diverge slightly. This prevents possible superior migration of the medial malleolus when the 4.0-mm screws are placed.
  - A 45° osteotomy cut is made from the superior medial malleolus that comes down to the junction of the tibial plafond.
  - The medial malleolus is gently pulled inferiorly to expose the talus.
  - The talus is inspected and any damaged surface is débrided with pickups, scalpel, and curette.

Pearls

- *Use intraoperative fluoroscopy for orientation if necessary.*
- *The ankle is distracted laterally at the time of the osteotomy to ensure that the medial talus is protected.*

Instrumentation/Implantation

- Oscillating saw
- Drill
- 4.0-mm cannulated screws

Step 3

- Osteochondral Autograft Transfer System (OATS) sizing rods are introduced for an accurate measurement of width (Fig. 9).
- One large core is desirable (Fig. 10A), but a second or even a third may be necessary (Fig. 10B).

Instrumentation/Implantation

- OATS instrumentation

Pearls

- *An oblong cyst allows two grafts (or even three) to be nested side by side. In a large cyst (around 20 mm), it is possible to nest three 7- to 8-mm grafts.*
- *For intimate fit, the recipient corer can be driven in such a manner that it takes a small amount of the first implanted core (this is uncommon).*
- *Grafts do not need to be proud or set lower relative to the surrounding articular surface; they should be flush.*
- *Larger grafts have more hyaline cartilage, fewer technical steps (as require fewer grafts), more robust graft, reduced concentration of loads, and improved pullout strength. Larger grafts are more difficult to contour, however.*
- *Perpendicular insertion should be done.*

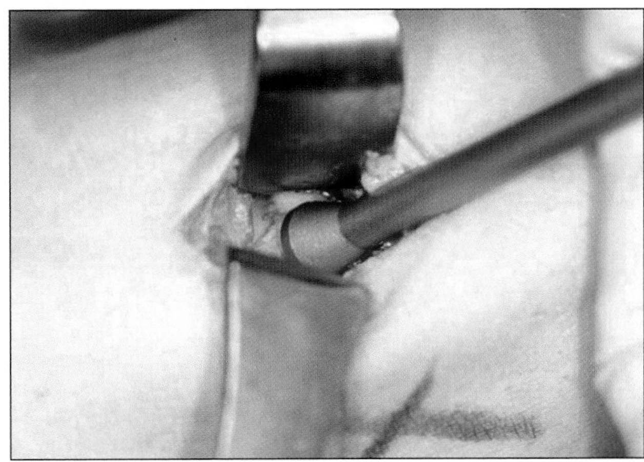

FIGURE 9

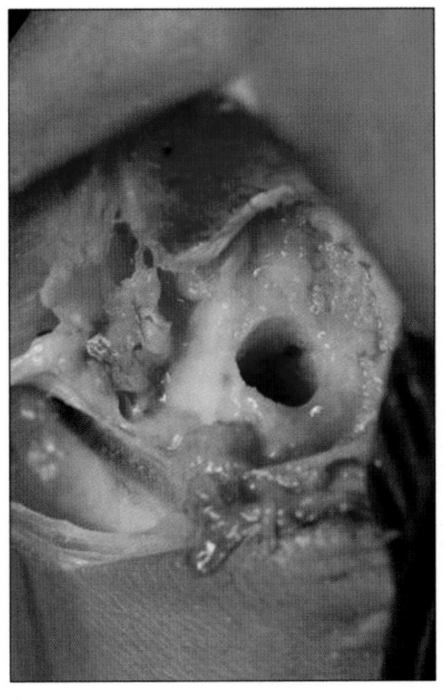

A

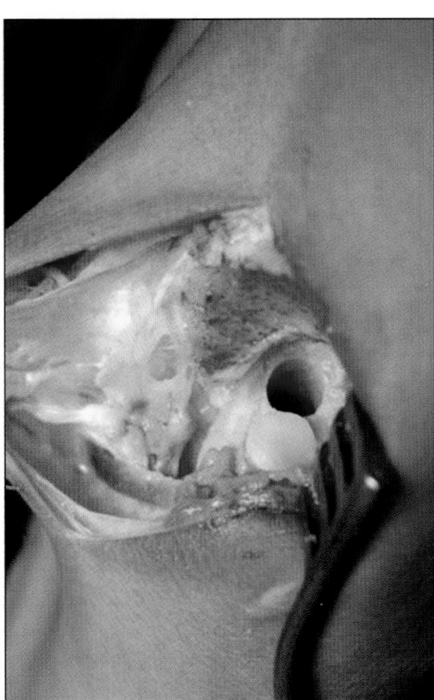

B

FIGURE 10

- The core/socket is 1 mm smaller than the graft.
- Once the depth and the width of the recipient hole are determined, the ankle joint is covered with a saline-dampened sponge as the grafts are obtained from the knee.

Pitfalls

- *Not fitting grafts with proper angular congruity*
- *Grafts not flush with surrounding articular surface*
- *A proud graft is subject to shear stress, micro-motion, subsidence, and fibrillation.*
- *A countersunk graft is subject to edge loading, fibrous overgrowth, and fibrillation.*
- *Flush is key but sometimes difficult to achieve.*

Instrumentation/ Implantation

- Standard arthroscopic tray for knee

Step 4

- The arthroscope is introduced through an anterolateral portal for the knee, followed by a routine inspection of the knee (Fig. 11).
- An appropriate-size donor tube from the OATS set is introduced (Fig. 12).
  - If the talar grafts that are required are from a "flat" area of the talus, the donor tube is positioned more vertical over the flat sulcus terminalis portion of the notch. The knee is partially extended to accommodate the vertical angle.
  - If graft that is required is more curved, then the donor tube is positioned along the corner of the lateral notch of the femoral trochlea.
- The donor tube is driven to a depth of 15 mm and twisted clockwise 90° under pressure, back, and then a full clockwise revolution.

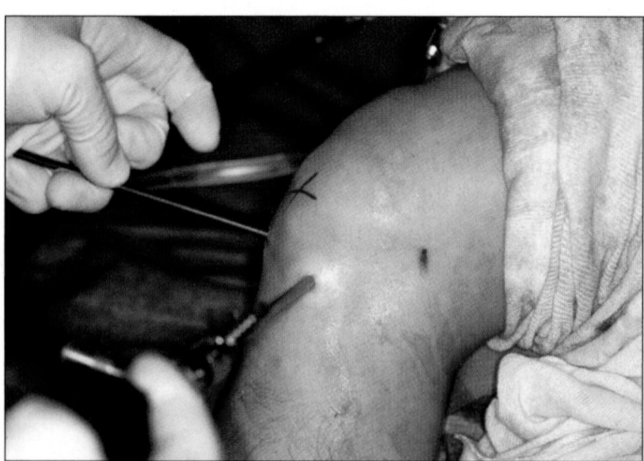

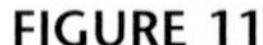

FIGURE 11

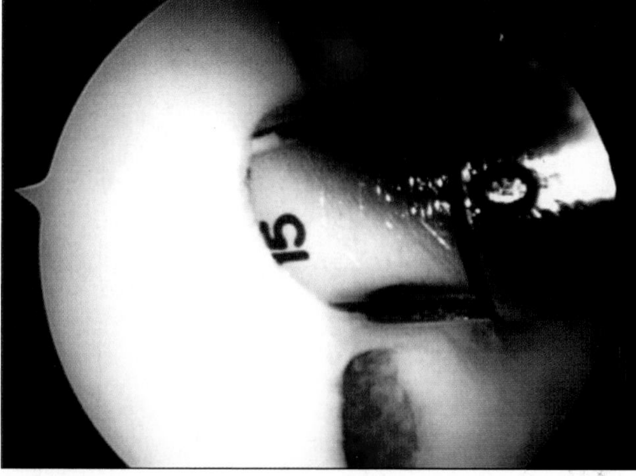

FIGURE 12

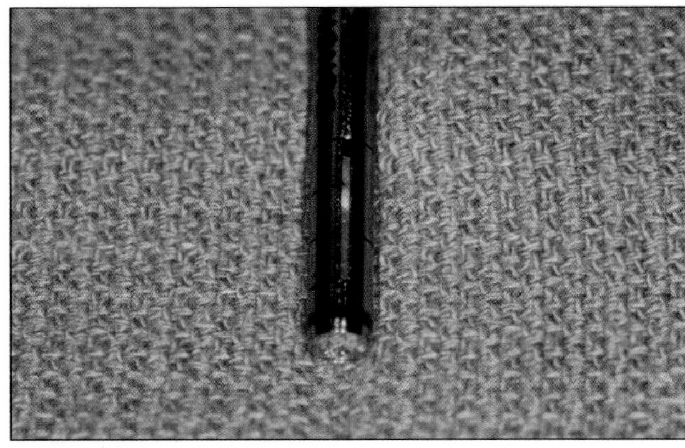

FIGURE 13

- The tube and graft are withdrawn. The graft is retrieved and inspected to make sure that it has an even cartilage surface area of good quality (Fig. 13).
- Backfilling the defect is not necessary.

Instrumentation/ Implantation

- Mosquito/small Kelly clamp

Step 5

- The cored osteochondral graft is extruded and measured.
- If 15 mm is harvested, it can be rongeured back to a tapered 12 mm to match the recipient hole in the talus. This makes it easier to introduce into the talar hole.
- The graft is held with a small Kelly or mosquito clamp and introduced into the talar hole in proper orientation for congruity.
- The graft is driven down until flush with the articular surface (Fig. 14).

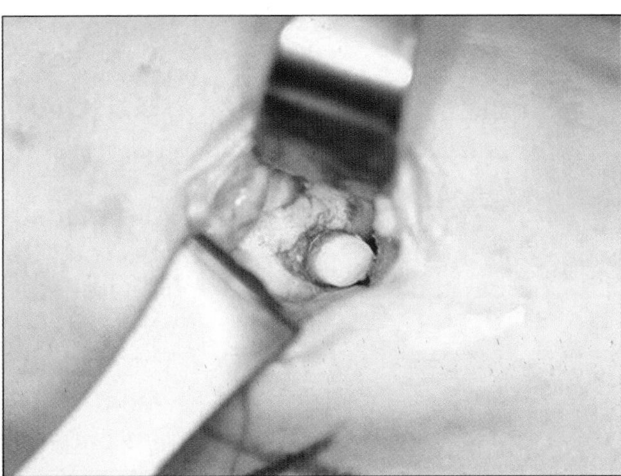

FIGURE 14

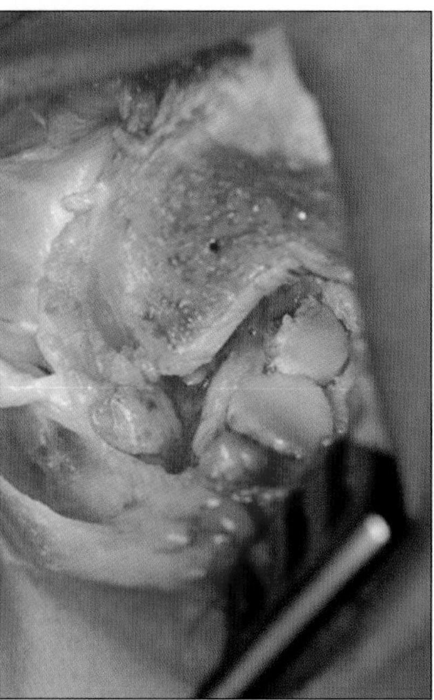

FIGURE 15

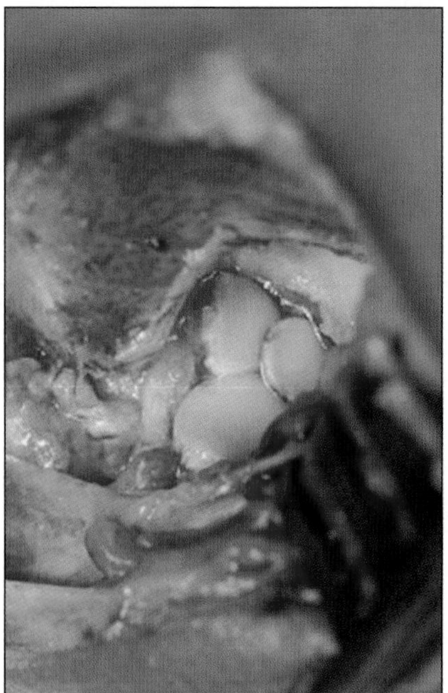

FIGURE 16

- Often, more than one graft is necessary to fill the void, and a second core is made (see Fig. 10B). In Figure 15, a second donor graft has been placed.
- Figure 16 demonstrates a case in which three donor grafts were necessary to treat the lesion.

- If a small cartilage edge protrudes, it may be trimmed with a scalpel.
- The medial malleolus is replaced if taken down initially.
- Closure is routine.
- A compression dressing is placed to the knee and the ankle. The ankle will also have a splint applied with the dressing.

PEARLS

- *The postoperative course is the same with and without a medial malleolar osteotomy.*

Postoperative Care and Expected Outcomes

- Pain management is necessary.
- This may be an outpatient procedure.
- The patient is kept non–weight bearing for 3–4 weeks in a splint or boot walker.
- The patient is then kept non–weight bearing for 3 weeks with no support.
- The patient is then allowed to bear weight in a boot walker for 3–4 weeks.
- Physical therapy and rehabilitation are begun.

Evidence

Hangody L, Fules P. Autologous osteochondral mosaicplasty for the treatment of full-thickness defects of weight-bearing joints: ten years of experimental and clinical experience. J Bone Joint Surgery [Am]. 2003;85(Suppl 2):25-32.

The technique described in this paper utilized an open knee arthrotomy for harvesting the graft and the use of multiple 4.5-mm or 6.5-mm diameter grafts. Good results were reported. (Level V evidence)

Hangody L, Kish G, Modis L, Szerb I, Gaspar L, Diozegi Z, Kendik Z. Mosaicplasty for the treatment of osteochondritis dissecans of the talus: two to seven year results in 36 patients. Foot Ankle Int. 2001;22:552-8.

This paper reported good to excellent results in 34 or 36 cases, with a 2- to 7-year follow-up. The technique described involves an open knee arthrotomy for graft harvesting and the nesting of multiple grafts. (Level I evidence)

Koh JL, Wirsing K, Lautenschlager I, Zhang LO. The effect of graft height mismatch on contact pressure following osteochondral grafting: a biomechanical study. Am J Sports Med. 2004;32:317-20.

The structure, stiffness, remodeling, and split-line characteristics of osteochondral autograft transplantation were studied in animal models with good results. The split-line pattern or tidemark discrepancy of the host versus graft tissue does not appear to matter as long as the graft is within 1 mm of congruity of the recipient tissue. (Level V evidence)

Robinson DE, Winson IG, Harries WJ, Kelly AJ. Arthroscopic treatment of osteochondral lesions of the talus. J Bone Joint Surg [Br]. 2003;85:989-93.

Drilling and débridement are reported to have a poor outcome in 53% of patients with large cystic osteochondral lesions. (Level I evidence)

Scranton PE, Frey CC, Feder KS. Outcome of osteochondral autograft transplantation for type-V cystic osteochondral lesions of the talus. J Bone Joint Surg [Br]. 2006;88:614-9.

In this retrospective study, 50 patients with large cystic type-V osteochondral lesions of the talus were reviewed. Osteochondral autograft transplantation was undertaken, and 90% of the patients had a mean good to excellent score using the Karlsson-Peterson Ankle Score. The mean follow-up was 36 months. A malleolar osteotomy was required in 26 of the patients. (Level I evidence)

Tol JL, Struijs PA, Bossuyt PM, Verhagen RA, van Dijk CN. Treatment strategies in osteochondral defects of the talar dome: a systematic review. Foot Ankle Int. 2000;21:119-26.

Electronic databases from 1966 to 1998 were reviewed. Thirty-two studies were reviewed for treatment strategies for OCD of the talus. The average highest success rate was reached by excision curettage and drilling (85%) and followed by excision and curettage (78%). Excision alone had a success rate of 38% and was not recommended. (Level V evidence)

PROCEDURE 34

Mosaicplasty with Bone-Periosteum Graft from the Iliac Crest for Osteochondral Lesions of the Talus

André Leumann, Victor Valderrabano, Robert Kilger, Christian Plaass, Geert I. Pagenstert, and Beat Hintermann

PITFALLS

- *The decision making on osteochondral lesions is difficult. Radiographically, asymptomatic osteochondral lesions also may be found. Therefore, specific evaluation is important.*
- *Unaddressed associated problems (e.g., ankle instability, malalignment) may be the cause of failure.*

Controversies

- Bone-periosteum grafting offers two advantages compared to normal mosaicplasty (e.g., from the knee joint): (1) no donor-site morbidity in an uninjured joint, and (2) the periosteum (with its pluripotent stem cells) has the potential to differentiate into fibrocartilage.
- The bone-periosteum plug is not covered by hyaline cartilage, however.

Indications

- Surgical treatment option for osteochondral lesions of Berndt and Harty grades III and IV (Berndt and Harty, 1959), and after failure of other surgical procedures
- Alternative grafting procedure for mosaicplasty (Hangody et al., 2003) to reduce donor-site morbidity (e.g., grafting from the knee joint) (Reddy et al., 2007)

Examination/Imaging

- Meticulous patient history and clinical examination is necessary.
  - Duration of symptoms
  - Preinjury level of sports and recreational activity
  - Character of pain, level of pain (visual analog scale)
  - Recurrent ankle sprains
  - Joint blocking, swelling, tenderness, feeling of giving way
  - Range of motion
  - Functional status (e.g., muscle strength, proprioception, and postural control)
  - Ligamentous ankle instability (anterior drawer test, lateral and medial talar tilt test)
  - Hindfoot alignment, footwear, and insoles
  - Patient's expectation (e.g., level of sports activities)
- Plain radiographs
  - Weight-bearing anteroposterior (Fig. 1A) and lateral (Fig. 1B) radiographs of the ankle often show the osseous defect.
  - Additionally, they provide further information on hindfoot alignment (Pagenstert et al., 2007), talocrural joint configuration (Frigg et al., 2007), joint degeneration (Valderrabano et al., 2006), and anterior or posterior ankle impingement syndrome. These factors have to be addressed at the same time (e.g., with supramalleolar osteotomy, calcaneal lengthening osteotomy, posterior tibial tendon reconstruction, peroneus longus–on-brevis transfer).
- Magnetic resonance imaging (MRI) shows the osteochondral defect by cartilage alterations, defects of the subchondral layer, and bone marrow edema, as well as by evidencing ligament ruptures or other pathologies (Hintermann, 2005; Raikin et al., 2007), as in the T_2-weighted image in Figure 2.

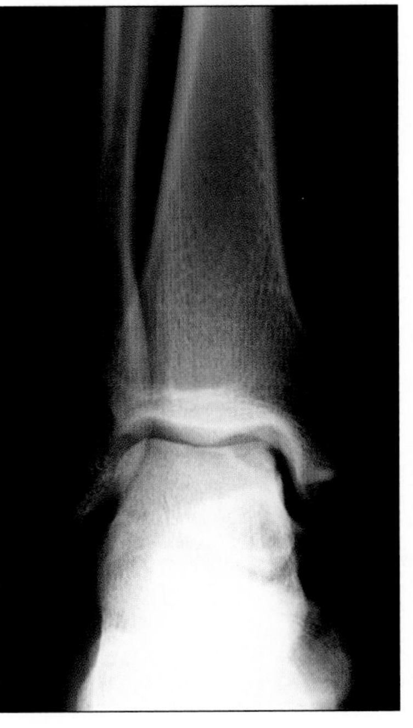

A

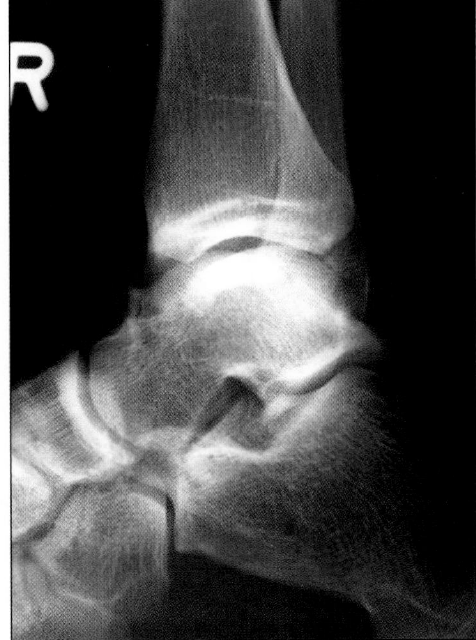

B

FIGURE 1

Treatment Options

- Other surgical procedures are based on the tissue that should be addressed (Verhagen et al., 2003).
  - Cartilage: microfracturing, autologous chondrocyte implantation (ACI), matrix-associated autologous chondrocyte implantation (MACI), autologous matrix-induced chondrogenesis (AMIC) (preferred); also débridement, antegrade drilling, refixation
  - Bone: cancellous bone grafting, retrograde or antegrade drilling (preferred); also refixation, débridement, AMIC, microfracturing
  - A combination of both: microfracturing, AMIC, débridement, refixation, antegrade drilling
- Besides harvesting at the iliac crest, other described possibilities are the proximal tibia, calcaneus, and talus (Kreuz et al., 2006).

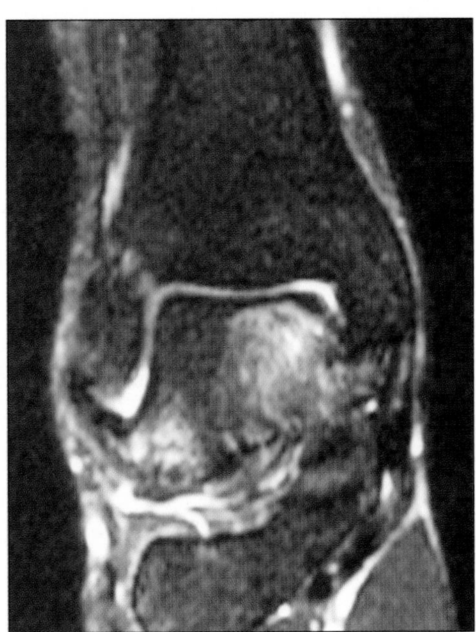

FIGURE 2

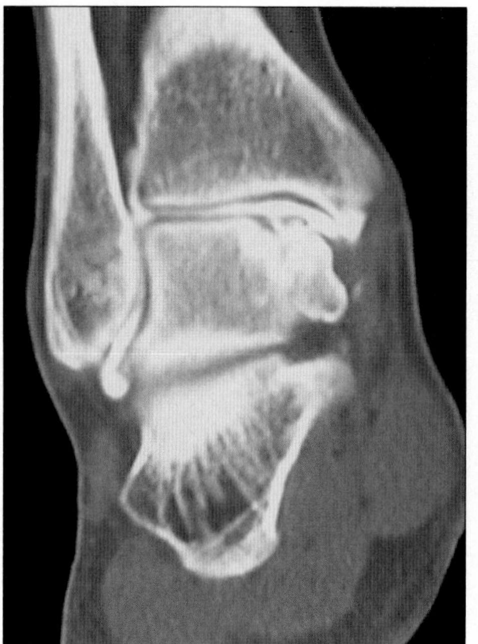

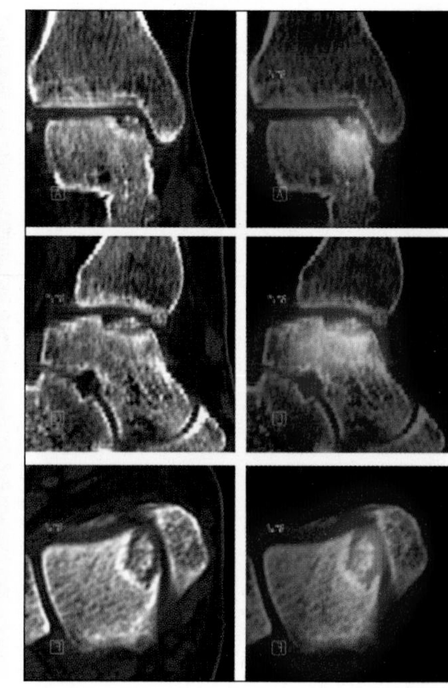

FIGURE 3 A B

- Computed tomography (CT) scanning
  - The CT scan is said to be equal in quality to MRI (Verhagen et al., 2005). It may show the osseous and cartilage (indirectly) lesions and possibly free bodies more exactly, but lacks the ability to give more information on the surrounding soft tissues (Fig. 3A).
  - Additional information on the activity of the lesion may be found by single-photon emission CT (Fig. 3B).

Surgical Anatomy

- Ankle biomechanics
  - The talocrural joint is the most congruent joint of the human joints.
  - The ligamentous function is very important and often insufficient in patients with osteochondral lesions (Hintermann et al., 2002).
- Anatomy of an osteochondral lesion (Fig. 4A)—three zones can be distinguished (Fig. 4B):
  - Cartilage: Compared to the knee joint, the ankle cartilage is 1–1.5 mm thinner and less elastic, and has chondrocytes that are more resistant to osteoarthritic damage.
  - Subchondral layer: The subchondral bone is essential for the stability of the cartilage. It fixes the cartilage stably to the bone.
  - Bone: Bone provides nutrition to the cartilage. Changes of the cancellous structure leading to cysts and sclerosis can be found.

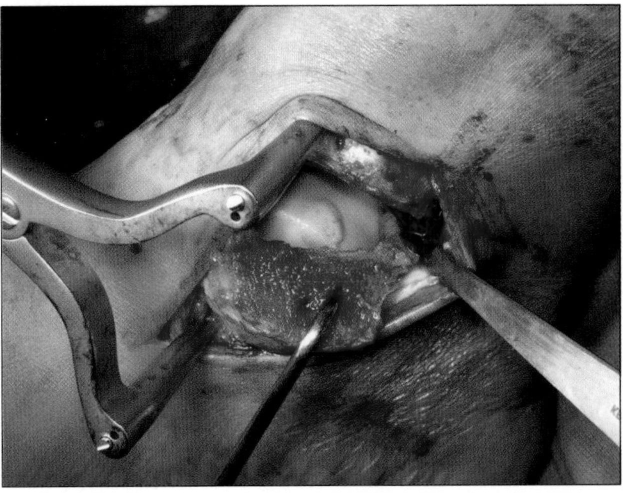

A

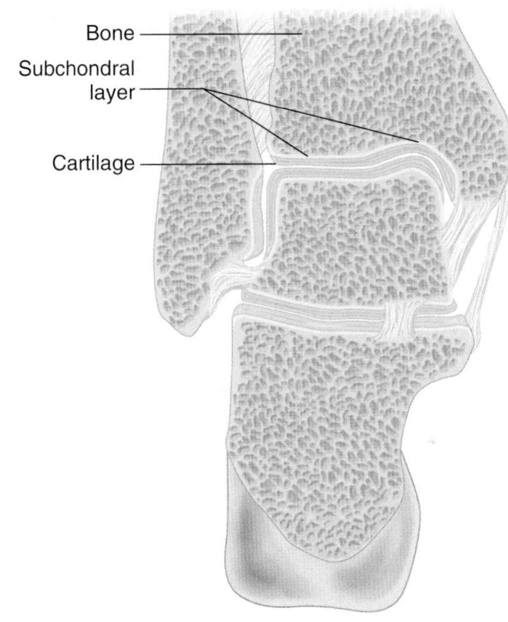

B

FIGURE 4

PEARLS

- *Removable knee holder facilitates the surgery after the arthroscopic evaluation.*

PITFALLS

- *Inappropriate draping may hinder proper harvest of the graft.*

Positioning

- Supine position
- Tourniquet at the ipsilateral thigh (350 mm Hg)
- Removable knee holder for the arthroscopy; should be removed before the mosaicplasty surgery
- Draping the iliac crest as an operative field
- Single injection of an antibiotic 30 minutes before surgery

Pearls

- *Medial approach to the ankle*
  - *Predrilling and prefixation with two AO 3.5-mm screws prior to osteotomy may help with anatomic reduction and fixation at the end of surgery.*
  - *A chevron-shaped osteotomy may achieve more primary stability.*
- *Lateral approach to the ankle*
  - *Instead of performing a fibular osteotomy, detachment of the lateral ligaments along the anterior border of the fibula allows dislocation of the talus anterolaterally sufficiently to expose the lesion.*
  - *Detachment of ligaments with a small bony piece will be beneficial for the healing process.*
  - *The use of a special spreader (Hintermann distractor; Newdeal, Lyon, France) facilitates anterolateral dislocation of the talus without hindering access to the talar dome.*

Pitfalls

- *Inappropriate osteotomy techniques may damage the cartilage.*
- *Lesion of the posteromedial neurovascular bundle and flexor tendons*

Portals/Exposures

- Arthroscopy is done by using a standard portal (e.g., anteromedial, anterolateral, anterocentral, or posterolateral)
- Medial approach for (postero)medial lesions
  - Fifty-eight percent are located on the medial mortise, mainly on the posteromedial aspect. Of these, 70% originate from an acute trauma.
  - These lesions can be accessed best by a medial malleolar osteotomy.
  - A 5-cm long, longitudinal incision over the anterior half of the malleolus gives rapid access to the bone (Fig. 5).
  - It is advised to protect the soft tissues with retractors: anteriorly, the anterior tibial tendon and branches of the saphenous nerve and vein; more posteriorly, the posterior tibial tendon and the bundle of posterior tibial nerve and vessels (Fig. 6A and 6B). (In Figure 6, mm = medial malleolus; * = deltoid ligament; solid arrow = anteromedial mini-arthrotomy; and dashed arrow = retractor positioned in the tibialis posterior tendon sheet protecting the tendons, nerve, and vessels.)
  - To prevent the cartilage from cracking, it is advised to perform the last cut of the osteotomy with a chisel (Fig. 7).
- Lateral approach for (antero)lateral lesions
- Forty-two percent are located on the lateral, mainly the anterolateral, mortise. Of these, 89% are of traumatic origin.
- A classic anterolateral ankle approach is often sufficient.
- Sometimes the anterior talofibular ligament has to be detached and the foot kept in plantar flexion (Fig. 8).

Controversies

- The lateral approach, by using an osteotomy of the fibula, requires extensive dissection of the tibiofibular ligaments and plating of the fibula at the end of surgery. As an alternative, dislocation of the talus anterolaterally is less invasive and, in our experience, it always allows enough exposure of the lateral dome of the talus for appropriate insertion of plugs.

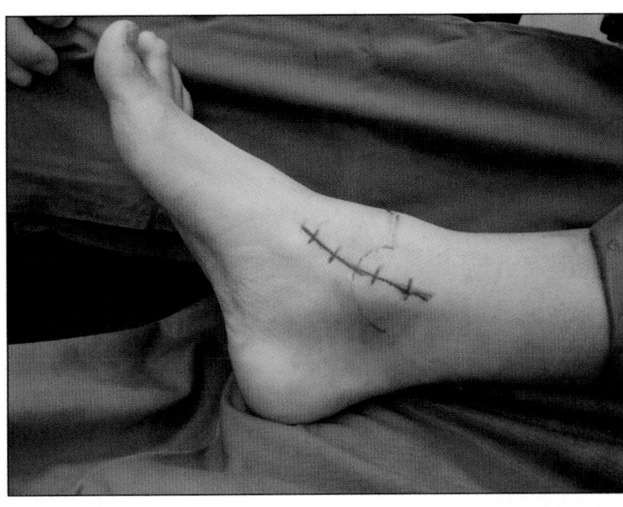

FIGURE 5

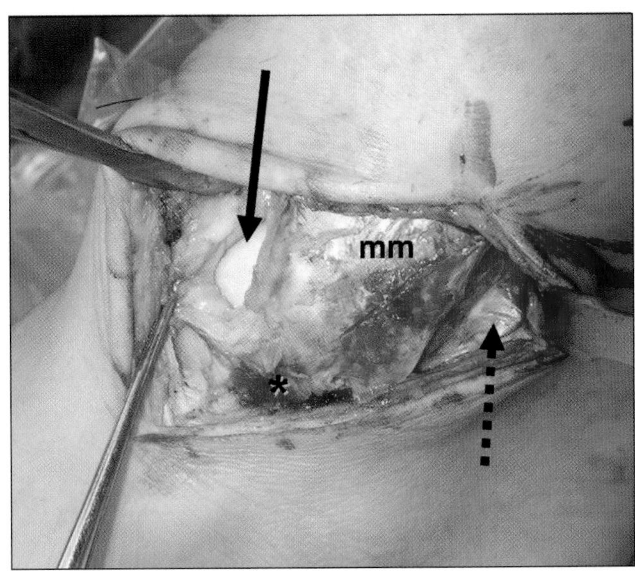

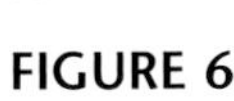

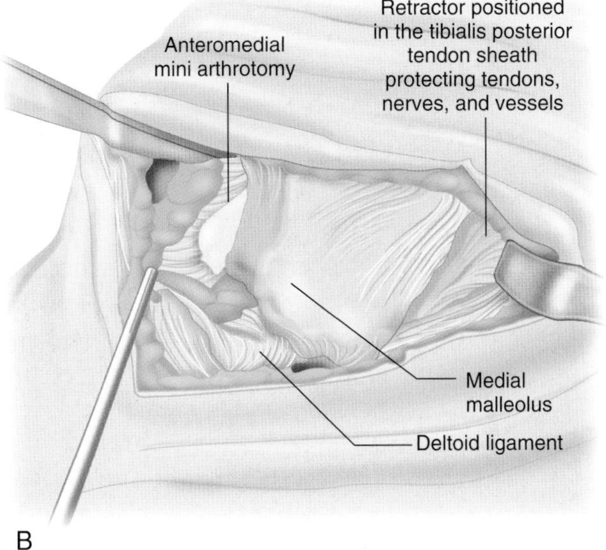

A B

FIGURE 6

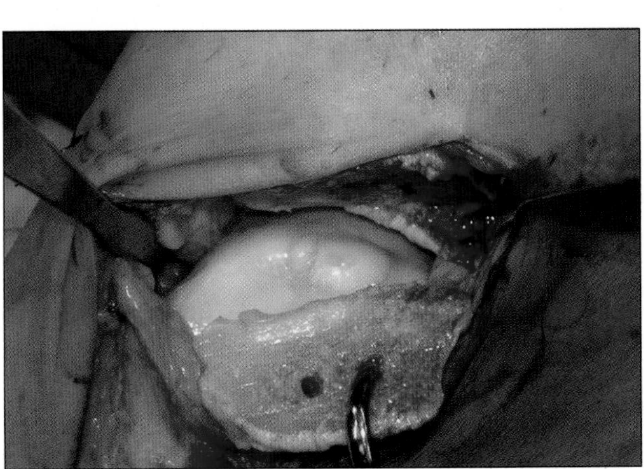

FIGURE 7

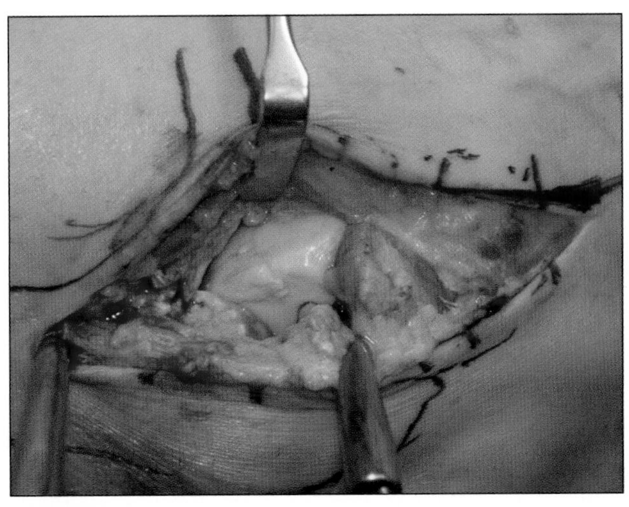

FIGURE 8

Procedure

Step 1

- Ankle arthroscopy is performed.
  - Diagnostic assessment of intra-articular structures, particularly cartilage condition and stability at the location of lesion
  - Functional testing with regard to ligamentous incompetence (Hintermann et al., 2002)
- We use a central portal to gain access to all compartments.
- Additionally, an anterolateral or anteromedial portal is used to insert the instruments.

Step 2

- Through a medial or lateral approach, the lesion is exposed at the talar dome.
- A cylindrical hole is drilled with the mosaicplasty instrument (diamond hollow drilling bit), aiming for minimal, but complete, resection (Fig. 9).
- The plug is removed by the handle.
- The hole should be inspected to determine whether, overall, all osseous lesions (cysts, sclerotic zones) were removed. If not, drill a bigger or an additional hole.
- The length of the plug is measured to determine the necessary length of the iliac plug (normally, 10–20 mm).

Step 3

- Exposure of the iliac crest
  - A 3- to 4-cm skin incision to the deep fascia is made, and hemostasis is obtained.
  - A sharp incision to the bone is made distally to the muscular insertion (e.g., along the lateral border).
  - The muscular insertion is meticulously separated from the periosteum, leaving it intact on bone.
- Harvesting of the plug
  - A bone plug is taken with an approximately 0.25-mm bigger diameter than the drill hole in the talus (Fig. 10).
  - Attention is paid not to damage the periosteal flap on the plug surface.

Step 4

- The cylindrical plug is inserted using a press-fit technique to achieve good primary stability (Fig. 11).
- The plug must be inserted à niveau. Edges, pins, and pikes may destroy the opposite cartilage and provoke "kissing lesions," accelerating the osteoarthritic process (Fig. 12).

Pearls

- *The use of CO_2 for arthroscopy helps to avoid swelling of soft tissues.*
- *Distraction of the ankle may be achieved by appropriate devices.*

Pitfalls

- *Too-extensive pressure from using a liquid to open the joint may result in swelling of the periarticular soft tissues.*

Pearls

- *To avoid development of substantial heat while drilling, cooling with water is essential to not damage the bone.*

Pitfalls

- *Inappropriate drilling may be the cause of failure—particularly not including the whole lesion or not drilling perpendicular to the direction of the drill system.*

Controversies

- To date, there is no evidence as to whether it is better to treat a large lesion with one big plug or several smaller plugs.
- Although not reported in most studies, there is evidence of higher donor-site morbidity at the knee joint than generally believed (Leumann et al., 2007). From that point of view, alternative use of a plug from the iliac crest is advised.

Pearls

- *The surface geometry of the selected graft should be as close as possible to that required by the location on the talus.*
- *Harvesting of a slightly longer plug is advised.*

Pitfalls

- *The use of a cannula that is not slightly oversized will result in insufficient press-fit of the graft, which may cause nonunion or malunion.*
- *Inappropriate application of force may cause fracture of the plug.*

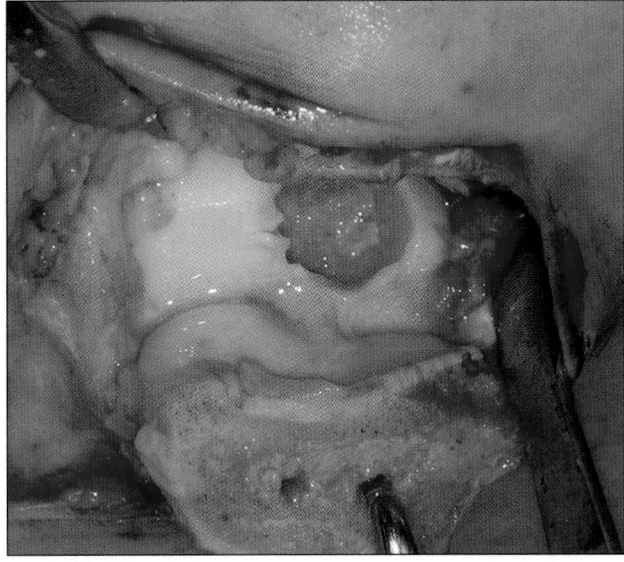

FIGURE 9

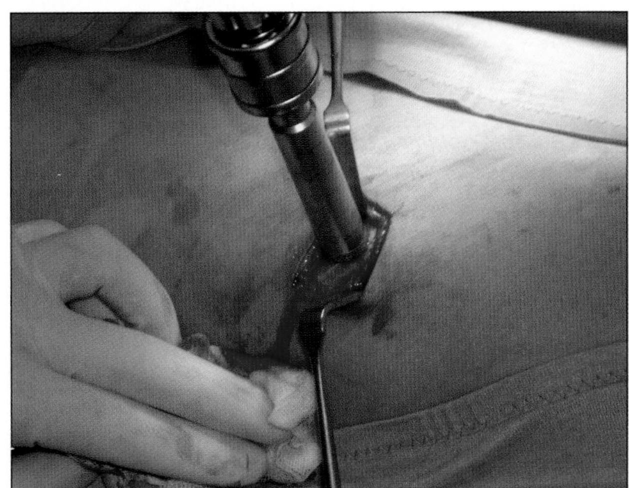

FIGURE 10

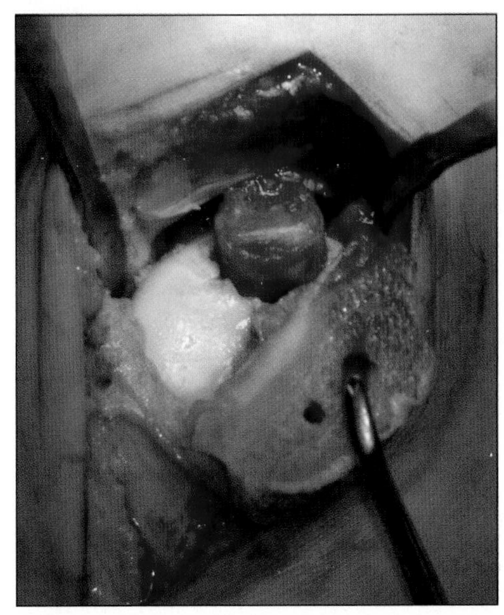

FIGURE 11

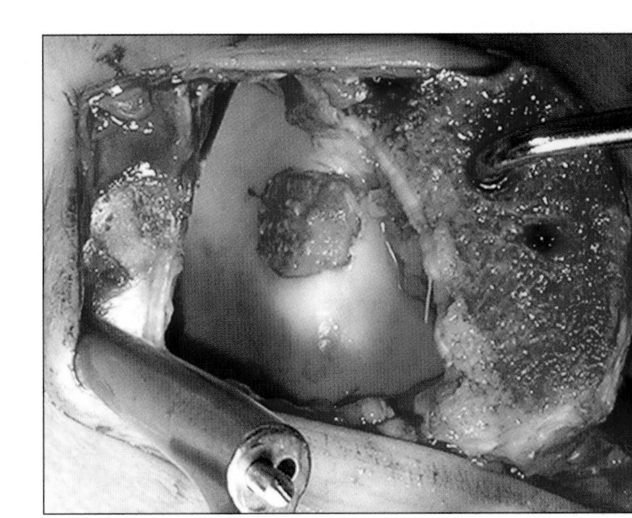

FIGURE 12

STEP 5

- Closure of medial arthrotomy
  - Anatomic reduction of the medial malleolus is achieved.
  - Fixation is accomplished by insertion of the two screws as prepared at the beginning.
  - Step-by-step wound closure is obtained.
- Closure of lateral arthrotomy
  - If done by fibular osteotomy, anatomic reduction and plate fixation are used.
  - If done by ligamentous detachment, the ligaments are reattached to the fibula by transosseous sutures or anchors.
  - Step-by-step wound closure is obtained.
- A slightly compressive dressing is applied.
- A splint is applied to keep the foot in neutral position

PEARLS

- *To augment healing, demineralized bone matrix may be added on the surface of the drilling hole (Fig. 13).*

PITFALLS

- *Inappropriate force application may result in fracture of the plug or destruction of the periosteal layer (e.g., the pluripotent stem cells).*
- *Insufficient stability through press-fitting may result in plug necrosis and recurrence of subchondral cyst formation.*

PEARLS

- *In the case of varus or valgus malalignment, supramalleolar and/or calcaneal osteotomy may be advised to get a well-balanced ankle joint.*

PITFALLS

- *Nonanatomic reconstruction of the bony geometry may result in degenerative disease.*
- *Insufficient restoration of joint stability may result in recurrence of the lesion.*

Controversies

- A suction drainage system is widely used. We do not use it on a regular basis, however, because we do not see any advantage for the use of such a device.

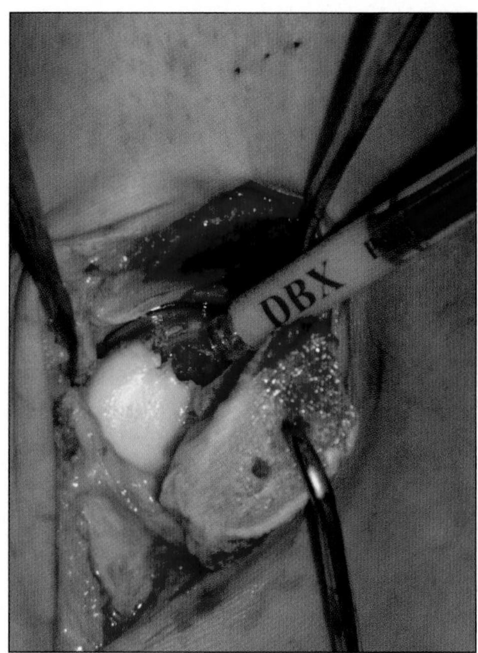

FIGURE 13

Postoperative Care and Expected Outcomes

- The patient is permitted 15-kg partial weight bearing for 8–12 weeks. Supportive cartilage nutrition (e.g., chondroitin sulfate, hyaluronic acid) is prescribed.
- A continuous passive motion machine is used, allowing for free range of motion.
- The patient is permitted active motion as tolerated from the beginning.
- When bony healing of the osteotomy and plugs has occurred (normally within 6–8 weeks) (Fig. 14), progressive loading of the ankle is permitted. Also, a rehabilitation program is started that includes, in addition to passive and active mobilization of the ankle joint, improvement of coordination and proprioception, and training of muscular strength.
- Protection by a walker or stabilizing shoe when walking is recommended for 12 weeks overall.
- Athletes should anticipate to return to sports in 9–12 months after their reconstruction.

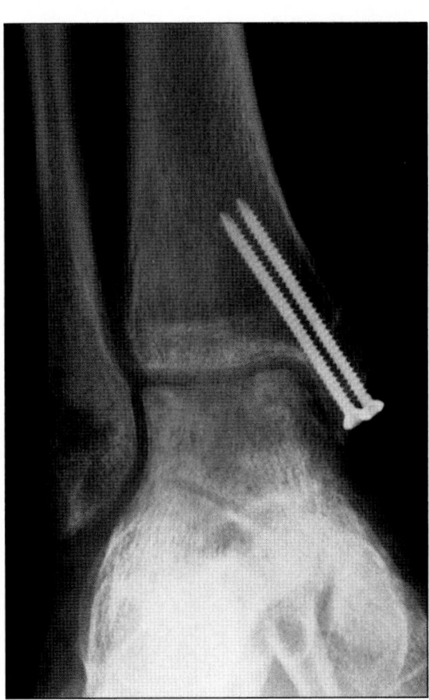

FIGURE 14

Pearls

- *Additional osteotomies (supramalleolar or calcaneal) and/or ligament reconstruction, if they are necessary, may change the postoperative rehabilitation program.*
- *Hardware removal is frequently necessary and can be considered after 6–8 weeks.*
- *If necessary, re-arthroscopy can be considered at the same time for scar shaving and débridement.*

Pitfalls

- *Too-aggressive rehabilitation and loading may result in delayed union/nonunion of plugs, excessive scar formation, or ligament incompetence.*
- *Complications include delayed wound healing and superficial or deep infection.*

Controversies

- No data are available giving advice as to what extent of sports activity after osteochondral treatment is advisable. Because most often young, sports-active patients are affected, early discussion and information on rehabilitation potential seems important.

Evidence

Berndt AL, Harty M. Transchondral fractures (osteochondritis dissecans) of the talus. J Bone Joint Surg [Am]. 1959;41:988-1020.

This study was the first publication on osteochondral lesions of the talus. It described four radiologic stages of ostechondral lesions and showed results of an early treatment rationale. (Level IV evidence)

Frigg A, Magerkurth O, Valderrabano V, Ledermann HP, Hintermann B. The effect of osseous ankle configuration on chronic ankle instability. Br J Sports Med. 2007;41:420-4.

This study described the importance of the osseous configuration of the talus for chronic ankle instability, a key factor in the pathomechanism of osteochondral lesions.

Hangody L. The mosaicplasty technique for osteochondral lesions of the talus. Foot Ankle Clin. 2003;8:259-73.

The inventor of the mosaicplasty, Laszlo Hangody, reported on the technique for mosaicplasty of the talus and his results in 63 patients. (Level IV evidence)

Hintermann B. What the orthopaedic foot and ankle surgeon wants to know from MR imaging. Semin Musculoskelet Radiol. 2005;9:260-71.

This overview article summarized indications and limitations of MRI in foot and ankle surgery. (Level V evidence)

Hintermann B, Boss A, Schäfer D. Arthroscopic findings in patients with chronic ankle instability. Am J Sports Med. 2002;30:402-9.

Ankle arthroscopy of 148 symptomatic chronic unstable ankles showed cartilage damage in 66% of ankles with lateral ligament injuries and 98% of ankles with deltoid ligament injuries. (Level IV evidence)

Kreuz PC, Steinwachs M, Erggelet C, Lahm A, Henle P, Niemeyer P. Mosaicplasty with autogenous talar autograft for osteochondral lesions of the talus after failed primary arthroscopic management: a prospective study with a 4-year follow-up. Am J Sports Med. 2006;34:55-63.

This study reported results of osteochondral autografting with grafts harvested on the ipsilateral talar articular facet implanted with a tibial wedge osteotomy. Best results were shown in patients without osteotomy. (Level III evidence)

Leumann A, Valderrabano V, Pagenstert G, Hintermann B. Reconstruction of talar osteochondral lesions with mosaicplasty from the knee joint. Presented at the GOTS-Kongress, Munich, Germany, June 23, 2007.

This report was a retrospective analysis of 11 cases treated with mosaicplasty from the knee joint with 58 months' follow-up, showing significant donor-site morbidity and limited functional and radiologic results. (Level IV evidence)

Pagenstert GE, Hintermann B, Barg A, Leumann A, Valderrabano V. Realignment surgery as alternative treatment of varus and valgus ankle osteoarthritis. Clin Orthop Relat Res. 2007;(462):156-68.

This study described a treatment rationale for malalignment, a factor that has to be addressed in osteochondral lesions. (Level IV evidence)

Raikin SM, Elias I, Zoga AC, Morrison WB, Besser MP, Schweitzer ME. Osteochondral lesions of the talus: localization and morphologic data from 424 patients using a novel anatomical grid scheme. Foot Ankle Int. 2007;28:154-61.

This study analyzed MRI of 424 patients, showing that 62% of lesions are localized medially and 34% laterally. Of all lesions, 80% were localized close to the equator: medially rather than behind and laterally rather than before the top of the mortise.

Reddy S, Pedowitz DI, Parekh SG, Sennett BJ, Okereke E. The morbidity associated with osteochondral harvest from asymptomatic knees for the treatment of osteochondral lesions of the talus. Am J Sports Med. 2007;35:80-5.

A case series of 15 patients treated with mosaicplasty with osteochondral transplantation from the asymptomatic ipsilateral knee to the talus demonstrated significant donor-site morbidity in 4 of the 11 patients available for follow-up, with a poor knee Lysholm score. (Level IV evidence)

Valderrabano V, Hintermann B, Horisberger M, Fung TS. Ligamentous posttraumatic ankle osteoarthritis. Am J Sports Med. 2006;34:612-20.

Of a cohort of 247 patients with end-stage ankle osteoarthritis, 12% (30 patients) showed ligamentous posttraumatic ankle osteoarthritis. The authors explained the process of pathologic biomechanical cartilage loading with long-standing chronic ankle instability leading to osteoarthritis. (Level IV evidence)

Verhagen RA, Maas M, Dijkgraaf MG, Tol JL, Krips R, van Dijk CN. Prospective study on diagnostic strategies in osteochondral lesions of the talus: is MRI superior to helical CT? J Bone Joint Surg [Br]. 2005;87:41-6.

This study showed in a case series of 103 patients that MRI and CT show no significant difference in diagnosing osteochondral lesions. (Level III evidence)

Verhagen RA, Struijs PA, Bossuyt PM, van Dijk CN. Systematic review of treatment strategies for osteochondral defects of the talar dome. Foot Ankle Clin. 2003;8: 233-42.

This review summarized all studies with different treatment modalities for osteochondral lesions and showed comparable results for mosaicplasty, microfracture, and drilling strategies. However, the level and amount of data are poor; no level I study has been published so far. (Level III evidence)

PROCEDURE 35

Arthroscopy of the Subtalar Joint

Carol Frey

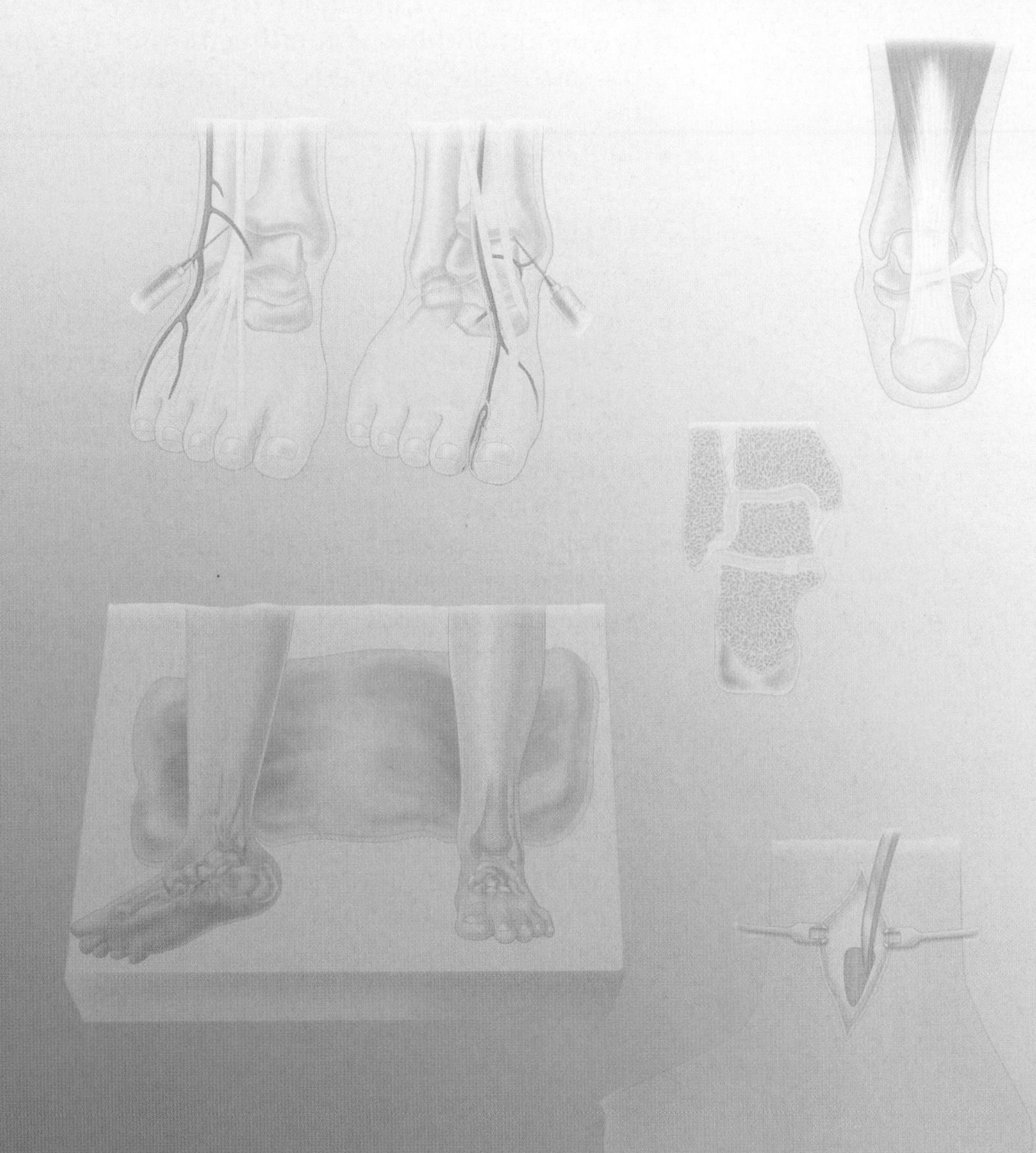

PITFALLS

- *The absolute contraindications to subtalar arthroscopy must be ruled out. These include localized infection leading to a potential septic joint and advanced degenerative joint disease, particularly with deformity. Relative contraindications include severe edema, poor skin quality, and poor vascular status.*

Controversies

- Instability
- Evaluation of coalition

Indications

- Chondromalacia
- Subtalar impingement lesions
- Osteophytes
- Lysis of adhesions with posttraumatic arthrofibrosis
- Synovectomy
- Removal of loose bodies
- Débridement and treatment of osteochondral lesions
- Retrograde drilling of cystic lesions
- Removal of a symptomatic os trigonum
- Evaluation and excision of fractures of the anterior process of the calcaneus and lateral process of the talus
- Subtalar fusion

Examination/Imaging

Physical Examination

- Motion of the subtalar joint is best tested by holding the left heel in the right hand and vice versa, then using the opposite hand to hold the forefoot and move the foot from inversion to eversion. In the normal subtalar joint, this motion should be smooth and painless.
- It should be noted that, although inversion and eversion are primarily coming from the talocalcaneal (subtalar) joint, they are not limited to that joint. Furthermore, subtalar motion is not pure inversion and eversion. Therefore, exact measurements are difficult using standard techniques.
- When pathology exists in the subtalar joint, there may be swelling or stiffness in the joint. This is not specific to one diagnosis.
- Subtalar stiffness and pain indicates pathology in and around the subtalar joint but is not specific to one diagnosis.
- Relief of symptoms with injection of local anesthetic directly into the sinus tarsi confirms the diagnosis of pain or dysfunction in the sinus tarsi (Fig. 1). Differential injections may be required to confirm pathology in the subtalar joint.
- Pathology of the interosseous ligaments of the subtalar joint usually is associated with focal pain over the lateral entrance to the sinus tarsi. Patients often have slight restriction and discomfort with passive subtalar motion.

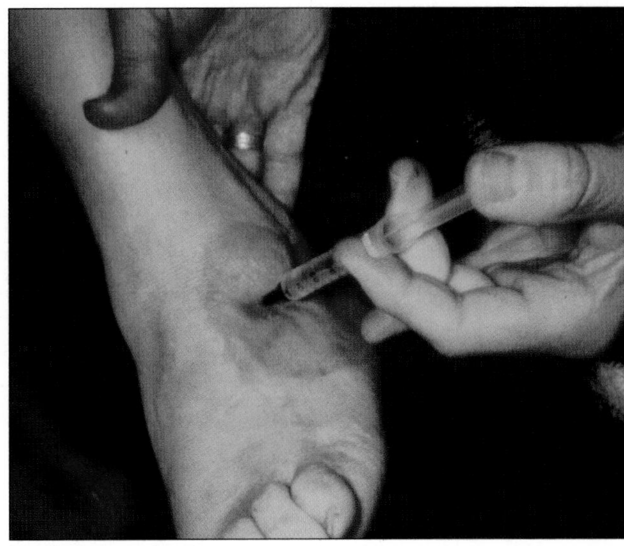

FIGURE 1

Treatment Options

- Injection of anesthetic agent or corticosteroid
- Foot orthosis, including a UCBL
- Anti-inflammatory medication
- Ankle brace with a hindfoot lock
- Cast
- Peroneal tendon–strengthening exercises

Imaging

- Anteroposterior (AP), lateral, and modified AP views of the foot are necessary to identify the subtalar joint.
- The lateral and posterior process are better seen on hindfoot oblique views.
- The 45° oblique foot film shows the anterior portion of the subtalar joint.
- Borden's view shows the posterior facet of the subtalar joint (Fig. 2). This view is obtained by rotating the foot medially 45° with dorsiflexion. The x-ray beam is pointed at the lateral malleolus and angled 10° cephalad. Different views are obtained by changing the angle of the x-ray beam from 10° to 40°.

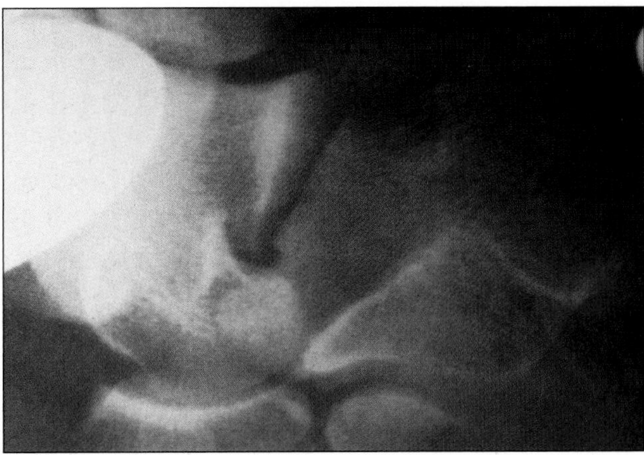

FIGURE 2

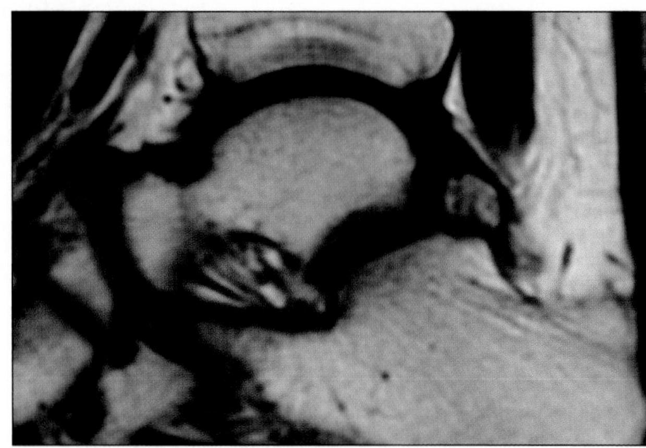
A

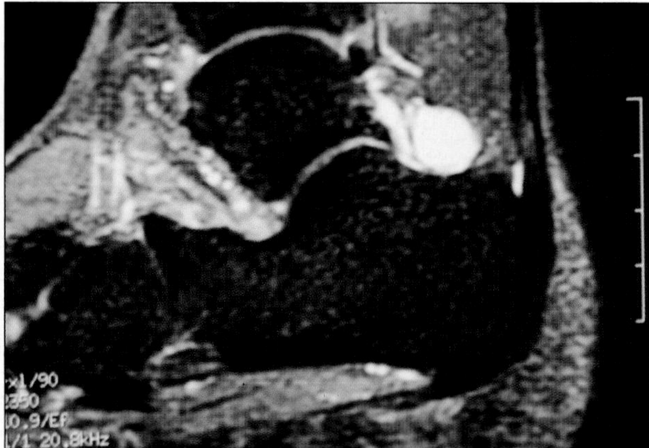
B

FIGURE 3

- Computed tomography (CT) scans in the coronal plane are best for visualizing the talar body or posterior and lateral process of the talus. CT can be used to show intra-articular pathology (Fig. 3A).
- CT scans in the transverse or sagittal planes are best to visualize the talar neck and dome.
- Magnetic resonance imaging (MRI) may detect chronic inflammation or fibrosis within the subtalar joint (Fig. 3B). Ligament injury, bone contusions, osteochondral lesions, chondral injury, impingement, synovitis, and fibrous or cartilagenous coalitions can be well demonstrated on MRI.

Surgical Anatomy

- For arthroscopic purposes, the subtalar joint is divided into anterior (talocalcaneal-navicular) and posterior (talocalcaneal) articulations (Fig. 4).
- The anterior and posterior articulations are separated by the tarsal canal, which has a large lateral opening called the sinus tarsi.
- Within the tarsal canal and sinus tarsi, the interosseous talocalcaneal ligament, the medial and intermediate roots of the inferior extensor retinaculum, the cervical ligament, fatty tissue, and blood vessels are found (Fig. 5). The lateral ligamentous support of the subtalar joint consists of the lateral talocalcaneal ligament, the posterior talocalcaneal ligament, the lateral root of the inferior extensor retinaculum, and the calcaneofibular ligament.

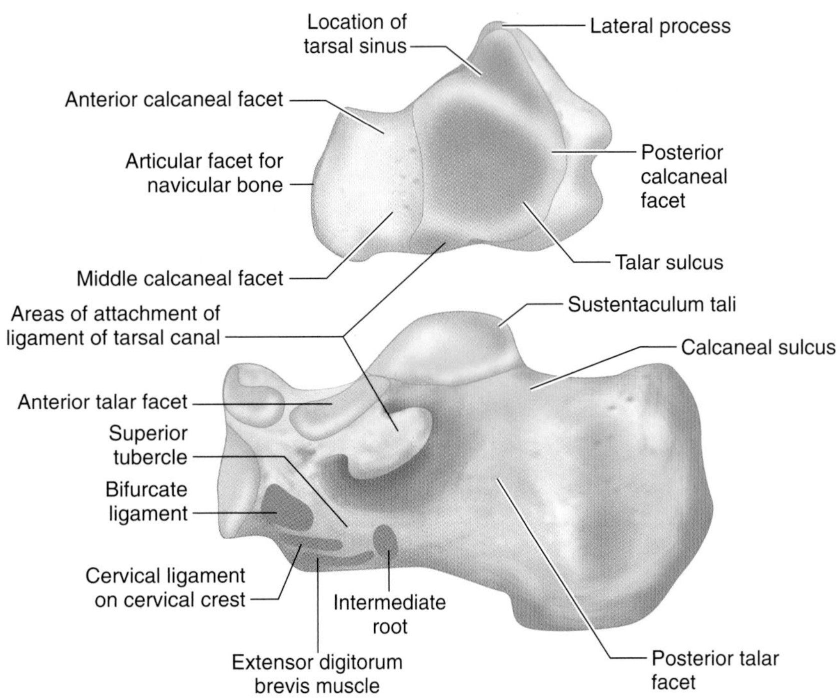

FIGURE 4

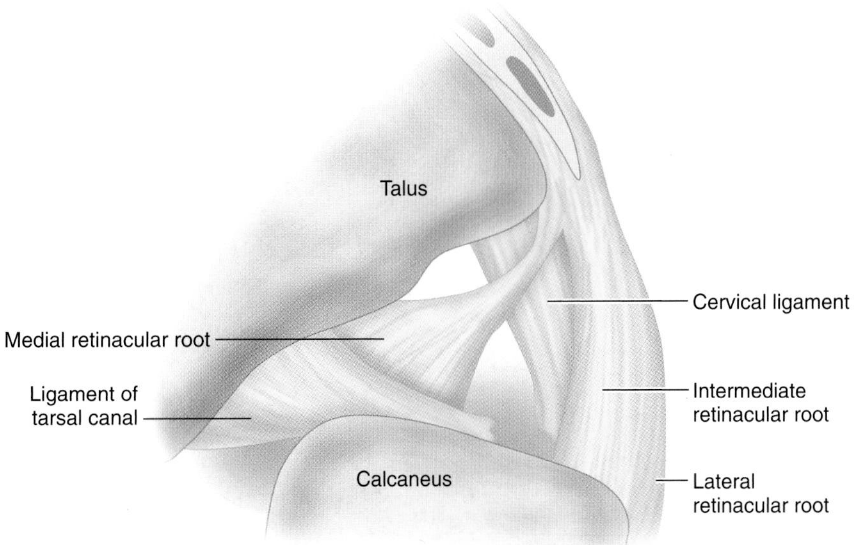

FIGURE 5

- The anterior subtalar joint is generally thought to be inaccessible to arthroscopic visualization because of the thick interosseous ligament that fills the tarsal canal. Because of this, the region normally has no connection with the posterior joint complex.
- The posterior subtalar joint has a synovial lining. This joint has a posterior capsular pouch with small lateral, medial, and anterior recesses.

Equipment

- Bean bag for positioning

Positioning

- The patient is placed in the lateral decubitis position with the operative extremity draped free. Padding is placed between the lower extremities, as well as under the contralateral extremity to protect the peroneal nerve (Fig. 6).
- A thigh tourniquet is recommended.

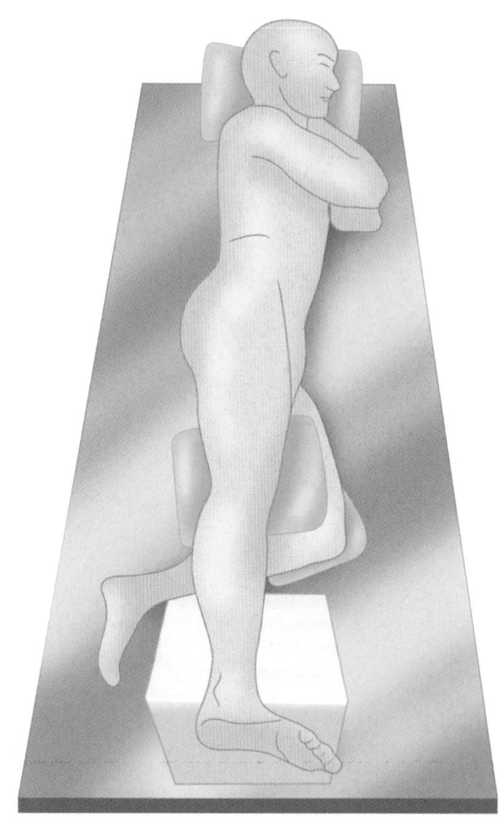

FIGURE 6

Portals/Exposures

Lateral Approach

- Three standard portals are recommended for visualization and instrumentation of the subtalar joint (Fig. 7). The anatomic landmarks for lateral portal placement include the lateral malleolus, the sinus tarsi, and the Achilles tendon.
- Careful dissection and portal placement help avoid the superficial peroneal nerve, as well as its branches, with placement of the anterior portal and the sural nerve and peroneal tendons with placement of the posterior portal.
- The anterior portal is established approximately 1 cm distal to the fibular tip and 2 cm anterior to it.
- The middle portal is just anterior to the tip of the fibula, directly over the sinus tarsi.

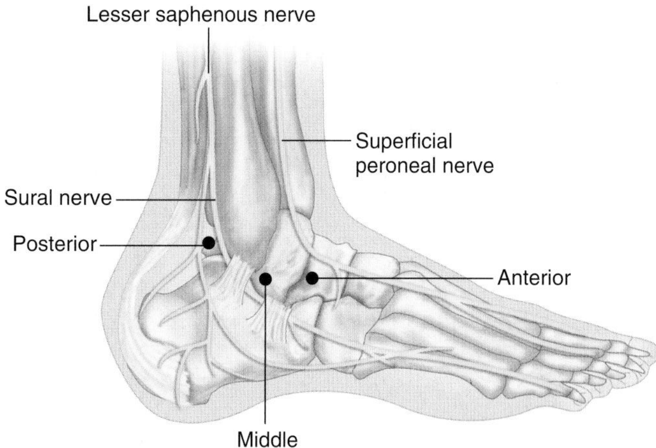

FIGURE 7

- The posterior portal is at or approximately one finger-width proximal to the fibular tip and 2 cm posterior to the lateral malleolus.
- The posterior portal is usually safe when placed behind the saphenous vein and sural nerve and anterior to the Achilles tendon. With placement of the posterior portal, care must be taken to avoid the sural nerve.

Posterior Approach

- Subtalar arthroscopy can be performed using a posterolateral and posteromedial portal (Fig. 8A–C). This two-portal endoscopic approach to the hindfoot with the patient in the prone position provides better access to the medial and lateral aspects of the posterior subtalar joint.

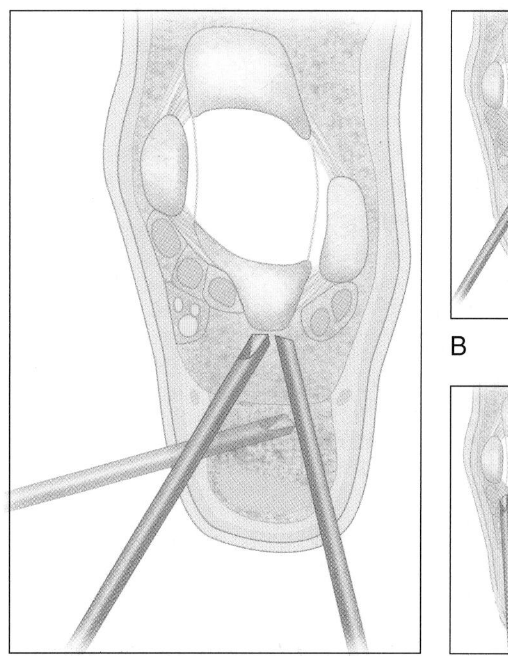

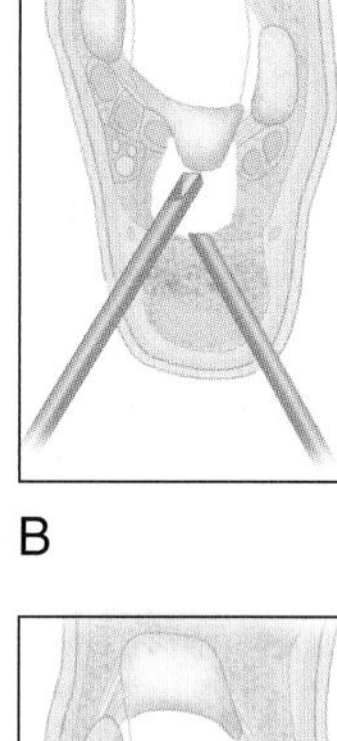

B

C

FIGURE 8 A

- The main difference between the two techniques is that the lateral approach for subtalar arthroscopy is a true arthroscopy technique in which the arthroscope and the instruments are placed within the joint, whereas the two-portal posterior technique (using a posterolateral and posteromedial portal) starts as an extra-articular approach.
- With the two-portal posterior technique, first a working space is created adjacent to the posterior subtalar joint by removing the fatty tissue overlying the joint capsule and the posterior part of the ankle joint.
- The joint capsule is then partially removed in order to be able to inspect the joint from outside-in with the arthroscope positioned at the edge of the joint without actually entering the joint space.
- The maximum size of the intra-articular instruments depends on the available joint space.

Procedure

Step 1

- Local, general, spinal, or epidural anesthesia can be used for this procedure.
- The anterior portal is identified first with an 18-gauge spinal needle, and the joint is inflated with a 20-ml syringe.
- A small skin incision is made, and the subcutaneous tissue is gently spread using a straight mosquito clamp.
- A cannula with a semiblunt trocar is then placed, followed by a 2.9-mm 30° oblique arthroscope.
- The middle portal is placed under direct visualization using an 18-gauge spinal needle and outside-in technique.
- The posterior portal can be placed at this time using the same direct visualization technique. The trocar is placed in an upward and slightly anterior manner.

Step 2

- Diagnostic subtalar arthroscopy examination begins with the arthroscope viewing from the anterior portal (Fig. 9A).
  - With the arthroscope in the anterior portal, the ligaments that insert on the floor of the sinus tarsi are visualized. In Figure 9A, the ligaments that insert on the floor of the sinus tarsi have been débrided.

Pearls

- *The best portal combination for the evaluation and débridement of pathology in the sinus tarsi is the arthroscope in the anterior portal and the instruments placed in the middle portal.*
- *One can débride torn interosseous ligaments and synovitis, remove loose bodies, and lyse adhesions. A radiofrequency wand is a useful tool to access the hard-to-reach spots in the sinus tarsi and subtalar joint.*

Instrumentation/Implantation

- 2.9-mm arthroscope with a camera with a wide-angle lens
- Arthroscopic pump
- High-flow system
- Small joint instrumentation
- 18-gauge spinal needle
- Straight mosquito clamp
- Radiofrequency wand

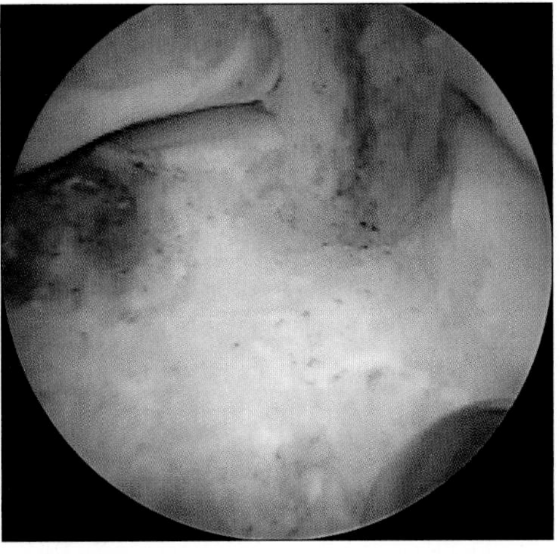
A

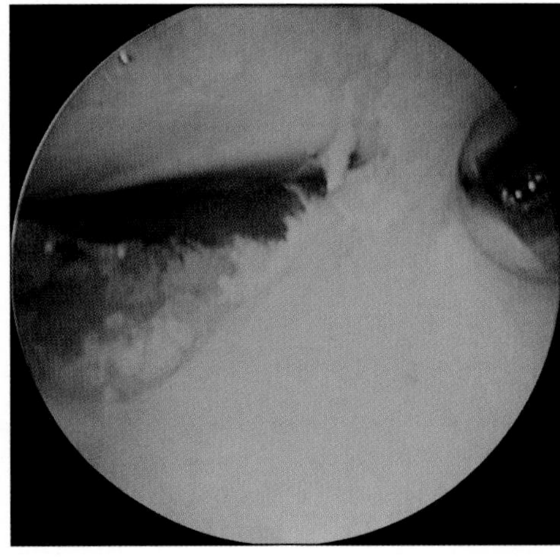
B

FIGURE 9

Pearls

- *The best portal combination for evaluation and removal of the os trigonum is the arthroscope in the anterior portal and the instrumentation in the posterior portal.*
- *The asymptomatic os trigonum (Steida's process) can be débrided with a burr or shaver and removed through an arthroscopic portal using a standard arthroscopic grasper.*
- *Rarely, it is necessary to enlarge the portal for delivery of the os trigonum.*

  - It is easy to get disoriented, as the ligaments are closely packed and cross over one another in the sinus tarsi.
- More medially, the deep interosseous ligament is observed to fill the tarsal canal.
- The arthroscope should now be slowly withdrawn and the arthroscopic lens rotated to view the anterior process of the calcaneus (Fig. 9B).
- The arthroscopic lens is then rotated in the opposite direction to view the anterior aspect of the posterior talocalcaneal articulation (Fig. 10).

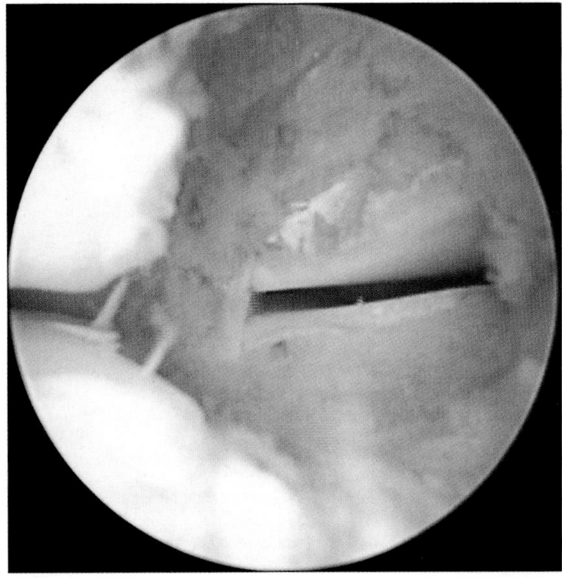

FIGURE 10

- Next, the anterolateral corner of the posterior joint is examined and reflections of the lateral talocalcaneal ligament and the calcaneofibular ligament are observed (Fig. 11). The lateral talocalcaneal ligament is noted anterior to the calcaneofibular ligament.
- The arthroscopic lens may then be rotated medially and the central articulation between the talus and the calcaneus observed (Fig. 12; synovitis is seen on the left). The posterolateral gutter may be seen from the anterior portal.
- It is often possible to advance the scope along the lateral and posterolateral gutter and visualize the posterior pouch and Stieda's process (os trigonum) (Fig. 13).

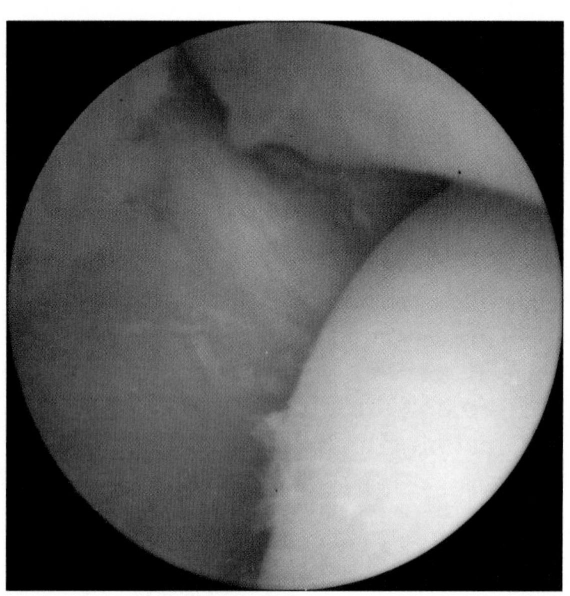

FIGURE 11

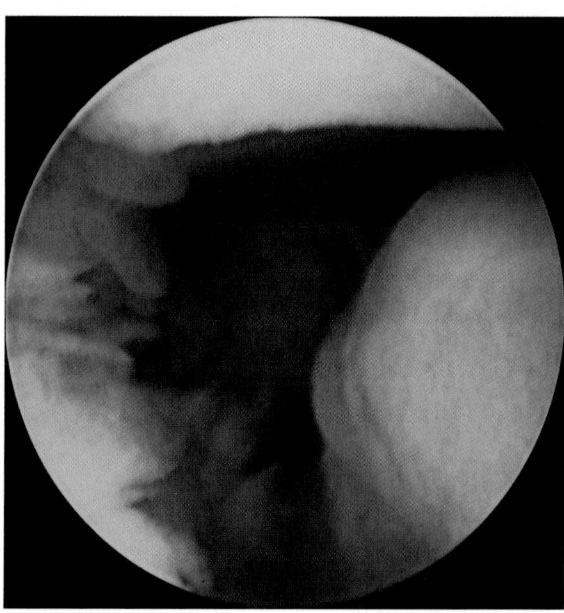

FIGURE 12

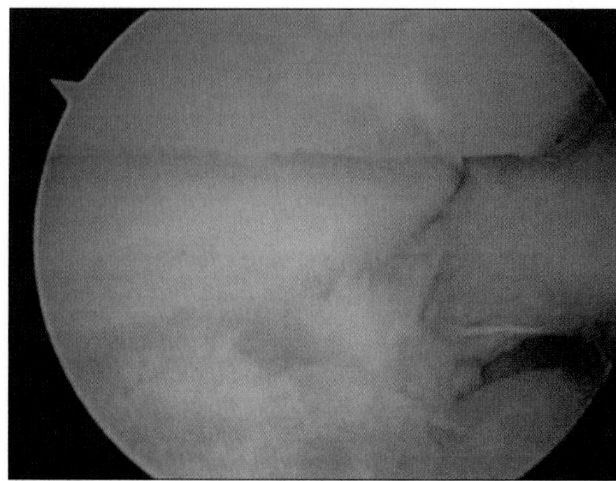

FIGURE 13

Step 3

- The arthroscope is switched to the posterior portal.
  - From this view, the interosseous ligament may be seen anteriorly in the joint.
  - As the arthroscopic lens is rotated laterally, the lateral talocalcaneal ligament and calcaneofibular ligament reflections again may be seen.
- The central talocalcaneal joint may then be seen from this posterior view and the posterolateral gutter examined (Fig. 14). Adhesions are seen on the posterolateral capsule in Figure 14.
- The posterolateral recess, posterior gutter, and posterolateral corner of the talus are visualized (Fig. 15).
- The posteromedial recess and posteromedial corner of the talocalcaneal joint can be seen from the posterior portal (Fig. 16).

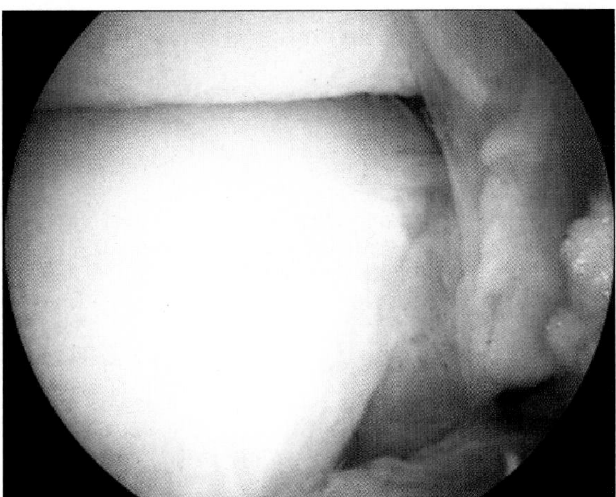

FIGURE 14

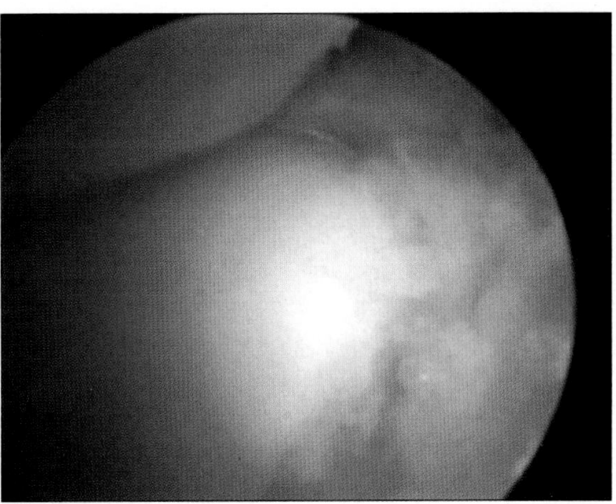

FIGURE 15

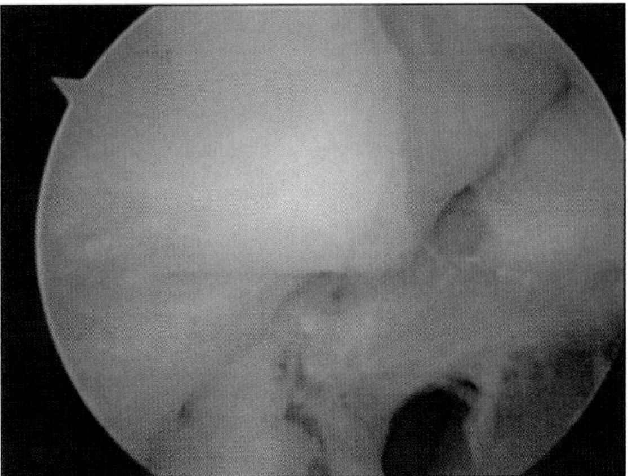

FIGURE 16

Postoperative Care and Expected Outcomes

- After completing the procedure, the portals are closed with sutures.
- A compression dressing is applied from the toes to the midcalf. Ice and elevation are recommended until the inflammatory phase has passed.
- The patient is allowed to ambulate with the use of crutches, and weight bearing is permitted as tolerated.
- The sutures are removed approximately 10 days after the procedure.
- The patient should begin gentle active range-of-motion exercises of the foot and ankle immediately after surgery. Once the sutures are removed, if indicated, the patient is referred to a physical therapist for supervised rehabilitation.

Evidence

Cugat R, Cusco X, Garcia M, Samitier G, Seijas R. Posterosuperior osteochondritis of the calcaneus: case report. Arthroscopy 2007;23:1025.

Osteochondritis of the posterior facet of the calcaneus is a relatively uncommon injury, and this report described the second in the literature. Débridement of the osteonecrotic area was performed, followed by microfracture using the Steadman technique. Arthroscopic excision and débridement have shown good to excellent results in 75–80% of cases on the talar surface. (Level I evidence)

Frey C, Feder K, Chow H. Arthroscopy of the subtalar joint: clinical outcomes. Foot Ankle Int. 2009 (in press).

In this study of 126 cases followed for over 2 years, a significant improvement was noted using both the American Orthopaedic Foot and Ankle Society (AOFAS) and Karlsson-Peterson Ankle Scores. The average preoperative AOFAS score was 67.3 and the average postoperative score was 84.07. The average preoperative Karlssen-Peterson score was 59.09 and the average postoperative score was 81.41. (Level I evidence)

Frey C, Feder KS, DiGiovanni C. Arthroscopic evaluation of the subtalar joint: does sinus tarsi syndrome exist? Foot Ankle Int. 1999;20:185-91.

The authors demonstrated a success rate of 94% good and excellent results in the treatment of various types of subtalar pathology using arthroscopic techniques. Of the 14 patients who had a preoperative diagnosis of sinus tarsi syndrome, all the diagnoses were changed at the time of arthroscopy. The most common finding in these cases was a tear of the interosseous ligaments. Surgical removal of the contents of the lateral half of the sinus tarsi improved or eradicated symptoms in roughly 90% of cases of patients with sinus tarsi pain/dysfunction. (Level I evidence)

Goldberger MI, Conti SF. Clinical outcome after subtalar arthroscopy. Foot Ankle Int. 1998;19:462-5.

The authors retrospectively reviewed 12 patients who underwent subtalar arthroscopy for symptomatic subtalar pathology with nonspecific radiographic findings. The preoperative diagnoses were subtalar chondrosis in nine patients and subtalar synovitis in three patients. At 17.5 months' (average) follow-up, the postoperative AOFAS hindfoot score was 71 (range 51–85) compared to a preoperative score of 66 (range, 54–79). All patients stated that they would have the surgery again. (Level I evidence) van Dijk CN, Scholten PE, Krips R. A 2-portal endoscopic approach for diagnosis and treatment of posterior ankle pathology. Arthroscopy 2000;16:871-6.

The authors described the two-portal endoscopic approach to the subtalar joint, and subtalar arthroscopy using a posterolateral and posteromedial portal. The authors believe that the two-portal endoscopic approach to the hindfoot with the patient in the prone position provides better access to the medial and lateral aspects of the posterior subtalar joint. (Level I evidence)

Williams MM, Ferkel RD. Subtalar arthroscopy: indications, technique, and results. Arthroscopy 1998;14:373-81.

The authors reported on the 32-month (average) follow-up of 50 patients with hindfoot pain who underwent simultaneous ankle and subtalar arthroscopy. Preoperative diagnoses included degenerative joint disease, sinus tarsi dysfunction, and os trigonum. Good to excellent results were noted in 86% of the patients. Overall, less favorable results were noted with associated ankle pathology, degenerative joint disease, increased age, and increased activity level of the patient. No operative complications were reported. (Level I evidence)

PROCEDURE 36

Modified Brostrom Procedure for Lateral Ankle Laxity

Glenn B. Pfeffer

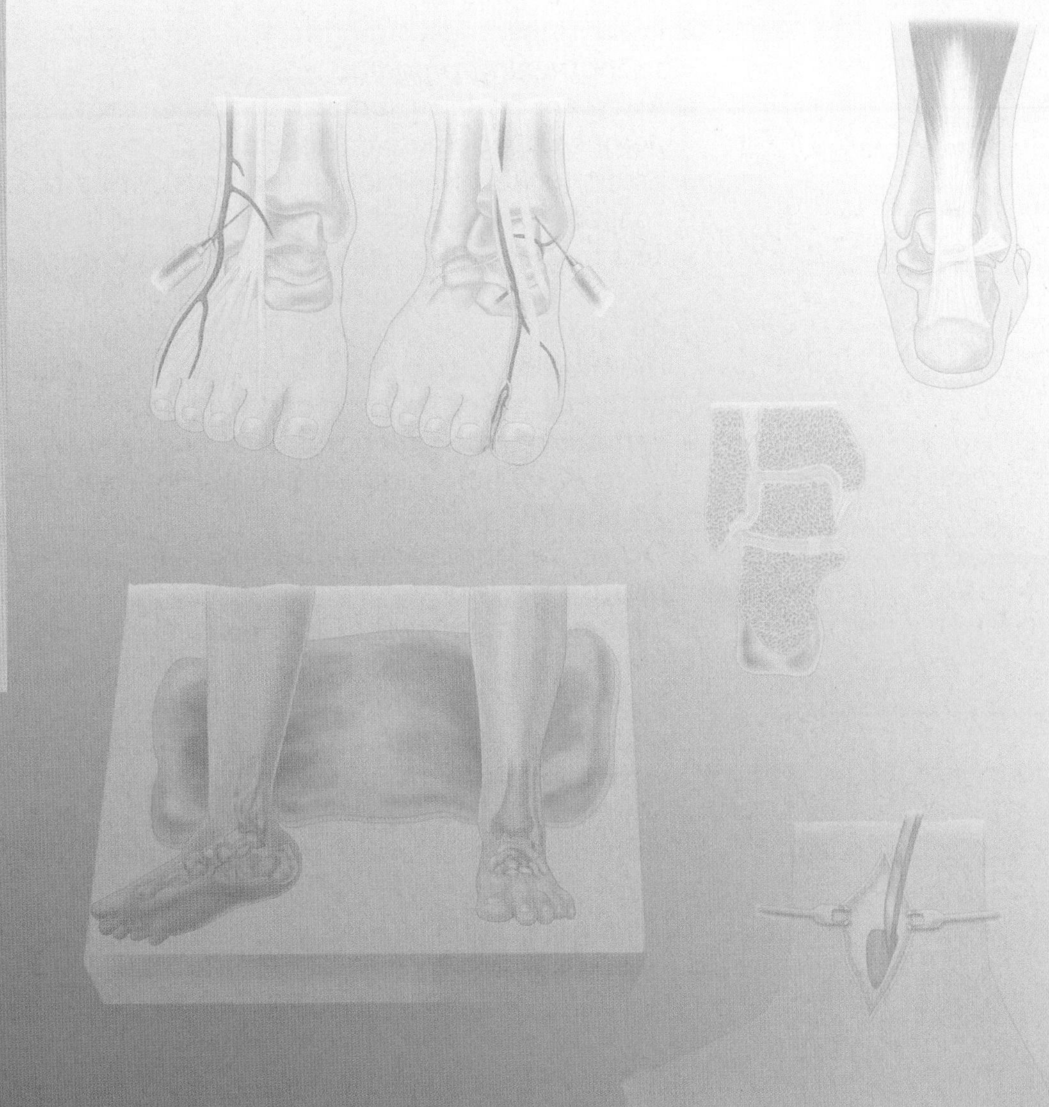

Indications

- Symptomatic chronic laxity of the lateral ankle with repeated sprains
- Limitation of activity
- Failure of an appropriate rehabilitation program

Examination/Imaging

- Document a cavovarus foot, with hindfoot varus or forefoot valgus, which predisposes a patient to repeated sprains.
- Evaluate peroneal strength, and the need for a strengthening program.
- Assess for ankle or subtalar joint line tenderness, and peroneal tenderness or dislocation.
- Assess for subtalar motion (patients with a tarsal coalition have a high incidence of ankle laxity).
- Test for generalized ligament laxity (positive findings include passive dorsiflexion of the fifth metacarpophalangeal joint to 90°, ability to appose the thumb to the volar forearm, and hyperextension of the elbow or knee beyond 0°) (Fig. 1A and 1B).
- Perform manual anterior drawer and talar tilt tests (with or without radiographic documentation) (Fig. 2A and 2B).
- Obtain weight-bearing anteroposterior, lateral, and mortise views of the ankle.
- Bilateral comparative stress views may be helpful if the diagnosis is in question. These views can be performed fluoroscopically in the operating room, after the patient has received anesthesia, to confirm which ligaments need repair (Fig. 3A and 3B).
- Magnetic resonance imaging (MRI) is essential if chronic peroneal, ankle, or subtalar joint pathology is suspected. Otherwise, MRI is not helpful in diagnosing dynamic laxity.

Pitfalls

- *Ankle laxity is often part of a triad that includes peroneal tendinopathy and intra-articular pathology. Always consider these associated conditions. Isolated ankle laxity with repeated sprains does not usually cause persistent chronic pain. Peroneal tendinopathy, lateral impingement, or an osteochondral lesion will.*
- *Athletes who weigh more than 200 lbs may require an additional procedure to augment the modified Brostrom repair.*
- *If the patient has heel varus, a Dwyer closing wedge osteotomy must be performed at the time of the Brostrom reconstruction. Forefoot varus may also require simultaneous correction, although this is much less common.*
- *A brief ankle arthroscopy can be performed during the same surgery just prior to a Brostrom repair. A prolonged arthroscopy causes too much extravasation of fluid, and the ligament repair should be done on a subsequent day.*

Controversies

- Physical therapy is commonly prescribed to a patient with ankle laxity in an attempt to avoid surgery. If the patient already has good peroneal strength, there probably is little benefit.

Pearls

- *The anterior drawer test rotates the talus forward around the intact medial axis of the deltoid ligament complex (except on very rare occasions when the deltoid is also lax). This rotation is most easily appreciated if the examiner, seated in front of the patient, uses his or her right hand for the left foot, and left hand for the right foot.*

Pitfalls

- *Nonpathologic ligamentous laxity is common. Numeric values for stress tests should not be used to determine which patients require surgery.*

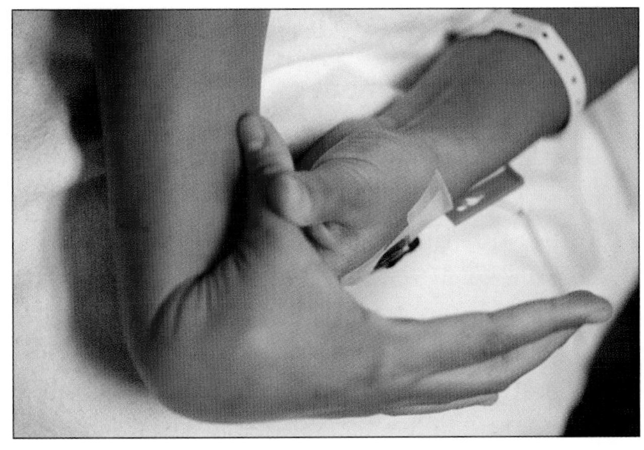
A

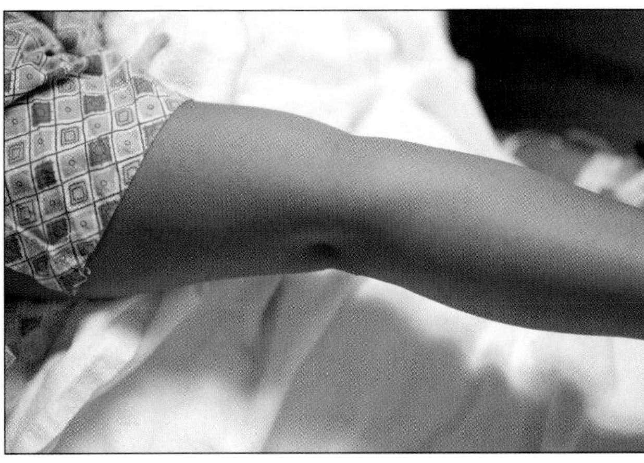
B

FIGURE 1

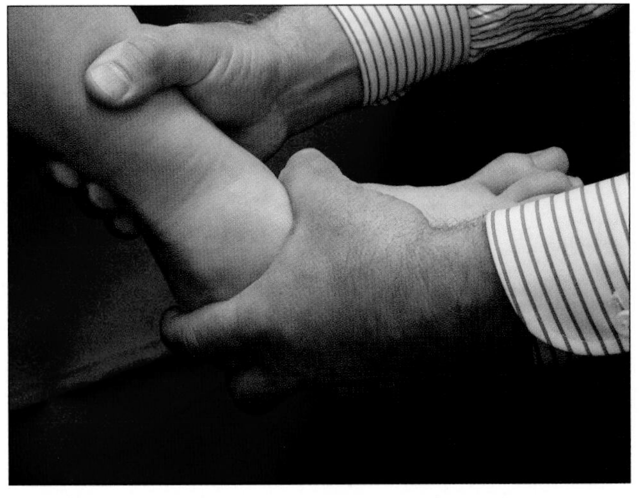
A

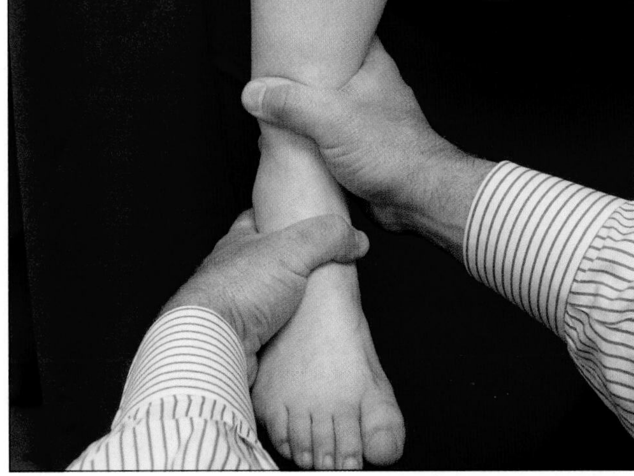
B

FIGURE 2

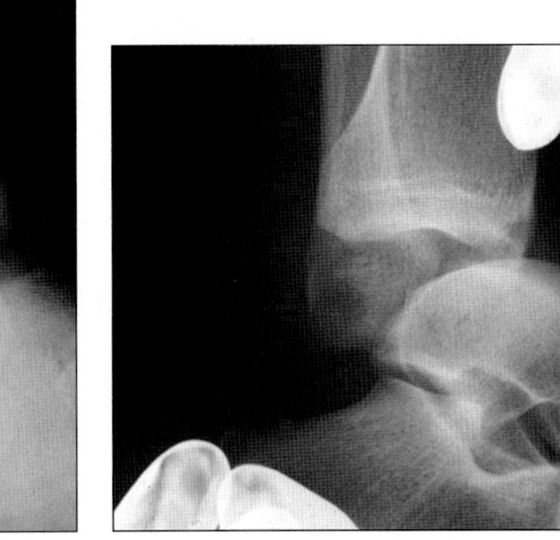
A B

FIGURE 3

Surgical Anatomy

- The anterior talofibular ligament (ATFL) originates 1 cm proximal to the distal tip of the fibula and inserts into the lateral talar body just beyond the articular surface (Fig. 4).
  - The ligament is not discrete; it is contiguous with the joint capsule as a discrete capsular thickening.
- The calcaneofibular ligament (CFL) is a discrete extra-articular structure (see Fig. 4).
  - It originates just inferior to the ATFL on the fibula and travels to the calcaneus, where it inserts 15 mm distal to the subtalar joint.
  - The ligament travels obliquely, in a plantar and posterior direction, and forms a variable 90–135° angle with the ATFL.

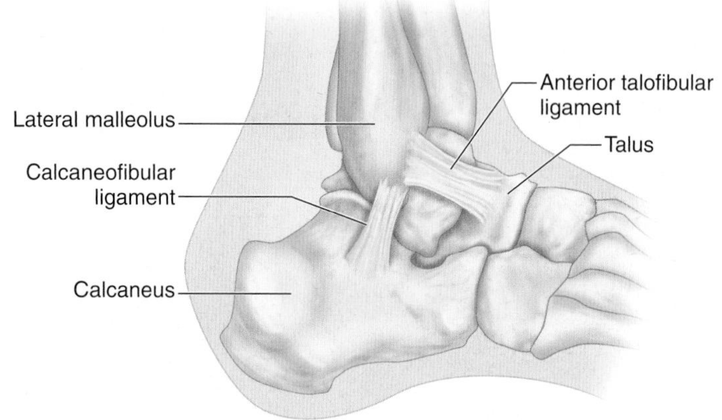

FIGURE 4

Positioning

- The patient is in a lateral position.
- A femoral-sciatic or popliteal block is used.
- A calf or thigh tourniquet allows adequate exposure of the lateral ankle.

Portals/Exposures

- Make a curvilinear incision 1 cm anterior to the fibula (Fig. 5A and 5B).

Procedure

Step 1

- The extensor retinaculum is dissected off of the joint capsule.
  - The retinaculum is often difficult to dissect out as a discrete layer. It is most easily isolated 2 cm proximal to the tip of the fibula (Fig. 6A and 6B).
  - Tag the retinaculum with a suture.

Pearls

- *The lateral branch of the superficial peroneal nerve may be injured during the approach, or inadvertently sewed into the repair.*
- *If the peroneal tendons are abnormal and require surgical correction, use a longitudinal incision that extends obliquely across the distal fibula from posterior to anterior.*
- *Varus of the heel should be corrected with a Dwyer osteotomy. Two incisions work best, unless the peroneal tendons also need surgery. In that case, make one long incision along the posterior border of the peroneal sheath, curving anteriorly distal to the fibula.*

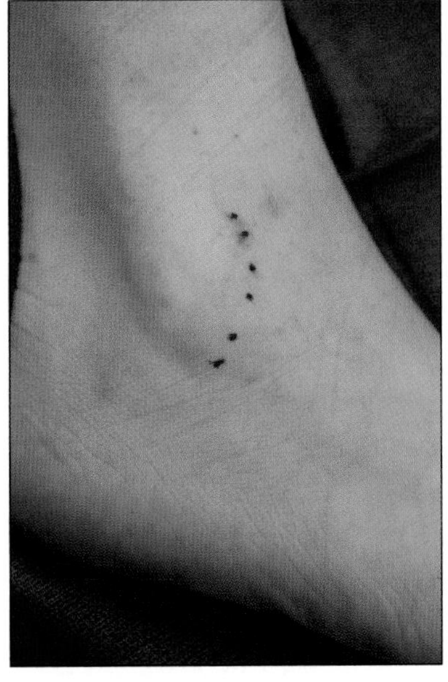

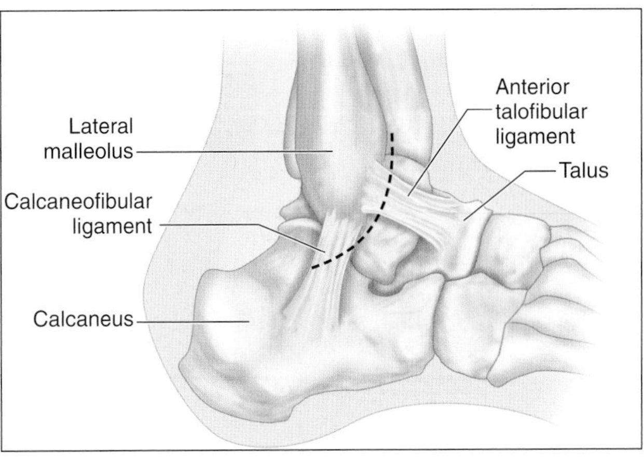

A B

FIGURE 5

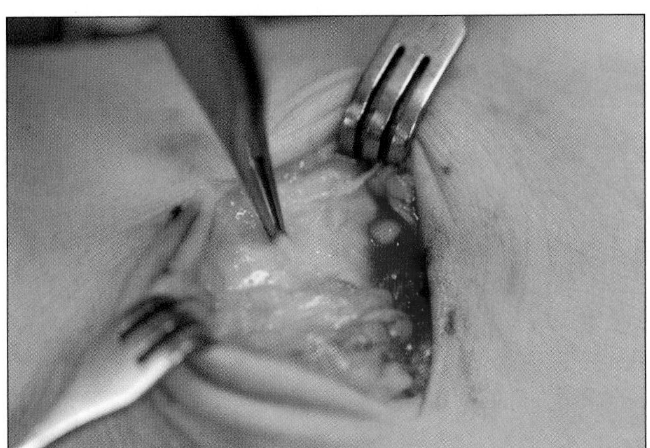

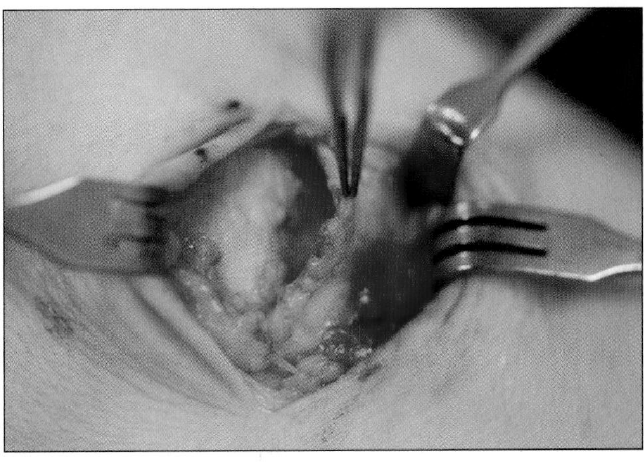

A B

FIGURE 6

PEARLS

- *Reinforcement of the ligament repair with the retinaculum is a key part of the procedure. While the ligaments may be attenuated, a robust retinaculum can almost always be found.*

PEARLS

- *There is almost always sufficient ligamentous tissue present to perform a Brostrom procedure, unless the patient has had a prior surgical repair.*

PITFALLS

- *If the capsular incision is made too anterior to the fibula, it is possible to inadvertently enter the subtalar joint instead of the ankle.*

STEP 2

- Open 2 cm of the peroneal tendon sheath anterior to the tip of the fibula. Inspect the tendons (Fig. 7).
- Pierce the joint capsule with a small knife blade at the level of the ankle joint, 3-5 mm anterior to the fibula.
  - Leave a sufficient cuff of tissue on the fibula for the repair (Fig. 8).
  - There is no need to detach the capsule from the fibula, which would then require reattachment with drill holes or suture anchors.
- Place a small hemostat beneath the capsule and ATFL and exit just above the peroneal tendons (Fig. 9). Divide the capsule and the ATFL (Fig. 10A and 10B).
- The ATFL can usually be identified as a discrete area of capsular thickening (Fig. 11).

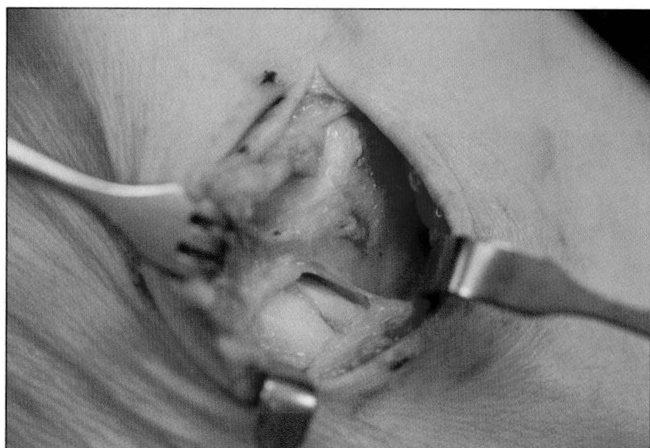

FIGURE 7

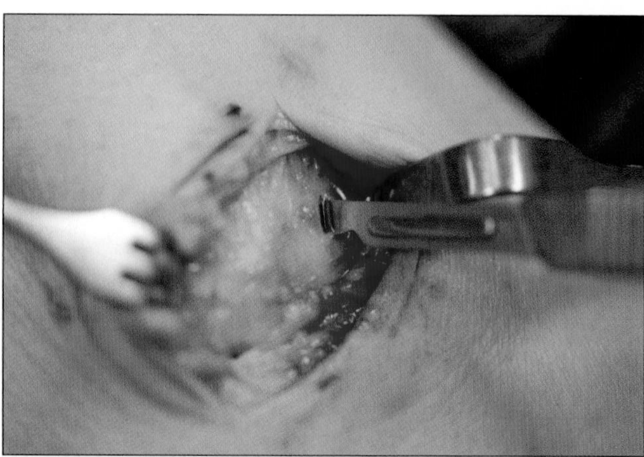

FIGURE 8

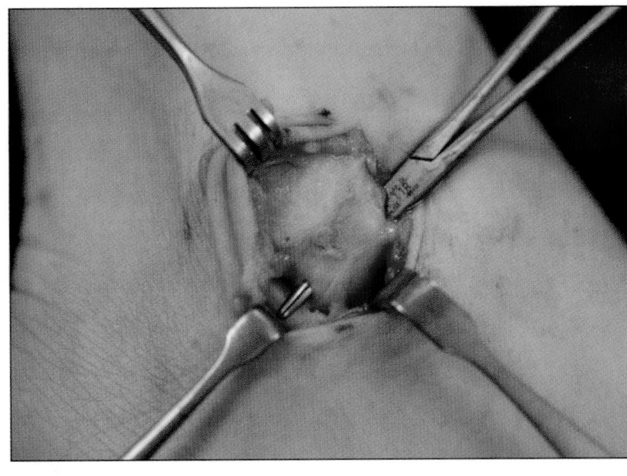

FIGURE 9

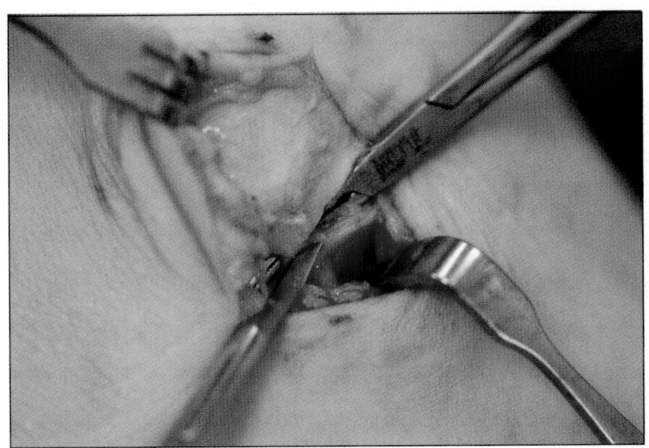

A

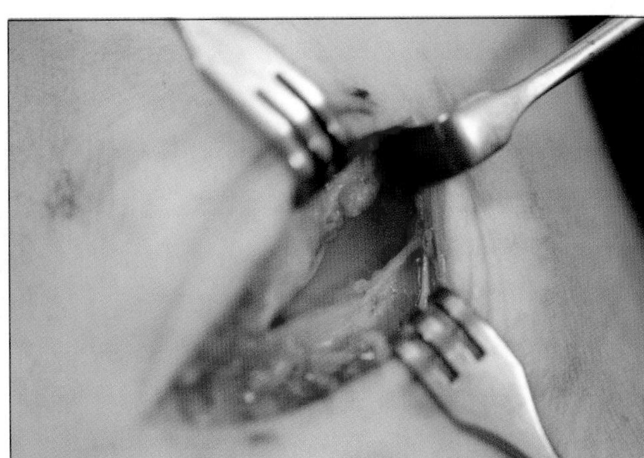

B

FIGURE 10

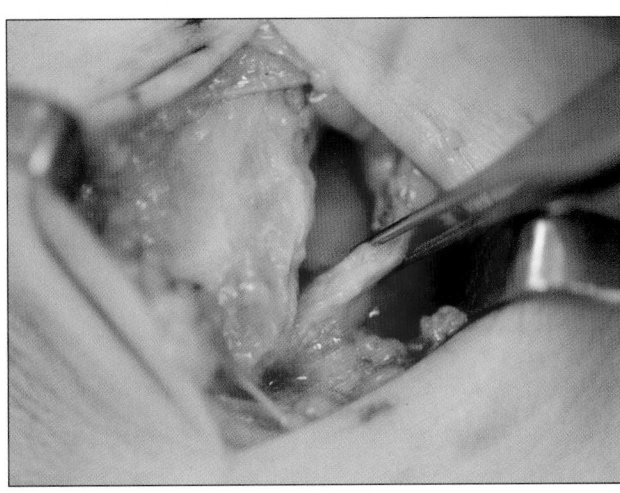

FIGURE 11

Pearls

- *If the CFL has been avulsed off of the calcaneus, it can be reattached with a small suture anchor. The cortical bone at the insertion site should first be roughened with a low-speed 3-mm burr.*

Step 3

- If the CFL requires repair, retract the peroneal tendons with a small Ragnell retractor and expose the ligament (Fig. 12 is an expanded view of the CFL).
- Divide the attenuated ligament midsubstance and excise 2–3 mm (Fig. 13).
- Place two figure-of-8, 2-0 Ethibond sutures into the ends of the ligament.
- Tag the suture ends with a small hemostat.

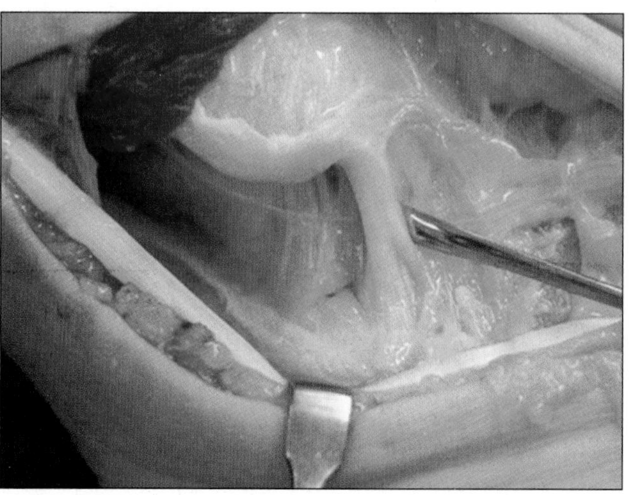

FIGURE 12

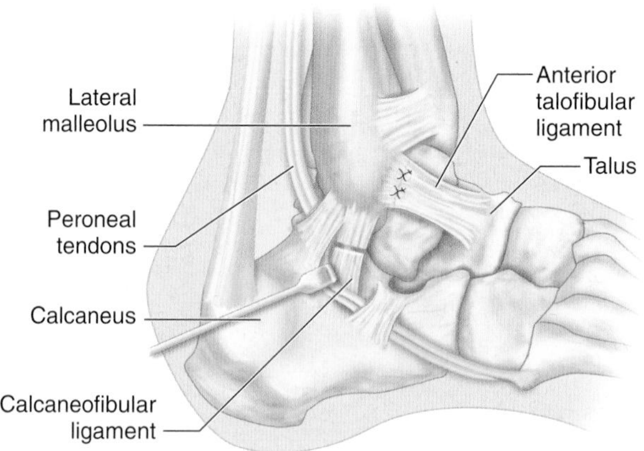

FIGURE 13

Step 4

- Reef the ATFL/capsule with several 2-0 PDS sutures. Usually three or four sutures are required.

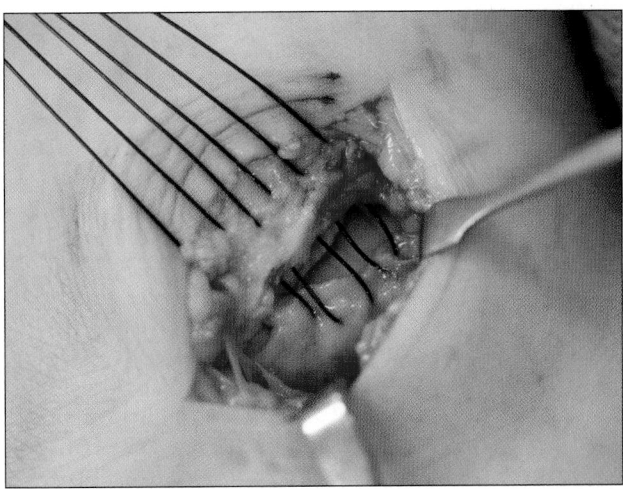

FIGURE 14

- The sutures are placed in a vest-over-pants fashion, so that the distal flap will lie deep.
- Tag the suture ends with a hemostat (Fig. 14).

STEP 5

- Place the foot on a small bump of sterile towels so the heel is floating and places no pressure on the repair.
- An assistant should hold the foot in eversion, with the ankle in neutral or slight dorsiflexion. Tie the sutures sequentially, starting with the CFL.
- Bring the extensor retinaculum snugly over the repair and sew it down to the fascia and periosteum of the lateral fibula, using a 0 or 2-0 Vicryl suture (Fig. 15).
- Deflate the tourniquet. Obtain hemostasis, and perform a layered closure of the skin (Fig. 16). Place a three-sided short-leg splint.

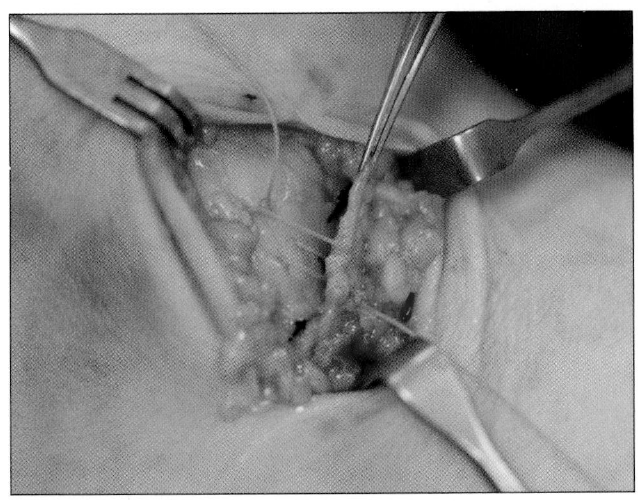

FIGURE 15

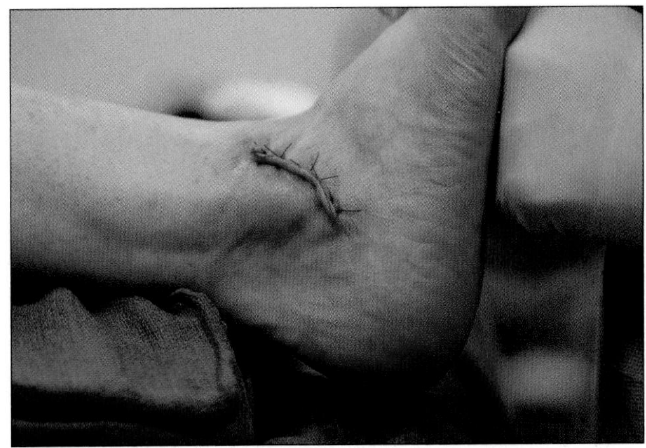

FIGURE 16

Postoperative Care and Expected Outcomes

- The sutures are removed at the first postoperative visit, 10–12 days after surgery.
- A short-leg non–weight-bearing cast is placed in 0-5° of dorsiflexion and slight eversion.
- The cast is removed at 3–4 weeks after surgery, depending on the quality of the repair, and the patient is allowed to weight bear as tolerated in an air stirrup brace that is worn at all times.
- Swimming and a stationery bike can be started in the splint at 4–6 weeks postoperatively. Physical therapy starts at 6 weeks. The brace is worn for normal activities until 8 weeks after surgery. Gradual return to unrestricted activity occurs at 10–12 weeks.
- An excellent outcome with few failures can be expected.

Evidence

Brostrom L. Surgical treatment of chronic ligament ruptures. Acta Chir Scand. 1966;132:551-65.

The original description of a simple anatomic reefing of the attenuated lateral ankle ligaments. (Level IV evidence)

DiGiovanni BF, Fraga C, Cohen BE, Shereff MJ. Associated injuries found in chronic lateral ankle instability. Foot Ankle Int. 2000;21:809-15.

This study of 61 patients documented the high incidence of peroneal tendon and intra-articular ankle pathology with chronic ligamentous laxity. (Level IV evidence)

DiGiovanni CW, Brodsky A: Current concepts: lateral ankle laxity. Foot Ankle Int. 2006;27:854-66.

A superb review of the topic.

Gould N, Seligson D, Gassman J. Early and late repair of lateral ligaments of the ankle. Foot Ankle. 1980;1:84-9.

A series of lateral ligament repairs using the inferior extensor retinaculum for reinforcement. (Level IV evidence)

Hamilton W, Thomson F, Snow S. The modified Brostrom procedure for lateral ankle instability. Foot Ankle. 1993;14:1-7.

These authors widely popularized the use of the modified Brostrom procedure with this study. (Level IV evidence)

PROCEDURE 37

Lateral Ankle Ligament Reconstruction Using Plantaris Autograft

Geert I. Pagenstert, Victor Valderrabano, and Beat Hintermann

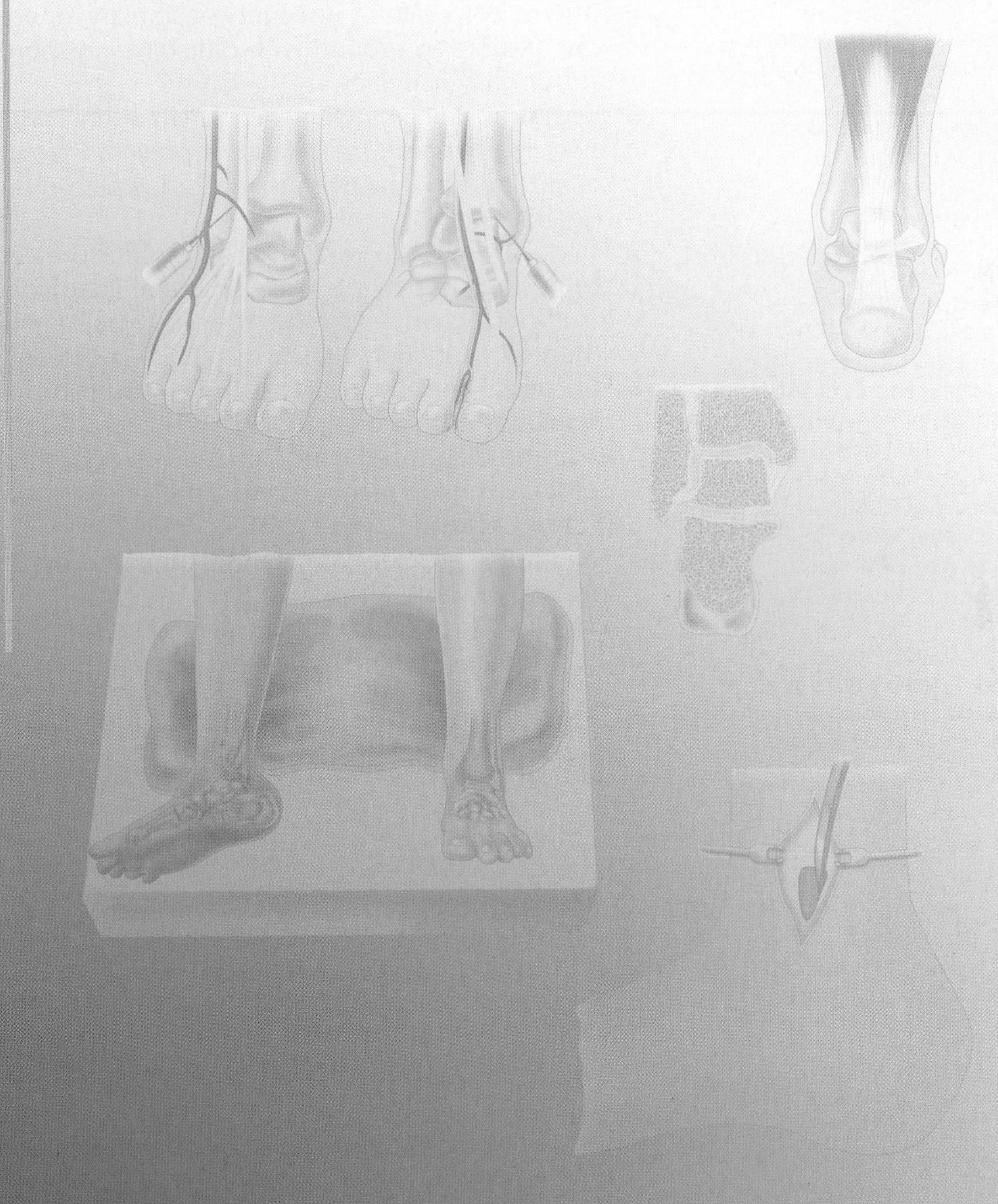

Pitfalls

- *Significant heel varus and/or muscle dysbalance will doom isolated lateral ligament reconstruction to failure and have to be addressed in the same surgical setting.*

Controversies

- Use of stress radiographs to indicate surgery is controversial because positive stress radiographs correlate poorly with symptomatic ankle instability. However, stress radiographs are used to document ligamentous insufficiency and to direct reconstructive treatment (Hintermann et al., 1992).
- Reconstructive procedures using tenodesis procedures or the tip or the posterior edge of the fibula prevent subtalar rotation and posterior fibula motion with ankle dorsiflexion (Burks and Morgan, 1994; Hintermann et al., 1995). This tight lateral ankle construct changes the physiologic center of rotation of the ankle, disturbing the coupling mechanism between leg and foot and thereby causing subtalar and ankle arthritis (Krips et al., 2002).

Indications

- Symptomatic chronic lateral ankle instability with insufficient local tissue (ligament remnants, extensor retinaculum)
- Failed primary lateral ankle ligament repair

Examination/Imaging

- Diagnosis and treatment are based on typical history and clinical findings.
- Patients complain of insecurity, instability, and giving way on uneven ground with difficulties in sports and/or daily activities.
- We test ankle laxity with the patient sitting and the lower leg hanging free. This will prevent involuntary stabilization by reactive peroneal muscle contraction (Fig. 1A and 1B).
- The talar tilt test (Fig. 2) and/or anterior drawer sign are positive in patients with structural ligament insufficiency, whereas these tests may be negative when only functional ankle instability is present.
- Functional ankle instability is likely caused by damaged mechanoreceptors in the lateral ligaments. It can be diagnosed with gait analysis or prolonged peroneal muscle reaction time on electromyography (Konradsen and Ravn, 1990).
- The finding of laxity may be documented by stress inversion or anterior drawer films.
  - A talar tilt of more than 5° difference from the contralateral uninjured ankle is usually considered pathologic (Hintermann et al., 1992).
  - Anterior subluxation of over 6 mm is usually considered pathologic (Hintermann et al., 1992).

Treatment Options

- Acute lateral ankle sprains may be sufficiently managed by functional rehabilitation (Pijnenburg et al., 2000), and surgery does not significantly improve results (Kerkhoffs et al., 2007).
- Anatomic ligament repair is indicated after failed nonoperative treatment. The Brostrom repair is the established repair technique (Brostrom, 1966). The extensor retinaculum may be used for augmentation and additional subtalar stabilization (Gould, 1987).
- In cases of insufficient ligament remnants, numerous other techniques exist for ligament reconstruction using plantaris grafts in addition to the procedure that is described here (Anderson, 1985; Segesser and Goesele, 1996).

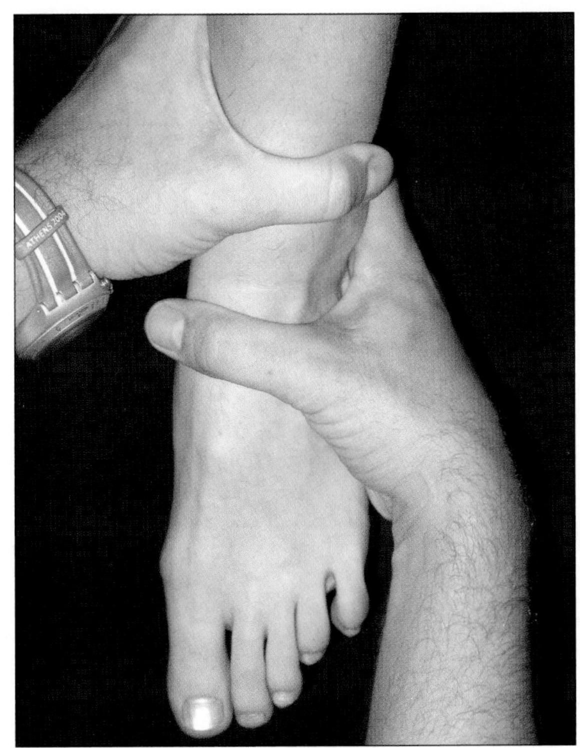

A

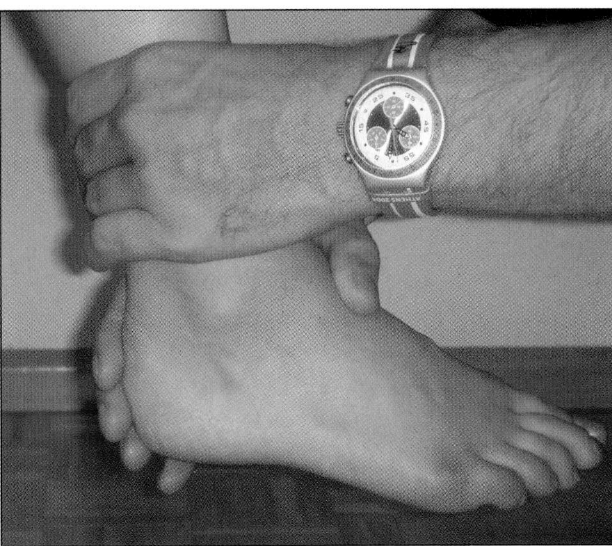

B

FIGURE 1

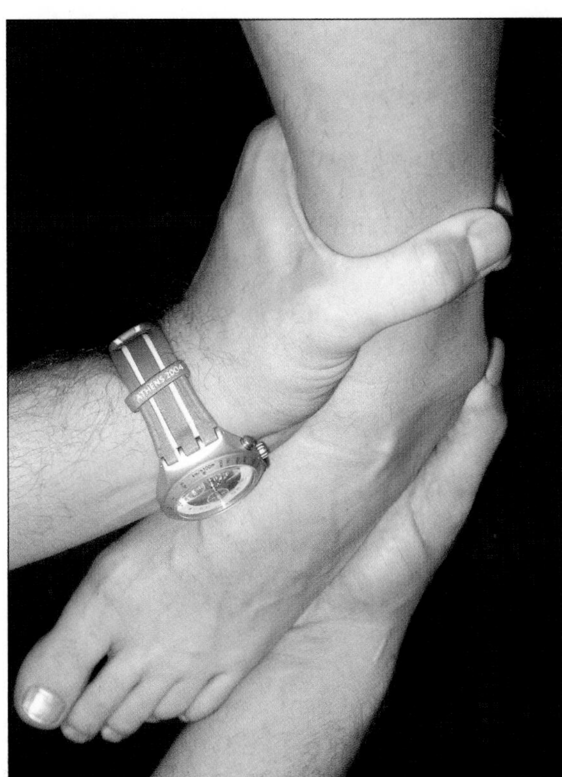

FIGURE 2

Surgical Anatomy

- Anterior tibiofibular ligament (ATFL)
  - This ligament blends with the anterior capsule of the ankle.
  - It originates at the anterior edge of the fibula, just lateral to the articular cartilage of the lateral malleolus. The center of attachment lies 10 mm proximal to the tip of the fibula when measured along the long axis of the fibula (Fig. 3A).
  - The insertion on the talus begins directly distal to the articular surface, and the center is 18 mm proximal to the subtalar joint (Burks and Morgan, 1994).
  - The ATFL is the first ligament restriction to supination of the foot.
- Calcaneofibular ligament (CFL)
  - Contrary to popular belief, the CFL does not originate at the apex of the tip of the lateral malleolus. Its attachment on the anterior edge of distal fibula is centered 8.5 mm from the distal tip just below the origin of the ATFL. The ligament courses medially, posteriorly, and inferiorly from its fibular origin to the calcaneal insertion (Fig. 3B).
  - The calcaneal insertion begins 13 mm distal to the subtalar joint, with its proximal edge on a line nearly perpendicular to the subtalar joint (Burks and Morgan, 1994).
  - The CFL resists ankle and subtalar joint supination, restricting inversion and internal rotation of the subtalar joint. Strain in the CFL increases with dorsiflexion when it becomes more vertically oriented, and takes over the role of the lateral collateral ligament of the ankle. Chronic insufficiency of the CFL is combined typically with a positive talar tilt test.

Positioning

- The patient is placed supine with a wedge under the ipsilateral hip so that the toes point to the ceiling. Draping includes the calf for optional plantaris tendon grafting (Fig. 4).
- The leg is exsanguinated with an Esmarch bandage and a thigh tourniquet is inflated.
- After arthroscopy is completed, the table is tilted medially to facilitate the lateral approach.

Pearls

- *We typically perform an ankle arthroscopy prior to the reconstruction to allow arthroscopic talus tilt and anterior drawer tests. Associated intra-articular pathologies (scar tissue impingement, osteochondral flake fractures, etc.) can be evaluated, documented, and addressed.*

Equipment

- The use of an ankle traction device that is fixed to the surgeon's belt may facilitate distraction during arthroscopy.

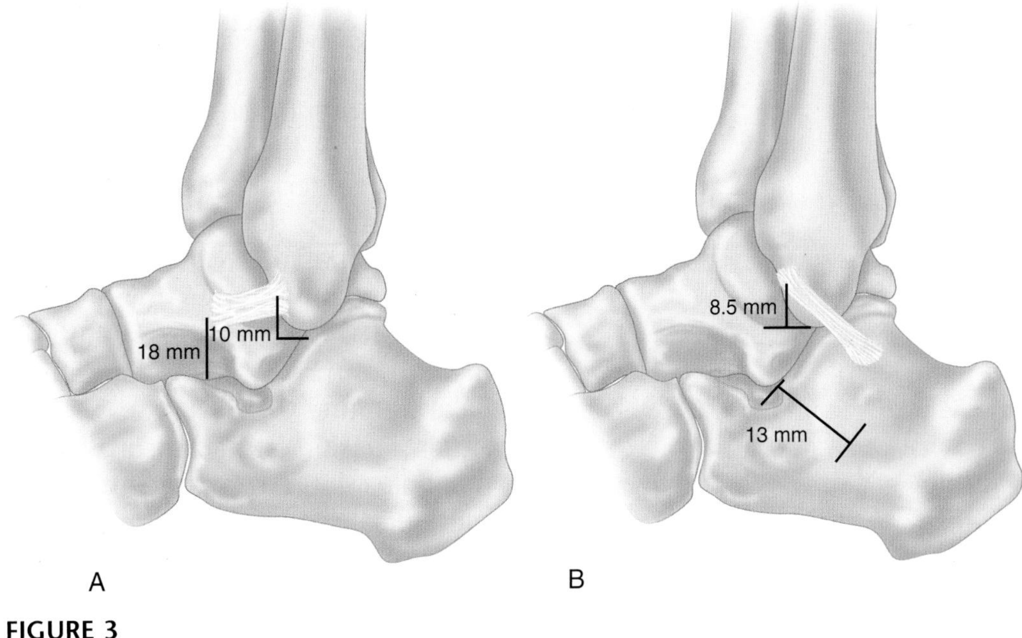

FIGURE 3

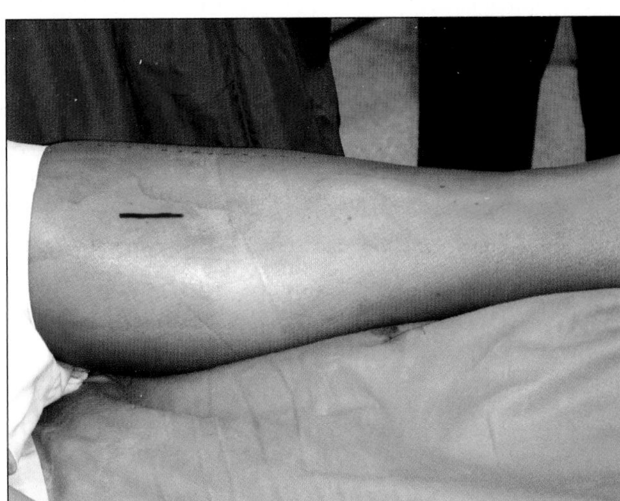

FIGURE 4

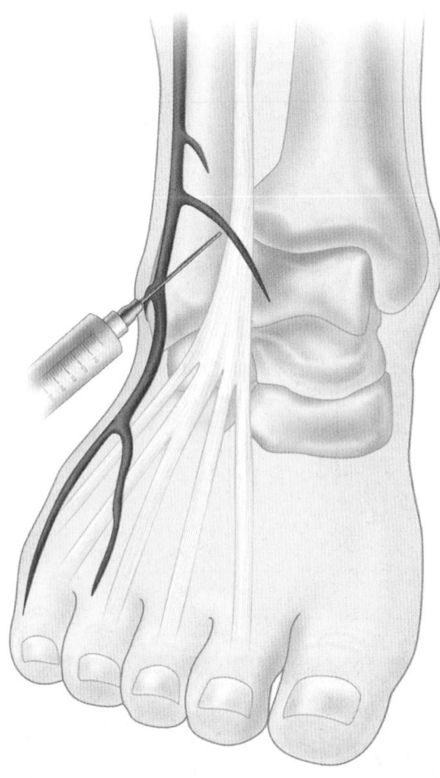

Portals/Exposures

- Arthroscopy with manual distraction is performed via a single anterior portal between the tibialis anterior and extensor hallucis longus tendons.
- The skin is incised and the soft tissues are divided by a blunt clamp down to the ankle capsule.
- An additional anteromedial portal, at the soft spot medial to the anterior tibial tendon, is placed if needed for débridement of anterior impingement, fixation, removal, or microfracturing of osteochondral flake fractures (Fig. 5).
- A skin incision is made from the tip of the lateral malleolus 4–6 cm toward the base of the fifth metatarsal with the foot held in plantar flexion (Fig. 6).

PEARLS

- *With plantar flexion of the ankle, the superficial peroneal nerve can be seen as a prominent line that crosses the anterior ankle from lateral-proximal to medial-distal. The nerve is avoided during portal placement.*
- *Dorsiflexion of the ankle during trocar insertion minimizes the risk of iatrogenic cartilage injury.*

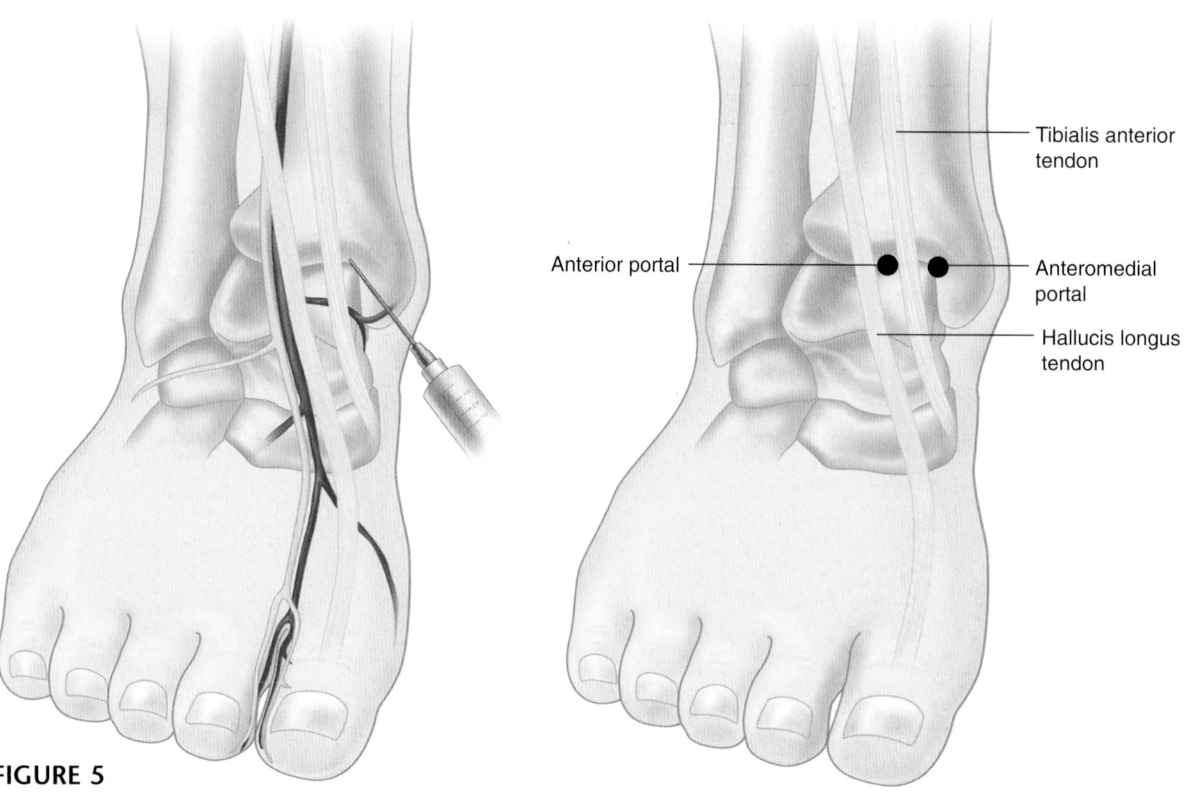

FIGURE 5

Pitfalls

- *During lateral skin incision, the sural nerve is identified and retracted as it runs 1 cm posterior around the lateral malleolus and courses further distally close to the base of the fifth metatarsal bone.*

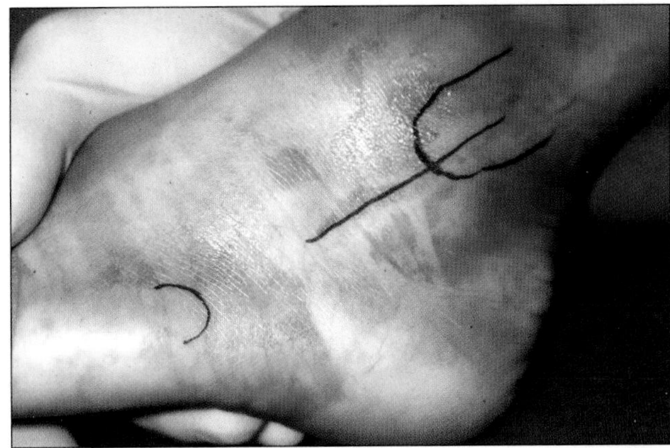

FIGURE 6

Procedure

Pearls

- *Excessive subtalar motion and scarred ligaments may cause painful sinus tarsi syndrome associated with ankle instability. Débridement of the sinus tarsi during lateral ankle reconstruction may prevent pain and impingement that may otherwise persist despite gained stability.*

Step 1: Lateral Ankle Preparation

- The sinus tarsi is probed with the forceps, and all scar tissue within the sinus is débrided.
- The ankle is opened anteriorly and parallel to the possible remnants of the ATFL, and a blunt retractor is placed on the neck of the talus. The peroneal tendons within their sheath are retracted posteriorly to uncover the distal insertion of the CFL. In Figure 7, the sinus tarsi was débrided, insufficient remnants of the ATFL are present, the talus is dislocated anteriorly.
- The ATFL, CFL, and extensor retinaculum are evaluated for possible Brostrom-Gould repair.
  - If the local tissue remnants are less than 50%, we use a free plantaris tendon graft.
  - In patients with failed previous repair, tendon graft augmentation is routinely done.

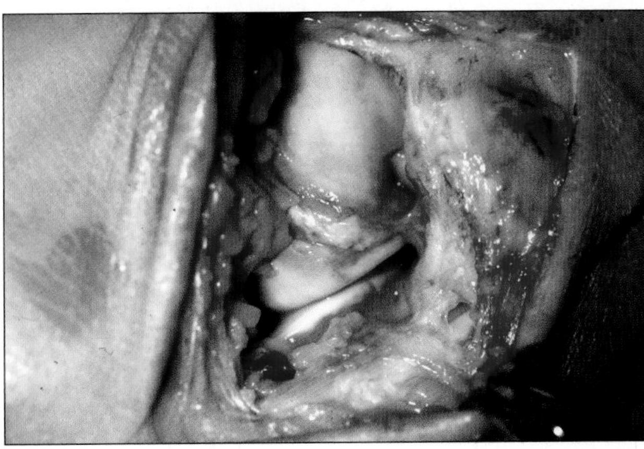

FIGURE 7

Step 2: Harvesting of Plantaris Tendon Autograft (Pagenstert et al., 2006)

- A 2-cm longitudinal skin incision is made (see Fig. 4) at the medial border of the triceps surae 30 cm proximal to the medial malleolus.
- Subcutaneous blunt dissection to the fascia is performed, protecting the saphenous nerve and vein (Fig. 8).
- Again, a 2-cm longitudinal incision is made in the fascia to allow the surgeon's finger to enter the intermuscular space between the soleus and gastrocnemius muscles (Fig. 9A). The only rigid tubular structure that is palpable at this muscular interspace is the plantaris tendon (Fig. 9B).

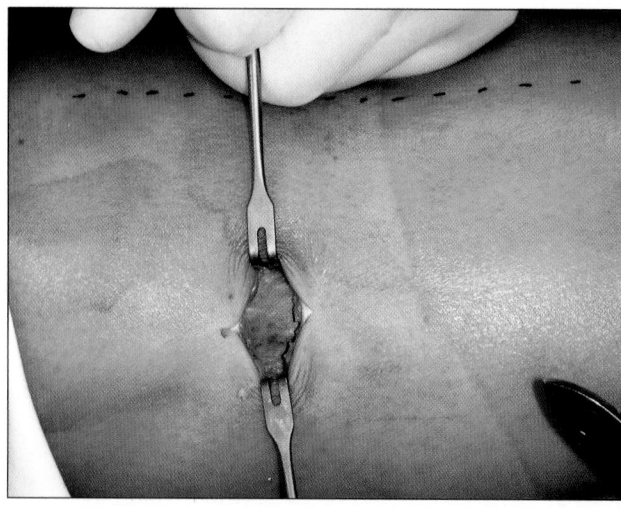

FIGURE 8

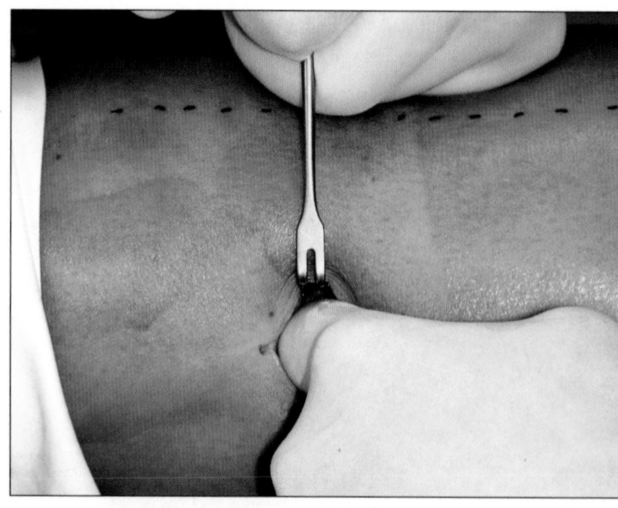

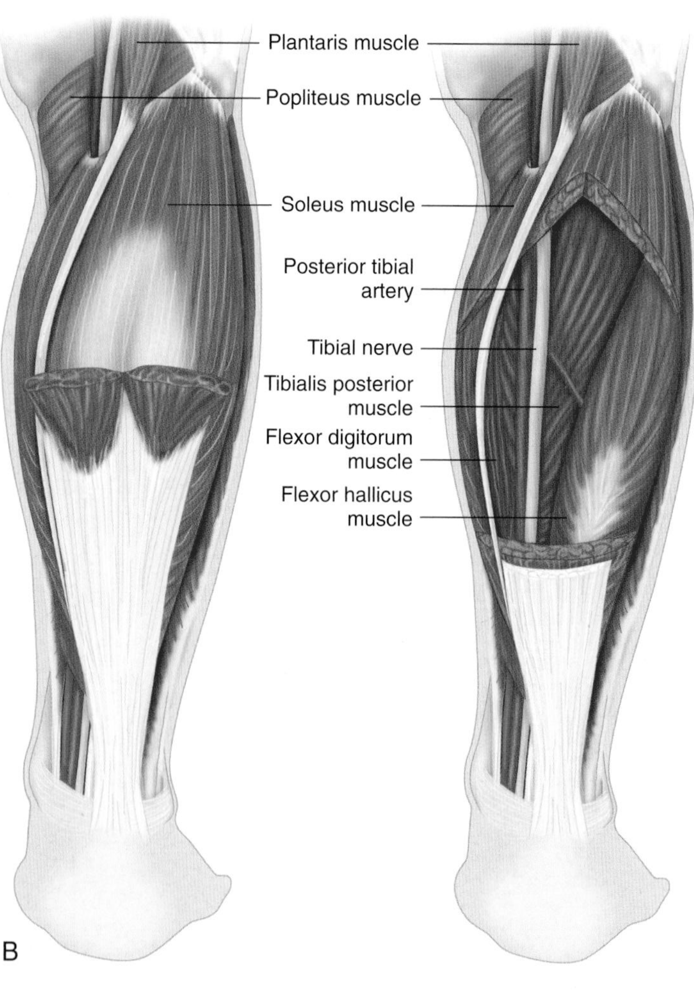

A

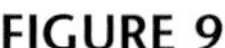
FIGURE 9

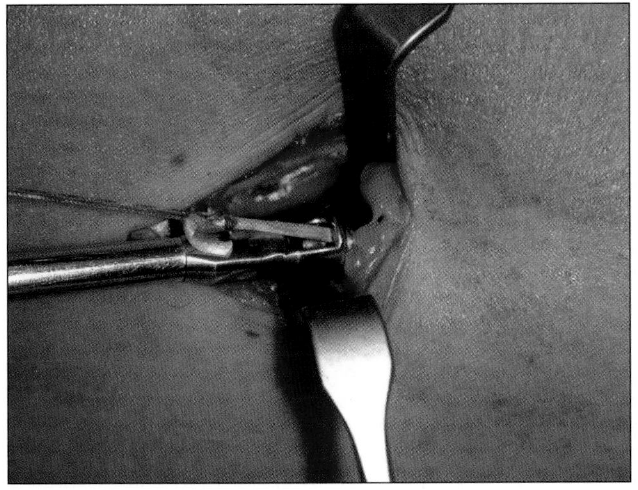

FIGURE 10

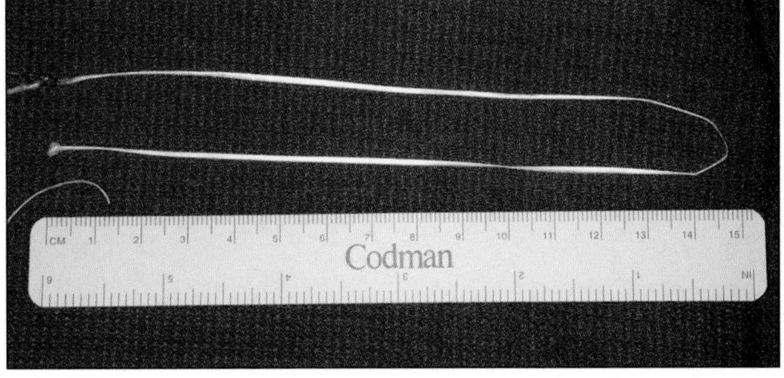

FIGURE 11

Instrumentation/ Implantation

- A tendon harvester is needed for blunt dissection and closed cutting of the tendon at its distal insertion.

- The tendon is developed with the finger or a nerve retractor and anchored with a no. 0 suture.
  - The tendon stripper is used for blunt dissection and cutting as distal as possible (Fig. 10). An additional skin incision is not needed.
  - The tendon is stored in a wet sponge for later use; a graft of 30 cm is usually available (Fig. 11).
- Wound closure is performed with a subcuticular running stitch and Steri-Strips to achieve a favorable cosmetic result.

Pearls

- *Graft selection often depends on the preference of the surgeon. However, the plantaris tendon has the highest tensile strength per cubic millimeter and leaves no functional donor-site deficit (Bohnsack et al., 2002).*
- *Harvesting of the plantaris with a single incision at the proximal calf increases the surgical viability of the graft until reimplantation (Pagenstert et al., 2006).*
- *Traditional plantaris harvesting with an incision at the medial calcaneus may cause scar formation, which may irritate the foot in shoes. This scar is prevented by the proximal harvesting procedure (Pagenstert et al., 2006).*

Pitfalls

- *Due to its variable distal insertion (at the Achilles, tuber, bursa, septum, etc.), the plantaris tendon is not found in up to 20% of cases if the traditional harvesting procedure at the medial calcaneus is used (Anderson, 1985; Segesser and Goesele, 1996).*

Controversies

- Cadaver and MRI studies have demonstrated an absence of the plantaris tendon in 6–7% of cases (Harvey et al., 1983; Saxena and Bareither, 2000; Daseler and Anson, 1943). Therefore, alternative tendon grafting may be needed (i.e., fourth extensor digitorum tendon) (Hintermann and Renggli, 1999).
- The use of peroneal tendons as autograft for lateral reconstruction is paradoxical because preservation of these tendon functions is crucial for dynamic lateral ankle stabilization.

Pitfalls

- *With absent ligament remnants, precise knowledge of anatomic insertion locations is the key to reconstructive techniques (Burks and Morgan, 1994).*

Step 3: Lateral Ankle Reconstruction (Hintermann and Renggli, 1999)

- Bony tunnels 3.2 mm in diameter are placed around the anatomic insertions of the ATFL and CFL.
- Two tunnels 10 mm deep are drilled into the anterior aspect of the fibula 7 and 13 mm proximal to the distal tip (Fig. 12).
  - These tunnels are placed just at the bony border with the fibular cartilage.
  - The two tunnels join each other within the fibula at a depth of 10 mm.
- From the posterolateral aspect of the fibula, an additional tunnel is drilled to meet the anterior tunnels (see Fig. 12). A reduction clamp is inserted and swiveled through the drill holes to smoothen the sharp edges of the osseous channels and assure its continuity (Fig. 13).

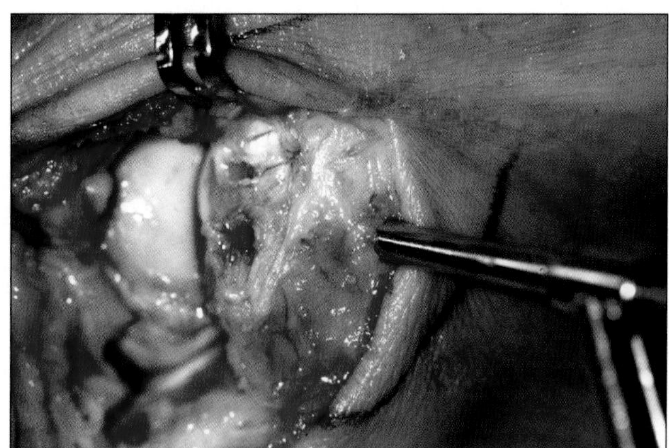

FIGURE 12

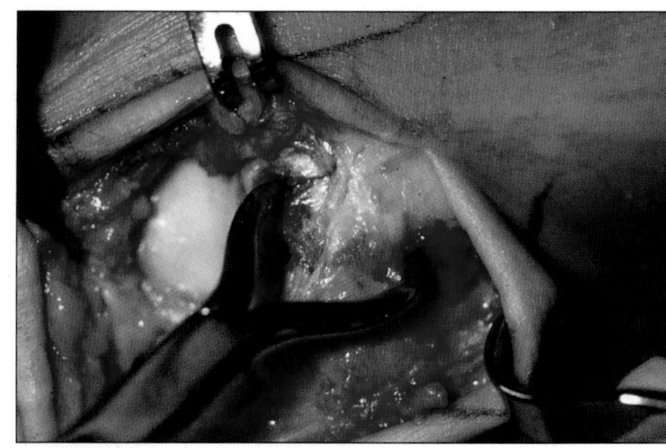

FIGURE 13

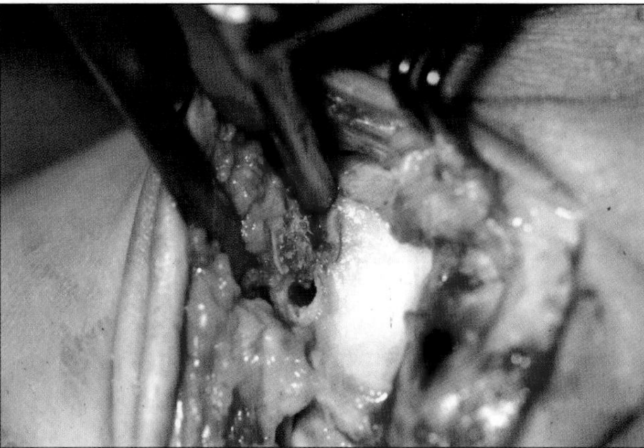

FIGURE 14

- Two tunnels are drilled in the talus in the same fashion 14 and 22 mm cranial to the subtalar joint, just distal to the cartilaginous surface of the talus, with a craniocaudal distance of 6–8 mm to each other (Fig. 14). Convergence of the channels should occur approximately 18 mm cranial to the subtalar joint.
- Two converging holes are produced parallel to the posterior facet of the calcaneus at the insertion site of the CFL, approximately 13 mm distal to it, on a line perpendicular to the subtalar joint (Fig. 15). During the procedure, the peroneal tendons are gently retracted.

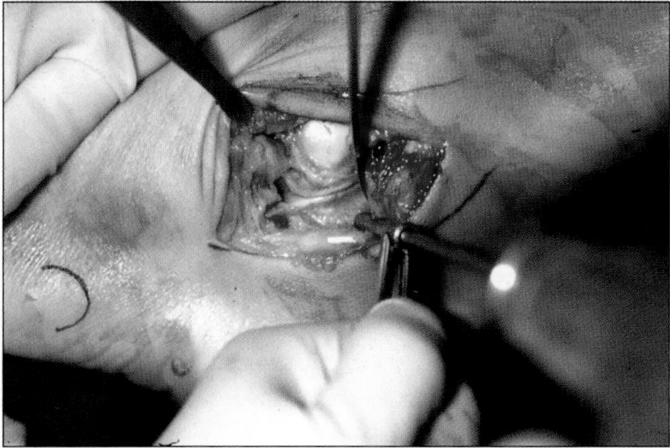

FIGURE 15

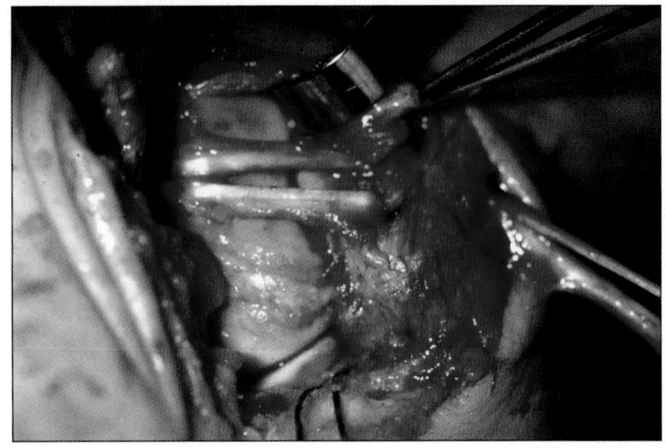
A

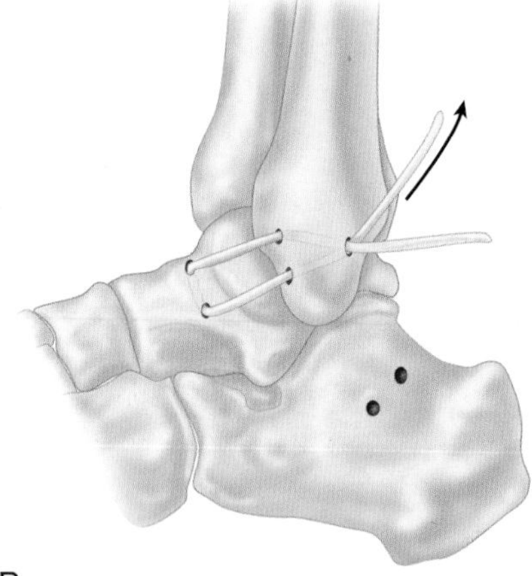
B

FIGURE 16

- The plantaris tendon graft is directed through the holes as shown in Figures 16, 17, and 18, with the foot held in supination and dorsiflexion, and sutured to itself and the periosteum while holding the tendon under tension (Fig. 19).
- The construct is then checked for evenly distributed tension and unimpeded ankle and subtalar joint mobility. If beneficial, small interference screws may be used to enhance construct rigidity.
- No. 0 absorbable suture is used to fix the remnants of the fibula ligaments and/or extensor retinaculum to the reconstruction.
- The skin is closed in layers, and a compressive dressing and neutral brace are applied.

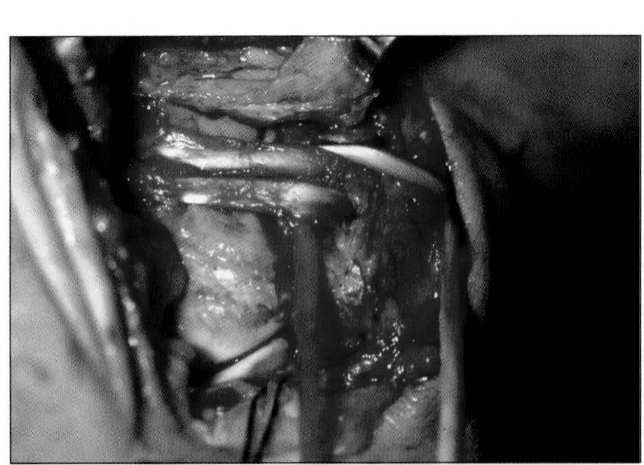
A

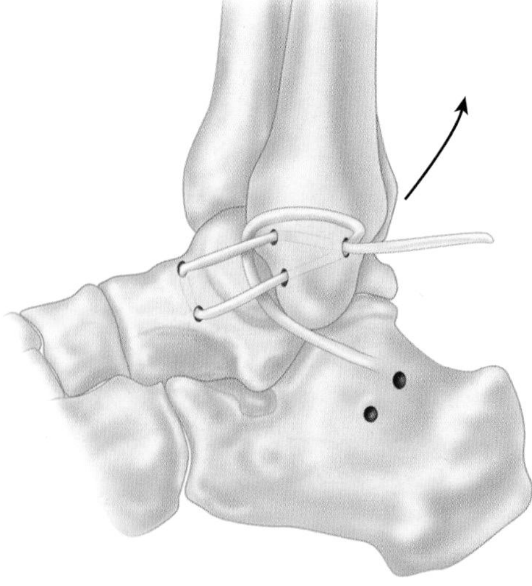
B

FIGURE 17

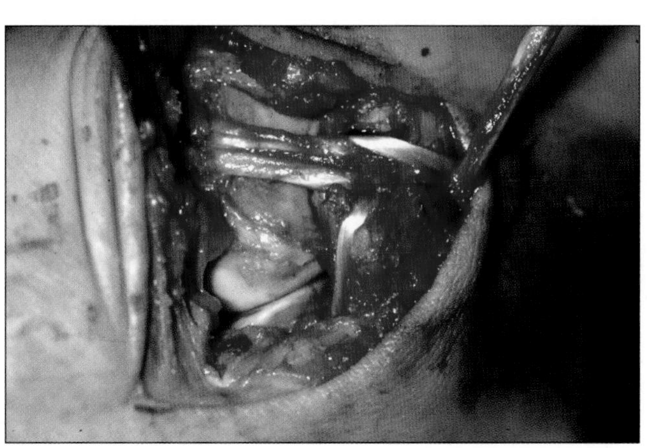
A

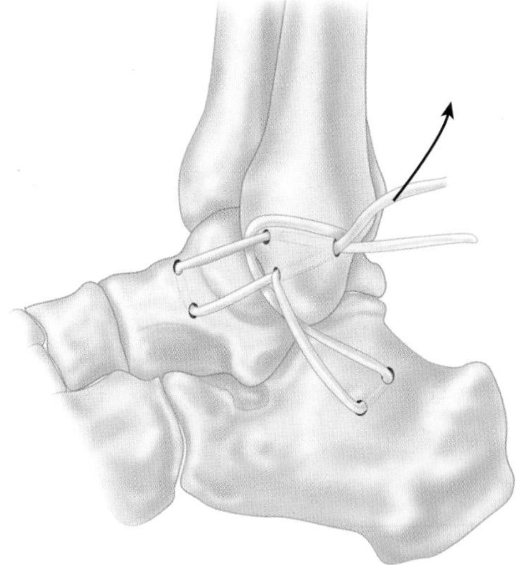
B

FIGURE 18

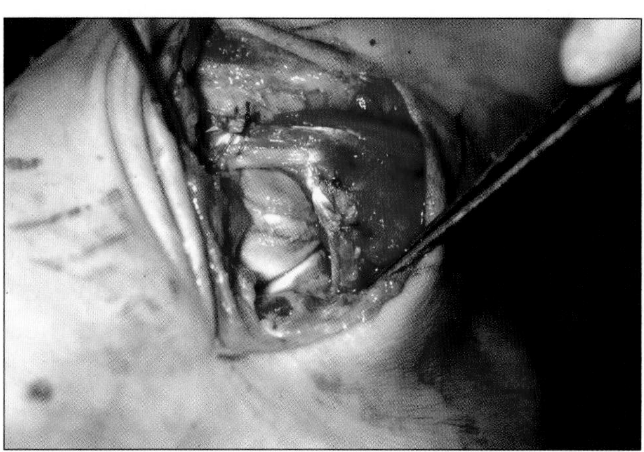

FIGURE 19

Postoperative Care and Expected Outcomes

Postoperative Care

- The lower leg is immobilized in a removable soft cast with the ankle in neutral for 2–4 weeks at night.
- Cautious range of motion for dorsiflexion and plantar flexion is allowed after 2–3 days, with isometric training of all lower leg muscles. Eversion and inversion, and supination and pronation, are permitted 4–6 weeks postoperatively.
- Orthopedic boots or semirigid ankle braces preventing eversion, inversion, and excessive dorsiflexion and plantar flexion can be used; gradual weight bearing as tolerated is allowed after 2–3 days, and always reached after 10 days.

- Return to work ability is allowed for sedentary workers after 10 days, and for heavy laborers after 4–6 weeks. Heavy laborers may use rigid protective footwear continuously. Sports activity is started at 4–6 weeks. Again, ankle braces should be worn, and gradually discarded.
- Return to full sports activity depends on the individual, but generally occurs at 6–12 weeks from the operation.

Outcomes

- Over a period of 10 years in 52 ankles (48 patients, 30 males and 18 females), a free plantaris tendon graft was used for anatomic ligament reconstruction as described above (Hintermann and Renggli, 1999).
  - The average age at operation was 28.6 years (range 16–46).
  - Three patients had had a ligament repair before. All remaining patients had undergone prolonged conservative management before the operation.
- A total of 45 patients (49 ankles) were controlled with an average follow-up of 8.5 years (range 6–15 years). Three patients could not be located.
  - Forty-four patients (98%) had no limitations of sports or everyday activity.
  - Twelve patients reported that inconstant discomfort or mild swelling at the ankle was present after running or walking for more than 1 hour. Eleven of these patients showed no evidence of structural laxity at clinical testing and stress radiographs.
  - One patient reported mild insecurity playing soccer, with inconstant pain at the lateral ankle after an additional ankle sprain since the time of surgery. This patient had a positive anterior drawer sign and stress radiographs.
- Range of motion for dorsiflexion and plantar flexion was unrestricted compared to the uninjured site. In two patients, supination (inversion) of the subtalar joint was mildly restricted compared to the uninjured site.
- At the latest follow-up, 41 patients (44 ankles) undertook their previous sports at their preoperative level. Three patients (4 ankles) had changed their previous sport and/or level for other reasons. One patient (one ankle) was not practicing sport as he did before surgery.
- Two patients had marked varus of the hindfoot, and a Dwyer osteotomy to reconstitute the normal hindfoot alignment was added.

Evidence

Anderson ME. Reconstruction of the lateral ligaments of the ankle using the plantaris tendon. J Bone Joint Surg [Am]. 1985;67:930-4.

This study described the authors' technique of lateral ankle reconstruction using the plantaris tendon harvested at the calcaneal tuber. (Level IV evidence [case series])

Bohnsack M, Surie B, Kirsch IL, Wulker N. Biomechanical properties of commonly used autogenous transplants in the surgical treatment of chronic lateral ankle instability. Foot Ankle Int. 2002;23:661-4.

This in vitro study examined biomechanical properties of the peroneus brevis tendon, Achilles tendon, plantaris tendon, fascia lata, periosteal strip, ATFL, and CFL.

Brostrom L. Sprained ankles—VI. Surgical treatment of "chronic" ligament ruptures. Acta Chir Scand. 1966;132:551-65.

This study described the author's technique of direct lateral ankle repair. (Level IV evidence [case series])

Burks RT, Morgan J. Anatomy of the lateral ankle ligaments. Am J Sports Med. 1994;22:72-7.

This is a descriptive anatomic study with implications for tenodesis procedures.

Daseler EH, Anson BH. The plantaris muscle: an anatomical study of 750 specimens. J Bone Joint Surg. 1943;25:822-7.

This is a descriptive anatomic study of the plantaris muscle.

Gould N. Repair of lateral ligament of ankle. Foot Ankle. 1987;8:55-8.

This study described the author's technique of direct lateral ankle repair with extensor retinaculum augmentation. (Level IV evidence [case series])

Harvey FJ, Chu G, Harvey PM. Surgical availability of the plantaris tendon. J Hand Surg [Am]. 1983;8:243-7.

This is a descriptive anatomic study of the plantaris muscle.

Hintermann B, Holzach P, Matter P. [Injury pattern of the fibular ligaments: radiological diagnosis and clinical study]. Unfallchirurg. 1992;95:142-7.

This study compared different methods to evaluate lateral ankle instability. Stress radiographs and manual testing with and without general anesthesia were compared to each other in 76 subjects. (Level II evidence [prognostic study])

Hintermann B, Sommer C, Nigg BM. Influence of ligament transection on tibial and calcaneal rotation with loading and dorsi-plantarflexion. Foot Ankle Int. 1995;16:567-71.

This is a biomechanical in vitro study of the effect of sequential ligament transection on the rotational movement of the tibia and the calcaneus.

Hintermann B, Renggli P. [Anatomic reconstruction of the lateral ligaments of the ankle using a plantaris tendon graft in the treatment of chronic ankle joint instability]. Orthopade. 1999;28:778-84.

This study described the authors' technique of lateral ankle reconstruction using the plantaris tendon. (Level IV evidence [case series])

Kerkhoffs GM, Handoll HH, de Bie R, Rowe BH, Struijs PA. Surgical versus conservative treatment for acute injuries of the lateral ligament complex of the ankle in adults. Cochrane Database Syst Rev. 2007;(2):CD000380.

This study was a meta-analysis of randomized, controlled clinical trials of existing treatment strategies for acute ruptures of the lateral ankle ligaments. (Level I evidence [review of level I studies])

Konradsen L, Ravn JB. Ankle instability caused by prolonged peroneal reaction time. Acta Orthop Scand. 1990;61:388-90.

This study compared peroneal reaction time of functional unstable ankles in 15 subjects with that of healthy controls. (Level III evidence [case-control study])

Krips R, Brandsson S, Swensson C, van Dijk CN, Karlsson J. Anatomical reconstruction and Evans tenodesis of the lateral ligaments of the ankle: clinical and radiological findings after follow-up for 15 to 30 years. J Bone Joint Surg [Br]. 2002;84:232-6.

This study compared the outcome of 54 subjects with anatomic reconstruction and 45 subjects with Evans tenodesis. (Level III evidence [retrospective comparative study])

Pagenstert GI, Hintermann B, Knupp M. Operative management of chronic ankle instability: plantaris graft. Foot Ankle Clin. 2006;11:567-83.

This study described the authors' technique of lateral ankle reconstruction using the plantaris tendon harvested at the proximal calf. (Level IV evidence [case series])

Pijnenburg ACM, van Dijk CN, Bossuyt PMM, Marti RK. Treatment for lateral ankle ligament ruptures: a meta-analysis. J Bone Joint Surg [Am]. 2000;82:761-73.

This study was a meta-analysis of randomized, controlled clinical trials of existing treatment strategies for acute ruptures of the lateral ankle ligaments. (Level I evidence [review of level I studies])

Saxena A, Bareither D. Magnetic resonance and cadaveric findings of the incidence of plantaris tendon. Foot Ankle Int. 2000;21:570-2.

This is a descriptive anatomic study of the plantaris muscle.

Segesser B, Goesele A. [Weber fibular ligament-plasty with plantar tendon with Segesser modification]. Sportverletz Sportschaden. 1996;10:88-93.

This study described the authors' technique of lateral ankle reconstruction using the plantaris tendon harvested at the calcaneal tuber. (Level IV evidence [case series])

PROCEDURE 38

Salvage of a Failed Lateral Ligament Repair

Glenn B. Pfeffer

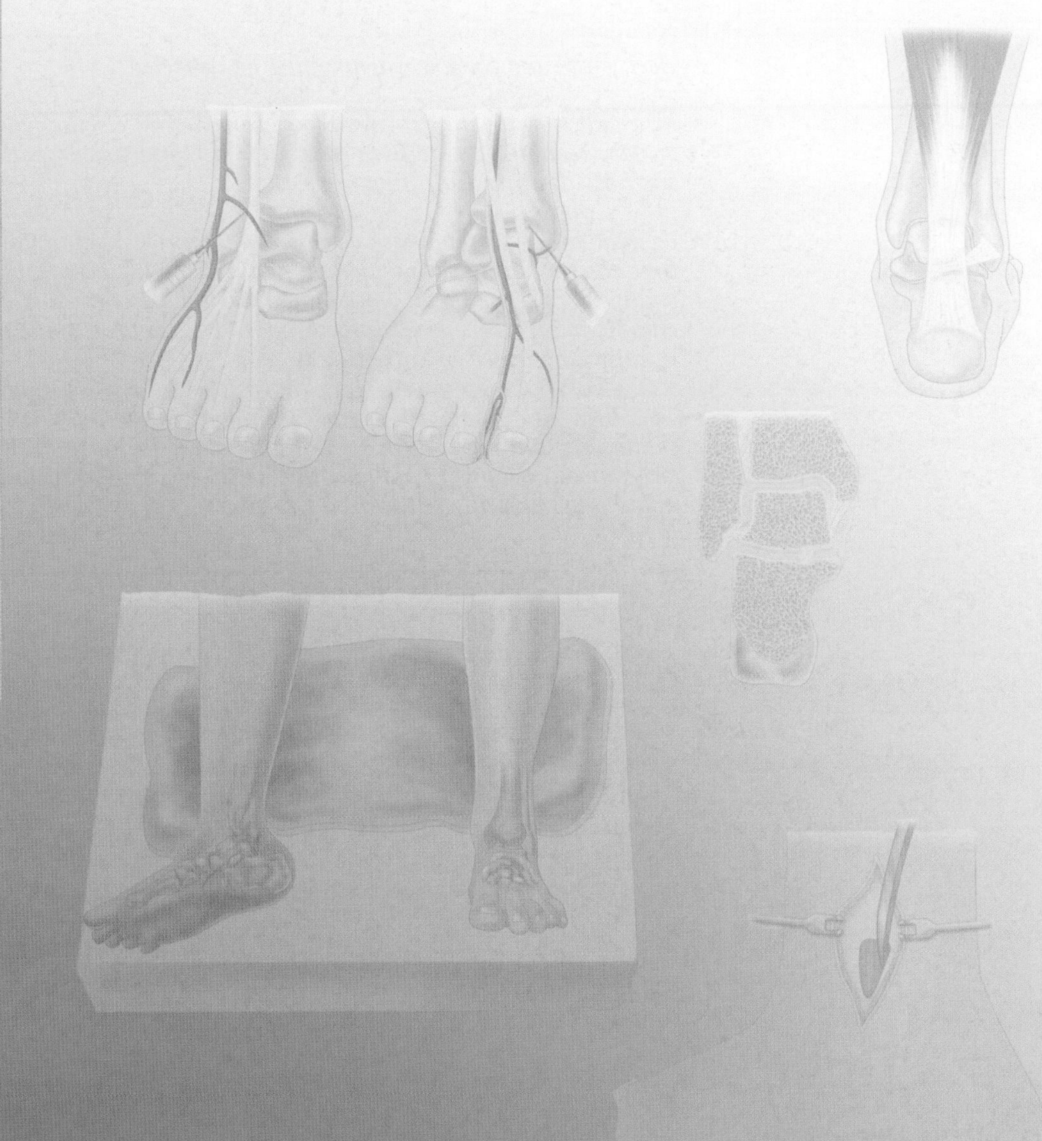

Indications

- Persistent symptomatic lateral ankle laxity following a lateral ligament procedure
- Failure of a physical therapy program that emphasizes peroneal strength, proprioception, and range of motion
- Inability to return to sports, even with the use of a brace

Pitfalls

- *Heel varus and forefoot valgus must be corrected.*
- *In a patient with a high cavus foot, consider an electromyogram or nerve conduction study to rule out a hereditary neuropathy such as Charcot-Marie-Tooth disease.*
- *Exclude all other sources of chronic symptoms before assuming that chronic laxity is the problem. Have the patient's symptoms changed since the index procedure? Does the patient complain of chronic pain, frequent sprains, or both? Persistent, chronic pain is usually not caused by ankle laxity alone.*
- *The differential diagnosis includes complex regional pain syndrome, traumatic surgical neuroma, superficial peroneal nerve entrapment, peroneal tendinopathy, ankle or subtalar arthritis, ankle impingement, generalized hyperlaxity, and medial ankle laxity.*

Controversies

- Semitendinosus or gracilis autograft is a viable option, but requires an additional surgical procedure.
- Several surgical reconstructions use all or part of the patient's peroneus brevis tendon. The brevis is the major dynamic stabilizer of the lateral ankle and should not be used.
- In a patient with generalized hyperlaxity, allograft tissue is probably preferable.
- An anatomic reconstruction that follows the normal course of the lateral ligaments will minimize loss of ankle and subtalar motion.

Treatment Options

- See Procedure 36 on the modified Brostrom procedure.

Examination/Imaging

- See Procedure 36 on the modified Brostrom procedure.
- Carefully evaluate subtalar motion. A stiff subtalar joint contributes to repeated inversion sprains. It is very difficult to distinguish gross varus laxity of the ankle from normal subtalar motion without fluoroscopic evaluation (Fig. 1).

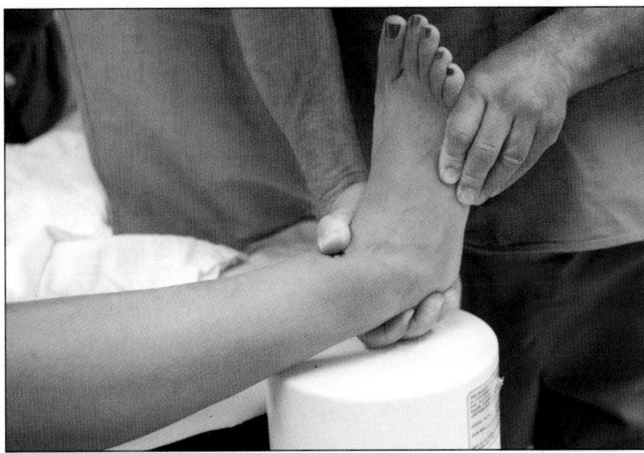

FIGURE 1

- A gastrocnemius contracture may be present, which predisposes to inversion sprains.
- Test for medial ankle laxity (see Procedure 40).
- Obtain four radiographic views of the ankle, including a standing mortise view.
- Patients with a failed Brostrom procedure should have stress radiographs preoperatively.
- Magnetic resonance imaging should be obtained on all patients.

Surgical Anatomy

- The anterior talofibular ligament (ATFL) arises from the inferior oblique segment of the anterior border of the lateral malleolus, approximately 1 cm proximal to the tip (Fig. 2).
  - The ATFL inserts on the body, not the neck, of the talus, just anterior to the lateral malleolar articular surface.

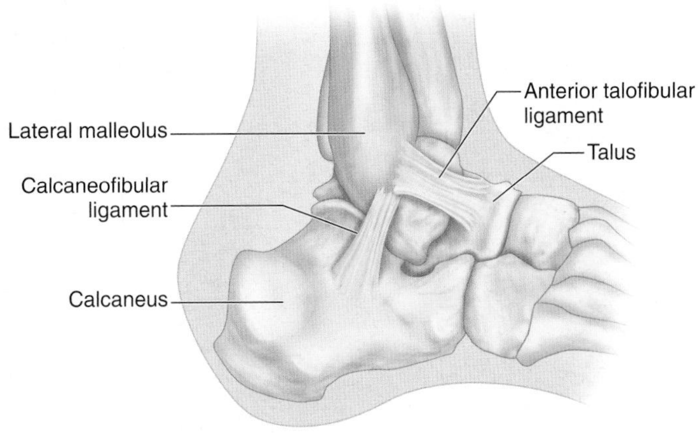

FIGURE 2

- The distance to the insertion is 1.5–2 cm directly anterior to the leading edge of the lateral malleolus.

- The calcaneofibular ligament (CFL) arises from the lower segment of the *anterior border* of the lateral malleolus, just below the ATFL. It is 2–3 cm in length.
  - The CFL inserts on a small tubercle on the lateral calcaneus, 15 mm distal to the subtalar joint. The insertion site is highly variable.
  - The ligament creates a 90–135° angle with the ATFL. Obliquity of the ligament is dependent on heel position; it is increased with valgus and decreased with varus.

Positioning

- The patient is in a lateral position.
- A femoral-sciatic or popliteal block is used.
- A calf or thigh tourniquet allows adequate exposure of the lateral ankle.

Portals/Exposures

- The surgical exposure is often dictated by previous incisions (Figs. 3 and 4).
- The ideal incision extends obliquely across the distal fibula. This incision can be extended over the calcaneal tuberosity to perform a calcaneal osteotomy.

PEARLS

- *If an ankle arthroscopy is required preoperatively, it can usually be done with the patient in the lateral position. The lax ankle ligaments negate the need for distraction of the joint.*

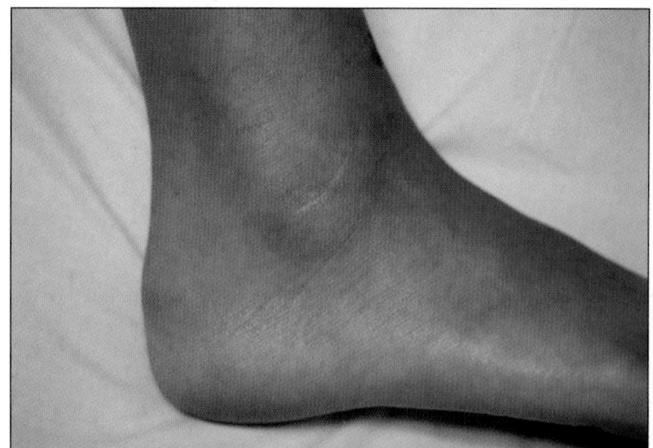

FIGURE 3

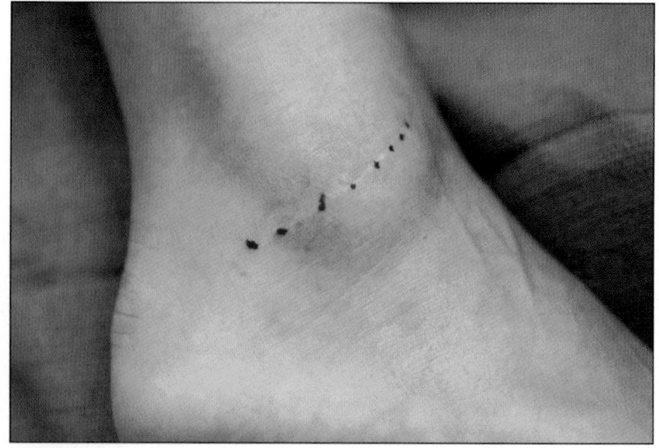

FIGURE 4

Instrumentation

- This procedure uses an Arthrex Biotenodesis screw set.

Procedure

Step 1

- Loupe magnification is helpful.
- Keep the skin flaps full thickness.
- Identify the lateral branch of the superficial peroneal nerve, which is invariably bound down in scar tissue. Protect the sural nerve at the inferior edge of the incision.
- Place a small hemostat beneath the remnants of the joint capsule and ATFL. Divide the structures with a #15 blade (Fig. 5).
- Remove old sutures while preserving as much of the capsule and ligamentous structures as possible.
- Débride all scar tissue and osteophytes. Try to locate and preserve the anatomic origins and insertions of the ATFL and CFL.
- Open the peroneal sheath to the level of the ankle joint. Leave an adequate cuff of tissue on the poster fibula for closure. Inspect the tendons for tears or synovitis (Fig. 6).

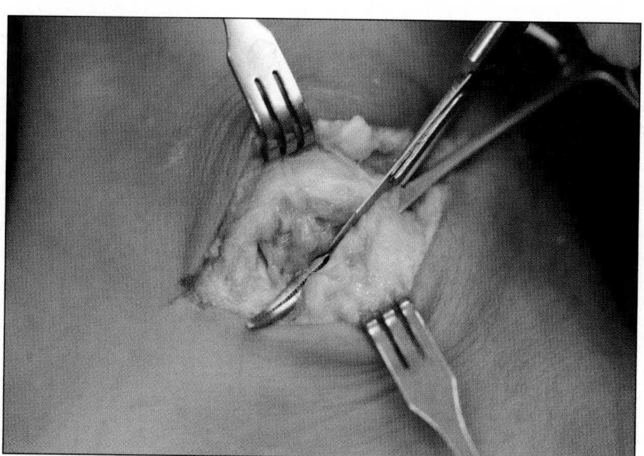

FIGURE 5

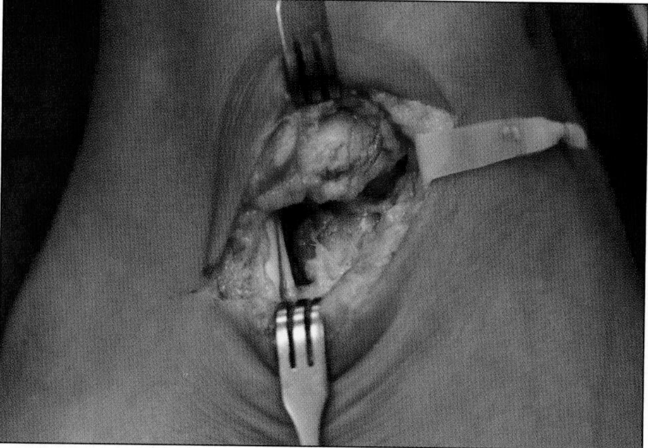

FIGURE 6

Step 2

- Place a 2-0 nonabsorbable suture into the ends of a semitendinosus allograft.
  - Size the graft using the Arthrex Biotenodesis screw set.
  - Sew a 2-0 Fiberwire baseball stitch into each end of the graft.
  - Apply 10 lbs of stretch to the graft for at least 15 minutes (Fig. 7).
- Identify the insertion site for the ATFL, which is on the body, not the neck, of the talus, just anterior to the lateral malleolar articular surface. The distance to the insertion is 1.5–2.0 cm directly anterior to the leading edge of the lateral malleolus.
- Place a guide pin from the Arthrex Biotenodesis set into the talus (Fig. 8). Confirm its position by direct inspection and fluoroscopy.
- Create a tunnel with the appropriate drill bit to a depth of 22 mm (Fig. 9).
- Secure one end of the semitendinosus graft using (in this case) a 5.5-mm biotenodesis screw (Fig. 10).

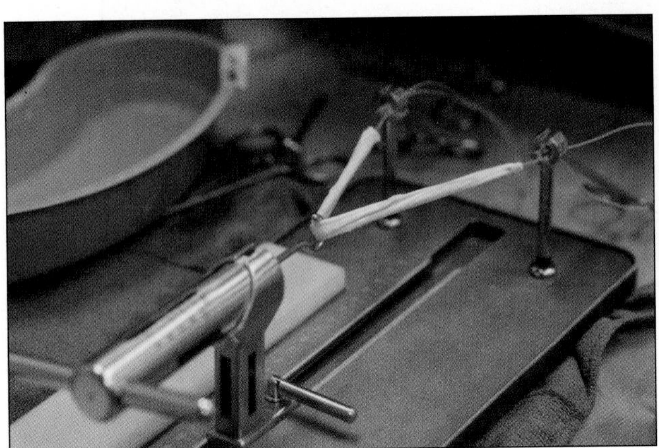

FIGURE 7

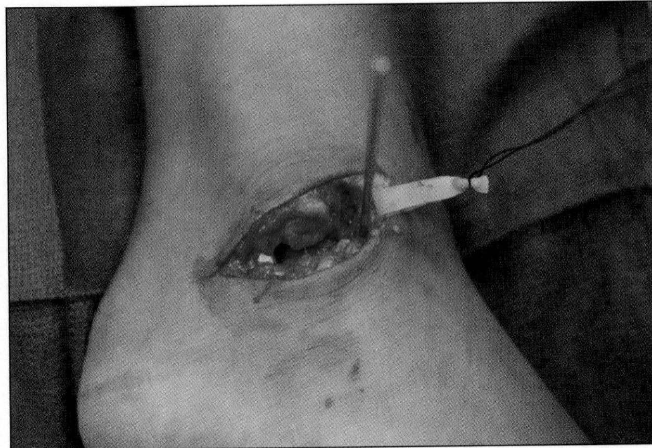

FIGURE 8

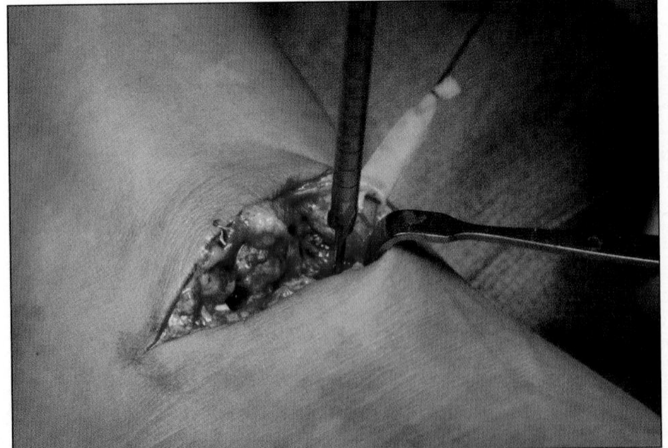

FIGURE 9

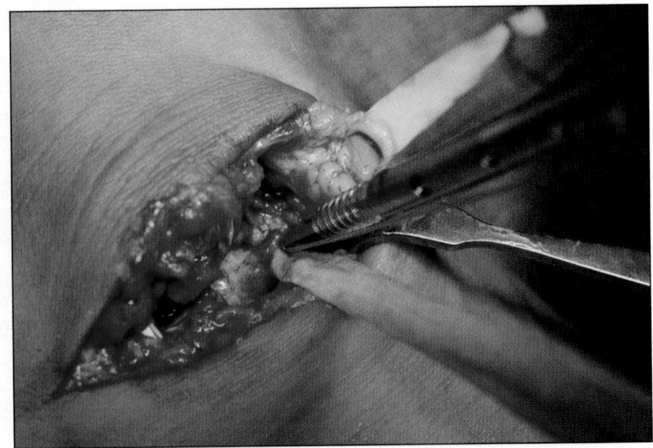

FIGURE 10

Pearls

- *If a suture anchor is present in the fibula, it is usually possible to drill around it, or move it out of the way as the drill bit advances. Start with small drill bits and progressively increase in size.*
- *The first drill hole can be placed into the exact location of the ATFL origin. The second drill hole is usually at the tip of the fibula, which is slightly posterior to the anatomic CFL origin.*

Step 3

- Elevate the periosteum off of the distal fibula and locate the origins of the ATFL and CFL.
- Protect the peroneal tendons.
- Drill an Arthrex guide wire through the fibula from distal to proximal (Fig. 11).
- Using a 5-mm drill bit, create two bony tunnels that converge at the posterior fibula. Join the tunnels using a small curette (Fig. 12A and 12B).

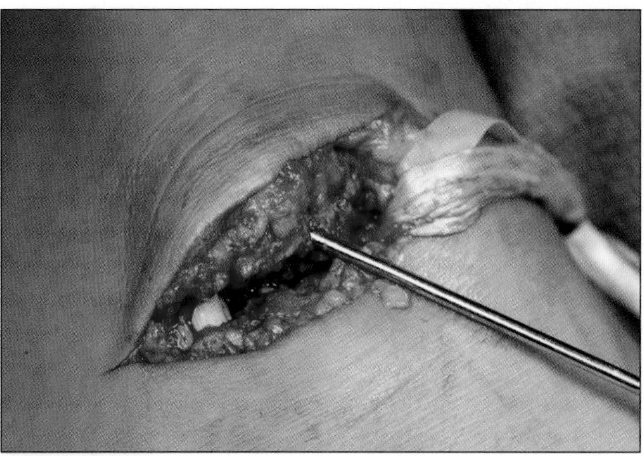

FIGURE 11

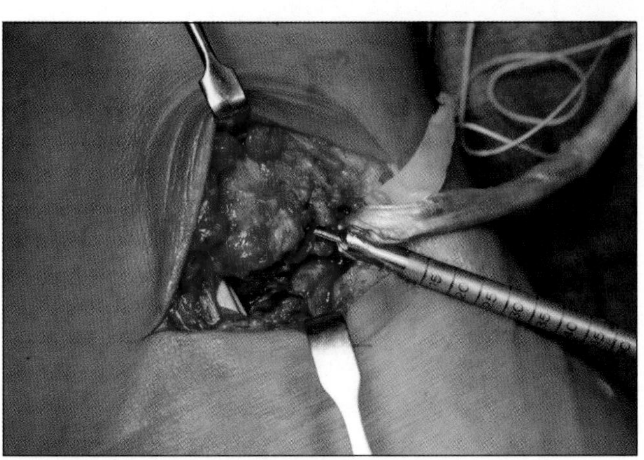

A

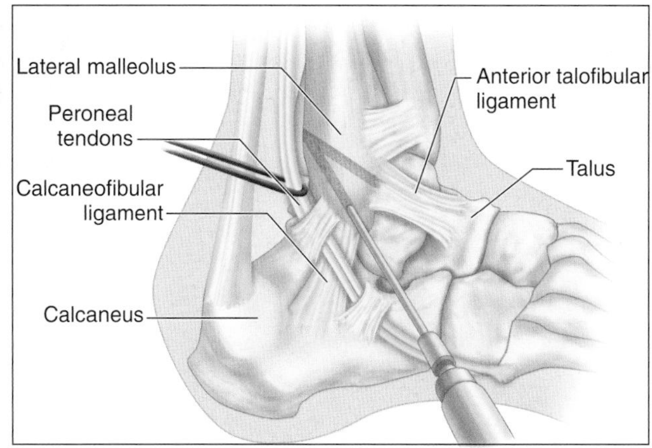

B

FIGURE 12

PEARLS

- *The CFL arm of the graft can be tensioned by measuring the graft, cutting it to appropriate length, and placing the biotenodesis screw. Another option is to cut the graft to an appropriate length, exchange the Fiberwire for a 0 Vicryl suture, pass the graft through the calcaneus from lateral to medial with a Keith needle, and pull the suture through the medial skin. Use the suture to appropriately tension the graft, place a biotenodesis screw, and cut the suture subcutaneously.*

STEP 4

- Pass the graft through the fibula from anterior to posterior (Fig. 13) and then out the tip (Fig. 14). A suture passer can be used. Another option is to pass a narrow metal suction tip through the tunnel, suck up the suture ends attached to the graft, and draw them out the other end.
- The insertion of the CFL is highly variable. Use the remnant of the CFL to locate the correct site for the drill hole in the calcaneus.
- If the ligament cannot be found, hold the ankle and subtalar joints in neutral and place an Arthrex guide wire into the calcaneus, 15 mm distal to the subtalar joint line and just posterior to the longitudinal axis of the fibula. Angle the guide wire posterior-medially. Drill the calcaneal tunnel using the 5.5-mm Arthrex cannulated bit and exit through the medial cortex (Fig. 15).

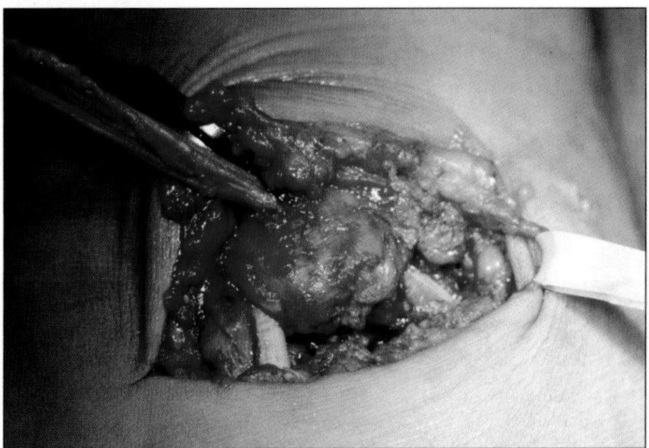

FIGURE 13

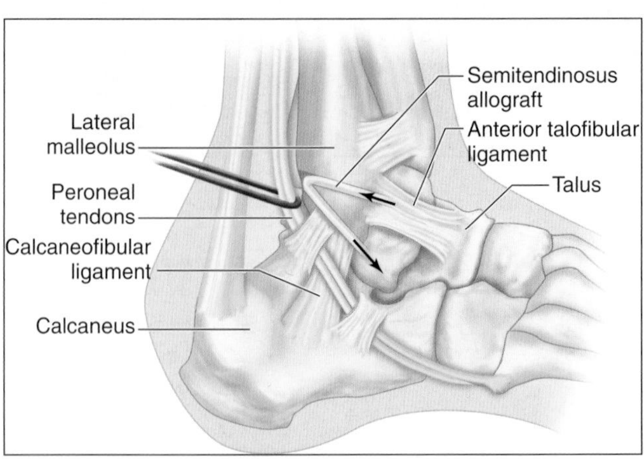

FIGURE 14

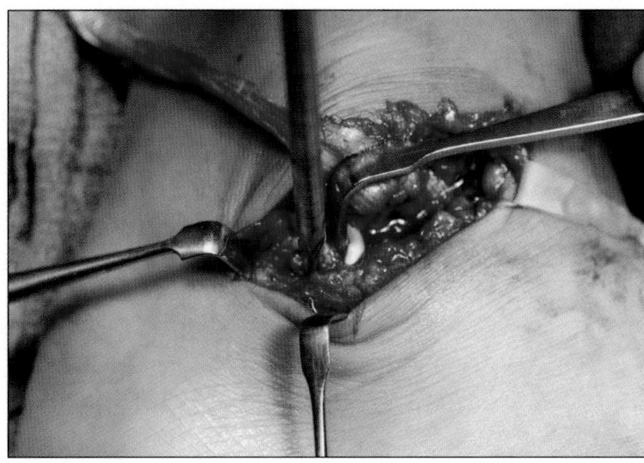

FIGURE 15

- Place the ankle in neutral and the subtalar joint halfway between neutral and maximal eversion. Hold this position until the graft is secured to the calcaneus.
- Tighten the graft starting with the ATFL arm, followed by the segments within the fibula.
  - Place the ankle on a towel bump that floats the heel, so as not to stretch the graft.
  - Place a 2-0 Vicryl suture into the tendon and periosteum where the graft enters and exits the bone.
  - Cut the calcaneofibular arm of the graft to the appropriate length (Fig. 16). Secure the graft snugly into the calcaneus with 5.5-mm biotenodesis screw, making sure to pass the graft deep to the peroneal tendons (Fig. 17).

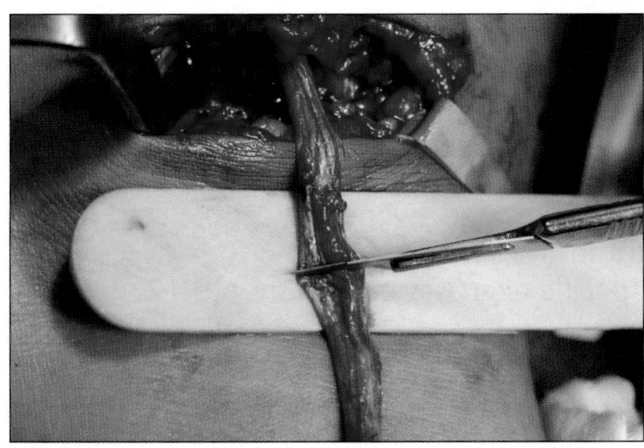

FIGURE 16

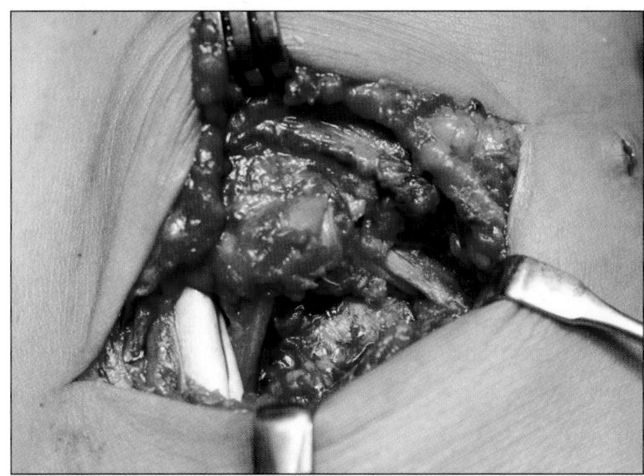

FIGURE 17

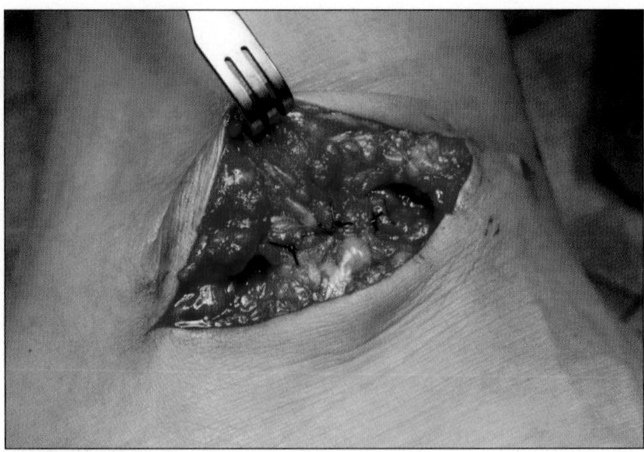

FIGURE 18

  - Check the range of motion of the ankle and subtalar joints.
  - Close the peroneal sheath with interrupted 3-0 nonabsorbable sutures.
- Advance the extensor retinaculum onto the fibula. Sew it snugly down to the periosteum using a O Vicryl absorbable suture (Fig. 18).
- Deflate the tourniquet. Close the wound in layers. Apply a three-sided plaster splint.

Postoperative Care and Expected Outcomes

- The sutures are removed at the first postoperative visit, 12 days after surgery. A short-leg non–weight-bearing cast is applied.
- The patient can use a short-leg non–weight-bearing cast boot at 1 month postoperative. At that time, start a home program of ankle and subtalar motion.
- Allow the patient to start weight bearing in a well-fitted ankle stirrup brace 6 weeks after surgery, at which point a formal physical therapy program is started.
  - Focus on peroneal strength, range of motion, and proprioception.
  - A stationary bike and swimming can be started at this point in the stirrup.
  - Sports-specific exercises can be started 12 weeks after surgery.
- Discontinue the ankle stirrup 8 weeks after surgery. Continue to use a soft velcro or lace-up ankle brace for the next month and during sports for the next 6 months.

- An excellent result can be obtained with this technique. If overtightening of the CFL arm of the graft is avoided, most patients will be able to return to full sports activity.

Evidence

Anderson ME. Reconstruction of the lateral ankle ligaments of the ankle using the plantaris tendon. J Bone Joint Surg [Br]. 1985;71:300-3.

In this study of nine patients with chronic lateral laxity who underwent an anatomic surgical reconstruction using a plantaris tendon autograft, the authors emphasized the advantages of using the plantaris tendon and not sacrificing the peroneus brevis. (Level IV evidence)

Coughlin MJ, Schenck RC. Comprehensive reconstruction of the lateral ankle for chronic instability using a free gracilis graft. Foot Ankle Int. 2004;25:231-41.

This study assessed the results in 29 patients of primary lateral ligament reconstruction using an autograft gracilis tendon. Ankle range of motion was not affected by the procedure, and all patients had a good to excellent result. (Level IV evidence [retrospective study])

DiGiovanni CW, Brodsky A. Current concepts: lateral ankle instability. Foot Ankle Int. 2006;27:854-66.

A superb review of the literature on lateral ankle instability.

Paterson R, Cohen B, Taylor D. Reconstruction of the lateral ligament of the ankle using semi-tendinosis graft. Foot Ankle Int. 2000;21:313-9.

In this study of 26 patients who had the ATFL reconstructed with a semitendinosus autograft and drill holes in the bone, the authors recognized that their technique did not address subtalar instability. (Level IV evidence [retrospective study])

PROCEDURE 39

Lateral Ankle Reconstruction with the Fourth Extensor Digitorum Communis Tendon

Edmund H. Choi and Andrew K. Sands

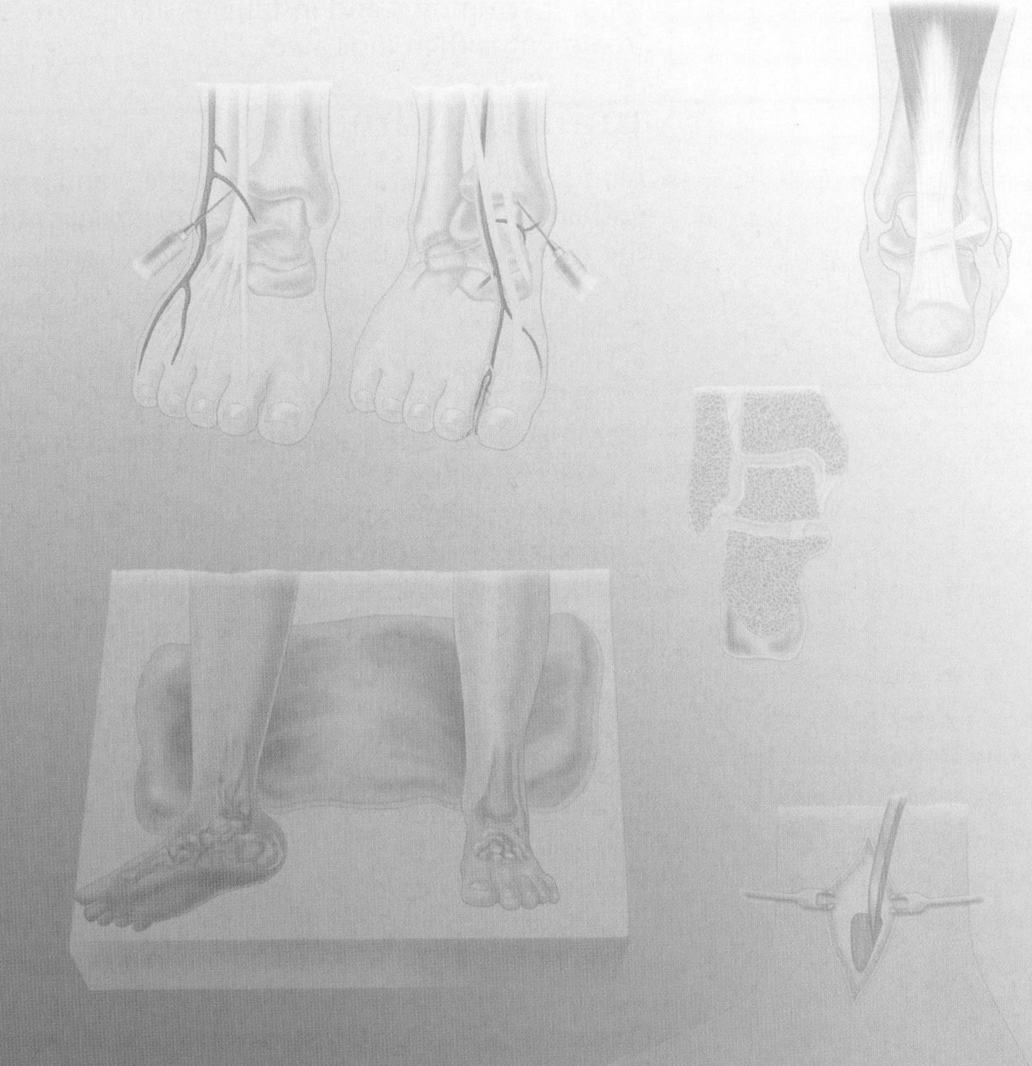

Indications

- Persistent lateral ankle instability that is refractory to nonoperative treatment or presenting with one of the following:
  - Early degenerative arthritis
  - Varus tilt in the ankle mortise
  - Normal eversion strength
- If eversion strength is not normal, instability cannot be reliably judged and nonoperative treatment, (including physical therapy and bracing) should be tried. If symptoms and instability still persist, surgical treatment is then indicated.

Examination/Imaging

- Along with a careful history and the standard foot and ankle examination, observe for malalignment of the foot that may predispose to lateral ankle instability, such as hindfoot varus and cavus malalignment.
  - Hindfoot varus/cavus foot causes stress at the ankle, which causes ankle instability. In fact, failure to recognize and treat these problems is the major cause of failure.
  - Cavus malalignment can be corrected at the time of ankle reconstruction.
- Check for generalized ligamentous laxity.
  - Hypermobility can be assessed by the Beighton scoring system.
  - Although not clinically accurate, the anterior draw and talar tilt stress can be performed to examine the integrity of the anterior talofibular ligament (ATFL) and the calcaneofibular ligament (CFL), respectively.
  - Sometimes a complete rupture of the ATFL may present with a sulcus sign at the anterior margin of the fibula. Palpate along the peroneal sheath, and also test the peroneal strength.
- Propioception can be tested with a modified Romberg test where the patient is asked to stand on one leg with the hands folded over the chest and the eyes closed. Another method is by measuring passive joint position with a Biodex dynamometer.
- Decide by physical examination and stress radiographs where instability is.
  - If there is isolated ankle joint instability, plan to reconstruct only the ankle. If there is ankle plus subtalar joint instability, then reconstruct both the ankle and subtalar joints.

- There is no sense in reconstructing the subtalar joint if that area is not unstable. If this is done, it unnecessarily locks up the hindfoot, preventing full functional hindfoot range of motion.
- Obtain plain radiographs.
  - Weight-bearing anteroposterior and lateral views of the foot/ankle should be evaluated for degenerative changes as well as alignment.
  - Stress views can also be taken. In the mortise view, both an anterior drawer stress and talar tilt stress can be examined radiographically. The anterior draw should measure less than 10 mm or within 3–5 mm of the opposite side. A talar tilt of more than 10° (or more than 5° compared to the opposite side) is consistent with laxity.
- Magnetic resonance imaging is not useful in acute injuries or in dynamic ankle instability.

Treatment Options

- Immobilization
- The "rest, ice, compression, and elevation" (RICE) protocol
- Physical therapy with a focus on propioception training, muscle strengthening, and weight bearing with an ankle support (i.e., lace-up ankle supports).

Surgical Anatomy

- The ATFL originates 1 cm proximal to the tip of the lateral malleolus (Fig. 1).
  - The ligament averages 7.2 mm in length and inserts into the talus just distal to the articular surface, 18 mm proximal to the subtalar joint.
  - The ATFL is contiguous with the joint capsule and may not be easily defined in cases of chronic injuries.
  - The ATFL stretches with plantar flexion.

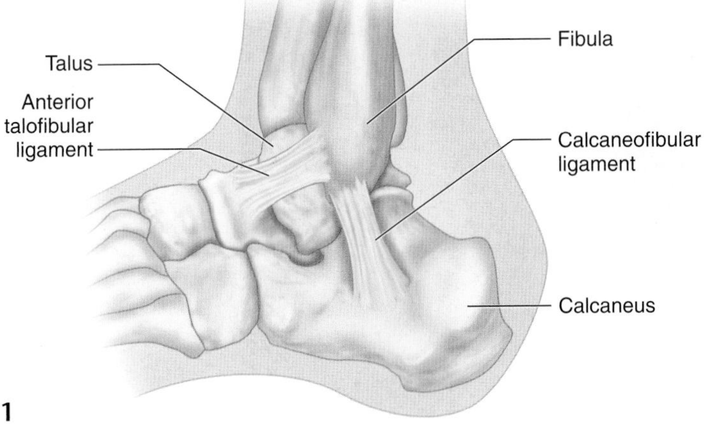

FIGURE 1

- The CFL originates adjacent to the ATFL, approximately 8 mm proximal to the tip of the fibula, and courses posterior and distal to the calcaneus (see Fig. 1).
  - The CFL inserts onto the calcaneus 13 mm distal to the subtalar joint.
  - The CFL ligament is an extracapsular ligament and makes up the floor of the peroneal sheath.
  - The CFL stretches with dorsiflexion.
- Neurovascular injury concerns are both anterior to the fibula, where superficially, the superficial peroneal nerve lies, and posterior to the fibula, where the sural nerve and short saphenous vein lie.

Equipment

- Curettes
- Lamina spreaders with and without teeth
- Osteotomes
- Periosteal elevators
- Spade retractors, Hohmann retractors, and curved Creigo elevators
- Tendon harvestors

Positioning

- Supine position with the ankle propped on a soft roll padding and a large ipsilateral bump under the buttock
- Utilization of tourniquet placed on the upper calf

Portals/Exposures

- Incision 1
  - A curvilinear incision is made centered over the fibula approximately 4 cm above the distal tip (Fig. 2).
  - The incision is carried down along the fibula to the tip and then curved forward to the calcaneocuboid joint. This allows exposure of the distal fibula and sinus tarsi.
- Incision 2
  - On the anterior ankle (see Fig. 2), allows access to the lateral extensor tendon for extensor digitorum communis (EDC) tendon harvest, and to the lateral talus.

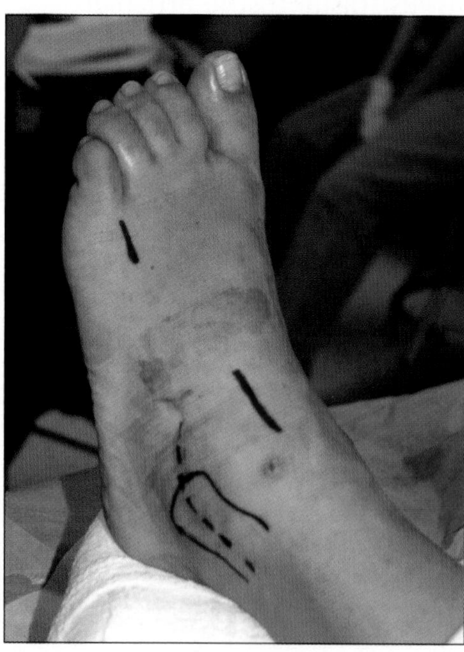

FIGURE 2

- Incision 3
  - On the distal dorsal lateral foot (see Fig. 2), allows access to the EDC tendon distally.
- Decide if the ankle or subtalar joint or both are unstable. If reconstruction of both joints is planned, inferior incision extension is needed. If just the ankle is to be reconstructed, as in this case, only a superior incision is needed.
- If equinus is present, a calf lengthening is required and can be done before the ankle reconstruction is done.

Procedure

Step 1: Exposure of the ATFL

- Expose the anterior border of the distal fibula. Sharply dissect off the soft tissue that is the remnant of the ATFL and the anterolateral soft tissue of the ankle. This soft tissue is usually attenuated, and it should be preserved as it is flipped distally.
- The ankle joint is now exposed and can be explored and irrigated.
- The remaining soft tissue on the distal fibula is then elevated laterally. This would include the insertion remnant of the ATFL as well as the periosteum of the fibula. These two flaps are closed "pants over vest" for the Brostrum-type reconstruction.
- A sharp-edged chisel is used to make a trough along the anterior edge of the distal fibula (Fig. 3).

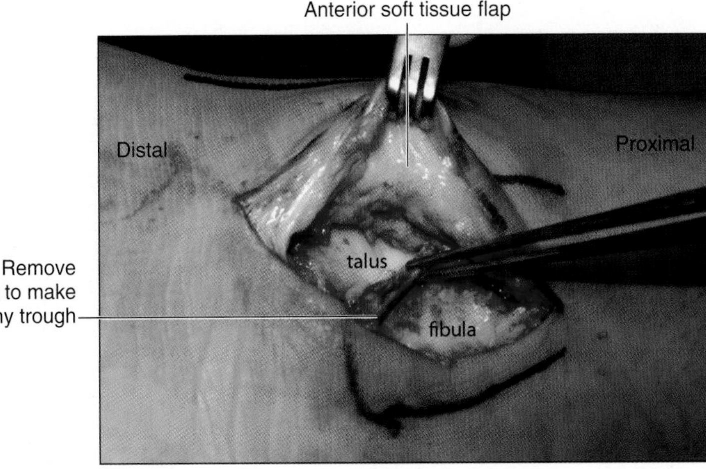

FIGURE 3

Pearls

- *If this is a revision of a previously failed repair, there may be retained hardware (suture anchor). These can be left in place and the new anchors placed to avoid the retained anchors (Fig. 10A and 10B).*
- *If both ankle and hindfoot instability exist, and a double reconstruction is to be done, then the tendon can be passed along the CFL to the calcaneus after it exits the posterior fibula tunnel, and secured at the calcaneus. This full anatomic repair replaces both the ATFL and CFL.*

Pitfalls

- *If EDC autograft is harvested, the toe from which it is taken can droop. Usually the extensor digitorum brevis (EDB) is sufficient to lift the toe and give it enough resistance to bending. All that is needed is enough force to allow socks to be placed on the foot. Anatomic variation sometimes shows that certain patients are missing their fifth EDB. Harvesting the fifth EDC can lead to complete loss of fifth toe dorsiflexion. For this reason, the fifth EDC should not be taken.*

Step 2: Preparation of the Graft Site

- An incision is made over the dorsolateral foot along the lateral border of the talar neck.
- The extensor tendons are retracted and the sinus tarsi is entered. The lateral aspect of the talar neck is exposed.
- A drill hole is made through the superolateral base of the talar neck from dorsal to plantar.

Step 3: Harvesting the EDC Tendon

- The EDC of the fourth toe is identified at the base of the toe.
- A tendon harvester is used from distal to proximal (Fig. 4). The harvester appears in the dorsolateral incision and the tendon graft is released in the front of the ankle.
- The graft should be wrapped in a moist lap pad until it is implanted.

Step 4: Reconstruction of ATFL with EDC Graft

- Pass the EDC tendon through the talar tunnel and loop it back on itself (Fig. 5A–C). Secure it with suture. Place a suture anchor in the corner of the talar lateral neck base. Secure the tendon there with the suture anchor suture.
- Pass the tendon subcutaneously along the periosteum from the dorsal incision at the talus to the lateral incision at the anterior fibula (Fig. 6A and 6B).

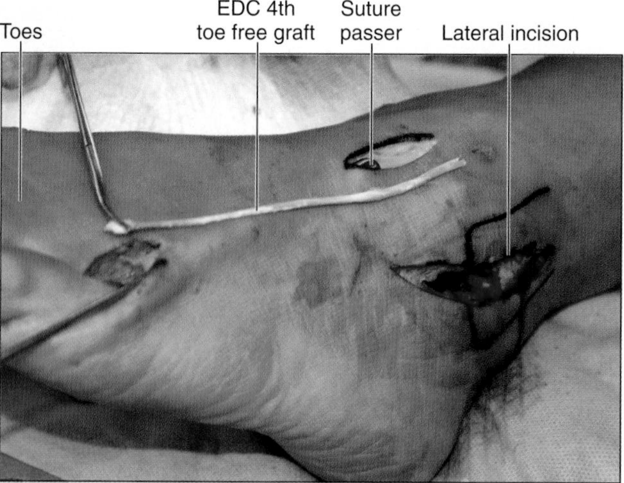

FIGURE 4

Anterior lateral incision

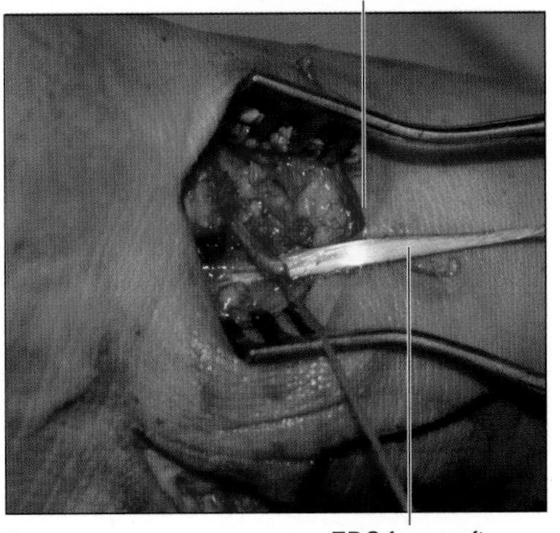

A EDC free graft

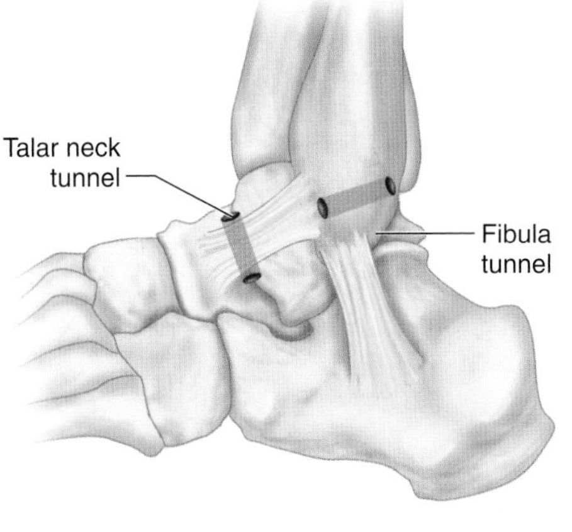

B

1st loop

C

FIGURE 5

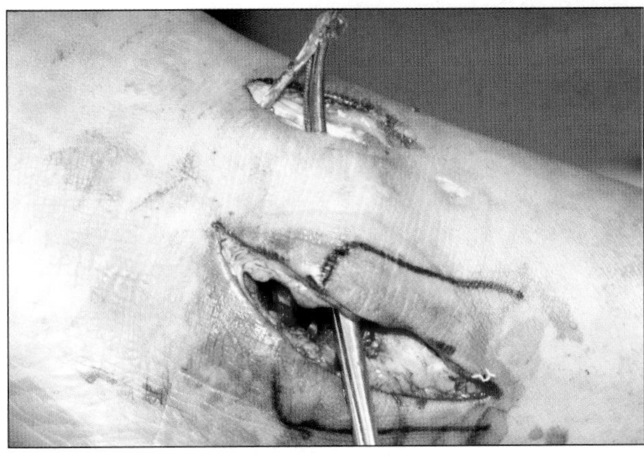

A

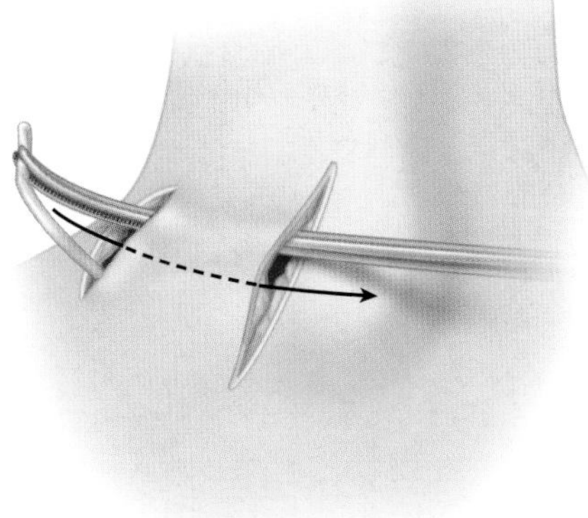

B

FIGURE 6

Controversies

- Autograft versus allograft: one could, instead of using autograft, use allograft of various types.

- Make a drill hole from the anterior to the posterior fibula at the anatomic insertion of the ATFL (see Fig. 5B). Pass the harvested tendon from anterior to posterior through the fibular tunnel, starting where the ATFL inserted on the fibula (Fig. 7A and 7B). Then, if length allows, pass the tendon back on itself (Fig. 7C).
- Place the ankle and hindfoot in neutral position and tension the graft.
- Secure with suture and a suture anchor placed within the trough. Do not cut the attached suture.
- Pull the distal flap (the ATFL remnant along with the extensor digitorum brevis and anterior ankle soft tissue) proximally and secure with the suture anchor (Fig. 8A). Do not cut the suture.
- Pull the proximal periosteal flap distally over the distal flap (Fig. 8B) in a "pants-over-vest" fashion. Pass the suture anchor suture up through this flap and secure (Fig. 8C). Supplement the repair with extra sutures as needed (Fig. 9).

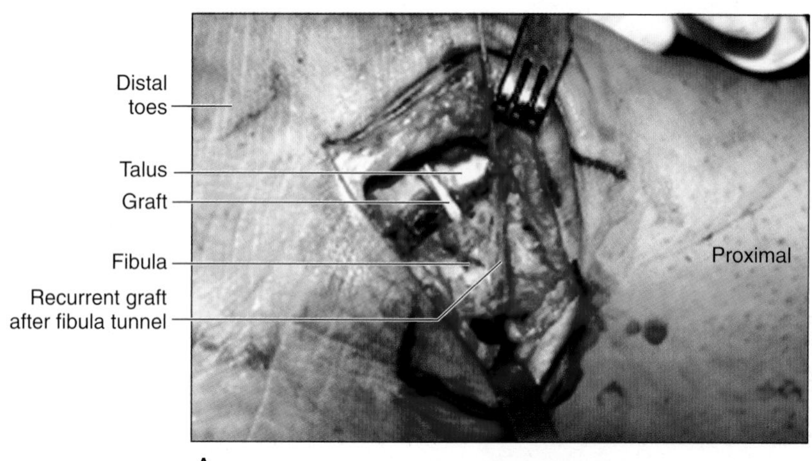

A

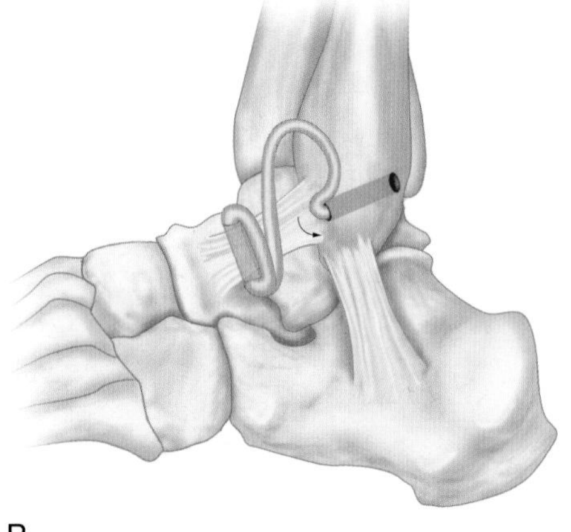

B

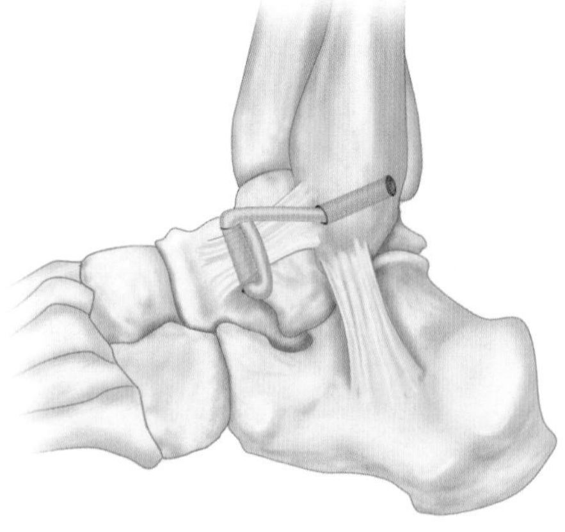

C

FIGURE 7

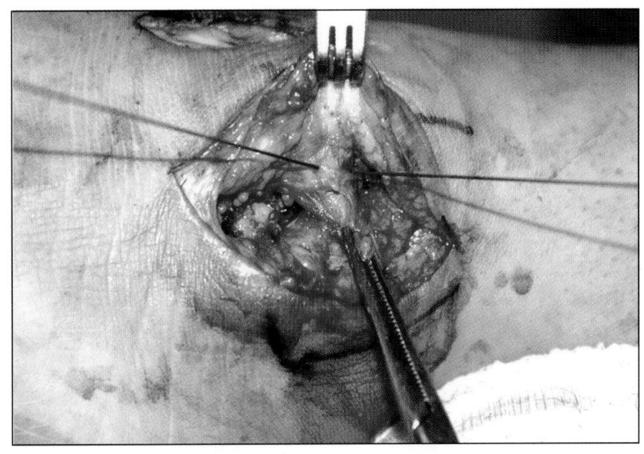
A

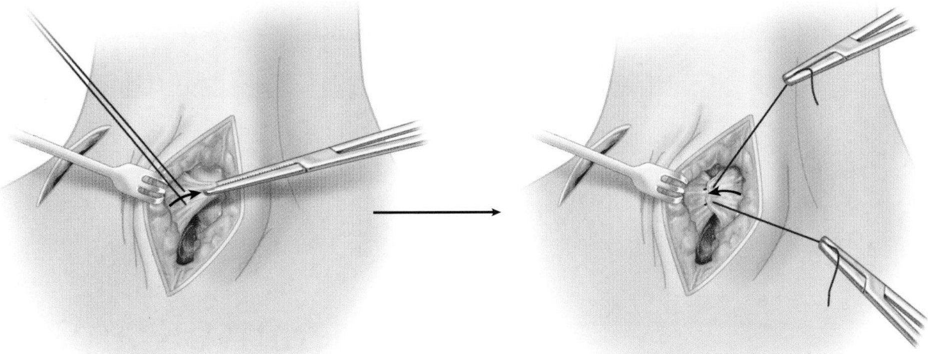
B

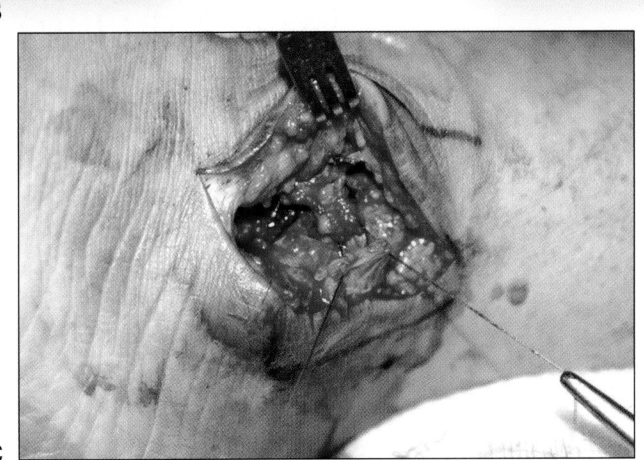
C

FIGURE 8

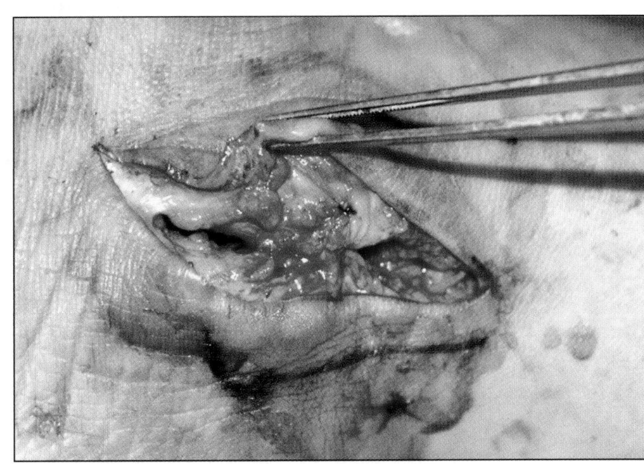

FIGURE 9

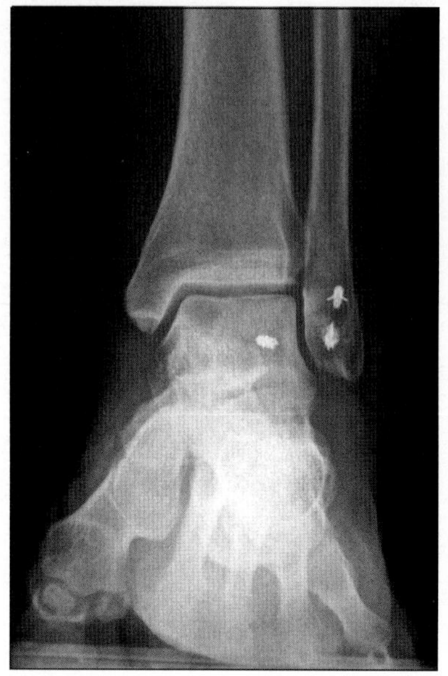

A

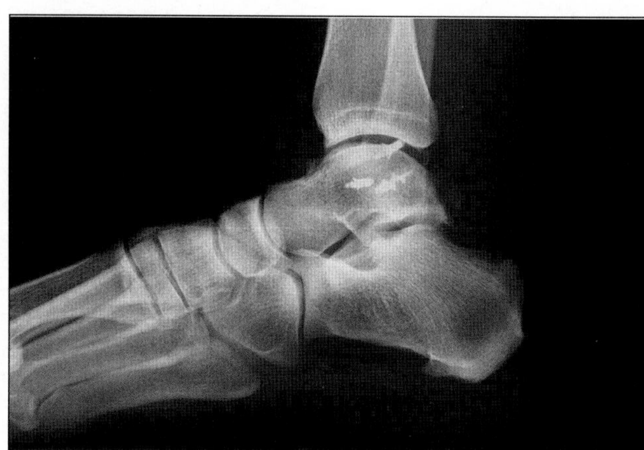

B

FIGURE 10

Postoperative Care and Expected Outcomes

- The postoperative three-sided short-leg splint is removed at 2 weeks, at which point the patient is allowed to bear weight with the assistance of a cam walker boot. Gentle bone motion is started at this point.
- At 6–8 weeks, patients are started on active and passive range of motion, toe intrinsic exercises, and gait training. Then they are started on strengthening of ankle dorsiflexion, plantar flexion, eversion, and inversion.
- Full athletic activity is permitted at 6 months.
- Use of an ankle brace is encouraged during the 3-month postoperative period and thereafter as needed.

Evidence

Burks RT, Morgan J. Anatomy of the lateral ankle ligaments. Am J Sports Med. 1994;22:72-7.

The authors peformed a cadaveric study of the anterior talofibular ligament and the calcaneofibular ligament. (Level V evidence [cadaveric study])

Colville MR. Surgical treatment of the unstable ankle. J Am Acad Orthop Surg. 1998;6:368-77.

The author presented a review of surgical treatment of lateral ankle instability as well as tendon graft procedures. (Level V evidence [author review])

DiGiovanni CW, Brodsky A. Current concepts: lateral ankle instability. Foot Ankle Int. 2006;27:854-66.

The authors presented a review of lateral ankle instability, including published series of anatomic repairs. (Level V evidence [review article])

Hazratwala K, Best A, Kopplin M, Giza E, Sullivan M. A radiographic investigation to determine the safety of suture anchor systems for pediatric modified Brostrom ankle ligament reconstruction. Am J Sports Med. 2005;33:435-8.

The authors performed a radiographic study to measure the distance of the suture anchors to the physis in skeletally immature patient who underwent a modified Brostrom ankle ligament reconstruction. (Level V evidence [radiographic study])

Messer TM, Cummins CA, Ahn J, Kelikian AS. Outcome of the modified Brostrom procedure for chronic lateral ankle instability using suture anchors. Foot Ankle Int. 2000;21:996-1003.

The authors reviewed 22 patients who underwent modified Brostrom procedure using suture anchors. Follow-up averaged 34.5 months, and outcome was determined by functional outcome scores and Karlsson-Peterson ankle function scores. (Level IV evidence [case series])

Van Dijk CN. Management of sprained ankle. Br J Sports Med. 2002;36:83-4.

Van Dijk CN, Bossuyt PM, Marti RK. Medial ankle pain after lateral ligament rupture. J Bone Joint Surg [Br]. 1996;78:562-7.

The authors reviewed 30 consecutive patients with operative repair of acute ruptures of lateral ligaments who also presented with medial ankle pain. The authors presented their arthroscopic findings during the lateral complex repair. (Level IV evidence [case series])

PROCEDURE 40

Ligament Reconstruction for Chronic Medial Ankle Instability

Beat Hintermann

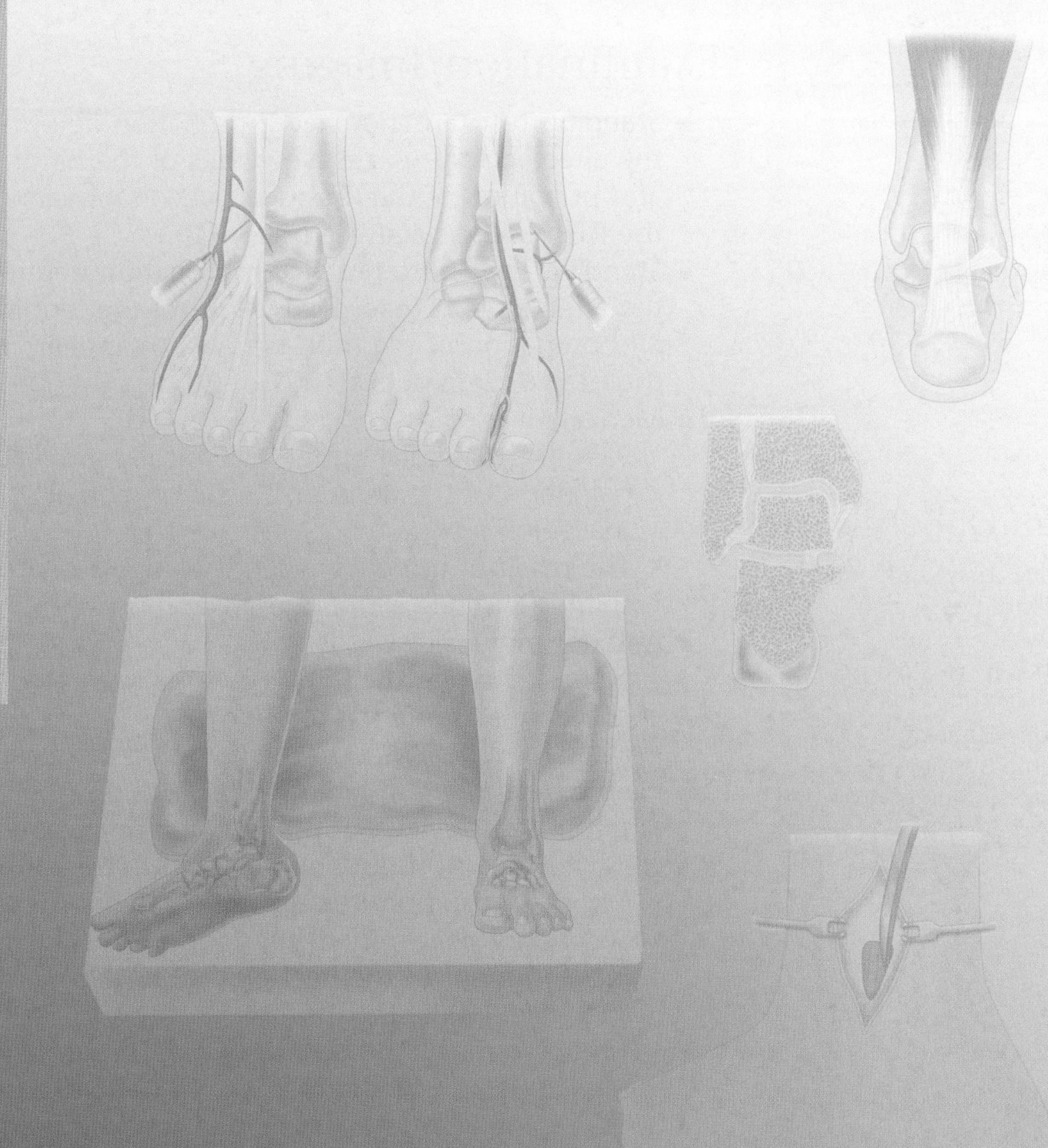

Pitfalls

- *Incompetent deep deltoid ligament (e.g., stage 4 PT dysfunction)*
- *Fixed pronation deformity (e.g., talocalcaneal coalition)*
- *Paralytic foot (e.g., loss of PT muscle power)*
- *End-stage osteoarthritis of the ankle joint*

Controversies

- Supple acquired flatfoot with loss of PT function
- Valgus malalignment of the heel not addressed by calcaneal osteotomy

Treatment Options

- Shoe modifications and orthotics with medial arch support
- Physical therapy to strengthen the PT muscle
- Proprioceptive training
- Ankle arthrodesis may be advised for incompetence of the deep deltoid ligament.

Indications

- Chronic medial ankle instability based on patient's feeling of "giving-way," especially toward medial, when walking on even ground, downhill, or downstairs
- Pain at the anteromedial aspect of the ankle, and sometimes pain in the lateral ankle, especially during dorsiflexion of the foot
- Progressive pronation deformity
- Secondary tendinosis of posterior tibial (PT) tendon

Examination/Imaging

- Standing test (anterior view): pronation deformity of the affected foot (excessive valgus of the hindfoot and pronation of the foot; Fig. 1A) disappears when the PT muscle is activated (Fig. 1B).
- Standing test (posterior view): pronation deformity of the affected foot (excessive valgus of the hindfoot and pronation of the foot; Fig. 2A) disappears when the PT muscle is activated (Fig. 2B).
- Medial ankle pain
  - Pain in the medial gutter, as typically provoked by palpation of the anterior border of medial malleolus
  - The result of underlying synovitis due to chronic shifting of talus within the ankle mortise
- Anterior drawer test
  - Increased when the foot is externally rotated (as compared to internal rotation)
  - Highly sensitive test for medial ankle instability
- Plain weight-bearing radiographs, including anteroposterior views of the foot and ankle and lateral view of the foot, should be obtained to rule out
  - Old bony avulsion fractures
  - Secondary deformity of the foot (e.g., valgus malalignment of the heel, and dislocation at the talonavicular joint)
  - Tibiotalar malalignment (e.g., medial gapping of the joint due to incompetence of deltoid ligament)
- Stress radiographs may be helpful to discern an incompetence of the deltoid ligament in treatment of acute ankle fractures (Tornetta, 2000), but they are not helpful in chronic conditions (Miller and Soames, 1998).
- Computed tomography scans may be initiated to detect a talocalcaneal coalition, or bony fragmentation that involves the articular surfaces.

- Magnetic resonance imaging may reveal an injury to the deltoid ligament, particularly in acute conditions, and may also show pathologic conditions of the PT tendon.
- Ankle arthroscopy is used to evaluate the stability of the ankle and discern associated intra-articular lesions (e.g., to the cartilage).

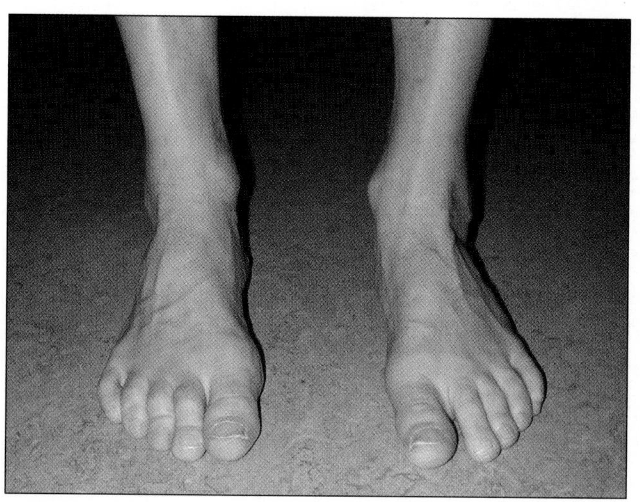
A

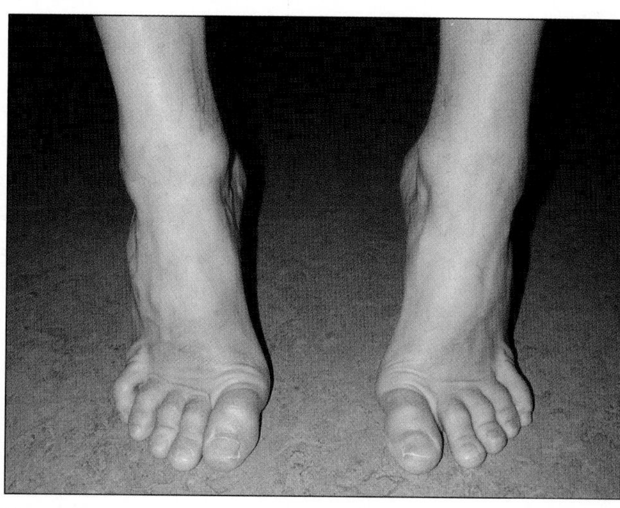
B

FIGURE 1

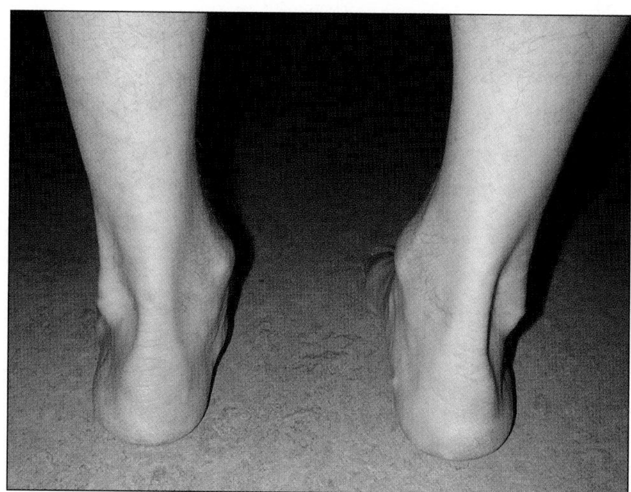
A

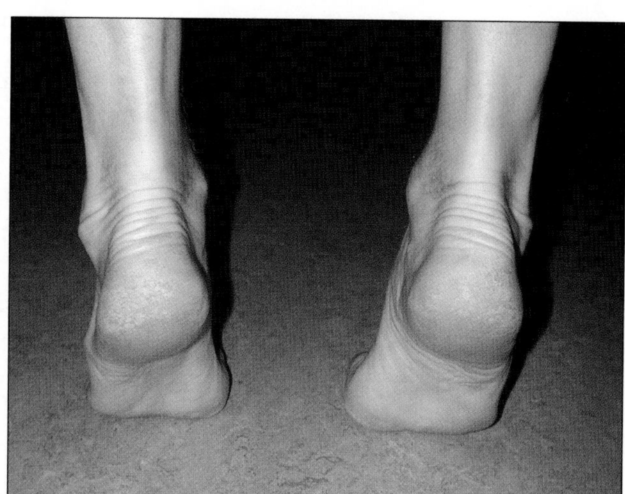
B

FIGURE 2

Surgical Anatomy

- The deltoid ligament is a multibanded complex with superficial and deep components (Fig. 3A) (Boss and Hintermann, 2002; Harper, 1987; Milner and Soames, 1998).
- It may be wise to differentiate the superficial and deep portions of the deltoid complex with respect to the joints they are spanning.
  - The superficial ligaments cross two joints: the ankle and the subtalar joints.
  - The deep ligaments cross only one joint, the ankle joint, although differentiation is not always absolutely clear.
- The three superficial and more anterior bands (Fig. 3B) are the tibionavicular ligament (TNL), tibio-spring ligament (TSL), and tibiocalcaneal ligament (TCL). There are three deep bands constituting the anterior, intermediate, and posterior tibiotalar ligaments (TTL).
- As the tibioligamentous portion of the superficial deltoid has a broad insertion on the spring ligament (Spring L in Fig. 3B), this ligament complex may interplay with the deltoid ligament in the stabilization of the medial ankle joint, and thus functionally not be separated from it.

Positioning

Pearls

- *Use of a knee holder that does not fix the leg will facilitate its removal after arthroscopy.*

- The patient is placed in supine position with the feet at the edge of the table.
- A commercially available knee holder is used to support the distal femur and get the foot into a hanging position (Fig. 4).
- This allows for free movement of the foot while arthroscopy is done prior to open reconstruction.
- After the arthroscopy, the knee holder is removed, leaving the foot on the table.
- A tourniquet is placed at the ipsilateral thigh.

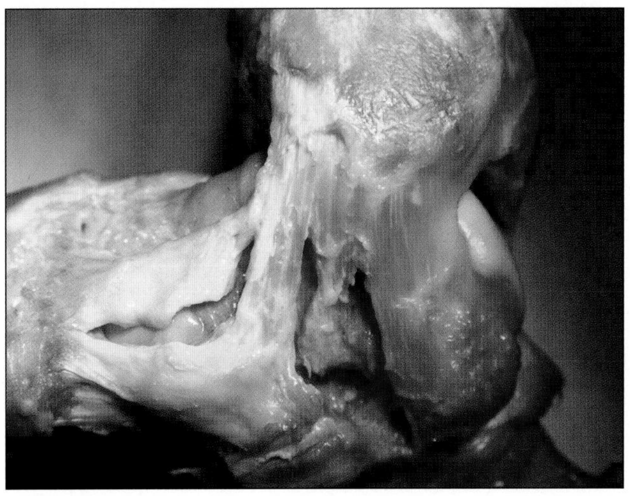

A

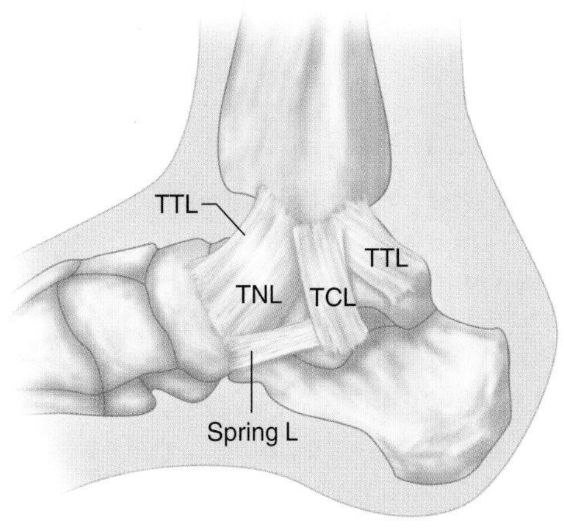

FIGURE 3 B

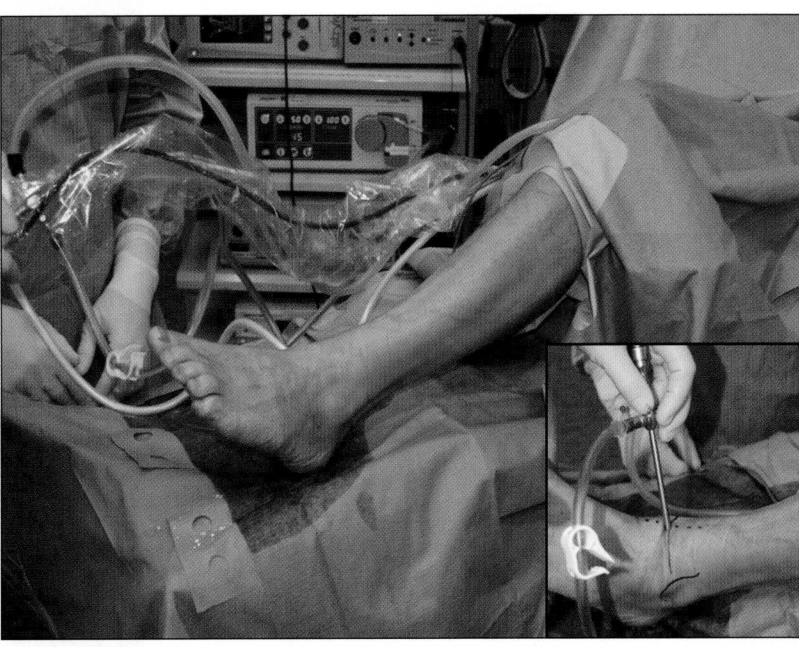

FIGURE 4

Pearls

- *The PT tendon sheath is opened to assess the condition of tendon.*
- *The spring ligament is assessed while distracting the PT tendon with a hook.*
- *The superficial fascia is carefully separated from the anterior bundles of the deltoid.*

Pitfalls

- *Overlooking a lesion of the spring ligament*

Controversies

- In the case of a strictly proximal lesion to the deltoid ligament without clinical appearance of PT tendinosis, extended exposure of the PT tendon and spring ligament may not be necessary.

Portals/Exposures

- An anteromedial approach is used for ankle arthroscopy (Hintermann et al., 2002) (Fig. 5).
- Medially, a gently curved incision of 3–5 cm is made, starting 1 cm cranially of the tip of the medial malleolus and extending toward the medial aspect of the navicular bone (see Fig. 5).
- In the case of an additional instability of the lateral ankle ligaments, as found in the clinical investigation and confirmed by the arthroscopy, a lateral approach to the ankle is additionally performed to explore the anterior talofibular and calcaneofibular ligaments (Fig. 6).
- In the case of pre-existing valgus and pronation deformity (e.g., when a valgus and pronation deformity is also present on the contralateral, asymptomatic foot), and/or in the case of a severe attenuation or defect of the tibionavicular, tibio-spring, and/or spring ligaments, the lateral incision is lengthened distally.

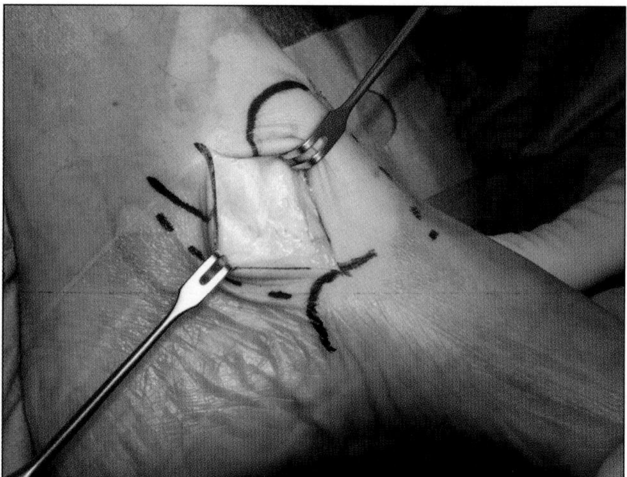

FIGURE 5

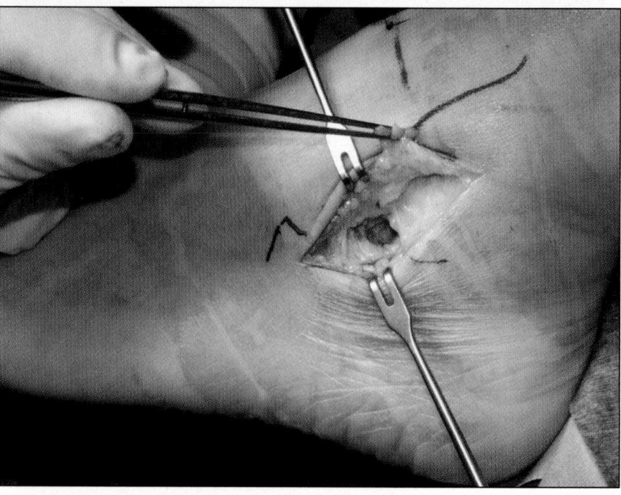

FIGURE 6

PEARLS

- *If distended, the interval between the tibio-spring and tibiocalcaneal ligament is closed by a duplication suture.*

PITFALLS

- *The naked bony area beneath the detached superficial deltoid ligament is not roughened carefully*
- *Insufficient reattachment of the deltoid ligament to the bone of the medial malleolus*

Procedure

STEP 1: RECONSTRUCTION OF SUPERFICIAL DELTOID LIGAMENT (INCLUDING SPRING LIGAMENT) (SEE VIDEO 1)

- Chronic ruptures of the superficial deltoid ligament, involving the tibionavicular and spring ligaments, are classified as noted below (Hintermann et al., 2004, 2006).
  - Type I: proximal
    - Involves the tibionavicular and tibio-spring ligaments (occasionally the spring ligament)
    - Found in 71% of patients (Hintermann et al., 2004)
  - Type II: intermediate
    - Involves the tibionavicular and tibio-spring ligaments (occasionally the spring ligament)
    - Found in 10% of patients
  - Type III: distal
    - Involves the tibionavicular and spring ligaments
    - Found in 19% of patients
- Type I chronic rupture of superficial deltoid ligament
  - The anterior border of the medial malleolus is exposed by a short longitudinal incision between the tibionavicular and tibio-spring ligaments, where usually a small fibrous septum without adherent connective fibers between the two ligaments is present (Fig. 7).

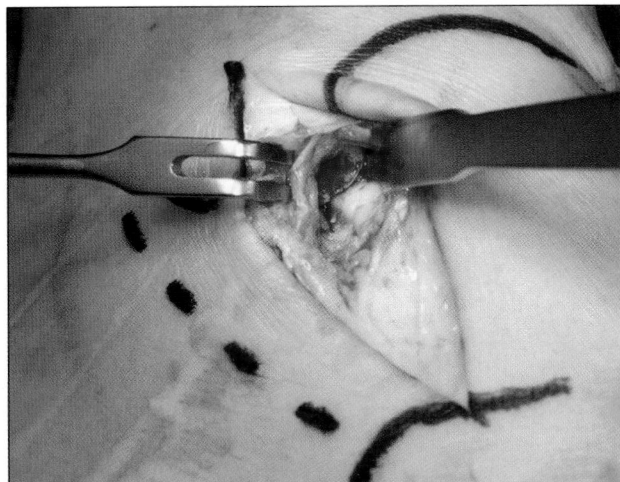

FIGURE 7

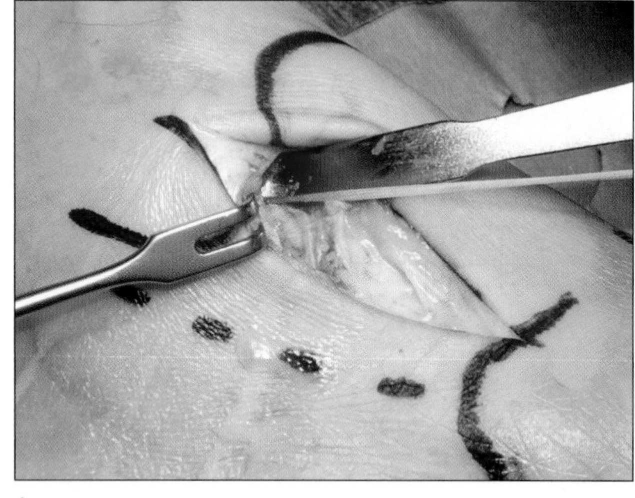
A

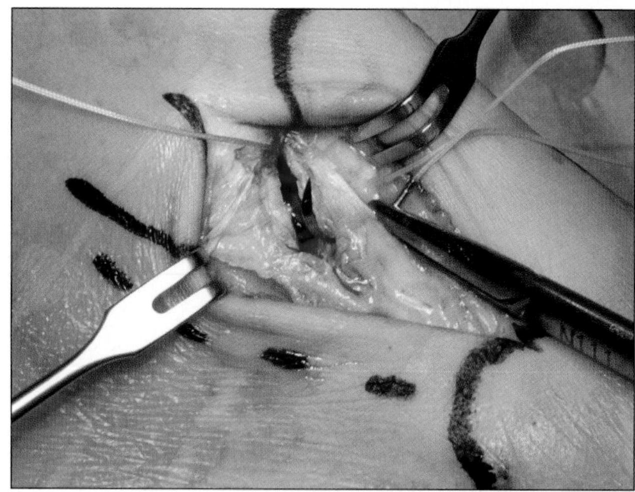
B

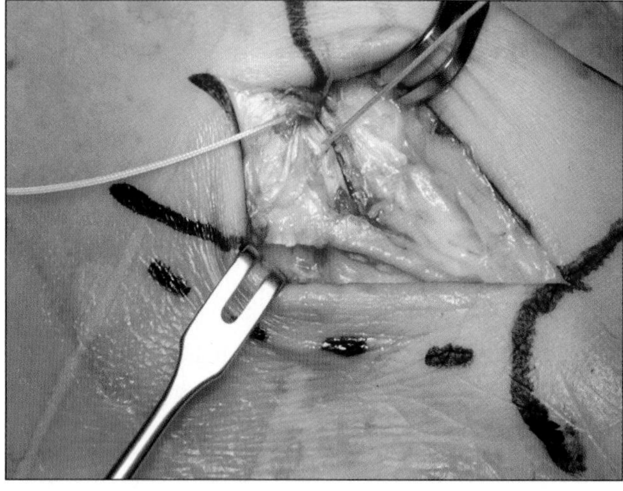
C

FIGURE 8

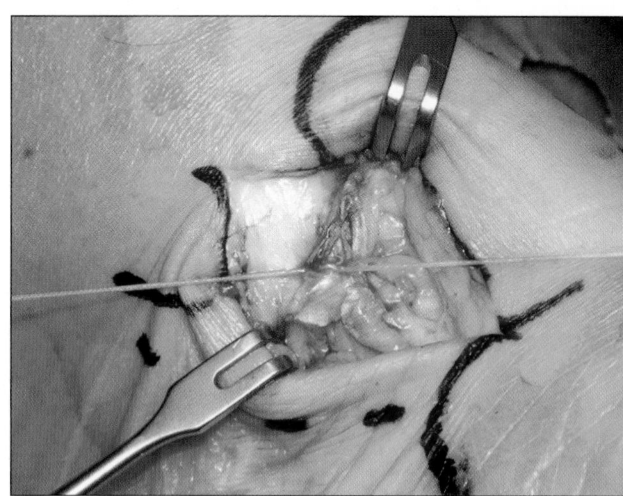
A

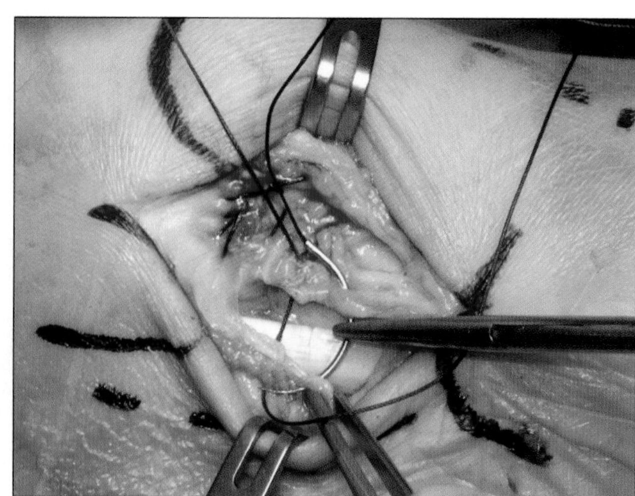
B

FIGURE 9

- After roughening of the medial aspect of the medial malleolus, an anchor (Panalock) is placed 6 mm above the tip of the malleolus (Fig. 8A) that serves for refixation of the tibionavicular and tibio-spring ligaments to the medial malleolus, and to shorten both the tibionavicular and tibio-spring ligaments (Fig. 8B and 8C).
- Additional 0 resorbable sutures are used to refix the tibionavicular and tibio-spring ligaments (Fig. 9A and 9B).

- Type II chronic rupture of superficial deltoid ligament
  - The scarred, insufficient ligament (Fig. 10) is divided into two flaps: The deep flap remains attached distally, whereas the superficial flap remains attached to the medial malleolus.
  - Two anchors (Panalock) are placed 6 mm above the tip of the malleolus (Fig. 11A), and one anchor (Panalock) is placed at the superior edge of the navicular tuberosity (Fig. 11B).
  - The two anchors serve for refixation of the deep flap to the medial malleolus (Fig. 11C), and the single anchor for fixation of the superficial flap to the navicular tuberosity (Fig. 11D), thereby creating a strong and well-tightened ligament reconstruction (Fig. 11E).
  - The second superior anchor on the medial malleolus also serves for reattachment of the tibionavicular ligament (Fig. 11F).

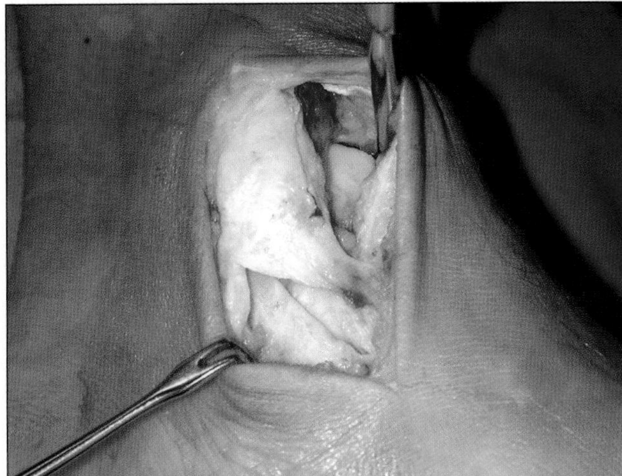

FIGURE 10

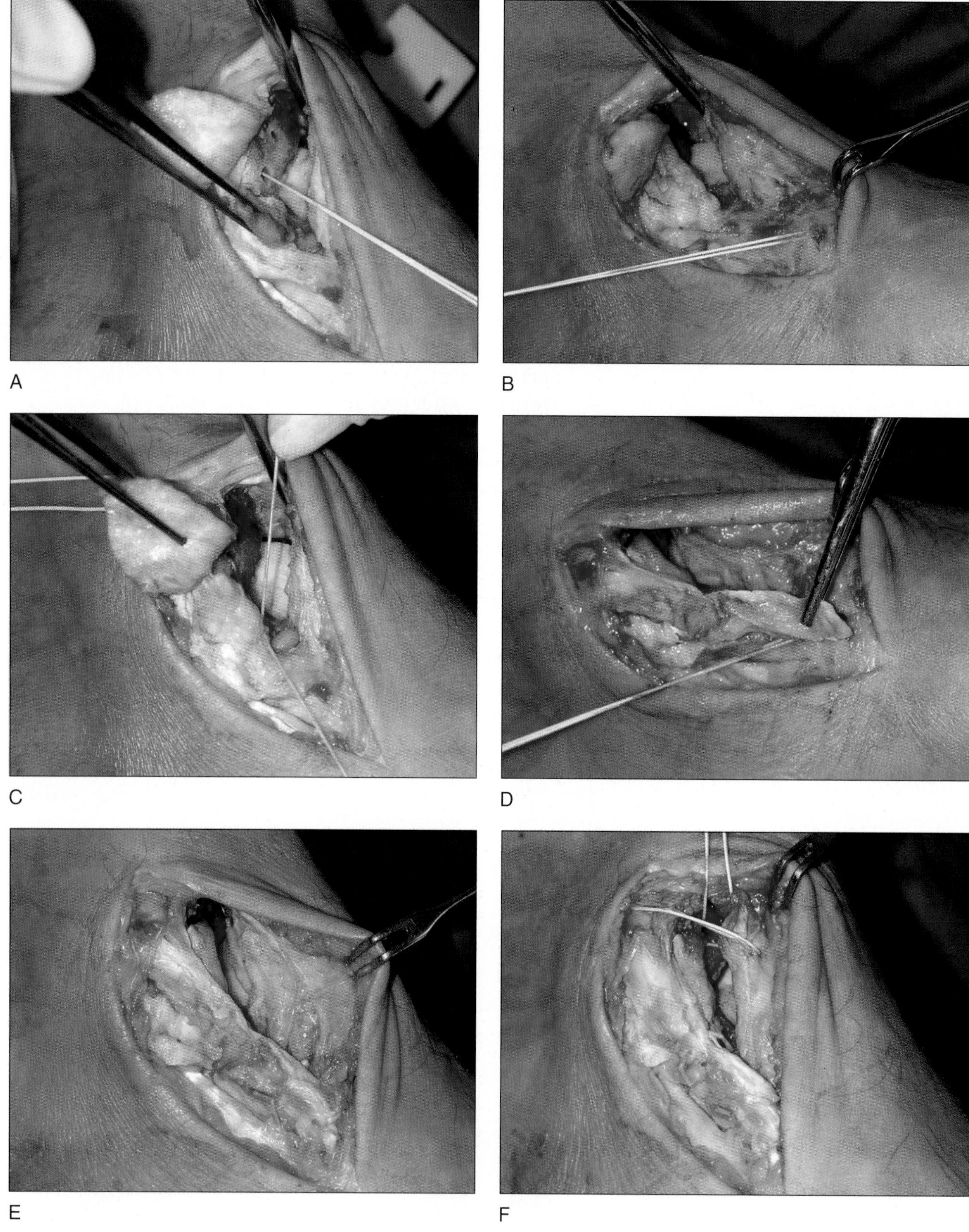

FIGURE 11

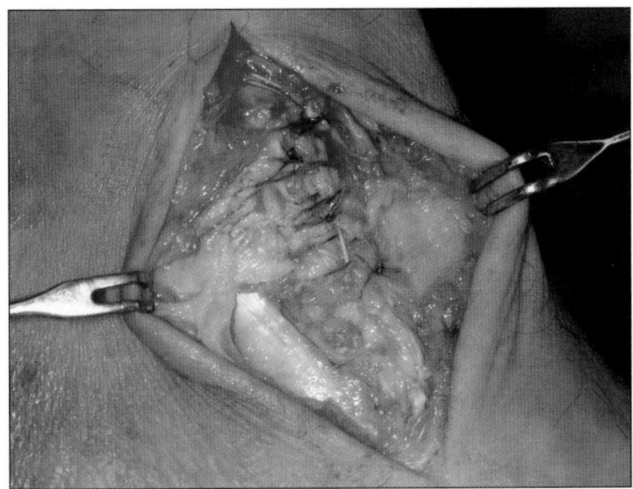

FIGURE 12

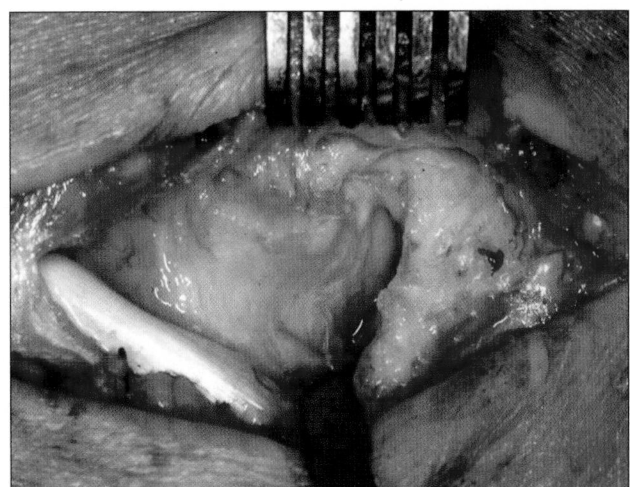

FIGURE 13

- Additional 0 resorbable sutures are used to further stabilize the reconstructed tibionavicular and tibio-spring ligaments (Fig. 12).

- Type III chronic rupture of superficial deltoid ligament
  - If necessary, the tear is débrided (Fig. 13).
  - Then, two nonabsorbable sutures are placed in the spring ligament (Fig. 14A). If the tibionavicular ligament is completely detached from its insertion, an anchor (Panalock) is also placed at the superior edge of the navicular tuberosity.
  - After having tightened the sutures (Fig. 14B), additional 0 resorbable sutures are used to further stabilize the reconstructed tibionavicular and spring ligaments.

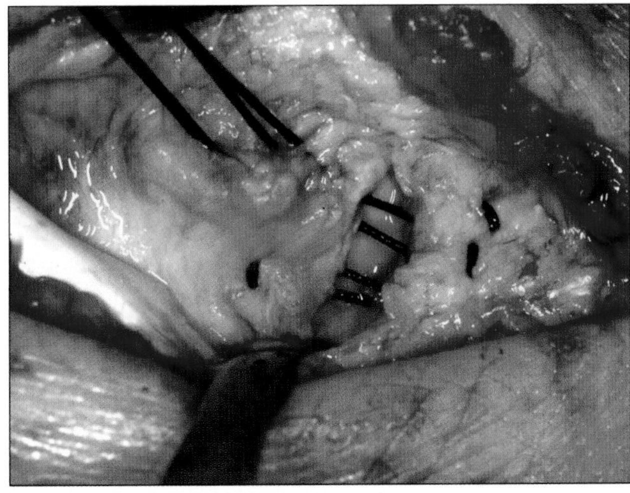

A

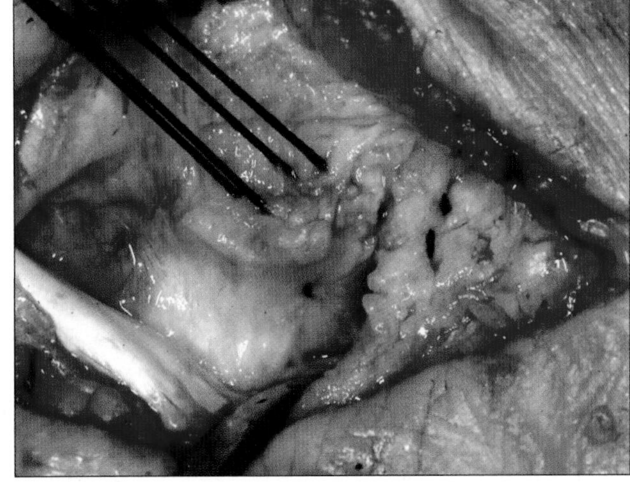

B

FIGURE 14

Pearls

- *Reconstruction of the peroneal tendon sheath may improve postoperative function.*

Pitfalls

- *Nonanatomic tenodesis for lateral ligament reconstruction may result in loss of subtalar motion and thus alter hindfoot biomechanics.*

Controversies

- Although concomitant lateral instability is still controversial, it was found in our practice to be present in about 75% of cases, mostly in the case of type I lesions of the deltoid ligament.

Step 2: Lateral Ankle Ligament Reconstruction

- Approximately 75% of patients with chronic medial ankle instability were found to have an associated avulsion of the anterior talofibular ligament that resulted in a complex rotational instability of the talus within the ankle mortise (Hintermann et al., 2004).
- If the condition of the anterior talofibular ligament and calcaneofibular ligament allows an adequate primary repair, these ligaments are reconstructed by shortening and reinsertion (Fig. 15A and 15B).
- When no substantial ligamentous material is present, augmentation with a free plantaris tendon graft is performed (Pagenstert et al., 2006).

Step 3: PT Tendon Reconstruction

- The PT tendon is meticulously inspected during surgery, especially in the case of a type II or type III lesion of the anterior deltoid ligament.
- If there is some degeneration of the tendon, débridement of the tendon is performed.
- If there is an elongation of the tendon, shortening of the tendon is considered.
- If there is an accessory bone (os tibiale externum), reattachment of the bone with the tendon insertion is considered; the PT tendon can additionally be tightened if the bone is reattached more distally to the navicular bone (Knupp and Hintermann, 2005).
- A transfer of the flexor digitorum tendon might be considered in the case of a diseased or ruptured tendon. This is, however, very seldom the case.

Step 4: Lateral Lengthening Osteotomy of Calcaneus

- This repair is considered in the case of a pre-existing valgus and pronation deformity of the foot (e.g., when a valgus and pronation deformity is also present on the contralateral, asymptomatic foot), and/or in the case of a severe attenuation or defect of the tibionavicular, tibio-spring, and/or spring ligaments.
- Calcaneal osteotomy is performed along and parallel to the posterior facet of the subtalar joint, from lateral to medial, preserving the medial cortex intact (Fig. 16A and 16B) (Hintermann and Valderrabano, 2003).
- As the osteotomy is widened (Fig. 17A), the pronation deformity of the foot is seen to disappear (Fig. 17B).

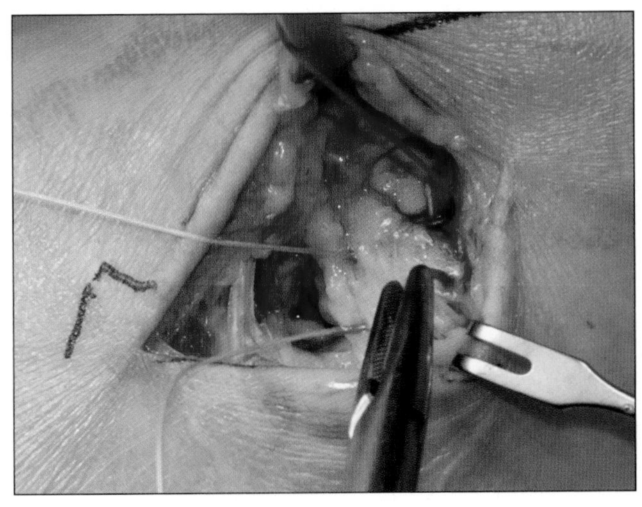

A

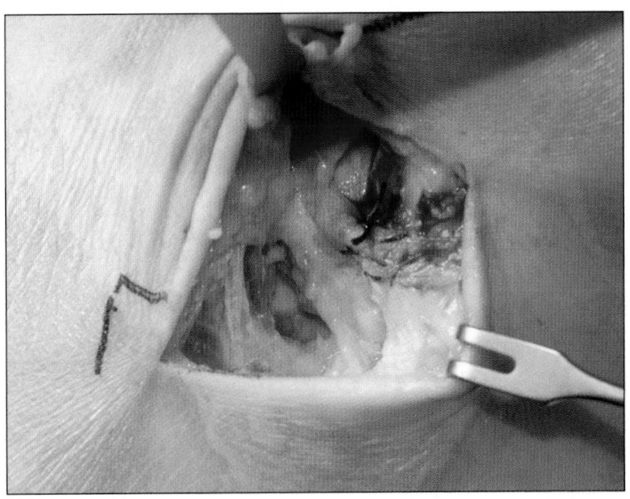

B

FIGURE 15

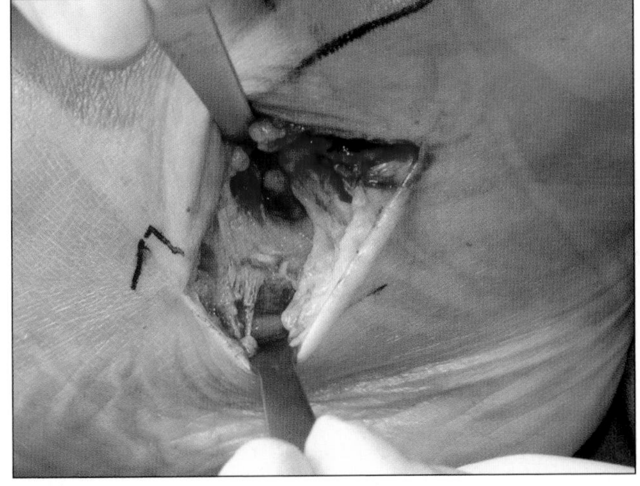

A

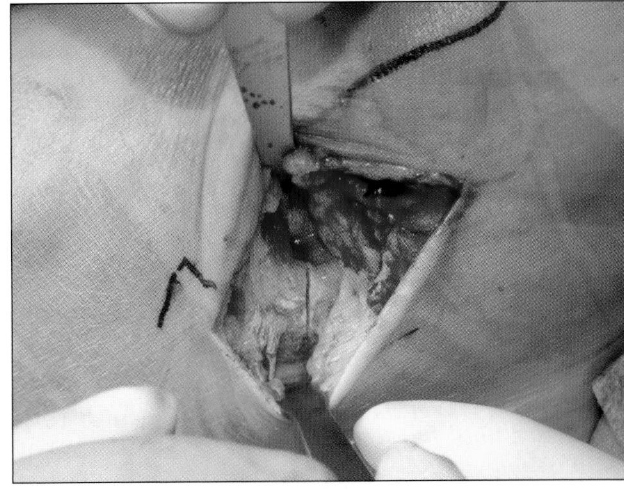

B

FIGURE 16

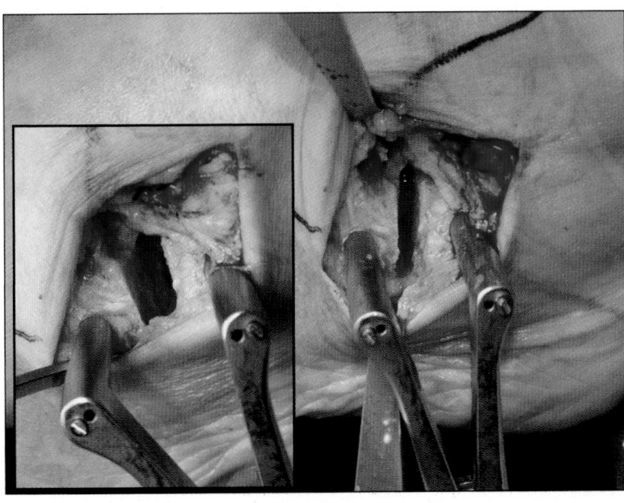

A

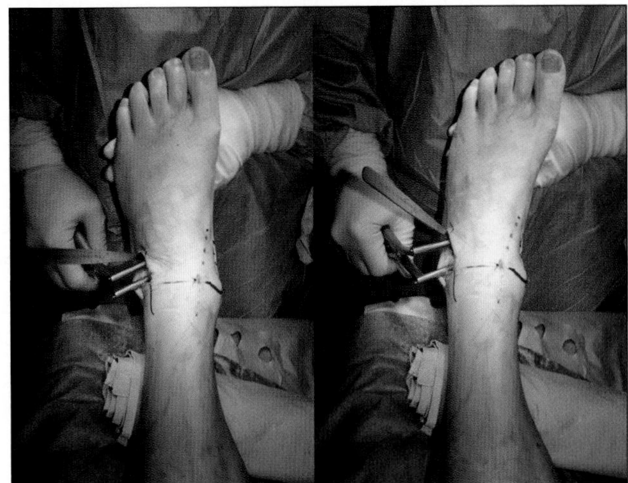

B

FIGURE 17

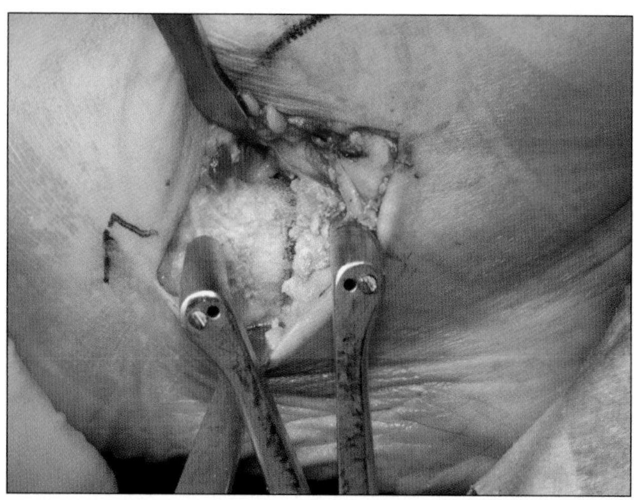

FIGURE 18

- A tricortical graft from the iliac crest is fashioned to the length required and placed into the osteotomy site (Fig. 18).

Pearls

- *Isometric training of the PT muscle may be beneficial for regaining proper function.*
- *Medial heel support may be advised until full recovery of muscular control.*

Pitfalls

- *Early return to physical activities prior to restoration of muscular balance may result in chronic overload of reconstructed ligaments, thereby causing failure.*

Controversies

- Early full weight bearing may be beneficial for muscular recovery (Valderrabano et al., 2004). Therefore, we prefer cast immobilization that allows the patient full weight bearing as tolerated, usually after 2 weeks.

Postoperative Care and Expected Outcomes

- The foot is protected by a plaster cast for 6 weeks, and full weight bearing is allowed as soon as pain-free loading is possible.
- A rehabilitation program starts after plaster cast removal. It includes passive and active mobilization of the ankle joint, training of muscular strength, and protection by a walker or stabilizing shoe when walking.
- A walker or stabilizing shoe may be recommended to be used for 4–6 weeks after plaster cast removal, depending on regained muscular balance of the hindfoot. Afterward, we still recommend that the patient use it for walks on uneven ground, for high-risk sports activities, and for professional work outside.
- Athletes should anticipate return to sports in 8–12 months after reconstruction of medial ankle ligaments.
- Figures 19 and 20 show the same patient seen in Figures 1 and 2 at 9 months postoperative. The pronation deformity of the affected foot has been corrected, as seen on a standing test in anterior (Fig. 19A and 19B) and posterior (Fig. 20A and 20B) views.

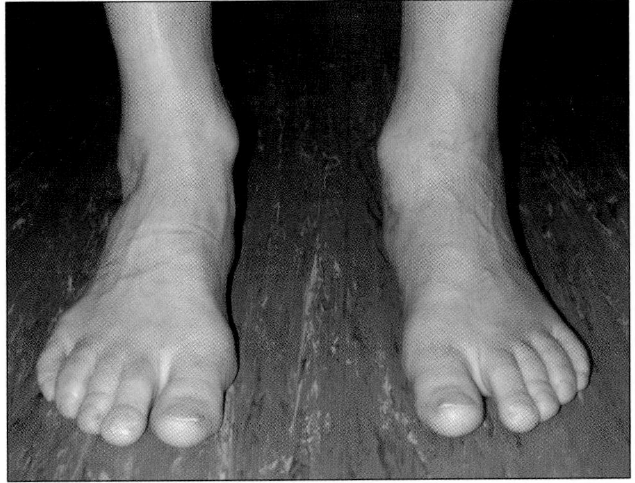

A

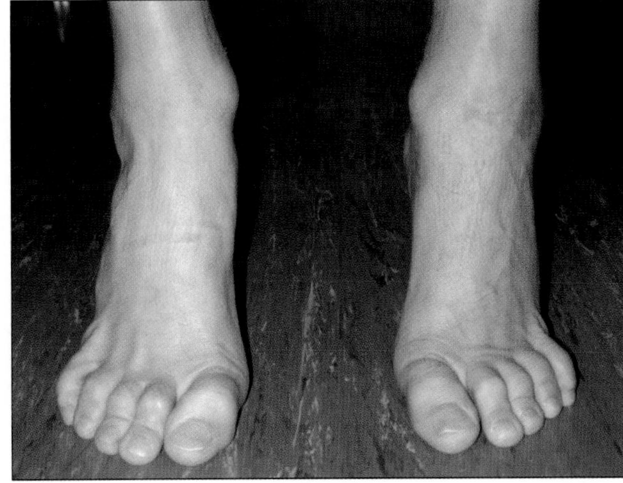

B

FIGURE 19

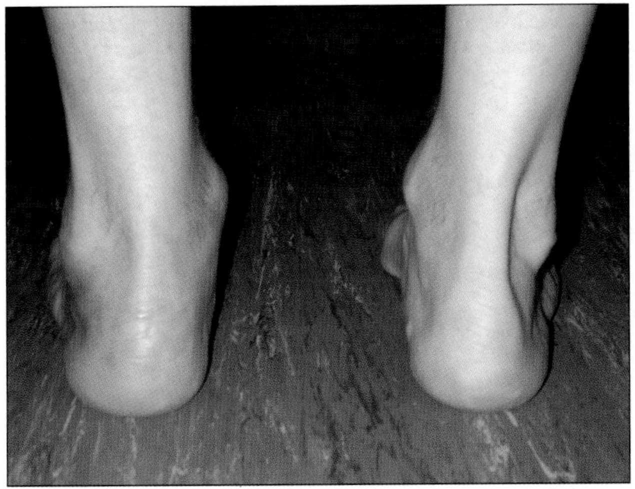

A

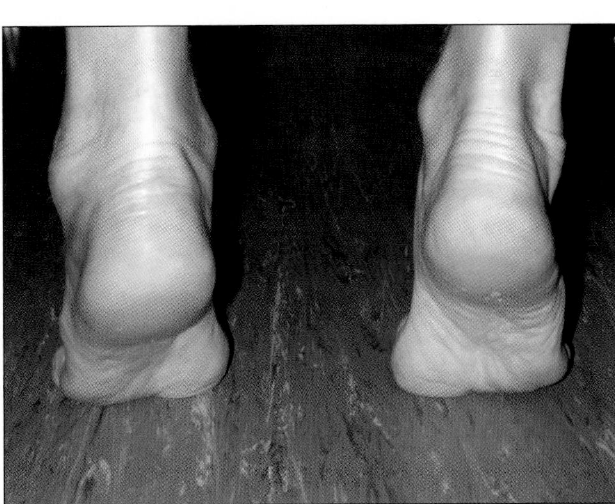

B

FIGURE 20

Evidence

Boss AP, Hintermann B. Anatomical study of the medial ankle ligament complex. Foot Ankle Int. 2002;23:547-53.

A descriptive anatomic study of the deltoid ligament complex.

Harper MC. Deltoid ligament: an anatomical evaluation of function. Foot Ankle. 1987;8:19-22.

A descriptive anatomic study and functional analysis of the deltoid ligament complex.

Hintermann B. Medial ankle instability. Foot Ankle Clin. 2003;8:723-38.

The author presented an elaboration of the entity known as "medial ankle instability" based on data from a case series. (Level IV evidence [case series])

Hintermann B, Boss A, Schäfer D. Arthroscopic findings in patients with chronic ankle instability. Am J Sports Med. 2002;30:402-9.

This prospective study of 152 patients presented evidence that there are more associated structural lesions in the unstable ankle joint than generally expected. This may explain the high incidence of long-term problems. (Level IV evidence [prospective case series])

Hintermann B, Knupp M, Pagenstert GI. Deltoid ligament injuries: diagnosis and management. Foot Ankle Clin. 2006;11:625-37.

This study presented a summary of experience with medial ankle instability based on data from a case series. (Level IV evidence [case series])

Hintermann B, Valderrabano V. Lateral column lengthening by calcaneal osteotomy. Techn Foot Ankle Surg. 2003;2:84-90.

A description of the principles and technique of lateral column lengthening by this surgical technique.

Hintermann B, Valderrabano V, Boss AP, Trouillier HH, Dick W. Medial ankle instability—an exploratory, prospective study of 52 cases. Am J Sports Med. 2004;32:183-90.

The authors reported the results of a study of 54 patients with medial ankle instability, elaborating a rationale for this entity. (Grade 1 recommendation; Level IV evidence [prospective case series])

Knupp M, Hintermann B. Reconstruction in posttraumatic combined avulsion of an accessory navicular and the posterior tibial tendon. Techn Foot Ankle Surg. 2005;4:113-8.

A description of the principles and surgical technique for this reconstruction.

Milner CE, Soames RW. The medial collateral ligaments of the human ankle joint: anatomical variations. Foot Ankle Int. 1998;19:289-92.

A descriptive anatomic study of the deltoid ligament complex.

Pagenstert GI, Hintermann B, Knupp M. Operative management of chronic ankle instability: plantaris graft. Foot Ankle Clin. 2006;11:567-83.

A description of the principles and surgical technique for this procedure.

Tornetta P III. Competence of the deltoid ligament in bimalleolar ankle fractures after medial malleolar fixation. J Bone Joint Surg [Am]. 2000;82:843-8.

The authors presented evidence from a case series of a persisting medial ankle instability after medial malleolar fracture, indicating that there often may be more complex injuries to the medial ankle than generally believed. (Level IV evidence [descriptive case series])

Valderrabano V, Hintermann B, Wischer T, Fuhr P, Dick W. Recovery of the posterior tibial muscle after late reconstruction following tendon rupture. Foot Ankle Int. 2004;25:85-95.

The authors presented evidence from a case series indicating that muscle power may be restored, to some extent, after a long-standing rupture of the posterior tibial tendon. (Grade 1 recommendation; Level IV evidence [prospective case series])

PROCEDURE 41

Exosectomy for Haglund's Disease

Alexej Barg and Beat Hintermann

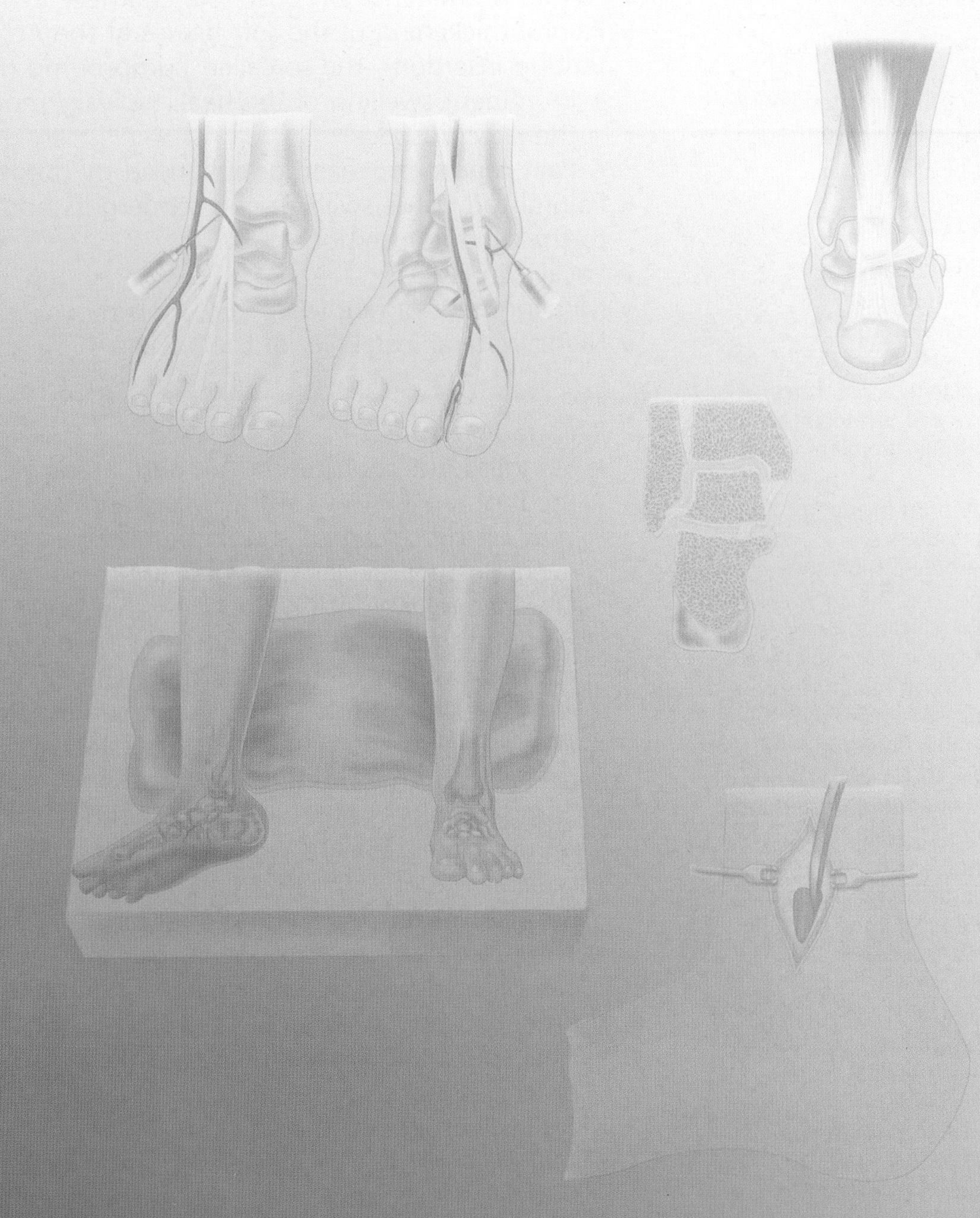

Pitfalls

- *Isolated subcutaneous bursitis*
- *Local infections*
- *Peripheral vascular diseases*

Controversies

- Symptomatic intratendinous heel spurs
- Chronic rupture/intratendinous lesion of Achilles tendon

Treatment Options

- Conservative treatment
  - Nonsteroidal anti-inflammatory drugs, immobilization, restriction of sports activities, ice, physical therapy (e.g., stretching), shoe modifications (e.g., heel lifts)
  - Peritendinous injections of local anesthetics
  - Extracorporeal shock-wave therapy
- Endoscopic calcaneoplasty
  - Endoscopic calcaneoplasty is an alternative minimally invasive technique with comparable outcome results (van Dijk et al., 2001).
  - It is a demanding procedure requiring adequate surgical experience, with some possible technical difficulties (e.g., enough bone must be removed to prevent impingement).
  - Comparative studies show that the important anatomic structures (Achilles tendon, plantaris tendon, sural nerve) are at risk in both open and endoscopic resection for Haglund's disease.
  - Further clinical and laboratory studies are needed to determine the long-term results and the value of endoscopic calcaneoplasty.

Indications

- Haglund's disease refractory to conservative measures
- Symptomatic retrocalcaneal bursitis
- Chronic pain symptoms
- Persistent limitation of sports activities

Examination/Imaging

Physical Examination

- Painful prominence on posterolateral heel
- Painful thickening of the soft tissues at the Achilles tendon insertion—the so-called pump bump (Fig. 1)
  - Prominent swelling of the heel, typically more on the lateral aspect
  - Pain can be provoked or enhanced by tiptoeing
- Painful soft tissue swelling and tenderness posterior to the tendon insertion
- Local skin lesions
- Misalignment of hindfoot
- Medial/lateral instability of the ankle

Imaging

- Plain radiographs
  - Standard anteroposterior (AP) and lateral views of the foot, an AP view of the ankle, and an axial view of the calcaneus should be obtained to assess overall osteoarticular structures and deformities.
  - On a lateral weight-bearing view (Fig. 2), Haglund's calcaneal deformity may be present as a marked osseous prominence of the tuber calcanei with swelling of soft tissues. As shown in Figure 2, the Achilles tendon inserts distally (star) and is deflected by the prominence (arrow).
  - The deformity is often associated with retrocalcaneal bursitis which causes the pathologic appearance of Kager's fat pad, also known as the pre-Achilles fat pad (Ly and Bui-Mansfiels, 2004).
  - The prominent posterosuperior calcaneal tuberosity can be measured by using parallel pitch lines, described by Pavlov et al. (1982).
  - Heel spurs, and intratendinous ossification processes can also be detected on lateral view.
- Magnetic resonance imaging (MRI)
  - MRI findings may include significantly increased signal intensity and thickening at the insertion area of the Achilles tendon. Further signs are Haglund's deformity associated with calcaneal marrow edema and distended retrocalcaneal and Achilles bursitis. The sagittal MRI in Figure 3 shows increased signal intensity at the insertion area of the Achilles

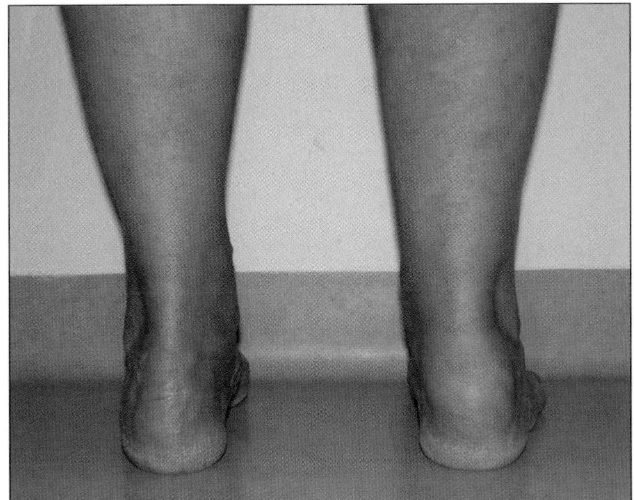

FIGURE 1

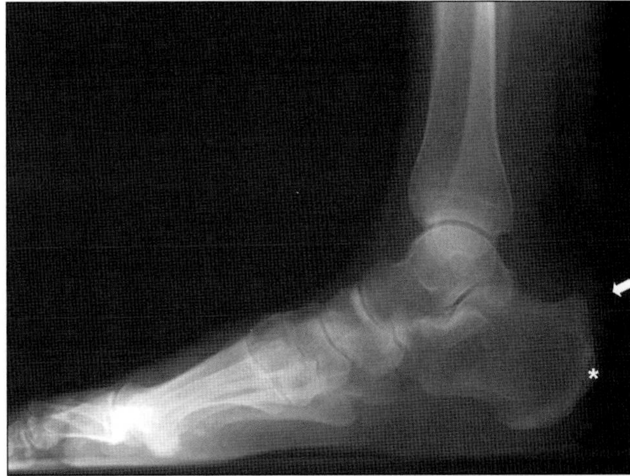

FIGURE 2

tendon associated with retrocalcaneal bursitis (arrow). A prominent posterosuperior calcaneal tuberosity (Haglund's deformity) and concomitant edematous bone marrow (star) are also visible.

- MRI also allows for the assessment of pathologic processes and disorders of the Achilles tendon (Rosenberg et al., 2000).

- Sonography
  - Sonography may be helpful to detect pathologic changes at the distal Achilles tendon and chronic retrocalcaneal and subcutaneous bursitis, as is often present in Haglund's disease (Sofka et al., 2006).
  - A high-frequency, linear, 13-MHz transducer should be used for examining the retrocalcaneal region. A 7.5-MHz transducer is not suitable as the diagnostic sensitivity is only 50%.

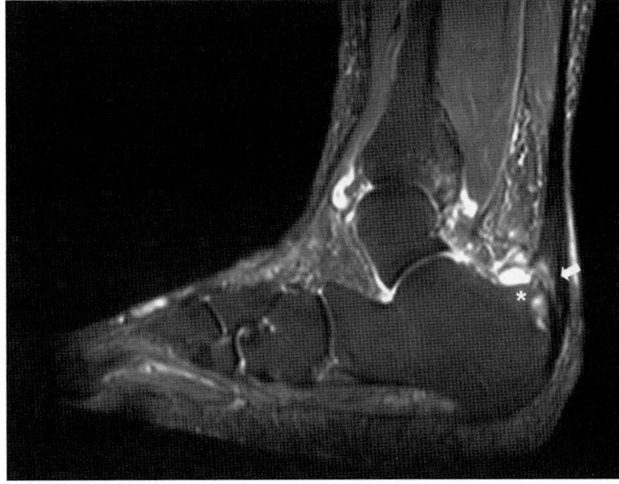

FIGURE 3

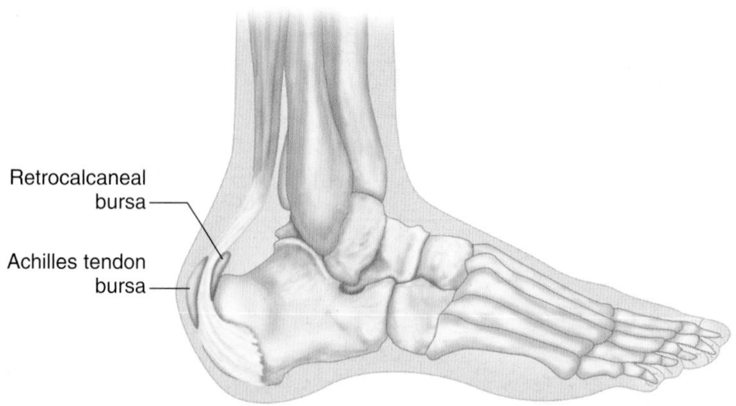

FIGURE 4

Surgical Anatomy

- The Achilles tendon serves as the insertion of the musculus triceps surae—the largest of the calf muscles—which is innervated by the tibial nerve. The Achilles tendon is the largest tendon, with the highest resistance, in the human body.
- The distal insertion of the Achilles tendon measures approximately 1 × 2 cm, and is located approximately 2 cm distal of the superoposterior edge of the calcaneal tuberosity.
- Two bursas are associated with the insertion area of the Achilles tendon (Fig. 4): the subcutaneous bursa (Achilles tendon bursa) between the tendon and the skin, and the retrocalcaneal bursa between the Achilles tendon and the calcaneus. Both can be involved in the inflammatory process.
- The vascular supply to the Achilles tendon can be divided into two parts.
  - The first part (distal) has its origin from the calcaneus and consists of small interosseous arterioles.
  - The second part (proximal) emanates from the intramuscular arterial branches.
  - Because of this two-part blood supply, there is an area of relative avascularity located 2–6 cm proximal to the calcaneal insertion.

Pearls

- *It can be useful to position and disinfect the contralateral lower leg for comparison of clinical appearance and radiologic details (calcaneal tuberosity).*

Pitfalls

- *If the operative foot does not hang over the edge of the table, it is forced into a plantar-flexion position.*

Positioning

- General or regional anesthesia
- Prone positioning of patient on operating table with radiolucent lower extremity support (Fig. 5); the foot should hang over the edge of the table

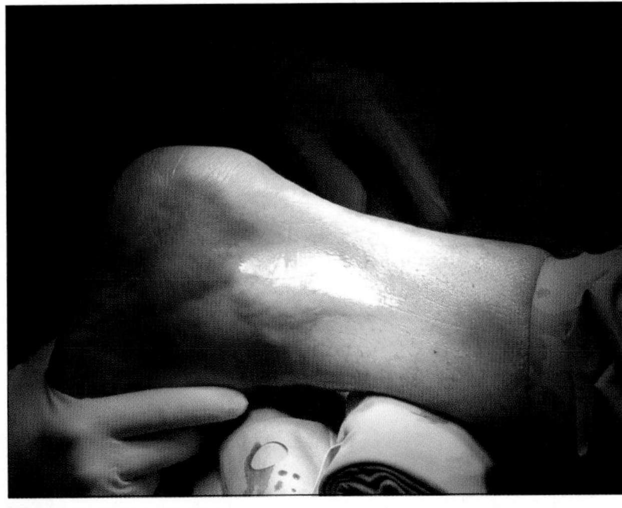

FIGURE 5

- Higher positioning of the operative lower leg on a stable radiolucent cushion with the knee in slight flexion
- Free draping of the whole limb
- Tourniquet at the thigh of the ipsilateral leg

Portals/Exposures

- Landmarks include
  - Lateral malleolus: subcutaneous distal end of the fibula
  - Achilles tendon with its insertion into the calcaneus
- Skin incision
  - Make a 3- to 4-cm longitudinal incision approximately 1 cm lateral to the posterior edge of the calcaneal tuberosity (Fig. 6).
  - The sural nerve should run more anteriorly to the incision; however, attention should be paid so as not to damage it.

Pearls

- *Plantar flexion of the foot will remove tension on the Achilles tendon and facilitate exposure of the calcaneal tuberosity.*

Pitfalls

- *Injuries to the branches of the sural nerve*

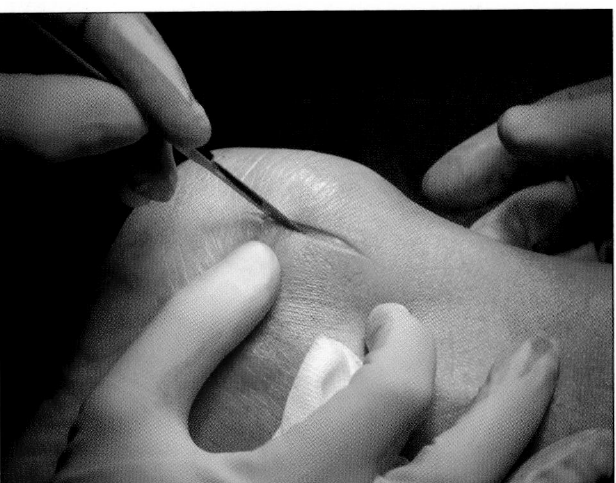

FIGURE 6

- Exposure
  - Perform sharp dissection to the bone.
  - Expose the retrocalcaneal bursa (Fig. 7); the tendon can be held medially by a small Hohmann retractor (Fig. 8) to get a better view of the posterior aspect of the calcaneal tuberosity.
  - Expose the tuber calcanei (Fig. 9).
  - Expose the Achilles tendon.
  - Expose the subcutaneous bursa.

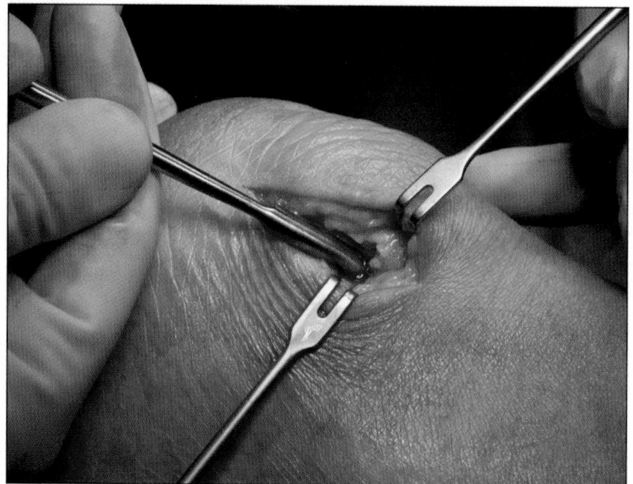

FIGURE 7

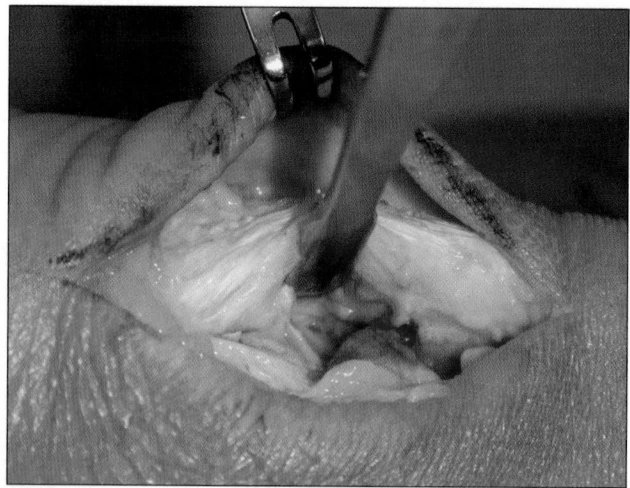

FIGURE 8

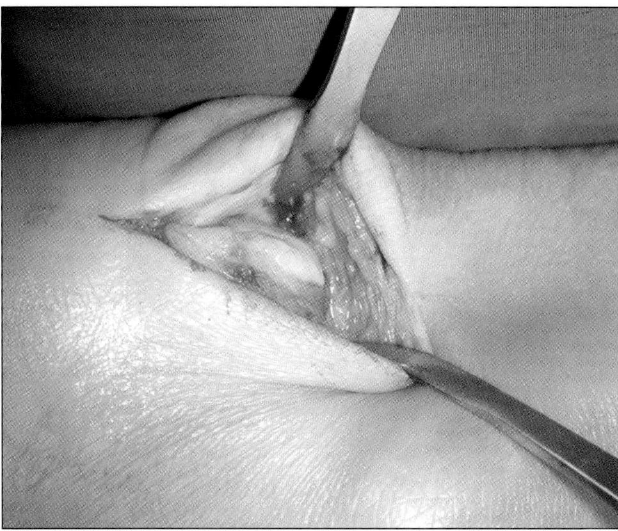

FIGURE 9

Controversies

- An alternative longitudinal posterior approach is advised in the presence of a symptomatic osseous heel spur or intratendinous ossification. The longitudinal incision is made through all soft tissue layers to the calcaneal tuberosity, separating the distal tendon in the medial center (Fig. 10A). This allows revision of the tendon and exosectomy through the same approach, while medial and lateral slips of tendon remain intact (Fig. 10B).
- An alternative medial approach may facilitate exposure of the calcaneal tuberosity; however, wound healing and disturbance of scar will be more critical as the heel is more prominent on the medial side.

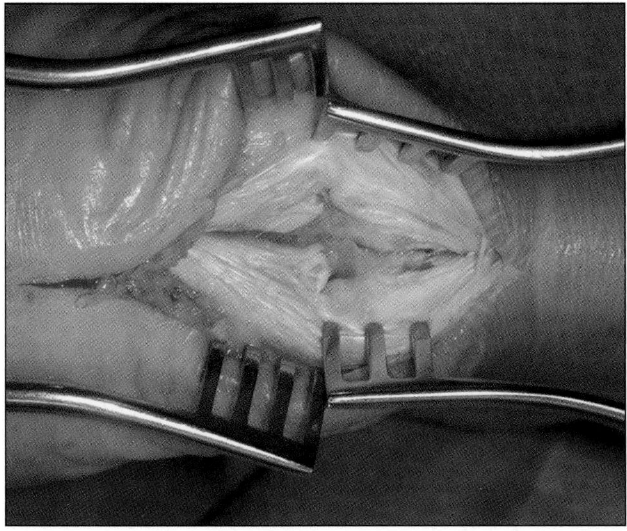

A

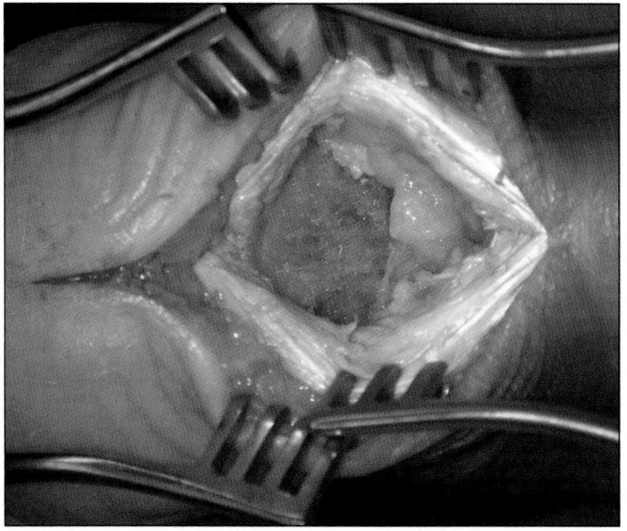

B

FIGURE 10

Pitfalls

- *Skin necrosis following too-aggressive resection of the subcutaneous bursa*

Controversies

- The debate continues as to whether the retrocalcaneal bursa should be removed. We do not do so routinely; rather, we remove it only in cases of significant inflammatory scar formation between tendon and bone.

Pearls

- *To avoid postoperative hematoma formation, the bony resection area can be covered by a film of bone wax.*

Pitfalls

- *Remaining sharp bony edges and insufficient bony resection distally may be a source of recurrent irritation syndrome.*
- *Too-aggressive resection (e.g., too-horizontal bone resection) may weaken the calcaneal tuberosity and provoke stress fracture.*

Procedure

Step 1

- Soft tissue débridement and bursectomy
  - Achilles tendon: in the case of inflammatory scarring along this tendon, perform careful débridement of the distal tendon.
  - Subcutaneous bursa: in the case of inflammatory changes, perform careful resection, paying attention not to damage the skin layer.

Step 2

- Resect the Haglund's tuberosity using a saw or wide chisel (Fig. 11), taking care to make a sharp resection distally to the insertion area of the tendon.
- Smoothen the resection surface with a rongeur to get a flat resection area (Fig. 12).
- Check the resection under fluoroscopy (Fig. 13)

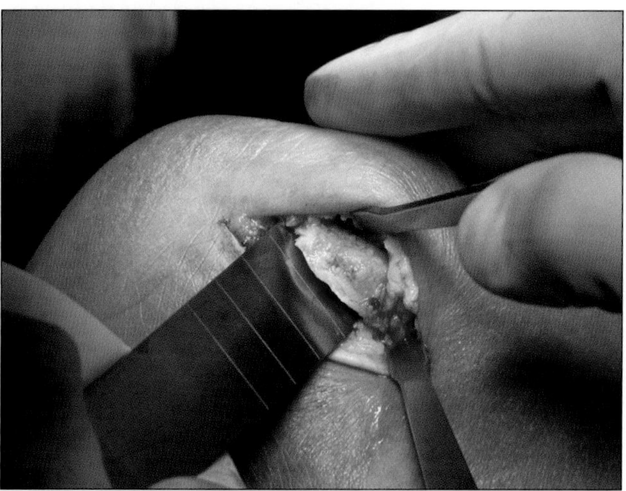

FIGURE 11

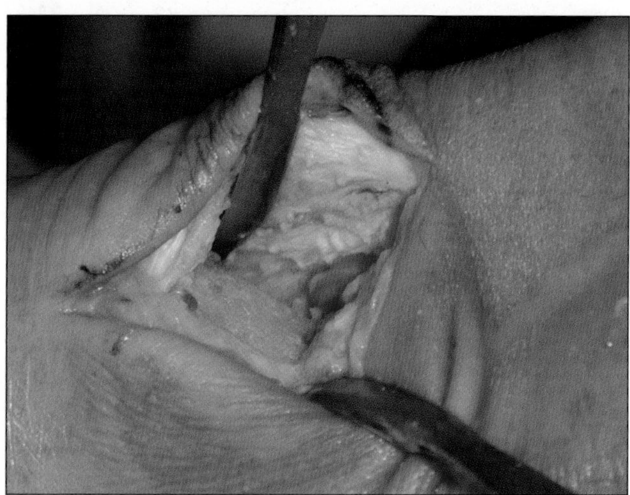

FIGURE 12

Controversies

- The debate continues as to whether the Achilles tendon should be detached by 1–2 mm at its cranial insertion area. We routinely do so on the lateral edge in the presence of a large lateral prominence of the calcaneal tuberosity.
- In vitro studies have shown that detaching of up to 60% of its insertion does not decrease the pullout force of the Achilles tendon (Kolodziej et al., 1999).

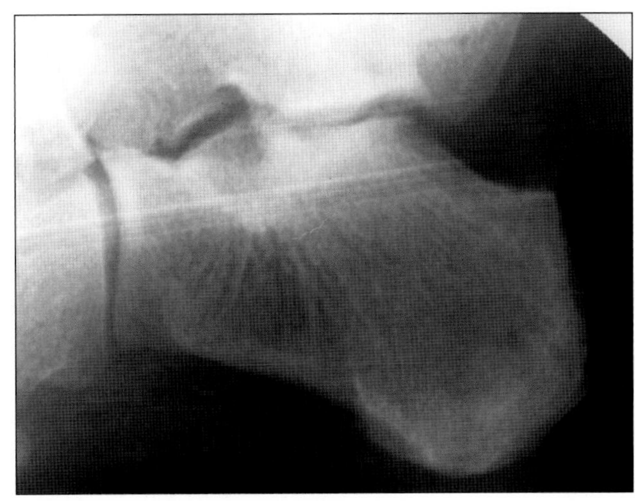

FIGURE 13

PEARLS

- *Transosseous reattachment of the lateral border of the distal Achilles tendon may smooth the posterolateral edge of the calcaneal tuberosity and increase primary stability of the wound.*

PITFALLS

- *Inappropriate skin closure may provoke scar formation with local discomfort.*

Controversies

- The use of drainage is still controversial; we do not use it on a routine basis, thereby experiencing fewer instances of hematoma formation or wound-healing problems.

STEP 3

- The incision is closed with interrupted resorbable 0 sutures for subcutaneous closure, and interrupted nonabsorbable 3-0 sutures for skin readaption.
- The wound is dressed with compresses and a bandage, and a splint is applied.

Postoperative Care and Expected Outcomes

- Immobilize the foot in a splint at 10–15° of plantar flexion until wound healing is complete, usually for 2 weeks.
- The patient is placed in a walking Scotchcast cast or walker (VACOped) for an additional 4 weeks, with weight bearing as tolerated. If a removable walker is used, active motion without weight bearing is allowed.
- A rehabilitation program is then begun. It includes passive and active mobilization of the ankle joint, training of muscle strength, and local measures to decrease local swelling.
- Athletes should anticipate to return to sports in 6–9 months after their exosectomy.

PEARLS

- *Bicycling on a home trainer may be started upon complete wound healing.*

Pitfalls

- *Wound infection, fistula formation → meticulous surgical revision with complete removal of the suture material (second wound closing)*
- *Rupture of the Achilles tendon → open tendon suture*
- *Lesion of the sural nerve → local revision*

Controversies

- There is no evidence that early mobilization improves muscular function and thereby allows patients to return to sports activities earlier. The same is true for percutaneous exosectomy (van Djik et al., 2001).

Evidence

Kolodziej P, Glisson RR, Nunley JA. Risk of avulsion of the Achilles tendon after partial excision for treatment of insertional tendonitis and Haglund's deformity: a biomechanical study. Foot Ankle Int. 1999;20:433–7.

The authors performed a biomechanical study addressing the influence of Achilles tendon detaching on weakness of tendon pullout force.

Lohrer H, Nauck T, Dorn NV, Konerding MA. Comparison of endoscopic and open resection for Haglund tuberosity in a cadaver study. Foot Ankle Int. 2006;27:445–50.

This controlled laboratory study evaluated both methods for resection of Haglund's deformity. Tuberosity resection and iatrogenic injury of surrounding anatomic structures were evaluated. (Level III evidence)

Ly JQ, Bui-Mansfiels LT. Anatomy of and abnormalities associated with Kager's fat pad. AJR Am J Roentgenol. 2004;182:147–54.

An extensively illustrated pictorial atlas describing various diseases associated with abnormal appearance of Kager's fat pad.

Pavlov H, Heneghan MA, Hersh A, Goldman AB, Vigorita V. The Haglund syndrome: initial and differential diagnosis. Radiology. 1982;144:83–8.

The authors described a measurement method for Haglund's deformity using parallel pitch lines. This measurement was determined in 10 symptomatic feet and 78 control feet. (Level IV evidence)

Rosenberg ZS, Beltran J, Bencardino JT, for the Radiological Society of North America. MR imaging of the ankle and foot. Radiographics. 2000;20:S153–79.

This outstanding review described MRI as a helpful modality for assessment of pathologic conditions of the foot and ankle.

Sofka CM, Adler RS, Positano R, Pavlov H, Luchs JS. Haglund's syndrome: diagnosis and treatment using sonography. HSSJ. 2006;2:27–9.

This is a case report of Haglund's disease diagnosed clinically, confirmed radiographically, more specifically evaluated with sonography, and treated with sonography-guided retrocalcaneal bursal injection. (Level IV evidence)

Van Dijk CN, van Dyk GE, Scholten PE, Kort NP. Endoscopic calcaneoplasty. Am J Sports Med. 2001;29:185–9.

This clinical study described clinical results after endoscopic calcaneoplasty in 20 patients undergoing 21 procedures. All patients were unresponsive to conservative treatment before. (Level IV evidence)

PROCEDURE 42

Haglund's Deformity: Open and Arthroscopic Treatment

Carol Frey

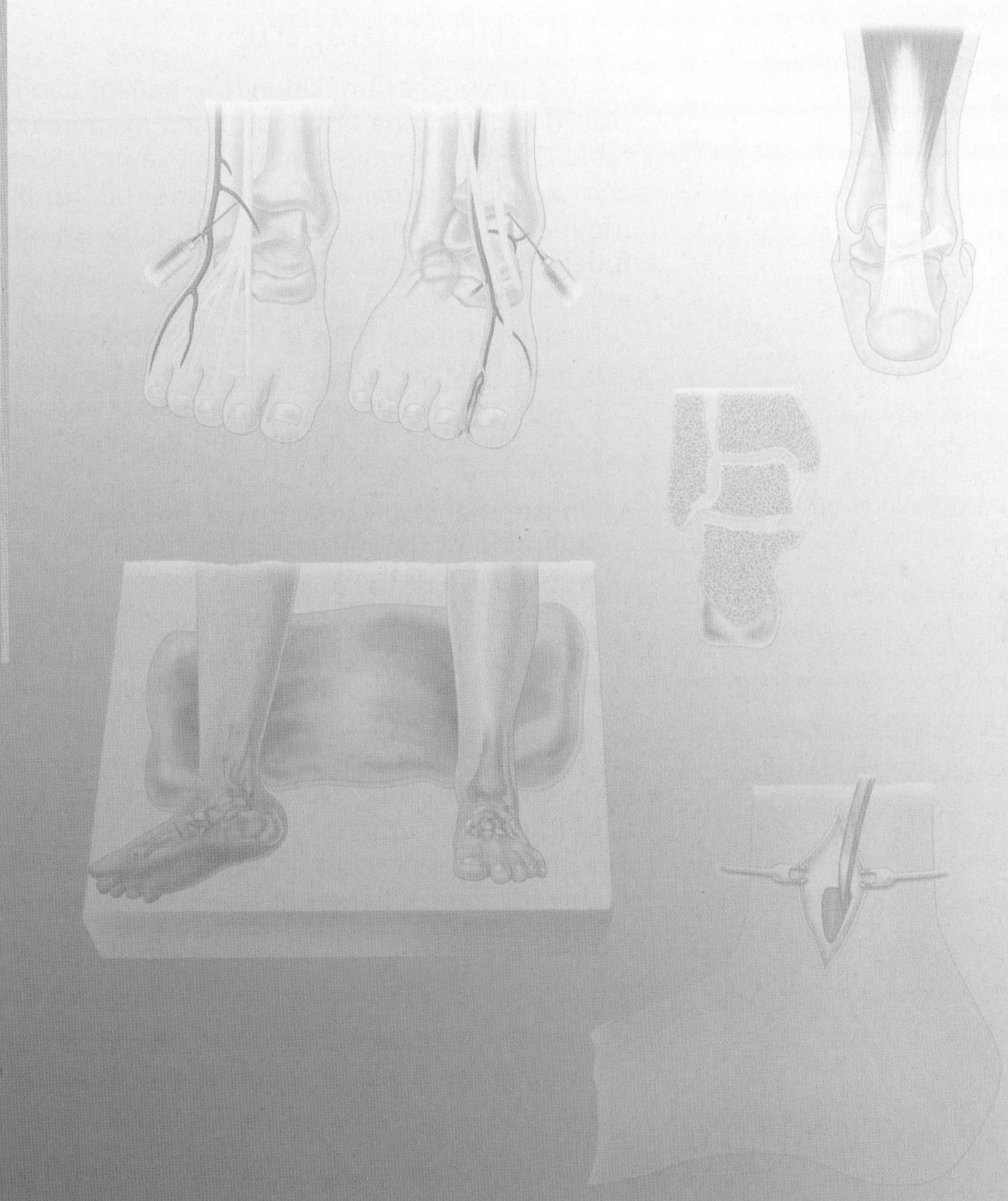

Open and Arthroscopic Treatment

PITFALLS

- *This type of treatment is contraindicated in patients with infection, open wound, blister, and a dysvascular extremity.*
- *Avoid the patient with minimal symptoms who wants a cosmetic improvement.*

Indications

- Painful bone prominence in the retrocalcaneal region of the posterior calcaneus
- No relief with 6 months of conservative treatment

Examination/Imaging

- For the physical examination, the patient can be placed in the prone position on the examination table. The foot should rest in the examiner's hand, and the index finger and thumb are used to palpate the medial and lateral aspects of the posterosuperior tuberosity of the calcaneus.
  - When the bursa is inflamed, a soft mass is felt bulging on both sides of the Achilles tendon that is painful when palpated.
  - Dorsiflexion of the foot, which compresses the bursa between the tendon and the bone, also causes pain.
  - On external inspection, loss of the skin lines due to distention of the retrocalcaneal bursa may be present.
  - In severe cases, erythema and warmth may be seen.
  - Signs of retrocalcaneal bursitis differ from those of insertional Achilles tendinosis, in which there is tenderness several centimeters proximal to the tendon insertion, as well as at the insertion.
- Plain, weight-bearing radiographs of the foot will help to rule out other causes of hindfoot pain, such as a stress fracture, chronic infection, or tumor.
  - No radiologic criterion has been absolutely reliable when used for the diagnosis of Haglund's disease, and none is a predictor for preoperative symptoms or postoperative outcome.
  - Lateral radiographs will reveal a thin strip of fat between the Achilles tendon and the bone proximal to the insertion of the tendon.
  - The anterior aspect of the Achilles tendon should be sharply outlined throughout its extent by the pre-Achilles fat pad (PAFP).
  - Retrocalcaneal bursitis is indicated when shape definition of the retrocalcaneal recess is lost and the lucency of the PAFP is replaced by soft tissue density (Fig. 1).

Treatment Options

- Nonsteroidal anti-inflammatory medication.
- Heel lifts, soft heel counters, and a backless shoe.
- Running athletes should decrease mileage and stop training on hills and hard surfaces.
- Tight calf muscles, tight hamstrings, or a cavus foot may be associated and should be stretched.
- A cavus foot may require a custom orthotic device.
- Most patients respond to conservative treatment in the first 6 months.

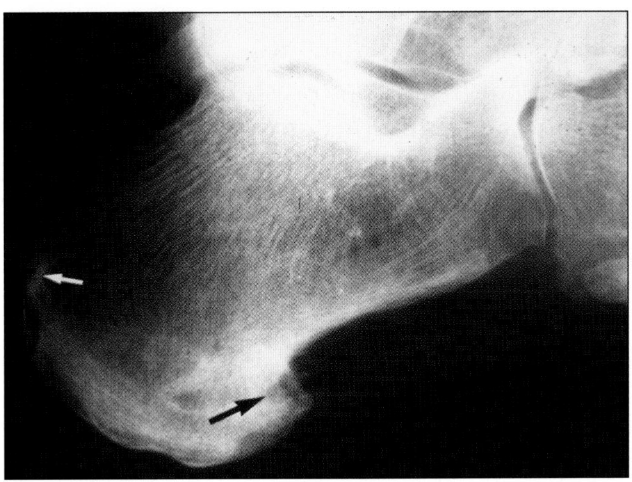

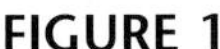
FIGURE 1

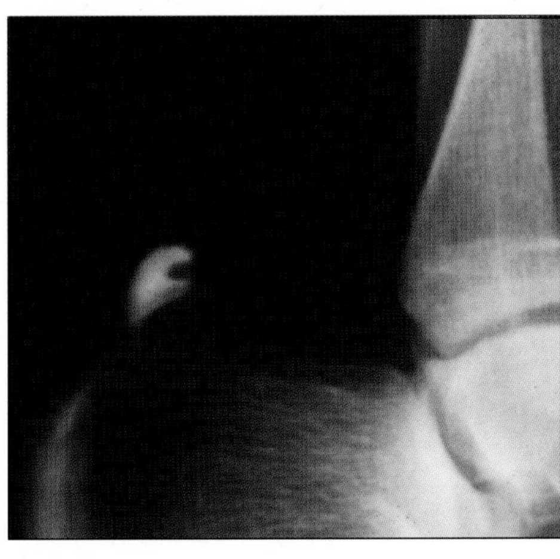

FIGURE 2

- The distended, fluid-filled bursa often projects above the calcaneus and into the PAFP.
- Look for erosion of the cortex of the posterior superior aspect of the calcaneus with chronic bursitis (white arrow in Fig. 1). Black arrow shows plantar enthesopathy.

• Achilles tendinosis is noted by a thickening of the tendon and loss of the sharp anterior interface with the PAFP.

• The anatomy of the bursa can be seen with bursography (Fig. 2), but this is not recommended.

■ On magnetic resonance imaging (MRI), the retrocalcaneal bursa is a potential space that is most clearly demarcated when inflamed (Fig. 3). MRI is only recommended in those cases in which making a diagnosis is difficult.

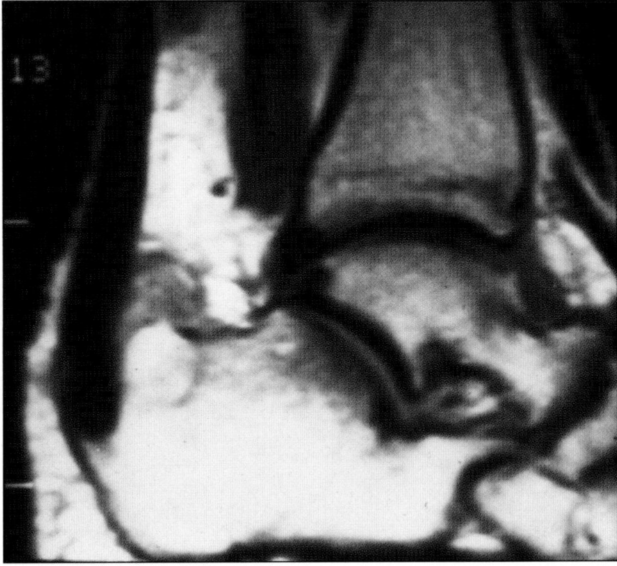

FIGURE 3

Surgical Anatomy

- The retrocalcaneal bursa is a consistently present structure that sits atop the posterosuperior aspect of the calcaneus (Fig. 4).
  - The normal bursa has a volume of 1–1.5 ml.
  - The bursa is horseshoe shaped. The average length of the bursa legs is 22 mm, measured from the most superior aspect of the bursa arch to the most inferior aspect of the bursa legs (Fig. 5).
  - The average width of the bursa legs is 4 mm and the average width of the bursa body is 8 mm. The entire bursa has an average thickness of 4 mm, as measured from side to side.
- The Achilles tendon does not insert at the superior aspect of the calcaneus, but significantly more inferiorly in the apophyseal portion of the calcaneus.
  - The Achilles tendon sweeps backward and away from the tibia to meet the inclined calcaneus obliquely and form an acute angle.

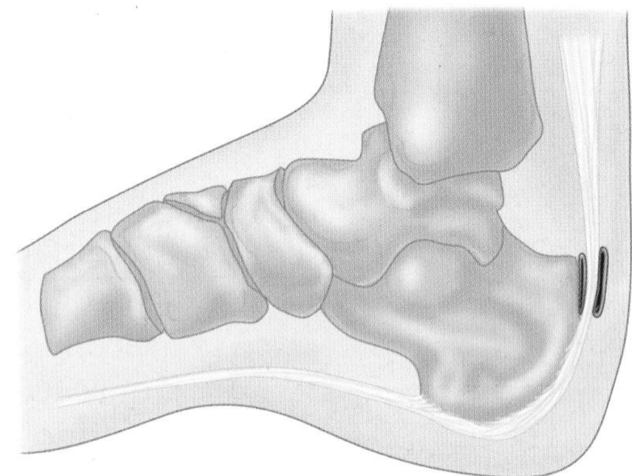

FIGURE 4

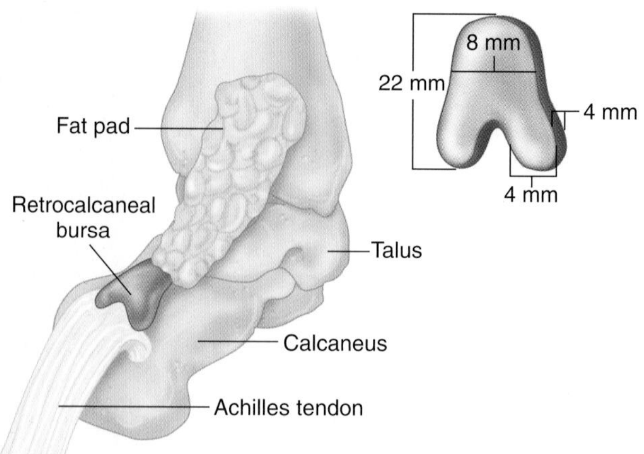

FIGURE 5

Positioning

- For open treatment, the patient is placed in the prone position with a bolster under the distal leg (Fig. 6).
- For arthroscopic treatment, the patient is placed into the prone position, with a bump under the ankle.

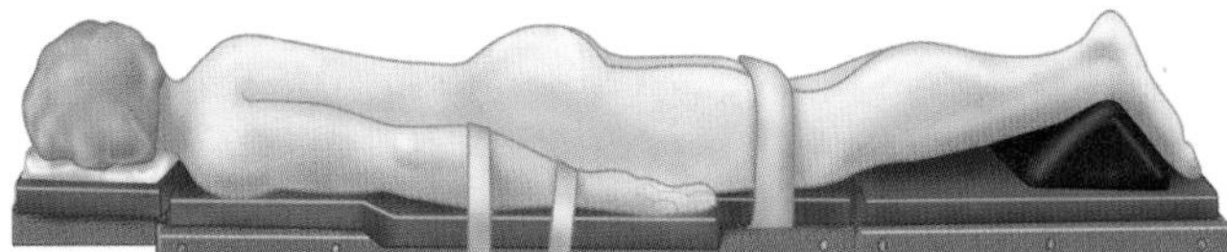

FIGURE 6

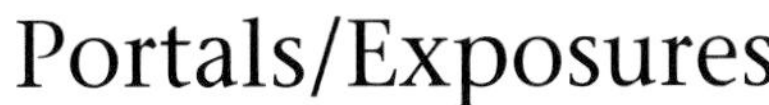

Portals/Exposures

- For open treatment, an 8-cm longitudinal incision is made just anterior to the Achilles tendon on the lateral aspect of the heel (Fig. 7A and 7B).
- The retrocalcaneal area and the superior aspect of the calcaneus are exposed by a combination of blunt and sharp dissection, being careful to avoid the sural nerve, which lies approximately 6 mm anterior to the lateral border of the Achilles tendon (Fig. 8).
- The sural nerve should be protected by retracting it anteriorly with the subcutaneous tissues.
- The incision is carried down to the bone, making sure that the insertion site of the Achilles tendon is adequately exposed.

A

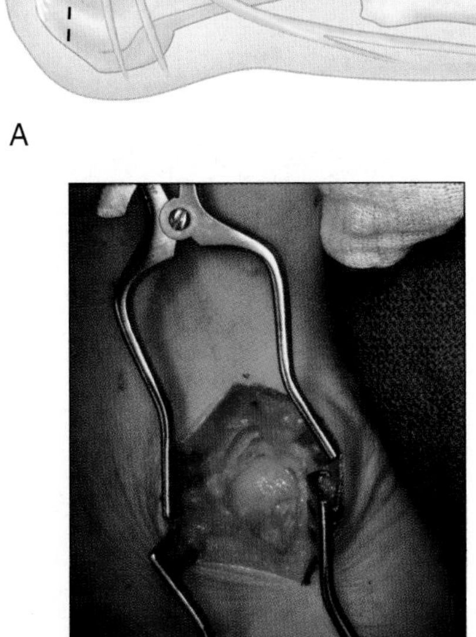

B

FIGURE 7

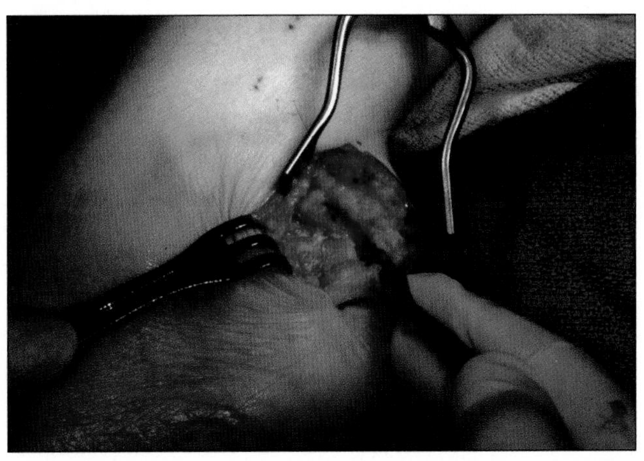

FIGURE 8

Pearls

- *Removal of the bursa tissue is not as important as adequate decompression of the posterior calcaneal prominence.*
- *To successfully decompress the retrocalcaneal space, adequate bone must be removed. Bone can be removed up to the insertion site of the Achilles tendon.*
- *Do not leave a spike of bone near the insertion of the tendon, because it may become painful and a source of irritation to the tendon.*

Pitfalls

- *It is possible to remove too much distal bone and cut into the insertion of the Achilles tendon. This could allow the tendon to avulse later. Careful exposure of the insertion site should help avoid this pitfall.*

Procedure: Open Treatment

Step 1

- If there is inflammation of the retrocalcaneal bursa, the bursa tissue should be removed with sharp and blunt dissection.
- Decompression of the posterior calcaneal prominence (Haglund's deformity), is carried out using an oblique osteotomy of the superior angle of the calcaneus (Fig. 9A and 9B), starting approximately 1.5 cm anterior to the posterior border of the calcaneus and angling downward to the insertion of the Achilles tendon (approximately 2 cm distal onto the superior margin of the calcaneus).
  - The osteotomy is carried out with a micro-sagittal saw, keeping perpendicular to the longitudinal axis of the calcaneus (Fig. 9C).
  - A ridge of bone is always left at the insertion site of the Achilles tendon and must be carefully removed with a small curette and micro-reciprocating rasp. By resection of bone down to the insertion site of the Achilles tendon, adequate decompression can usually be obtained (Fig. 10A and 10B).
  - In the case of a very large calcaneal prominence, the lateral margin of the Achilles tendon may be raised to allow for the prominence to be removed.

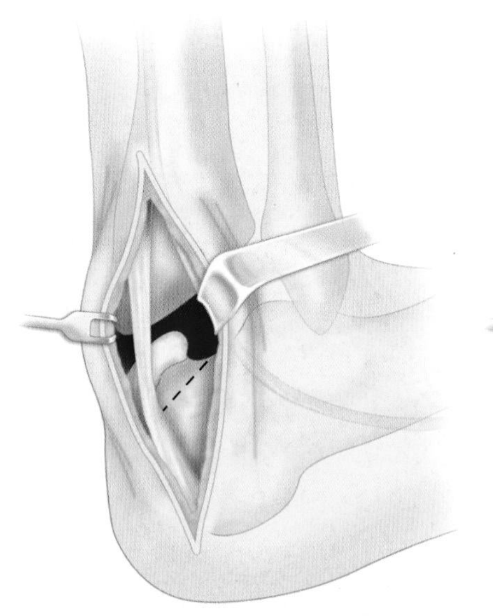

A

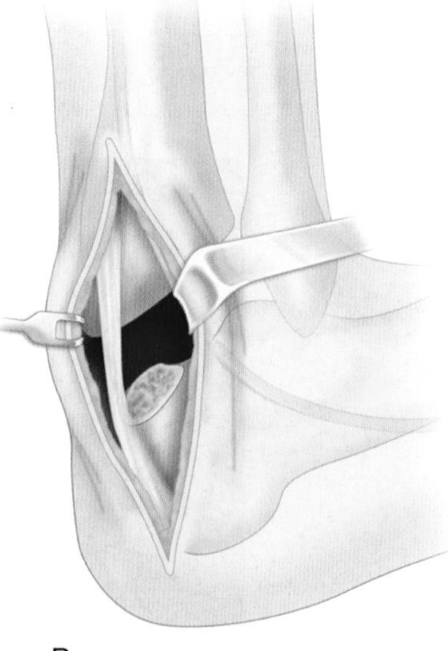

B

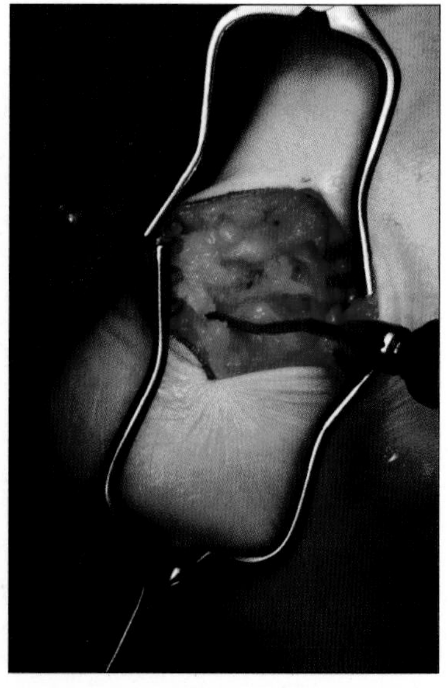

C

FIGURE 9

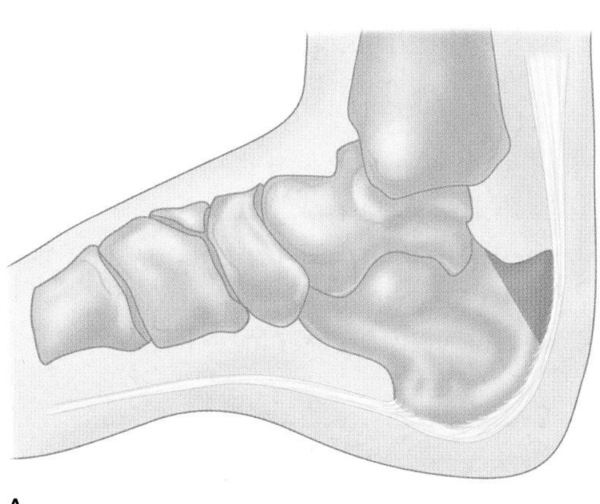
A

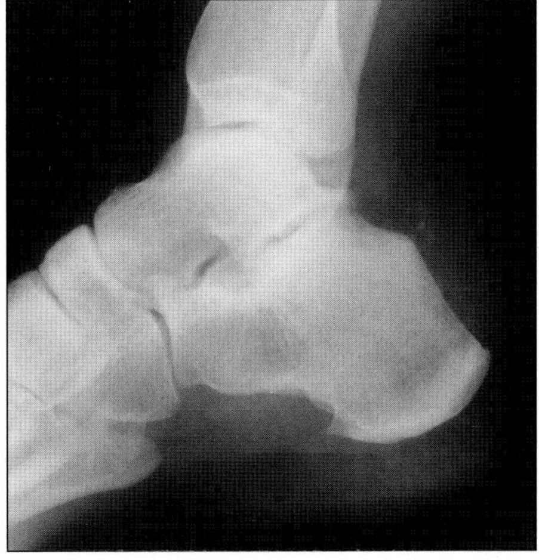
B

FIGURE 10

Instrumentation/ Implantation

- Micro-sagittal saw
- Small curette
- Micro-reciprocating rasp
- Standard foot tray

The margin of the tendon attachment may be repaired with suture anchors or a tenodesis screw. In Figure 11, the posterior prominence has been removed and a nonstrangulating stitch is used to reattach the damaged Achilles tendon. A tenodesis screw is being used in this case.

- If the medial ridge cannot be adequately reached, a medial incision can be added, but this is rarely necessary.

■ The area of calcaneal prominence is palpated repeatedly through the overlying skin to make sure that all ridges and spikes are removed.

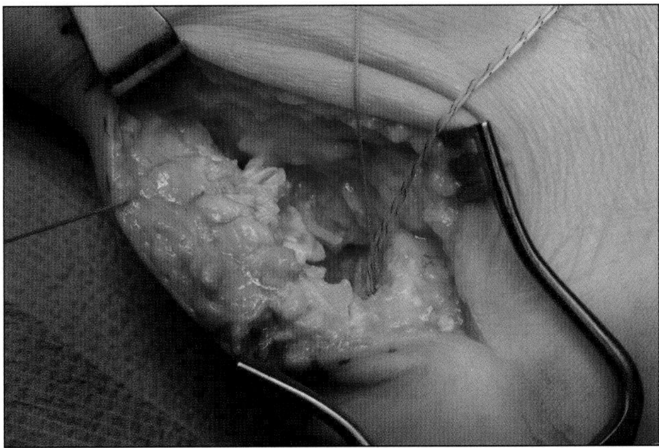

FIGURE 11

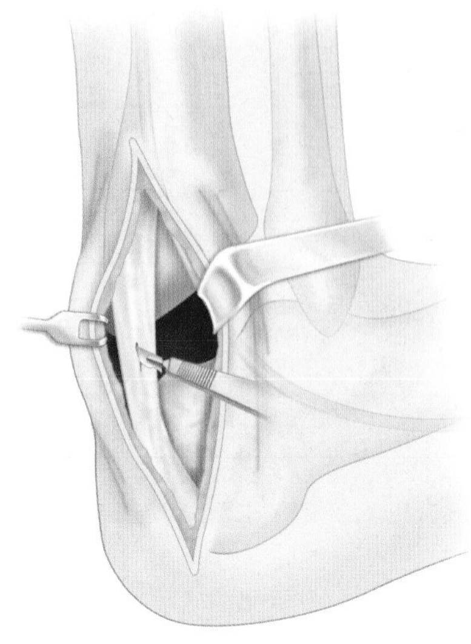

FIGURE 12

Step 2

- The Achilles tendon should be inspected for tendinosis. A longitudinal incision is carefully made with a scalpel in the anterior 50% of the tendon (Fig. 12).
- This may reveal necrotic areas that require débridement.
- After débridement, the area is repaired with buried nonabsorbable 3-0 suture.
- The wound is closed routinely in layers.

Pearls

- *It is usually safe to raise as much as 2 cm of the Achilles tendon insertion to remove the appropriate amount of bone.*

Pitfalls

- *The location of even a small portal in the area of the sural nerve (lateral portal) or the calcaneal branches of the lateral plantar nerve (medial portal) can cause a long period of postoperative tenderness aggravated by a firm heel counter on a shoe.*

Instrumentation/ Implantation

- 2.9-mm arthroscope
- Synovial shaver

Procedure: Arthroscopic Treatment

Step 1

- The medial and lateral borders of the Achilles tendon are palpated. The posterosuperior aspect of the calcaneus is also readily located. The Achilles tendon inserts on the posterior margin of the calcaneus, approximately 2 cm to its posterosuperior margin.
- Medial and lateral portals are placed just above the superior aspect of the calcaneus, medial and lateral to the Achilles tendon (Fig. 13A and 13B).
  - The medial portal is made under direct visualization by introducing an 18-gauge spinal needle just proximal to the superomedial border of the os calcis.
  - Care must be taken when making the medial portal, because the calcaneal branch of the lateral plantar nerve is at risk for injury in this region.
- A 2.9-mm arthroscope and small joint instrumentation are used interchangeably through these ports.
- The arthroscope, with a blunt trocar, is introduced into the bursa after making a skin incision just proximal to the superolateral border of the os calcis.
- A full-radius synovial shaver is used to remove the bursa.

Step 2

- When the Haglund's deformity is detected (Fig. 14A), a small acrominizer or abrader is used to remove it.

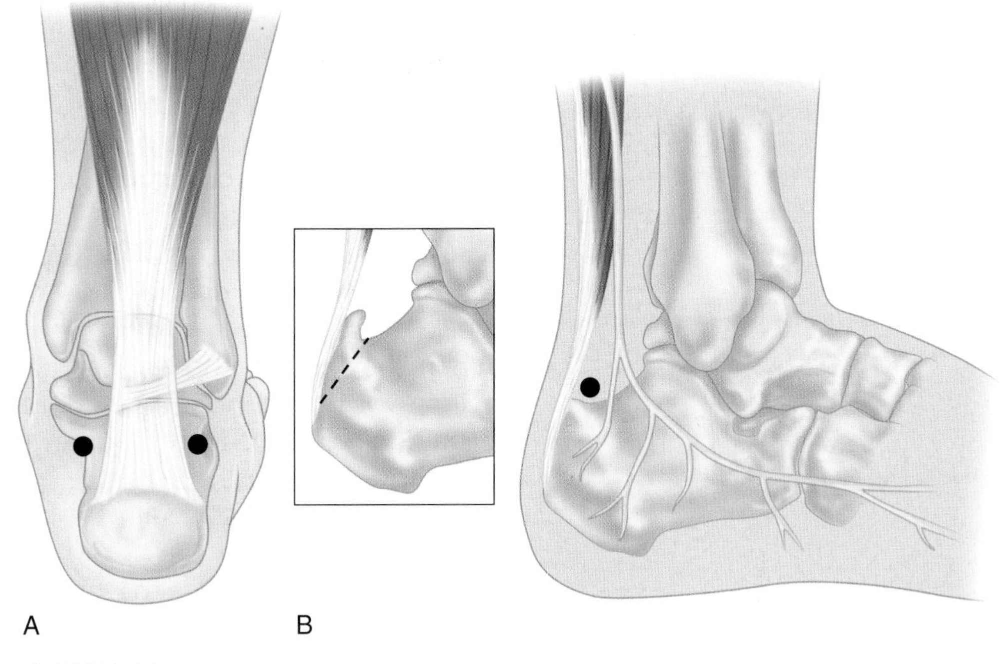

FIGURE 13

- The deformity is removed starting at the posterosuperior aspect of the calcaneus and proceeding inferiorly 2–4 cm to the superior attachment site of the Achilles tendon (Fig. 14B).
- After the Haglund's deformity is removed, it is important to dorsiflex the ankle to check for further impingement (Fig. 14C).

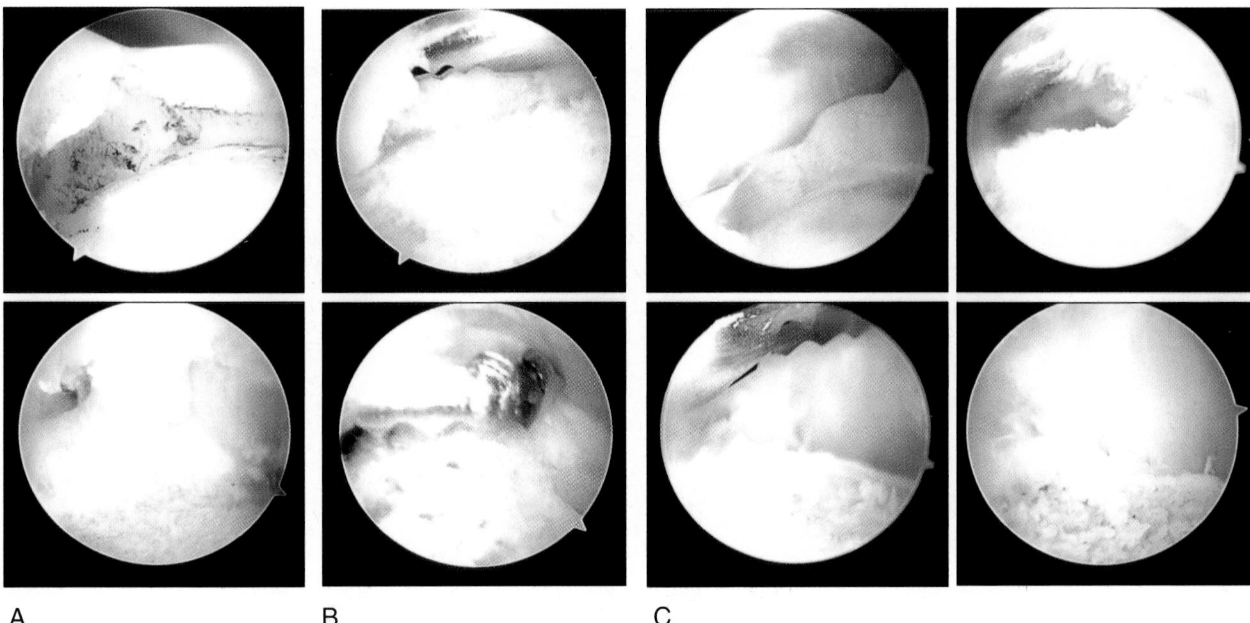

FIGURE 14

PEARLS

- *A review of the literature indicates that 73–97% good to excellent results have been reported with the open procedure.*

Postoperative Care and Expected Outcomes

- The patient is placed into a short-leg, non–weight-bearing cast with the foot in mild plantar flexion for the first 1–2 weeks, depending on the involvement of the Achilles tendon.
- A short-leg walking cast with the foot gradually repositioned up to neutral is used for the next 2 weeks.
- When the cast is removed, the patient is placed into a shoe with a $^{7}/_{16}$-inch, tapered internal heel lift that is gradually reduced to $^{3}/_{16}$ of an inch, and this is worn for 3 months.
- General muscle conditioning is begun when the cast is removed.
- The recovery period for the open operative technique can be 3–6 months. After that period, full activity may be resumed.

Evidence

Frey C, Rosenberg Z, Shereff M, Kim H. The retrocalcaneal bursa: anatomy and bursography. FAIJ. 1992;13:203-7.

In this paper, the anatomic characteristics of the retrocalcaneal bursa were noted from latex bursal models and correlated well with the findings at bursography. The size, capacity, and configuration of the bursa were measured and recorded. (Level V evidence)

Sammarco GJ, Taylor AL. Operative management of Haglund's deformity in the non-athlete: a retrospective study. FAIJ. 2000;19:724-9.

This study reported the results of 39 feet that underwent excision of the posterior calcaneal tuberosity and reattachment of the Achilles tendon with bone anchors. The investigators reported a rate of 97% excellent or good results with an average of 3 years of follow-up. (Level I evidence)

Van Dijk CN, van Dyk E, Scholten P, Kort NP. Tendoscopic calcaneoplasty. Am J Sports Med. 2001;29:185-9.

In this study, removal of an inflamed retrocalcaneal bursa along with a prominent posterosuperior aspect of the calcaneus was associated with good or excellent results in 80% of the patients. The authors reported excellent visualization of the space from both the medial and the lateral portal. (Level I evidence)

PROCEDURE 43

Intra-articular Calcaneus Fractures

Matthew DeOrio and Mark E. Easley

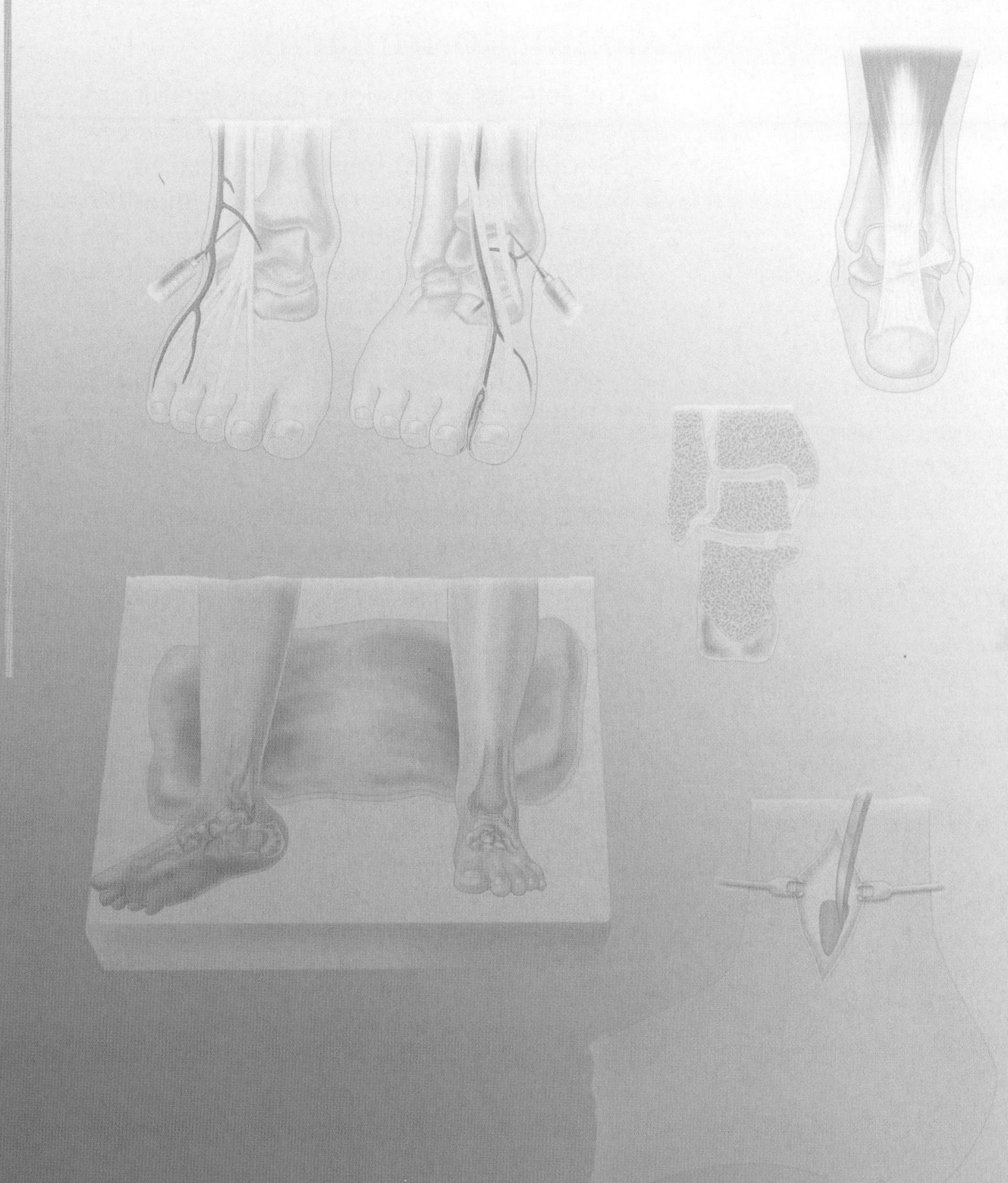

Pitfalls

- *When the soft tissues allow, operative treatment should be performed within 2–3 weeks from injury, before the fracture heals in a malunited position.*
- *Operative treatment should be delayed until a positive skin wrinkle test is observed (the skin should wrinkle with ankle dorsiflexion and hindfoot eversion) and pitting edema has resolved.*

Controversies

- Relative contraindications:
  - Peripheral vascular disease
  - Type 1 diabetes mellitus
  - Medical comorbidities/life-threatening injuries preventing surgery
  - Soft tissue compromise/massive edema
  - Nonambulatory patients

Treatment Options

- Closed treatment
- Open reduction and internal fixation (ORIF)
- Minimally invasive surgery: closed reduction and internal fixation with limited skin incisions; especially applicable to tongue-type fractures (intra-articular fractures exiting the posterior calcaneal tuberosity), for which the Essex-Lopresti maneuver can be employed
- Closed reduction and external fixation

Indications

- Nonoperative management is indicated for nondisplaced calcaneal fractures or extra-articular calcaneal fractures with near-physiologic hindfoot alignment (computed tomography [CT] confirmation is recommended).
- Operative treatment of calcaneus fractures is indicated for displaced intra-articular and open calcaneal fractures.

Examination/Imaging

- The soft tissue envelope about the hindfoot must be amenable to surgery: edema and fracture blisters (at the operative site) must have resolved.
- Plain foot and ankle radiographs should be obtained (anteroposterior, lateral, oblique foot; Harris axial heel view; Broden's view; ankle series to rule out concomitant ankle fracture).
  - The lateral foot radiograph in Figure 1 demonstrates posterior facet depression.
  - The mortise view of the ankle in Figure 2 illustrates lateral calcaneal wall displacement with resultant widening of the heel.
- Associated lower back pain and tenderness necessitate lumbar spine radiographs given the association of calcaneal and lumbar spine fractures.
- Preoperative fine-section CT is mandatory and defines the intra-articular (posterior facet) fracture pattern, as shown in the posterior facet's intra-articular comminution in Figure 3A–C.
  - The fracture pattern is determined on the coronal images, using the Sanders classification.
  - Sagittal and axial images provide further detail of the fracture pattern.

Surgical Anatomy

- Relevant vascular anatomy
  - A lateral soft tissue flap of hindfoot skin and subcutaneous tissue must be elevated directly from the calcaneus in the lateral extensile approach.
  - This flap receives its blood supply from the laterally located calcaneal, malleolar, and tarsal arteries (Fig. 4A).
  - The commonly used extensile L-shaped incision to the calcaneus respects the vascular anatomy (angiosomes) of the flap.

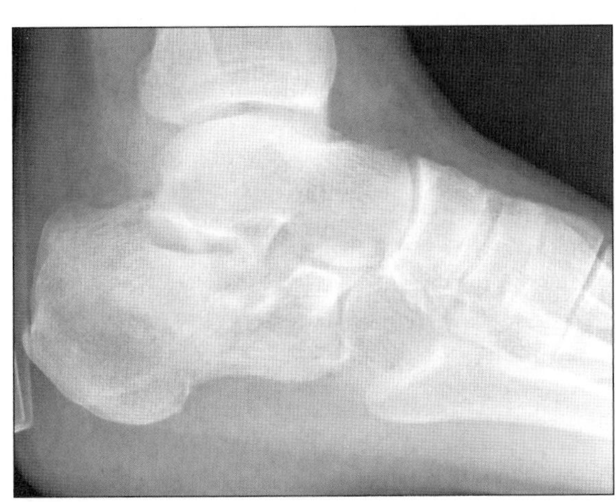

FIGURE 1

FIGURE 2

A

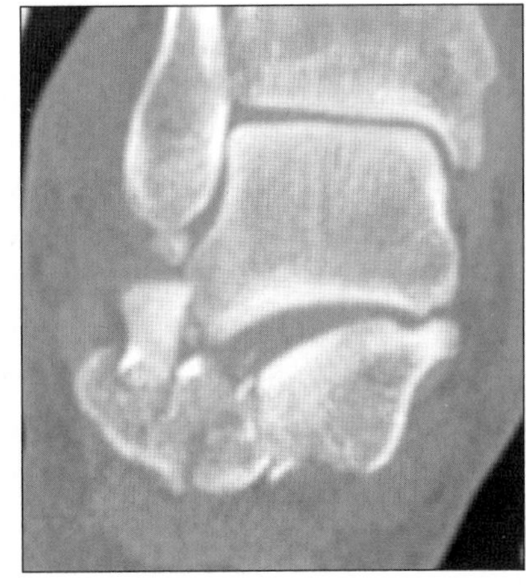

B

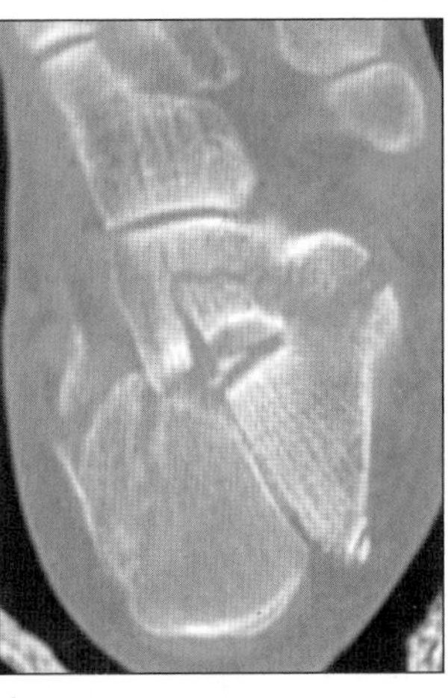

C

FIGURE 3

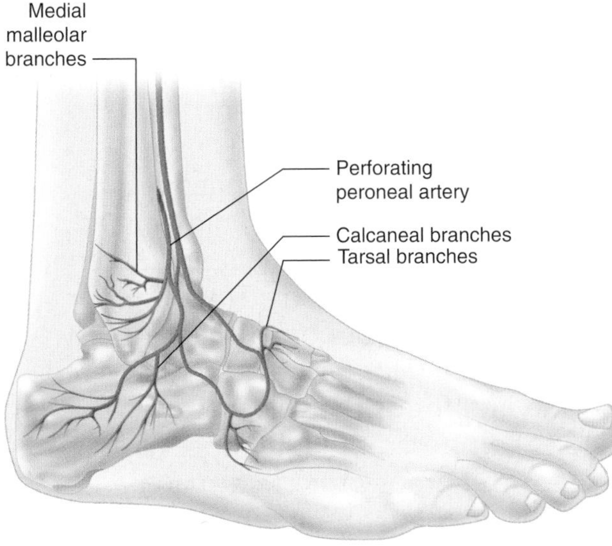

A

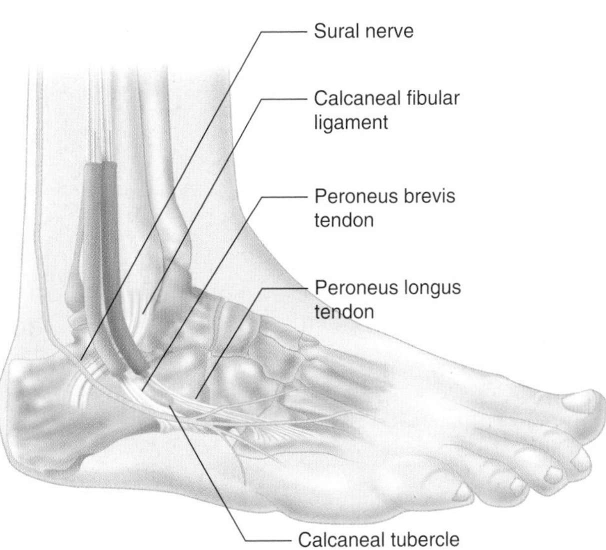

B

FIGURE 4

- Relevant lateral structures to be protected in the lateral extensile approach to the calcaneus (Fig. 4B)
  - The peroneal tendons and sural nerve are both elevated with the lateral soft tissue flap during exposure. The lateral wall includes the peroneal tubercle, which bisects a groove for the peroneus brevis and longus tendons; the brevis tendon courses anterior to the tubercle.
  - The calcaneofibular ligament attaches posterior to the peroneal tubercle and lies deep to the tendons. Typically, the calcaneofibular ligament is elevated with the lateral soft tissue flap from the calcaneus (despite this, ankle instability is rare following surgical management of calcaneus fractures).
  - The sural nerve courses parallel and posterior to the peroneal tendons before passing superficially at the inferior peroneal retinaculum to course along the lateral border of the foot.
- Relevant osseous anatomy
  - Comminuted, intra-articular fractures of the calcaneus typically fracture into four distinct fragments (Fig. 5): (1) sustentaculum tali ("constant fragment"), (2) lateral wall fragment (typically with the lateral posterior facet articular surface attached), (3) anterior process fragment, and (4) posterior tuberosity.
  - The "constant fragment" includes the sustentaculum tali and its middle facet. The medial ligamentous structures, including the interosseous talocalcaneal, medial talocalcaneal, and deltoid ligament complex, typically maintain the position of the fragment relative to the talus and ankle, hence the name "constant fragment."
- Articular surfaces
  - The superior surface (Fig. 6A) includes the calcaneal tuberosity and anterior, middle, and posterior facets. In 60% of patients, the anterior and middle facets are confluent. The posterior facet is the largest and supports the talar body.
  - The anterior surface (Fig. 6B) is entirely covered with cartilage and forms the calcaneocuboid joint.
- The heel pad is composed of highly specialized adipose tissue with fibrous septa that may be disrupted with high energy trauma.

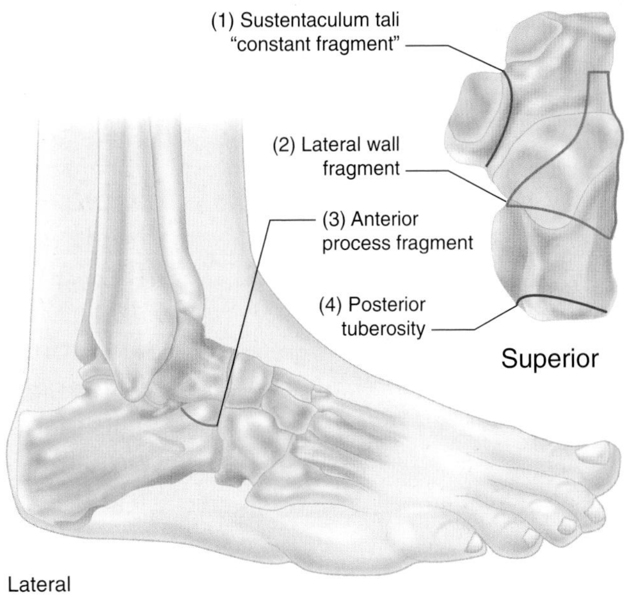

FIGURE 5

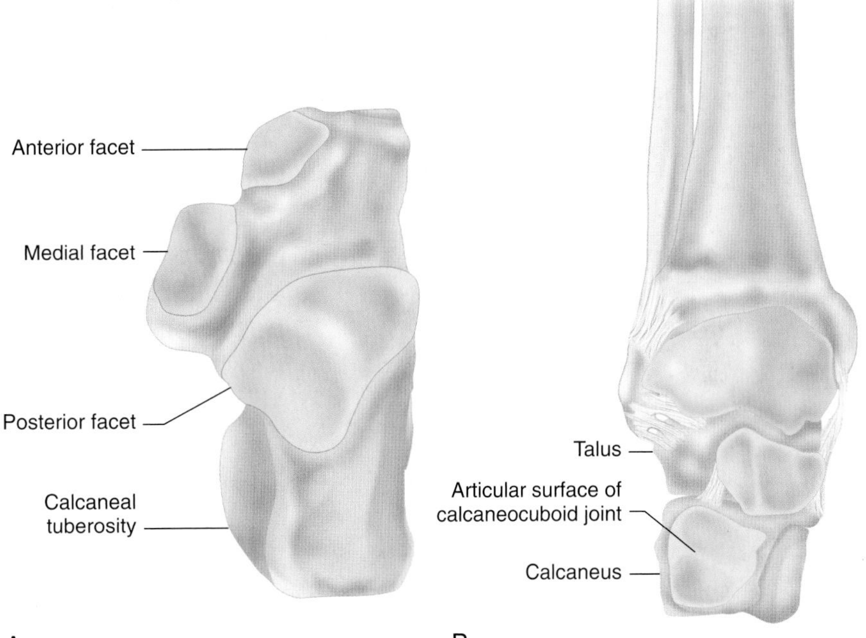

FIGURE 6

> **PEARLS**
>
> - *The patient may be positioned prone with the lower extremities externally rotated and supplemental armboards augmenting the operating table's width to allow simultaneous surgical approaches to bilateral calcaneal fractures.*

Positioning

- ORIF using the extensile lateral L-shaped approach may be performed with the patient positioned in the prone or lateral position.
- We favor a full lateral decubitus position with the patient's torso safely secured within a beanbag and the operative extremity carefully supported on a well-padded bump of folded sheets or towels.
- The knee is flexed, and the heel of the patient rests at the posterior corner of the operating table.

Pitfalls

- *Scissor the legs with the operative extremity posterior to improve access to the fracture and unobstructed fluoroscopic visualization.*
- *A radiolucent operative table is recommended.*
- *An axillary roll is recommended.*

Equipment

- Beanbag
- Protective padding below contralateral limb and axilla to protect the peroneal nerve and brachial plexus, respectively
- Fluoroscopy (mini or standard C-arm)
- Thigh-level pneumatic tourniquet

Portals/Exposures

- The calcaneus is approached through an extensile lateral approach.
  - The vertical limb of the incision is made approximately 2 cm proximal to the tip of the fibula and halfway between the anterior border of the Achilles tendon and the posterior border of the fibula.
  - The corner of the incision may be rounded or fashioned at a right angle.
  - The plantar limb of the incision is made just proximal and parallel to the demarcation between the thickened skin of the plantar heel and the thinner skin of the lateral heel.
- The sural nerve is protected, and subperiosteal elevation of all tissue off the lateral aspect of the calcaneus is performed.
  - The calcaneofibular ligament is elevated with the flap, along with the peroneal tendons within their sheath.
  - The full-thickness flap is then retracted using a "no-touch" technique with 0.062-inch Kirschner wires (K-wires) placed up the fibular shaft, in the talar neck, and in the cuboid (Fig. 7), exposing the lateral wall. An additional wire may be placed in the talar body if there is difficulty visualizing the posterior facet.
- A short Schanz pin is placed into the posterior aspect of the calcaneal tuberosity or the posteroinferior corner of the calcaneus to use as a joystick for the reduction of the tuberosity.

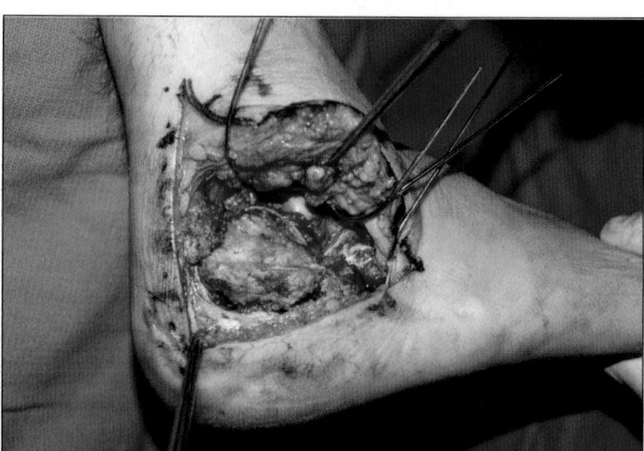

FIGURE 7

Pearls

- *Identify the sural nerve at the most proximal and distal aspects of the wound. Once it is identified and protected, sharp dissection may be carried down to bone with the scalpel blade.*
- *Determine during the approach whether the peroneal tendons have been dislocated anteriorly from the injury (this may also be evident on the preoperative CT scan). The tendons will need to be reduced and the superior peroneal retinaculum repaired prior to wound closure.*

Procedure

Step 1: Fracture Reduction

- The thin lateral wall is either reflected or removed and placed on the back table (Fig. 8A and 8B).
  - Irrigation of the wound and removal of organized clots will expose the fracture lines in the posterior facet.
  - The articular surface of the posterior facet is elevated, and the depressed articular fragments are visualized and rotated out of the body of the calcaneus (Fig. 9). Loose articular fragments may be removed and placed on the back table in a moist gauze.
- To mobilize the fracture fragments, restore calcaneal height, and initiate the correction of varus malalignment, a periosteal elevator is placed into the "primary fracture line"—the fracture common to most intra-articular calcaneal fractures, between the calcaneal tuberosity and sustentacular ("constant") fragment. The elevator is used to lever the tuberosity fragment down and medial to reposition it below the sustentaculum tali.

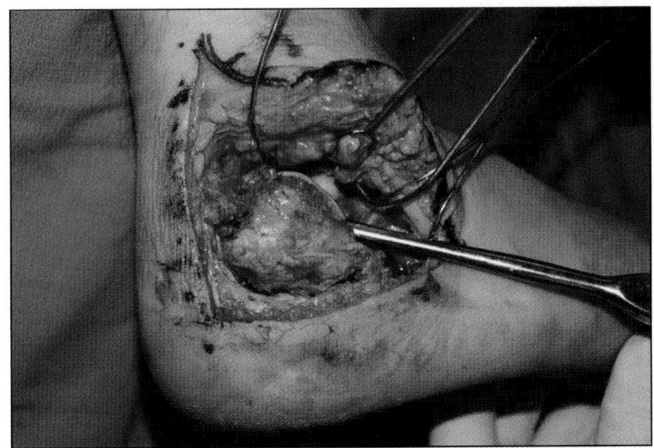

A

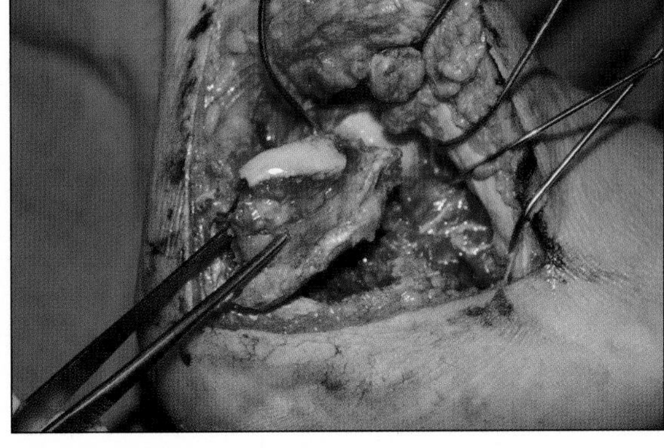

B

FIGURE 8

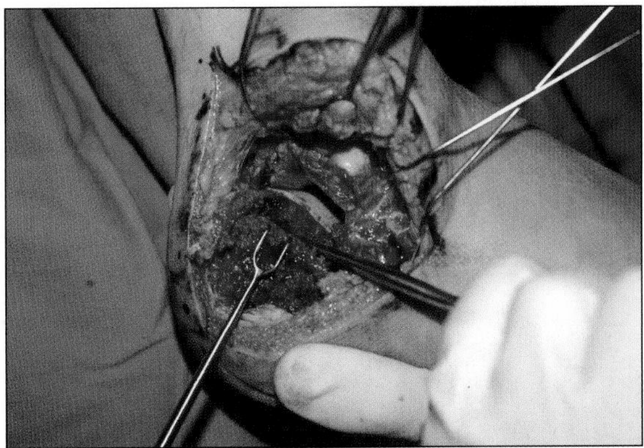

FIGURE 9

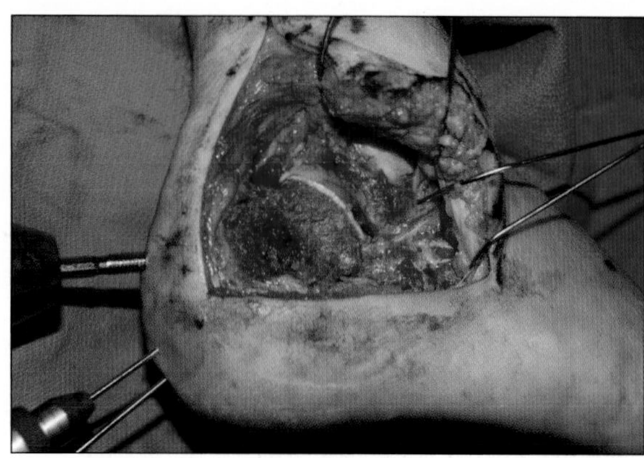

A

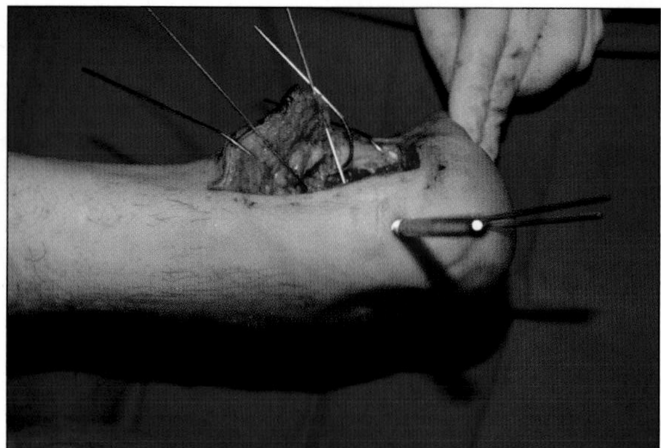

B

FIGURE 10

PITFALLS

- *Avoid using dissection scissors other than at the proximal and distal aspects of the wound when locating the sural nerve. A sharp knife will preserve a full-thickness flap for superficial wound closure and a thick periosteal layer for deep wound closure.*

Instrumentation

- Use a no-touch technique to elevate the lateral flap by avoiding forceps on the lateral skin flap. A sharp two-pronged skin hook placed deep to the periosteum is useful to retract the subperiosteal flap.

  - Once the fragments have been mobilized, a Schanz pin may be placed in the calcaneal tuberosity to be used to lever the tuberosity into proper position relative to the constant fragment (Fig. 10A and 10B).
  - One or two K-wires should then be placed from the medial tuberosity across the reduced primary fracture line into the constant fragment, without blocking subsequent reduction of the lateral articular and wall fragments. If greater support is required, the K-wires may be driven into the talar body. (However, care must be taken to avoid breaking these wires during the remainder of the procedure, since they will be nearly impossible to retrieve from the talus.)
  - Confirm tuberosity positioning and reduction of the medial wall with a Harris axial heel view. Frequently, it may take several attempts at reduction to anatomically reduce the medial calcaneal wall. Figure 11A demonstrates malreduction of the medial wall, which has been corrected in Figure 11B.
- Once the medial wall is reduced and the height of the calcaneus has been re-established, the articular fragments may be reduced to the medial sustentacular fragment. These have been cleared of all clots to allow for anatomic reduction.
  - If there is more than one superolateral articular fragment, these may be assembled on the back table with K-wires (Fig. 12) or bioabsorbable pins, then subsequently reduced as a unit to the medial sustentacular fragment.

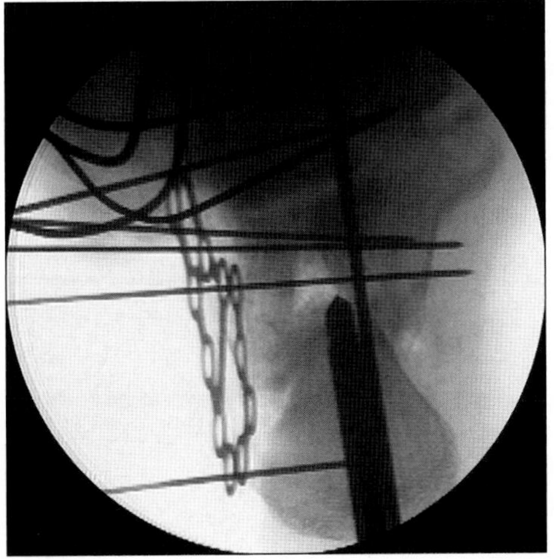

A

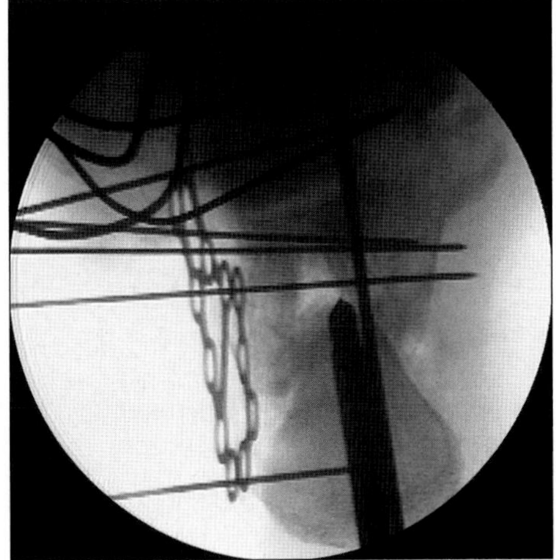

B

FIGURE 11

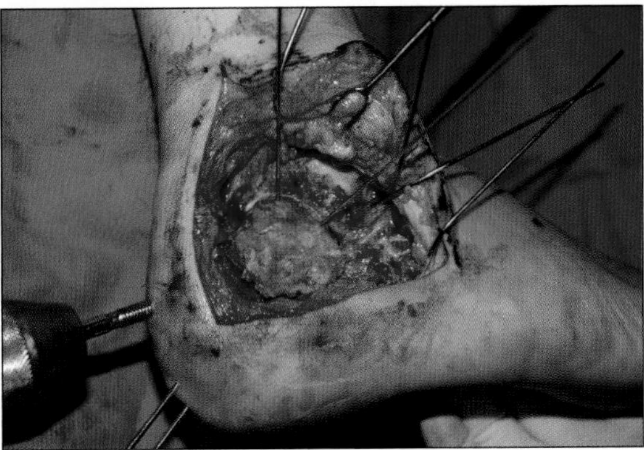

FIGURE 12

Pearls

- *Aggressively mobilize the primary fracture line before attempting reduction (particularly if the fracture is more than 10–14 days old).*
- *When placing a Schanz pin from a lateral direction, remember that the calcaneus has assumed a varus position and therefore aim the Schanz pin slightly cephalad rather than perpendicular to the heel.*
- *Do not proceed with further fracture reduction until the medial calcaneal wall (primary fracture line) is anatomically reduced.*
- *If the articular reduction is difficult, occasionally the lateral wall fragments may need to be temporarily reassembled to guide the articular reduction.*
- *In simple terms, the Broden's view is a mortise view of the ankle angled into the articulating plane of the subtalar joint.*

  - The lateral articular fragments should be secured to the constant fragment with a minimum of two pins to prevent rotation of the articular segment (however, these pins must be placed outside of the intended path for final screw fixation of the articular fragments).
  - Should the lateral wall include a superolateral articular segment of the posterior facet that is one with the lateral wall fragment, the articular and lateral wall reduction is performed simultaneously.
- Anterior reduction of the lateral articular fragment (with or without a lateral wall fragment attached) must also be confirmed with the anatomic restoration of the angle of Gissane (fracture reduction between the anterior aspect of the lateral articular fragment and the anterior process fragment). This step in the reduction re-establishes the proper relationship between the anterior and posterior calcaneal fragments. Reduction is confirmed on a lateral fluoroscopic image.

PITFALLS

- *To restore the articular congruity of the posterior facet, do not reduce the fragments to the talar articular surface. This may lead to over-reduction of the posterior facet and varus positioning of the articular fragment. The facet should be visualized and reduced to the medial (constant) articular fragment.*

- Posterior facet reduction should be confirmed not only under direct visualization, but also with a Freer elevator to obtain tactile feedback of the articular congruency, as well as with intraoperative fluoroscopic Broden's views (Fig. 13).

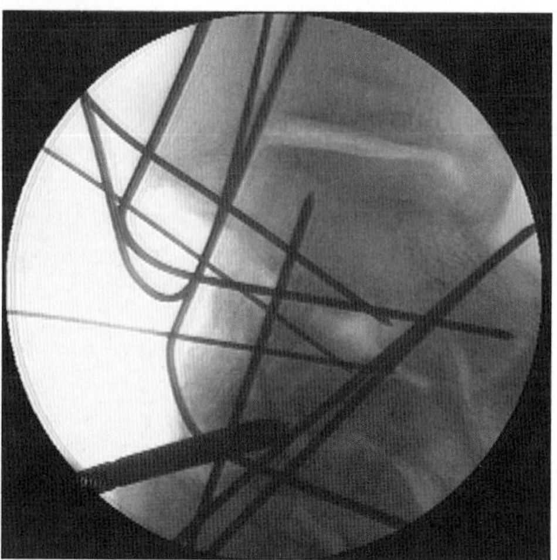

FIGURE 13

- The articular fragments are secured to one another with a lag screw placed from the lateral fragment into the constant fragment. Alternatively, the lateral wall fragment may be reduced, a lateral plate applied, and the lag screw for the articular fragments placed through the superior plate (see Step 2).

STEP 2: PLATE AND SCREW PLACEMENT

- Bone graft may be packed into the fracture, into the space formerly occupied by the displaced articular fragments (Fig. 14), but is not essential.
- The lateral wall fragments are anatomically reduced relative to the lateral articular and anterior fragments and provisionally fixed with K-wires.

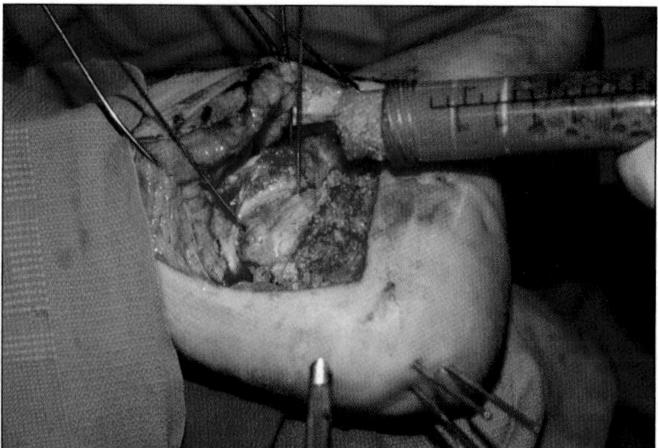

FIGURE 14

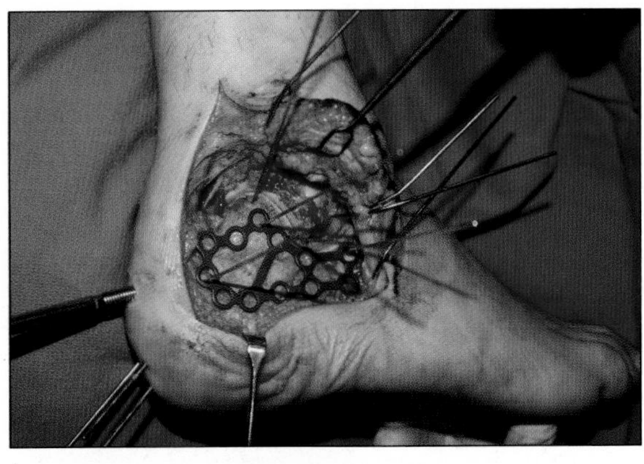

A

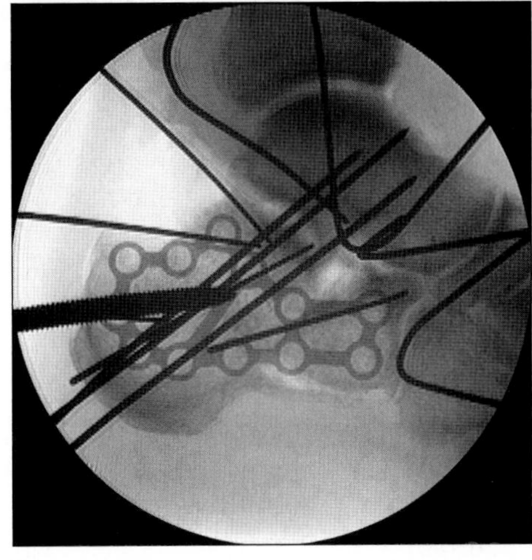

FIGURE 15 B

- Most surgeons prefer to use a multihole lateral plate designed specifically for the calcaneus (Fig. 15A and 15B); several plate designs are commercially available.
- The articular fragments may be secured with lag screw(s) either above or through the plate.
  - For fixation of the articular fragments, 3.5-mm cortical lag screws are aimed slightly distal and plantar from the lateral cortex into the sustenacular fragment.
  - Fully threaded screws placed in standard lag fashion may allow for better purchase in the subchondral bone of the articular fragments.
- Further stabilization of the calcaneus fracture is obtained with screws placed through the plate.
  - Several screws are placed in the anterior and tuberosity fragments; typically, screws placed directly inferior to the posterior facet have poor purchase (we generally leave these holes open).
  - Cortical screws are usually possible for the anterior process; cancellous screws may provide better purchase in the tuberosity fragment.

Pearls

- *During articular fixation, direct the lag screws for the posterior facet in a slightly distal and plantar direction to capture the sustentacular (constant) fragment and avoid the articular surface of the posterior facet. (The surgeon may wish to carefully place a finger of the nondrilling hand on the medial aspect of the sustentaculum tali to serve as a guide.)*

Pitfalls

- *If provisional K-wires were placed across the subtalar joint, they must be avoided during drilling or screw placement. If a wire breaks, it may not be possible to retrieve it from the talus.*

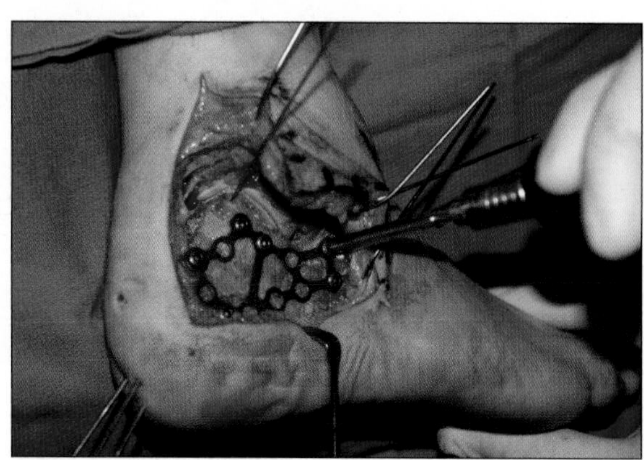
A

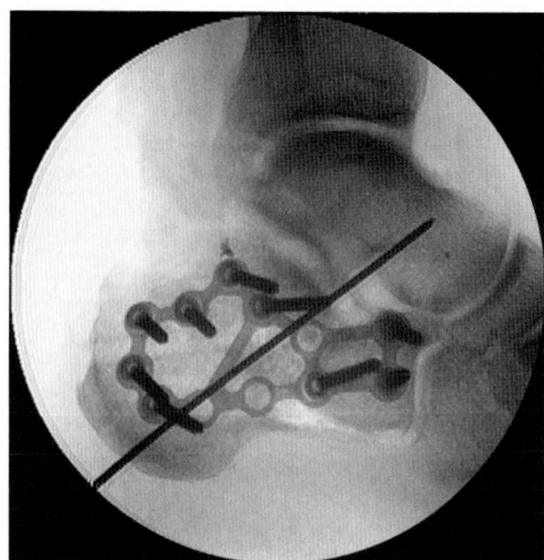
B

FIGURE 16

- Once the plate is secured to the anterior, sustentacular, and tuberosity fragments, the provisional K-wires may be removed (Fig. 16A and 16B).

Step 3: Repair of Peroneal Tendon Dislocation

- Occasionally, a high-energy calcaneal fracture displaces the peroneal tendons with the lateral calcaneal wall enough to disrupt the superior peroneal tendon retinaculum, leading to peroneal tendon dislocation.
  - Typically, peroneal tendon dislocation can be diagnosed on preoperative physical examination. When the superior peroneal retinaculum is disrupted, the tendons are subluxated or dislocated anterior to the fibula (Fig. 17).

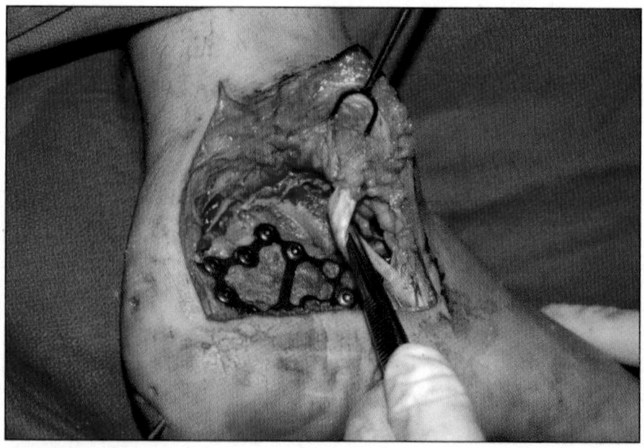
FIGURE 17

Controversies

- There are studies that both support and refute the use of bone graft or bone graft substitutes. In cases of severe comminution, we typically add cancellous allograft bone with or without a platelet-rich product.

Pitfalls

- *Remember to look for potential peroneal tendon dislocation preoperatively, both clinically and on preoperative CT scanning.*

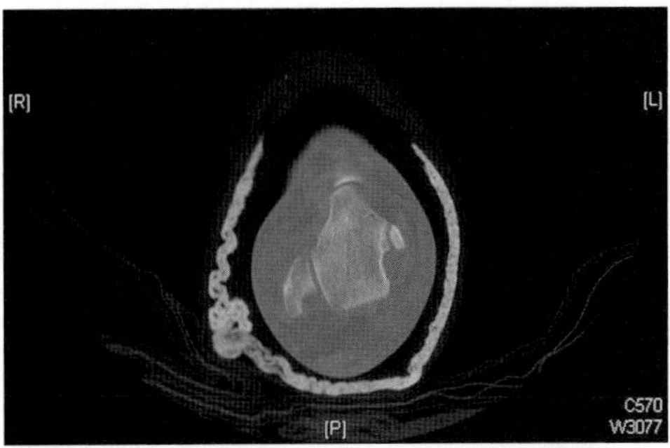

A

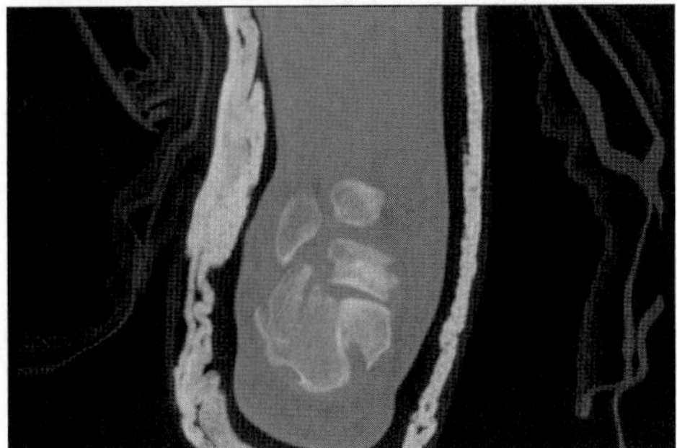

B

FIGURE 18

- This can be visualized on preoperative axial (Fig. 18A) and coronal (Fig. 18B) CT scans.
- A recommended routine is to check peroneal tendon reduction when ORIF of the calcaneal fracture is complete.

■ Following ORIF of the calcaneal fracture into its anatomic alignment, the subfibular recess is restored, allowing for reduction of the peroneal tendons.
  - The vertical limb of the incision is taken slightly more proximally, the sural nerve is protected, and the vacant fibular groove is visualized with the tendons dislocated anteriorly (Fig. 19A and 19B).

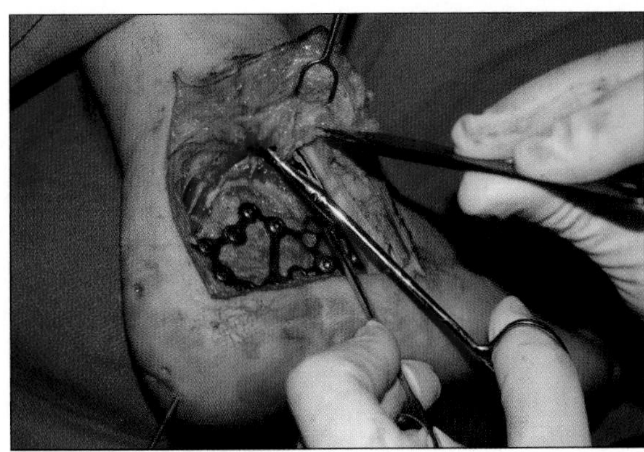

A

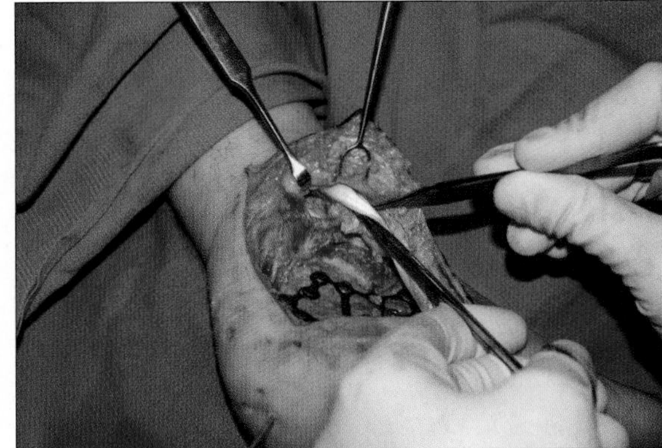

B

FIGURE 19

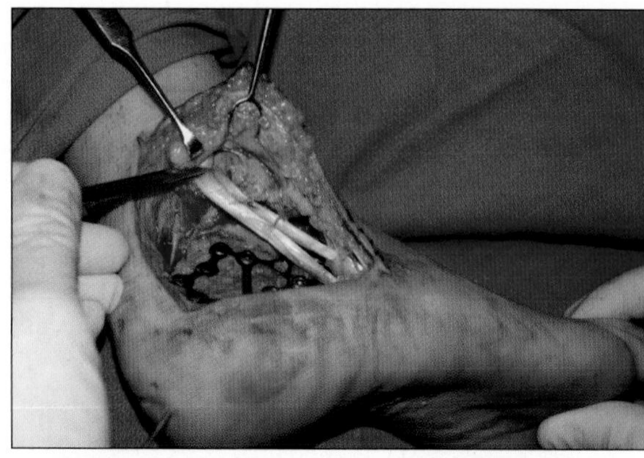

A

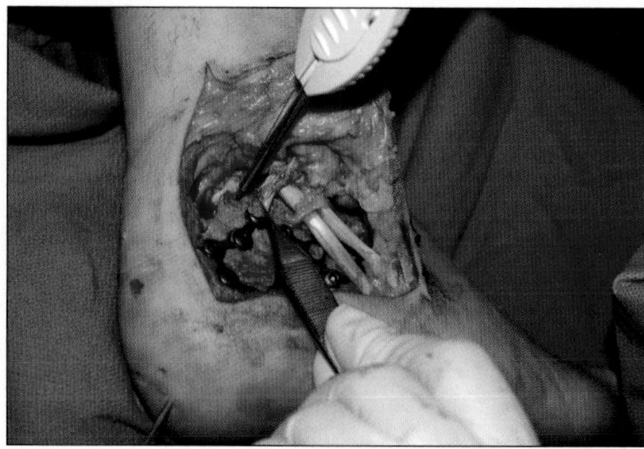

B

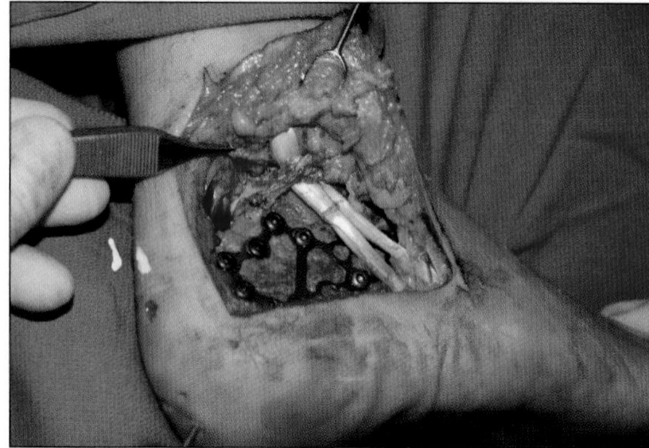

C

FIGURE 20

- The tendons are carefully separated from the soft tissues, elevated for exposure without damaging the integrity of the soft tissue flap, and reduced into the fibular groove.
- Retinacular tissue and periosteum are then utilized to reconstruct at least a portion of the superior peroneal retinaculum (a suture anchor may be used) (Fig. 20A–C).

Step 4: Wound Closure

- The wound is closed using 2-0 Vicryl sutures by reapproximation of the deep periosteal layer over a deep suction drain that is brought either through the lateral skin anterior to the Achilles tendon (posterior to the sural nerve) or out the distal aspect of the foot (dorsal to the sural nerve).
  - The deep layer is reapproximated first at the proximal and distal aspects of the wound to decrease tension at the apex of the wound (Fig. 21).
  - The skin is closed with 4-0 nylon interrupted Allgower-Donati sutures (Fig. 22).

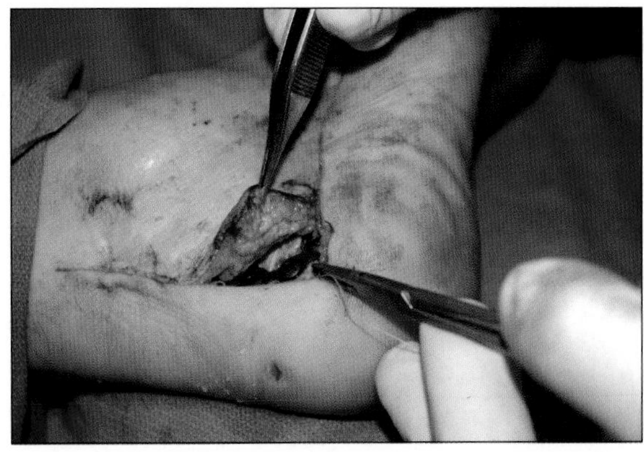

FIGURE 21

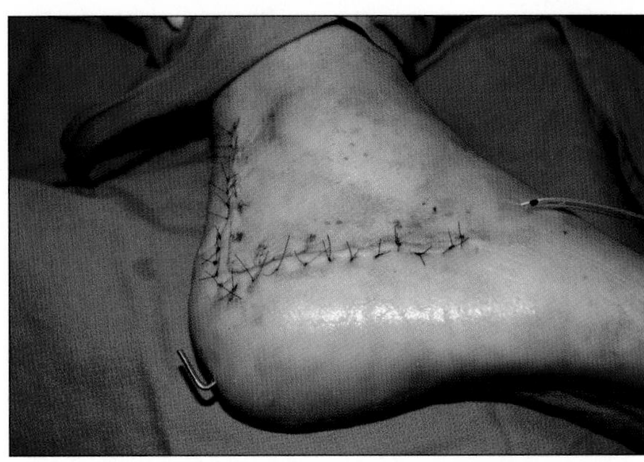

FIGURE 22

- A sterile dressing is placed on the wound. With the hip and knee flexed to allow the ankle to be easily positioned in a neutral position, a posterior/sugar tong splint is applied over adequate padding.
- With the suction drain functioning, the tourniquet is let down after wound closure.

Pearls

- *Skin tension at the corner of the wound may be minimized by progressively closing the incision from the ends of the wound to the corner.*
- *Maintaining the tourniquet until the dressing and splint are applied and the drain is functioning reduces the potential for deleterious hematoma formation.*
- *The Allgower-Donati suture places the knot of the suture away from the lateral flap of skin and subcutaneous tissue, theoretically decreasing ischemic pressure from the knot (see Fig. 22).*

Pitfalls

- *To prevent potential skin necrosis, the skin edges should not be pinched with the forceps and the tourniquet time should not exceed 2.5 hours (preferably <2 hours).*

Postoperative Care and Expected Outcomes

- We routinely remove the skin sutures between 2 and 3 weeks, but may delay suture removal for up to an additional 3 weeks if necessary.
- If calcaneal fracture fixation was deemed stable, we recommend a removable boot so that the patient can perform range-of-motion exercises for the ankle and foot, provided the wound is healed. If there is any concern regarding the wound, immobilization in a short-leg cast is preferred and sutures remain until the 6-week follow-up appointment.
- Progressive weight bearing is allowed at 10–12 weeks, if radiographs suggest adequate fracture consolidation.
- Figure 23 shows postoperative radiographs including a Broden's view (Fig. 23A), Harris axial heel view (Fig. 23B), and lateral view (Fig. 23C) demonstrating anatomic reduction of the posterior facet, medial wall, and Böhler's angle, respectively.

Pearls

- *Wound healing is often delayed following ORIF of calcaneal fractures. Without evidence for infection, continued immobilization and protective weight bearing typically lead to progression toward satisfactory wound healing.*
- *Function may be enhanced with early range of motion of the ankle and foot while continuing strict non–weight-bearing status, provided the wound and fracture are stable.*

Pitfalls

- *A wound that fails to improve or exhibits signs of infection should prompt early infection workup, irrigation and débridement, and infectious disease and plastic surgery consultation in select cases.*
- *Weight bearing should be restricted until satisfactory fracture healing is suggested on postoperative radiographs.*

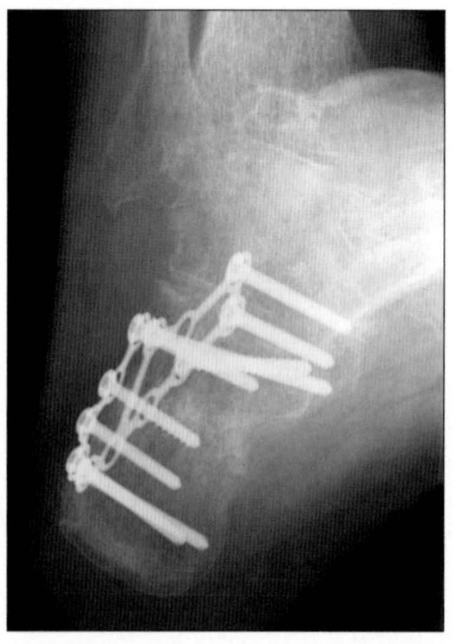
A

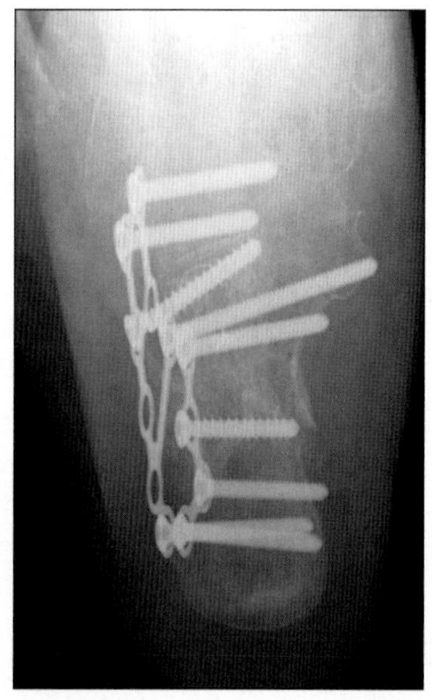
B

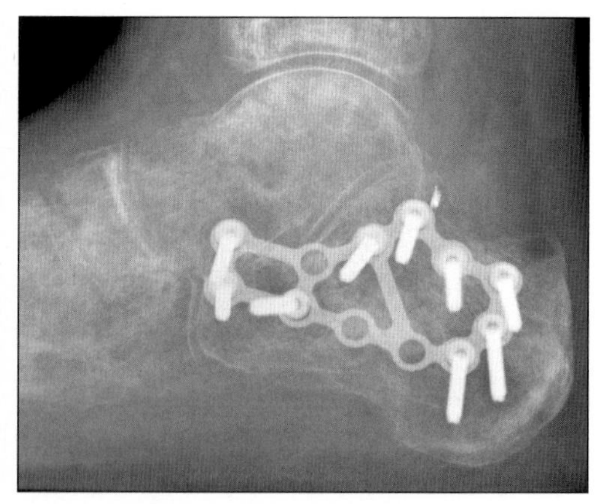
C

FIGURE 23

Evidence

Aldridge JM 3rd, Easley M, Nunley JA. Open calcaneal fractures: results of operative treatment. J Orthop Trauma. 2004;18:7-11.

In this study, all patients were treated with intravenous antibiotics, tetanus prophylaxis, and immediate and repeat irrigation and débridement. Definitive fracture reduction was performed at an average of 7 days after injury (range 0–22 days). For the patients with Gustilo type II and type III open calcaneal fractures, there was an 11% complication rate with higher-than-expected health-related quality-of-life indices. The treatment group did not reflect as high a complication rate for open calcaneal fractures as previously reported, and the results support previous claims that definitive hardware placement at the time of initial irrigation and débridement probably is not warranted: Definitive fracture stabilization can and should wait until soft tissue coverage is fully assessed.

Bajammal S, Tornetta P 3rd, Sanders D, Bhandari M. Displaced intra-articular calcaneal fractures. J Orthop Trauma. 2005;19:360-4.

This study was designed to determine the effect of operative treatment compared with nonoperative treatment on the rate of union, complications, and functional outcome after intra-articular calcaneal fracture in adults.

Buckley R, Tough S, McCormack R, Pate G, Leighton R, Petrie D, Galpin R. Operative compared with nonoperative treatment of displaced intra-articular calcaneal fractures: a prospective, randomized, controlled multicenter trial. J Bone Joint Surg [Am]. 2002;84:1733-44.

Without stratification of the groups, the functional results after nonoperative care of displaced intra-articular calcaneal fractures were equivalent to those after operative care in this study. However, after unmasking the data by removal of the patients who were receiving workers' compensation, the outcomes were significantly better in some groups of surgically treated patients. Patients who were not receiving workers' compensation and were managed operatively had significantly higher satisfaction scores ($p = .001$). Women who were managed operatively scored significantly higher on the Short Form-36 than did women who were managed nonoperatively ($p = .015$). Patients who were not receiving workers' compensation and were younger (less than 29 years old) and had a moderately lower Böhler angle (0–14°), a comminuted fracture, a light workload, or an anatomic reduction or a stepoff of ≤2 mm after surgical reduction ($p = .04$), scored significantly higher on the scoring scales after surgery compared with those who were treated nonoperatively.

Herscovici D Jr, Widmaier J, Scaduto JM, Sanders RW, Walling A. Operative treatment of calcaneal fractures in elderly patients. J Bone Joint Surg [Am]. 2005;87:1260-4.

Open reduction appears to be an acceptable method of treatment for displaced calcaneal fractures in elderly patients.

Howard JL, Buckley R, McCormack R, Pate G, Leighton R, Petrie D, Galpin R. Complications following management of displaced intra-articular calcaneal fractures: a prospective randomized trial comparing open reduction internal fixation with nonoperative management. J Orthop Trauma. 2003;17:241-9.

This study determined that complications occur regardless of the management strategy chosen for displaced intra-articular calcaneal fractures and despite management by experienced surgeons. Complications were a cause of significant morbidity for patients. Outcome scores in this study tended to support ORIF for calcaneal fractures. However, ORIF patients were more likely to develop complications. Certain patient populations (worker's compensation and Sanders type IV) developed a high incidence of complications regardless of the management strategy chosen.

Huang PJ, Huang HT, Chen TB, Chen JC, Lin YK, Cheng YM, Lin SY. Open reduction and internal fixation of displaced intra-articular fractures of the calcaneus. J Trauma. 2002;52:946-50.

The authors recommended that Sanders type II and type III fractures be treated with ORIF. Despite the results of type IV fractures being significantly worse than those of type II and type III fractures, the authors also recommended ORIF for type IV fractures to restore the hindfoot architecture and the subtalar joint, if possible. When the disrupted subtalar joint is so comminuted that it is beyond the surgeon's ability to reconstruct, primary subtalar arthrodesis should be performed in addition to ORIF.

Longino D, Buckley RE. Bone graft in the operative treatment of displaced intraarticular calcaneal fractures: is it helpful? J Orthop Trauma. 2001;15:280-6.

The authors found no objective radiographic or functional benefit to the use of bone graft supplementation in the operative treatment of displaced intra-articular calcaneal fractures.

Sanders R, Fortin P, DiPasquale T, Walling A. Operative treatment in 120 displaced intraarticular calcaneal fractures: results using a prognostic computed tomography scan classification. Clin Orthop Relat Res. 1993;(290):87-95.

To evaluate the results of this study, a classification for intra-articular calcaneal fractures was developed based on standardized coronal and transverse CT scans of both feet. Excellent or good clinical results occurred in 58 of 79 (73%) type II fractures, 21 of 30 (70%) type III fractures, and 1 of 11 (9%) type IV fractures. When excellent and good clinical results were compared by year, a distinct learning curve appeared (1987, 27%; 1988, 54%; 1989, 74%; 1990, 84%). Despite an improved outcome for type II and III fractures with increasing surgical experience, the results of operative intervention in type IV fractures were no better, even after 4 years.

PROCEDURE 44

Calcaneus Open Reduction and Internal Fixation with Extensile Lateral Incision

Christina Kabbash and Andrew K. Sands

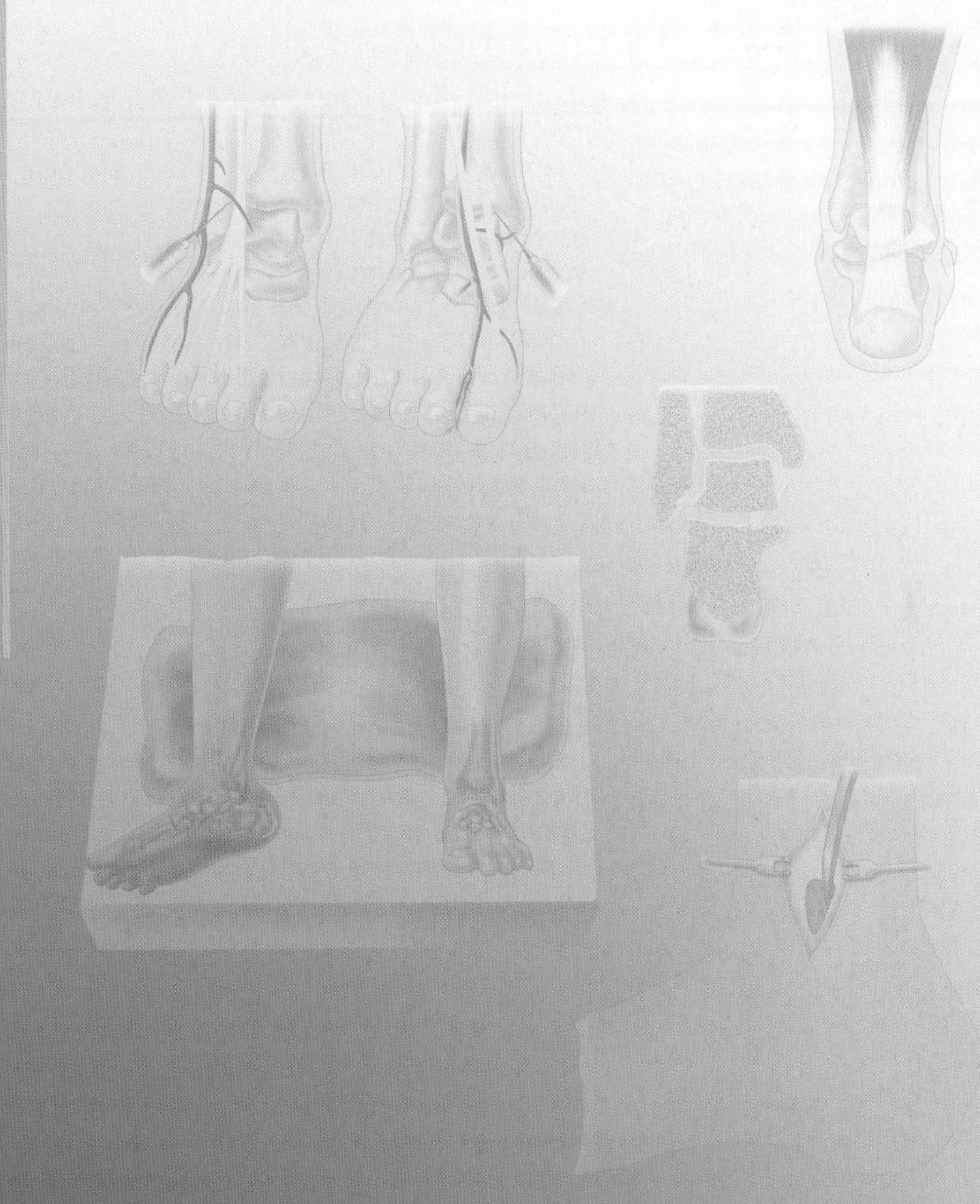

Andrew K. Sands would like to acknowledge the assistance of Edmund Choi, MD with this chapter.

Pitfalls

- *Contraindications include vascular insufficiency, poorly controlled diabetes, age, smoking, and noncompliant patients.*
- *Relative contraindications may include various medical comorbidities, including uncontrolled diabetes and heart disease.*

Controversies

- Use of a foot pump to decrease edema prior to operative intervention

Indications

- Intra-articular calcaneal fractures with 2-mm or more gap or stepoff of the posterior facet, and, intra-articular calcaneal fractures with Böhler's angle less than 15° on lateral radiographs of the foot or ankle
- Surgical intervention with an extended lateral incision may be performed urgently before swelling occurs, or in 2–3 weeks with the resolution of swelling and fracture blisters.

Examination/Imaging

- A thorough physical examination should be performed.
  - Examination of the foot for closed calcaneal fractures often reveals significant swelling, ecchymoses, and fracture blisters that may be serous or serosangineous.
  - Open fractures often indicate greater energy of impact: 10% of calcaneal fractures are associated with spine fractures and 25% with additional lower extremity fractures. Open fractures are typically medial, although they may be lateral or plantar.
  - Pain with passive motion of the toes may indicate an impending compartment syndrome, which may be confirmed by monitoring deep plantar and calcaneal compartment pressures. Late signs of compartment syndrome include pallor, paresthesias, and loss of pulses.
- Plain radiographs
  - Lateral, Harris, and oblique (Broden) views of the calcaneus and foot should be obtained in both the injured and contralateral feet.
  - Lateral radiographs may show fractures of the calcaneus associated with flattening of Böhler's angle, normally 25–40°, and loss of calcaneal pitch (Fig. 1A).
    - Böhler's angle is formed by the intersection of a line from the highest part of the calcaneal tuberosity to the highest part of the posterior facet and a line from the highest point of the posterior facet to the highest point of the posterior process of the calcaneus (Fig. 1B).
  - Harris views may show fractures through the posterior facet, widening of the calcaneus with lateral wall impingement, and loss of calcaneal height.

Treatment Options

- Closed calcaneal fractures may be treated nonoperatively with bulky Jones dressings and splinting for comfort.
  - The foot should be kept level avoiding a dependent position. Early foot and ankle range-of-motion exercises should be initiated as soon as tolerated (at 1–3 weeks) to decrease stiffness, and cool Epsom soaks may further reduce the swelling. Weight bearing is started at 3 months.
  - Complications associated with nonoperative protocols include subtalar stiffness and pain, loss of foot dorsiflexion, widening of the heel, peroneal dislocation, lateral wall impingement, and difficulty walking on uneven ground.
  - Operative treatment of closed fractures with an extensile lateral incision may be performed immediately, or with resolution of swelling and fracture blisters. Percutaneous or mini-open reduction techniques should be performed within the first week, while the fracture fragments are still easily mobilized. Some surgeons utilize lateral incisions over the sinus tarsi, or medial incisions, which are not discussed here.
- Open fractures should be emergently irrigated and débrided.
  - Repeat irrigations and débridements should be performed as needed.
  - If primary closure is not an option, then a preliminary reduction may be obtained and held with Kirschner wires until definitive fixation and wound closure are performed.

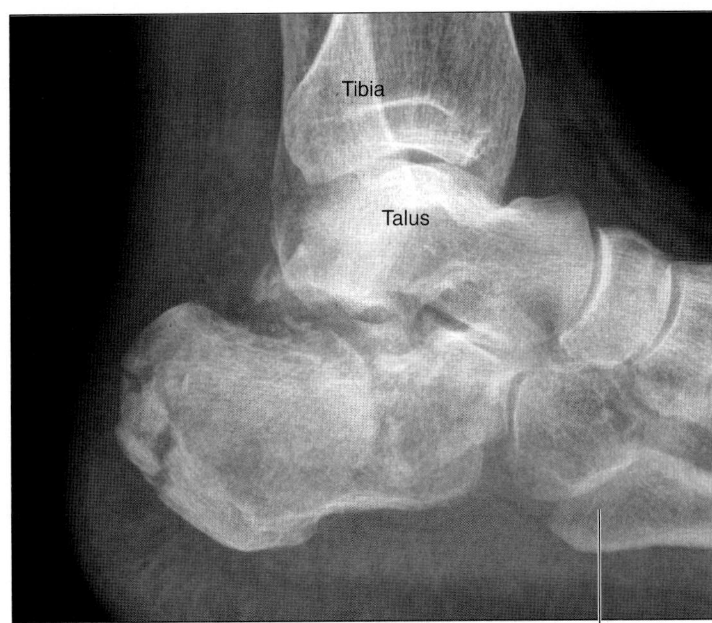

A

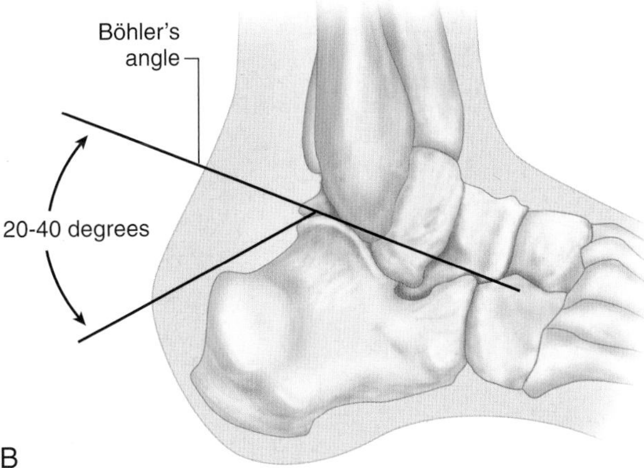

B

FIGURE 1

- Oblique views may demonstrate fractures of the calcaneocuboid joint.
- Anteroposterior Broden's views with the foot internally rotated 20° and plantar flexed 10–40° will show the posterior facet.

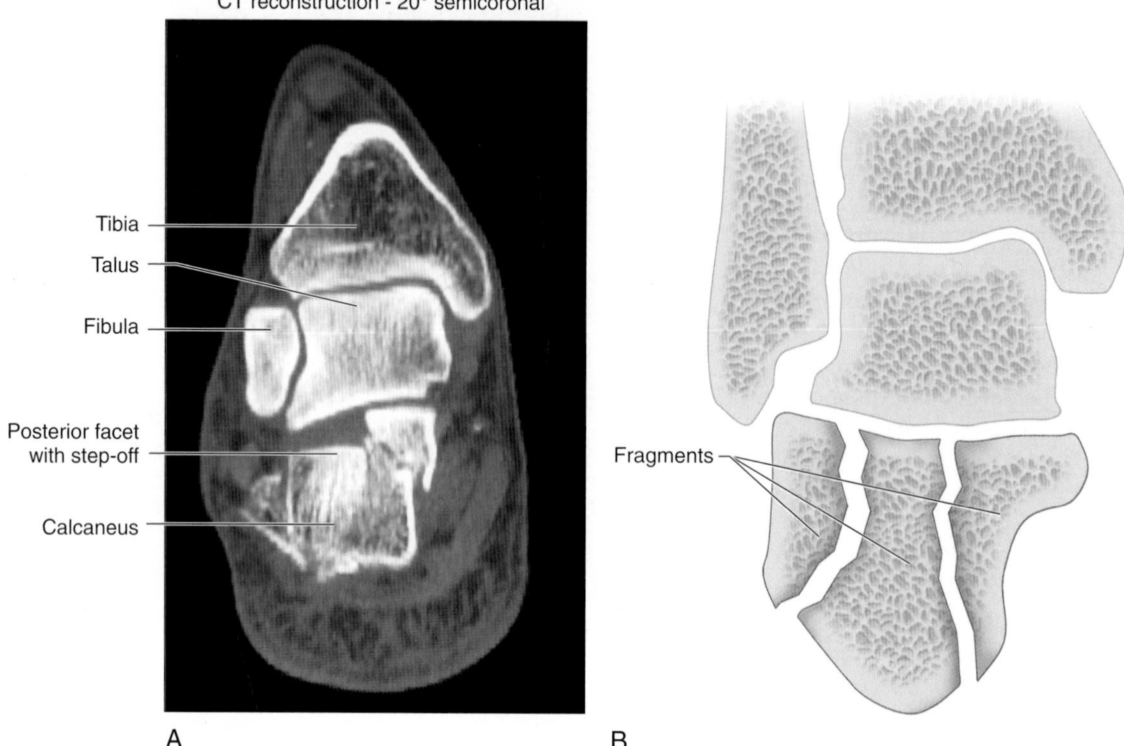

FIGURE 2

- Computed tomography
  - One-millimeter axial cuts with large overlap should be obtained with the following reconstructed views oriented:
    - Perpendicular to the posterior facet to visualize gapping or step-off and identify the constant fragment containing the sustentaculum tali (Fig. 2A and 2B).
    - Parallel to the plane of the floor to obtain cuts perpendicular to the calcaneocuboid joint.
    - Sagittal views to visualize the orientation of the fracture fragments of the posterior facet (Fig. 3).

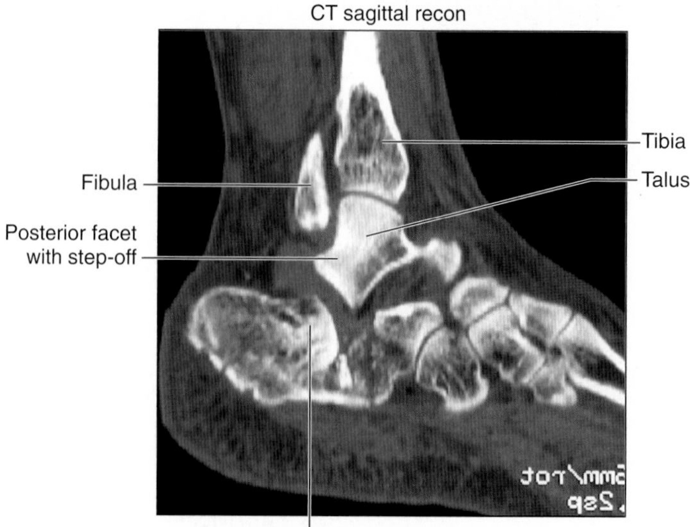

FIGURE 3

Surgical Anatomy

- The peroneal tendons and sural nerve cross the lateral aspect of the calcaneus and are often exposed or at risk with the lateral extensile incision.
- The peroneal tendons emerge from the peroneal tendon sheath at the inferior and posterior aspect of the fibula (Fig. 4A). The peroneus brevis then inserts on the styloid of the fifth metatarsal, while the peroneus longus crosses under the cuboid on the way to its insertion on the base of the first metatarsal.
- The sural nerve often courses just posterior to the peroneal tendons and then along the lateral aspect of the foot (Fig. 4B). The sural nerve is often encountered in both the proximal and distal arms of the extensile incision. When transected, it is best to cut the nerve as proximally as possible to avoid a stump neuroma.

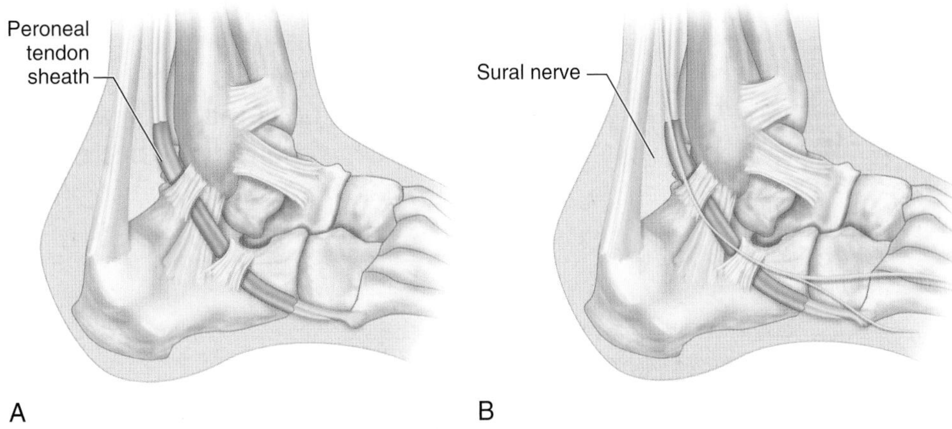

FIGURE 4

PEARLS

- *Position the down leg such that it does not interfere with fluoroscopic visualization.*
- *While a large C-arm allows for increased resolution, it may be difficult to obtain Harris and oblique views. In contrast, a mini C-arm allows for greater flexibility but with decreased resolution and a smaller field.*

Equipment

- An operating room table with a radiolucent extension
- Lateral decubitus hip positioners
- Foam blocks
- Either a large C-arm or a mini C-arm
- Thigh tourniquet

Positioning

- The patient is placed in a lateral decubitus position.
- An axillary roll is placed along with extra padding under the knee/peroneal nerve of the down leg, with additional padding between the knees.
- A thigh tourniquet is applied.
- Utilization of pillows or large foam blocks between the legs allows for a stable surface.
- If a large C-arm is used, it is positioned anteriorly.

Portals/Exposures

- An extensile lateral incision is used. Elements of the anatomy are marked preoperatively (Fig. 5A and 5B).
    - The distal fibula is outlined as well as the entire calcaneus.
    - With respect to the calcaneus, careful attention is paid to the posterior, plantar, calcaneocuboid, lateral neck, and sinus tarsi.
    - The approximate course of the peroneal tendons and sural nerve is detailed as well.
    - The incision is marked starting at the level of the ankle joint, then coursing just anterior to the Achilles tendon along its insertion on the tuber, and curving anteriorly along the plantar surface of the calcaneus. If the calcaneocuboid joint requires reduction, the distal aspect of the incision may veer superiorly to better expose the calcaneocuboid joint.

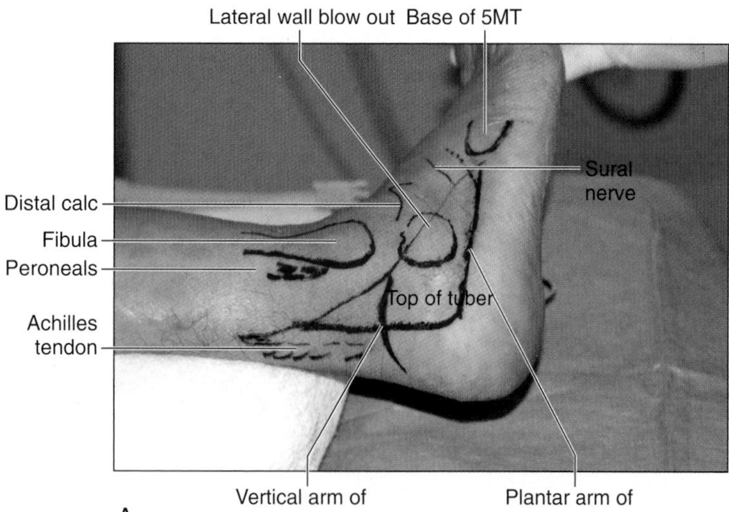

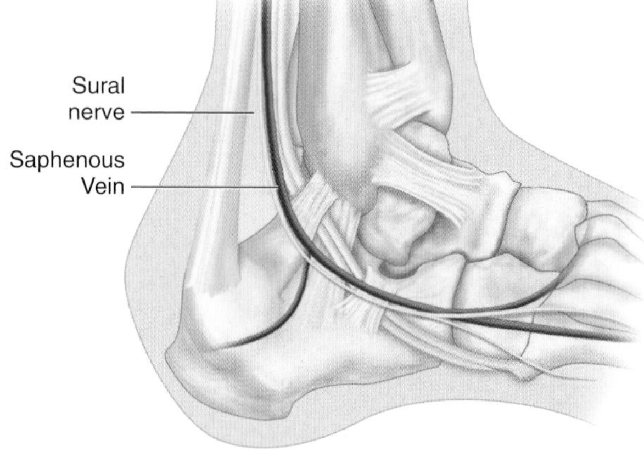

FIGURE 5

Controversies

- With an extensile lateral exposure, restoration of Böhler's angle and anatomic reduction of the posterior facet have both been shown to be associated with improved outcomes. However, percutaneous and mini-incision techniques have also demonstrated good or equal results with approximate anatomic reductions, possibly due to less soft tissue trauma and scar formation.

- Make a longitudinal incision parallel and just anterior to the Achilles tendon and its insertion on the calcaneus starting at the level of the ankle joint and curving anteriorly at the plantar aspect of the calcaneus.
- The incision is then extended distally along the plantar aspect of the calcaneus, to just past the calcaneocuboid articulation. The incision is made sharply through the skin and then is carried down to bone over the tuber.
- Careful dissection is made at the proximal and distal aspects of the incision to avoid transection of the peroneal tendons and sural nerve.

Pearls

- *The sural nerve is often encountered on both arms of the incision and should be protected. Curving the incision anteriorly to expose the calcaneocuboid joint increases the risk of sural nerve transection in the distal arm. Rounding out the corner decreases the incidence of wound dehiscence and necrosis in this area.*
- *The advantage of the extensile incision is adequate visualization of the distal calcaneus, the calcaneocuboid joint, sinus tarsi, and posterior facet with decreased skin tension during the reduction.*
- *Kirschner wires may be drilled into the talus and fibula and bent to allow for adequate retraction of the thick lateral flap. Care must be taken when using this technique as it can injure the lateral flap.*

Procedure

Step 1

- Starting at the rounded corner, a thick flap is sharply raised off of the lateral wall of the calcaneus until the sinus tarsi, neck, and posterior facet are visualized.
- 1.6-mm Kirschner wires (K-wires) may be drilled into the talus and bent to retract this flap. Fracture-associated peroneal tendon displacement may be noted during the approach.

Pearls

- *Avoid elevators with sharp edges. If the sural nerve is transected, trace it proximally and transect to avoid a painful distal neuroma.*

Pitfalls

- *Mobilization of the peroneal tendons may be difficult. Dissection of the peroneal tendons distally may be required.*
- *If possible, avoid placing the incision through fracture blisters as this may increase the risk of perioperative infection.*

Step 2

- The lateral wall is either reflected on a periosteal hinge or removed and set aside in saline for later replacement. Soft tissues are sharply removed with a scalpel or rongeur to allow adequate visualization of the posterior facet.
- The fracture fragments are identified and loosened with either osteotomes or Cobb elevators to allow for their manipulation and reduction.

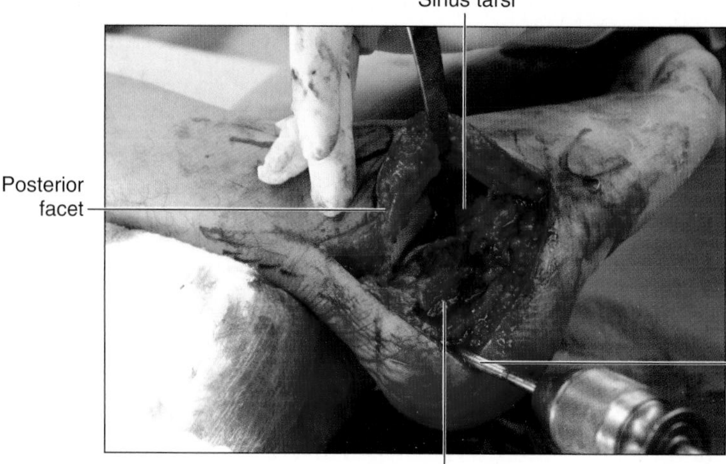

FIGURE 6

Instrumentation/Implantation

- Scalpel
- Cobb elevator
- K-wires

Pearls

- *Fracture fragments must be adequately identified and mobilized to allow for reduction. Mark the lateral wall orientation prior to removal.*

Pitfalls

- *Fracture fragments may have increased comminution, osteoporotic bone, or old fractures with partial healing*

- A 5.0-mm Schanz half-pin is inserted into the lateral aspect of the posterior tuber (Fig. 6).
- Longitudinal traction and a valgus force are applied to the Schanz pin to correct for the varus malpositioning and widening of the heel; 1.6-mm K-wires are inserted to hold the reduction.

Step 3

- The reconstruction is started distally. If the fracture has extended into the calcaneocuboid joint, it is addressed with the distal calcaneus. K-wires are used for provisional fixation.
- The angle of Gissane is addressed by pushing down on the distal calcaneus while elevating the posterior facet.
- The posterior facet is then reconstructed. The lateral and middle fragments are restored to the medial sustentacular part of the joint.
- K-wires may be partially drilled into fragments to joystick them into place. Once a fragment is reduced, the K-wire may be advanced until it is flush by grasping the other end to allow stacking of comminuted fragments. The Schanz pin is removed (Fig. 7).

Instrumentation/Implantation

- 5.0-mm Schanz half-pin
- T-handle chuck
- Osteotomes
- Cobb elevator
- Freer elevator

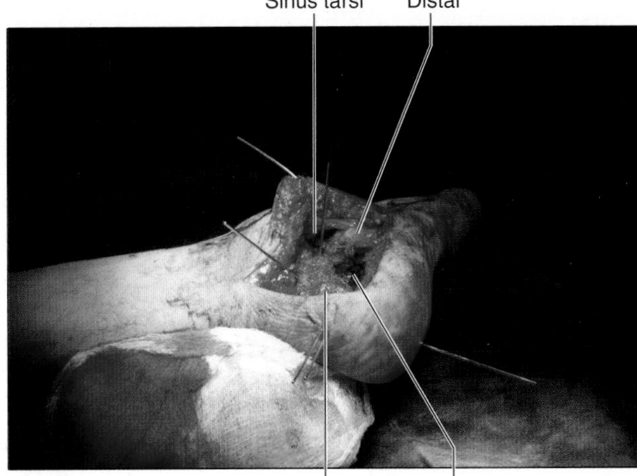

FIGURE 7

Pearls

- *Removal of fat from the sinus tarsi and distraction of the subtalar joint with blunt lamina spreaders will usually allow improved visualization. If visualization is still inadequate, a thin elevator may be passed over the articular surface to confirm reduction.*
- *Rebuild the posterior facet starting with the most medial fragment in continuity with the sustentaculum. Use of a dental pick may help reduce the smaller fragments.*

Pitfalls

- *Loss of articular cartilage may make anatomic reduction difficult. Calcaneocuboid comminution may make it difficult to restore and maintain Böhler's angle.*

Instrumentation/Implantation

- Blunt lamina spreader
- Dental pick
- 1.6-mm K-wires
- Ronguer

Controversies

- Comminution of the posterior facet may make anatomic reduction impossible. It is controversial whether to procede with a primary subtalar fusion or plate and screw fixation in this situation. The order of fixation is also controversial. Some surgeons prefer to start with reduction of the posterior facet. However, it may be more difficult to adequately visualize the posterior facet if the neck is not reduced first.
- Locking versus nonlocking plates: There was no difference in load to failure with either plate in cadaver bones or sawbones.

Controversies

- The need to fill the void with bone morphogenetic protein (BMP), bone graft, or bone graft substitutes is highly controversial. Some surgeons advocate filling the void with bone cement with/without antibiotics and having the patient bear weight at 3 weeks. Other surgeons may not utilize bone graft or BMP at all.

Step 4

- Autologous bone graft or bone graft substitutes may be packed into the void prior to replacing the lateral wall (Fig. 8).
- After the lateral wall is replaced, an appropriate-sized calcaneal plate is applied to the lateral aspect of the calcaneus and contoured accordingly (Fig. 9A and 9B). At least one of the screws through the plate should lag the sustentaculum tali constant fragment.

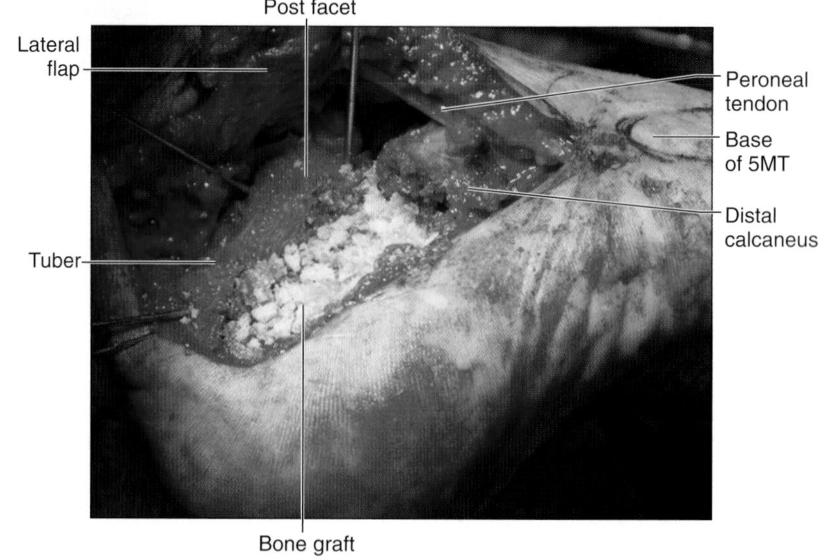

FIGURE 8

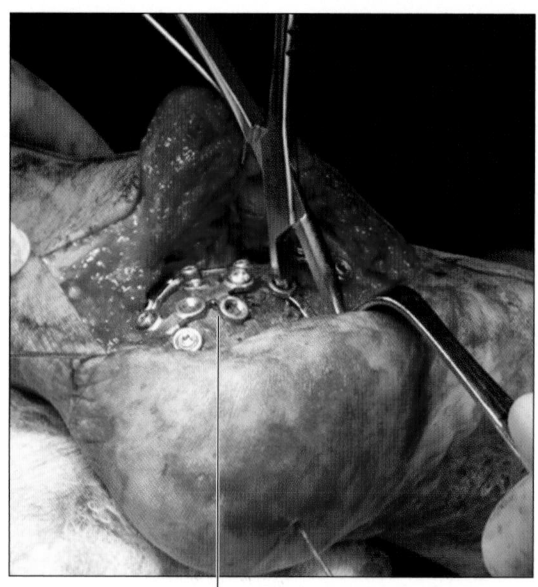

A

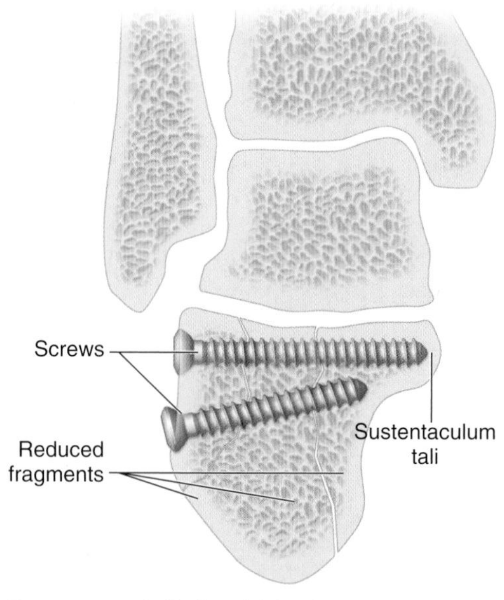

B

FIGURE 9

Pitfalls

- *Blanching of the skin indicates increased skin tension. If advancement of the deep layers of the flap is insufficient to obtain a tension-free skin closure, "pie crusting" of the skin may be performed.*

Step 5

- The goal is to obtain a tension-free closure of the skin and subcutaneous tissues to limit the potential for corner necrosis and dehiscence.
- The deep fascial layer of the flap is closed with an absorbable braided 0 suture from either end of the incision, advancing the flap with each stitch. This ensures that the corner will close and be tension free.
- The subcutaneous tissues and skin are closed as per surgeon preference.
- Sterile dressings and a three-sided splint with the foot in neutral are applied.

Postoperative Care and Expected Outcomes

- The operative dressing is left intact for 2 weeks and removed at the first postoperative visit.
- A cam boot is placed. Early active range-of-motion exercises are shown, especially hindfoot motion.
- The patient is non–weightbearing with two crutches or a walker for 6–12 weeks until there is resolution of swelling and evidence of consolidation is present on lateral radiographs.
- Improvement will continue over a 2-year period.
- The most common postoperative complication is tissue necrosis and wound dehiscence of the corner area. There is also a 5% infection rate for closed calcaneal fractures with open reduction and internal fixation. This infection rate is increased with open calcaneal fractures.
- Sural nerve transection or retraction may result in postoperative paresthesias.
- Painful hardware, malreduction, or subtalar arthritis may require later arthrodesis or removal of hardware.

Evidence

Aldridge JM 3rd, Easley M, Nunley JA. Open calcaneal fractures: results of operative treatment. J Orthop Trauma. 2004;18:7–11.

This was a retrospective review of 19 consecutive patients with open calcaneal fractures treated with initial débridement and then definitive fracture reduction 7 days later. Follow-up averaged 26.2 months, and outcome was determined by American Orthopaedic Foot and Ankle Society (AOFAS) Ankle-Hindfoot scores, clinical examinations, and radiographs. (Level IV evidence [case series])

Benirschke SK, Kramer PA. Wound healing complications in closed and open calcaneal fractures. J Orthop Trauma. 2004;18:1–6.

This was a retrospective cohort review of 341 closed calcaneal fractures during a 6-year period and 39 open calcaneal fractures during an 11-year period that were treated with open reduction and internal fixation using an extensile lateral approach. The rate of infection in each group was assessed. (Level III evidence [retrospective cohort])

Berry GK, Stevens DG, Kreder HJ, McKee M, Schemitsch E, Stephen DJ. Open fractures of the calcaneus: a review of treatment and outcome. J Orthop Trauma. 2004;18:202–6.

This was a retrospective review of 29 patients with open calcaneal fractures. Follow-up averaged 49 months, and outcome was assessed with AOFAS Ankle-Hindfoot scores, Baltimore Painful Foot Scores, and Short Form-36 (SF-36) scores. (Level IV evidence [case series])

Bibbo C, Patel DV. The effect of demineralized bone matrix-calcium sulfate with vancomycin on calcaneal fracture healing and infection rates: a prospective study. Foot Ankle Int. 2006;27:487–93.

This was a prospective study of 33 displaced intra-articular calcaneal fractures treated by open reduction and internal fixation with demineralized matrix–calcium sulfate with vancomycin. Follow-up averaged 22.4 months, and outcome was assessed radiographically and clinically. (Level II evidence [prospective case series])

Buckley R, Tough S, McCormack R, Pate G, Leighton R, Petrie D, Galpin R. Operative compared with nonoperative treatment of displaced intra-articular calcaneal fractures: a prospective, randomized, controlled multicenter trial. J Bone Joint Surg [Am]. 2002;84:1733–44.

This was a randomized controlled trial of operative versus nonoperative treatment of displaced intra-articular calcaneus fractures in 319 patients who were followed for 2 years. Outcomes were determined by SF-36 scores and clinical and radiographic examination. (Level I evidence [randomized controlled trial])

Buckley RE, Meek RN. Comparison of open versus closed reduction of intraarticular calcaneal fractures: a matched cohort in workmen. J Orthop Trauma. 1992;6: 216–22.

This was a retrospective cohort study of 17 intra-articular calcaneal fractures treated operatively and 17 cases that were treated nonoperatively. Follow-up averaged 6.3 years and 5.4 years for the two groups, respectively. Outcome was assessed clinically. (Level III evidence [retrospective cohort])

Heier KA, Infante AF, Walling AK, Sanders RW. Open fractures of the calcaneus: soft tissue injury determines outcome. J Bone Joint Surg [Am]. 2003;85:2276–82.

This was a retrospective review of 503 open calcaneus fractures treated at one institution. Follow-up averaged 55 months, and outcome was determined by AOFAS scores and clinical examination. (Level IV evidence [case series])

Herscovici D Jr, Widmaier J, Scaduto JM, Sanders RW, Walling A. Operative treatment of calcaneal fractures in elderly patients. J Bone Joint Surg [Am]. 2005;87:1260–4.

This was a retrospective review of 44 fractures undergoing operative treatment. Follow-up averaged 44 months, and outcome was determined by SF-36 scores and clinical and radiographic examination. (Level IV evidence [case series])

Myerson MS, Juliano PJ, Koman JD. The use of a pneumatic intermittent impulse compression device in the treatment of calcaneus fractures. Mil Med. 2000;165:721–5.

This was a retrospective review of 55 patients treated with preoperative intermittent foot compression devices and then subsequent operative treatment. Outcome was determined by postoperative swelling examination and compartment pressure measurements. (Level IV evidence [case series])

Redfern DJ, Oliveira ML, Campbell JT, Belkoff SM. A biomechanical comparison of locking and nonlocking plates for the fixation of calcaneal fractures. Foot Ankle Int. 2006;27:196–210.

This was a cadaveric study of 10 pairs of cadaver feet re-created to have calcaneus fractures in which one foot was treated with a nonlocking plate and the other was treated with a locking plate. Outcome was determined by number of cycles to failure when cyclically loaded. (Level V evidence [cadaveric study])

Richter M, Gosling T, Zech S, Allami M, Geerling J, Droste P, Krettek C. A comparison of plates with and without locking screws in a calcaneal fracture model. Foot Ankle Int. 2005;26:309–19.

This was a sawbone study of seven pairs of feet re-created to have calcaneus fractures in which one set was treated with a plate without locking screws and another set was treated with a plate with locking screws. Outcome was determined by measurement of displacement upon cyclic loading. (Level V evidence [sawbone study])

Schildhauer TA, Bauer TW, Josten C, Muhr G. Open reduction and augmentation of internal fixation with an injectable skeletal cement for the treatment of complex calcaneal fractures. J Orthop Trauma. 2000;14:309–17.

This was a prospective cohort study of 30 patients treated with calcium phosphate cement augment after open reduction and internal fixation. Follow-up was 6 weeks, and outcome was measured by a calcaneal scoring system. (Level II evidence [prospective cohort])

Seibert CH, Hansen M, Wolter D. Follow-up evaluations of open intra-articular fractures of the calcaneus. Arch Orthop Trauma Surg. 1998;177:442–7.

This was a retrospective review of 35 patients treated for open intra-articular calcaneus fractures. Follow-up averaged 44 months, and outcome was determined by a modified Merle d'Aubigné functional score and a Zwipp radiographic score. (Level IV evidence [case series])

Thordarson DB, Bollinger M. SRS cancellous bone cement augmentation of calcaneal fracture fixation. Foot Ankle Int. 2005;26:347–52.

This was a retrospective review of 15 patients treated with open reduction and internal fixation and calcium phosphate cement augmentation for calcaneus fractures. Follow-up averaged 13 months for nine patients and less than 6 months for the remaining six patients. Outcome was determined by radiographic and clinical examination. (Level IV evidence [case series])

Thordarson DB, Greene N, Shepard Long House, Perlman M. Facilitating edema resolution with a foot pump after calcaneus fracture. J Orthop Trauma. 1999;13: 43–6.

This was a randomized control trial of 28 patients undergoing operative treatment for calcaneus fractures, with one group using a preoperative foot pump and other group not using a foot pump. Outcome was determined by volumetric changes of the foot. (Level I evidence [randomized control trial])

Thordarson DB, Krieger LE. Operative versus nonoperative treatment of intra-articular fractures of the calcaneus: a prospective randomized trial. Foot Ankle Int. 1996;17:2–9.

This was a randomized control trial of 30 patients who received operative versus nonoperative treatment of the calcaneus fractures. Follow-up averaged 17 and 14 months, respectively. Outcome was determined by a functional scoring system. (Level I evidence [randomized control trial])

Thornton SJ, Cheleuitte D, Ptaszek AJ, Early JS. Treatment of open intra-articular calcaneal fractures: evaluation of a treatment protocol based on wound location and size. Foot Ankle Int. 2006;27:317–25.

This was a retrospective review of the treatment of 29 patients with open calcaneus fractures. Outcome was determined by postoperative clinical examination. (Level IV evidence [case series])

Varela CD, Vaughan TK, Carr JB, Slemmons BK. Fracture blisters: clinical and pathological aspects. J Orthop Trauma. 1993;7:417–27.

This was a retrospective review of 51 patients who developed fracture blisters over a 3½-year period in four institutions. Blisters were examined clinically and pathologically. (Level IV evidence [case series])

PROCEDURE 45

Osteotomies for the Correction of Varus Ankle

Markus Knupp, Geert I. Pagenstert, Victor Valderrabano, and Beat Hintermann

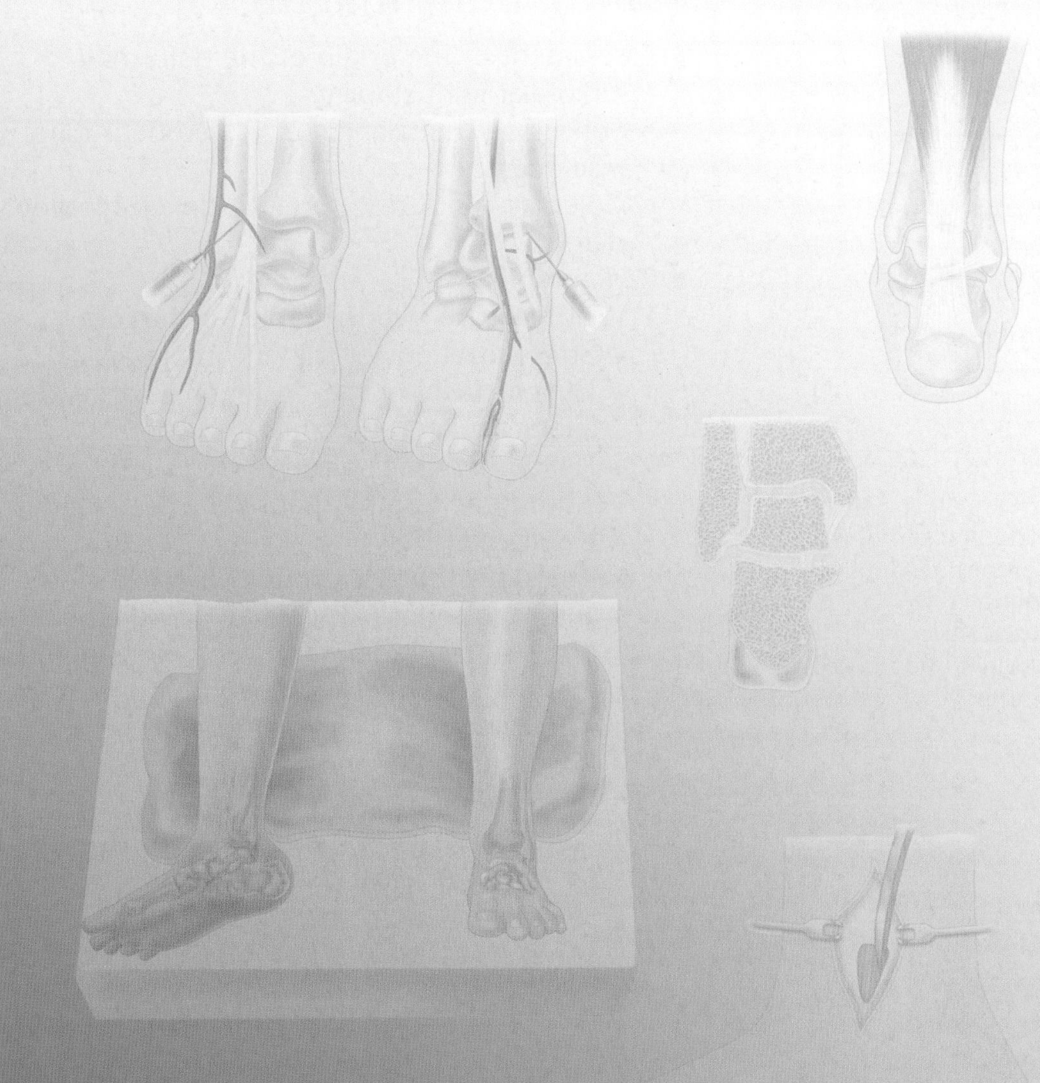

Pitfalls

- *Severe hindfoot instability ("floppy hindfoot")*
- *Severe vascular or neurologic deficiency in the affected extremity*
- *Neuropathic disorders (Charcot foot)*

Controversies

- Altered bone quality (medication, large cysts, osteopenia/osteoporosis)
- Age (>70 years)
- Insulin-dependent diabetes
- Tobacco use
- Rheumatic disease

Treatment Options

- Conservative treatment: shoe modifications, braces, physical therapy (peroneal tendon strengthening)
- Fusion or total ankle replacement in advanced stages of osteoarthritis

Indications

- Corrections of malaligned ankles with medial osteoarthritis
- Corrections of malunions after distal tibial fractures
- Realignment prior to total ankle replacement or fusion
- Corrections after malpositioned ankle fusions
- Osteochondritis dissecans (OCD) lesions

Examination/Imaging

- Assessment of the origin of the deformity
  - Tibiotalar joint stability
  - Soft tissue dysbalance (e.g., peroneus longus/brevis insufficiency)
  - Coleman block test: forefoot-driven hindfoot deformity?
- Radiographs
  - Weight-bearing radiographs of the foot
    - Stress reactions of the fifth metatarsal?
    - Hyperactivity of the posterior tibial tendon with talonavicular subluxation?
    - Flexed first metatarsal?
  - Weight-bearing radiographs of the ankle (including the Saltzman view)
    - Amount of the deformity: Figure 1 shows anteroposterior (AP) (Fig. 1A) and lateral (Fig. 1B) preoperative radiographs of a varus deformity in the tibiotalar joint with beginning joint space narrowing on the medial side of the ankle joint.
    - Extent of the degeneration (Takakura score).

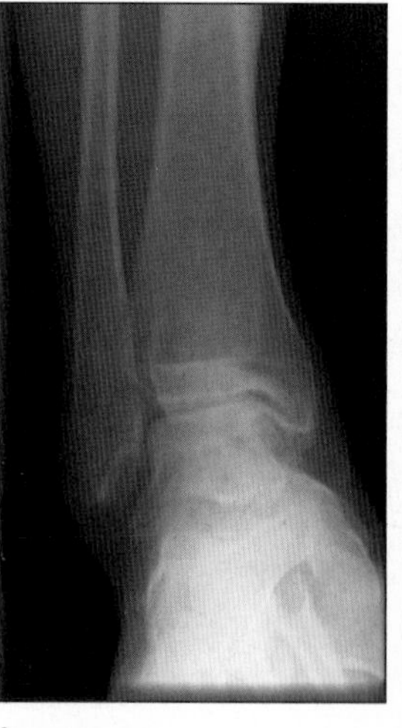
A

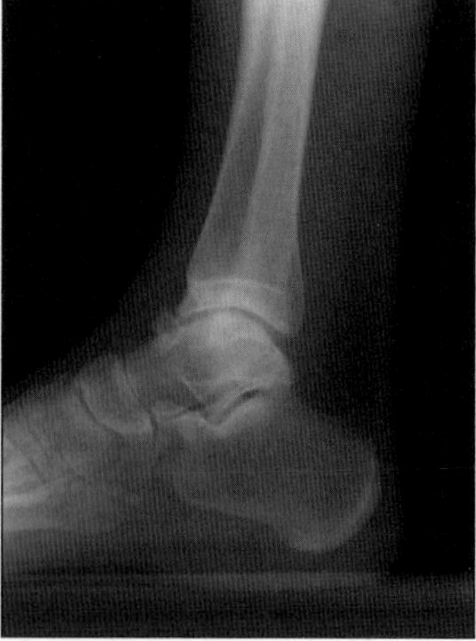
B

FIGURE 1

- Computed tomography scan, magnetic resonance imaging: not needed routinely
  - OCD lesions
  - Peroneal tendon disorder
  - Assessment of the ligaments (e.g., lateral insufficiency may indicate scarred/tight deltoid)

Surgical Anatomy

- Lateral approach (Fig. 2)
  - The sural nerve and the short saphenous vein run dorsal to the line of the incision and are usually not seen during this procedure.
    - In Figure 2, the sural nerve is running posterior to the incision line.
    - Sometimes the short saphenous vein can be seen running along the posterior border of the lateral malleolus before the limb is exsanguinated.
  - Extended proximal dissection may require exposure of the branches of the superficial peroneal nerve.
  - Cauterization of some of the branches of the peroneal artery, which lie deep to the medial surface of the distal fibula, may be necessary.
  - The proximal border of the syndesmosis marks the height of the fibula osteotomy.
- Lateral approach to the calcaneus
  - The sural nerve runs together with the short saphenous vein and may be located right under skin incision.
  - The peroneal tendons run superior to the incision under the superior and inferior peroneal retinaculum.

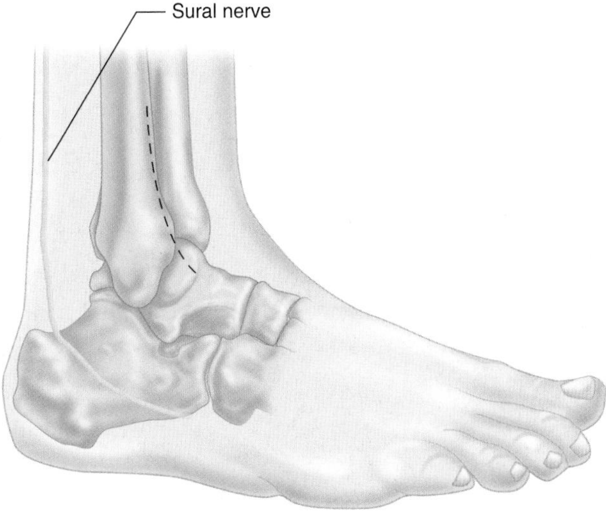

FIGURE 2

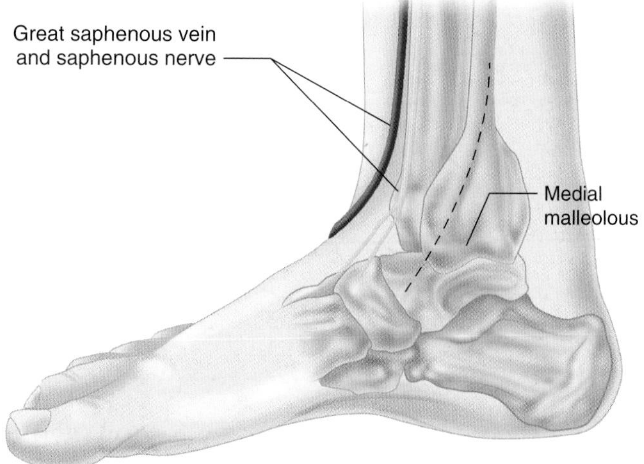

FIGURE 3

- Medial approach (Fig. 3)
  - The great saphenous vein and the saphenous nerve usually lie anterior to the incision.
  - The posterior tibial tendon runs immediately posterior to the medial malleolus under the tendon sheet.
- Anterior approach
  - The neurovascular bundle (deep peroneal nerve and the dorsalis pedis artery) lies lateral to the incision.
  - The ankle joint is covered by an extensive fat pad that contains a venous plexus requiring partial cauterization.

Positioning

- Lateral approach
  - The patient is placed in a lateral decubitus position or supine with a sandbag under the buttock of the affected limb.
  - After exsanguinating the leg, a pneumatic tourniquet is inflated on the thigh.
- Calcaneal osteotomy
  - The patient is placed supine on the operating table with a sandbag under the buttock.
  - Additionally, a support can be placed on the opposite iliac crest in order to tilt the table away from the surgeon to improve access.
- Medial approach
  - Place the patient supine on the operating table. The natural external rotation of the leg usually exposes the medial malleolus (Fig. 4).

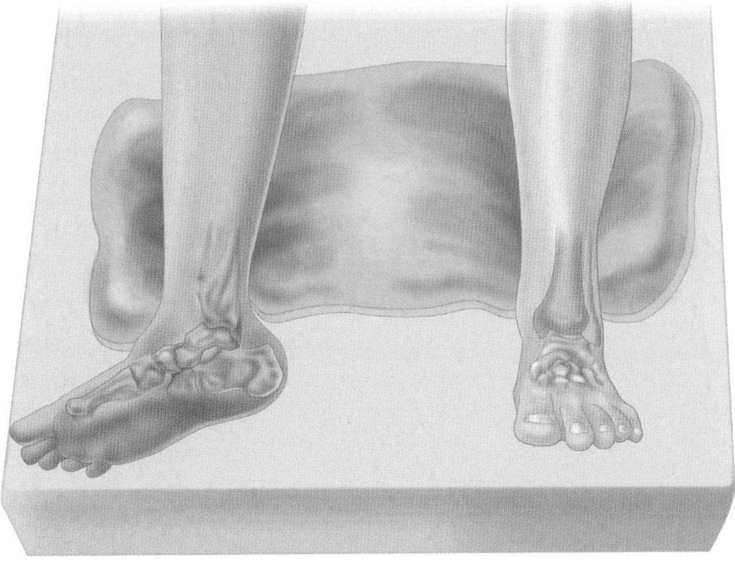

FIGURE 4

- Alternatively, the knee may be held in a slightly flexed position and the hip externally rotated.
- The limb is exsanguinated and the tourniquet inflated.

■ Anterior approach
- The patient is placed in a supine position with the heel at the edge of the table, allowing the surgeon to stand at the end of the operating table by the heel (Fig. 5).
- The limb is then exsanguinated and the thigh tourniquet inflated.

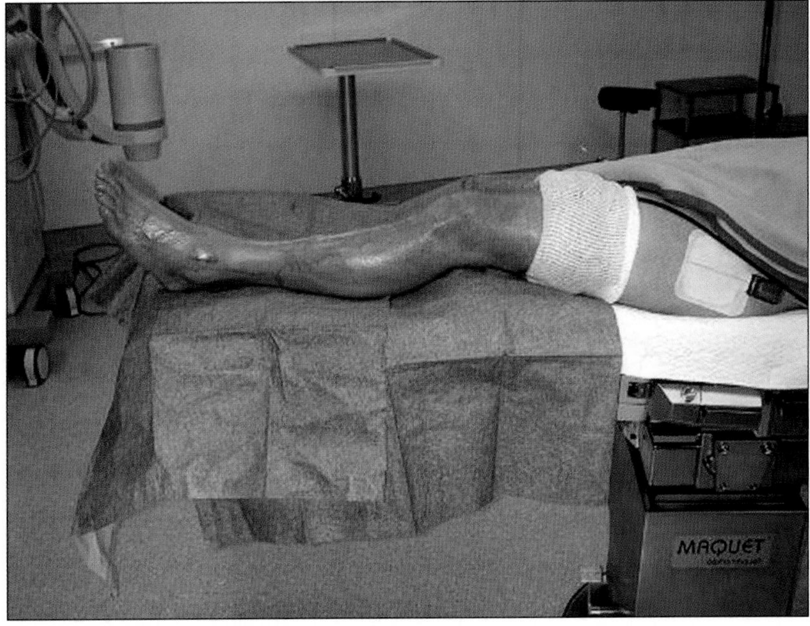

FIGURE 5

Portals/Exposures

- Lateral approach
  - A 10-cm longitudinal, slightly curved incision is made along the anterior margin of the distal fibula (see Fig. 2). If the incision needs to be extended distally, it is curved forward to end just distal and anterior of the lateral malleolus.
  - The fibula and the tibia are then exposed laterally without stripping the periosteum to avoid devascularization of the bone.
  - At the distal end of the incision, the anterior syndesmosis is exposed.
- Approach for the calcaneal osteotomy
  - A slightly curved incision is used to expose the lateral aspect of the calcaneus. The incision is placed about 1 cm posterior to the peroneus longus tendon, taking care not to damage the lateral dorsal cutaneous branch of the sural nerve.
  - The periosteum is then stripped from the lateral wall.
- Medial approach
  - A 10-cm longitudinal incision is made beginning over the medial malleolus and extending proximally over the distal tibia (see Fig. 3).
  - The skin flaps are mobilized, taking care not to damage the long saphenous vein and the sapheous nerve, which run together along the anterior border of the medial malleolus. The posterior tibial tendon is in danger during this procedure as it lies immediately posterior to the medial malleolus, and therefore needs to be exposed.
  - The tendon sheath is incised and the tendon retracted posteriorly in order to expose the posterior surface of the distal tibia. The distal tibia is then exposed without stripping of the periosteum.
- Anterior approach
  - A longitudinal incision is made between the tendons of the anterior tibial tendon and the extensor hallucis longus tendon, starting 10 cm proximal to the joint, about midway between the malleoli (Fig. 6). Care should be taken not to cut the skin incision too deeply to avoid damage to the underlying neurovascular bundle (deep peroneal nerve and dorsal pedis artery).

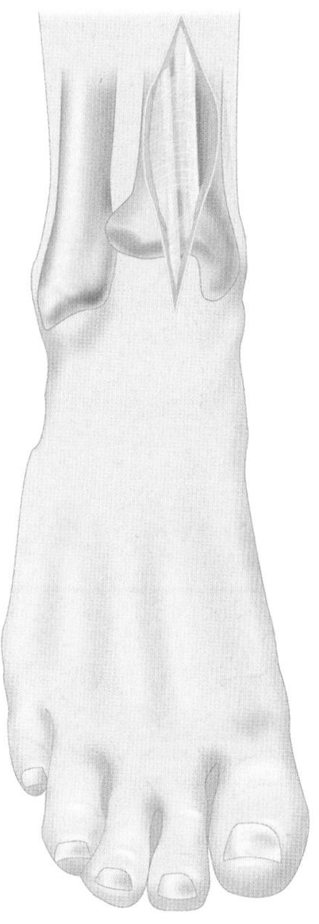

FIGURE 6

- After identifying the neurovascular bundle and retracting it laterally, the extensor retinaculum is cut in line with the skin incision between the anterior tibial tendon and the extensor hallucis longus tendon. The anterior tibial tendon is retracted medially and the tendon of the extensor hallucis longus laterally without opening the tendon sheaths.
- The anterior surface of the tibia can now be exposed after incising the remaining soft tissues longitudinally. The joint is usually covered by fatty tissue containing a venous plexus. As the approach for osteotomies is usually extra-articular, the joint itself is not exposed; however, sometimes it is necessary to cauterize some of the veins in the distal part of the incision.
- Now the distal tibia is exposed. Care is taken that the retractors on the medial side are placed beneath the posterior tibial tendon, which lies immediately posterior to the medial malleolus.

Procedure: Lateral Closing Wedge Osteotomy

Step 1

- In most cases in which a varus deformity is addressed with a lateral closing wedge osteotomy, the fibula needs to be shortened in order to preserve the congruency in the ankle joint. The shortening can be done by simple bone block removal or a Z-shaped osteotomy (Fig. 7). In Figure 7, the bone blocks that need to be removed for the shortening are highlighted.
- The length of the Z-osteotomy of the fibula is about 8–10 cm starting distally on the height of the anterior syndesmosis.
  - Kirschner wires (K-wires) can be placed on the height of the transverse cuts to be able to fluoroscopically check the localization of the osteotomy.
  - The osteotomy is done with an oscillating saw.
- After the fibula has been mobilized, bone blocks that are sized according to the amount of the planned shortening need to be resected on both ends.

Pearls

- *Due to the surrounding soft tissue, it may be easier to direct the proximal cut anteriorly and the distal cut posteriorly.*

Pitfalls

- *Simple bone block removal as opposed to the Z-osteotomy may lead to malpositioning (particularly rotational malunion) and provides less primary stability.*

Step 2

- The distal tibia is exposed anteriorly without stripping of the periosteum; consequently, K-wires are placed according to the preoperative planning (Fig. 8). Unless the deformity is located proximal to the supramalleolar area, the wires are directed from proximal of the anterior syndesmosis to the area of the former growth zone on the medial side.
- After fluoroscopic verification of the location of the wires (Fig. 9), the periosteum is incised and carefully mobilized with a scalpel or raspatorium.
- The osteotomy is then performed using an oscillating saw.

Pearls

- *Placing the wires in such a manner that they cross on the height of the medial cortex will prevent the saw from cutting a trough the entire bone and thereby preserve the medial cortex as a hinge.*

Pitfalls

- *Deformity correction in posttraumatic cases needs to be done at the center of rotation and angulation in order to avoid translational malpositioning.*
- *Great care needs to be taken not to accidentally cut the posterior tibial tendon. In some posttraumatic cases with extensive scarring on the posteromedial aspect of the ankle, it may be necessary to expose the tendon through a mini-incision in order to protect it.*

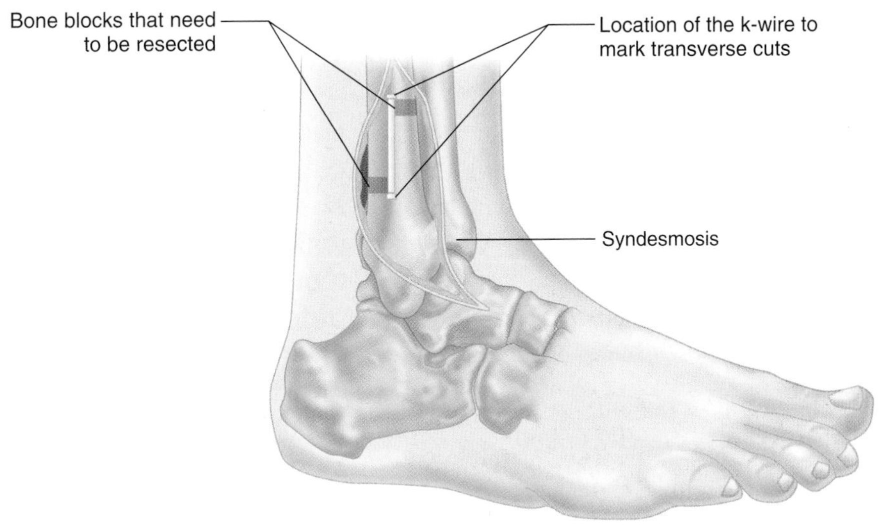

FIGURE 7

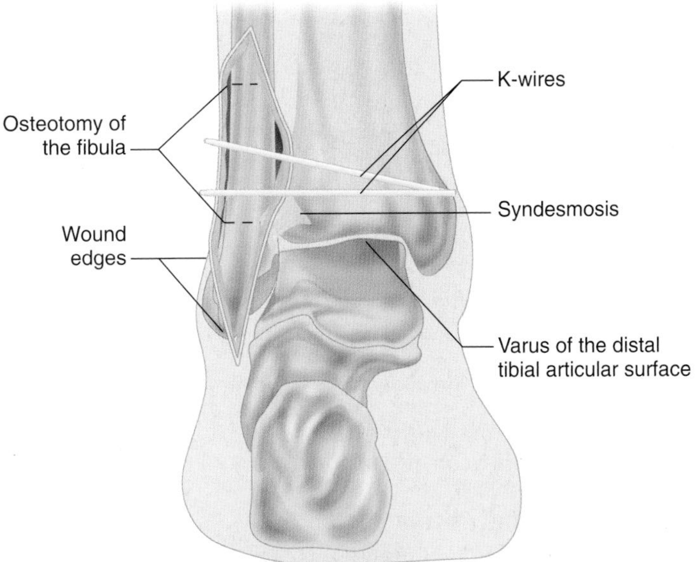

FIGURE 8

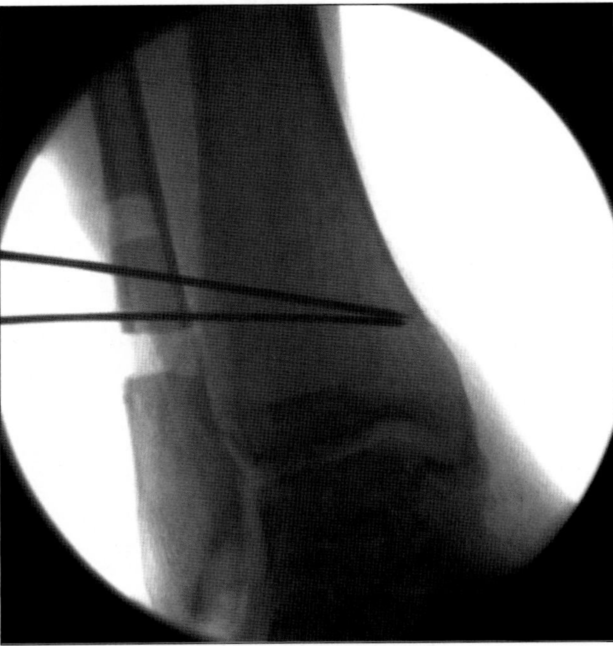

FIGURE 9

PEARLS

- *In order to get proper compression on the osteotomy, a tension device can be used. Alternatively, excentric drilling of the proximal screws will provide some compression.*
- *In rare cases the syndesmosis needs to be mobilized. For this purpose, the proximal attachment of the anterior syndesmosis is released from the tibia (anterior tibial tubercle of Tillaux-Chaput). The tubercle is mobilized using a chisel. After positioning of the fibula, it is reattached either with a screw and washer or with transosseous sutures.*
- *Use the image intensifier to verify that the correction is only done in the desired plane (e.g., simple varus corrections: only the frontal plane) and no accidental flexion or extension was added.*

PITFALLS

- *Osteotomy of the entire tibia: loss of the hinge on the medial side bears the risk of malpositioning (rotational/ translational) and secondary dislocation. Additional fixation (e.g., second plate in a second plane) should be considered.*

Instrumentation/ Implantation

- Plates that provide angular stability should be used in order to achieve good primary stability and prevent secondary dislocation.

STEP 3

- The osteotomy is then closed and the correction secured with a plate (Fig. 10). Care is taken to apply compression on the osteotomy when placing the plate.
- Next the periosteum is closed over the osteotomy with 2–0 absorbable sutures.
- Now the position of the fibula needs to be determined under the fluoroscan. Once the joint appears congruent, the fibula is secured with screws or a third tubular plate.
- Finally, the subcutaneous tissues and the skin are closed with interrupted sutures.
- Figure 11 shows AP (Fig. 11A) and lateral (Fig. 11B) radiographs 6 months after a lateral closing wedge osteotomy.

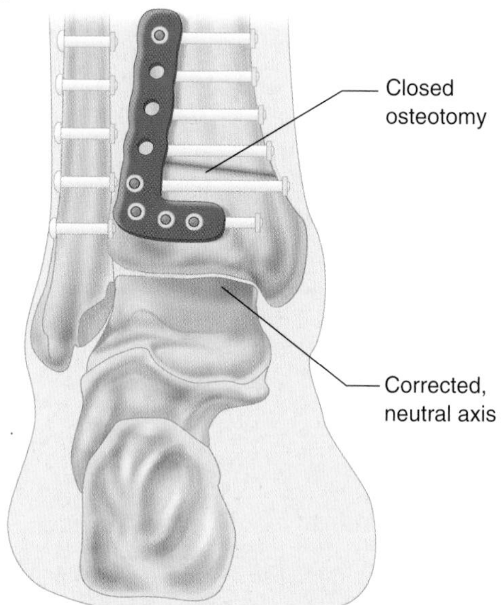

FIGURE 10

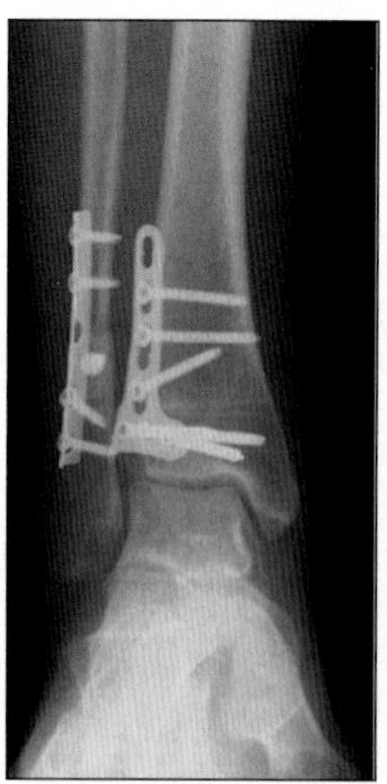

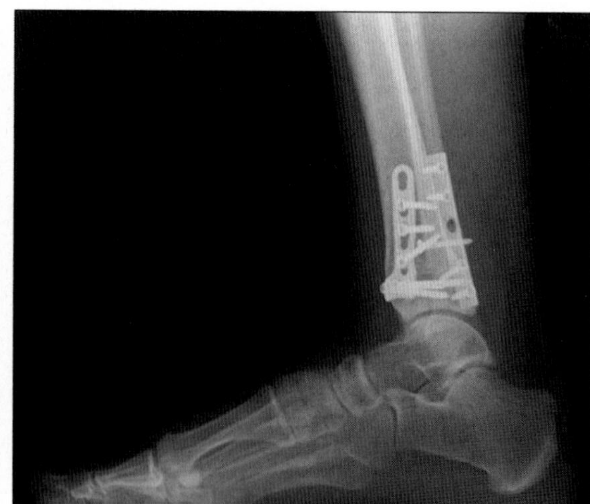

A B

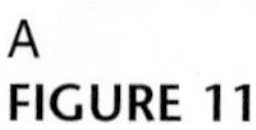

FIGURE 11

PEARLS

- *The cuts of the calcaneal osteotomy can be completed with an osteotome to avoid soft tissue damage.*
- *Tight soft tissue structures on the medial side may prevent mobilization. In these cases, the osteotomy can be mobilized with a distracter, such as a wide laminar spreader.*

PITFALLS

- *The skin over the calcaneal tuberosity is only slightly mobile; therefore, extensive displacement of a calcaneal osteotomy may put tension on the suture line and thereby interfere with wound healing. In these cases, removal of a larger bone wedge should be considered.*

Procedure: Z-Osteotomy of the Calcaneus

- Two Hohmann retractors are placed, one distally/plantarward in order to protect the plantar structures and one proximally on top of the posterior part of the tuberosity. This allows good exposure of the lateral calcaneal wall.
- Four K-wires are then used to mark the edges of the wedge to be removed. The horizontal part of the osteotomy is about 2 cm long and parallel to the plantar fascia.
  - The anterior vertical cut is made slightly anterior to the tuberosity.
  - The posterior cut is placed in the posterior half of the concavity of the tuberosity; care is taken not to place it too far posteriorly in order to avoid interference with the insertion of the Achilles tendon.
- The osteotomy is performed with an oscillating saw, taking care not to damage the medial soft tissue structures. The bone wedge is removed (Fig. 12) and the osteotomy mobilized.

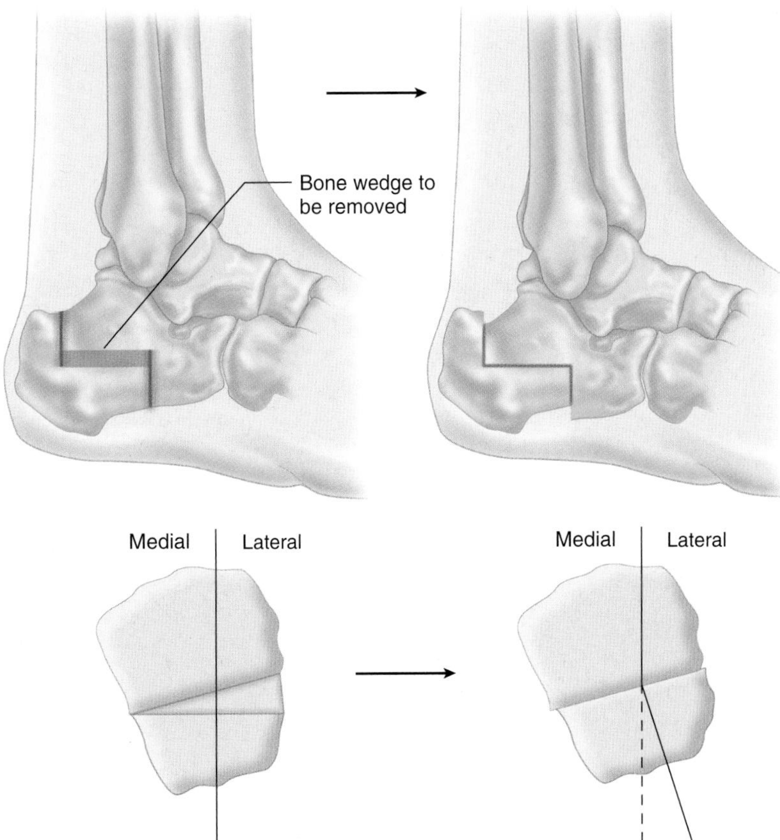

FIGURE 12

- After lateralization of the tuberosity and closing of the gap, the osteotomy is secured with a K-wire. The result is checked under the fluoroscan as well as clinically and finally fixed with a cannulated screw.
- The subcutaneous tissues and the skin are closed with interrupted sutures.

Procedure: Medial Opening Wedge Osteotomy

Step 1

- The plane of the osteotomy is determined under image intensification, and a K-wire is placed from the medial cortex into the area of the former growth plate, or on the height of the deformation in the case of a malunion (Fig. 13).
- The periosteum is then carefully incised at the level of the osteotomy and elevated from the bone using a scalpel or a raspatorium. Subsequently, the osteotomy is done using a wide saw blade.
- Now the correction can be done according to the preoperative planning. The gap can be filled with allograft (Tutoplast Spongiosa; Tutogen Medical GmbH, Neunkirchen, Germany) or iliac crest bone. Alternatively, plates with an integrated spacer (Puddu-plate; Arthrex, Naples, FL) may be used.

Pearls

- *Use a wide saw blade to avoid an uneven surface of the osteotomy.*

Instrumentation/ Implantation

- Alternatively, a chisel can be used instead of the oscillating saw. This will diminish the heat production during the cut.

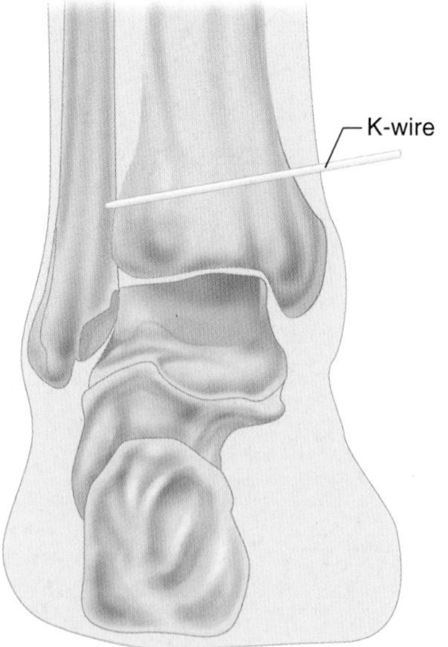

FIGURE 13

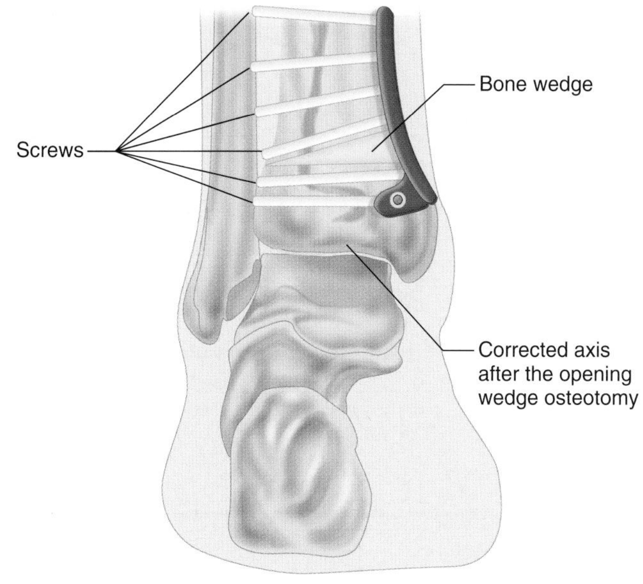

FIGURE 14

Pitfalls

- *If the tendon sheath of the posterior tibial tendon is closed too tightly, painful restrictions may result.*

Step 2

- Fixation of the correction is done with a plate similar to the lateral side (Fig. 14) (see Lateral Closing Wedge Osteotomy, Step 3).
- The tendon sheath of the posterior tibial tendon is adapted with 2–0 absorbable sutures, and the subcutaneous tissues and skin are closed with interrupted sutures.

Postoperative Care and Expected Outcomes

- Elevation of the leg and a compressive dressing and splint are maintained for 2 days.
- A short-leg non–weight-bearing cast is used for 6–8 weeks.
- If radiologic signs of consolidation are found after 6 weeks, partial weight bearing is allowed for an additional 2 weeks.
- A rehabilitation program for strengthening, gait training, and range of motion is begun 8 weeks postoperatively, with gradual return to full activities as tolerated.
- Reduction of radiologic and clinical signs of osteoarthritis with pain reduction and functional improvement can be expected.
- Potential complications
  - Over- or undercorrection: an overcorrection of 2–3° is recommended by most authors for asymmetric osteoarthritis.
  - Lateral impingement under the fibula after extensive correction: consider correction of the fibula.

Evidence

Cheng YM, Huang PJ, Hong SH, Liu SY, Liao CC, Chiang HC, Chen LC. Low tibial osteotomy for moderate ankle arthritis. Arch Orthop Trauma Surg. 2001;121:355–8.

This study evaluated 18 patients with primary and posttraumatic varus arthritis of the ankle joint. All patients were treated with an anteromedial opening wedge osteotomy in combination with a fibula osteotomy. (Level IV evidence)

Harstall R, Lehmann O, Krause F, Weber M. Supramalleolar lateral closing wedge osteotomy for the treatment of varus ankle arthrosis. Foot Ankle Int. 2007;28:542–8.

The authors presented their results on lateral closing wedge osteotomy, which was done in nine patients, finding pain relief and improved function. (Level IV evidence)

Knupp M, Horisberger M, Hintermann B. A new Z-shaped calcaneal osteotomy for 3-plane correction of severe varus deformity of the hindfoot. Tech Foot Ankle Surg. 2008;7:90-5.

Description of the Z-osteotomy in detail, with preliminary results in 18 consecutive patients. (Level IV evidence)

Malerba F, De Marchi F. Calcaneal osteotomies. Foot Ankle Clin. 2005;10:523–40.

A description of the operative technique of the scarf-shaped calcaneal osteotomy. (Level V evidence)

Pagenstert G, Hintermann B, Barg A, Leumann A, Valderrabano V. Realignment surgery as alternative treatment of varus and valgus ankle osteoarthritis. Clin Orthop Relat Res. 2007;(462):156–68.

The authors presented their data on corrective osteotomies in posttraumatic asymmetric osteoarthritis of the ankle joint. Of the 35 cases, 13 patients had a varus deformity that was treated with medial opening wedge osteotomy in seven cases and with lateral closing wedge osteotomy in six cases. (Level IV evidence)

Takakura Y, Takaoka T, Tanaka Y, Yajima H, Tamai S. Results of opening-wedge osteotomy for the treatment of a post-traumatic varus deformity of the ankle. Bone Joint Surg [Am]. 1998;80:213–8.

The authors evaluated five posttraumatic cases of varus osteoarthritis in the ankle joint. All patients were treated with a medial opening wedge osteotomy in combination with an oblique fibula osteotomy. (Level IV evidence)

Takakura Y, Tanaka Y, Kumai T, Tamai S. Low tibial osteotomy for osteoarthritis of the ankle: results of a new operation in 18 patients. J Bone Joint Surg [Br]. 1995;77:50–4.

The authors presented 18 cases of primary osteoarthritis in the tibiotalar joint with a varus malalignment of the hindfoot. Five were treated with a dorsolateral closing wedge, 1 with an oblique wedge, and 12 with an anteromedial opening wedge osteotomy. (Level IV evidence)

Weil LS Jr, Roukis TS. The calcaneal scarf osteotomy: operative technique. J Foot Ankle Surg. 2001;40:178–82.

The authors reported on 22 cases in which a Z-shaped calcaneal scarf osteotomy was performed in a fashion similar to that described in this chapter. The osteotomy was carried out in patients with acquired adult flatfoot deformity as an alternative treatment to a double osteotomy of the calcaneus (e.g., a medial displacement calcaneal osteotomy and an Evans procedure). (Level IV evidence)

PROCEDURE 46

Tarsal Tunnel Syndrome

Carol Frey

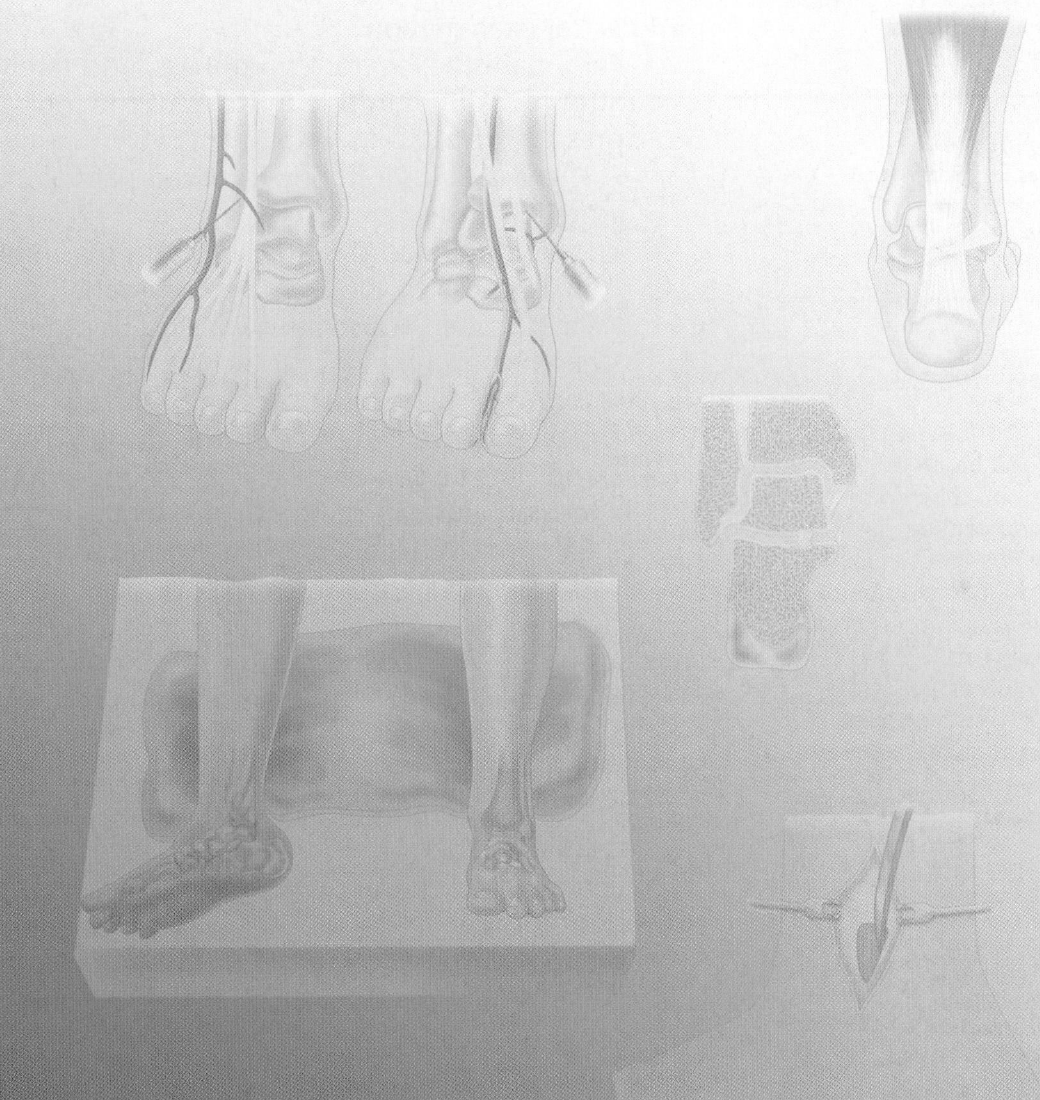

PITFALLS

- *Failure to remove a space-occupying lesion.*
- *Failure to note that a patient has a significant valgus deformity of the hindfoot that can contribute to the nerve pathology.*
- *Failure to rule out stress fracture of the calcaneus, inflammatory arthritis, herniated disc, plantar fasciitis, and peripheral neuropathy.*
- *In contrast to carpal tunnel syndrome, tarsal tunnel syndrome is less common, symptoms are more vague and intermittent, and diagnosis is more difficult.*

Controversies

- Patients with space-occupying lesions do the best.
- Decompression may not alter the condition of the nerves.
- Stabilization of the foot in a corrected position may be the only way to decompress and relieve tension on the nerve.
- Nerve decompression of the tarsal tunnel may not produce the long-term favorable results seen in other nerve decompressions.

Treatment Options

- Anti-inflammatory medication
- Shock-absorbing midsole in the shoes
- Rest
- For patients with increased valgus of the hindfoot, an orthotic device used to support the medial longitudinal arch and decrease stretch on the nerve may alleviate symptoms.

Indications

- Patient with a space-occupying lesion such as lipoma, ganglion cyst, neoplasm, varicosities, accessory flexor digitorum longus muscle, neurilemmoma, or exostosis in the tarsal tunnel
- Unresponsive to conservative treatment after 3 months of treatment
- If symptoms persist longer than 6 months

Examination/Imaging

- Physical examination
  - Pain, paresthesias, foot numbness, and rarely atrophy of the intrinsic muscles of the foot are present.
    - There is diffuse, poorly localized pain along the medial ankle.
    - Paresthesia and dysesthesia along the medial ankle and into the arch are common.
    - Pain is often worse after walking or other exercise and may occur at night.
    - Pain may be reproduced when the ankle is placed in the extremes of dorsiflexion. Eversion and dorsiflexion place the nerve under more tension and can bring out the symptoms.
    - Pain may radiate along the plantar aspect of the foot and may go up the calf, but will not radiate above the knee.
  - A positive Tinel's sign behind the medial malleolus is possible, but usually there is only percussive tenderness along the nerve.
  - Manual compression of the nerve in the tarsal tunnel may reproduce the symptoms after 30 seconds.
  - Percussion over the nerve may reproduce the symptoms.
  - Decreased sensation in the distribution of the tibial nerve on the plantar aspect of the foot may be present.
- Radiography
  - Standard anteroposterior and lateral radiographs of the foot are necessary to rule out bone pathology, but are usually normal.
  - Look for stress fractures of the calcaneus and exostosis in the region of the tarsal tunnel.

- Electromyography (EMG)
  - EMG is positive approximately 80% of the time. Look for a prolonged distal motor latency and fibrillation in the abductor hallucis.
  - A positive or negative EMG or nerve conduction study does not always correlate with intraoperative findings.
- Magnetic resonance imaging (MRI)
  - MRI is recommended in symptomatic children and in operative candidates.
  - MRI can identify space-occupying lesions, varicose veins, exostosis, accessory muscles, and ganglions. For example, MRI of the tarsal tunnel can reveal varicosities (Fig. 1A), flexor hallucis longus tenosynovitis (Fig. 1B), and neurilemmoma (Fig. 1C).
  - The information provided by MRI enhances surgical planning and indicates the extent of decompression required and the need to examine the contents of the tarsal tunnel fully.

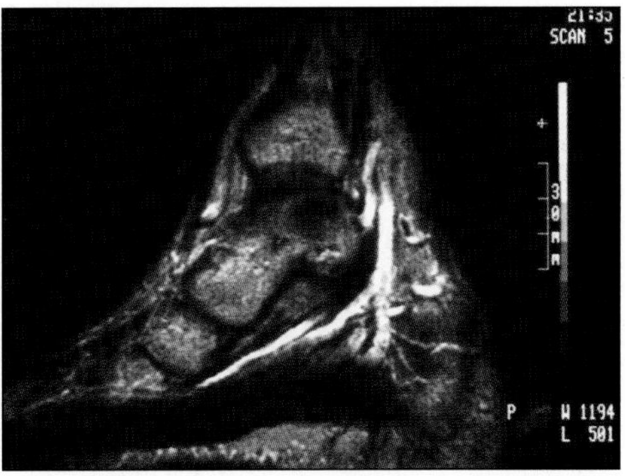

A

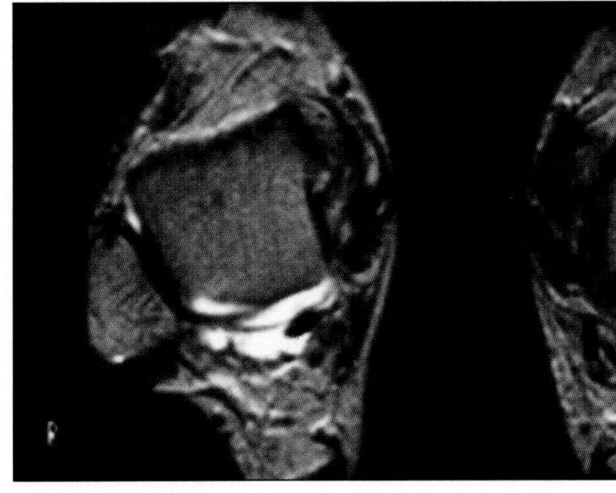

B

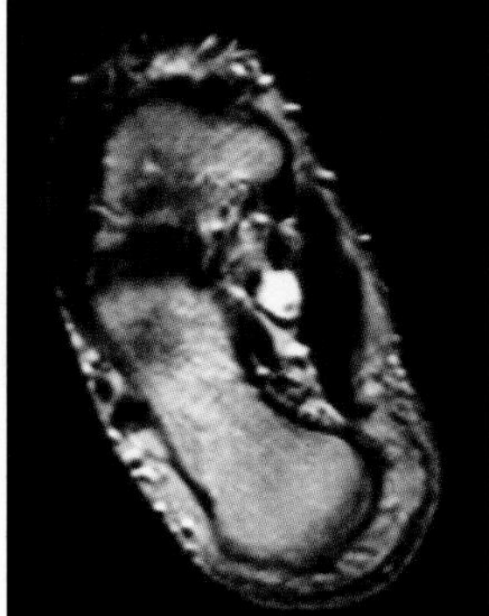

C

FIGURE 1

Surgical Anatomy

- The medial ankle tendons and the posterior tibial neurovascular bundle pass through the tarsal tunnel.
  - The tunnel extends from the level of the medial malleolus to the plantar aspect of the navicular bone (Fig. 2).
  - The tunnel has an osseous floor and a roof that is formed by the deep fascia of the leg, the flexor retinaculum, and distally the abductor hallucis muscle (Fig. 3A).

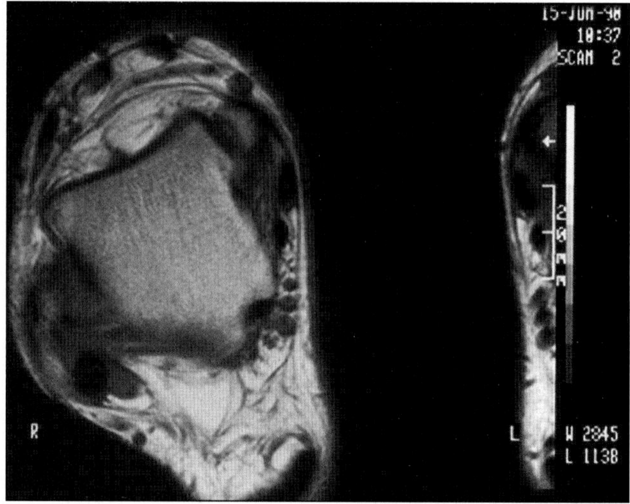

FIGURE 2

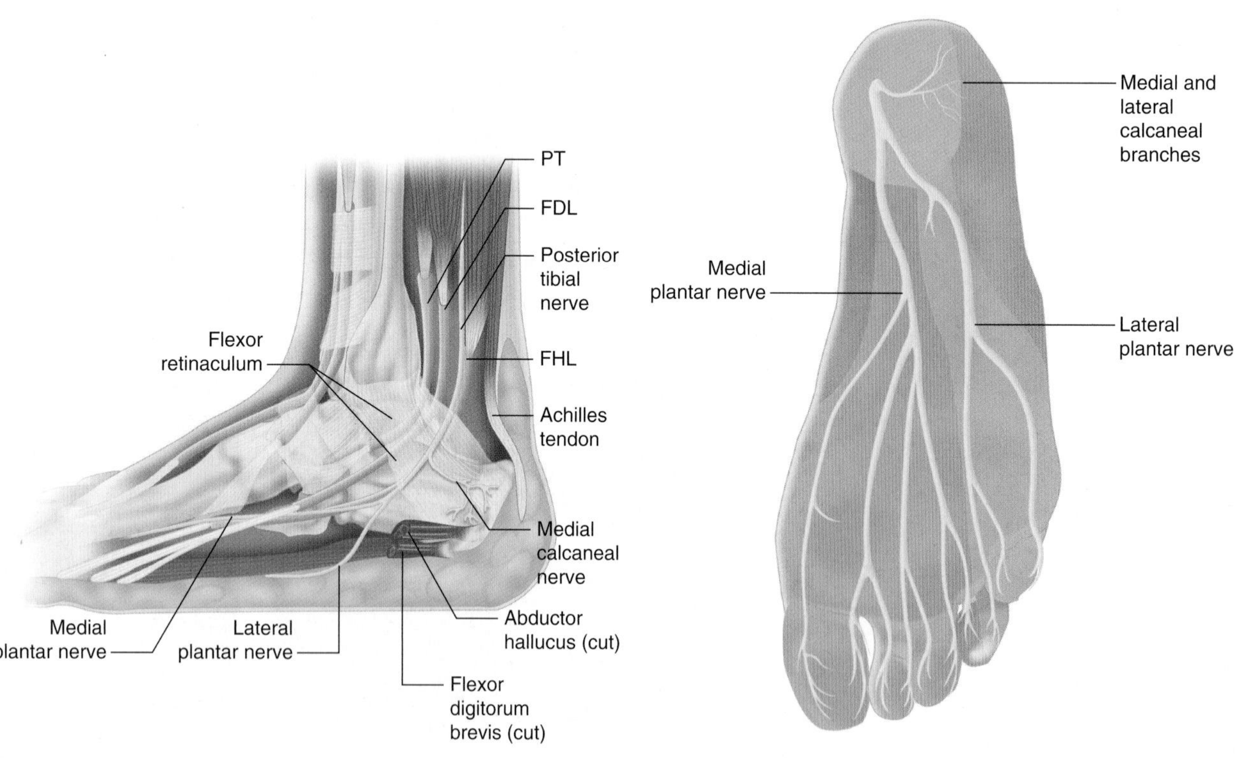

FIGURE 3

- The tunnel is divided into two parts: upper tibiotalar tunnel and lower talocalcaneal tunnel.

- The flexor retinaculum is a thick continuation of the deep fascia and extends in a fanlike pattern from the medial malleolus to the medial surface of the calcaneus, enclosing the tendons and neurovascular structures that pass through the tarsal tunnel.
  - The proximal and distal borders of the flexor retinaculum blend proximally with the deep fascia of the leg and distally with the dorsal aponeurosis of the foot.
  - Compressive lesions may be observed proximal to the flexor retinaculum, under the deep fascia of the leg and distal under the abductor hallucis muscle.
- The medial calcaneal nerve arises beneath the flexor retinaculum or proximal to it with equal frequency. Bifurcation into the medial and lateral plantar nerves typically occurs beneath the flexor retinaculum.
- The medial plantar nerve is in close proximity to the flexor hallucis longus tendon, posteromedial to it.
- The lateral plantar nerve is between the abductor hallucis and the quadratus plantar muscles and then travels lateral along the sole of the foot inferior to the quadratus plantar muscle and superior to the flexor digitorum brevis muscle (Fig. 3B).
  - The first branch of the lateral plantar nerve supplies the abductor digiti quinti and deep sensory innervation.
  - The nerve runs deep to the deep fascia of the abductor hallucis and then runs lateral and transverse and superficial to the quadratus plantar muscle, on its way to innervate the abductor digiti quinti.

Positioning

- The patient is placed in the supine position, with a bump under the opposite hip.
- A thigh tourniquet is utilized.
- General or regional anesthesia may be used.

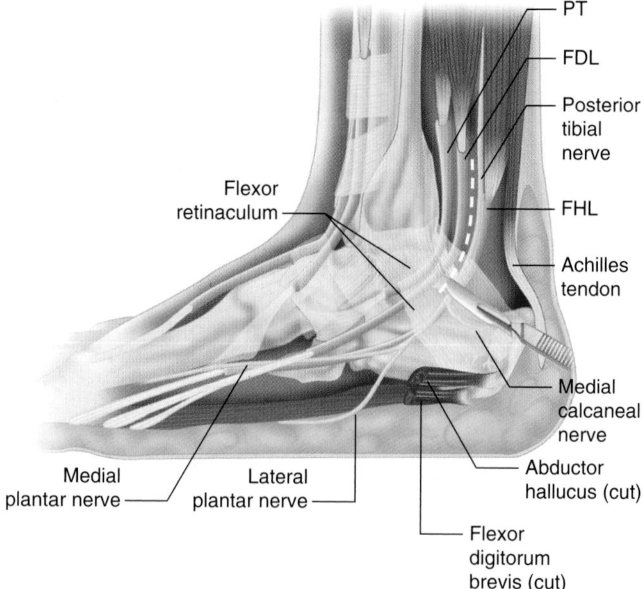

FIGURE 4

Instrumentation

- Bipolar electrocautery
- Pneumatic thigh tourniquet
- Loupe magnification if smaller branches are involved
- Standard foot/soft tissue tray

Controversies

- The first branch of the lateral plantar nerve is best exposed by superior retraction of the abductor hallucis, and in some cases the muscle must be mobilized or divided to adequately expose the nerve.
- The medial calcaneal nerve innervates the plantar medial aspect of the heel and lies superficial to the abductor hallucis.
- If there is valgus of the heel, the medial calcaneal nerve may be involved in the entrapment.

Portals/Exposures

- The posterior tibial nerve is exposed through a curved medial incision that extends from above the medial malleolus to the superior margin of the abductor hallucis muscle.
- The incision is centered over the tarsal tunnel (Fig. 4).

Procedure

Step 1

- An incision begins 6 cm above the tip of the medial malleolus and extends along the distal course of the nerve. This is approximately 2 cm posterior to the medial malleolus. Distally, it follows the course of the lateral plantar nerve as it courses plantar and more anterior.
- Dissection is made through the skin, and careful dissection is made down to the flexor retinaculum and crural fascia.
- The posterior tibial nerve, artery, and vein are present in a sheath that exists posterior to the sheaths of the posterior tibial and flexor digitorum longus tendons.
- The nerve is identified above the retinaculum. This is usually a safe level to begin identification of the nerve.
- The flexor retinaculum is incised with curved, blunt-tipped scissors (Fig. 5A). Alternatively, a smooth elevator may be passed deep to the retinaculum and a sharp release used (Fig. 5B).

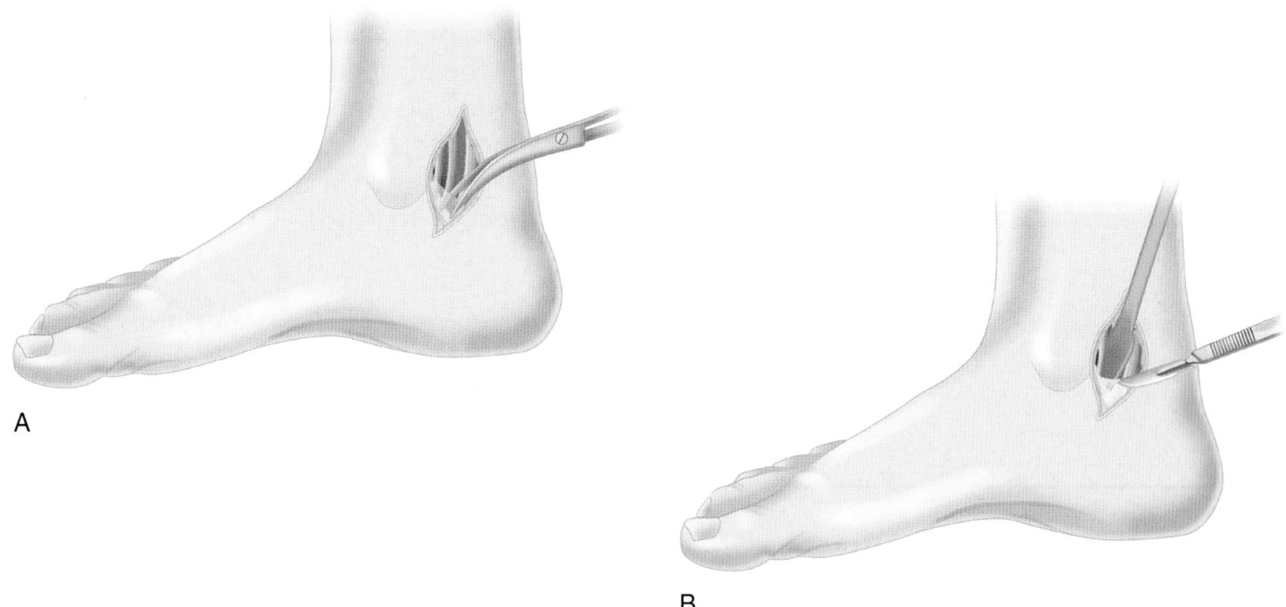

FIGURE 5

- Any space-occupying lesions, such as the neurilemmoma causing tarsal tunnel syndrome shown in Figure 6, are excised.
- The nerve may show thickening or fusiform dilation.

PEARLS

- *Internal neurolysis is avoided. It may lead to perineural fibrosis.*
- *The abductor hallucis is commonly a source of compression; it should be routinely released.*

Step 2

- The dissection is carried distally to the superior margin of the abductor hallucis.
- The posterior tibial nerve is traced distally and decompressed.
- Constricting vascular bands and varicosities may be present. They should be ligated.
- A simple release of the nerve is undertaken.

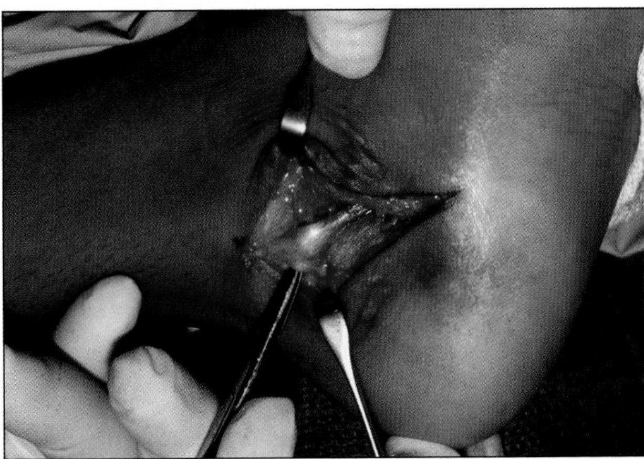

FIGURE 6

- Most commonly the nerve divides into the medial and lateral plantar nerves before it reaches the superior margin of the abductor hallucis (Fig. 7A–D).
- The lateral and medial plantar nerves should be released of investing fibrous bands that encircle the nerve and form compartments as the nerve courses to the plantar aspect of the foot.

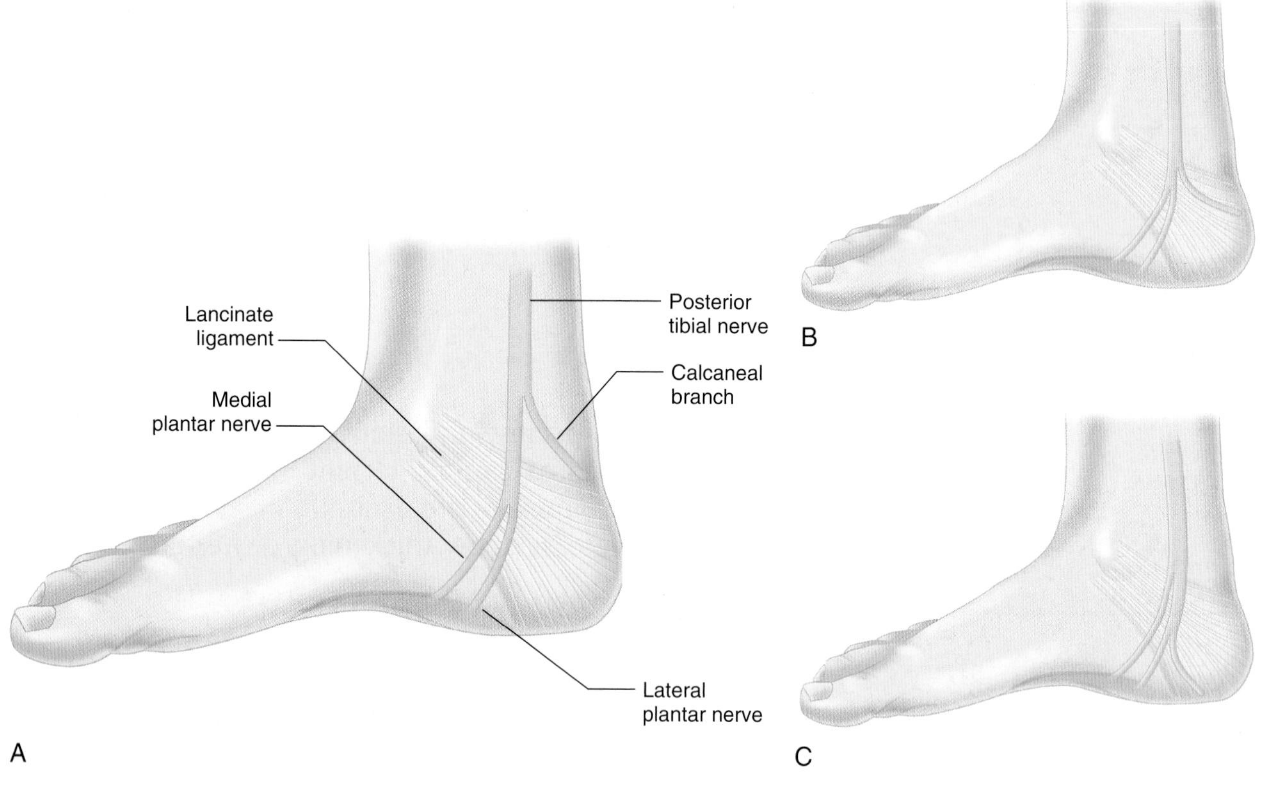

FIGURE 7

Step 3

- The muscle belly of the abductor hallucis is mobilized and retracted inferiorly with a small right-angle retractor (Fig. 8).
- Superior and deep fascia of abductor muscle are identified and sharply divided.
- The first branch of the lateral plantar nerve is seen deep to the abductor hallucis muscle in this location (Fig. 9), and care is taken to protect it.
- The muscle is then retracted superiorly along with the medial and lateral plantar nerves and their branches.
- The lateral plantar nerve and its first branch lie between the plantar quadratus and the flexor digitorum brevis. There may be fascial bands in this location that need to be released.
- The medial and lateral plantar nerves should have free passage into the plantar aspect of the midfoot. Manual probing should confirm this.

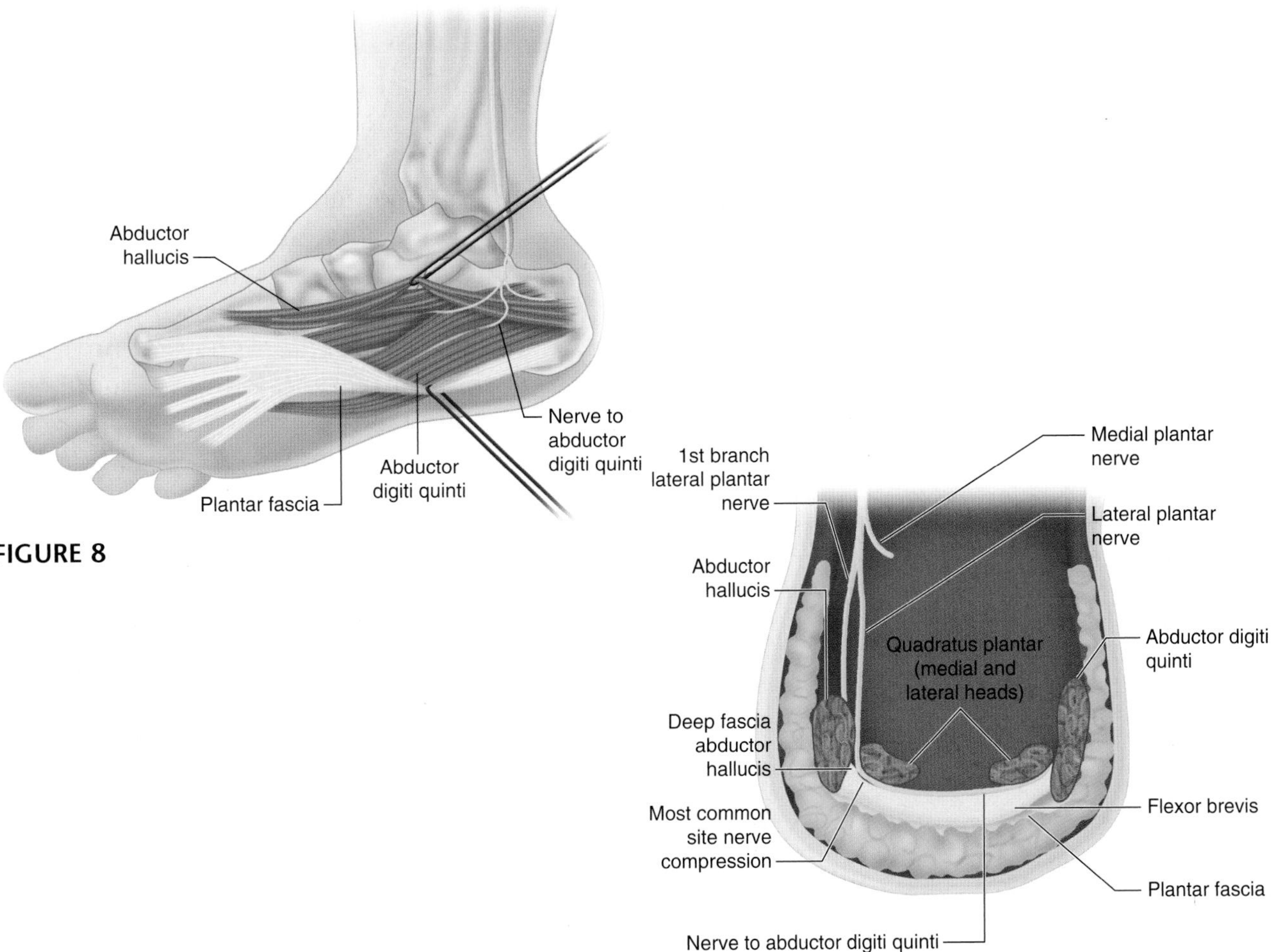

FIGURE 8

FIGURE 9

Step 4

- The tourniquet is deflated and hemostasis is obtained.
- The flexor retinaculum is not repaired.
- The subcutaneous layer is closed with 3–0 absorbable sutures.
- The skin is closed with 4–0 nylon.
- The patient is placed in a padded dressing with a posterior splint in neutral.

Postoperative Care and Expected Outcomes

- The patient should remain non–weight bearing during the inflammatory phase, approximately 7 days.
- Sutures are removed at 2 weeks, and gentle active range of motion and physical therapy modalities are started.
- The patient is kept in a walking boot for 2 additional weeks.
- The patient is advised to wear a night splint to prevent adhesions around the medial ankle structures.
- Outcome
  - Results indicate that the percussive tenderness, Tinel's sign, and abnormal nerve conduction studies will improve in 85% of patients.
  - Around 50% of patients will report nearly complete or complete resolution of symptoms.
  - If a specific cause or impinging lesion is identified, postoperative results are better.

Evidence

Frey C, Kerr R. Magnetic resonance imaging and the evaluation of tarsal tunnel syndrome. Foot Ankle Int. 1993;14:159–64.

In this study, 88% of the symptomatic patients had positive findings on MRI. MRI revealed an inflammatory or mass lesion in the tarsal tunnel in the majority of cases. There were 33 patients with 40 involved extremities in the study. (Level V evidence)

Gondring WH, Sheilds B, Wenger S. An outcome analysis of surgical treatment of tarsal tunnel syndrome. Foot Ankle Int. 2003;24:545–50.

The authors evaluated outcomes in 60 patients with tarsal tunnel syndrome. All the patients had preoperative findings of a positive Tinel's sign and abnormal nerve conduction studies. Postoperative results revealed 85% of patients had resolution of the Tinel's sign. In nerve conduction studies, 51% reported complete or near-complete subjective improvement in their symptoms. (Level I evidence)

Keck C. The tarsal-tunnel syndrome. J Bone Joint Surg [Am]. 1962;44:180–2.

This case report described the features of tarsal tunnel syndrome in a 20-year-old male army recruit. The syndrome was commonly misdiagnosed at the time this article was written. This is a classic article. (Level III evidence)

Kinoshita M, Ryuzo O, Morikawa J, Tsuyoshi J, Muneaki A. The dorsiflexion-eversion test for diagnosis of tarsal tunnel syndrome. J Bone Joint Surg [Am]. 2001; 83:1835–9.

The authors described a new diagnostic test in which the tibial nerve is compressed as it courses under the flexor retinaculum. The ankle is passively and maximally everted and dorsiflexed while all of the metatarsophalangeal joints are maximally dorsiflexed and held in position for 5–10 seconds. Local tenderness was intensified with this position in 42 of 43 feet. (Level V evidence)

Nagaoka M, Satou K. Tarsal tunnel syndrome caused by ganglia. J Bone Joint Surg [Br]. 1999;81:607–10.

The authors described 30 feet with tarsal tunnel syndrome secondary to a ganglion. Swellings that were not palpable were picked up on ultrasound. Most of the ganglions came from the talocalcaneal joint, and five were associated with a coalition of that joint. Surgical treatment was satisfactory in all but one patient. (Level III evidence)

PROCEDURE 47

Anterior Ankle Impingement

Carol Frey

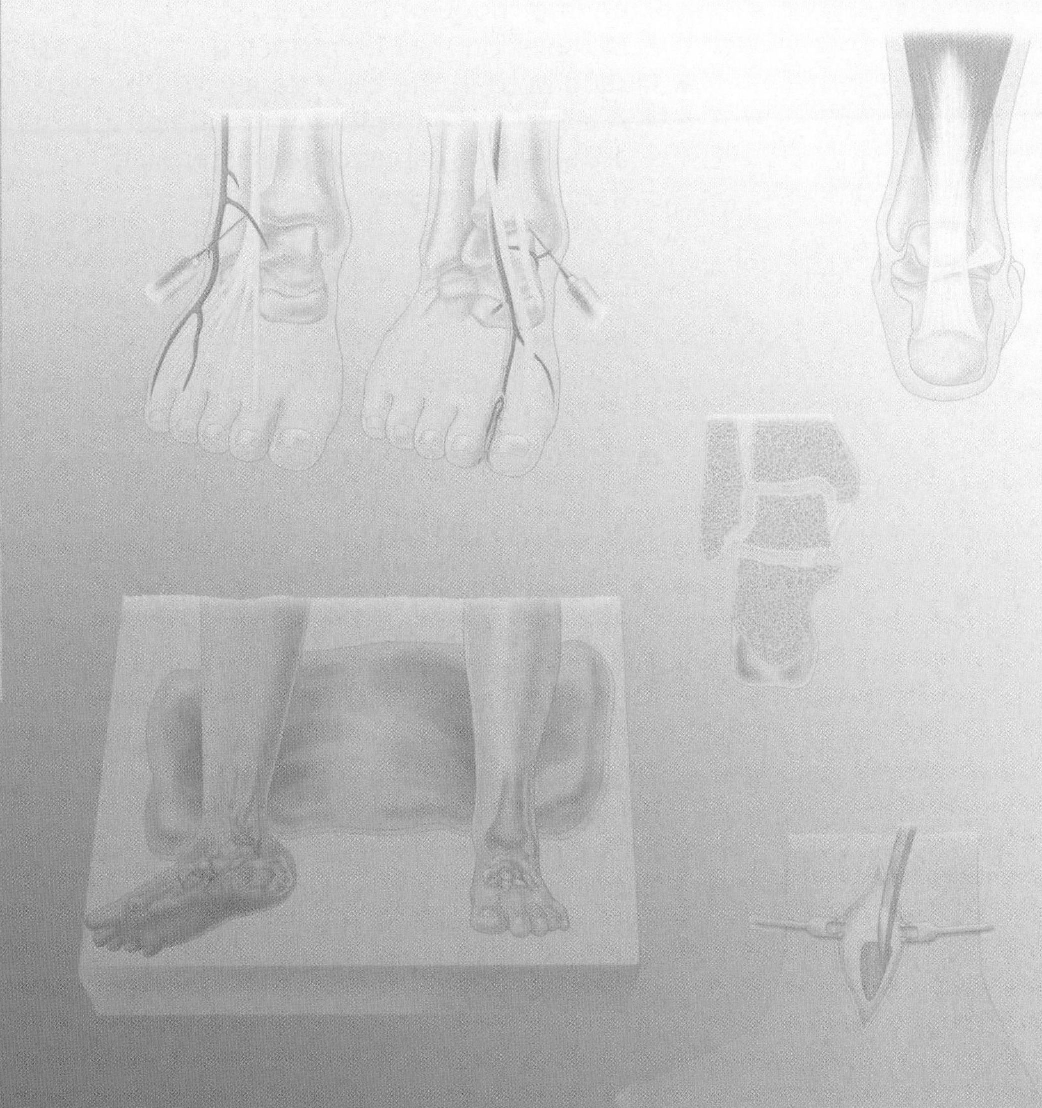

PITFALLS

- *Anterior tibial spurs are usually asymptomatic.*

Controversies

- Anterior spurs may be part of an early degenerative process in the ankle joint.

Treatment Options

- Heel lift
- Anti-inflammatory medication

Indications

- Painful anterior tibial spurs
- Persistent anterior ankle pain
- Loss of dorsiflexion

Examination/Imaging

- Physical examination will reveal anterior ankle pain, exacerbated by forced dorsiflexion of the ankle.
  - Localized tenderness may be present along the anterior ridge of the tibia.
  - Dorsiflexion may be restricted.
- Radiographs in the early stages may be negative.
  - A lateral radiograph may reveal the spur, as in the ankle with an anterior tibial spur with fragmentation seen in Figure 1.
  - A forced dorsiflexion lateral radiograph may confirm anterior impingement.
  - The talus may show secondary dorsal spur formation.
- Magnetic resonance imaging will often show cartilage hyperplasia and soft tissue reaction, in addition to the osteophyte.

Surgical Anatomy

- The distal tibia is concave in the sagittal plane and convex in the coronal plane.
- The anterior tibial rim is slightly convex with a medial notch, which recedes proximally for 3–5 mm, near the junction of the medial malleolus.
- The medial malleolus is about 2 cm anterior to the lateral malleolus.
- In any position, the tibial plafond covers only two thirds of the talar articular surface, as seen in the sagittal cross-section of a cadaver limb through the distal tibia and ankle joint shown in Figure 2.
- The superficial peroneal nerve and its branches are at risk with the placement and use of the anterolateral portal.
- The saphenous vein and nerve run along the anterior border of the medial malleolus and are near the anteromedial portal.

PEARLS

- *Noninvasive distraction is recommended for this procedure to allow for better access to the spur and to prevent cartilage damage.*

PITFALLS

- *Care must be taken not to excessively distract the joint as this will pull the synovium and capsule tight up against the spur and make visualization and access difficult.*

Positioning

- A standard arthroscopic set-up for an ankle arthroscopy is utilized (Fig. 3).
- A tourniquet is recommended.

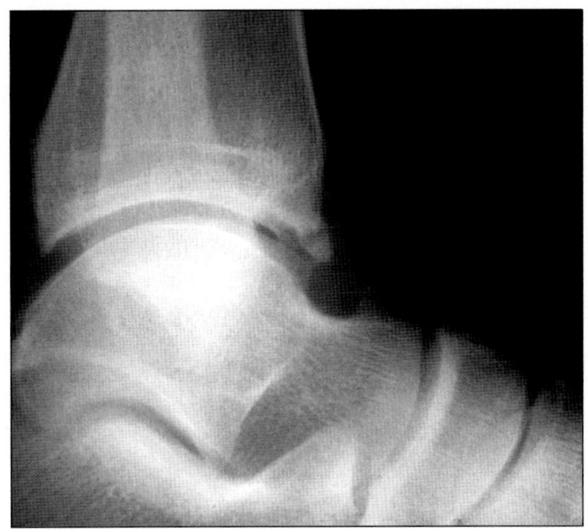

FIGURE 1

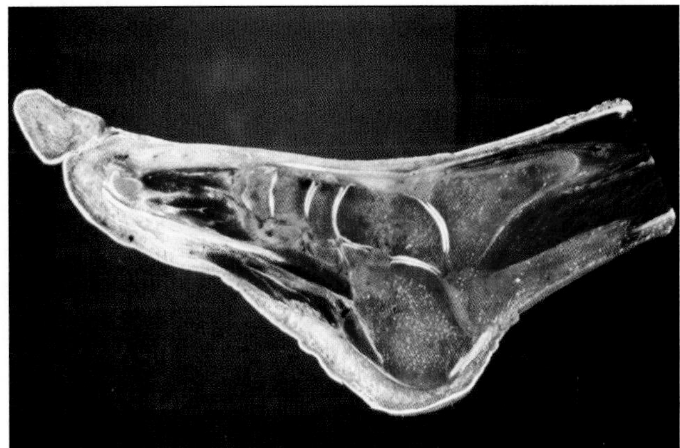

FIGURE 2

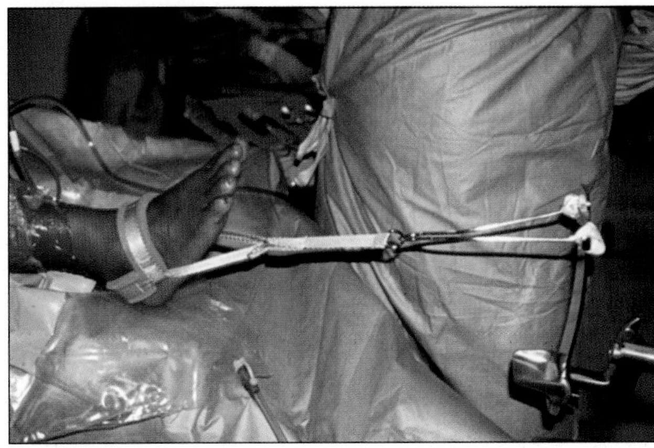

FIGURE 3

PEARLS

- *Dorsiflexion and plantar flexion may be necessary to visualize the impinging structures.*
- *Excessive synovium is cleared away with a 4.0-mm full-radius power shaver or radiofrequency wand.*
- *Posterior portals are not necessary for the removal of anterior spurs on the talus and tibia.*

PEARLS

- *Interchangeable cannulas are useful to maintain arthroscopic portal access and decrease extravasation of fluid, as well as prevent unnecessary trauma to the soft tissues from repeated instrument placement.*

Portals/Exposures

- Mark the anatomic landmarks, including structures at risk: superficial peroneal nerve and saphenous nerve.
- The anterolateral and anteromedial portals are utilized for the treatment of anterior ankle impingement (Fig. 4).
  - The anterolateral portal is placed just lateral to the peroneus tertius, entering the joint between the fibula and the talus just distal to the joint line.
  - The anteromedial portal is located at the level of the joint line just medial to the tibialis anterior tendon.

Procedure

STEP 1

- A 2.7-mm arthroscope, high-flow system, and an arthroscopic pump are utilized for this procedure.
- Excessive synovium is cleared away with a full-radius power shaver or radiofrequency wand.
- The spur is visualized and removed with a 4.0-mm power burr.
  - Figures 5 and 6 show arthroscopic views of two ankles with spurs at the anterior ridge of the distal tibia, before (Fig. 5A and Fig. 6A) and after (Fig. 5B and Fig. 6B) débridement.
- The acrominizer works well for removal of the exostosis.

Instrumentation/Implantation

- 20-ml syringe
- 18-gauge spinal needle
- #11 blade
- Noninvasive distractor
- Straight mosquito clamp
- 2.9-mm oblique, wide-angle 30° video arthroscope
- CHP camera with compatible light source
- Video/TV monitor
- High-flow infusion pump
- 3.5-mm arthroscopic full-radius shaver
- Radiofrequency wand
- Acrominizer (burr)
- Rasp
- Blunt trochar/cannula

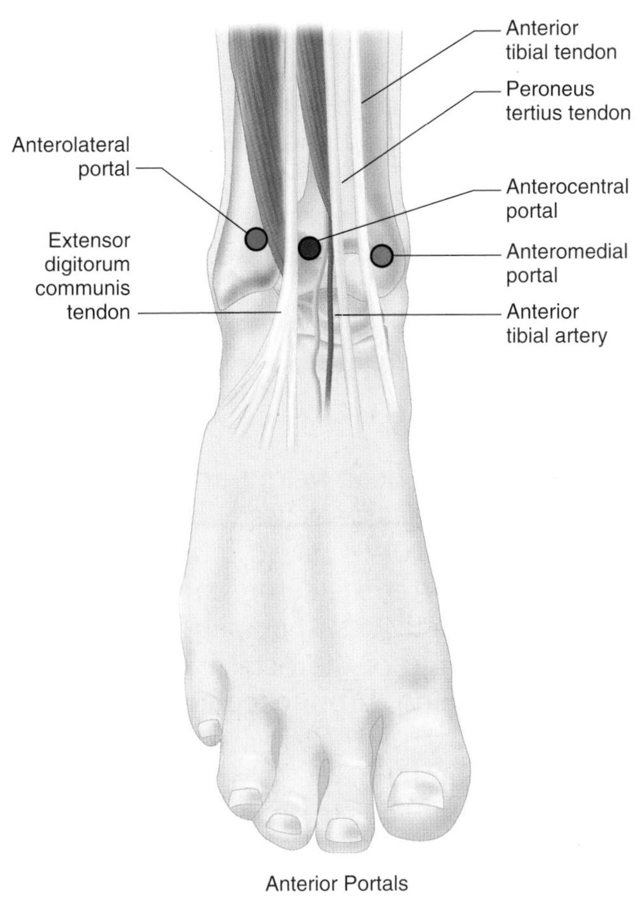

FIGURE 4

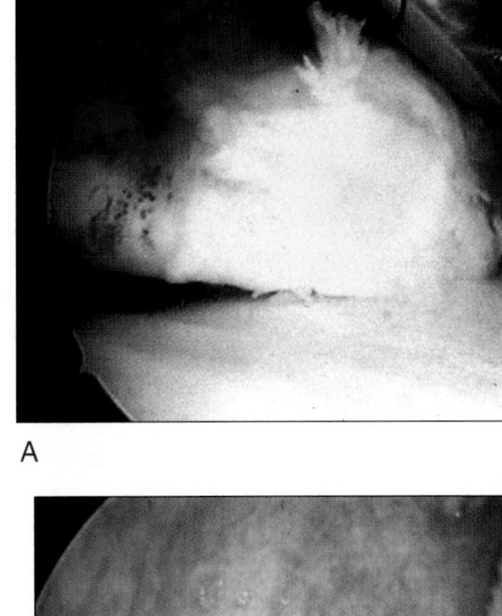

A

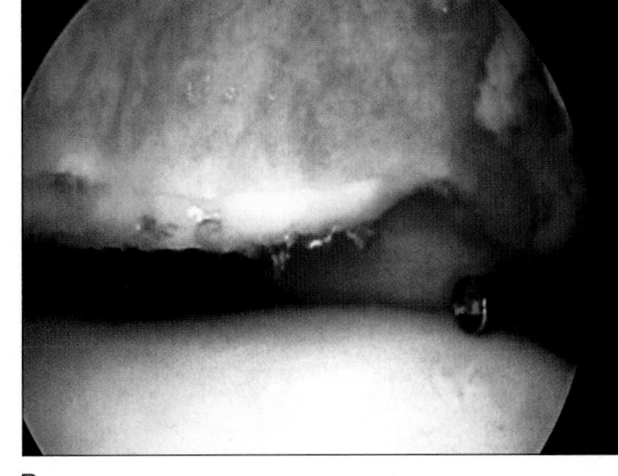

B

FIGURE 5

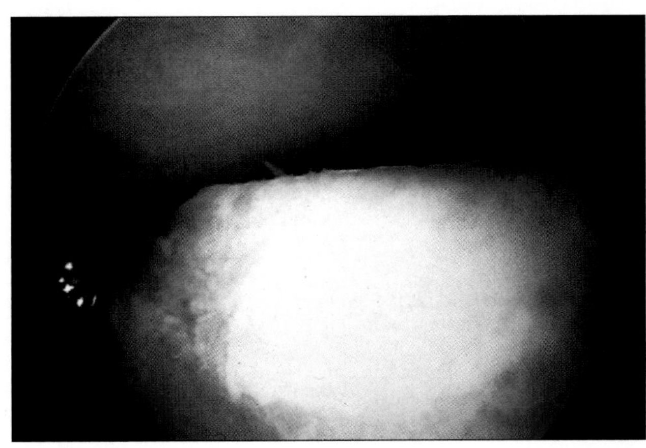

A

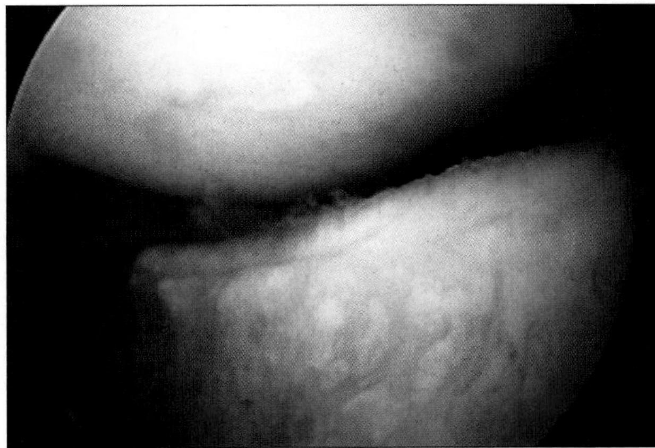

B

FIGURE 6

Instrumentation/ Implantation

- Small curettes
- Small grasping forceps, probes, baskets

Step 2

- Once the spur is removed, the anterior surface is smoothed with a full-radius shaver or a curette.
- Care must be taken to inspect the joint for loose bodies.
- The patient is placed into a bulky dressing with or without a cryotherapy unit incorporated into the dressing.

Postoperative Care and Expected Outcomes

- The patient is allowed to bear weight at 5 days, when the inflammation has decreased.
- Sutures are removed at 10–14 days.
- Physical therapy starts after the sutures are removed with range-of-motion activities, therapeutic modalities, and stretching of the Achilles. This is followed by strengthening, proprioception, and closed chain activities.
- Patients with anterior impingement, with and without fragmentation, will take approximately 6 weeks to recover postoperatively.
- Patients with arthritic changes in the ankle joint will take approximately 12 weeks to recover.

Evidence

Branca A, DiPalma L, Bucca C, Visconti CS, DiMille M. Arthroscopic treatment of anterior ankle impingement. Foot Ankle Int. 1997;18:4183–8.

The authors reported improvement in all stages of anterior impingement after arthroscopic treatment. Overall, they reported 63% good results and 24% fair results. (Level I evidence)

Scranton PE, McDermott JE. Anterior tibiotalar spurs: a comparison of open versus arthroscopic debridement. Foot Ankle. 1992;13:124–9.

In this study, the authors compared open versus arthroscopic techniques for the removal of anterior tibiotalar spurs. They found the operative time similar. Recovery time was shorter for the arthroscopic group. They also present a classification system that grades the degree of spur formation. (Level I evidence)

Van Dijk CN, Tol SL, Verheyen CC. A prospective study of prognostic factors concerning the outcome of arthroscopic surgery for anterior ankle impingement. Am J Sports Med. 1997;25:737–45.

The authors reported that the degree of arthritic changes present at the time of arthroscopic surgery was a better predictor of outcome than the size and location of the spur. Ninety percent of the patients without joint space narrowing had good to excellent results at 2-year follow-up. Only 50% of those with joint space narrowing had good to excellent results. (Level I evidence)

PROCEDURE 48

Lateral Calcaneal Lengthening Osteotomy for Supple Adult Flatfoot

Victor Valderrabano, André Leumann, Hans-Peter Kundert, and Beat Hintermann

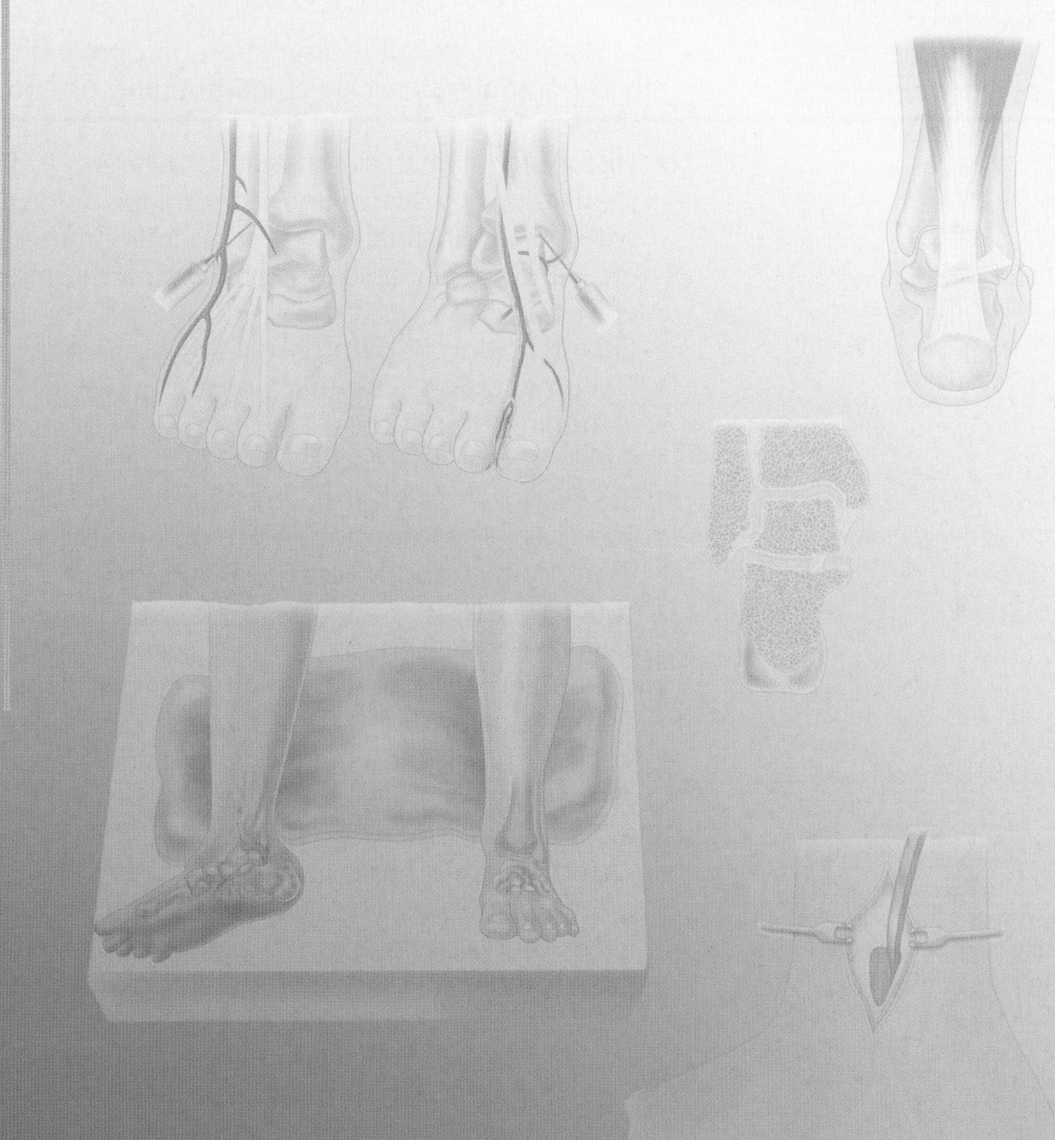

Indications

- Posterior tibial tendon insufficiency (PTTI), stage II to II-III
- Medial ankle instability
- Both must be accompanied by
  - Supple pes planovalgus et abductus deformity with forefoot pronation and subfibular impingement
  - Preserved subtalar and talonavicular joints

Examination/Imaging

- The standard clinical examination of a patient requiring a lateral calcaneal lengthening osteotomy includes:
  - History for differential diagnosis between PTTI (female, >40 years of age, continuous deformity with posterior tibial [PT] tendon inflammation, etc.) and medial ankle instability (trauma history, etc.)
  - Quantification of pain (visual analogue scale, 0–10)
  - Documentation of tender points
  - Flattening of arch
  - Swelling over PT tendon (Fig. 1)
  - Pes planovalgus et abductus deformity (Fig. 2A)
  - Too-many-toes sign (abductus deformity)
  - PT tendon strength test (weakness)
  - Functional tests
    - Single heel-rise test
    - Double heel-rise test: hindfoot valgus while on tiptoes as evidence for PTTI (Fig. 2B)
  - Ankle instability tests (lateral: inversion stress test, drawer test; medial: eversion stress test)
- Radiologic assessment includes:
  - Weight-bearing radiographs
    - Anteroposterior (AP) view of the foot: abductus deformity; subluxation of talonavicular joint; pathologic AP talus–first metatarsal angle (Fig. 3A); bunion deformity
    - Lateral view of the foot: flatfoot deformity; plantar subluxation of talonavicular joint; pathologic lateral talus–first metatarsal angle (Fig. 3B)
    - AP view of the ankle joint: valgus deformity; quantification of hindfoot alignment angle; involvement of ankle joint with medial joint laxity; lateral fibular impingement (Fig. 3C)

Pitfalls

- *Calcaneal lengthening osteotomy is not indicated in cases of:*
  - *Rigid pes planus et abductus deformity (PTTI stage III or IV)*
  - *Osteoarthritis of the subtalar and/or Chopart joints*
  - *Isolated valgus deformities without abductus component*

Controversies

- It has been postulated that lateral column lengthening osteotomy will cause overload in the calcaneocuboid joint and thus lead to degenerative disease (Philipps, 1983). More recent work, however, did not prove increased joint pressure (Benthien et al., 2007). We also did not see any degenerative disease over time in our patients with a follow-up to 12 years.

Treatment Options

- Myerson's calcaneal medial sliding osteotomy: indicated for correction of isolated hindfoot valgus deformity
- Hintermann's lateral calcaneal lengthening osteotomy: osteotomy along and parallel to the posterior subtalar joint facet
- Evans' osteotomy: 10 mm proximal to the calcaneocuboid joint between the middle and anterior subtalar joint facets; commonly done in children for congenital flatfoot
- Hansen's calcaneocuboidal interposition arthrodesis: arthrodesis with lateral column lengthening effect

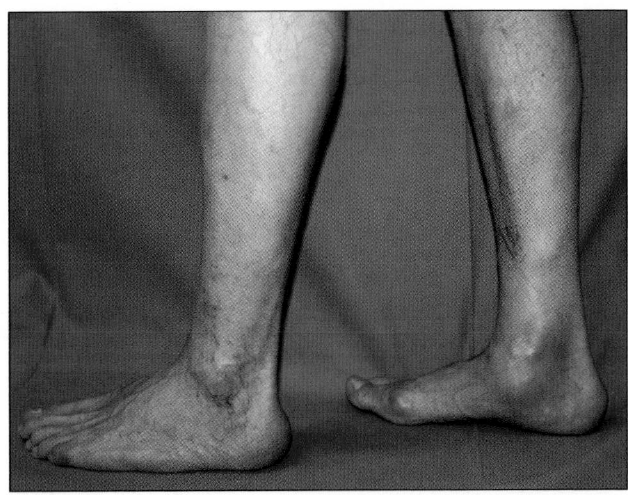

FIGURE 1

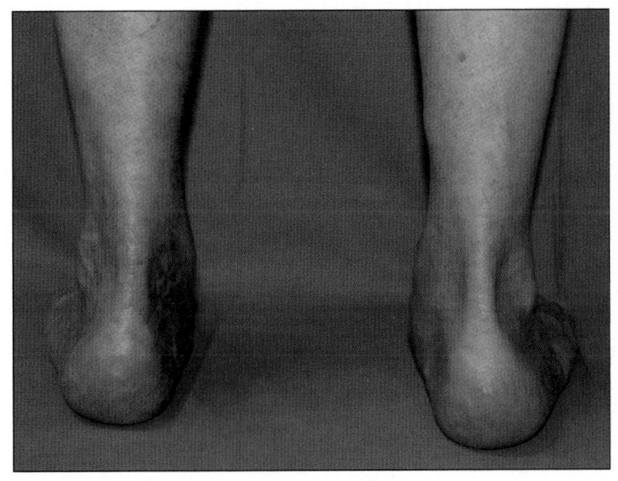

A

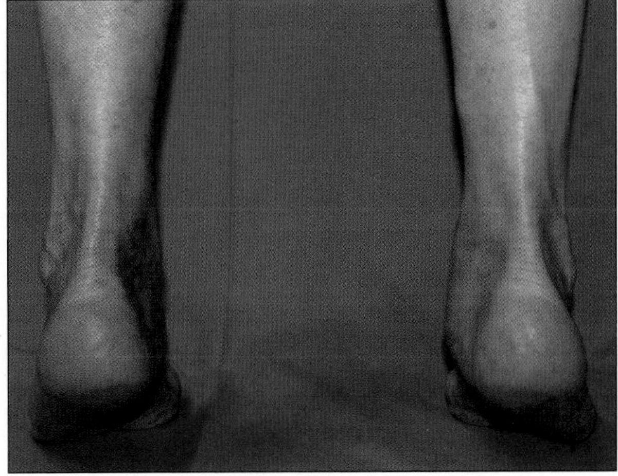

B

FIGURE 2

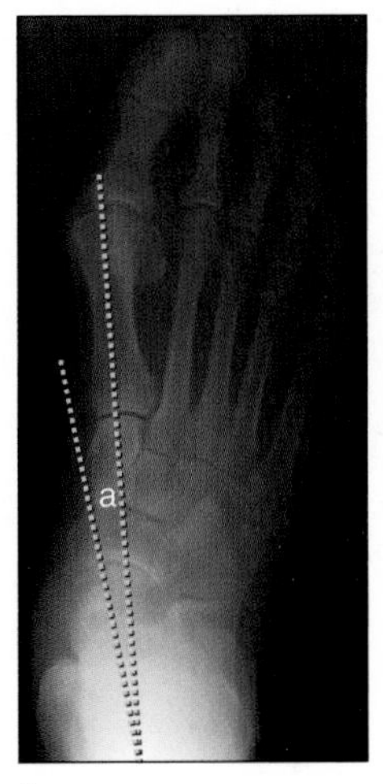

A

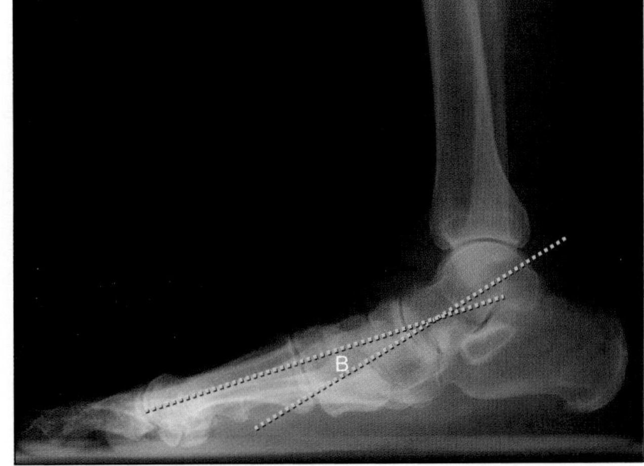

B

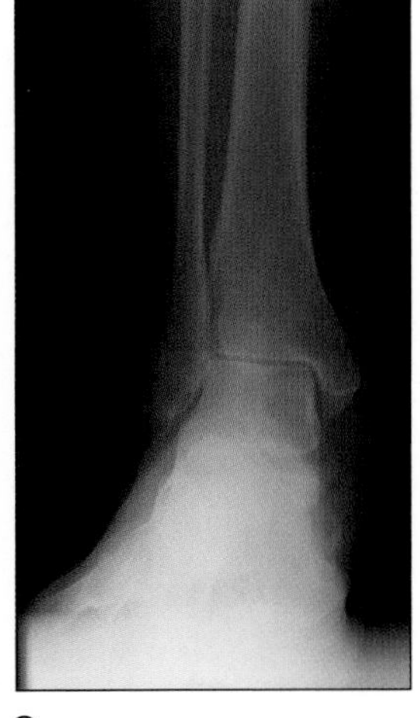

C

FIGURE 3

- Magnetic resonance imaging: detection of tendon degeneration, ligament involvement (spring ligament, deltoid ligament), and possible chondral and osteoarthritic hindfoot changes
- Computed tomography (CT) scan: assessment of possible osseous defects, impingements (sinus tarsi, calcaneofibular), and osteoarthritis

Surgical Anatomy

- Lateral hindfoot anatomy (Fig. 4A)
  - Sinus tarsi
  - Peroneal tendons
  - Sural nerve
  - Posterior subtalar joint facet
  - Anterior process of the calcaneus
- Medial midfoot anatomy (Fig. 4B)
  - Spring ligament
  - Flexor tendons
  - Neurovascular structures

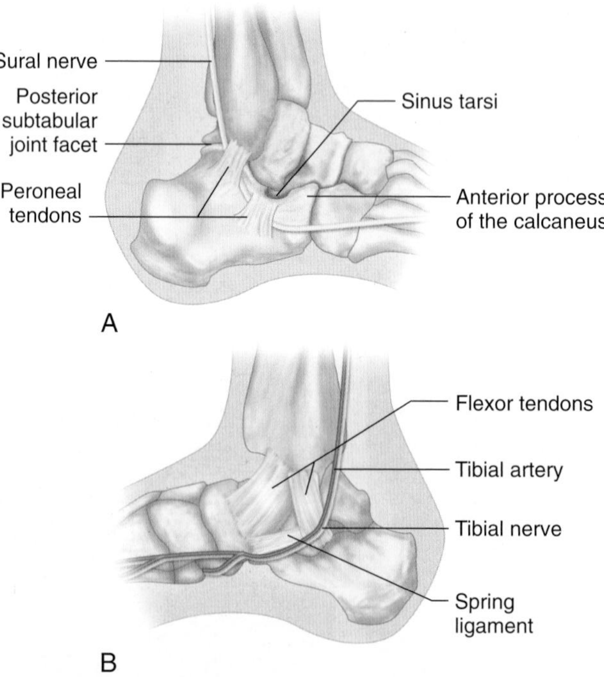

FIGURE 4

Positioning

- Supine position with wedge underneath the ipsilateral hip, placing the leg and foot in internal rotation
- Heel at the edge of the table
- Tourniquet at the thigh (350 mm Hg)
- Free draping of the ipsilateral iliac crest for harvesting an autograft
- Preparation of a sterile covered fluoroscan for intraoperative radiographic imaging

PEARLS

- *Landmarks: tip of fibula, peroneal tendons, sinus tarsi, calcaneocuboid joint*

PITFALLS

- *Injury to sural nerve and peroneal tendons*

Portals/Exposures

- Make a slightly curved 5-cm incision starting at the tip of fibula and following the peroneal tendons to the anterior process of the calcaneus.

Procedure

STEP 1

- Expose the sinus tarsi with an incision above the peroneal tendons.
- Position a small Hohmann retractor into the sinus tarsi to retract the soft tissues dorsally.
- Perform a subperiosteal exposure of the calcaneal neck with a raspatorium and position a small Hohmann retractor, protecting the peroneal tendons and sural nerve (Fig. 5).
- Identify the anterior border of the posterior subtalar joint facet.

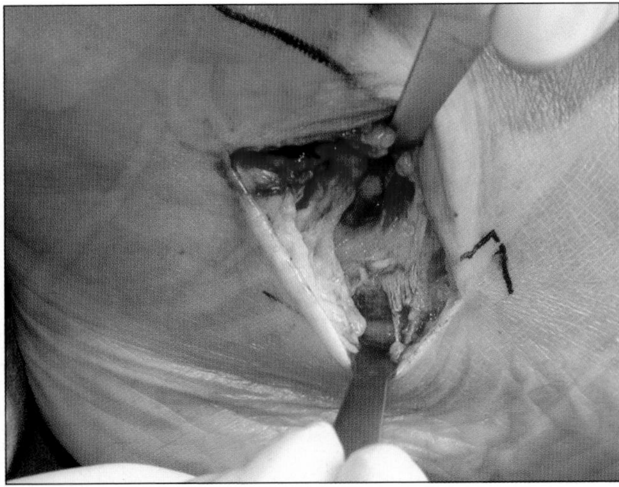

FIGURE 5

Pearls

- *Use a spreader at the osteotomy site to define the intraoperative amount of lateral column lengthening.*

Pitfalls

- *Avoid osteotomy of the medial calcaneal cortex.*
- *Dislocation of bone graft because of critical bone quality (e.g., osteoporotic bone)*

Instrumentation/ Implantation

- Retractors
- Spreader
- Oscillating saw
- Osteotome

Step 2

- Perform an osteotomy along and parallel to the posterior facet with the oscillating saw, from lateral to medial, leaving the medial cortex intact (Fig. 6).
- Insert two 2.5-mm Kirschner wires approximately 5 mm anterior and posterior to the planned osteotomy, and insert a double-pin distractor (Hintermann distractor; Newdeal, Lyon, France) (Fig. 7).
- Open the osteotomy with the distractor (Fig. 8A) until the forefoot abductus and medial longitudinal arch seem to be restored (Fig. 8B).
- Measure the gap (usually 8–12 mm) and harvest a corresponding tricortical iliac crest wedge autograft (alternative: use an allograft wedge such as Tutoplast).
- Insert the graft into the osteotomy site and remove the spreader (Fig. 9).
- With intrinsic compression, usually no internal fixation is necessary. However, a 3.5-mm cortical screw from anterior to posterior across the graft may prevent the graft from plantar dislocation, especially in osteoporotic bone.
- Check the correction and positioning of the graft and screw with fluoroscan (Fig. 10A and 10B).
- Irrigate the wound, and perform subcutaneous and skin closure.

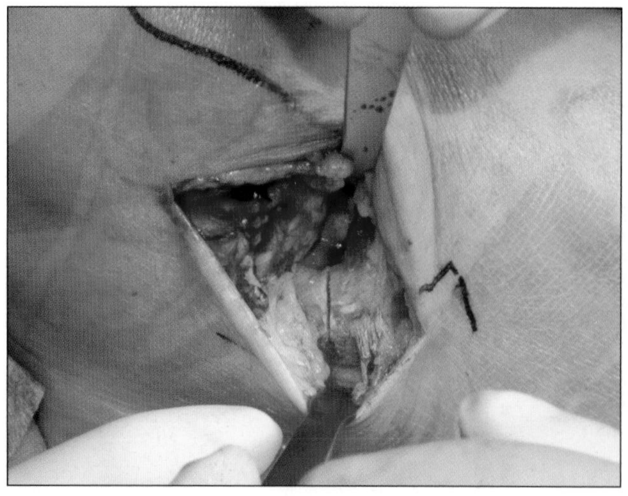

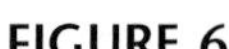

FIGURE 6

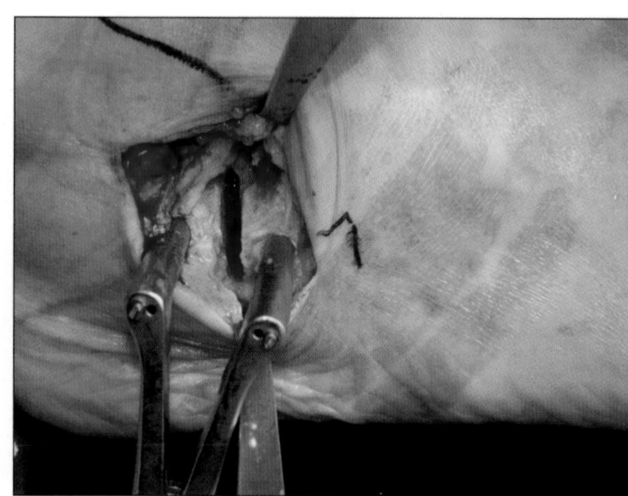

FIGURE 7

Controversies

- Level of the osteotomy
  - A more distal osteotomy, as proposed by Evans, may cause instability of the anterior process of the calcaneus with a tendency to rise up, thereby causing incongruency at the calcaneocuboid joint. A complete osteotomy is also needed in this procedure because of its relationship to the center of rotation of the talonavicular joint.
  - Osteotomy through the sinus tarsi, as described here, permits an incomplete osteotomy and keeps the complex capsular and ligamentous structures intact, which ensures stability of the anterior process of the calcaneus and preservation of congruency at the calcaneocuboid joint.
- Potential damage to the intermediate and anterior joint facets of the subtalar joint by the osteotomy was claimed to be a potential reason for degenerative disease. However, we found no such complication in any of our patients. A specific trial (20 patients) with CT scan controls 2 years after surgery did not show any degenerative disease at the subtalar joint.

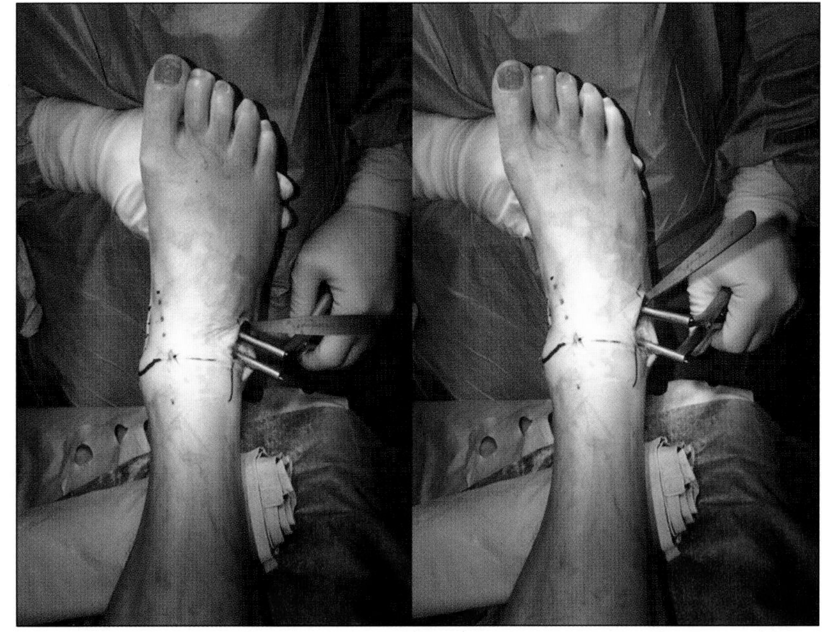

A B

FIGURE 8

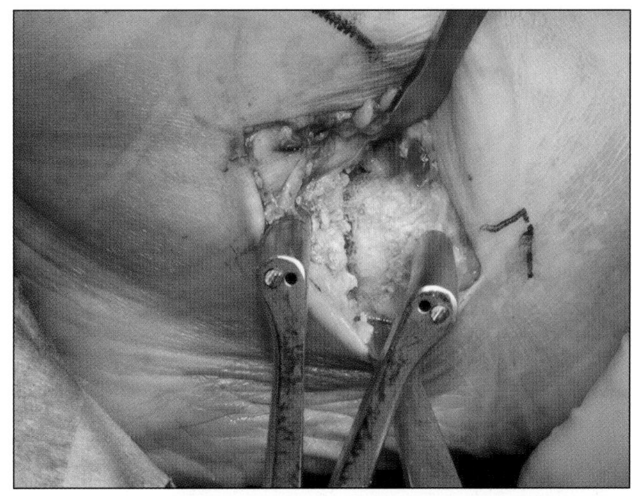

FIGURE 9

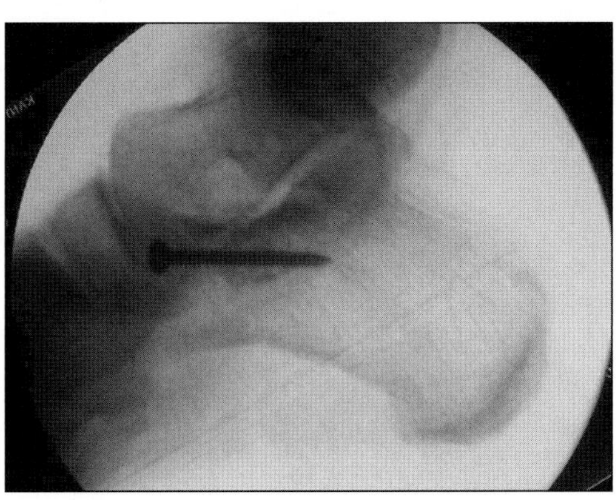

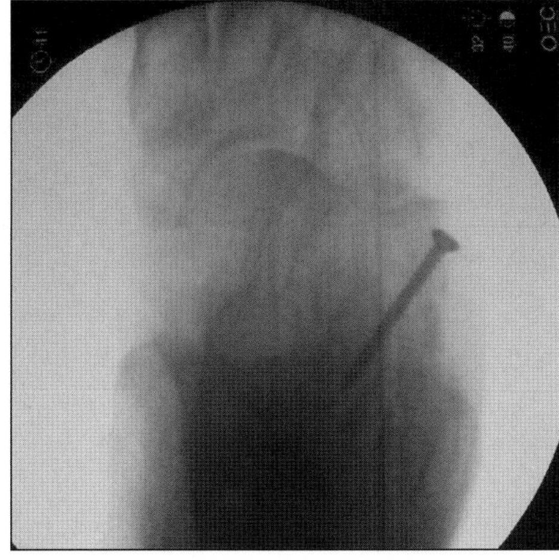

A B

FIGURE 10

Controversies

- PTTI and medial ankle instability require medial soft tissue reconstruction after lateral calcaneal lenghthening osteotomy.

Pearls

- *Compliant patients with normal body mass index and no risk factors (smoking, diabetes) may be treated functionally in a removable boot or orthosis.*

Pitfalls

- *Infection*
- *Migration of the inserted graft*
- *Malunion*
- *Nonunion*
- *Hardware failure*
- *Sural nerve problems*
- *Peroneal tendon lesions/ dysfunction*
- *Complex regional pain syndrome*

Step 3

- In cases of PTTI and medial ankle instability, medial soft tissue surgical procedures are subsequently performed, including:
  - PT tendon reconstruction
  - Flexor digitorum longus tendon transfer
  - Deltoid ligament repair
  - Spring ligament repair

Postoperative Care and Expected Outcomes

- The patient is maintained in a lower leg cast or lower leg orthosis (e.g., Vacoped) for 6 weeks with 15 kg partial weight bearing and antithrombosis prophylaxis.
- Radiographic follow-up is done at 6 weeks postoperative for assessment of bony union. Rule out graft collapse, malunion, and hardware failure.
- Thereafter, start an intensive physical therapy program.

Evidence

Arangio GA, Chopra V, Voloshin A, Salathe EP. A biomechanical analysis of the effect of lateral column lengthening calcaneal osteotomy on the flat foot. Clin Biomech. 2007;22:472–7.

This three-dimensional multisegment biomechanical model study showed that a 10-mm lateral column lengthening calcaneal osteotomy reduced the excess force on the medial arch in adult flatfoot and added a biomechanical rationale to this clinical procedure.

Benthien RA, Parks BG, Guyton GP, Schon LC. Lateral column calcaneal lengthening, flexor digitorum longus transfer, and opening wedge medial cuneiform osteotomy for flexible flatfoot: a biomechanical study. Foot Ankle Int. 2007;28:70–7.

In this in vitro biomechanical study of 12 cadaver specimens (physiologically loaded) with radiographic and pedobarographic evaluation, lateral column lengthening increased lateral forefoot pressures in a severe flatfoot model. An added medial cuneiform osteotomy provided increased deformity correction and decreased pressure under the lateral forefoot. (Level IV evidence)

Hintermann B, Valderrabano V, Kundert HP. Lengthening of the lateral column and reconstruction of the medial soft tissue for treatment of acquired flatfoot deformity associated with insufficiency of the posterior tibial tendon. Foot Ankle Int. 1999;20:622–9.

This was a study of 19 patients treated with lengthening of the proximal lateral column by calcaneal osteotomy and reconstructing the medial soft tissue. (Level IV evidence)

Phillips GE. A review of elongation of os calcis for flat feet. J Bone Joint Surg [Br]. 1983;65:15–8.

Between 1959 and 1974, the late Dillwyn Evans treated severe symptomatic flatfoot by elongating the os calcis. The long-term follow-up of 20 of these patients with a total of 23 feet was presented in this study 7–20 years after the operation. At review, 17 of the 23 feet showed very good or good results, and it was concluded that this is a useful procedure for severe cases of flatfoot that appears to stand the test of time. (Level IV evidence)

PROCEDURE 49

Single Medial Approach for Triple Arthrodesis

Jeroen De Wachter and Beat Hintermann

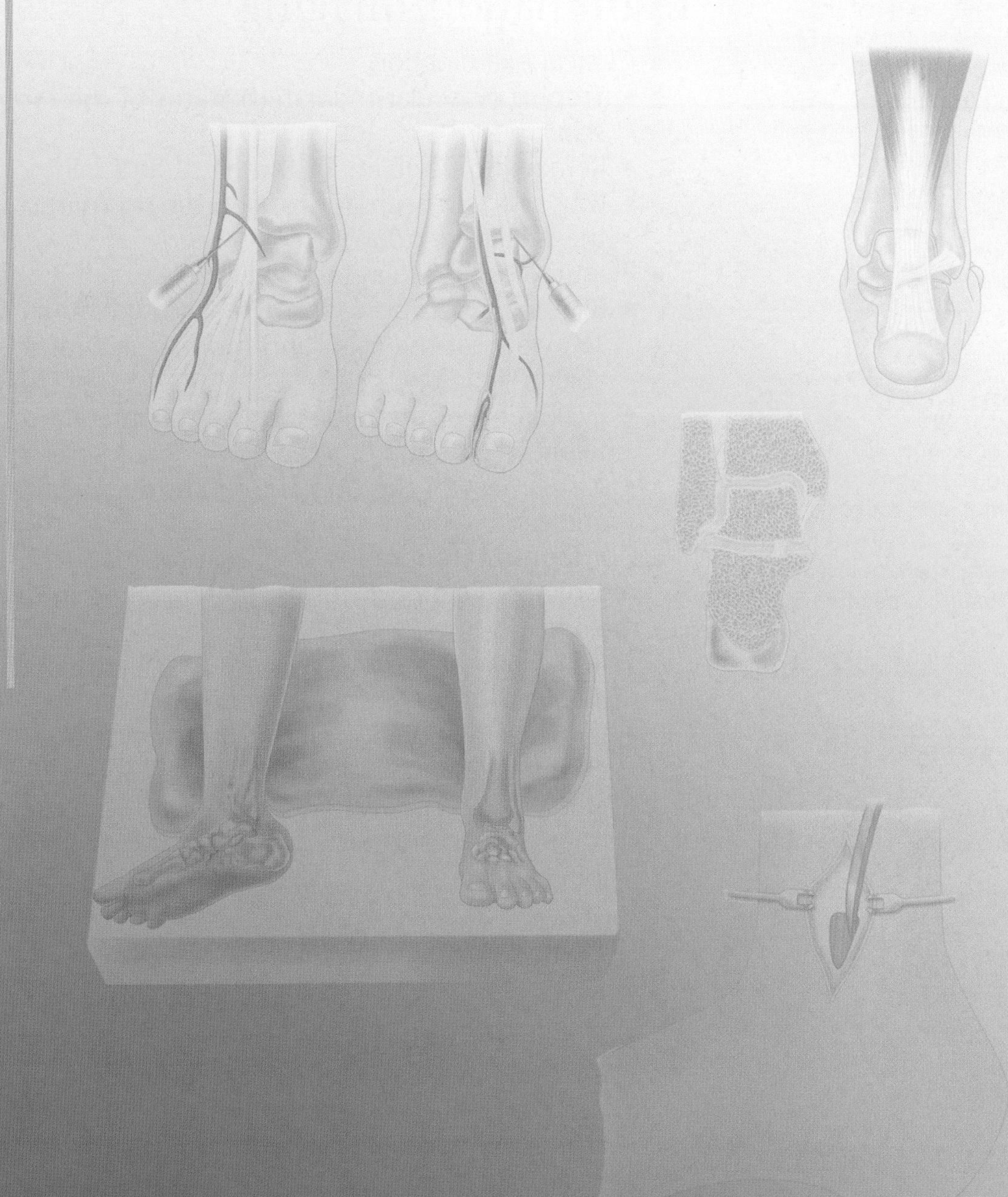

Pitfalls

- *Acute or chronic infection of the foot is an absolute contraindication for a triple arthrodesis.*

Controversies

- Vascular insufficiency of the lower leg and foot should be assessed and addressed before proceeding to hindfoot surgery.
- Unless the calcaneocuboid joint shows clear clinical and/or radiographic signs of arthritic changes, this joint should not be fused while doing a standard triple arthrodesis procedure.

Treatment Options

- Orthotics and shoe modifications can be used to relieve pain if surgical correction is not advised.
- No true surgical alternatives exist for treating a painful rigid adult flatfoot.
- In the case of involvement of the tibiotalar joint (valgus arthritis of the ankle joint), additional ankle joint replacement may be considered, if medial ankle instability remains preserved.

Indications

- Symptomatic rigid pes planus (valgus-abductus) of the adult not responding to conservative treatment:
  - End-stage posterior tibial tendon disease
  - Tarsal coalitions
  - Inflammatory or posttraumatic arthritis of the hindfoot
  - Sequelae of a neuromuscular disease

Examination/Imaging

- Clinical examination
  - Trophic (vascular-mediated) status of the foot and skin
  - Remaining flexibility in the hind- and midfoot
  - Muscular strength and/or shortening (particularly the Achilles tendon)
- Plain radiographs (weight bearing)
  - Bilateral anteroposterior (Fig. 1A) and lateral (Fig. 1B) views of the foot, and mortise view of the ankle (Fig. 2)
  - Evaluation of the talocalcaneal, talometatarsal, and talonavicular angles
  - Assessment of the degree of joint degeneration and bone density
- Computed tomography (CT) scan or magnetic resonance imaging (MRI) is rarely needed in decision making.
  - MRI may help to assess avascular necrosis of involved bones, particularly of the talar body.
  - CT scan may help in better understanding extremely complex hindfoot deformities.
  - Single-photon emission CT or bone scan may help to assess the arthritic changes of the involved joints.

Surgical Anatomy

- The deltoid ligament is divided into two main layers:
  - The anterior superficial layer (Fig. 3A) consists of the tibionavicular, tibio-spring, and tibiocalcaneal ligaments, and it stretches from the anterior aspect of medial malleolus toward the navicular bone, the spring ligament, and the sustentaculum tali of the calcaneus.
  - The posterior deep layer (Fig. 3B) consists of three bundles, and it runs from the posterior colliculus of the medial malleolus posteriorly and distally to the talus.

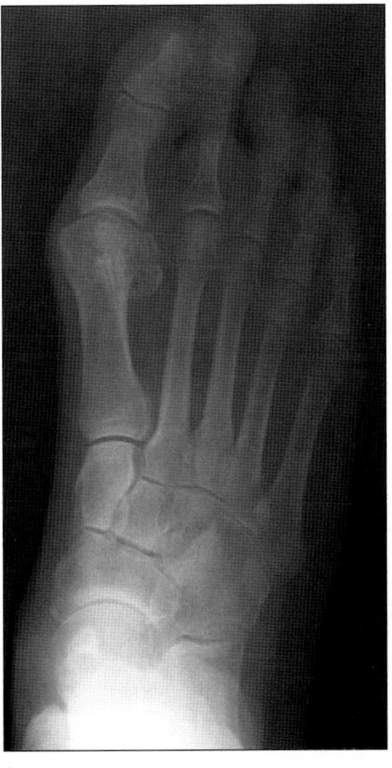

A

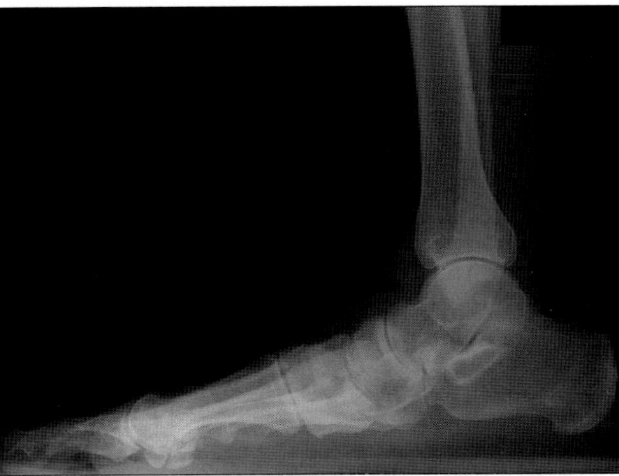

B

FIGURE 1

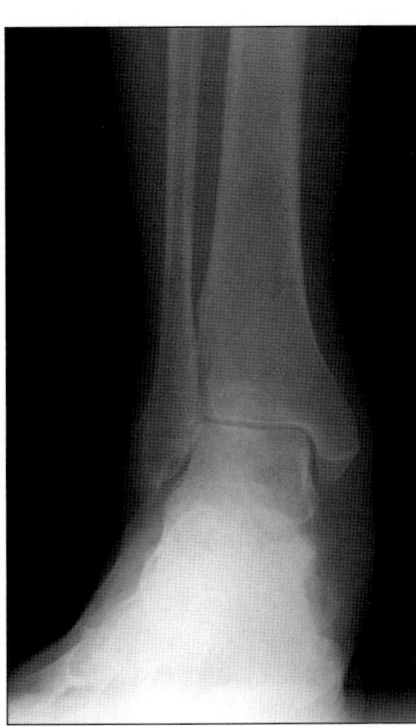

FIGURE 2

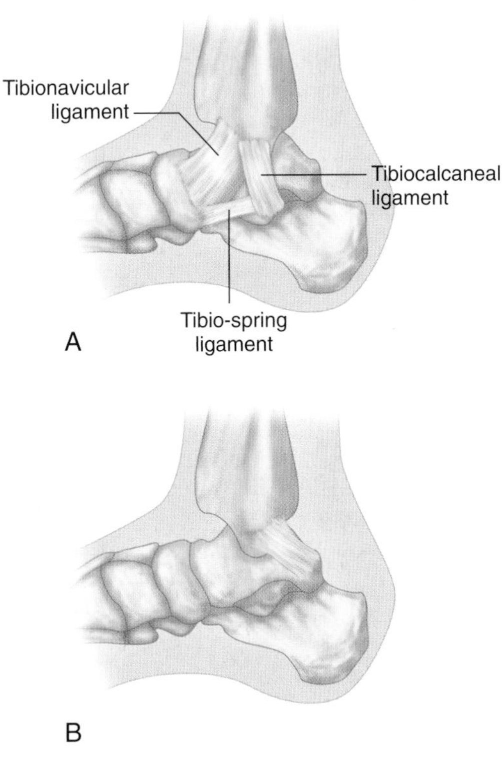

FIGURE 3

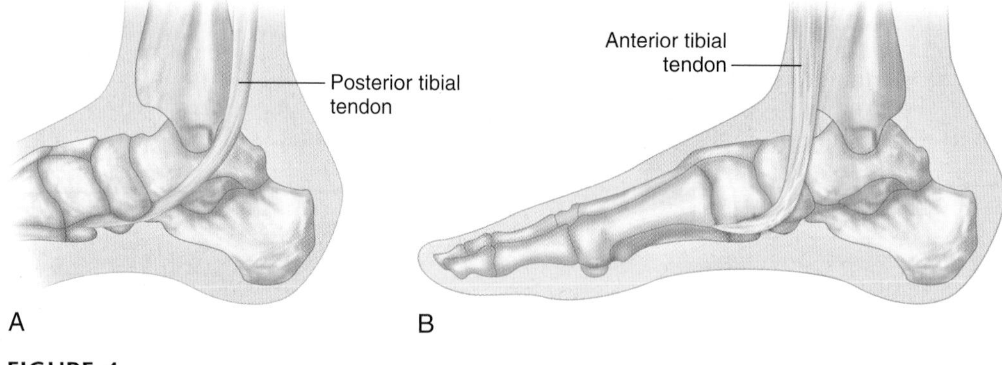

FIGURE 4

- The posterior tibial tendon runs behind the medial malleolus, and inserts on the medioplantar aspect of the navicular bone (Fig. 4A).
- The anterior tibial tendon runs dorsally over the talonavicular joint to insert at the medial aspect of medial cuneiform bone (Fig. 4B).
- The talonavicular joint can be palpated just behind the navicular tubercle.

PEARLS

- *If an Achilles tendon lengthening procedure is deemed necessary, the extended leg can be lifted 60° ceilingward by an assistant while the surgeon performs the lengthening.*
- *The same leg-lifting maneuver allows the surgeon to visually control the correction of hindfoot valgus during surgery.*
- *Drape the ipsilateral iliac crest free if autologous bone grafting is suspected to be necessary.*

Positioning

- The patient is placed in supine position.
- A tourniquet is placed at the thigh.
- The C-arm, or better a fluoroscan, is placed at the same side as the operated foot, to obtain easy fluoroscopic control during surgery.

PEARLS

- *Keep the dissected layers of the deltoid ligament intact while performing arthrotomy of the talonavicular and subtalar joints.*

PITFALLS

- *Extending the incision too posteriorly puts the deep tibiotalar layers of the deltoid ligament at risk.*

Portals/Exposures

- A longitudinal 6-cm skin incision is made starting at the navicular tubercle along the superior border of the posterior tibial tendon, paying attention to not expand over the longitudinal axis of the tibia (Fig. 5).
- The posterior tibial tendon sheath is opened and the tendon is inspected; in the case of any tendinitis, the tendon is excised.
- A partial superior release of the tendon at the level of its insertion on the navicular provides better visualization of the deeper structures.
- The talonavicular and subtalar joints are exposed by a horizontal cut above the posterior tibial tendon (Fig. 6).

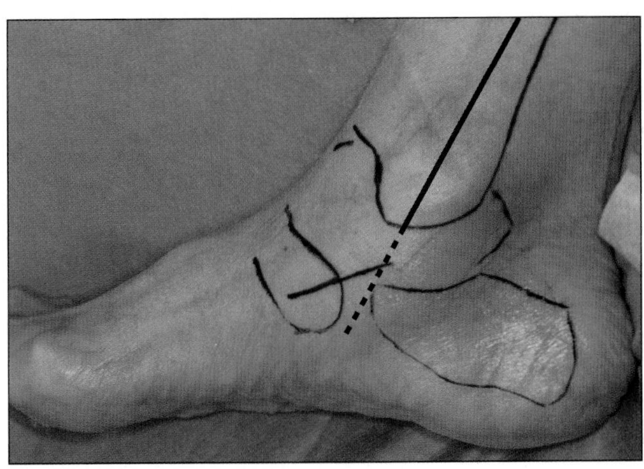

FIGURE 5

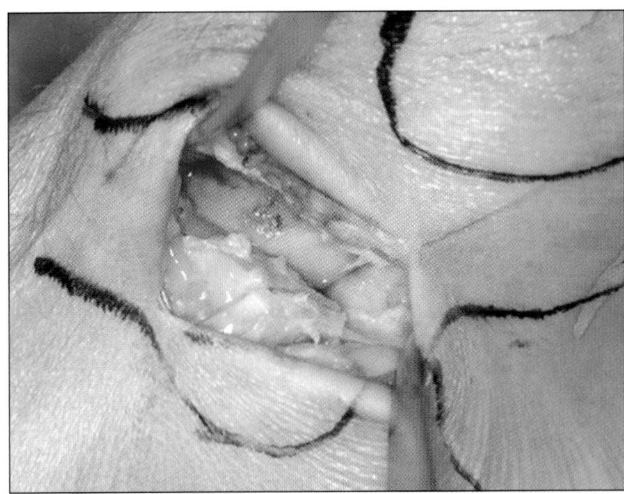

FIGURE 6

Procedure

Step 1

- Two 2.5-mm Kirschner wires (K-wires) are first placed in the dorsomedial aspect of the navicular bone and in the talar neck.
  - The talonavicular joint is exposed by opening the spreader; dissection of the talonavicular ligament may help to open the joint (Fig. 7).
  - The talonavicular joint surfaces are denuded of their cartilage using a chisel and a curette (Fig. 8).
  - The bony surfaces are feathered with a small chisel or drilled with a 2.5-mm drill bit in order to break the subchondral plate and get good bleeding bone.
  - The spreader is removed but the two K-wires are left in place.

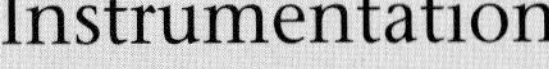

Instrumentation

- A special distractor using two Kirschner wires may help to spread the talonavicular and subtalar joints.

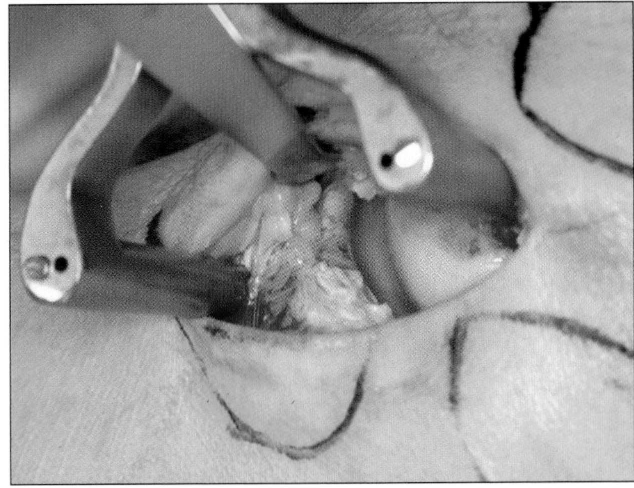

FIGURE 7

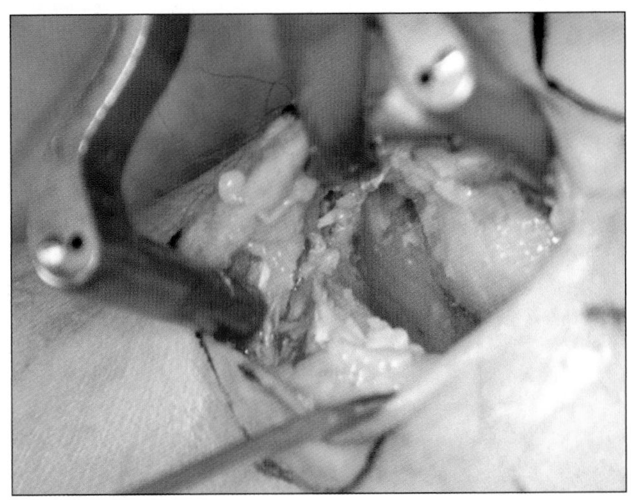

FIGURE 8

- The sustentaculum tali is exposed by using a small Hohmann retractor, and a 2.5-mm K-wire is put in place.
- The spreader is put in place using the K-wires on the talar neck and sustentaculum tali (Fig. 9)
  - The subtalar joint is exposed by opening the spreader; dissection of the interosseous ligament using a chisel may help to open the joint (Fig. 10).
  - After visualization, the anterior, middle, and posterior facets of the calcaneus and the undersurface of the talus are denuded of their cartilage using a chisel and a curette. The interosseous ligament is removed carefully, and the bone of the sinus tarsi is roughened (Fig. 11).
  - The bony surfaces are feathered with a small chisel or drilled with a 2.5-mm drill bit in order to break the subchondral plate and get good bleeding bone.

Pearls

- *As the navicular joint surface is concave, the K-wire should be placed distally enough in the navicular in order not to penetrate the articular surface at its deepest concavity.*
- *If deemed necessary, (autologous) bone grafts can be inserted after preparing the joint surfaces. We routinely use a commercially available osteoinductive bone matrix substance to fill any gaps left after joint preparation (Fig. 12).*

Pitfalls

- *Insufficient cartilage removal at the utmost lateral side of the talonavicular joint will prevent proper joint reduction in the first place and will jeopardize future bony fusion.*
- *It is of utmost importance not to damage the deep deltoid ligament (e.g., the tibiotalar ligaments: pickups are used to mark the deltoid ligament fibers). Overzealous cutting of its deep fibers can lead to a progressive ankle valgus instability with a potentially disastrous evolution.*

Controversies

- Unless decided otherwise preoperatively, the calcaneocuboid joint is left untouched. If it needs to be fused, it can easily be reached and denuded through the talonavicular joint space.

Instrumentation/Implantation

- We use a special joint distractor with two long hollow legs. Two 2.5-mm K-wires can be placed through these legs into the respective bones of the joint to be distracted.

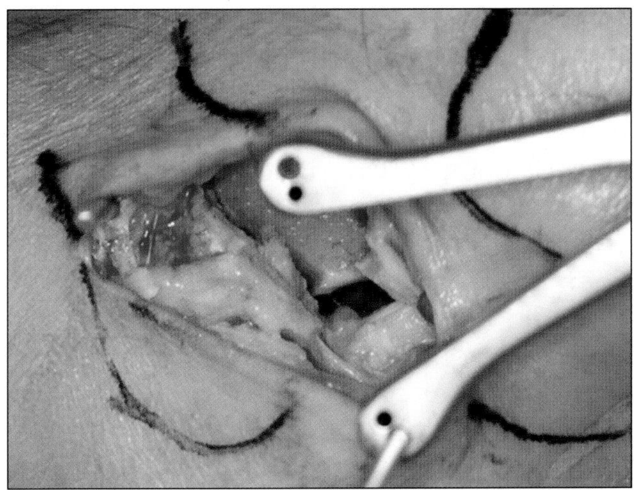

FIGURE 9

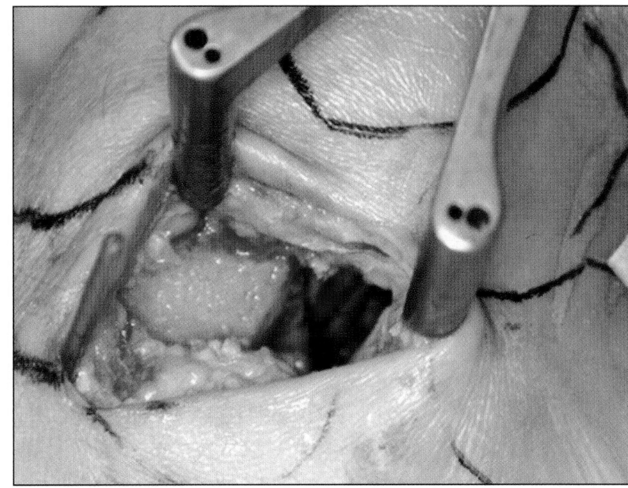

FIGURE 10

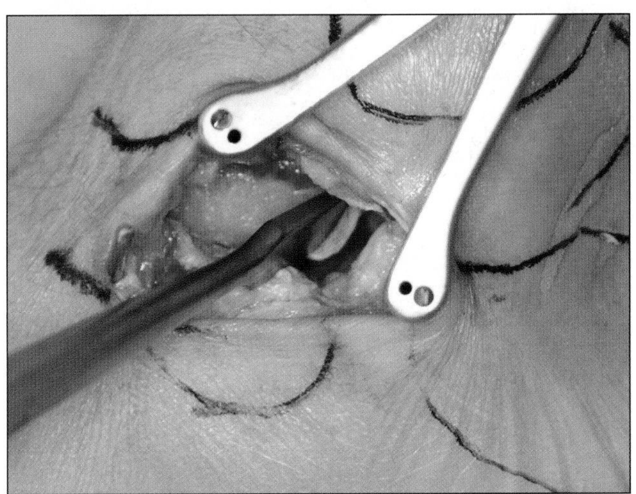

FIGURE 11

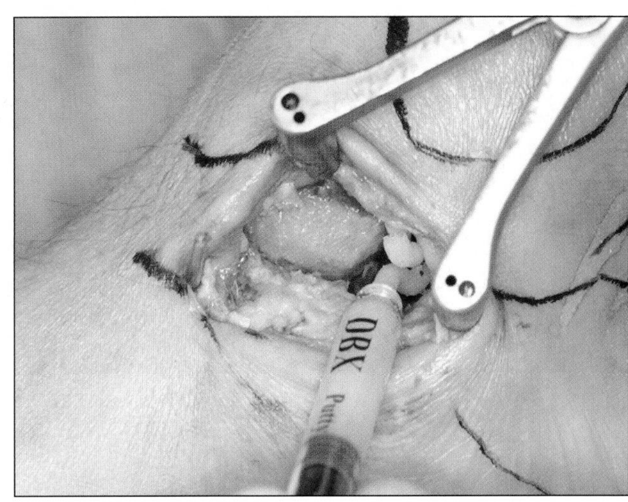

FIGURE 12

Step 2

- Prior to fixation of the triple arthrodesis, appropriate reduction of the foot (i.e., correction of the plano-valgo-abductus) is mandatory.
- Step-by-step reduction is performed as follows:
  - The ankle is held in the neutral 90° position.
  - The talonavicular joint is reduced to restore the correct joint congruency.
  - The heel is held in neutral varus-valgus with the talus being reduced on top of the calcaneus, thereby restoring their correct relationship (i.e., talocalcaneal angle of 30°).
- Guiding K-wires are used, first to transfix the talonavicular joint (Fig. 13A–C) and then the subtalar joint (Fig. 13D).

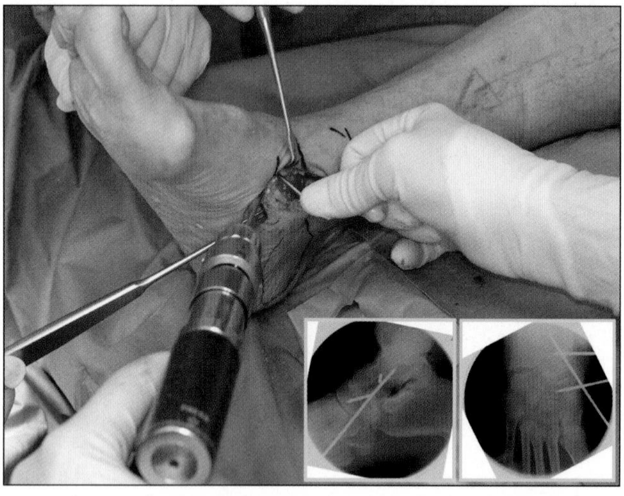
A

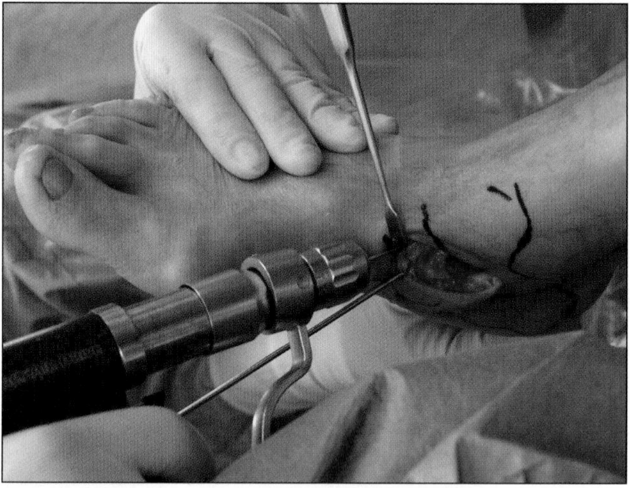
B

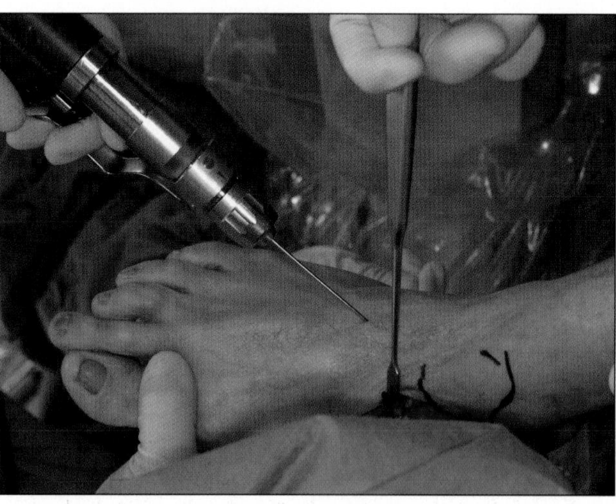
C

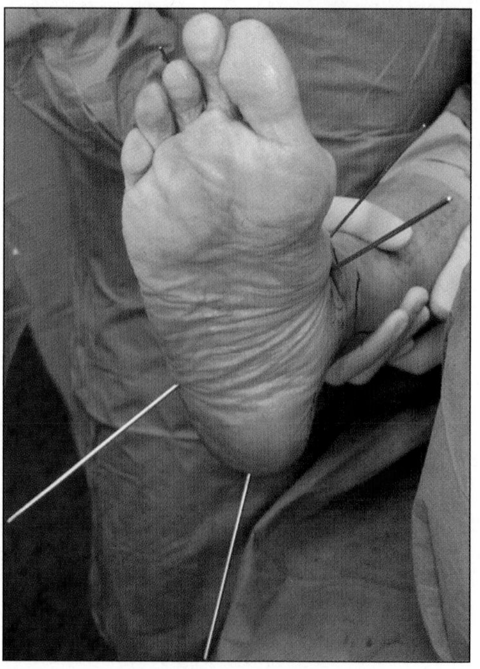
D

FIGURE 13

Pearls

- *Use the K-wires in the talus and the navicular as "joysticks" for easier manipulation of the bones during the reduction maneuver, particularly to get appropriate correction in the frontal plane (e.g., to correct the supination deformity of the forefoot) (Fig. 17A–C).*

Pitfalls

- *During the reduction maneuver of the talonavicular joint, always keep the forefoot in a pronated position, since a fixed forefoot supination (after fixation of the triple arthrodesis) is detrimental in the long run.*

Instrumentation/ Implantation

- A minimum thickness of 6.5 mm is needed for the large screws, usually partially threaded. The smaller screws should be 4.0 mm or more, depending on bone sizes.
- In severely osteoporotic bone, fully threaded screws may allow for stronger fixation.

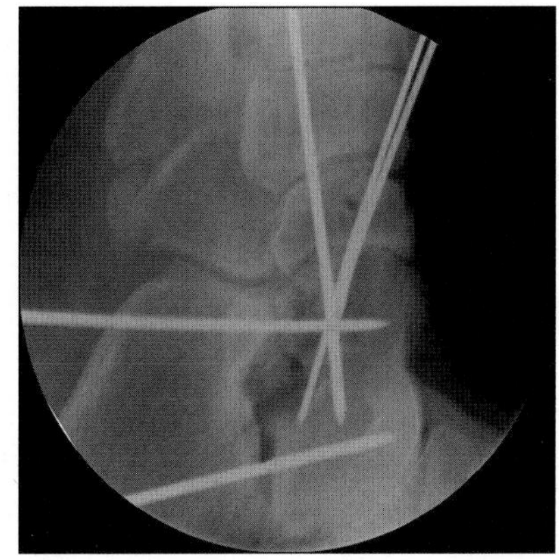
A

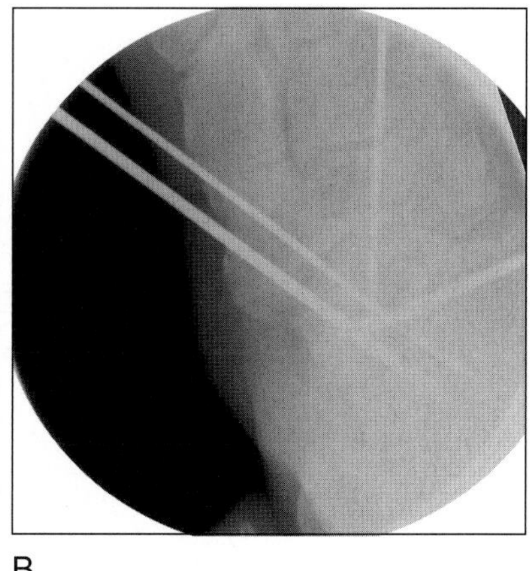
B

FIGURE 14

- Fluoroscopy is used for control (Fig. 14A and 14B).
- Fixation should be mechanically strong and biomechanically sound:
  - Three talonavicular screws are used, spread from medial to lateral on the navicular side and converging toward each other on the talar side.
    - One large screw starts at the navicular tubercle (Fig. 15A).
    - The two other (smaller) screws start at the dorsum of the navicular.
  - The subtalar joint is also fixed with two large screws.
    - One screw goes from the tuber calcanei through the posterior facet into the talar body (Fig. 15B).
    - A second screw goes from the plantar lateral side of the calcaneus (approximately 1 cm proximal to the calcaneocuboid joint) toward the talar head dorsomedially.

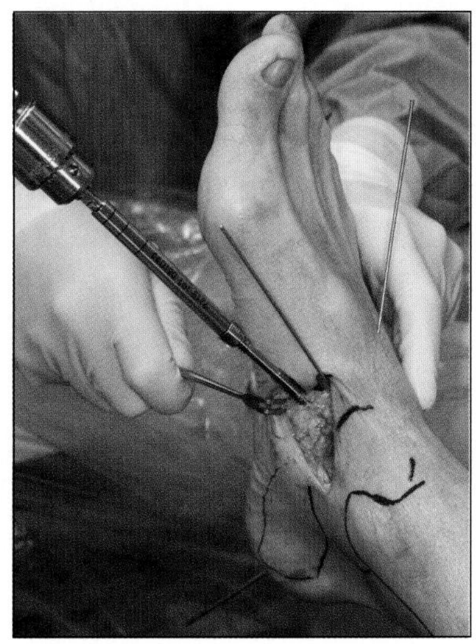
FIGURE 15 A

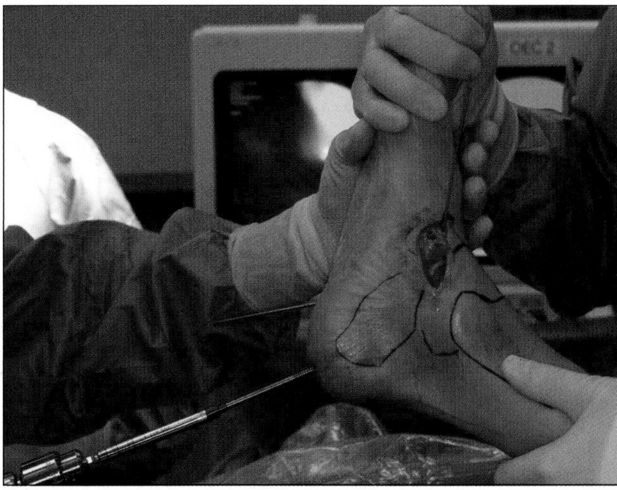
B

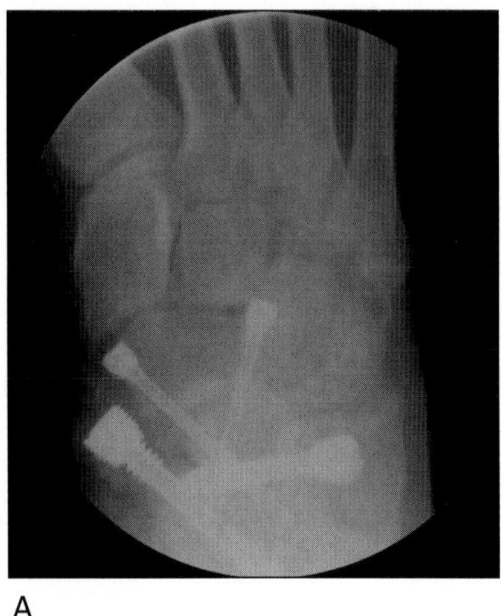

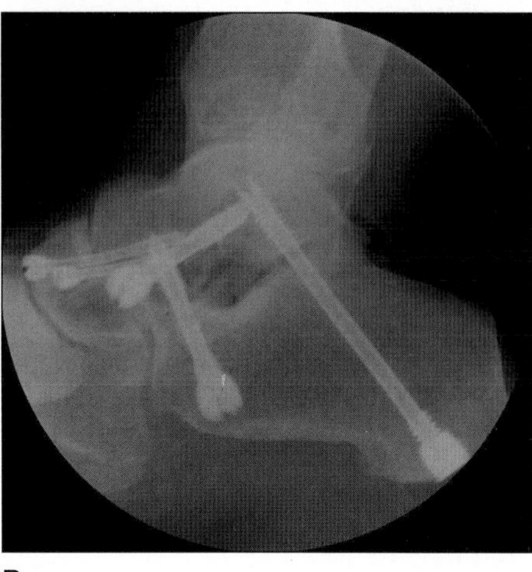

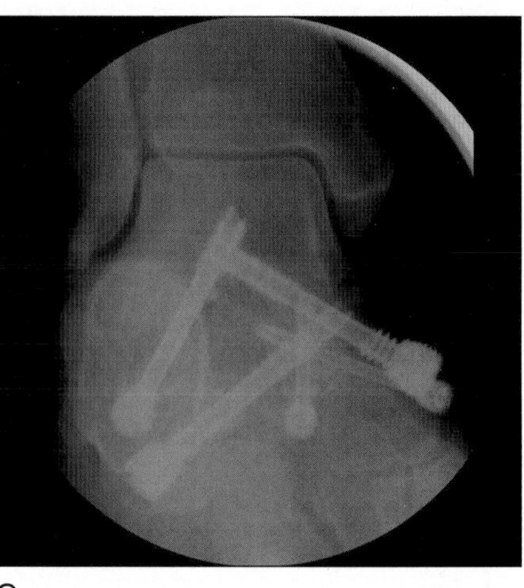

A B C

FIGURE 16

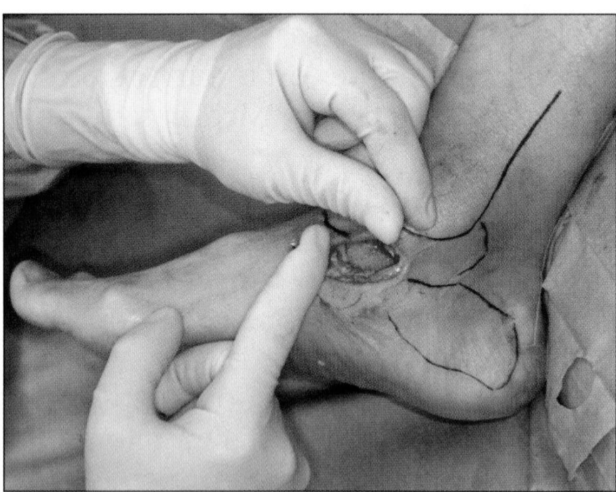

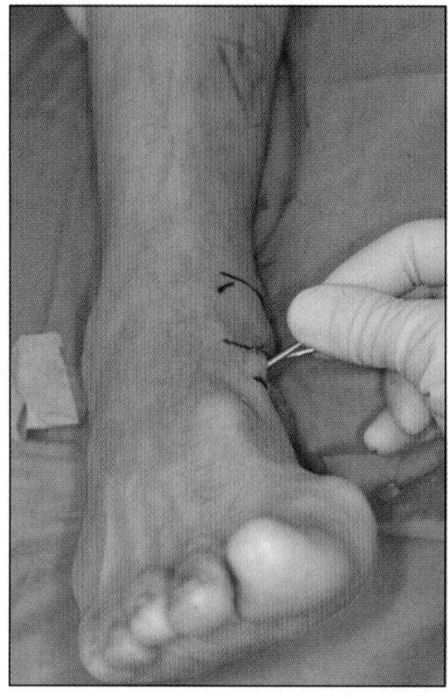

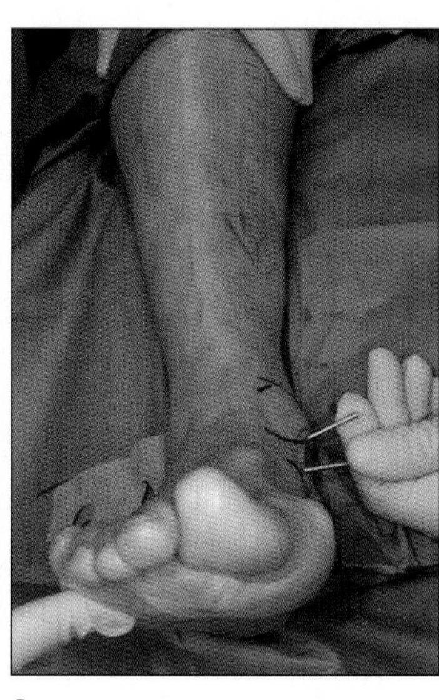

A B C

FIGURE 17

- Fluoroscopic control of the correct reduction and proper positioning of the hardware is mandatory (Fig. 16A–C).
- If any residual Achilles tendon shortening persists, an additional percutaneous Achilles tendon lengthening ("triple cut") or a mini-open gastrocnemius slide procedure is performed, depending on the shortening of the soleus.

Controversies

- Alternative fixation methods (staples, fewer screws, threaded K-wires) are possible, as long as the basic principles described above have been respected.
- In our experience, an Achilles tendon lengthening has been necessary in only a very limited number of cases.

Step 3

- The longitudinal incision of the capsule and ligaments from the navicular bone to the medial malleolus is closed by interrupted absorbable 2–0 sutures.
- The skin is closed with interrupted nonabsorbable 3–0 sutures (Fig. 18).

PEARLS

- *Careful closure of the capsular and ligamentous structures avoids postoperative swelling and increases the stability of the soft tissues.*

- A drain is not used routinely.
- A thick compressive dressing is applied (Fig. 19A and 19B), and the foot is placed in a reusable prefabricated splint (Fig. 20).
- The tourniquet is deflated.

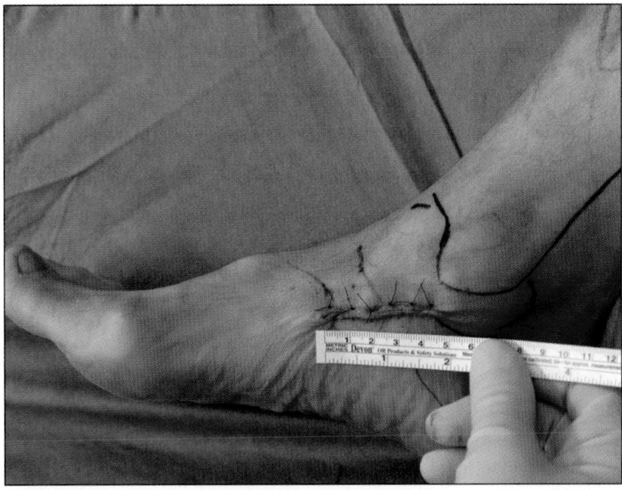

FIGURE 18

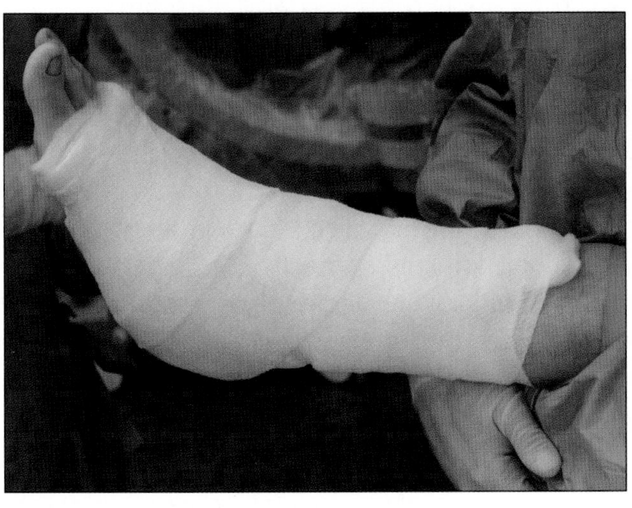

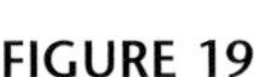

A

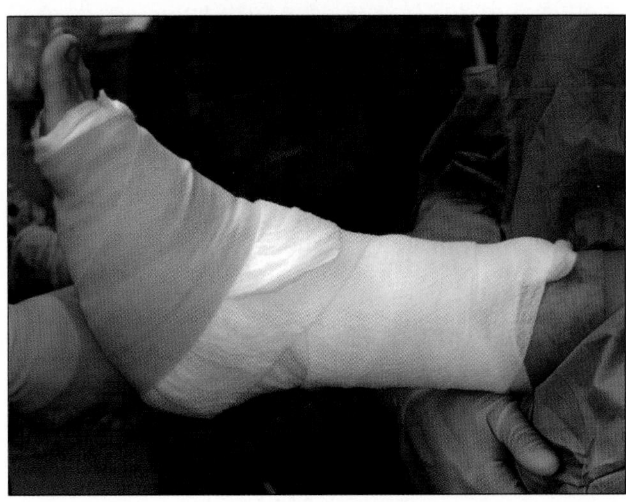

B

FIGURE 19

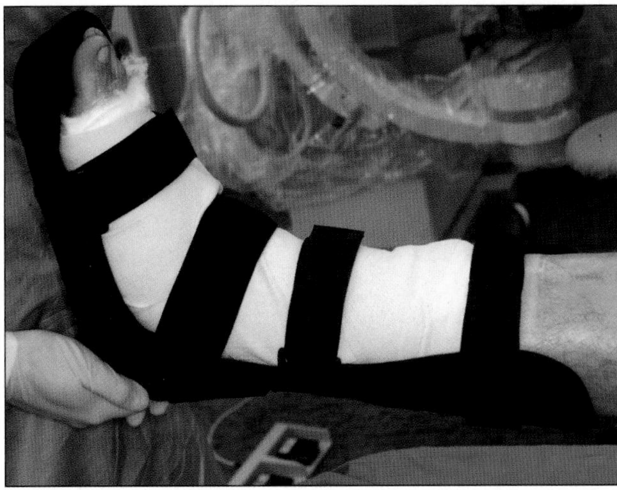

FIGURE 20

Controversies

- If no prefabricated splints are available, plaster of Paris casting is a valuable alternative (although more time consuming).

Pearls

- *General measures such as wearing compressive stockings and doing strengthening exercises of the lower leg are encouraged.*
- *Physical therapy for Achilles tendon stretching is necessary sometimes.*

Pitfalls

- *Make sure the postoperative casts support the position of the corrected hindfoot, rather than forcing the foot back into its preoperative malalignment.*
- *Potential complications include wound problems, infection (superficial or deep), malunion or nonunion of the fused joints, and late secondary arthritis of the adjacent joints.*

Controversies

- The recent literature on triple arthrodesis procedures supports our personal experience that fusing the calcaneocuboid joint routinely is not necessary, and should be done only in selected cases.

Postoperative Care and Expected Outcomes

- On the second postoperative day, the compressive dressings and prefabricated splint are replaced by a removable (synthetic) cast. This allows the use of an inflatable foot pump in case of substantial postoperative swelling.
- After subsidence of the swelling (mostly between days 6 and 14 postoperative), a below-the-knee walking cast is applied and left in place through the eighth postoperative week.
- Removal of the stitches should not be done before the 14th postoperative day; if the walking cast is applied earlier, the stitches may be left in place upon removal of the cast.
- Once the walking cast is applied properly, weight bearing is allowed as tolerated; usually full weight bearing is achieved after 10–14 days postoperatively.
- At 8 weeks, the cast is removed and standard radiographs are taken. If bony fusion is considered not to be sufficient, a removable walking cast is applied for another 4–6 weeks. If the fusion is considered to be sufficient, the patient is allowed free ambulation in custom shoes.
- At 4 months postoperative, final clinical and radiographic evaluation is carried out.
- Hardware removal—rarely necessary—is considered not earlier than 6 months after the initial triple arthrodesis surgery.
- A lasting pain-free and plantigrade foot is the final result in the majority of cases.

Evidence

Angus P, Cowell H. Triple arthrodesis: a critical long-term review. J Bone Joint Surg [Br]. 1986;68:260–5.

This study presented the outcome of 80 feet that underwent triple arthrodesis for severe hindfoot deformity. Average age at time of surgery was 14 years and 5 months. Main indications were cerebral palsy, clubfoot, polio sequelae, and tarsal coalitions. The patient's subjective rating was higher than the objective rating of the authors. Adjacent joint degeneration and residual deformity were common in this patient population. (Level IV evidence)

Astion D, Deland J, Otis J, Kenneally S. Motion of the hindfoot after simulated arthrodesis. J Bone Joint Surg [Am]. 1997;79:241–6.

This cadaver study showed that motion in the "triple-joint complex" is decreased to the greatest extent by fusing the talonavicular joint. A single fusion of the calcaneocuboid joint merely affects the motion in the other hindfoot joints.

Bednarz PA, Monroe MT, Manoli A 2nd. Triple arthrodesis in adults using rigid internal fixation: an assessment of outcome. Foot Ankle Int. 1999;20:356–63.

In this study, 57 adults underwent a total of 63 triple arthrodeses for hindfoot deformities of various etiologies. American Orthopaedic Foot and Ankle Society (AOFAS) Ankle-Hindfoot scores went from 28 to 81 points at 30 months postoperative. There was radiographic improvement of all hindfoot angles. Complications as well as secondary arthritis in the ankle did occur. (Level IV evidence)

Gellman H, Lenihan M, Halikis N, Botte MJ, Giordani M, Perry J. Selective tarsal arthrodesis: an in vitro analysis of the effect on foot motion. Foot Ankle. 1987;8:127–33.

In this study, 15 fresh cadaver feet underwent five different intertarsal arthrodeses. The authors presented the remaining degrees of range of motion in the nonfused ankle and hindfoot joints after these selective arthrodeses.

Graves S, Mann R, Graves K. Triple arthrodesis in older adults: results after long-term follow-up. J Bone Joint Surg [Am]. 1993;75:355–62.

In this study, 18 feet from 17 patients underwent triple arthrodesis. Average duration of follow-up was 42 months. Satisfaction rate was 14 of 17 patients. Complications included nonunion, adjacent joint secondary degeneration, infection, and early hardware removal. All 17 patients had less pain postoperatively. (Level IV evidence)

Jeng C, Tankson C, Myerson M. The single medial approach to triple arthrodesis: a cadaver study. Foot Ankle Int. 2006;27:1122–5.

This laboratory study proved that more than 90% of the cartilage of the subtalar, talonavicular, and calcaneocuboid joints can be removed by using a single medial incision. These results are comparable to two-incision (cadaver specimen) techniques.

Jeng C, Vora A, Myerson M. The medial approach to triple arthrodesis: indications and technique for management of rigid valgus deformities in high-risk patients. Foot Ankle Clin. 2005;10:515–21.

In this study, the authors reviewed 17 triple arthrodeses for rigid flatfoot, all operated on with a single medial approach. At a mean follow-up of 3.5 years after surgery, all 17 triple arthrodeses had fused. The authors advocated the medial approach to triple arthrodesis as a safe and reliable procedure with a predictable outcome. (Level IV evidence)

Pell R, Myerson M, Schon L. Clinical outcome after primary triple arthrodesis. J Bone Joint Surg [Am]. 2000;82:47–57.

This study presented the results of 132 triple arthrodeses in 111 patients with degenerative hindfoot deformities. Average duration of follow-up was 5.7 years. Overall satisfaction was excellent; average postoperative modified AOFAS Ankle-Hindfoot scale was 60.7 points. Eleven complications occurred in 10 patients. Secondary ankle arthritis was common in the study group, although no correlation existed with patient satisfaction. (Level IV evidence)

Sammarco V, Magur E, Sammarco G, Bagwe MR. Arthrodesis of the subtalar and talonavicular joints for correction of symptomatic hindfoot malalignment. Foot Ankle Int. 2006;27:661–6.

Sixteen double arthrodeses (subtalar and talonavicular joint) in 14 patients (indication: painful hindfoot deformity without calcaneocuboid joint involvement) were retrospectively reviewed with a minimum follow-up of 18 months. AOFAS Ankle-Hindfoot scores improved from 44.7 to 77 points; all patients were satisfied. Radiographically, secondary arthritic changes occurred in some of the adjacent joints. (Level IV evidence)

Sangeorzan BJ, Smith D, Veith R, Hansen ST. Triple arthrodesis using internal fixation in treatment of adult foot disorders. Clin Orthop Relat Res. 1993;(294):299-307.

Forty-four triple arthrodeses in 40 patients were evaluated at an average of 4.9 years, using outcome and function scales and radiographs. All radiographic angles improved. Two pseudarthroses, two unsatisfactory corrections, and no recurrences occurred. Thirty-four feet had good results, six had fair results, and there were four failures. (Level IV evidence)

Smith RW, Shen W, Dewitt S, Reischl SF. Triple arthrodesis in adults with non-paralytic disease: a minimum ten-year follow-up study. J Bone Joint Surg [Am]. 2004;86:2707-13.

In this study, the authors reviewed at a minimum follow-up of 10 years the outcome of 31 feet in 27 adults who had undergone triple arthrodesis for the treatment of painful hindfoot disease. Satisfaction rate was 93%, although only 41% of the patients could perform moderate activity with mild or no pain. The mean Short Form-36 (SF-36) score postoperatively was only 35.2 points; systemic inflammatory disease patients had significantly lower SF-36 scores. Severe arthrosis developed in a total of 20 adjacent joints. (Level IV evidence)

Wapner K. Triple arthrodesis in adults. J Am Acad Orthop Surg. 1998;6:188–96.

A general review on the indications, surgical technique, pitfalls, complications, and results of triple arthrodesis surgery in adults. (Level IV evidence)

Wulker N, Stukenborg C, Savory K, Alfke D. Hindfoot motion after isolated and combined arthrodeses: measurements in anatomic specimens. Foot Ankle Int. 2000;2:921–7.

In this cadaver study, the authors concluded that the talonavicular joint is the key articulation for hindfoot motion. Fusing it will greatly decrease hindfoot motion. Calcaneocuboid joint fusion had no significant influence on remaining hindfoot motion.

PROCEDURE 50

Triple Arthrodesis

Edmund H. Choi and Andrew K. Sands

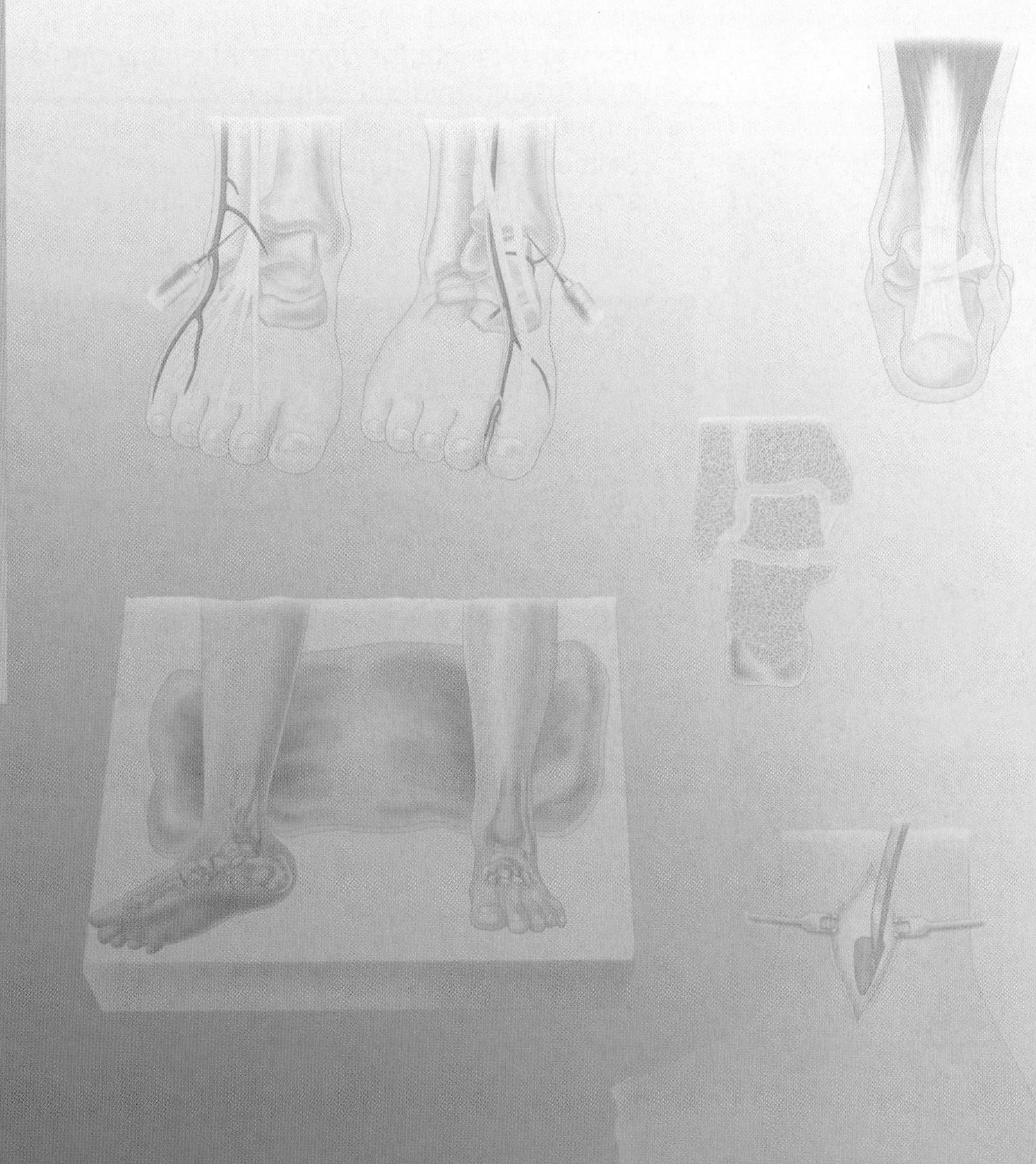

Treatment Options

- Nonoperative treatments include hindfoot and ankle bracing.
- Physical therapy and nonsteroidal anti-inflammatory drugs may help alleviate pain.

Indications

- Fixed hindfoot deformities
- Symptomatic hindfoot arthritis
- Salvage procedure of the foot

Examination/Imaging

- Weight-bearing physical examination reveals hindfoot range of motion, if any, and alignment.
- Weight-bearing radiographs are obtained in anteroposterior (AP) (Fig. 1A) and lateral (Fig. 1B) views to evaluate for degenerative changes in ankle hindfoot and midfoot joints.
- Computed tomography is helpful if evaluating for coalition or impingement if more advanced reconstruction options are to be eliminated.

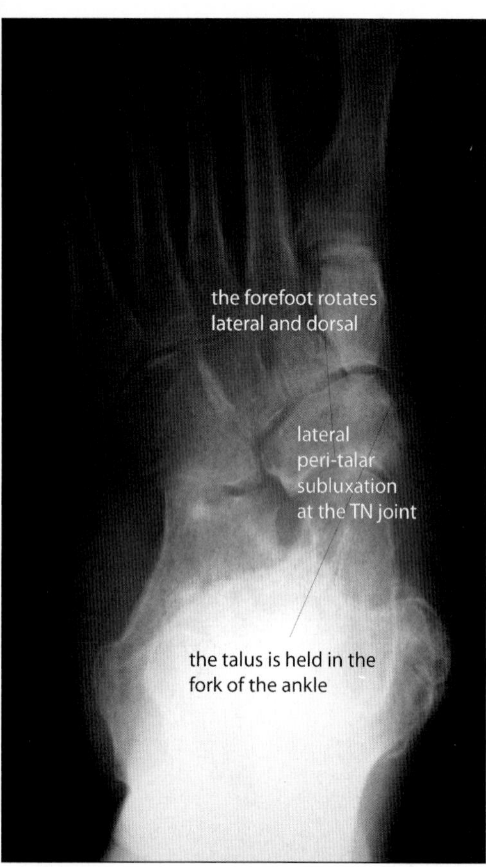

A

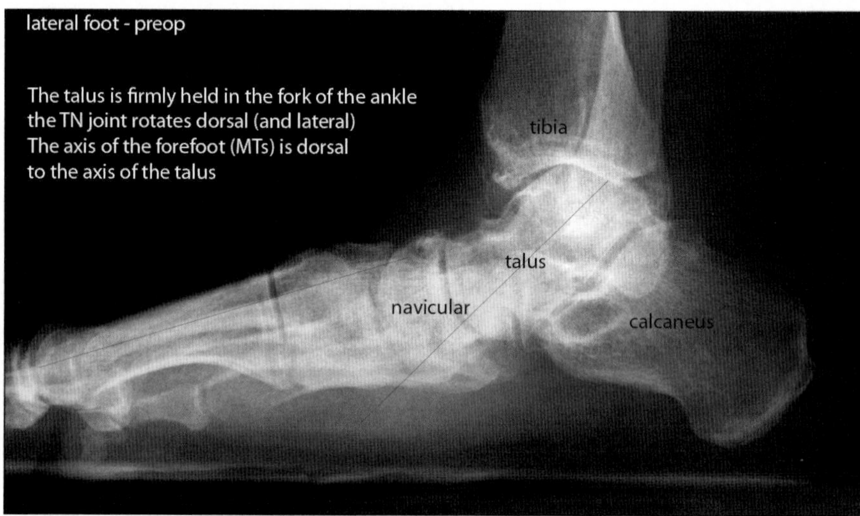

B

FIGURE 1

Surgical Anatomy

- The extensor digitorum brevis (EDB) originates on the superolateral surface of the calcaneus and branches to three tendons that insert to the lateral sides of the second, third, and fourth toes at the metatarsophalangeal joint level (Fig. 2A).
- The neurovascular (NV) bundle enters approximately 1.5 cm medial and distal to the anterior process of the calcaneus.

- Medial to the EDB is the peroneus tertius tendon, which originates from the distal third of the surface of the fibula and intermuscular septum and attaches to the dorsal surface of the base of fifth metatarsal (Fig. 2B).
- Lateral to the EDB are the peroneal tendons (Fig. 2C). Both the peroneus longus and brevis course through the common peroneal synovial sheath about 4 cm proximal to the lateral malleolus.

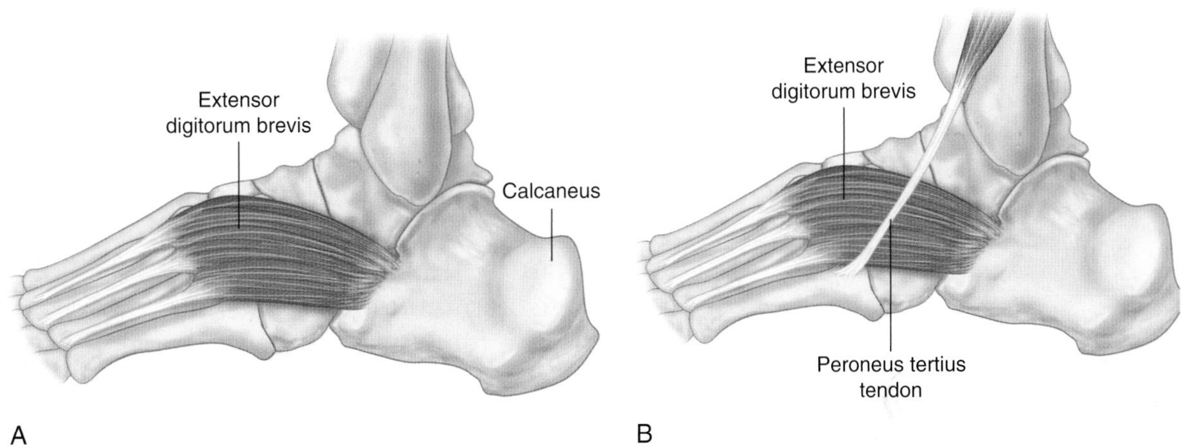

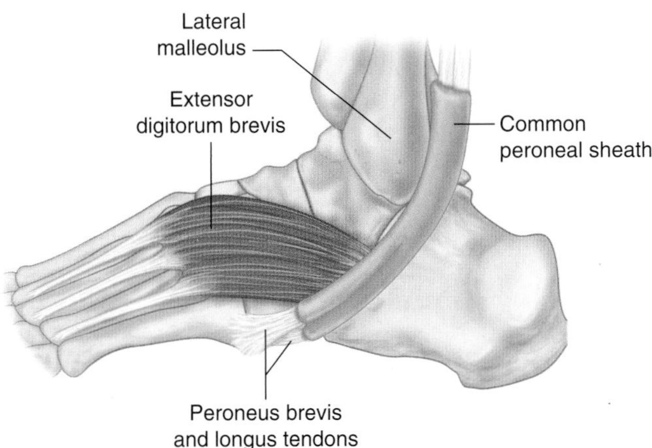

FIGURE 2

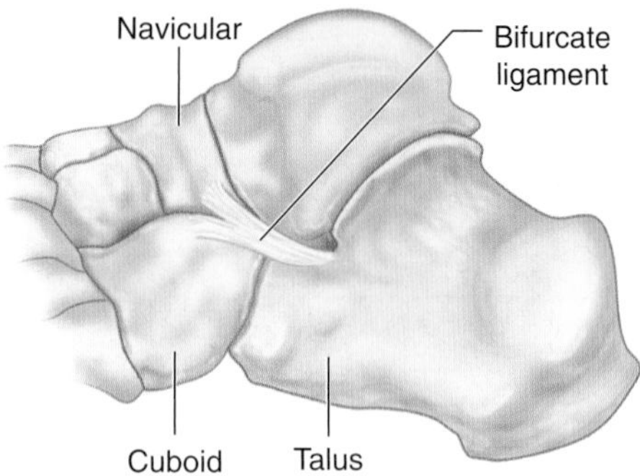

FIGURE 3

- The bifurcate ligament originates on the upper surface of the calcaneus and branches in a "Y" shape, with one branch inserting on the medial side of the cuboid and the other branch inserting on the lateral side of the navicular (Fig. 3).
- Often a coexisting equinus contracture will prevent reduction of the hindfoot to proper position. A calf or three-step tendo-Achilles lengthening is needed before the reduction and reconstruction can be carried out.

Equipment

- Lamina spreaders with and without teeth
- Distractor—cervical distractor with pins can be helpful in achieving reduction/positioning.

Positioning

- The patient is placed in supine position with the ankle propped on a soft roll padding.
- An ipsilateral bump rotates the foot to a more vertical position.
- A tourniquet is placed on the upper calf.

PEARLS

- *Avoid dorsal dissection above the talus neck to prevent injury to the blood supply to the talus.*
- *When débriding the posteromedial aspect of the joint, use a curette instead of the drill to avoid transecting the NV bundle.*
- *Flexing the great toe will result in movement of the flexor hallucis longus (FHL) tendon. This is helpful in determining the exact location of the NV bundle, which lies anteromedial to the FHL at the level of the subtalar joint.*

Portals/Exposures

- Two incisions are made: medial and lateral.
- The medial incision allows access to the talonavicular (TN) joint as well as to the anterior and middle facets of the talocalcaneal (TC) joint (Fig. 4A and 4B).
  - The posterior tibial tendon can be elevated; this allows access to the medial joints (Fig. 5A and 5B). However, since the posterior tibial tendon is often grossly pathologic, the tendon is resected.
  - The saphenous vein should be dorsal.
  - The proximal portion of the medial utility incision is used. This allows extension distally if an extended triple arthrodesis (which includes the midfoot) is needed.

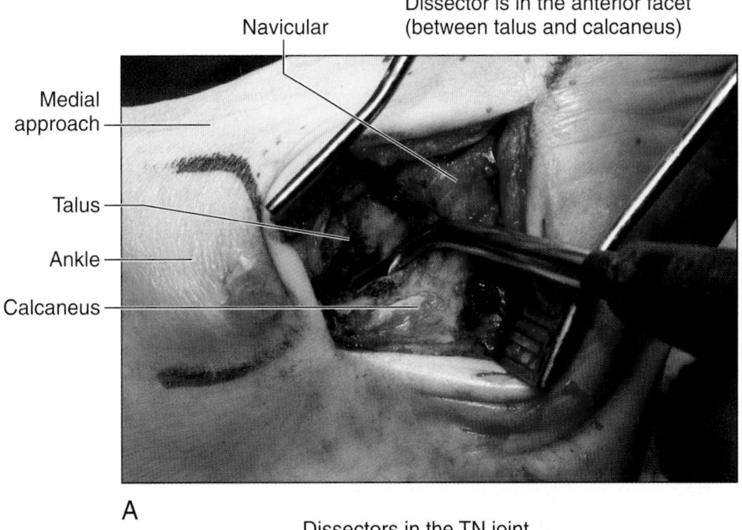

A

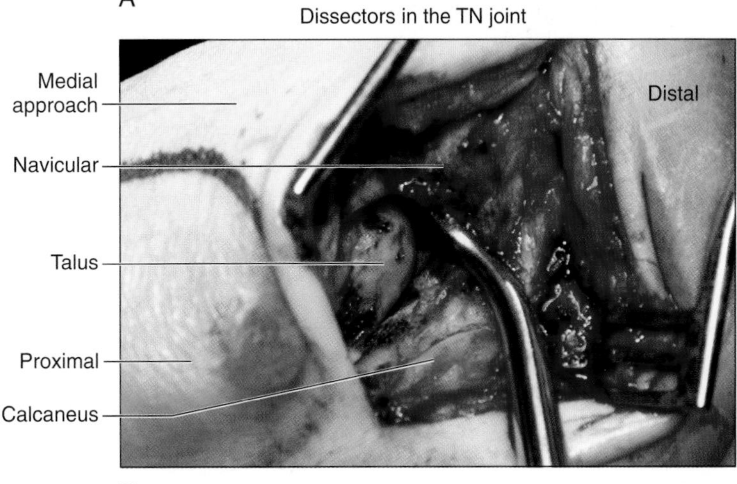

B

FIGURE 4

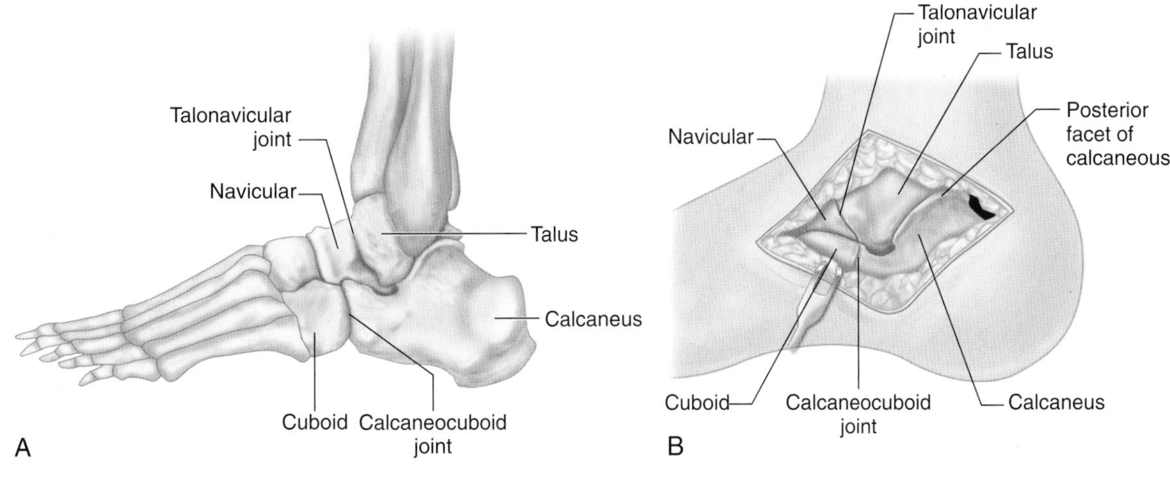

FIGURE 5

Controversies

- Choice of lateral incision—Ollier versus axial
  - Traditionally the Ollier incision was used. This incision is the oblique incision along the skinfolds approximately over the sinus tarsi, inferiorly bordered by the peroneals and superiorly bordered by the extensors. This incision is more cosmetically appealing but does not allow extension to the midfoot if needed. It can also make visualization of the CC joint more difficult. Finally, this transverse incision is more likely to result in injury to the sural or anterior sensory nerves.
  - The axial incision, in contrast, allows unlimited extension distally if needed. This incision is deepened between the EDB muscle belly (which is elevated superiorly) and the peroneals inferiorly. Access to the subtalar area, the CC joint, and the midfoot is easily obtained. Furthermore, the nerves course parallel to this incision, making sensory nerve injury less likely.

- The lateral incision allows access to the posterior facet of the TC joint, as well as the calcaneocuboid (CC) joint, the lateral part of the TN joint, and the anterior and middle facets of the TC joint (Fig. 6A–C).
  - The sinus tarsi should be débrided of all soft tissue, and can be later be packed with graft material to further aid in fusion.
  - The sural nerve courses approximately along the peroneal tendons before branching along the distal calcaneus. It is at risk with the lateral incision, especially if the Ollier incision is chosen.

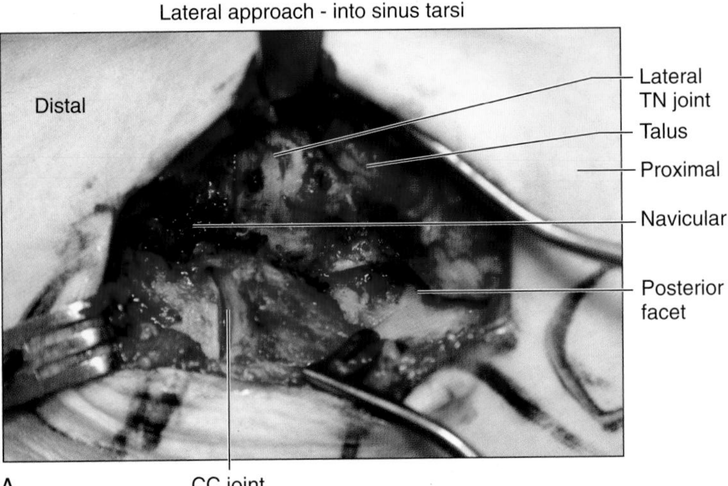

FIGURE 6

Pearls

- *Avoid excessive bone resection since this will decrease the subtalar joint height and will disrupt the articular relationship of the TN joint.*
- *Care should be taken to ensure excision of articular cartilage from the anterior, middle, and posterior subtalar facet.*
- *All of the nonarticular surfaces are decorticated.*

Pearls

- *An easy way to align the hindfoot is to place a fingertip into the sinus tarsi. The calcaneus is then pushed forward and distal, with careful attention not to rock the heel into varus or valgus. When properly aligned, the sinus tarsi is usually open enough to allow a fingertip to be placed in it.*
- *Correct not just the varus but also the internal rotation of the calcaneus underneath the talus when reducing the subtalar joint in the case of a planovalgus foot.*

Procedure

Step 1: Preparing the Joint Surfaces

- Each joint surface is denuded of articular cartilage carefully so as to not damage or deform the subchondral bony architecture (Fig. 7).
- The denuded surfaces are then carefully drilled with a series of small holes, extending into the subchondral bone and thereby enhancing fusion (Fig. 8A and 8B).
- The central area of each joint can be further prepared by making a cavity that is filled with bone graft. This acts as a shear-strain relief graft that ultimately further aids in fusion of the entire construct.

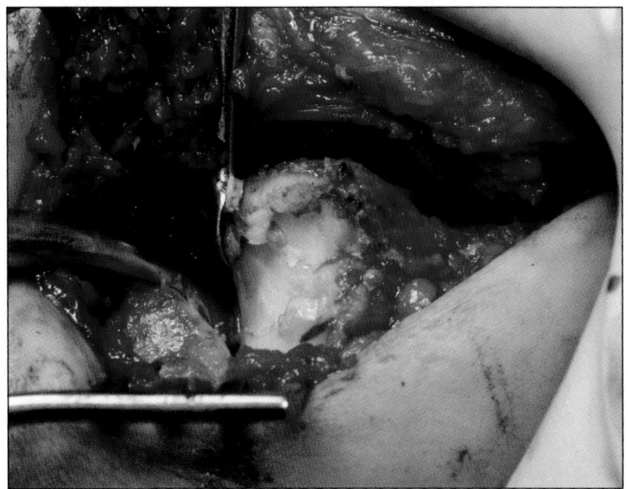

FIGURE 7

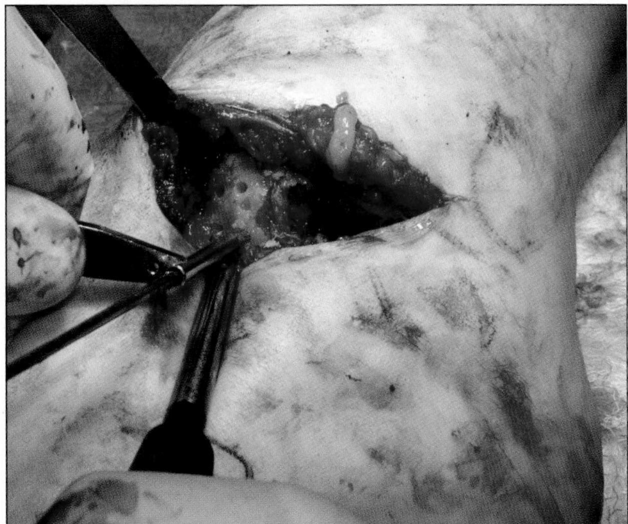

A

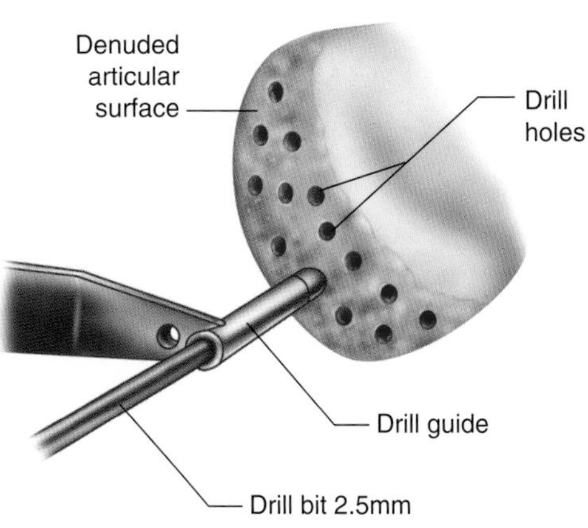

B

FIGURE 8

Step 2: Internal Fixation

- Align the TC joint. The hindfoot should be corrected to the desired alignment.
  - Once aligned, fixation across the subtalar joints is achieved by drilling from the heel into the talus, with one screw into the body and the other into the neck.
  - The body screw is placed from the lateral part of the inferior tuberosity into the central body.
  - The neck screw starts more medial (since the neck is medial) and is aimed at the central portion of the talar neck.
  - The subtalar joint should now be rigidly fixed in proper alignment.
- The Chopart region (TN and CC) can then be rotated into proper alignment. Often, hindfoot correction (subtalar joint) can lead to excessive supination of the forefoot. This is corrected through the Chopart joints.
- The TN joint is then fixed. Two screws are placed in a lag fashion from the navicular into the talus. If possible, crossed screws can also be used.
- The CC joint is more of an expansion joint and is not as important for stability in the fusion. Sometimes, one screw will suffice. It can be placed from the distal calcaneus process into the cuboid.

Pitfalls

- *After fixation of the subtalar joint, check the AP ankle view by fluoroscopy to make sure the screw is in the body and not in the lateral gutter, which is a common mistake.*
- *During fixation of the CC joint, the drill should be aligned with the axis of the foot and under the lateral malleolus. This allows the screw to go across the CC joint into the cuboid. If the angle of the drill is too high, it will miss the cuboid. For this reason and ease of insertion, staples are sometimes used at the CC joint.*

Controversies

- Screw technique for the TC joint (anterior to posterior vs. posterior to anterior)
  - Starting anteriorly from the dorsal talus into the calcaneus is one option, but this can be a problem as it can damage the dorsal blood supply to the talus. Since the plantar blood supply is already damaged by the fusion preparation, the talus could have problems (avascular necrosis) as well as fusion problems in other joints. It can also be performed posterior to anterior, starting from the heel pad and ending in the distal tibia.
  - The advantage of the former technique is better fixation due to longer threaded screws, while the disadvantage is the risk of ankle impingement from a screw too close to the talar head. The advantage of the latter technique is avoiding impingement by crossing the subtalar joint into the distal tibia. The disadvantage is using smaller threaded lag screws because the screws are going from a larger fragment of the calcaneus to a smaller fragment of the talus.
- Fixation (screws vs. staples): Screws are easier to control in their trajectory and the amount of compression placed. Staples cannot reliably provide compression across the joints. Whichever method is chosen, two fixation points across each joint are needed to prevent rotation or sliding, which would lead to nonunion at the fusion site.

STEP 3: BONE GRAFTING

- Allograft bone graft is placed into the remaining gaps of the subtalar joints.
- It is common to find a gap at the CC joint that will require bone grafting. This is in essence performing a lateral column lengthening.

Postoperative Care and Expected Outcomes

- The postoperative short-leg three-sided splint is removed at the first postoperative visit (2 weeks). A cam boot is placed and used for 6 weeks. Patient is kept non–weight bearing. Radiographs are taken at this point.
- At 6–8 weeks, weight-bearing status is progressed in the cam boot using a cane.
- Physical therapy is used only for gait training purposes and lower extremity rehabilitation.
- Figure 9 shows the 1-year postoperative appearance in the AP (Fig. 9A), lateral (Fig. 9B), and oblique (Fig. 9C) views.

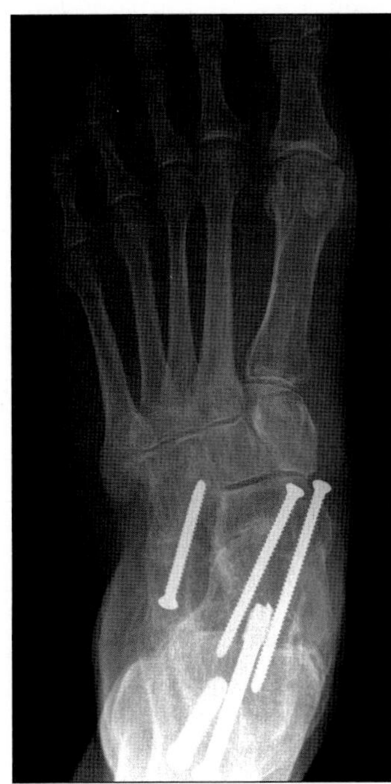
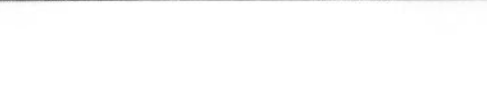
A

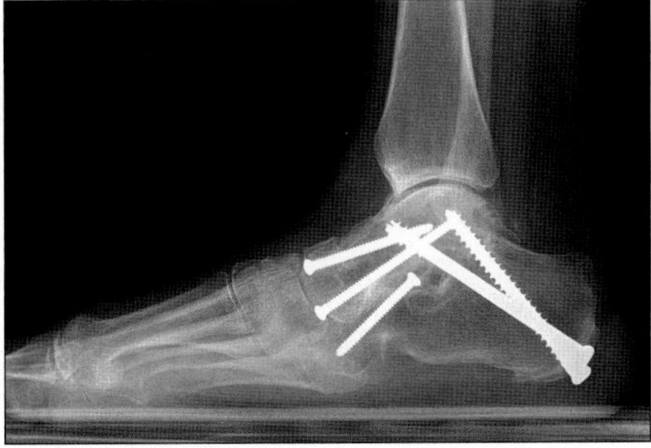
B

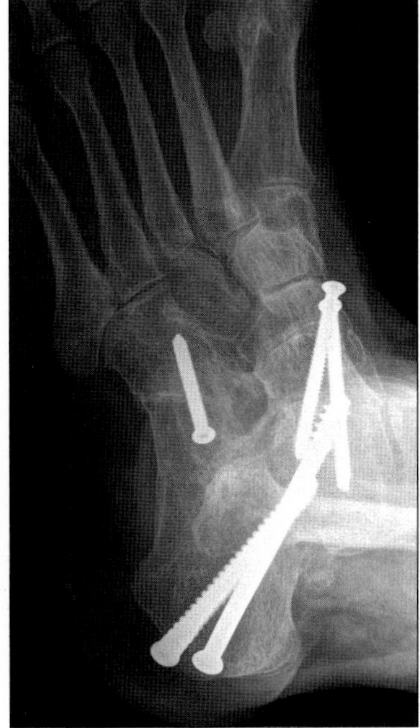
C

FIGURE 9

Evidence

Astion D, Deland J, Otis J, Kenneally S. Motion of the hindfoot after simulated arthrodesis. J Bone Joint Surg [Am]. 1997;79:241–6.

This study described a laboratory evaluation of 10 cadaveric foot specimens. The authors fused different subtalar joints and determined by three-dimensional magnetic resonance imaging which joint limited the motion of the triple joint complex. (Level IV evidence [case series])

Cracchiolo A, Cimino W, Lian G. Arthrodesis of the ankle in patients who have rheumatoid arthritis. J Bone Joint Surg [Am]. 1992;74:903–9.

This study was a retrospective review of cases of arthrodesis by internal fixation and external fixation. The authors determined the postoperative duration to fusion and the complication rates. (Level IV evidence [case series])

Graves SC, Mann RA, Graves KO. Triple arthrodesis in older adults: a long term follow-up. J Bone Joint Surg [Am]. 1993;75:355–62.

This study was a retrospective review of 17 patients. Follow-up averaged 3.5 years, and outcome was judged by patient pain scores, level of activity, shoewear, and patient satisfaction with appearance. (Level IV evidence [case series])

Haddad SL, Coetzee JC, Estok R, Fahrbach K, Banel D, Nalysnyk L. Intermediate and long-term outcomes of total ankle anthroplasty and ankle arthrodesis. J Bone Joint Surg [Am]. 2007;89:1899–905.

This study was a systematic review of 49 studies of ankle arthroplasty and 39 studies of ankle arthrodesis. The authors determined the intermediate outcomes of both procedures based on the American Orthopaedic Foot and Ankle Society scale system and revision rates. (Level III evidence [retrospective cohort])

Papa J, Myerson M, Girard P. Salvage, with arthrodesis, in intractactable diabetic neuropathic arthropathy of the foot and ankle. J Bone Joint Surg [Am]. 1993;75:1056–66.

This study was a retrospective review of 29 patients with diabetic neuropathy. Follow-up averaged almost 4 years, and the outcome was judged by physical examination. (Level IV evidence [case series])

Pell R, Myerson M, Schon L. Clinical outcome after primary triple arthrodesis. J Bone Joint Surg [Am]. 2000;82:47–57.

This study was a retrospective review of 160 patients. Follow-up averaged 5.7 years, and outcome was judged by patient satisfaction and physical examination. (Level IV evidence [case series])

Saltzman C, Fehrle M, Cooper R, Spencer E, Ponseti I. Triple arthrodesis: twenty-five and forty-four year average follow-up of the same patients. J Bone Joint Surg [Am]. 1999;81:1391–402.

This study was a retrospective review of 57 patients. Follow-up averaged 21 years, and outcome was judged by the Angus and Cowell assessment system. (Level IV evidence [case series])

Smith R, Shen W, DeWitt S, Reischl S. Triple arthrodesis in adults with non-paralytic disease: a minimum ten-year follow-up study. J Bone Joint Surg [Am]. 2004;86:2707–13.

This study was a retrospective review of 27 patients. Follow-up averaged 14 years, and outcome was judged by Short Form-36 scores, physical examination, and functional tests such as the 6-minute walk and 3-m up-and-go test. (Level IV evidence [case series])

Wetmore R, Drennan J. Long-term results of triple arthrodesis in Charcot-Marie-Tooth disease. J Bone Joint Surg [Am]. 1989;71:417–22.

This study was a retrospective review of 16 patients with Charcot-Marie-Tooth disease treated with triple arthrodesis. Follow-up averaged 21 years, and the outcome was judged by the Patterson clinical assessment system. (Level IV evidence [case series])

The Leg

SECTION IV

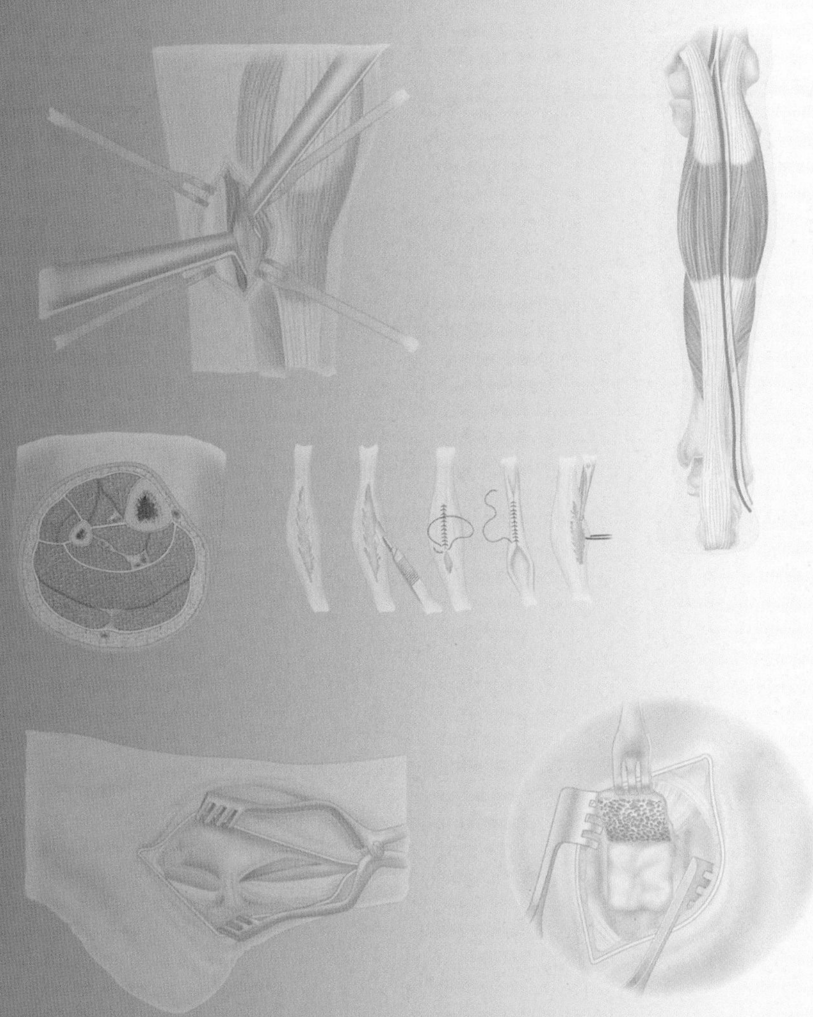

PROCEDURE 51

Treatment of Distal Achilles (Insertional) Degeneration and Associated Calf Tightness Plus Calcaneal Tuber Exostosis

Andrew K. Sands

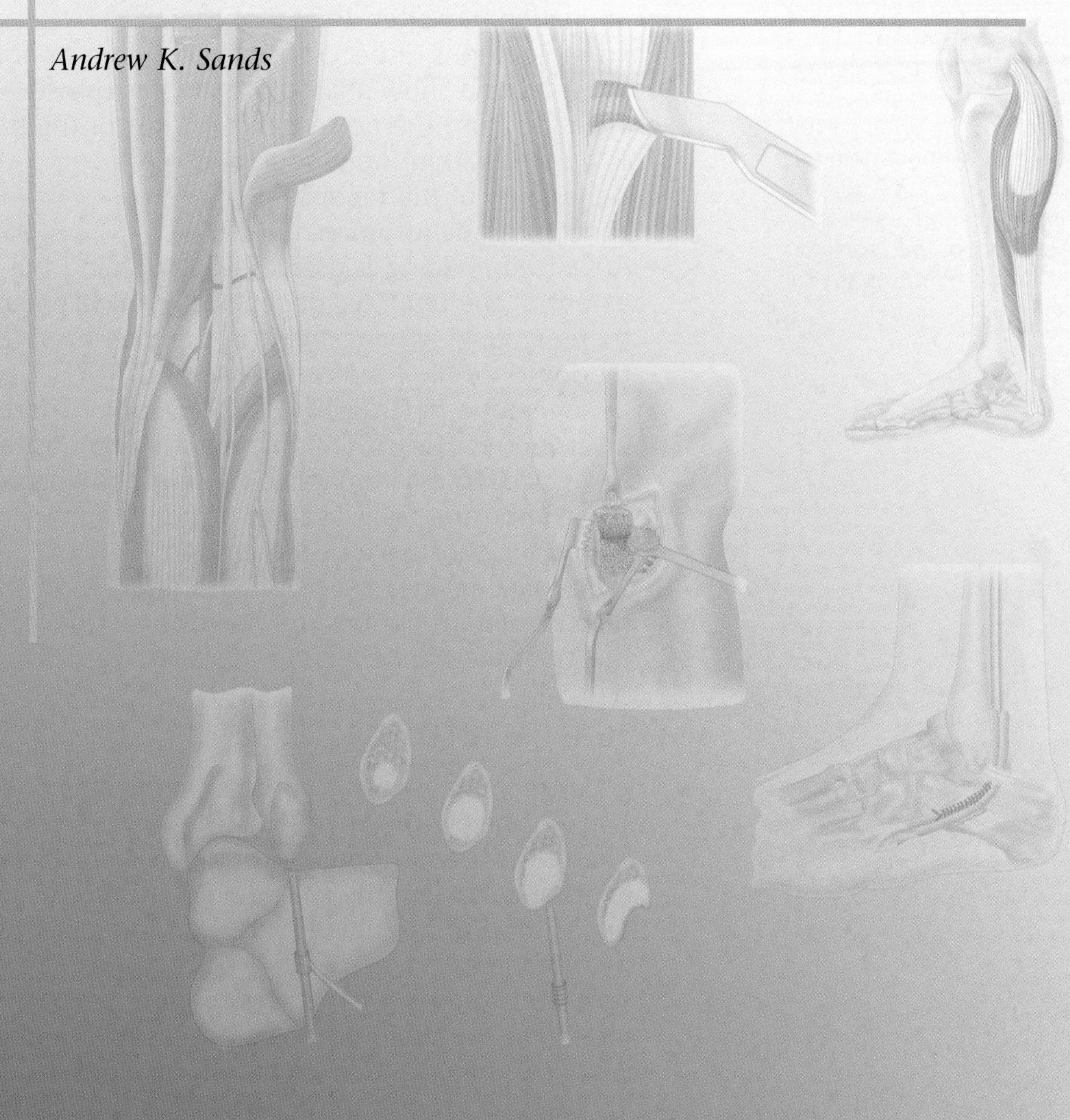

Andrew K. Sands would like to acknowledge the assistance of Edmund Choi, MD with this chapter.

Treatment Options

- Nonoperative treatment is often effective. Aggressive calf and hamstring stretching, ankle dorsiflexion night splinting, and physical therapy will often decrease the symptoms, although the bony prominence will often persist.
- Some perform the distal part of the procedure without doing the calf release, as they do not feel equinus contracture is an important part of the problem. Ignore the calf tightness at your own peril.

Indications

- Pain, deformity, and weakness of the Achilles tendon with maximum symptoms at the insertion onto the tuberosity

Examination/Imaging

- The area of maximum pain is the insertion of the Achilles onto the tuberosity. There may be swelling/enlargement of the area that is tender to touch. Shoewear and heels can cause problems. Equinus examination will often show tightness.
- Plain radiographs, especially the lateral foot or ankle view, will often show a large proximal exostosis originating from the posteroinferior area of the tuber. This bone is within the tendon and represents degeneration of the tendon.
- Magnetic resonance imaging (MRI)
  - Advanced imaging is useful in determining the extent of the tendon's degenerative involvement. If there is signal enhancement in the interior of the tendon on MRI, it indicates tendinous degeneration. Specifically, T_2-weighted or short tau inversion recovery (STIR) images will demonstrate an associated inflammation. T_1-weighted images will demonstrate calcification or bone formation within the substance of the tendon.
  - While axial images are helpful, sagittal reconstructions are best to view the tendon, and the associated degeneration distally.

Surgical Anatomy

- The gastrocnemius-soleus complex originates both above and below the knee (Fig. 1A and 1B).
  - The gastrocnemius muscles originate behind the femoral condyles. The soleus originates from the upper third of the tibia, fibula, and interosseous membrane.
  - They join to form the Achilles tendon, which inserts on the tuber of the calcaneus. The tendon is approximately 15 cm in length. It sends an aponeurosis around the tuberosity to the plantar aspect of the tuberosity, where it helps form the plantar ligaments.
- Blood supply of the tendon and the musculotendinous junction is derived from the posterior tibial artery (Fig. 2).

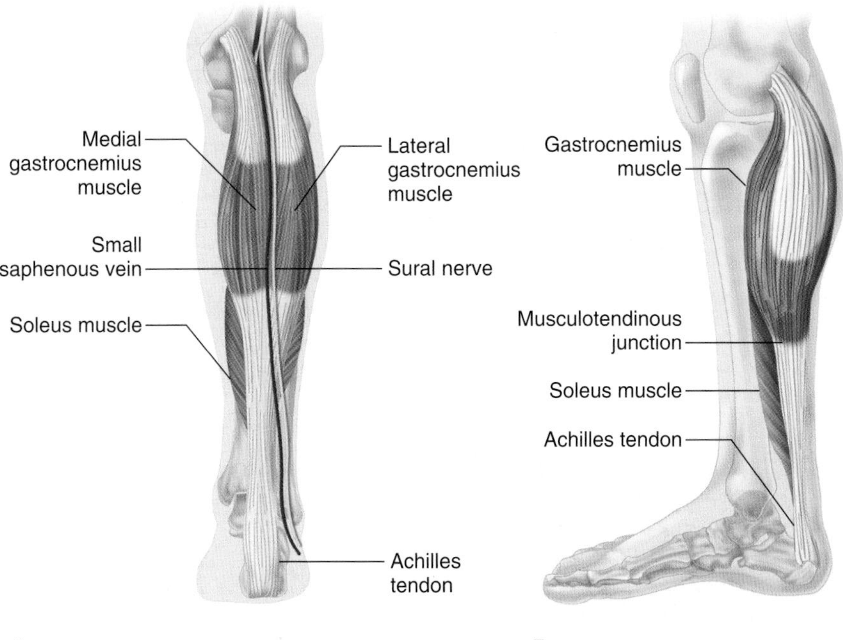

FIGURE 1

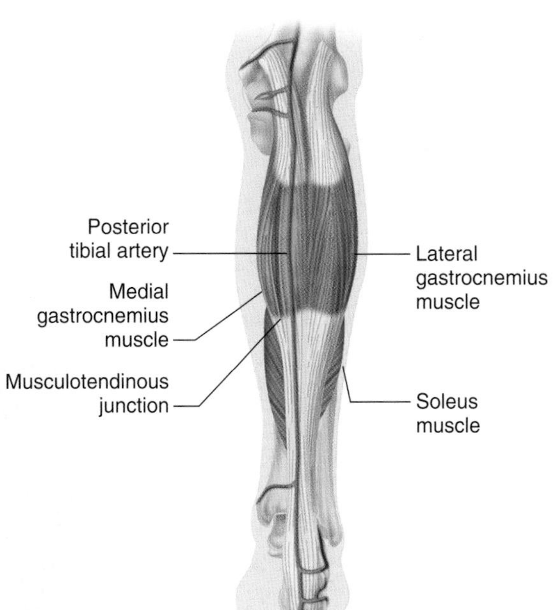

FIGURE 2

- The tendon-bone junction at the calcaneus derives its blood supply from mesosternal vessels that cross the paratenon.
- The watershed area is 2.5 cm proximal to the calcaneal insertion.

- The Achilles tendon lies directly posterior in the leg. The overlying skin and subcutaneous layer is very thin and prone to break down if injudicious dissection is done.
- The sural nerve passes superficial to the deep fascia of the posterolateral leg and onto the dorsolateral foot. The sural nerve runs lateral and anterior to the Achilles tendon at the level of the ankle joint (see Fig. 1A).

Positioning

- The patient is positioned prone on a prone spinal frame with a large bump (sterile) under the distal tibia to allow the ankle to dorsiflex.

Pearls

- *Make sure the patient is far enough up toward the head of the table so the foot is on the table and not hanging off the end. This allows for easy positioning of the ankle during the case.*

Equipment

- Spinal positioner—a Wilson frame works very nicely. The frame can be secured to the table. This is easier than using two linen rolls, which do not secure the patient as well or maintain position as well.

Portals/Exposures

- Two incisions are made: proximal and distal (Fig. 3).
- The proximal incision is made at the musculotendinous junction of the gastrocnemius, just medial to midline. This allows the sural nerve to be lateral to the field (Fig. 4A and 4B).
  - The sural nerve should still be identified and retracted gently to avoid traction injury to the nerve (Fig. 5).
  - The incision is carried down through the investing fascia, exposing the gastrocnemius muscle belly and the musculotendinous junction.

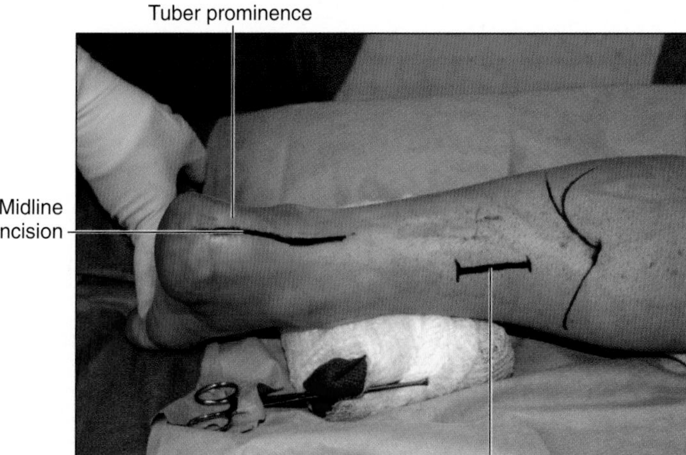

FIGURE 3

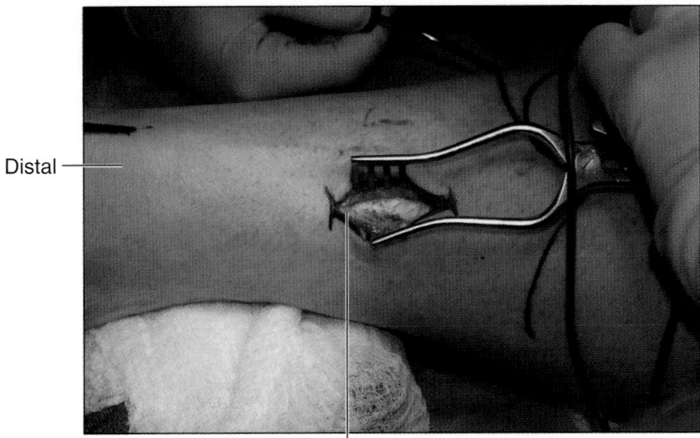

A Posteromedial calf incision at gastroc MT junction

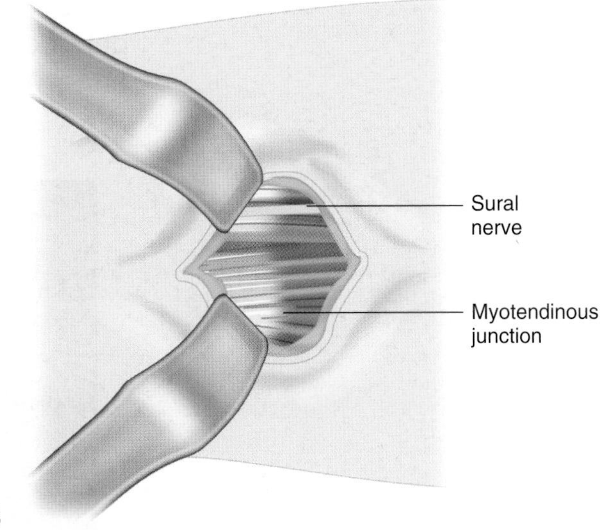

B

FIGURE 4

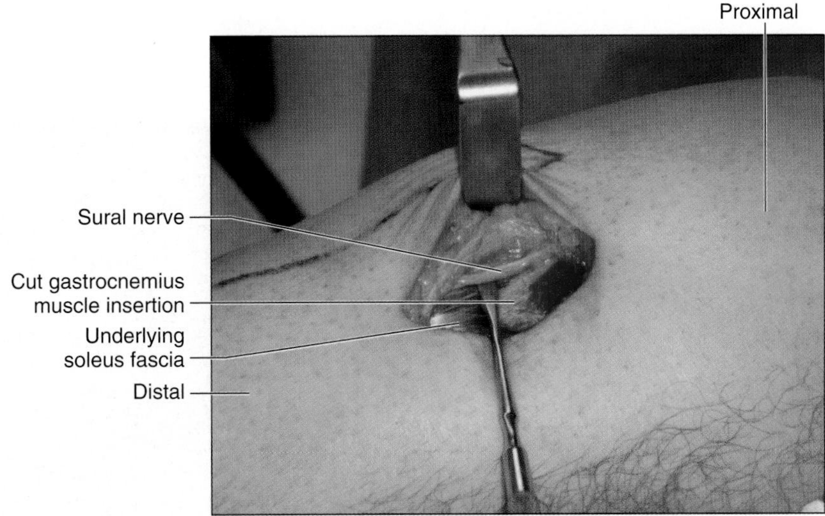

FIGURE 5

- The distal incision is made at the midline starting at the distal 3 cm of the Achilles tendon inferiorly around the tuberosity toward the plantar surface (Fig. 6). The dissection is carried through the central portion of the tendon to the pretendinous fat, without raising subcutaneous flaps. This protects the blood supply and helps prevent wound problems.
- The central tendon–splitting approach allows access to the tuberosity and the degenerative inner portion of the tendon (Fig. 7).
- The tendon dissection is carried medially and laterally along the subperiosteal plane, taking care not to detach the tendon. This allows access to the underside and central portion of the tendon for débridement of the degenerative portions, which are often yellowish in color and gritty in texture (Fig. 8).

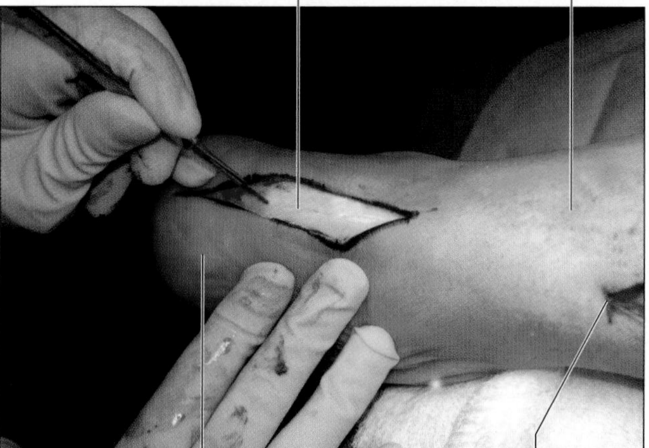

FIGURE 6

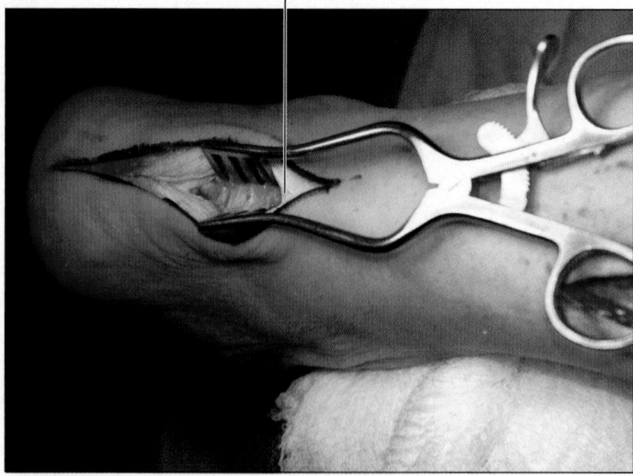

FIGURE 7

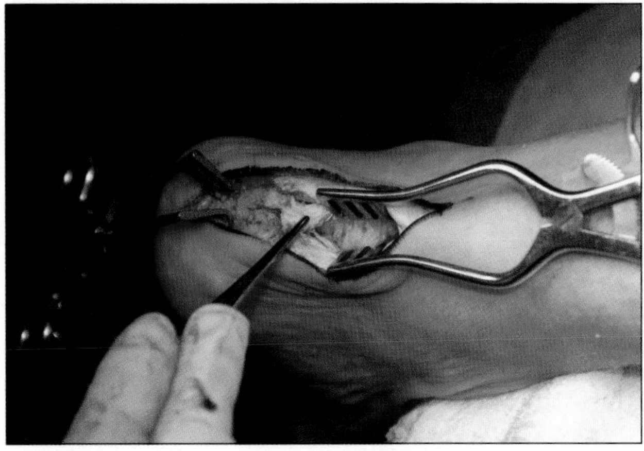

Pickup is holding yellowish disorganized scar tissue which does not look like organized collagen of healthy tendon tissue

FIGURE 8

Procedure

Step 1: Calf Lengthening

- Using the proximal approach, dissect down until the musculotendinous junction is exposed.
- The medial edge of the gastrocnemius tendon is identified, and an instrument or finger is placed under the gastrocnemius tendon between the gastrocnemius and the soleus.
  - Superficially, the soft tissue should be swept off of the exposed gastrocnemius tendon, thereby making sure the sural nerve is protected.
  - Deep retractors can then be placed, holding the soft tissue aside with the finger under the tendon.
- The entire width of the tendon is then exposed, allowing for release under direct visualization. This can be done with the cautery, adjacent to the surgeon's finger (Fig. 9).

Finger in gastrocnemius soleus interval. Gastrocnemius insertion released

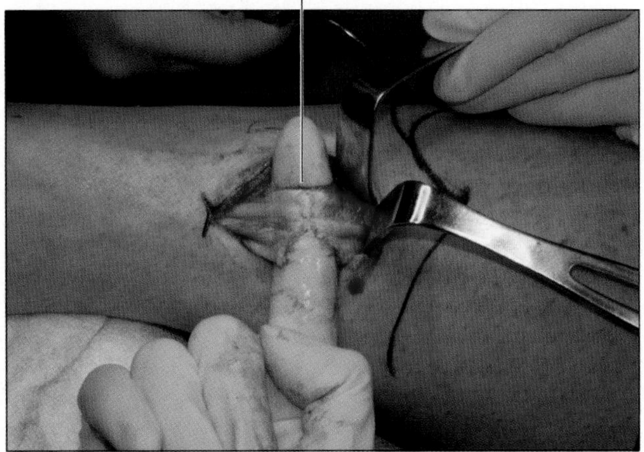

FIGURE 9

- The ankle is placed in neutral and the subcutaneous tissues are closed with the fascia in one layer.
- The skin is closed with monofilament rapidly absorbable suture in a running everted mattress suture.

Step 2: Reconstruction of the Distal Achilles

- The bony prominence of the calcaneal tuberosity is outlined and a back-cut with a curved osteotome is used to cut downward on the top of the tuberosity (Fig. 10). The remainder of the cut can be made from inferior to superior. The remainder of the bone can be removed using rongeurs.
- Once the surface is smoothed, a suture anchor is placed into the central inferior area of the tuberosity. The suture anchor should be placed tangential to the pull of the Achilles tendon.
- The Achilles tendon is then repaired full thickness side-to-side from proximal to distal using a 0 absorbable monofilament material (Fig. 11A and 11B).
- Distally, the anchored suture is woven proximally to augment the repair.
- A final purse-string suture (Fig. 12) is placed to close the tendon and the soft tissue.
- A few 00 braided absorbable sutures are placed to bring the subcutaneous layer together, but care should be taken not to strangulate the soft tissue.
- The skin is closed using running everted mattress suture of 000 absorbable monofilament.
- A fluffy dressing and three-sided plaster splint is then applied. This is overwrapped with Webril and elastic bandages. Make sure there is plenty of padding posteriorly.

Controversies

- Some have recommended using four suture anchors to hold the Achilles insertion in place. This is excessive, wasteful, and not necessary as failure with one suture is not common.

Achilles dissected medial and lateral exposing tuber back-cut with curved osteotome to prevent excessive removal of tuber

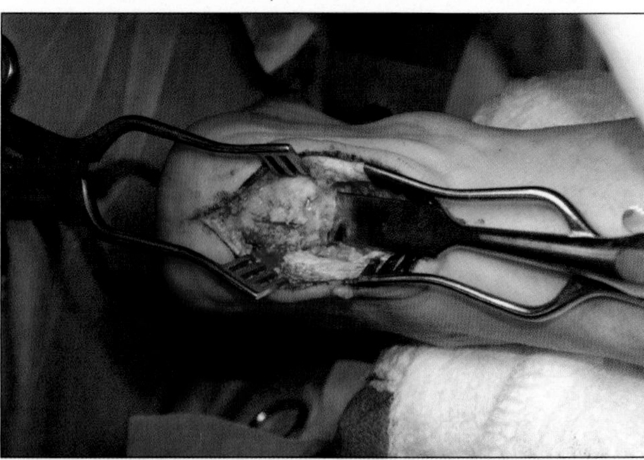

FIGURE 10

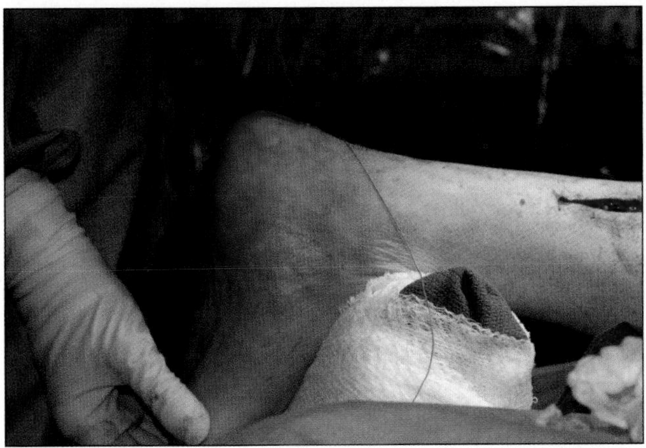

A

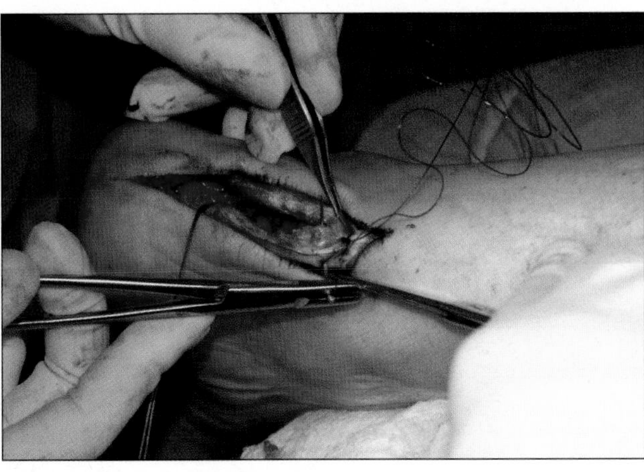

B

FIGURE 11

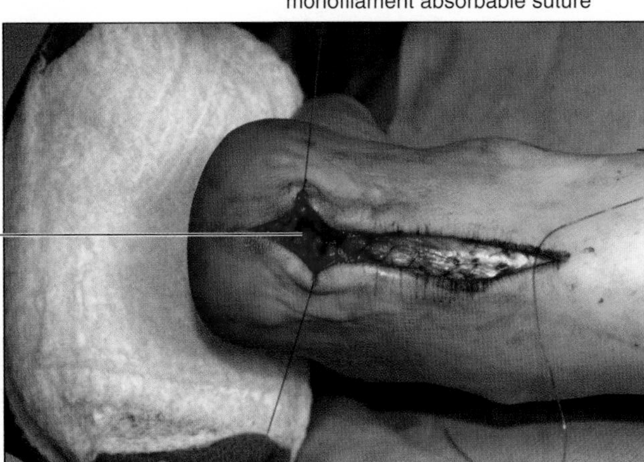

FIGURE 12

PEARLS

Proximal

- *As the last fibers are released, slight dorsiflexion pressure can be applied to the ankle. Once the tendon is completely released, the ankle dorsiflexes easily and a gap is noted in the gastrocnemius tendon.*
- *Closing the fascia helps prevent adherence of the skin to the cut tendon and makes for a more cosmetically pleasing result.*
- *Often, we place a lap pad into this wound and cover it with the stockinette while we work distally. When we come back proximally, the wound is usually dry without any bleeding.*

Distal

- *Use the knife side (not edge) along the bone in a filleting-type technique.*
- *If the tendon is completely degenerative and needs to be removed, the bailout is to resect it completely and do a flexor hallucis longus transfer (see Procedure 52).*

PITFALLS

- *The back-cut prevents more anterior propagation of the cut into the tuber.*
- *If the soft tissue is not cleared from the gastrocnemius tendon, the sural nerve is at risk.*

Instrumentation/Implantation

- Since the cortical bone has been removed, a screw-in type anchor is not recommended as these do not hold as well in cancellous bone. The expanding-arm type anchor holds better since the cortical bone has been removed with the bony prominence.

Postoperative Care and Expected Outcomes

- The three-sided splint is left in place for 2 weeks.
- When the patient is seen back in the office, the splint is removed and the wounds are checked. The leg can then be placed into a cam walker boot, which can be removed for washing.
- A 90° splint can be used for home/night/sleep use.
- At 6 weeks, gentle range of motion is started along with full weight bearing in the cam walker boot.
- At 12 weeks, a cushioned sneaker is used and formal physical therapy is started.
- The recovery after this reconstruction is long, and it often takes a year to return to full activity. Return to everyday activity can be expected at 5–6 months.

Evidence

Calder JD, Saxby TS. Surgical treatment of insertional Achilles tendinosis. Foot Ankle Int. 2003;24:119–21.

This study was a retrospective review of 52 operations. Follow-up was a minimum of 6 months. Outcome was determined by clinical examination. (Level IV evidence [case series])

Costa ML, Donell ST, Tucker K. Long-term outcome of tendon lengthening for chronic Achilles tendon pain. Foot Ankle Int. 2006;27:672–6.

This study was a retrospective review of 21 cases treated operatively. Follow-up averaged 7.5 years. Outcome was determined by pain scores and clinical examination. (Level IV evidence [case series])

Johnson KW, Zalavras C, Thordarson DB. Surgical management of insertional calcific Achilles tendinosis with a central tendon splitting approach. Foot Ankle Int. 2006;4:245–50.

This study was a retrospective review of 22 patients treated operatively. Follow-up averaged 34 months. Outcome was determined by American Orthopaedic Foot and Ankle Society (AOFAS) score, shoewear comfort, and return to work. (Level IV evidence [case series])

Maffulli N, Test V, Vapasso G, Sullo A. Calcific insertional Achilles tendinopathy: reattachment with bone anchors. Am J Sports Med. 2004;32:174–82.

This study was a retrospective review of 21 patients treated operatively. Follow-up averaged 48.4 months. Outcome was determined by VISA-A questionnaire. (Level IV evidence [case series])

Nicholson CW, Beret GC, Lee TH. Prediction of the success of nonoperative treatment of insertional Achilles tendinosis based on MRI. Foot Ankle Int. 2007;28:472–7.

This study was an MRI assessment of patients with nonoperative treatment after an average of 12 months. (Level IV evidence [case series])

Wagner E, Gould JS, Kneidel M, Fleisig GS, Fowler R. Technique and results of Achilles tendon detachment and reconstruction for insertional Achilles tendinosis. Foot Ankle Int. 2006;27:677–84.

This study was a retrospective review of 75 patients treated operatively. Follow-up averaged 47 months. Outcome was determined by patient subjective assessment. (Level IV evidence [case series])

Watson AD, Anderson RB, Davis WH. Comparison of results of retrocalcaneal decompression for retrocalcaneal bursitis and insertional Achilles tendinosis with calcific spur. Foot Ankle Int. 2000;21:638–42.

This study was a retrospective review of 16 cases of retrocalcaneal bursitis and 22 cases of calcific Achilles insertional tendinosis treated with decompression. Follow-up was at least 2 years. Outcome was determined by AOFAS scores, patient satisfication, duration until maximum symptomatic improvement, and radiographs. (Level III evidence [retrospective cohort])

Yodlowski ML, Scheller AD, Minos L. Surgical treatment of Achilles tendonitis by decompression of the retrocalcaneal bursa and the superior calcaneal tuberosity. Am J Sports Med. 2002;30:318–21.

This study was a retrospective cohort of 35 patients. Follow-up averaged 20 months. Outcome was determined by patient subjective assessment. (Level III evidence [retrospective cohort])

PROCEDURE 52

Achilles Tendon Reconstruction with Flexor Hallucis Longus Transfer Augmentation

Andrew K. Sands

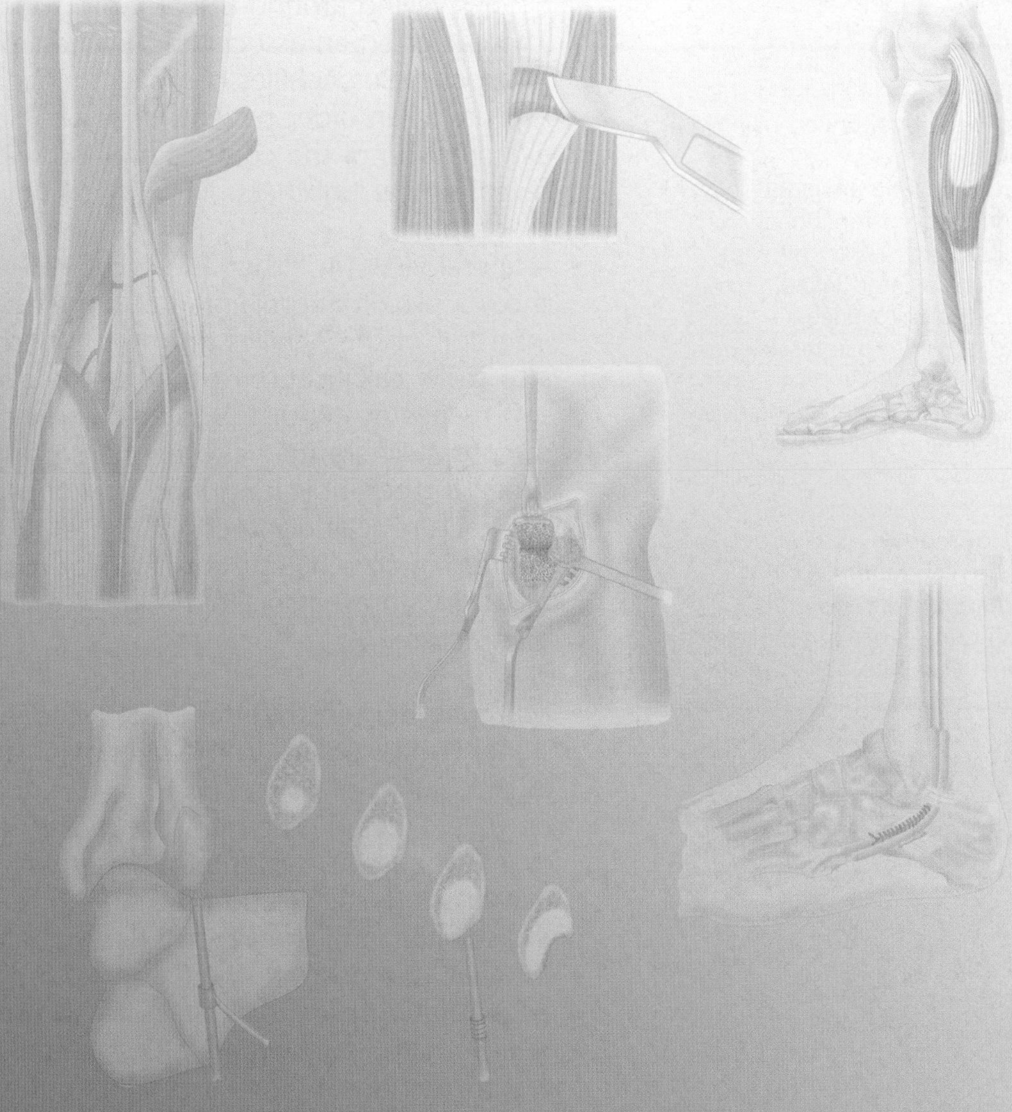

Andrew K. Sands would like to acknowledge the assistance of Edmund Choi, MD with this chapter.

Indications

- Symptomatic Achilles tendon disease (signal change on magnetic resonance imaging [MRI] within the tendon) or Achilles rupture in older individuals in whom end-to-end repair would lead to excessive tightness

Treatment Options

- Achilles ruptures
  - Nonoperative treatment can be done, but especially in older patients with degenerative tendons, the re-rupture rate is higher and the incidence of continued pain is higher.
  - Options include a weight-bearing cast or functional bracing/cam walker use with the ankle plantar flexed. Over 3 months, the ankle is brought out of plantar flexion back to neutral.
  - Some have advocated the use of ultrasound to check that the tendon ends are apposed.
  - Other techniques include fascia turndown, fascia lengthening, and use of allograft and various graft substitutes, either of human or animal source.
- Achilles tendinopathy
  - Cast or cam walker boot
  - Open débridement and tendo-Achilles lengthening at the gastrocnemius insertion

Examination/Imaging

- Examination of the Achilles tendon will often demonstrate pain and enlargement of the tendon itself or swelling around the tendon.
  - There is often an associated tightness of the gastrocnemius-Achilles complex. In the case of a rupture in an older patient (over age 38), examination of the contralateral leg will often reveal similar tightness.
- Radiographs
  - A lateral view (in either a foot or ankle series) may show a proximal projection of bone at the insertion of the Achilles onto the tuberosity. It may also show calcification within the tendon or in the soft tissues posterior to the ankle area (synovial sarcoma). There may also be plantar tuberosity spurs, further indicating long-standing equinus contracture (calf tightness).
  - There may also be a foot deformity (cavus or planus) with an associated Achilles equinus contracture.
- MRI
  - MRI may demonstrate tendinous degeneration by signal enhancement in the interior of the tendon. Inflammation of the tendon may be demonstrated on the T_2-weighted or short tau inversion recovery (STIR) images. T_1-weighted images will demonstrate calcification or bone formation within the substance of the tendon.
  - MRI will demonstrate the extent of the tendon degeneration proximal and distal to the rupture. While axial images are helpful, sagittal reconstructions are best to evaluate the tendon.

Surgical Anatomy

- The gastrocnemius-soleus complex originates both above and below the knee (Fig. 1A and 1B).
  - The gastrocnemius muscles originate behind the femoral condyles. The soleus originates from the

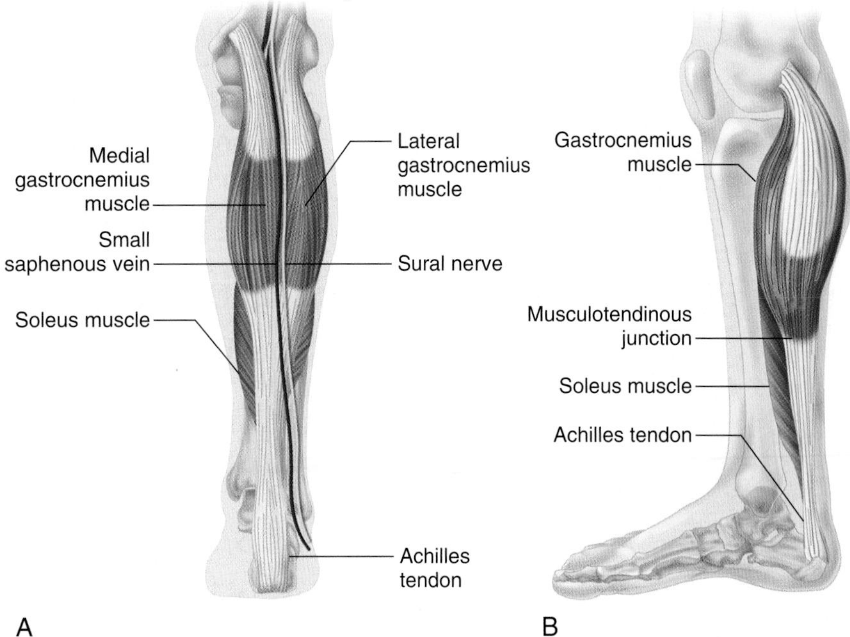

FIGURE 1

upper third of the tibia, fibula, and interosseous membrane.

- They join to form the Achilles tendon, which inserts on the tuber of the calcaneus. The tendon is approximately 15 cm in length. It sends an aponeurosis around the tuberosity to the plantar aspect of the tuberosity, where it helps form the planar ligaments.

- The Achilles tendon lies directly posterior in the leg. The overlying skin and subcutaneous layer is very thin and prone to break down if injudicious dissection is done.
- The sural nerve passes superficial to the deep fascia of the posterolateral leg and onto the dorsolateral foot. The sural nerve runs lateral and anterior to the Achilles tendon at the level of the ankle joint (see Fig. 1A).
- A straight medial approach allows for preservation of the subcutaneous blood supply (helping to avoid wound breakdown) and access to both the Achilles (and the degenerative portion) as well as the flexor hallucis longus (FHL) muscle belly and tendon.
- To expose the FHL, dissection is carried through the deep fascia layer, at which point the neurovascular (NV) bundle sits just medial to the FHL.

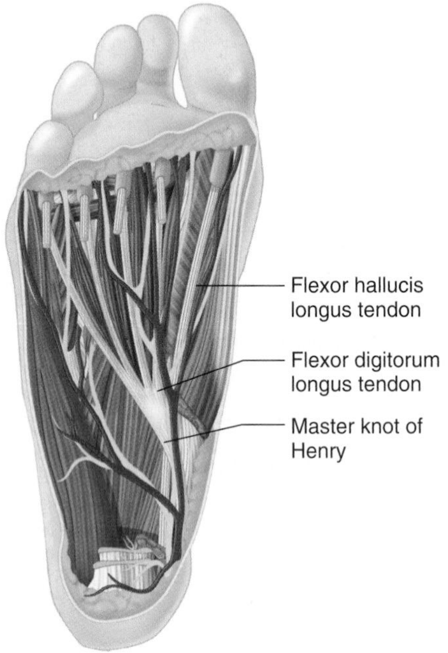

FIGURE 2

Pearls

- *A "super"-supine position makes the dual-incision approach easier.*
- *Cooperation with anesthesiology in keeping the blood pressure as low as is possible allows the procedure to be done without the use of the tourniquet, which allows for a decreased amount of anesthesia and less postoperative pain and bleeding.*

Pitfalls

- *Make sure the foot is fully on the bed and not hanging over the bottom. This allows for proper positioning of the ankle at the end of the case when the transfer is tensioned.*

Equipment

- Extra sheets allow for wider area and more stability.

- In the foot, the FHL tendon is found just deep to the flexor digitorum longus (FDL) tendon at the master knot of Henry, plantar medially in the midfoot (Fig. 2). These tendons also sit next to the NV bundle as they head distally into the forefoot. When the tendon is released at the master knot, care must be taken to avoid the NV bundle in the foot.

Positioning

- The patient is positioned supine with a large bump under the contralateral buttock.
- A thigh tourniquet is applied but not inflated, if possible.

Portals/Exposures

- Medial longitudinal incision—first incision
  - This incision is made just anterior to the anterior border of the Achilles profile and is carried from the midportion of the tuberosity superiorly approximately 20 cm (Fig. 3A and 3B). The incision is carried down through soft tissue in one step to maintain one thick layer from the skin through the paratenon. There is no subcutaneous dissection as this leads to wound problems.
  - Once the Achilles tendon is encountered, the tendon can be examined. The tendon should be débrided anteriorly. As the central portion of the tendon is seen, a degenerative yellow area can be débrided. This area is not normal collagen and should be excised. If the extent of the degenerative area requires it, full removal of the tendon may be necessary.
  - The fascia lies just anterior to the Achilles. The fascia is incised, exposing the underlying FHL muscle belly. The NV bundle is just superior/anterior to this, so care must be taken to avoid injury to it with a retractor.
  - The FHL muscle belly is followed distally until the FHL tendon is seen (behind the talus) (Fig. 4).

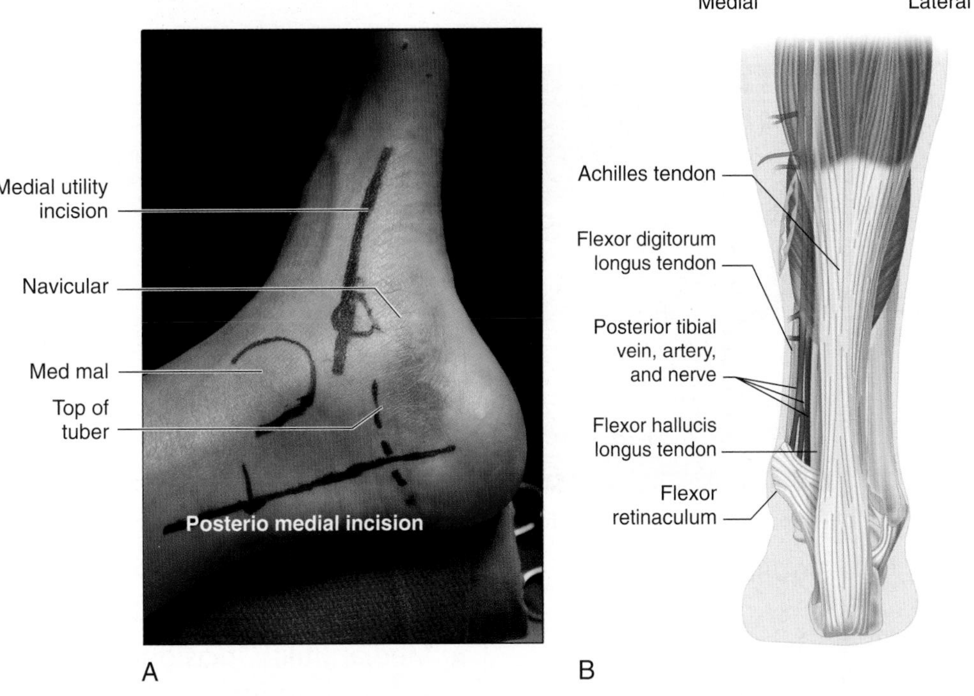

FIGURE 3

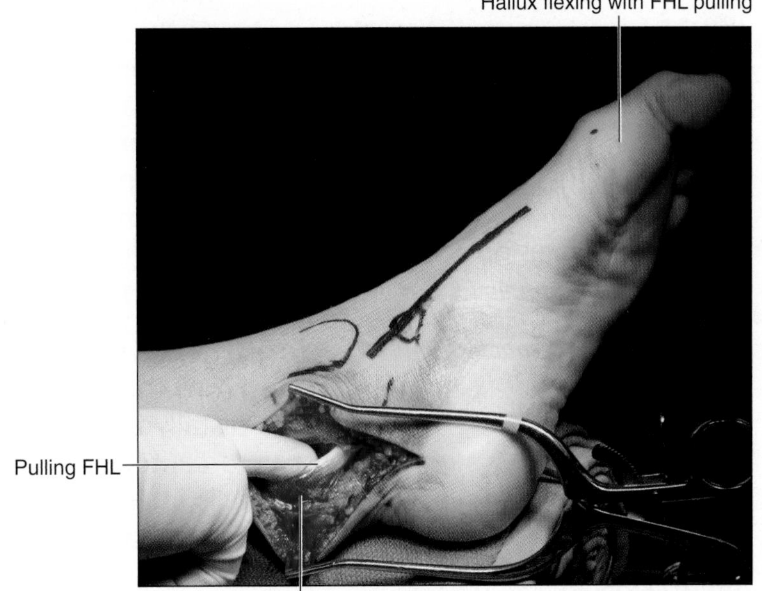

FIGURE 4

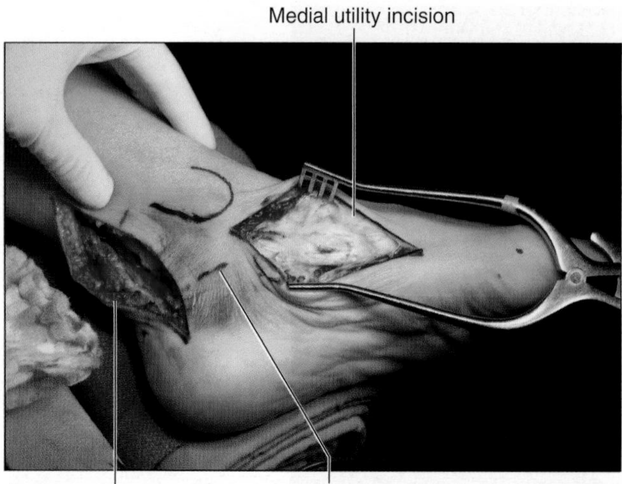

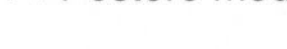

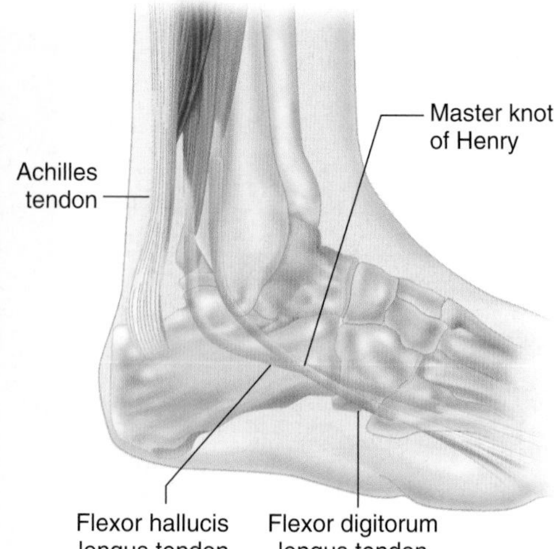

FIGURE 5

Pearls

Posteromedial incision

- *The fascia between the FHL muscle belly and the Achilles can be identified by noting the transverse nature of its fibers.*
- *If you are able to do this procedure without using a tourniquet, the pulse of the NV bundle is readily palpated after the fascial compartment is released.*

Medial utility incision

- *Slide a small clamp under the FDL tendon at the medial malleolus to keep some tension on the tendon as it is followed distally toward the master knot of Henry.*
- *Passively flex the hallux and the lesser toes separately to make sure the FDL and FHL are clearly identified. You can also pull the FHL at the posterior incision if further verification is needed.*

Pitfalls

- *There are many veins in the medial foot—go slowly and cauterize as you go.*

- Medial utility incision—second incision
  - A second incision is made to expose the master knot of Henry and the FHL tendon distally.
  - The incision starts 1 cm inferior to the medial malleolus (Fig. 5A and 5B). The incision is then carried distally over the prominence of the navicular and in line with the medial prominence of the first metatarsal. The distal extent of the incision is usually to the middle of the first metatarsal.
  - The incision is deepened proximally and the FDL tendon is identified behind the posterior tibialis tendon.

Procedure

Step 1: Harvesting the FHL Tendon

- From the second incision, follow the FDL tendon distally and deeper into the foot (Fig. 6), taking care to cauterize any small veins. The muscle layer usually falls inferiorly, and this plane can be followed.
- The master knot of Henry is then identified where the FDL crosses the FHL. These two tendons are connected with tight bands. Use a right-angle clamp to pull the FHL medially and mark it (Fig. 7).
- Side-stitch the FDL and FHL together using an absorbable monofilament suture. Then cut the FHL taking care to avoid the NV bundle, which is just adjacent to the master knot of Henry.
- Loop your finger around the posterior portion of the FHL tendon and pull it out through the posterior incision. Use a clamp to pull the tendon free (Fig. 8).

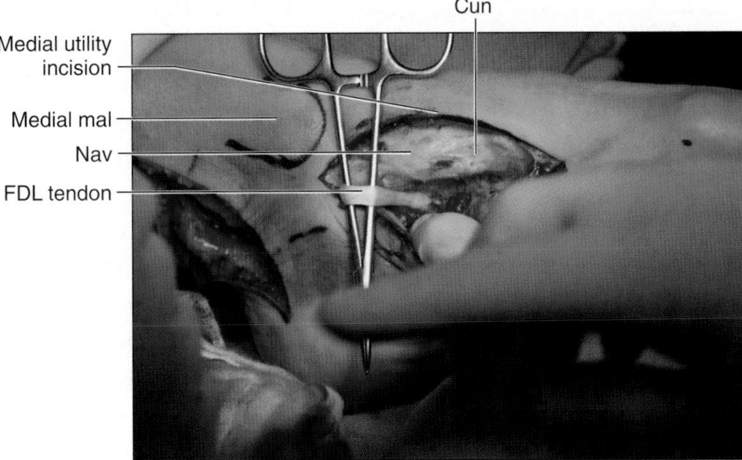

FIGURE 6

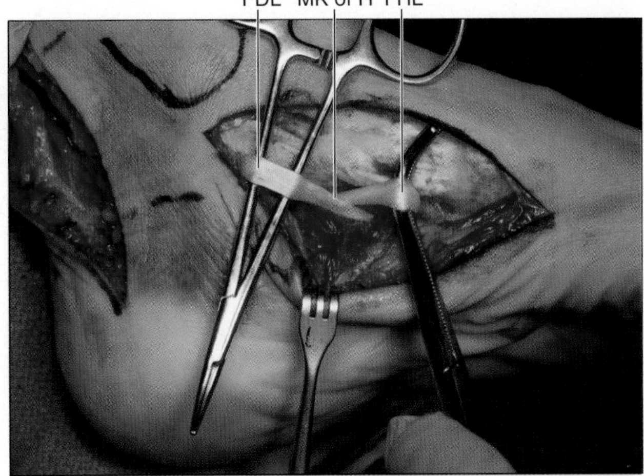

FIGURE 7

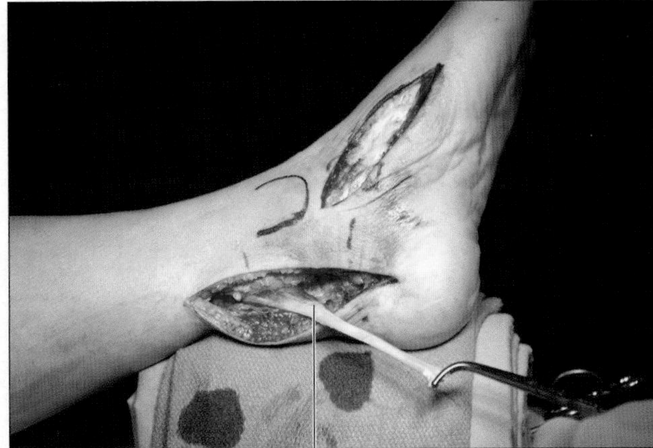

FIGURE 8

Pearls

- *When drilling the tunnel, dorsiflex the foot. This allows the superior part of the tunnel to be drilled farther away from the NV bundle.*

Pitfalls

- *Too-vigorous shaping of the tunnel or too-vigorous pulling of the tendon can cause breakout of the tunnel.*

Step 2: Preparing the Tunnel

- The dissection is carried inferiorly onto the tuber. The soft tissue is left in place adhering to the tuber.
- The superior part of the tunnel should be as posteriorly placed as possible to maintain mechanical advantage of the FHL. A 6.5-mm drill with a soft tissue protector is used to drill from the top of the tuber, inferiorly (Fig. 9).
- A second hole is then drilled from the midportion of the medial wall of the tuber, leaving as big a bridge as possible (Fig. 10). The two holes should meet if the drill has been aimed correctly.
- The tunnel can be enlarged and shaped using a curved curette.

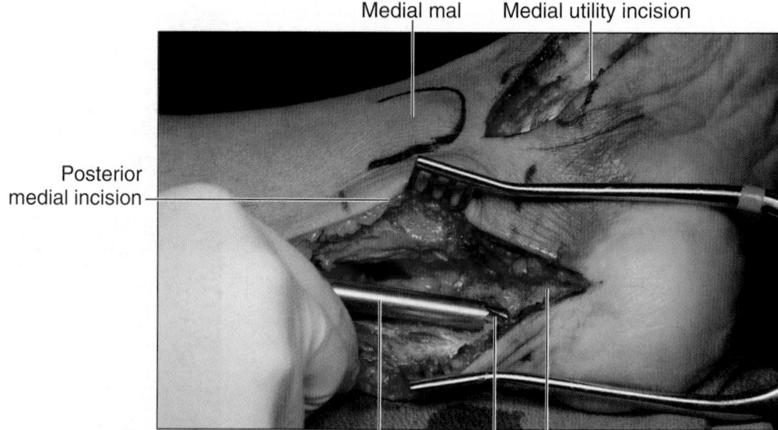

FIGURE 9

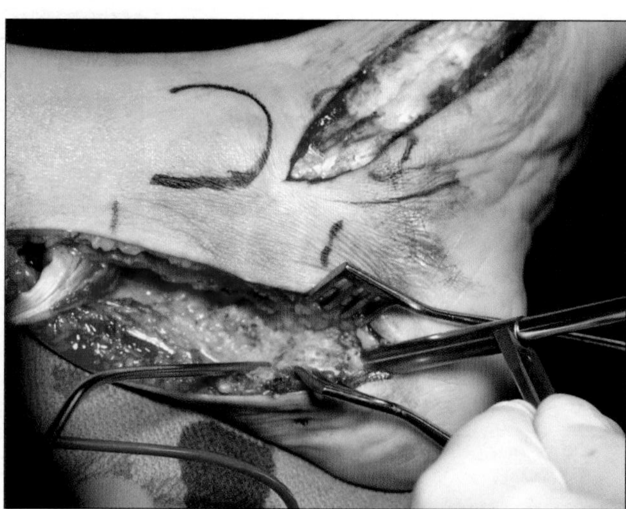

FIGURE 10

Controversies

- Releasing the tendon behind the talus and using an interference screw versus taking the tendon from the foot and putting it through a tunnel and looping it back on itself

Step 3: Preparing the Tendon

- Since we want the tendon to adhere to and not glide through the tuber, it is helpful to remove the paratenon from the FHL tendon.
- The distal most portion is grasped with a clamp and the side of a No. 15 blade is used to scrape the tendon and to fish-scale it distally.

Step 4: Passing the Tendon

- An easy way to pass the tendon is to pass a suture on its needle, blunt end first, up from below and out the top entrance.
- The non-needle end of the suture is clamped to prevent it from being pulled through the tunnel.
- The suture is carefully whip-stitched to the very end of the tendon, taking care not to cause bunching at the tip. The suture needle is then passed from superior to inferior, blunt end first.
- The tendon is carefully pulled from superior to inferior through the tunnel, taking care so as not to break the tunnel (Fig. 11).

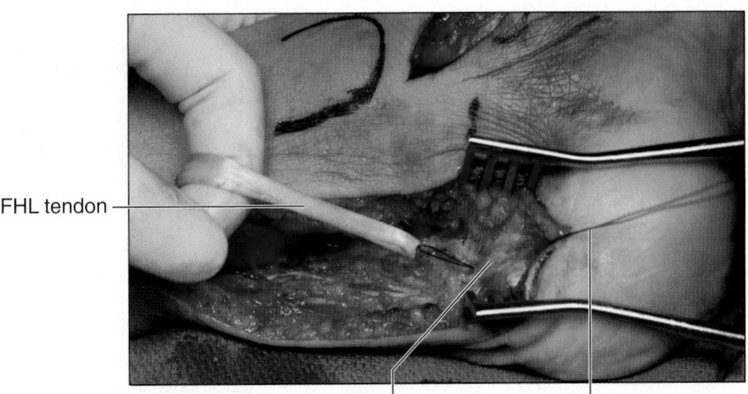

FIGURE 11

Controversies

- Setting the tension. Tension is set by the musculotendinous unit itself; however, some believe that maximum plantar flexion is needed for the transfer to be set properly.

Controversies

- Augmentation materials may be wrapped around the repair area. These materials may be of animal or human origin.

Step 5: Setting the Tension

- Place the ankle in neutral dorsiflexion/plantar flexion.
- Gently pull on the transfer and loop it back upon itself.
- Sew the two arms together and to the soft tissue around the tunnel, using a 0 absorbable monofilament suture (Fig. 12).
- The remaining Achilles (if present) is then side-stitched to the FHL tendon and muscle belly.

Step 6: Augmentation of Fixation

- A suture anchor is used in the tuber (at right angles to the line of pull) to augment the fixation (Fig. 13).
- The suture is then woven proximally to help hold the transfer in place, especially if the tunnel seems tenuous.

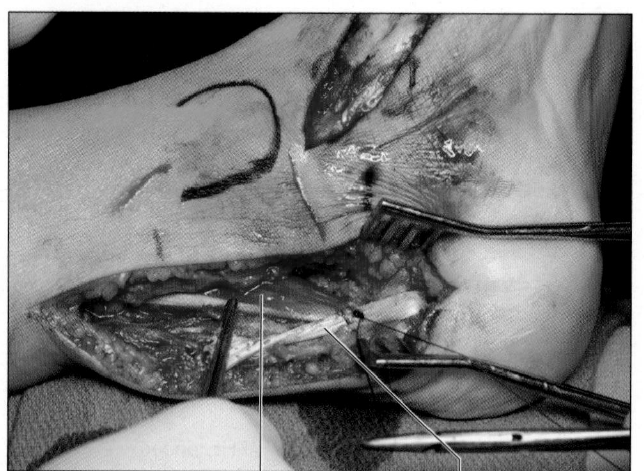

FIGURE 12

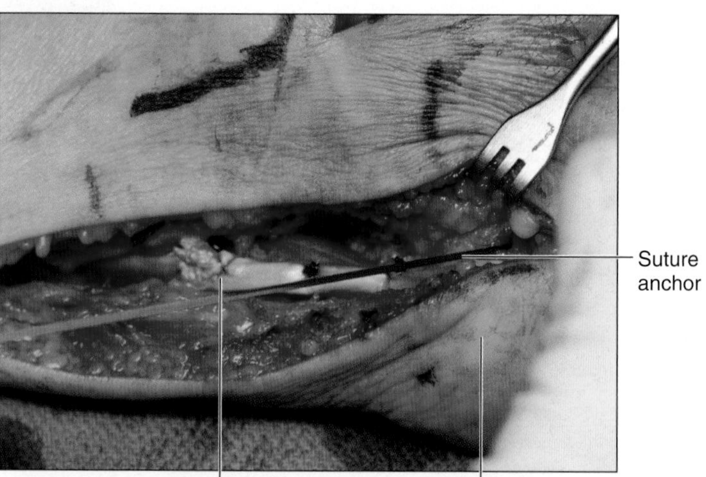

FIGURE 13

Step 7: Closure

- Care must be taken to maintain full thickness in both sides of the wound and to avoid including the NV bundle in the repair.
- The fascial layer over the FHL muscle belly is not closed. The subcutaneous tissue and skin are closed for both incisions.
- Bacitracin, Xeroform gauze, and sterile dressings are applied, and then a bulky dressing and Webril padding. A three-sided plaster splint is placed with the ankle in neutral (not plantar flexion). This is overwrapped with Webril and elastic bandages.
- This construct is left in place and not changed for 2 weeks.

Pearls

- *Cam boots can get dirty, so patients often can get an ankle "L" brace to wear at night for sleep while in bed or when they are relaxing around the house. They can leave the cam boot at the door to wear while they are out and about.*

Postoperative Care and Expected Outcomes

- Patients are discharged from the operating room non–weight bearing in the three-sided plaster splint.
  - They are told to keep the foot level on a chair or couch. They are NOT told to "elevate" the leg.
  - They can be up with assist devices but should limit the amount of time they are up and about with their leg dependent.
- At 2 weeks, the dressings are taken down and the foot is cleaned. The leg is then placed in a removable boot with the ankle at neutral. Non–weight bearing is maintained. Patients are started on gentle isometrics in the boot. They may remove the boot to wash.
- At 6 weeks patients are allowed to bear weight as tolerated and begin range-of-motion exercises, including making circles and dorsiflexion/plantar flexion. Formal physical therapy is started as well.
- At 12 weeks patients are placed into cushioned running sneakers and physical therapy is advanced as tolerated.
- Patients return to full normal activities in 4–6 months and competitive sports soon thereafter.

Evidence

Coull R, Flavin R, Stephens MM. Flexor hallucis longus tendon transfer: evaluation of postoperative morbidity. Foot Ankle Int. 2003;12:931–5.

This study was a retrospective review of 16 patients. Outcomes were determined by clinical and pedobarographic assessment. (Level IV evidence [case series])

Den Hartog BD. Flexor hallucis longus transfer for chronic Achilles tendonosis. Foot Ankle Int. 2003;24:233–7.

This study was a retrospective review of 26 patients. Follow-up averaged 35 months. Outcome was determined by American Orthopaedic Foot and Ankle Society (AOFAS) scores and clinical examination. (Level IV evidence [case series])

Elias I, Besser M, Nazarian LN, Raikin SM. Reconstruction for missed or neglected Achilles tendon rupture with V-Y lengthening and flexor hallucis longus tendon transfer through one incision. Foot Ankle Int. 2007;28:1238–48.

This study was a retrospective review of 15 consecutive patients treated operatively. Follow-up averaged 106 weeks. Outcome was determined by AOFAS score, Biodex isokinetic dynamometry, and clinical examination. (Level IV evidence [case series])

Hahn F, Maiwald C, Horstmann T, Vienne P. Changes in plantar pressure distribution after Achilles tendon augmentation with flexor hallucis longus transfer. Clin Biomech. 2008;23:109–16.

This study was a biomechanical assessment of 13 patients after augmentation with FHL transfer. Outcome was assessed clinically using pedobarography, gait assessment, and patient subjective assessment. Follow-up averaged 46 months. (Level IV evidence [case series])

Martin RL, Manning CM, Carcia CR, Conti SF. An outcome study of chronic Achilles tendinosis after excision of the Achilles tendon and flexor hallucis longus tendon transfer. Foot Ankle Int. 2005;26:691–7.

This study was a retrospective review of 56 operations. Follow-up averaged 3.4 years. Outcome was determined by AOFAS score and clinical examination. (Level IV evidence [case series])

Monroe MT, Dixon DJ, Beals TC, Pomeroy G, Crowley DL, Manoli A. Plantarflexion torque following reconstruction of Achilles tendinosis or rupture with flexor hallucis longus augmentation. Foot Ankle Int. 2000;21:324–9.

This study was a retrospective review of nine patients with tendon rupture or tendinosis who were treated operatively. Follow-up averaged 19 months. Outcome was determined by AOFAS scores, clinical examination, and Cybex isokinetic testing. (Level IV evidence [case series])

Wapner KL, Pavlock GS, Hecht PJ, Naselli F, Wallther R. Repair of chronic Achilles tendon rupture with flexor hallucis longus tendon transfer. Foot Ankle. 1993;14:443–9.

This study was a retrospective review of seven patients treated operatively. Follow-up averaged 17 months. Outcome was assessed with a questionnaire, clinical examination, and Cybex isokinetic testing. (Level IV evidence [case series])

Wilcox DK, Bohay DR, Anderson JG. Treatment of chronic Achilles tendon disorders with flexor hallucis longus tendon/augmentation. Foot Ankle Int. 2000;12:1004–10.

This study was a retrospective review of 20 patients. Follow-up averaged 14 months. Outcome was assessed by AOFAS scores, clnical examination, and Cybex isokinetic testing. (Level IV evidence [case series])

Wong MW, Ng VW. Modified flexor hallucis longus transfer for Achilles insertional rupture in elderly patients. Clin Orthop Relat Res. 2005;(431):201–6.

This study was a retrospective review of five patients older than 50 years. Follow-up averaged 28.8 months. Outcome was determined by AOFAS scores, clinical examination, and Cybex isokinetic testing. (Level IV evidence [case series])

PROCEDURE 53

Peroneal Tendon Tears: Débridement and Repair

Christina Kabbash and Andrew K. Sands

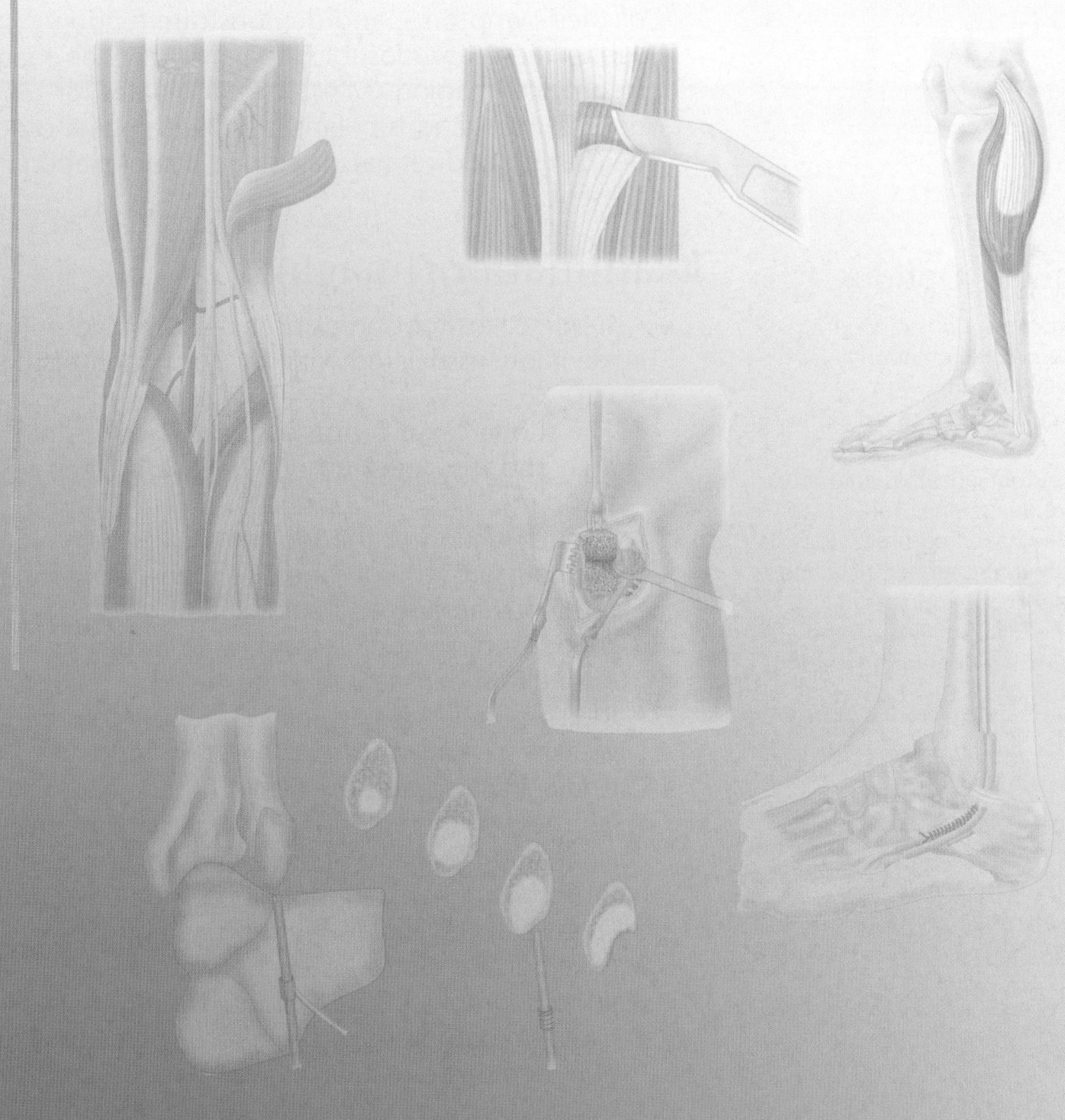

Andrew K. Sands would like to acknowledge the assistance of Edmund Choi, MD with this chapter.

Indications

- Typically presents with pain and swelling posterior to the fibula along the course of the peroneal tendons.
- There is often a history of an ankle sprain or repeated ankle sprains that never fully resolved.
- Activity modification, bracing, nonsteroidal anti-inflammatory drugs, ice, physical therapy, and possibly a 4- to 6-week trial of immobilization in a cast or cam walker should be attempted. Patients who do not improve, or experience a recurrence of their symptoms, and demonstrate tendon subluxation, pseudosubluxation, or tears on magnetic resonance imaging (MRI), are candidates for tendon débridement and tubularization, with fibula groove deepening and retinacular repair if subluxation is present.

Treatment Options

- Treatment options range from simple peroneal tendon tenosynovectomy with retinacular repair, to excision of the degenerative portion with tendon tubularization and fibula groove deepening. Various groove-deepening procedures have been described, including trap door, bone block, and intramedullary drilling of the fibula with subsequent tamping/indentation of the groove.

Examination/Imaging

- A subtle cavus foot predisposes to the inversion-type ankle injury associated with the formation of these tears.
  - The subtle cavus foot is associated with a high arch and the "peek-a-boo" heel sign when standing.
  - Circumduction of the foot may elicit pain along the course of the peroneal tendons, or peroneal tendon snapping and subluxation/pseudosubluxation, secondary to a torn or attenuated peroneal tendon sheath.
  - Resisted foot eversion may also elicit pain and/or weakness relative to the uninjured foot.
- Chronic ankle sprains are likely to have chronic tenderness of the anterior talofibular ligament, calcaneofibular ligament, and sinus tarsi and may have associated ankle instability as demonstrated by an anterior drawer sign. There may also be associated talar dome osteochondral injury.
- Plain radiographs of the weight-bearing foot/ankle
  - Lateral radiographs of the affected foot or ankle may demonstrate a cavus foot with an increased tarsal–first metatarsal angle, and a fibula that appears relatively posterior.
  - Three-dimensional views may demonstrate a fleck of bone if there was a traumatic tendon sheath avulsion.

- MRI
  - On T_2-weighted or short tau inversion recovery (STIR) sequences, observe for increased fluid signal within the sheath. T_1-weighted sequences will show retinacular tears and intrasubstance tendon degeneration.
  - Associated ganglion cysts or tendon sheath tears may also be visualized. Subluxated or dislocated tendons may also be detected/confirmed.

Surgical Anatomy

- The peroneus longus and brevis comprise the lateral compartment of the leg (Fig. 1).
  - The peroneus longus originates on the proximal fibula and inserts on the plantar aspect of the base of the first metatarsal and cuneiform, and acts to evert and plantar flex the foot.
  - The peroneus brevis originates from the distal half of the fibula and inserts in the tuberosity of the fifth metatarsal, where it acts to evert and dorsiflex the foot.
  - Both are innervated by the superficial branch of the peroneal nerve.
  - In the distal leg, the peroneus brevis can be recognized by its lower-lying muscle belly. At the level of the ankle joint, the peroneus longus runs posterior to the peroneus brevis within a fibular groove enclosed by a tendon sheath. Occasionally an accessory slip, or peroneus quartius, may also be found within the sheath.

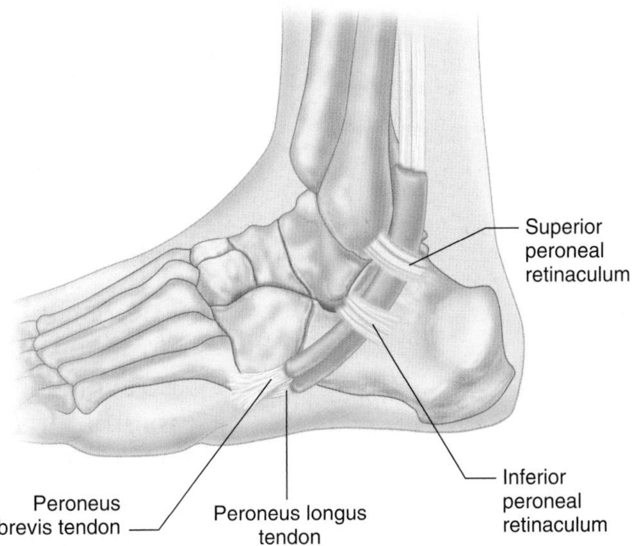

FIGURE 1

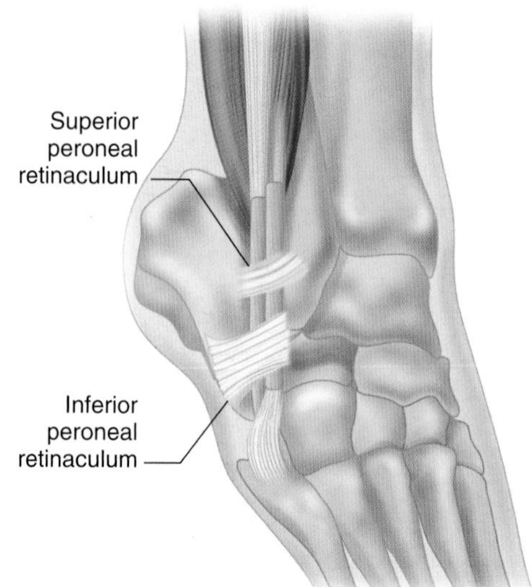

FIGURE 2

- The superior and inferior peroneal retinaculums prevent tendon dislocation or subluxation (Fig. 2).
  - The superior peroneal retinaculum runs from the fibula to the posterior calcaneal tuber.
  - The inferior peroneal retinaculum is an extension of the inferior extensor retinaculum of the foot.
- There is a common peroneal tendon sheath running from the level of the ankle joint to just inferior to the fibula, at which point it bifurcates along each tendon.
- The peroneus brevis is the tendon most frequently torn, with longitudinal tears occurring at the level of the distal fibula, likely due to traumatic subluxation over the edge of the fibular groove.
- The peroneus longus passes under the cuboid on the way to the base of the first metatarsal and may sustain injuries at this point. An os perineum may be found within the tendon as it passes around the cuboid, and there may be associated fractures or pathology due to injury at this point.

PEARLS

- *Ensure that the hip positioners do not limit hip flexion/extension that may be required for imaging.*
- *Keeping the blood pressure as low as possible with general anesthesia may avoid the need for tourniquet inflation during the procedure.*

Positioning

- The patient is positioned in the lateral decubitus position with an axillary roll and lateral hip positioners, peroneal padding under the down leg, a thigh tourniquet, and pillows or a foam block between the legs.
- A mini C-arm should be available for imaging if groove-deepening procedures will be performed.

Equipment

- Table with radiolucent extension
- Lateral hip positioners
- Axillary roll
- Foam padding
- Thigh tourniquet

Portals/Exposures

- A posterolateral incision is made starting 5 cm above the level of the ankle joint along the posterior aspect of the fibula, following the course of the peroneal tendons into the foot where they emerge from the inferior peroneal retinaculum.
- Landmarks include the inferior fibula, the superior border of the posterior tuber of the calcaneus, the calcaneocuboid articulation, and the tuberosity of the fifth metatarsal.

Procedure

Step 1: Exposure of the Peroneal Tendons

- Proximally, the incision is carried down to the fibula, where the peroneal tendons are identified (Fig. 3A and 3B). The superior peroneal retinaculum is kept intact. The tendons are traced down to where they exit the superior peroneal retinaculum and isolated and exposed distally.

Pearls

- *Eversion of the foot allows for increased tendon excursion for examination.*

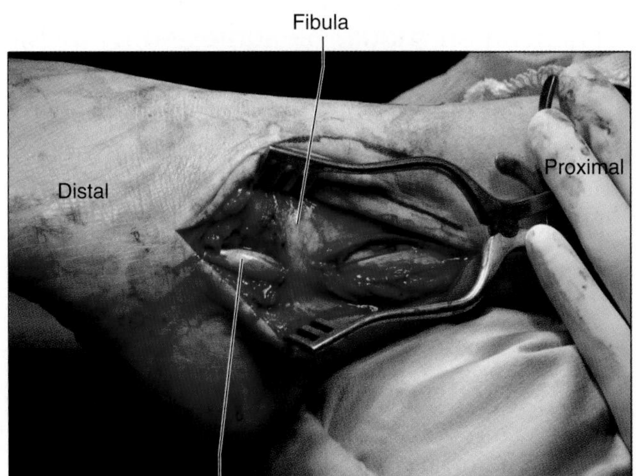

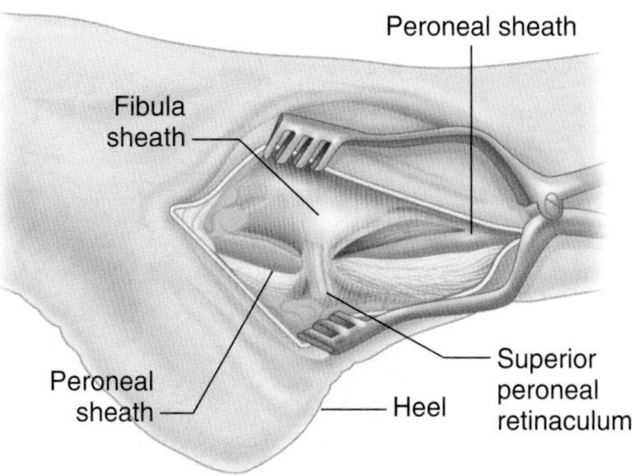

FIGURE 3

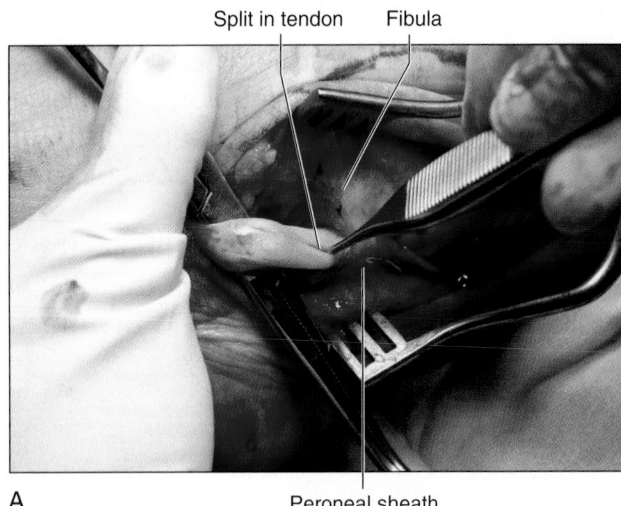

A

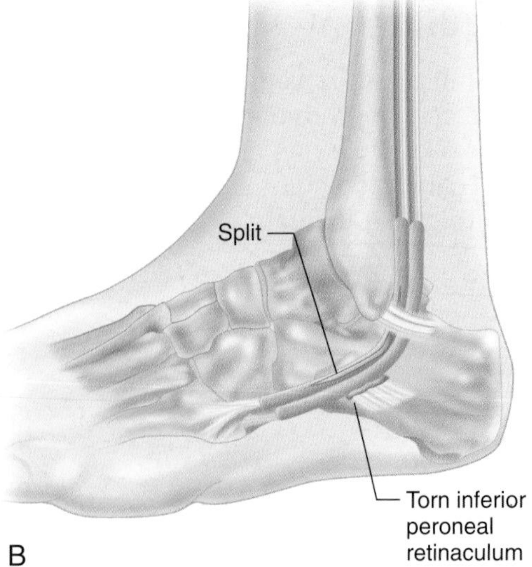

B

FIGURE 4

PITFALLS

- *A low-lying peroneus brevis muscle belly may predispose to subluxation. Muscle tissue may be débrided from the inferior aspect of the tendon if required.*

Controversies

- Repair with absorbable versus nonabsorbable suture

- Tenosynovectomy is performed as required.
- The foot is everted to allow adequate tendon excursion to isolate and examine each tendon for degeneration and tears (Fig. 4A and 4B).
- The superior retinaculum may be partially incised to allow for improved tendon visualization if required.

STEP 2: TENDON REPAIR

- Thickening of the tendon due to intrasubstance degeneration should be addressed by incising the tendon and excising degenerative tissue.
- Longitudinal tears and incisions can then be repaired by invaginating the split and closing the tear with a running 3-0 absorbable monofilament suture (clear PDS) (Fig. 5A and 5B and Fig. 6).

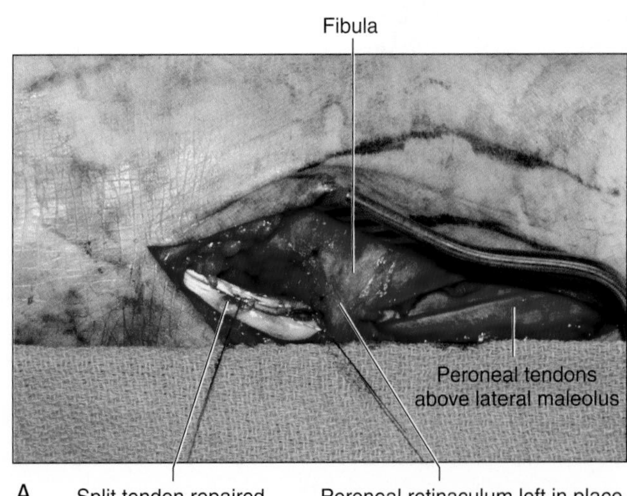

A

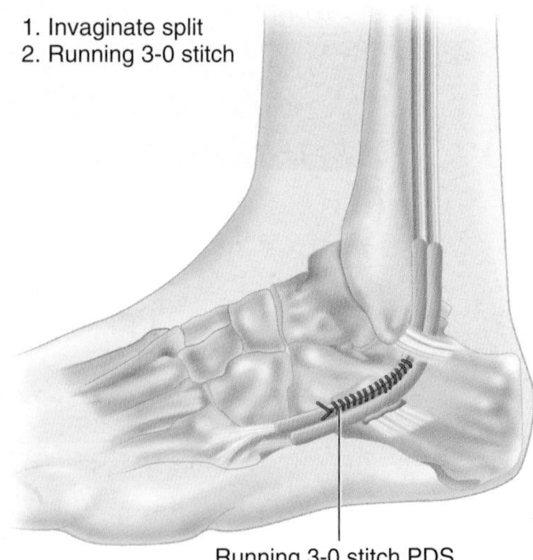

B

FIGURE 5

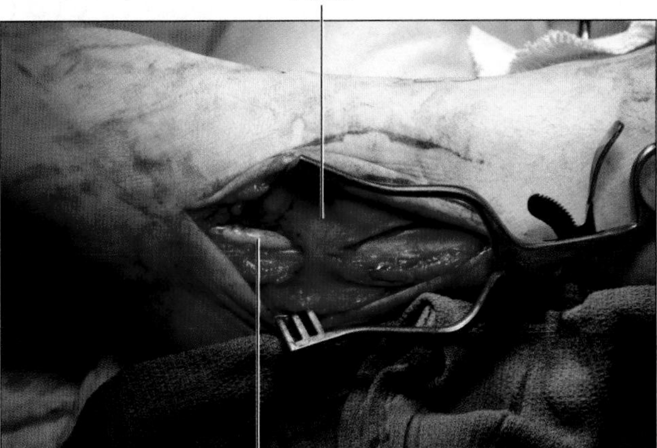

FIGURE 6

Pearls

- *The trap door technique both deepens the groove and provides a bony "shelf" to prevent subsequent subluxation. However, sharp bony edges should be filed or tamped to prevent further injury to the tendon.*

Controversies

- Some surgeons would argue that longitudinal tears due to traumatic or chronic subluxation necessitate a groove-deepening procedure. However, other surgeons may only perform this procedure if a shallow fibular groove is demonstrated on computed tomography or if an intraoperative subluxation can be demonstrated.

Step 3: Retinaculum

- If the superior peroneal retinaculum is ruptured or attenuated, a fibular groove-deepening procedure should be performed prior to the retinacular repair.
- If intact, the superior peroneal retinaculum is incised, leaving a small cuff of tissue on the fibula.
  - The peroneal tendons are dislocated from the peroneal groove to expose the posterior aspect of the fibula.
  - A 2.0-mm Kirschner wire is used to drill holes outlining a 4-cm box along the posterior aspect of the fibula. An osteotome is then used to connect the dots, leaving a posterior hinge intact.
  - A bone tamp depresses the "trap door," deepening the groove.
  - The tendons are relocated and the superior peroneal retinaculum is repaired to the bone and retinacular cuff using a 0 braided absorbable suture.
- If the tear is associated with instability due to a subtle cavus foot, a lateral tuberosity shift and a peroneus longus–to-brevis transfer may be required.

Step 4: Closure

- The skin and subcutaneous tissues are closed as per surgeon preference.
- Bacitracin and sterile dressings are applied to the wound.
- The foot is placed into a three-sided splint.

Postoperative Care and Expected Outcomes

- The operative dressing is removed at 2 weeks at the first postoperative visit.
- The patient is non–weight bearing for 6 weeks, at which time he or she is placed into a cam walker boot and progressed to weight bearing as tolerated, with initiation of gentle range-of-motion exercises.
- Cushioned running sneakers are initiated at 3 months.
- Full return to sports is at 6–8 months.
- Complications include superficial and deep infection, fracture of the fibula during the groove-deepening procedure, continued peroneal tendon pathology/tendon re-rupture, and a missed painful os peroneum syndrome.

Evidence

Dombek MF, Lamm BM, Saltrick K, Mendicino RW, Catanzariti AR. Peroneal tendon tears: a retrospective review. J Foot Ankle Surg. 2003;42:250-8.

This study was a retrospective review of 40 patients with operative repair. Follow-up averaged 13 months, and outcome was determined by patient subjective assessment and clinical examination. (Level IV evidence [case series])

Freccero DM, Berkowitz MJ. The relationship between tears of the peroneus brevis tendon and the distal extent of its muscle belly: an MRI study. Foot Ankle Int. 2006;27:236-9.

This study was a retrospective review of operative patients with tendon tears that were studied by sagittal MRI measurements. (Level IV evidence [case series])

Kollias SL, Ferkel RD. Fibular grooving for recurrent tendon subluxation. Am J Sports Med. 1997;25:329-35.

This study was a retrospective review of 11 consecutive patients treated with a fibular grooving procedure. Follow-up averaged 6 years. Outcome was determined by patient subjective assessment and clinical examination. (Level IV evidence [case series])

Krause E, Brodksy JW. Peroneus brevis tendon tears: pathophysiology, surgical reconstruction, and clinical results. Foot Ankle Int. 1998;19:271-9.

This study was a retrospective review of 20 patients treated by the senior author. Follow-up averaged 39 months. Outcome was determined by American Orthopaedic Foot and Ankle Society (AOFAS) scores and clinical examination. (Level IV evidence [case series])

Major NM, Helms CA, Fritz RC, Speer KP. MR imaging appearance of longitudinal split tears of peroneus brevis tendon. Foot Ankle Int. 2000;6:514-9.

This study was a retrospective MRI assessment of 22 patients with peroneus brevis tears. (Level IV evidence [case series])

Porter D, McCarroll J, Knapp E, Torma J. Peroneal tendon subluxation in athletes: fibular groove deepening and retinacular reconstruction. Foot Ankle Int. 2005;26:436-41.

This study was a retrospective review of 13 patients with operative treatment of peroneal tendon subluxation. Follow-up averaged 35 months, and outcome was determined by patient subjective assessment and clinical examination. (Level IV evidence [case series])

Redfern D, Myerson M. The management of concomitant tears of the peroneus longus and brevis tendons. Foot Ankle Int. 2004;25:695-707.

This study was a retrospective review of 28 consecutive patients treated operatively. Follow-up averaged 4.6 years. Outcome was assessed by AOFAS scores and clinical examination. (Level IV evidence [case series])

Saxena A, Cassidy A. Peroneal tendon injuries: an evaluation of 49 tears in 41 patients. J Foot Ankle Surg. 2003;42:215-20.

This prospective study examined 49 patients with operative treatment. Follow-up averaged 35.5 months. Outcome was determined by return to activity and AOFAS scores. (Level IV evidence [case series])

Steel MW, DeOrio JK. Peroneal tendon tears: return to sports after operative treatment. Foot Ankle Int. 2007;28:49-54.

This study was a retrospective review of 30 patients with operative repair of peroneal tendon tears. Follow-up averaged 31 months. Outcome was determined by questionnaire. (Level IV evidence [case series])

Title CI, Jung HG, Park BG, Schon LC. Peroneal groove deepening procedure: a biomechanical study of pressure reduction. Foot Ankle Int. 2005;6:442-8.

This was a biomechanical study of 12 cadaveric foot/ankle specimens. Outcome was determined by pressure measurements at various positions with groove-deepening procedure. (Level V evidence [cadaveric study])

PROCEDURE 54

Chronic Peroneal Tendon Subluxation-Dislocation

Marc Merian-Genast, James K. DeOrio, and Mark E. Easley

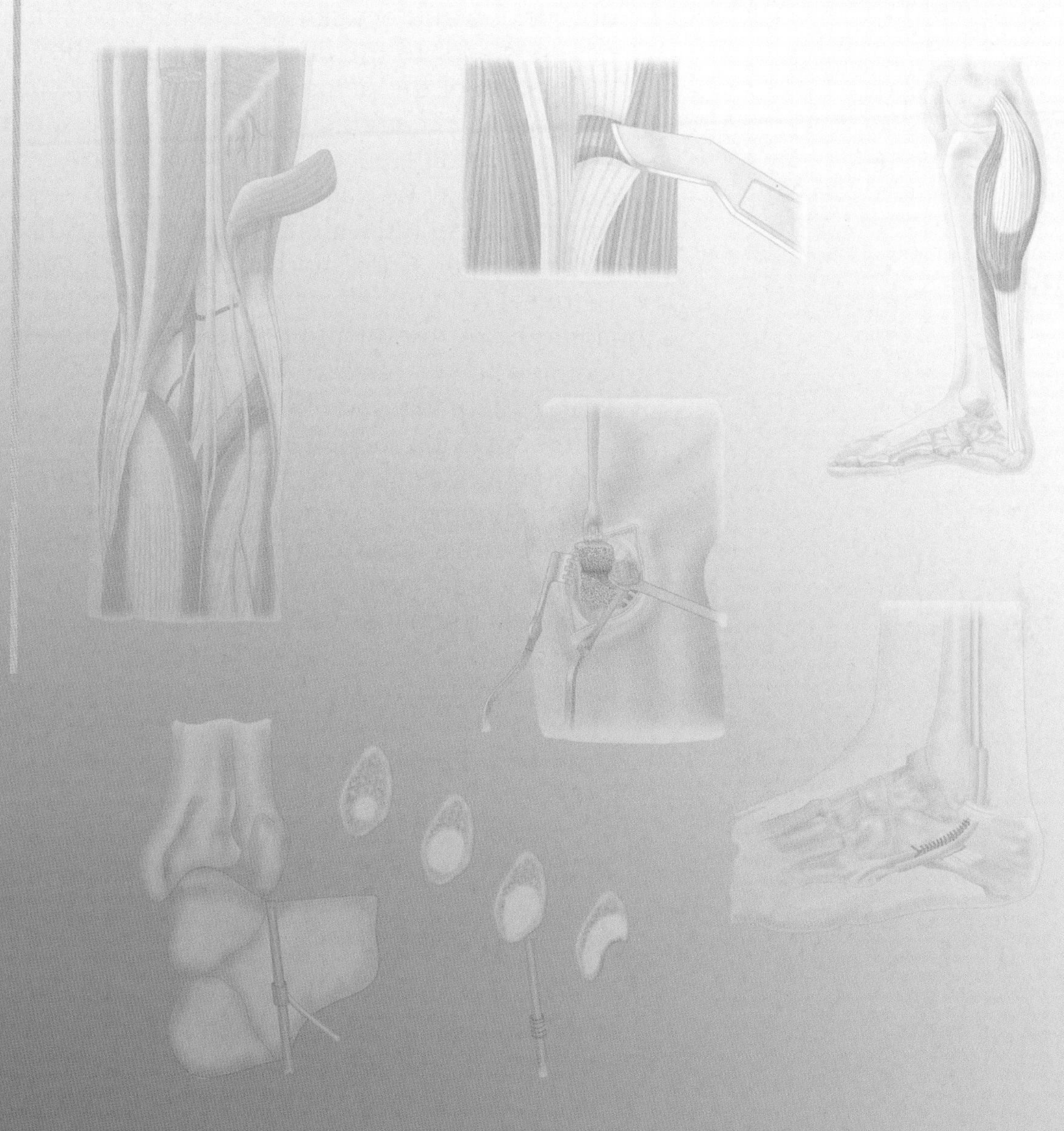

PITFALLS

- *Check for concomitant varus hindfoot alignment and lateral ankle instability that needs to be addressed during surgery.*

Treatment Options

- Nonsurgical treatment is an option for acute dislocation of the peroneal tendons, but has a success rate of only 50% (McGarvey and Clanton, 1996).
- Other techniques exist for operative treatment in addition to the groove deepening with periosteal flap procedure that is described here.

Indications

- Symptomatic chronic peroneal tendon subluxation-dislocation

Examination/Imaging

- Physical examination
  - When the ankle joint is passively circumducted, subluxation may be identified as a palpable "click" over the lateral malleolus. Resistance to active dorsiflexion and eversion of the foot may induce pain posterior to the fibula, and subluxation or dislocation of the peroneal tendon can occur.
  - With active circumduction of the foot, a subtle side-to-side difference of peroneal tendon excursion may be palpated.
  - An inability to dislocate the tendons does not rule out instability. Coexisting ankle instability and peroneal tendinopathy should be identified.
- Imaging helps to evaluate concomitant injuries and to confirm the diagnosis.
  - Plain radiographs should be taken in anteroposterior, lateral, and mortise views.
    - Often a normal, small flake of fibular cortex is pathognomonic for peroneal dislocation (Fig. 1).
    - Ankle stress views can be taken to evaluate concomitant ankle instability.
  - Magnetic resonance imaging is useful for assessment of the posterior fibular groove, and concomitant ligament and peroneal tendinopathy. Figure 2 shows insufficiency of the posterior fibular groove and the superior peroneal retinaculum on MRI.
  - Computed tomography (in uncertain cases) may be helpful to evaluate the posterior fibular groove.

Surgical Anatomy

- At the level of the ankle joint, the peroneal tendons run through a fibro-osseous tunnel (Fig. 3A). Note the position of the peroneal tendons in relation to the superior peroneal retinaculum and the calcaneofibular ligament. Figure 3B shows a transverse view of the fibro-osseous tunnel at the level of the ankle joint.
  - Anterior: the posterior surface of fibula develops a peroneal groove in 82% and a plantar convex surface in 18% (Edwards, 1988).

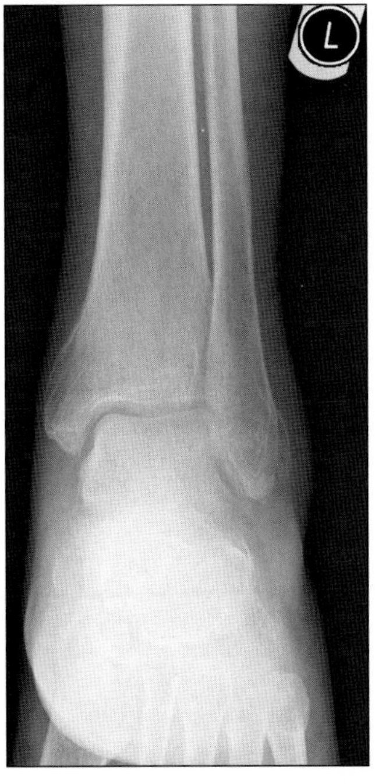

FIGURE 1

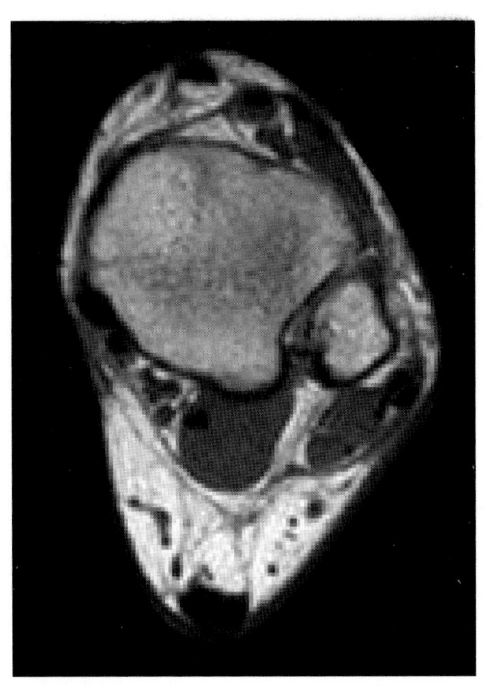

FIGURE 2

  - Medial: the calcaneal fibular ligament runs parallel to the superior peroneal retinaculum.
  - Posterior/lateral: the superior peroneal retinaculum (main primary stabilizer) originates from the posterolateral ridge of the distal 2 cm of the fibula and inserts on the calcaneus and/or the Achilles tendon sheath (Davis et al., 1994).
- The sural nerve runs subcutaneously just behind the lateral malleolus in direction of the peroneal tendons (see Fig. 3A).

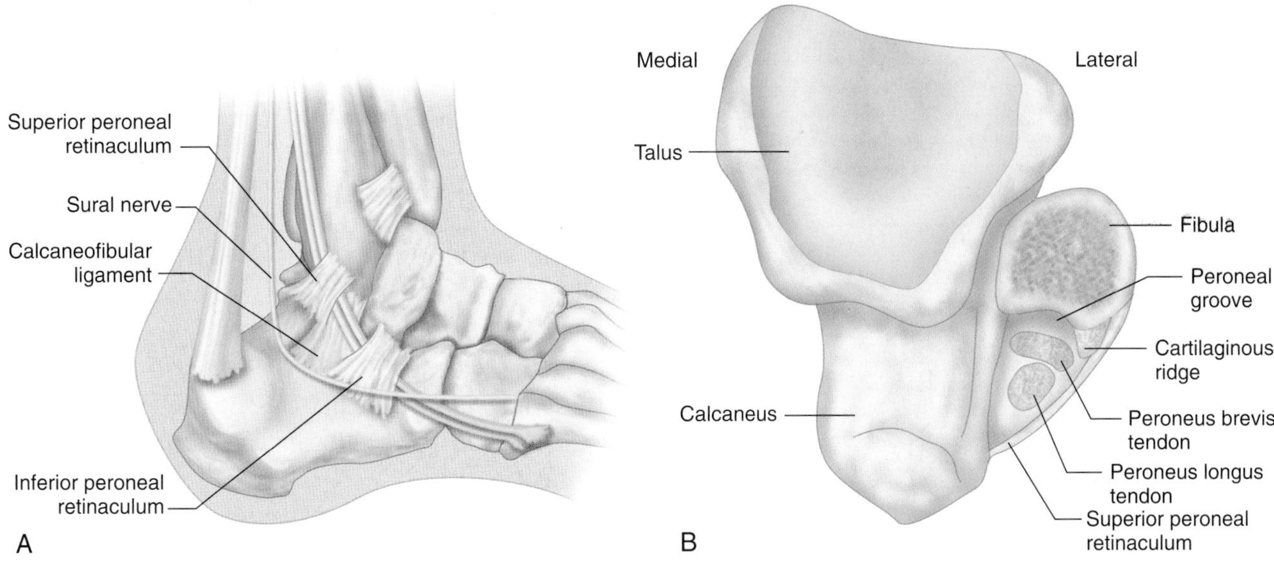

FIGURE 3

PITFALLS

- *Place a pillow between the knees, underneath the contralateral ankle and proximal fibula, to prevent pressure sores and common peroneal nerve compression (see Fig. 4).*

Positioning

- Lateral positioning of patient with a bean bag allows free range of motion at the ankle joint (Fig. 4).
- A thigh tourniquet (not a below-the-knee tourniquet) is used to allow free intraoperative peroneal tendon excursion.
- Drape up to the knee to have full exposure to the lower leg.

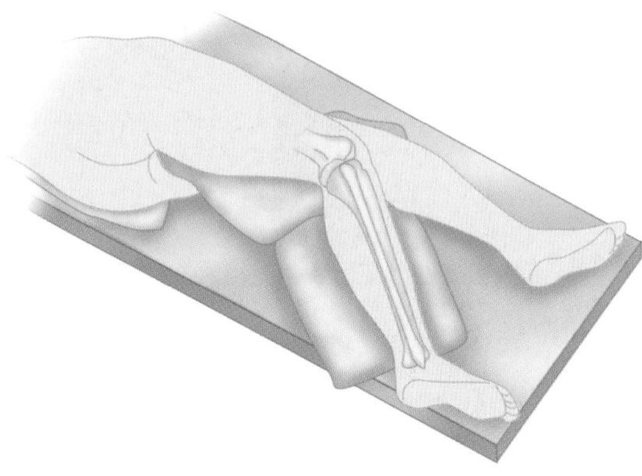

FIGURE 4

Equipment

- Bean bag

Controversies

- Alternatively, a prone position can be chosen.

PEARLS

- *In the case of concomitant peripheral tendon lesions (<50%), excise the redundant tissue and taper.*
- *In the case of central splits of the tendon, excise the edges and perform side-to-side repair (Fig. 6).*

PITFALLS

- *Care must be taken to watch for serpentine course of the sural nerve running through the operative exposure site.*

Portals/Exposures

- A 4- to 6-cm longitudinal incision is made over the posterior edge of the fibula, following the course of the peroneal tendons anteriorly 2 cm distal of the tip of the lateral malleolus.
  - Care should be taken not to injure the sural nerve. Once the sural nerve is identified, it should be retracted posteriorly.
  - Beware of the superficial peroneal nerve and its serpentine course.
- Develop full-thickness flaps and expose the peroneal tendon sheaths.
- Manipulate the ankle joint to observe the subluxation of the peroneal tendons and assess the competence of the superior peroneal retinaculum.
- Incise the peroneal tendon sheath, leaving a cuff of tissue at the posterior edge of the fibula. Peroneal tendons are assessed for split tears in association with subluxation-dislocation.
- The retromalleolar groove is assessed (Fig. 5). Note how flat the posterior groove of the fibula is in Figure 5.

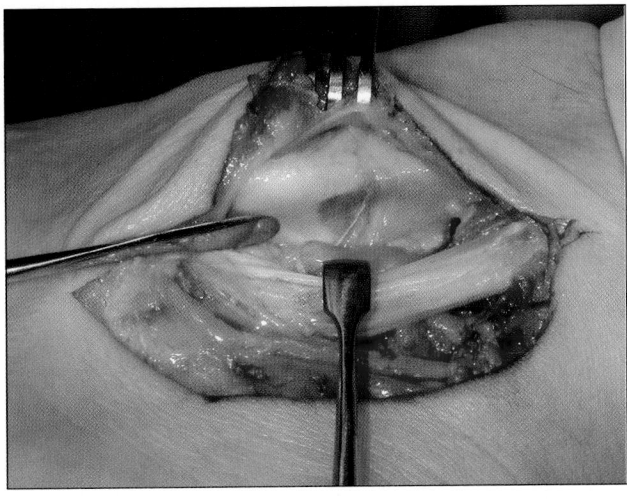

FIGURE 5

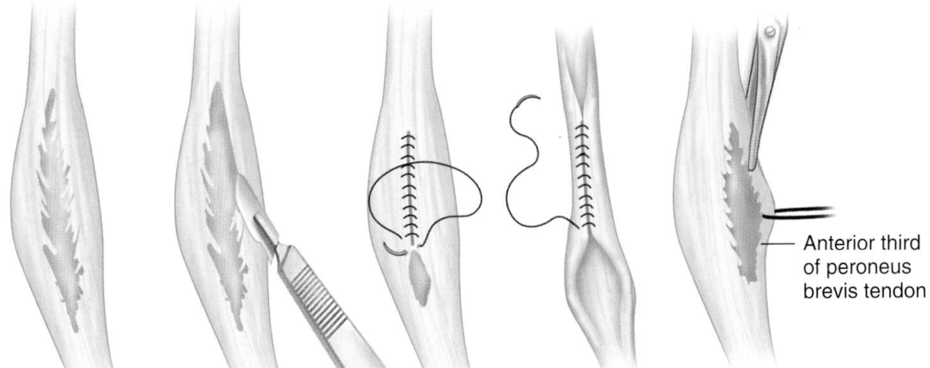

FIGURE 6

Procedure

Step 1

- Sharply elevate the cuff of the superior peroneal retinaculum, exposing the lateral cortex of the fibula.
- Roughen the lateral cortex to bleeding bone.
- Strip off the periosteum of the lateral cortex of the fibula to create a 1.5-cm² periosteal flap with the base just lateral to the original insertion of the superior peroneal retinaculum (Fig. 7).
  Excise redundant superior peroneal retinaculum tissue as necessary.

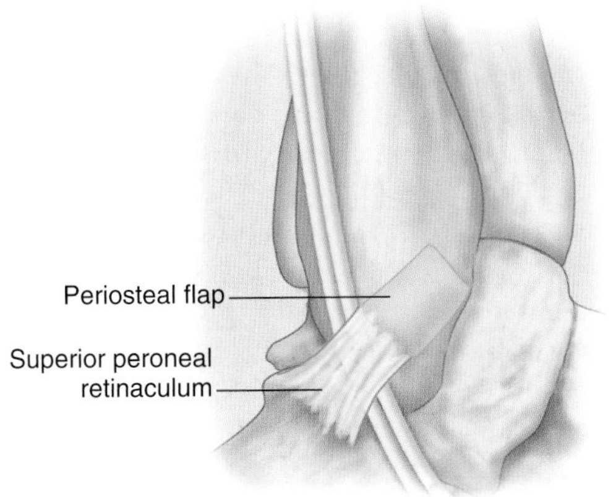

FIGURE 7

Pearls

- *Excise the low-lying peroneus brevis muscle belly or peroneus quartus to "make room" for the peroneal tendons (Fig. 8).*

Pitfalls

- *Do not roughen the lateral cortex too extensively as the groove-deepening procedure will weaken the bone as well, which results in an increased fracture risk to the bone laterally.*

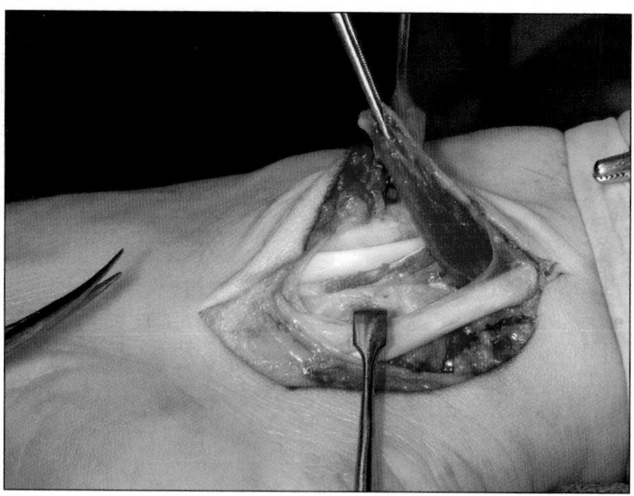

FIGURE 8

Step 2

- Place Hohmann retractors behind the medial edge of the fibula, thus reflecting the peroneal tendons posteriorly.
- Insert a 2-mm drill through the tip of the distal fibula just anterior to the calcaneofibular ligament (Fig. 9). Under fluoroscopic guidance, check the correct insertion site and direction of the drilling.
  - Weaken the posterior cancellous bone that supports the osteocartilaginous posterior aspect of the fibular groove by progressively increasing the size of the drills up to 7–8 mm, depending on the size of the fibula (Mendicino et al., 2001).
  - A small curette can be used to complete the removal of all the cancellous bone at the posterior aspect of the fibula.
- With a bone tamp (Fig. 10), impact the posterior fibular cortex, thus deepening the groove (Fig. 11) (Mendicino et al., 2001).

Pearls

- *Gradually impact the posterior cortex of the fibular groove in a distal-to-proximal direction. Impact the most distal part of the fibular groove in order to avoid a sharp bony ridge on which the peroneus brevis tendon might get injured.*

Pitfalls

- *Fracture and perforation of the posterior and lateral cortex of the fibula during the drilling and impacting process can result in violation of the periosteal covering and/or lateral wall insufficiency.*

Controversies

- Groove deepening (modified from Arrowsmith et al., 1983)
  - A posterior osteocartilaginous flap is detached from the retromalleolar groove from lateral to medial that includes the entire posterior surface of the fibula groove. The groove is deepened using a burr to remove underlying cancellous bone (Fig. 12A). The flap is placed onto the deepened cancellous surface (Fig. 12B).
  - This procedure exposes the tendons to cancellous bone of the lateral cortex of the fibula unless completely covered by the tendon sheath and retinaculum. Therefore, the superior peroneal retinaculum should be reattached with transosseous sutures to the fibula covering the cancellous bone.
  - Persisting sharp edges in the groove can result in a lesion and rupture of the peroneal tendons.

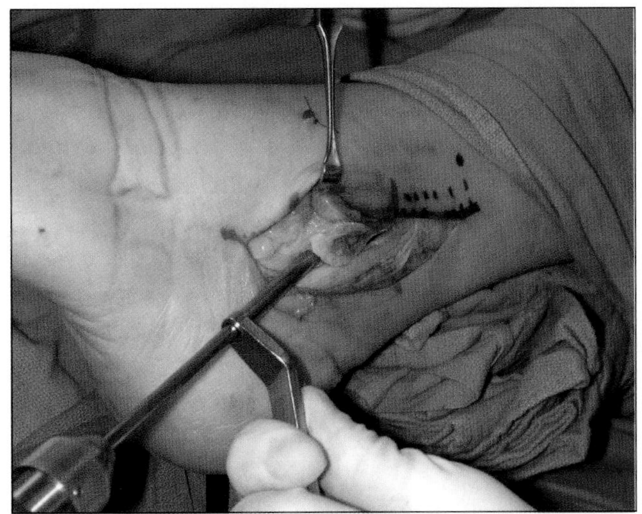

FIGURE 9

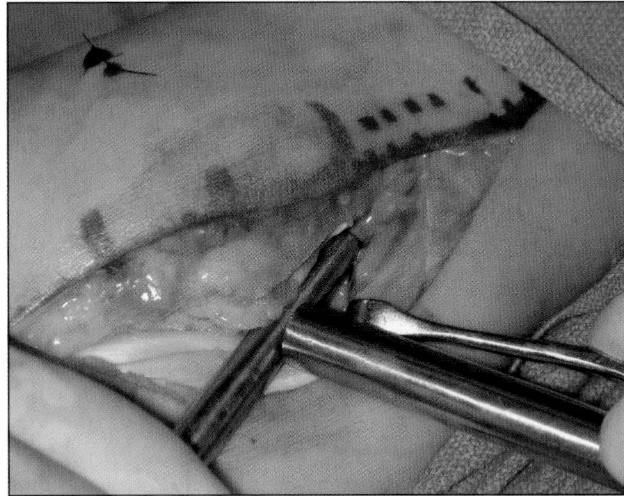

FIGURE 10

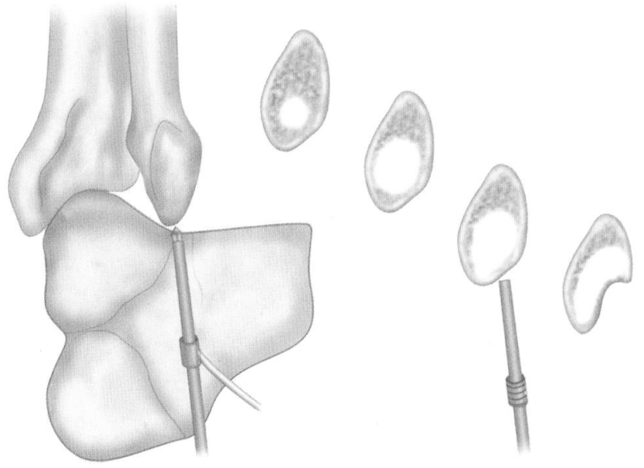

FIGURE 11

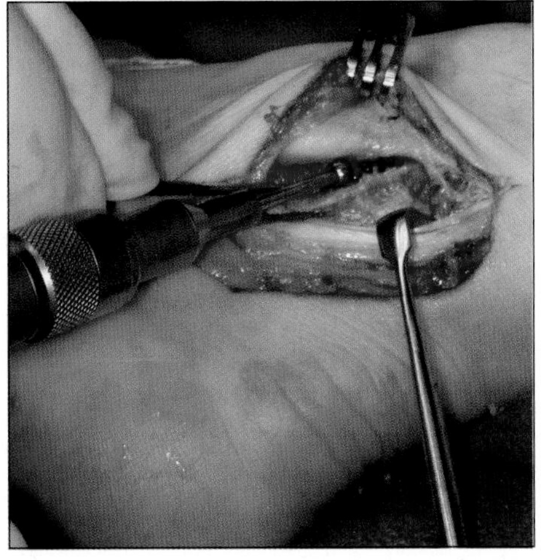

A

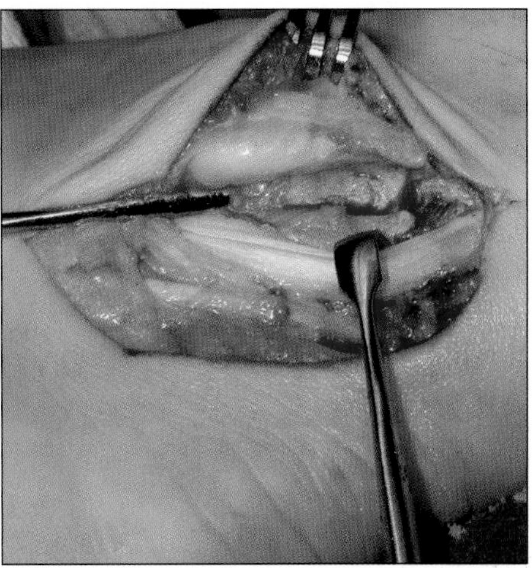

B

FIGURE 12

Pitfalls

- *Make sure that the peroneal tendons are not within the sutures of the periosteal flap and that they glide without any restraint in their sheath.*

Controversies

- Tissue transfer techniques have been proposed for augmentation of insufficient soft tissues of the superior peroneal retinaculum using a distally attached slip of Achilles tendon, peroneus brevis, or plantaris. Rerouting techniques have also been proposed, but a high rate of associated sural nerve injuries and ankle stiffness has been noticed (McGarvey and Clanton, 1996). These techniques are of historic interest only.

Step 3

- Use 1.6-mm Kirschner wires to create three tunnels in the posterolateral edge of the fibula. The tunnels run 4 mm anterior to the posterior edge to the previously roughened lateral cortex, where they exit.
- The Hohmann retractors are removed and the tendons allowed to glide back into the groove.
- Advance the superior peroneal retinaculum and secure to bone using 2-0 polyester (Ethibond) suture placed through the previously created bone tunnels (Fig. 13).
- The periosteal flap of the fibula is advanced posteriorly and oversewn to the posterior retinaculum, doubling the layer of the superior peroneal retinaculum repair (Fig. 14). A 2-0 polyglactin (Vicryl) suture is used.
- Irrigate the wound and then close the skin with 4-0 nylon suture.

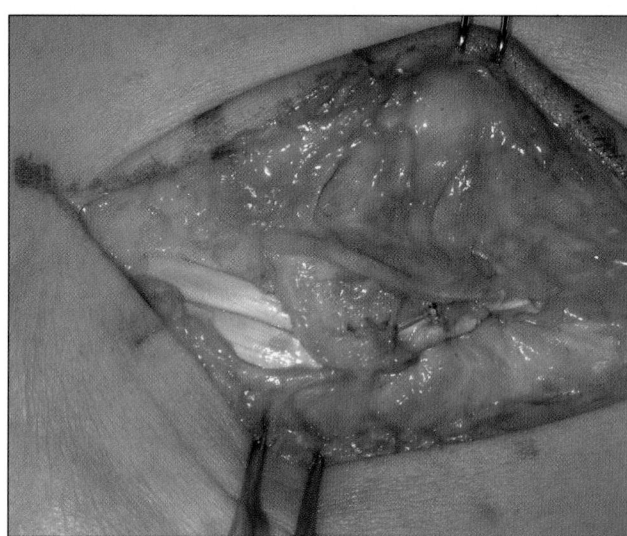

FIGURE 13

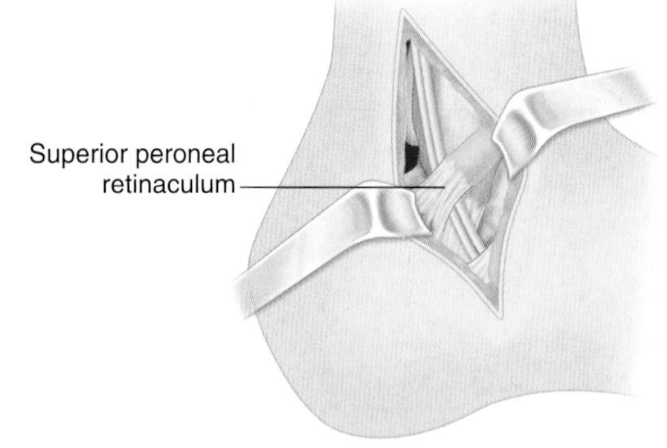

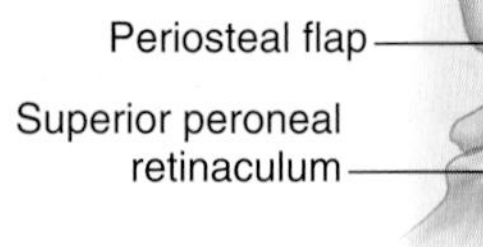

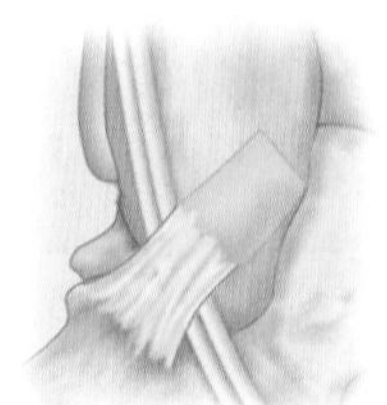

FIGURE 14

Postoperative Care and Expected Outcomes

- Place the foot in a non–weight-bearing short-leg cast in a slightly inverted position for the first 2 weeks postoperatively.
- After 2 weeks, apply a short-leg walking cast in neutral position for 4 more weeks and allow weight bearing as tolerated.
- Running and jogging with a brace are allowed at 8–10 weeks.
- At 8–10 weeks, peroneal strengthening is initiated.
- After completion of a progressive strengthening exercise program of the extrinsic foot muscles, cutting activities and skiing are allowed at 12 weeks.
- Outcome
  - Peroneal groove-deepening techniques in combination with reconstruction of the peroneal retinaculum have been generally successful. No recurrences have been reported. Most results are retrospective reports (Kollias and Ferkel, 1997; Karlsson et al., 1996).
  - Excellent results have been reported by Shawen and Anderson (2004) using the indirect groove-deepening technique. Twenty patients had no recurrence, and the report emphasized the minimal surgical dissection and morbidity with the indirect groove-deepening technique.
  - Ogawa et al. (2007) reported results in 15 patients using the indirect technique. There were no reoccurrence of subluxation or dislocation after a mean follow-up time of 13 months.

Evidence

There are no evidence-based trials for this topic due to the rare occurrence of this entity.

Arrowsmith SR, Fleming LL, Allman FL. Traumatic dislocations of the peroneal tendons. Am J Sports Med. 1983;11:142-6.

Study of the alternative surgical technique that directly deepened the groove after an osteochondral flap was elevated. (Level IV evidence [case series])

Davis WH, Sobel M, Deland J, Bohne WH, Patel MB. The superior peroneal retinaculum: an anatomic study. Foot Ankle Int. 1994;15:271-5.

Anatomic study of the superior peroneal retinaculum and its variable insertions.

Edwards M. The relations of the peroneal tendons to the fibula. Am J Anat. 1988;42:213-53.

Anatomic study of the peroneal tendons' course along the fibula.

Karlsson J, Eriksson BI, Swärd L. Recurrent dislocation of the peroneal tendons. Scand J Med Sci Sports. 1996;6:242-6.

Case series (15 patients) of the alternative surgical technique that directly deepened the groove after an osteochondral flap was elevated. (Level IV evidence [case series])

Kollias SL, Ferkel RD. Fibular grooving for recurrent peroneal tendon subluxation. Am J Sports Med. 1997;25:329-35.

Case series (11 patients) of the alternative surgical technique that directly deepened the groove after an osteochondral flap was elevated. (Level IV evidence [case series])

McGarvey W, Clanton T. Peroneal tendon dislocations. Foot Ankle Clin. 1996;1:325-42.

Review article of 265 reported cases in the literature. (Level III evidence)

Mendicino RW, Orsini RC, Whitman SE, Catanzariti AR. Fibular groove deepening for recurrent peroneal subluxation. J Foot Ankle Surg. 2001;40:252-63.

The first publication of the surgical technique using indirect groove deepening for chronic peroneal dislocation/subluxation.

Ogawa BK, Thordarson DB, Zalavras C. Peroneal tendon subluxation repair with indirect fibular groove deepening technique. Foot Ankle Int. 2007;28:1194-7.

Case series (15 patients) of the indirect fibular groove deepening technique. (Level IV evidence [case series])

Shawen SB, Anderson RB. Indirect groove deepening in the management of chronic peroneal tendon dislocation. Tech Foot Ankle Surg. 2004;3:118-25.

The surgical technique of indirect groove deepening is presented, with a brief review of preliminary results. (Level IV evidence)

PROCEDURE 55

Posterior Tibial Tendon Transfer for Footdrop

Aaron T. Scott and Mark E. Easley

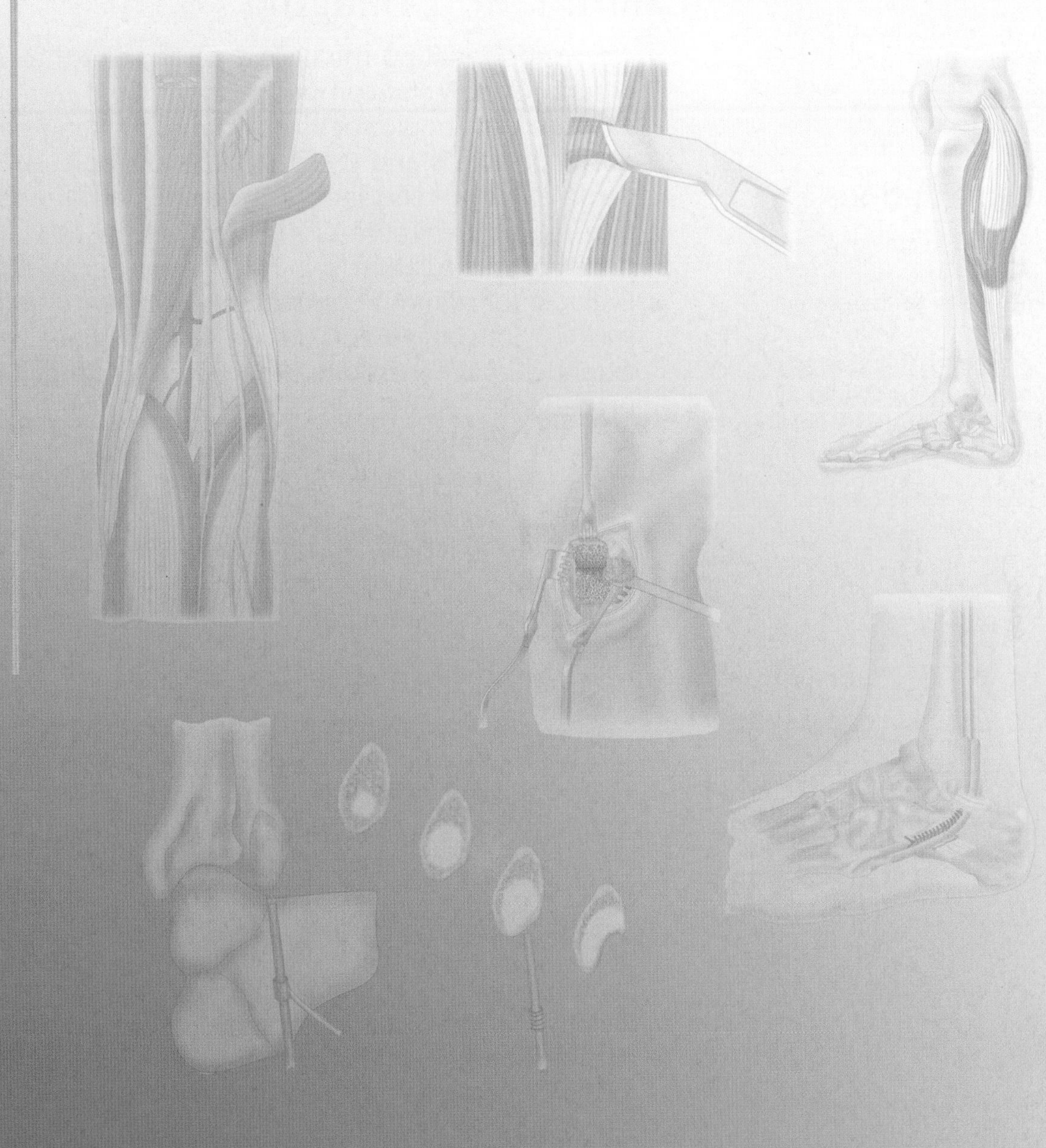

PITFALLS

- *Transfer of the posterior tibial tendon is contraindicated if there is a high likelihood of neurologic recovery (i.e., incomplete injury).*
- *Weakness of the gastrocnemius-soleus complex*
- *Insufficient vascularity*
- *Significant soft tissue scarring of the anterior ankle*

Treatment Options

- Nonoperative treatment in an ankle-foot orthosis
- Isolated transfer of the posterior tibial tendon
- Bridle procedure (triple tendon anastomosis) with or without insertion of the posterior tibial tendon into the middle cuneiform

Indications

- Flaccid footdrop following traumatic injury to the common peroneal nerve or peroneal division of the sciatic nerve
- Spastic footdrop seen in cerebral palsy
- Other indications may include footdrop associated with poliomyelitis, cerebrovascular accident, Charcot-Marie-Tooth disease, or leprosy

Examination/Imaging

- After substantiating the flaccid paralysis of the anterior and lateral compartments, motor examination should focus on strength testing of the posterior tibialis and the gastrocnemius-soleus complex. A prerequisite for posterior tibial tendon transfer is a minimum of 4/5 strength for this posterior musculature.
- Evaluate for equinus contracture. Inability to attain at least 10° of passive dorsiflexion with the knee extended will necessitate a heel cord lengthening procedure.
- Plain radiographs
  - Obtain anteroposterior (AP), lateral, and mortise views of the ankle.
  - Obtain AP, lateral, and oblique views of the foot.
  - Evaluate for any osseous or articular deformities that may require a concomitant osteotomy or arthrodesis.
- Electromyography/nerve conduction studies
  - These studies are useful for documenting the level of injury as well as the potential for nerve recovery.
  - They are not necessary if the injury was sustained greater than 1 year prior to evaluation and no functional improvement has been observed.

Surgical Anatomy

- Just proximal to the popliteal fossa, the sciatic nerve divides into the tibial nerve and the common peroneal nerve (Fig. 1A).
  - The tibial nerve provides motor input to the deep and superficial posterior compartments of the leg. Its function is essential to this procedure.
  - The common peroneal nerve, including its two terminal branches (the deep and superficial peroneal nerves), provides the motor innervation to the anterior and lateral compartments of the

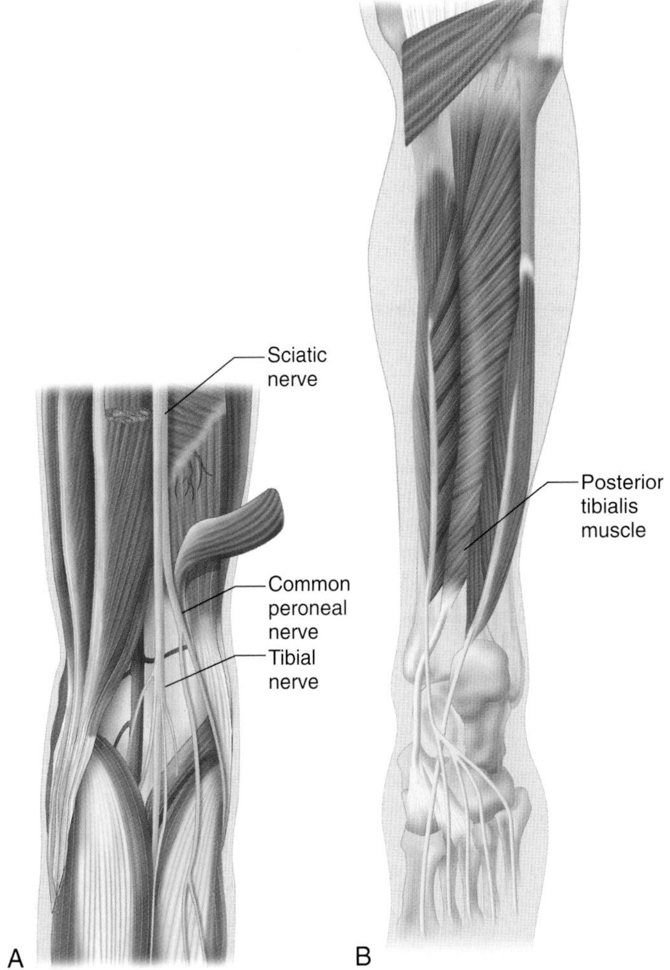

FIGURE 1

leg. Dysfunction of the common peroneal nerve leads to the development of footdrop.
  - The deep peroneal nerve runs between the tibialis anterior and the extensor hallucis longus and must be protected during anterior incisions.
- The posterior tibialis muscle arises from the posterior aspect of the interosseous membrane, tibia, and fibula (Fig. 1B). It travels posterior to the medial malleolus and has a broad insertion into the tuberosity of the navicular, all three cuneiforms, and the bases of the second through fourth metatarsals.

Positioning

- Postion the patient supine on the operating room table and apply a tourniquet to the upper thigh.
- The leg is exsanguinated using an Esmarch bandage, and the tourniquet is elevated to 300 mm Hg.

Portals/Exposures

- Up to seven separate incisions are utilized during the performance of this procedure. These are discussed separately during the appropriate stage of the technique.

Procedure

Step 1

- Extend the knee and dorsiflex the ankle to pre-tension the Achilles tendon.
- Carefully palpate the medial and lateral borders of the tendon, and insert a no. 11 scalpel blade vertically into the midline of the tendon approximately 2 cm proximal to its insertion. Insert the blade through the full thickness of the tendon and then turn the blade medially to transect half of the width of the tendon medially.
  - Figure 2 shows percutaneous tendo-Achilles lengthening in a patient with Charcot-Marie Tooth disease who is undergoing multiple other procedures in addition to the Achilles lengthening and posterior tibial tendon transfer.
- In a similar fashion, insert the no. 11 blade into the tendon approximately 2 cm distal to the musculotendinous junction, and proceed to transect the medial half of the tendon once again.
- The third incision is made midway between the first two incisions with the blade turned laterally after the vertical entrance wound to transect the lateral half of the tendon.
- The ankle is then dorsiflexed to eliminate the equinus deformity.

Pearls

- *Following percutaneous Achilles tendon lengthening or gastrocnemius recession, the toes should be evaluated for clawing. If clawing is present, tenotomies or tendon lengthening procedures should be performed.*

Step 2

- Two 3-cm incisions are created medially over the posterior tibial tendon. The first incision overlies the tendon's insertion on the navicular, with the second incision lying 8–10 cm proximal to the medial malleolus.
- The posterior tibial tendon is then sharply released from its insertion onto the navicular tuberosity and tagged with a heavy (no. 2) nonabsorbable suture (Fig. 3).
- Through the more proximal incision, the tendon is identified in its position deep to the flexor digitorum longus. With the assistance of a right-angled hemostat, the entire tendon is pulled in a retrograde fashion into the proximal posteromedial incision wound (Fig. 4).

Pearls

- *The opening created in the interosseous membrane must be large enough to accommodate the muscle belly of the posterior tibialis to allow adequate excursion of the transfer.*

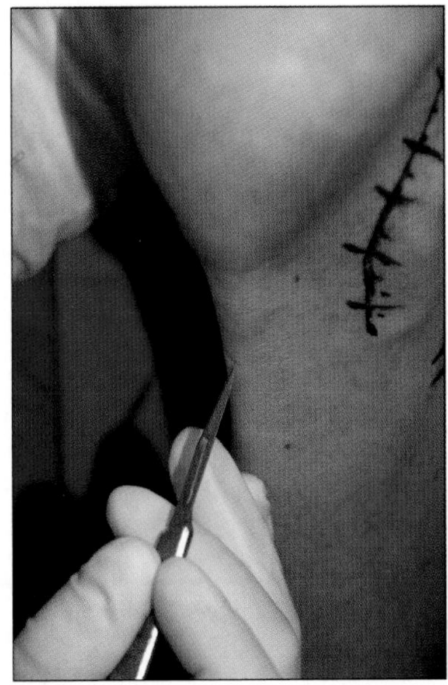

FIGURE 2

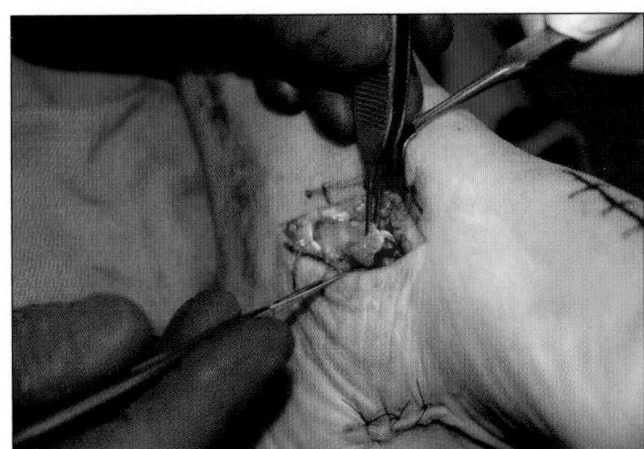

FIGURE 3

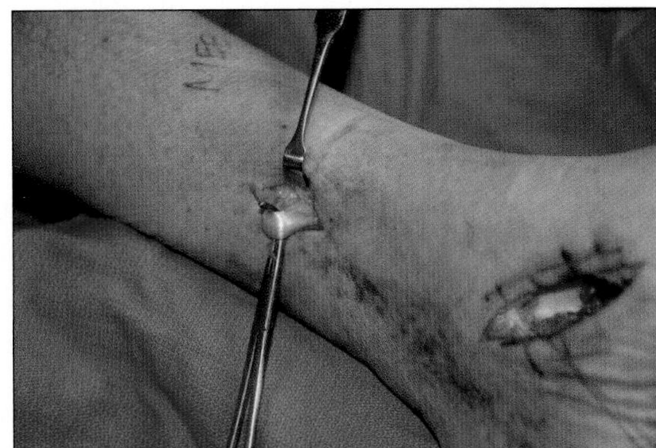

FIGURE 4

Step 3

- An additional anterolateral incision measuring 3 cm in length is created along the anterior border of the distal fibula approximately 3–5 cm above the anterior ankle joint.
- A large curved Kelly clamp is then passed through this anterolateral incision wound in a posteromedial direction until the interosseous membrane is reached. A large opening in the interosseous membrane is created by punching the tips of the clamp through the membrane and opening the jaws.
- The tips of the clamp are then brought into the proximal posteromedial wound, and the clamp is used to grasp the tag sutures of the tibialis posterior, which is subsequently pulled back into the proximal posteromedial wound, then passed through the interosseous membrane and out of the anterolateral wound along the previously created path (Fig. 5).

Step 4

- The next incision is made dorsally over the lateral cuneiform and measures 2–3 cm in length.
- The posterior tibial tendon is then passed subcutaneously from the anterior leg incision into the dorsal midfoot incision.
  - Using the Kelly clamp, a subcutaneous path is created in a retrograde fashion from the dorsal midfoot incision to the anterolateral incision, and the tag sutures are grasped with the tips (Fig. 6A).
  - The posterior tibial tendon is then pulled into the dorsal midfoot wound (Fig. 6B). (Note that our current method of fixation is demonstrated in a different surgical patient in Figure 6B through Figure 9.)
- Through this dorsal midfoot incision, a bony tunnel in the middle cuneiform is created from dorsal to plantar.
- The intraoperative fluoroscopic images in Figure 7 demonstrate the drill bit well positioned on the dorsal cortex of the lateral cuneiform (Fig. 7A) and the appearance following creation of the drill hole in the center of the lateral cuneiform (Fig. 7B).
- This tunnel should be of an appropriate diameter to accommodate the subsequent passage of the posterior tibial tendon.

Pearls

- *It is important that the passage of the posterior tibial tendon from the anterolateral wound to the dorsal midfoot wound occurs subcutaneously. Passage of the tendon deep to the extensor retinaculum will result in tethering and decreased dorsiflexion strength.*
- *When creating the dorsal-to-plantar drill hole in the midfoot, it is often helpful to use intraoperative fluoroscopy to verify that the drill is passing through the center of the lateral cuneiform.*
- *It is paramount that the ankle is maintained in neutral to 5° of dorsiflexion while implanting the transferred tendon into the lateral cuneiform. Failure to do so will result in recurrent equinus. However, overaggressive dorsiflexion may lead to a calcaneal gait pattern.*

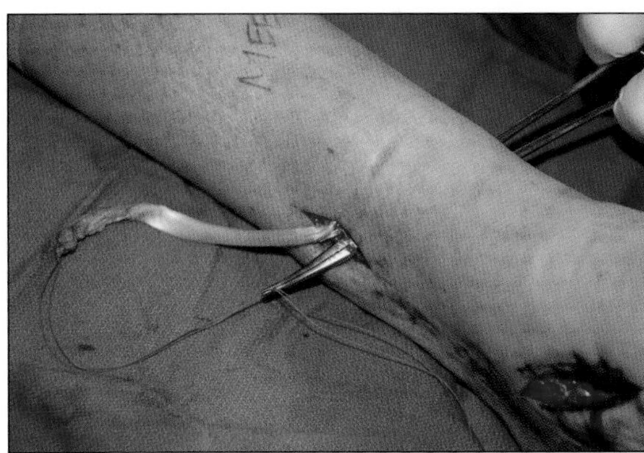

FIGURE 5

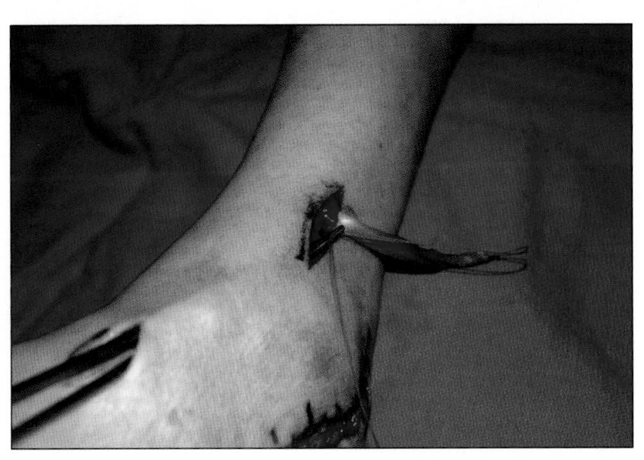

A

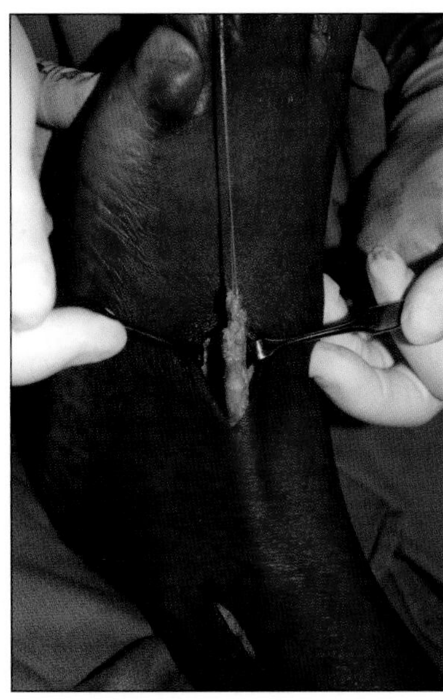

B

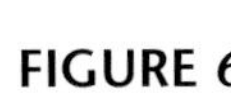

FIGURE 6

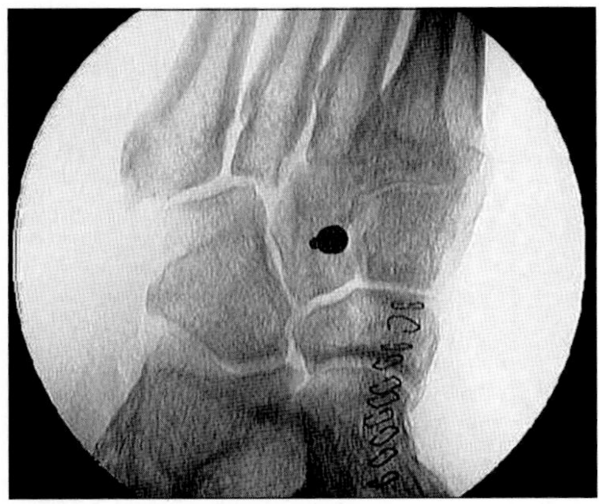

A

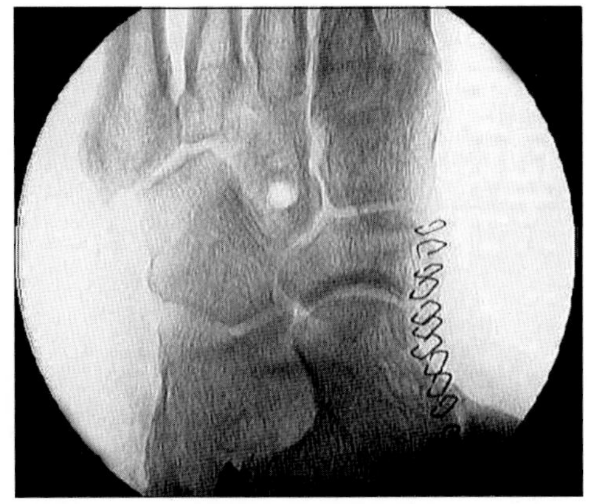

B

FIGURE 7

- The two limbs of the tag suture are attached to a free Keith needle, which is passed into the drill hole in the lateral cuneiform (Fig. 8A). The Keith needle is then pulled through the drill hole and out of the plantar surface of the foot, thus bringing the distal end of the posterior tibial tendon into the depths of the hole (Fig. 8B).
- This transferred posterior tibial tendon may be anchored to the middle cuneiform with the use of a bioabsorbable screw (Fig. 9) or tied over the plantar fascia through a separate plantar incision.

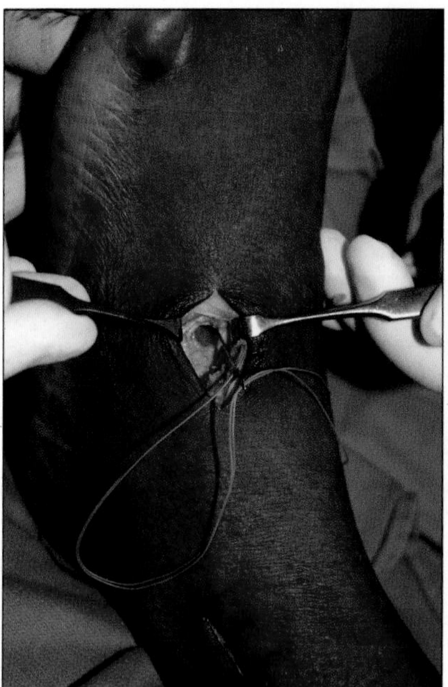

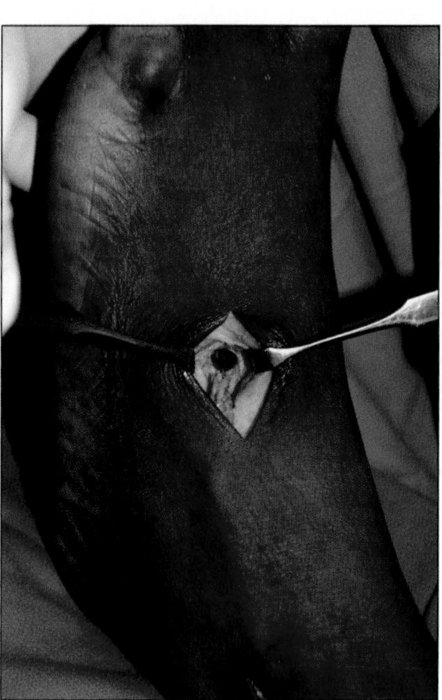

FIGURE 8 A B

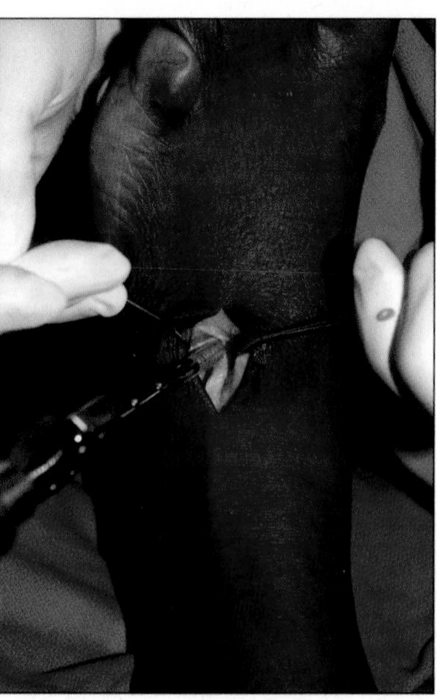

FIGURE 9

Step 5

- After thorough irrigation, the tourniquet is released and hemostasis is secured.
- All deep fascia is closed with 0 Vicryl suture, and all skin incisions are reapproximated using 3-0 Vicryl for the subcuticular layer and 3-0 nylon horizontal mattress sutures.
- Finally, the patient is placed in a well-padded short-leg plaster splint in maximal dorsiflexion.

Postoperative Care and Expected Outcomes

- The postoperative splint and sutures are removed at 3 weeks, and the patient is placed in a short-leg fiberglass walking cast. Full weight bearing is allowed following application of the cast.
- At 6 weeks postoperative, the cast is removed and the patient is placed in a cam walker. At this point, active dorsiflexion exercises are encouraged while plantar flexion of the ankle is prohibited.
- The cam walker is continued for an additional 12 weeks, at which point unrestricted range of motion is tolerated.
- Patients can be expected to attain 10–15° of active ankle dorsiflexion.

Evidence

Atesalp AS, Yildiz C, Komurco M, Basbozkurt M, Gur E. Posterior tibial tendon transfer and tendo-Achilles lengthening for equinovarus foot deformity due to severe crush injury. Foot Ankle Int. 2002;23:1103-6.

This study was a retrospective review of nine patients who underwent a posterior tibial tendon transfer (without an anastomosis of the peroneus longus or anterior tibialis) and Achilles lengthening for footdrop secondary to a crush injury sustained during an earthquake. At an average follow-up of 21 months, all patients were brace-free and there were no recurrences. (Level IV evidence [case series])

McCall RE, Frederick HA, McCluskey GM, Riordan DC. The Bridle procedure: a new treatment for equinus and equinovarus deformities in children. J Pediatr Orthop. 1991;11:83-9.

This study was a retrospective review of 128 posterior tibial tendon transfers performed on 101 pediatric patients, 80 of whom had an equinus or equinovarus deformity secondary to cerebral palsy. All transfers utilized the Bridle triple tendon anastomosis, but did not include anchoring of the posterior tibial tendon to the midfoot. Average follow-up was 5 years 9 months, with outcomes based on the need for postoperative bracing, gait patterns, plantigrade foot posture, and a neutral heel. (Level IV evidence [case series])

Mizel MS, Temple HT, Scranton PE, Gellman RE, Hecht PJ, Horton GA, McCluskey LC, McHale KA. Role of the peroneal tendons in the production of the deformed foot with posterior tibial tendon deficiency. Foot Ankle Int. 1999;20:285-9.

This retrospective review examined the results of posterior tibial tendon transfer in 10 patients with traumatic, common peroneal nerve palsies at an average follow-up of

74.9 months. The authors specifically evaluated each patient at final follow-up for collapse of the medial longitudinal arch and for a valgus hindfoot deformity, of which they found none. (Level IV evidence [case series])

Prahinski JR, McHale KA, Temple HT, Jackson JP. Bridle transfer for paresis of the anterior and lateral compartment musculature. Foot Ankle Int. 1996;17:615-9.

This study was a retrospective review of 10 highly active patients who underwent a Bridle posterior tibial tendon transfer with triple tendon anastomosis. At final follow-up, which averaged 61 months, 4 of 10 patients had returned to bracing, and 2 of these reported "an episode of acute tearing with dorsiflexion loss." Of the seven active-duty patients, three returned to duty. The authors concluded that a simple triple tendon anastomosis without insertion of the posterior tibial tendon into the middle cuneiform may stretch out over time, leading to unsatisfactory results in a highly active patient population. (Level IV evidence [case series])

Rodriguez RP. The Bridle procedure in the treatment of paralysis of the foot. Foot Ankle. 1992;13:63-9.

The author of this study modified the Bridle posterior tibial tendon transfer by inserting the distal end of the posterior tibial tendon into the middle cuneiform. The results of this procedure were then retrospectively reviewed with an average follow-up of 6.68 years. At final follow-up, all 10 patients (11 feet) were brace-free. (Level IV evidence [case series])

Schneider M, Balon K. Deformity of the foot following anterior transfer of the posterior tibial tendon and lengthening of the Achilles tendon for spastic equinovarus. Clin Orthop Relat Res. 1977;(125):113-8.

This study was a retrospective review of 24 cerebral palsy patients (29 feet) who underwent Achilles lengthening and simple anterior transfer of the posterior tibial tendon to the midfoot without triple tendon anastomosis. At final follow-up, a planovalgus deformity was seen in six feet, calcaneovalgus deformity in three feet, and calcaneovarus deformity in four feet. (Level IV evidence [case series])

PROCEDURE 56

Calf Lengthening for Equinus Contracture

Andrew K. Sands

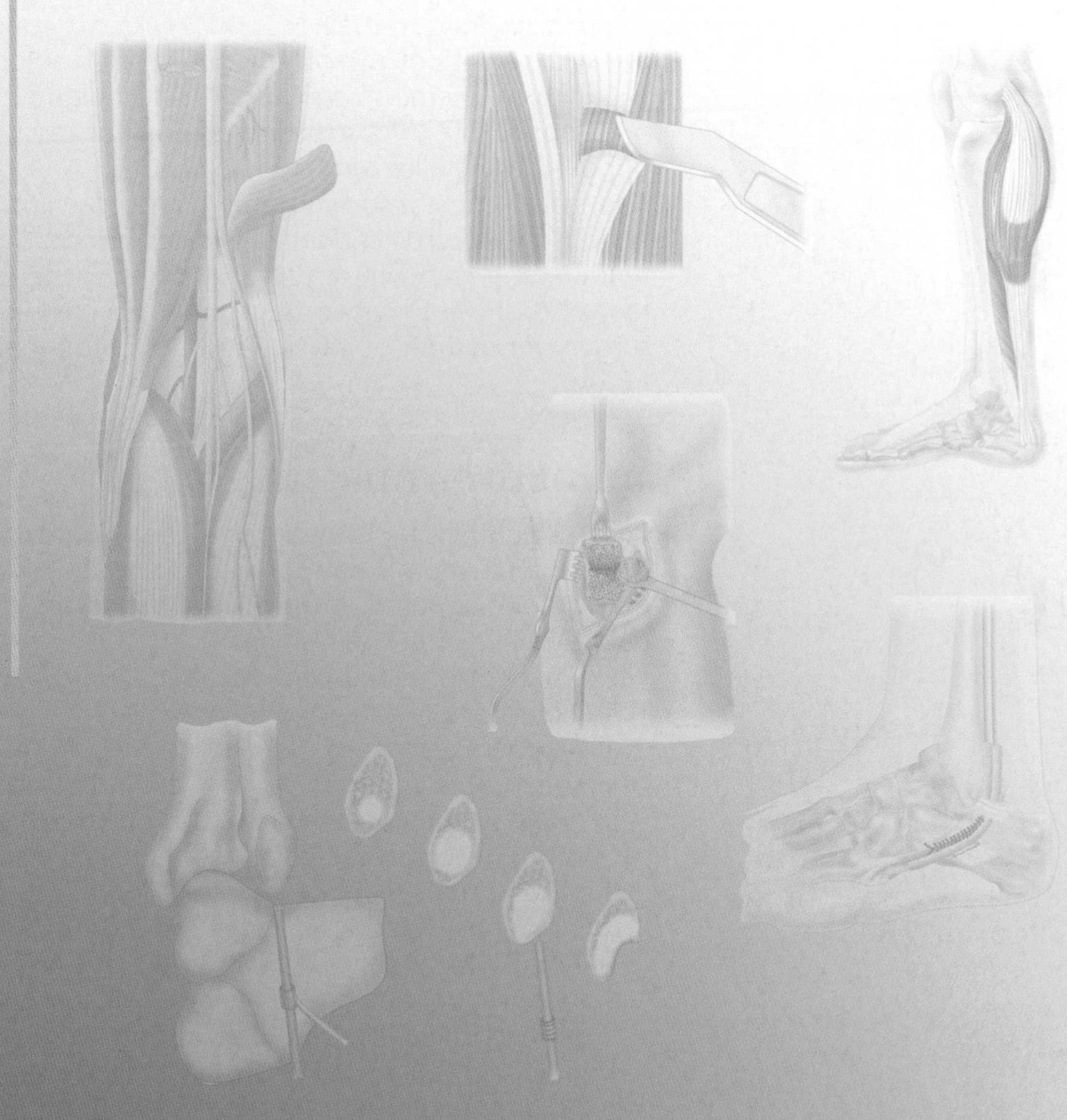

Andrew K. Sands would like to acknowledge the assistance of Edmund Choi, MD with this chapter.

Indications

- Equinus contracture/tight calf as an associated condition or a primary diagnosis.
- Most commonly seen in general orthopedic practice in flat or cavus feet.
- Associated with diabetes mellitus (DM) and has been shown to be an important causative factor in diabetic foot ulcers. It is also common in neuromuscular diseases such as cerebral palsy (CP). Often, CP or DM can be associated with an equinus contracture in the Achilles tendon itself.
- In cavus or flatfoot the contracture is often associated with "gastrocnemius" equinus. This technique is most applicable to gastrocnemius equinus (as opposed to Achilles tendon equinus).
- Can lead to heel pain syndrome/plantar fasciitis, Achilles insertional tendonitis, Achilles pain in the tendon, and calf pain or tear. Tightness of the calf may also prevent proper reduction in reconstructive surgery for flatfoot or cavus (either osteotomy or fusion).

Examination/Imaging

- Equinus contracture is found on clinical examination. If the examination is not done correctly the condition may go undiagnosed. It is important to follow this guideline in a stepwise fashion.
  - The patient is seated on an examination table and the knee is fully extended. (Since the gastrocnemius crosses three joints and the soleus only two, it is important to fully extend the knee to make sure the gastrocnemius is on stretch.)
  - Cup the heel with the contralateral hand, placing the thumb on the tarsonavicular (TN) joint. Using the ipsilateral hand around the forefoot, rock the TN joint into varus and valgus until you can find the neutral point of the TN joint. (This is important to prevent the ankle from dorsiflexing *around* the TN joint compared at the ankle. If the TN joint is everted, apparent dorsiflexion can occur at the TN joint instead of in the ankle.)
  - With the knee fully extended and the TN joint locked at neutral, gently dorsiflex the foot. If equinus is present, the ankle will remain in some degree of plantar flexion instead of coming into any amount of dorsiflexion.

- While maintaining the foot in the locked position with gentle dorsiflexion force, have the patient grasp under the knee and pull upward, releasing the tension on the gastrocnemius.
  - If the equinus contracture is a gastrocnemius equinus, the ankle should release and (more) dorsiflexion should be noted.
  - If the dorsiflexion does not increase then the equinus is not gastrocnemius equinus but rather a rigid "Achilles" contracture, which requires lengthening directly in the tendon.
- The examination can be repeated several times easily in a short time to confirm the diagnosis.

- Radiographs
  - Obtain weight-bearing films of the ankle.
  - Take care to make sure there is no bony block in the ankle preventing dorsiflexion or a capsule contracture that may also prevent dorsiflexion.

Surgical Anatomy

- The gastrocnemius-soleus complex originates both above and below the knee (Fig. 1A and 1B).
  - The gastrocnemius muscles originate behind the femoral condyles. The soleus originates from the upper third of the tibia, fibula, and interosseous membrane.

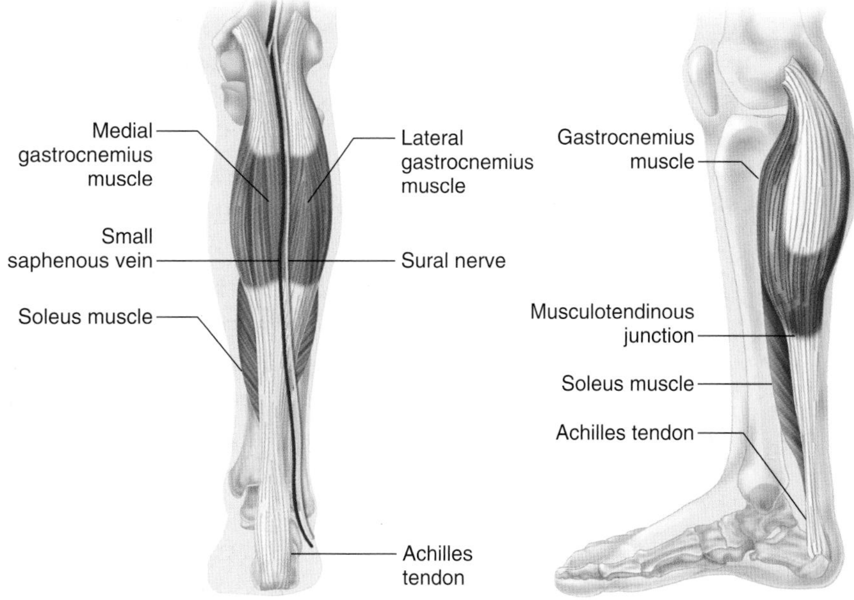

FIGURE 1 A B

- They join to form the Achilles tendon, which inserts on the tuber of the calcaneus. The tendon is approximately 15 cm in length. It sends an aponeurosis around the tuberosity to the plantar aspect of the tuberosity, where it helps form the planar ligaments.

- The sural nerve passes superficial to the deep fascia of the posterolateral leg and onto the dorsolateral foot. The sural nerve runs lateral and anterior to the Achilles tendon at the level of the ankle joint (see Fig. 1A).

Positioning

- The patient is placed in supine.
- Since this procedure is often done in conjunction with other reconstructive procedures, positioning also has to be done for those other procedures. However the medial approach makes it easy to release the gastrocnemius.
- If being done as an isolated procedure (as in calf lengthening for chronic heel pain syndrome), a "super"-supine position can be achieved by placing a large bump under the contralateral buttock. A towel bump can then be placed under the foot, allowing the calf to hang free. The topography can then be clearly visualized.

Portals/Exposures

- Surface topography allows the surgeon to find the gastrocnemius musculotendinous area. Mark the medial border of the tibia and find the outline of the gastrocnemius. Find a line approximately 1.5–2 finger-widths off of the tibia edge and mark a vertical line parallel to the tibial crest, across the gastrocnemius profile.
- If a more distal complete release of the gastrocnemius insertion is desired, shift your incision inferiorly. If the deep posterior incision is desired, the incision can be shifted superiorly.
- On the approach, note the deep investing fascia. Preserving this and closing it carefully helps to prevent adhesions between the skin and the muscle (a potential cosmetic problem of the procedure).
- Finding the gastrocnemius-soleus interval
  - Once below the investing fascia, lay your finger along the surface of the muscle at the tibial border. Carefully slide posteriorly and your finger

- should fall into the gap between the gastrocnemius and soleus.
- Sometimes it is easier to find this space if you move your finger a bit more proximally where the gap is more pronounced. The finger can then be slid distally to the insertion of the gastrocnemius onto the soleus/Achilles.

- The approach can also be done from posteriorly if the patient is face down. Care must be taken to approach a bit medially and to avoid the sural nerve as it exits at the musculotendinous junction.

Procedure

Instrumentation/ Implantation

- Retractors
- Curved blade AO/Cobb elevator
- Head light

Step 1: Prepping the Gastrocnemius Release

- The skin is incised and the incision is deepened straight to the investing fascia without raising flaps or elevating the subcutaneous layer off of the fascia (Fig. 2).
- Once the fascia is incised, the blunt dissection can then be carried medially and laterally under the fascia. Care should be taken to keep the superficial layer full thickness. This aids in closure and wound healing.

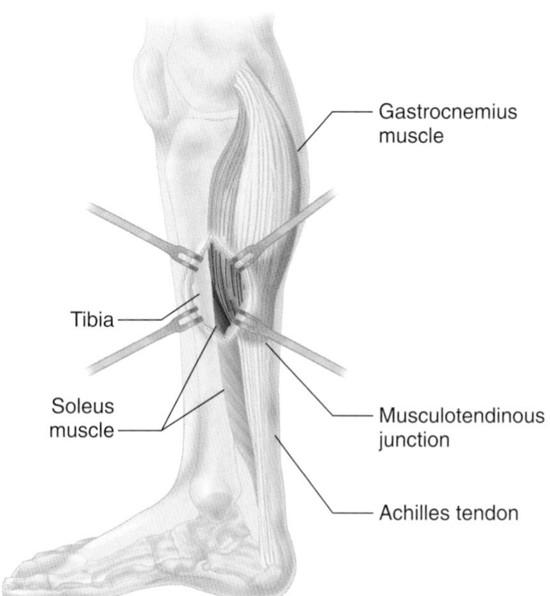

FIGURE 2

- The interval between the gastrocnemius and soleus is developed (see Surgical Anatomy section) and deep retractors are placed (Fig. 3A and 3B). Various types of retractors can be used.
  - Kocher-Langenbach oral surgery tongue retractors—skinny deep blades that come as a nested set (Fig. 4).
  - Adolescent vaginal speculum—placing one blade on each side of the insertion retracts the soleus deep and the soft tissue layer superficial (Fig. 5A and 5B).
- The curved or Cobb elevator is used to lift the soft tissue off of the superficial side of the insertion (and with it the sural nerve). The insertion should be clearly visualized on both the deep and superficial sides from medial to lateral.

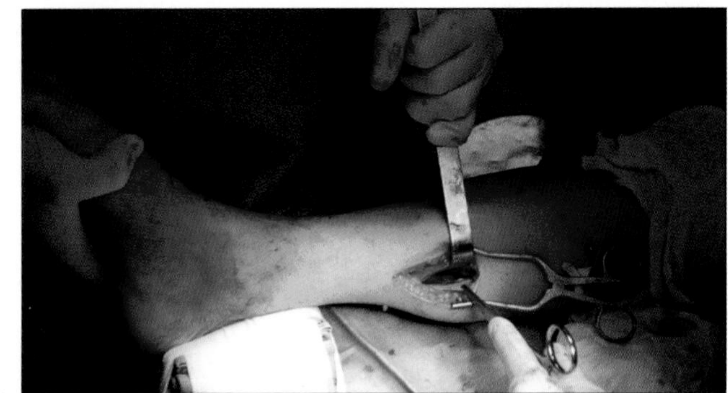

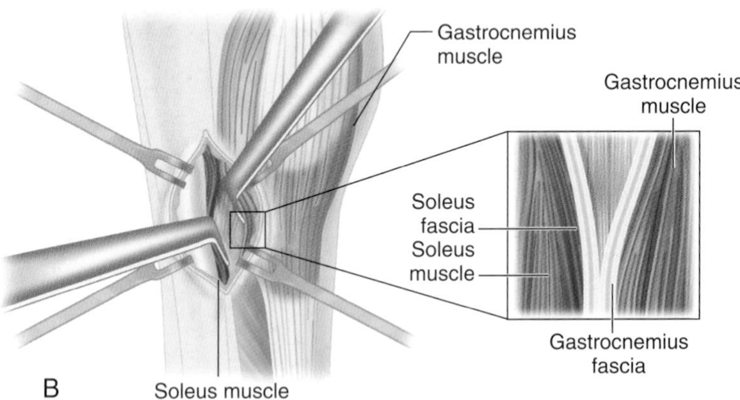

FIGURE 3

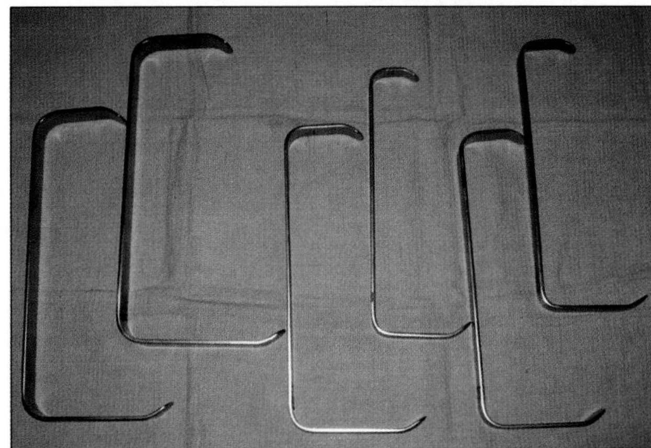

FIGURE 4

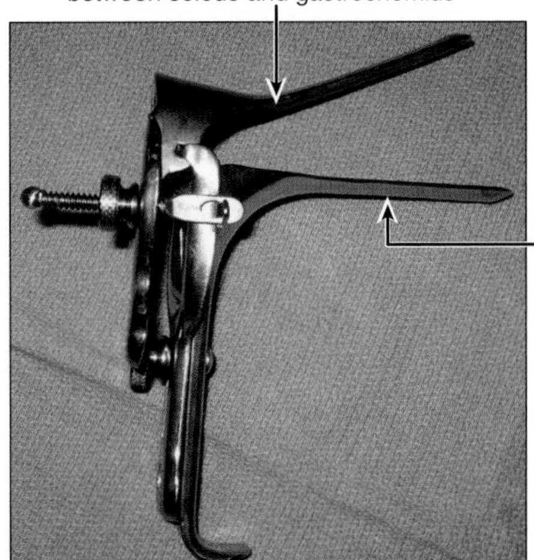

A

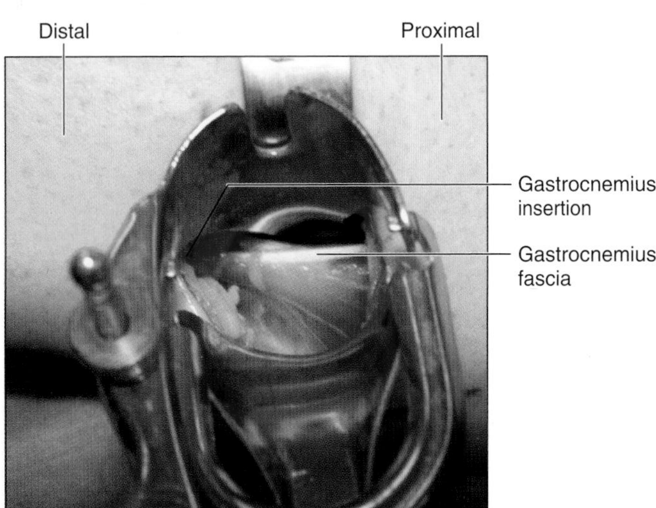

B

FIGURE 5

Instrumentation/ Implantation

- Long-handled scalpel with No. 15 blade

Step 2: Gastrocnemius Release

- A long-handled No. 15 blade is used to score the insertion from lateral to medial (Fig. 6A and 6B). If care is taken, there should be no damage to the muscle itself, decreasing the likelihood of bleeding.
- Once the insertion is released (Fig. 7), the ankle is gently dorsiflexed. The gap should be clearly seen and the equinus contracture should be released.
- If the alternative procedure is being done (behind the tendon insertion to preserve the muscle belly), care is taken to not cut into the muscle belly while incising the tendon. Dorsiflexion of the ankle leads to separation of the tendon layer and lengthening/ stretching of the muscle fibers.
- As this procedure is often done in conjunction with other procedures, closure is left until the end of the operation. A lap pad can be packed into the wound and left in place until closure. This has the added benefit of hemostasis.

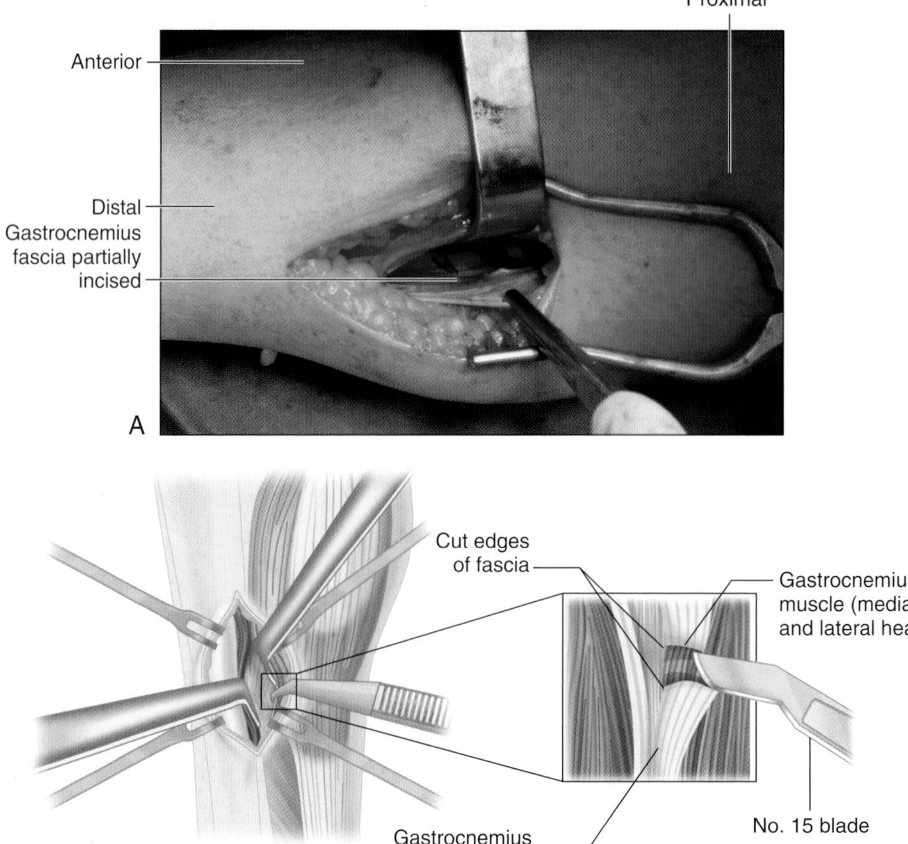

FIGURE 6

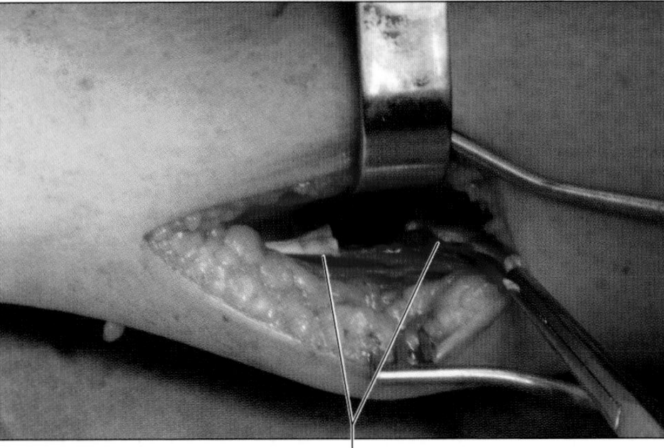

FIGURE 7

Pitfalls

- *Sural nerve injury*
  - *If the soft tissue is not fully retracted from the superficial layer, sural nerve injury can result. While there is no functional deficit, numbness on the lateral hindfoot can be an annoyance to the patient. Sometimes, overeager retraction can cause injury to the nerve.*
  - *Blind cutting of the most lateral area from the medial incision can lead to sural injury. Preoperative patient education should always include possible sural nerve injury.*
- *Deep vein injury with copious bleeding: The gastrocnemius mucle belly may have venous structures that can cause bleeding into the surgical field. Packing the wound with a lap pad can often stop the bleeding without having to use the cautery. Deep cautery should be done carefully as injury to the sural nerve can result.*
- *Adhesions between cut tendon or muscle and skin: Care should be taken in closure of the deep investing fascia layer. Overeager dissection, especially between the skin and the deep investing fascia, can lead to adhesions and adverse cosmetic results (although not adverse functional results). Taking care to not dissect the subcutaneous space or to lift the fat off of the deep investing fascia, and careful closing of the deep investing fascia, can help to minimize this potential problem. In short, go directly from skin to muscle and keep your fingers out of the wound until you are below the fascia.*

Step 3: Closure

- In the past, tacking sutures were placed on the now-lengthened tendon ends. Since these probably cut out and do not serve any structural purpose, these sutures are not needed.
- Instead the first layer to be closed is the deep investing fascia. A running 2-0 braided absorbable suture is used to close this layer while taking care to not create dead space by dissecting the subcutaneous fat off of the fascia.

Postoperative Care and Expected Outcomes

- The ankle should be kept in neutral position. If a splint is being applied for associated procedures, the ankle is usually in the correct position.
- The postoperative course for calf lengthening usually follows that of any associated procedures, and when these other procedures are ready for physical therapy, so too is the calf lengthening.
- If the calf lengthening is done alone, the splint can be left in place with the ankle in neutral for 2 weeks. After this the patient can be given a cane and started on physical therapy.
- The most important part of the postoperative care then is the night ankle "L" splint. Since the relaxed sleeping position is plantar flexion of the ankles and feet, the deformity could return. Patients should be kept in this splint for sleep for 3 months with occasional use for longer if needed.

- Physical therapy should concentrate on calf and hamstring stretching with a daily home exercise stretching program.

Controversies

- It is theoretically possible to overlengthen the calf/gastrocnemius-soleus complex and be left with a calcaneus posture. There have been anecdotal reports of this, although it is rare. If the leg is splinted and the 90° night "L" splint is used, it is less likely as the calf has a chance to heal down in the proper position and length/tension. If physical therapy and aggressive stretching are started too soon, the calf may be more susceptible to overstretching.
- Strength is decreased in the leg in the immediate postoperative period and for a year or so afterward. The strength is usually regained after that, but the bilateral symmetry is often never regained. Most leg power comes from the more proximal muscles, so deficit is rarely noted, but in some high-performance athletes, calf lengthening should be deferred while they are competing at the highest levels, unless their symptoms prevent it.

Evidence

Baddar A, Granata K, Damiano DL, Carmines DV, Blanco JS, Abel MF. Ankle and knee coupling patients with spastic diplegia: effects of gastrocnemius-soleus lengthening. J Bone Joint Surg [Am]. 2002;84:736-44.

This study was a retrospective review of 34 patients treated operatively with a gastrocnemius and soleus recession. Outcome was determined by gait analysis, electromyography, and physical examination. (Level IV evidence [case series])

Borton DC, Walker K, Pirpiris M, Nattrass GR, Graham HK. Isolated calf lengthening in cerebral palsy: outcome analysis of risk factors. J Bone Joint Surg [Br]. 2001;83:364-70.

This study was a retrospective review of 195 CP cases using percutaneous lengthening, open Z-lengthening of the tendo-Achilles and lengthening of the gastrocnemius-soleus aponeurosis. Follow-up averaged 6.9 years. Outcome was determined by physical examination and radiographic assessment. (Level IV evidence [case series])

DiGiovanni CW, Kuo R, Tejwani NM, Price R, Hansen ST, Cziernecki J, Sangeorzan B. Isolated gastrocnemius tightness. J Bone Joint Surg [Am]. 2002;84:962-70.

This prospective study evaluated the maximal ankle dorsiflexion in 34 consecutive patients with midfoot or forefoot pain, as well as the difference in dorsiflexion with the knee extended or flexed. (Level IV evidence [case series])

Pinney SJ, Hansen ST, Sangeorzan BJ. The effect on ankle dorsiflexion of gastrocnemius recession. Foot Ankle Int. 2002;23:26-9.

This study was a retrospective review of 20 consecutive patients treated operatively. Follow-up was 55 days. Outcome was determined by dorsiflexion measurements. (Level IV evidence [case series])

Pinney SJ, Sangeorzan BJ, Hansen ST. Surgical anatomy of the gastrocnemius recession (Strayer procedure). Foot Ankle Int. 2004;25;247-50.

This study was a retrospective review of 33 consecutive patients treated operatively. Surgical measurements were made to assess risk of sural nerve injury and release site from the gastrocnemius muscle belly. (Level IV evidence [case series])

Sammarco GJ, Bagwe MR, Sammarco VJ, Magur EG. The effects of unilateral gastrosoleus recession. Foot Ankle Int. 2006;27:26-9.

This study was a retrospective review of 40 patients treated operatively. Follow-up averaged 25.3 months. Outcome was determined by American Orthopaedic Foot and Ankle Society scores, subjective questionnaire, and physical examination. (Level IV evidence [case series])

Tashjian RZ, Appel AJ, Banerjee R, DiGiovanni CW. Anatomic study of the gastrocnemius-soleus junction and its relationship to sural nerve. Foot Ankle Int. 2003;24:473-6.

This study evaluated 15 cadaveric limbs to assess the relationship of the sural nerve to the gastrocnemius-soleus junction. (Level V evidence [cadaveric study])

Tashjian RZ, Appel AJ, Banerjee R, DiGiovanni CW. Endoscopic gastrocnemius recession: evaluation in a cadaver model. Foot Ankle Int. 2003;24:607-13.

This study evaluated 15 cadaveric limbs to determine the accuracy of incision placement during gastrocnemius recession. (Level V evidence [cadaveric study])

PROCEDURE 57

Proximal Tibia Bone Graft

Andrew K. Sands

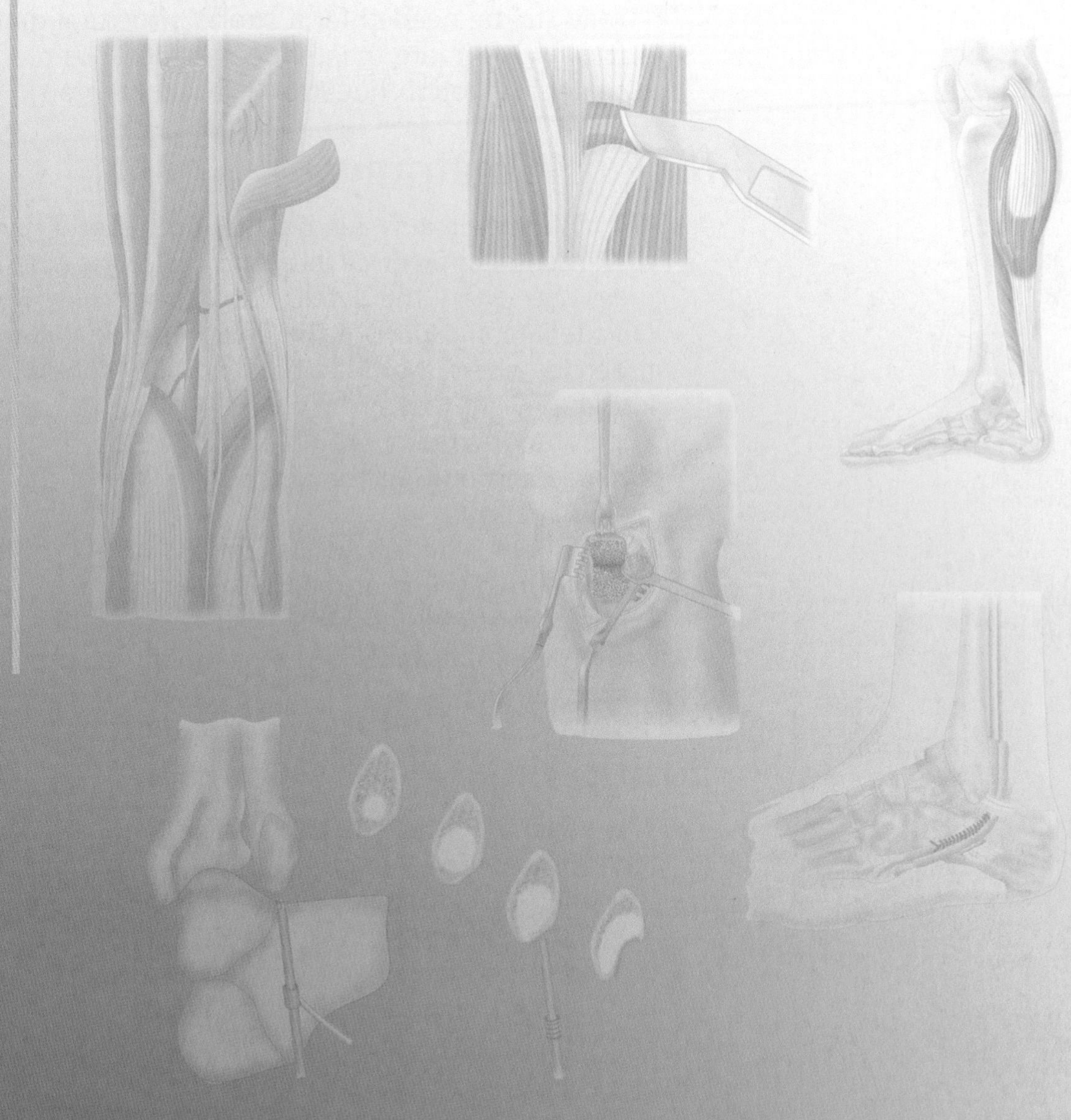

Andrew K. Sands would like to acknowledge the assistance of Edmund Choi, MD with this chapter.

Treatment Options

- Traditional iliac crest bone autograft technique
- Commercially available bone allograft

Indications

- Reconstruction procedures (fusions) require some form of bone graft. Despite great hope for non-autograft sources, the "gold standard" continues to be autograft. This technique uses the proximal tibia as the source.
- The advantages of the proximal tibia site are:
  - It is usually draped into the field already.
  - It avoids the pain and potential blood loss associated with the pelvic donor site. Pelvic bone may still be needed for a strong structural graft.
  - It can yield more than enough cancellous graft material (though not strong structural graft).

Surgical Anatomy

- The tibial tubercle is a large, oblong elevation where the anterior surfaces of the condyles of the tibia meet and where the patella tendon attaches (Fig. 1).
- On the lateral aspect of the tibial tubercle is Gerdy's tubercle, where the distal bands of the iliotibial band insert.
- The anterior crest of the tibia starts at the tibial tubercle and ends at the anterior margin of the medial malleolus.
- The anterior crest is sinuous and prominent in the proximal two thirds of the tibia, whereas it is rounded in the distal third.
- The anterior crest provides attachment for the deep fascia.

Positioning

- The patient is usually positioned for the reconstructive procedure.
- If possible, an ipsilateral bump internally rotates the leg, allowing easier access.
- If needed, the table can be rolled for graft harvesting, then rolled back afterward.

Portals/Exposures

- The tibial tubercle, joint line, and proximal fibula should be identified (Fig. 2). This makes it easy to find Gerdy's tubercle at the proximal lateral tibia.
  - The iliotibial band can also be followed distally to the insertion onto Gerdy's tubercle. The tubercle is subcutaneous and easily palpated.

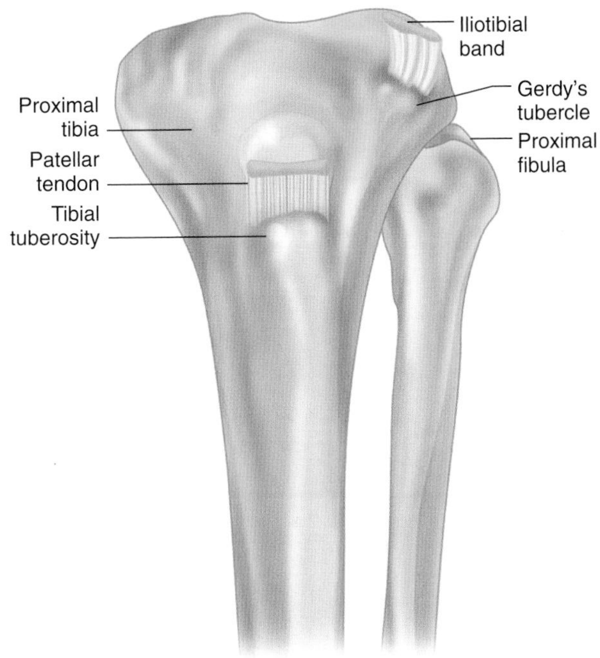

FIGURE 1

- Care must be taken to avoid confusing one of these other prominences with Gerdy's tubercle however.

■ Once the subcutaneous tissue is incised, the iliotibial band fibers are clearly visible and can be followed distally to the insertion point.

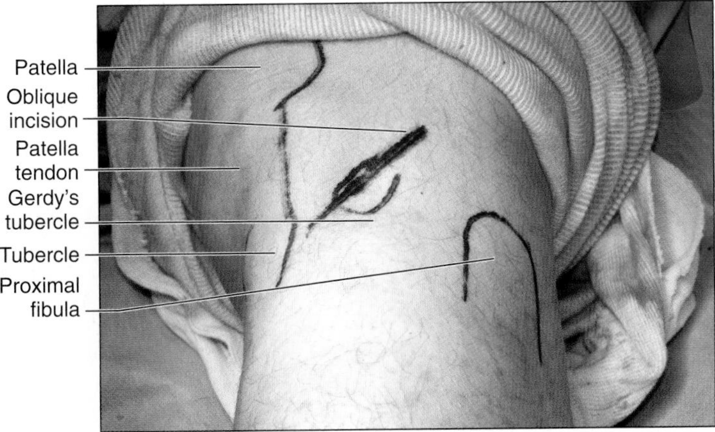

FIGURE 2

Procedure

Step 1: Prepping the Proximal Tibial Donor Site

- Once the incision is marked (from landmarks as outlined above), an incision is made through the skin into the subcutaneous space and Gerdy's tubercle is exposed (Fig. 3A).
- Hemostasis and deeper dissection can be accomplished with the electric cautery.
- The tubercle is identified and outlined with the marker (Fig. 3B). The distal, medial, and lateral margins are incised using the cautery.
- A curved ½-inch osteotome is used to carefully go through the cortex on the medial, distal, and lateral aspects of the tubercle.
  - The curve should be directed toward the center of the "lid."
  - The "lid" is then very slowly and carefully lifted. The proximal cortex is still within the fibers of the iliotibial band and either deforms or cracks but does not displace.
- The "lid" is then rotated upward and retracted.

Step 2: Harvesting the Proximal Tibial Site

- Underlying cancellous graft is then harvested (Fig. 4A and 4B).
- A lap pad corner can be left in the donor site. This aids in hemostasis and allows further harvesting if more graft is needed.
- Once adequate graft has been harvested and placed into the fusion site, the donor site can be stuffed with surgicel and gelfoam (Fig. 5A and 5B).

Pearls

- *Occasionally pause during graft harvesting and stuff the donor site with a lap pad corner. It will soak up marrow fluid, which can be mixed with the graft.*

Pitfalls

- *Care must be taken on the approach to not injure the iliotibial band fibers. If a self-retaining retractor (Wheatlander) is placed and lifted up slightly, the subcutaneous tissue is lifted off of the underlying iliotibial band fibers. It can then be divided and cauterized without danger to the iliotibial band fibers.*
- *When incising the soft tissue over the tubercle, the distal incision should not be made too far into the muscle of the anterior compartment.*
- *When opening the "lid," make sure to divide the cortex completely and gently lift the "lid" to avoid fracture into the joint.*

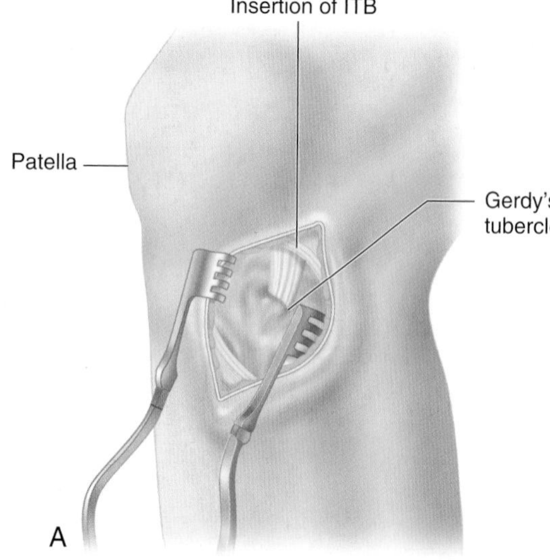

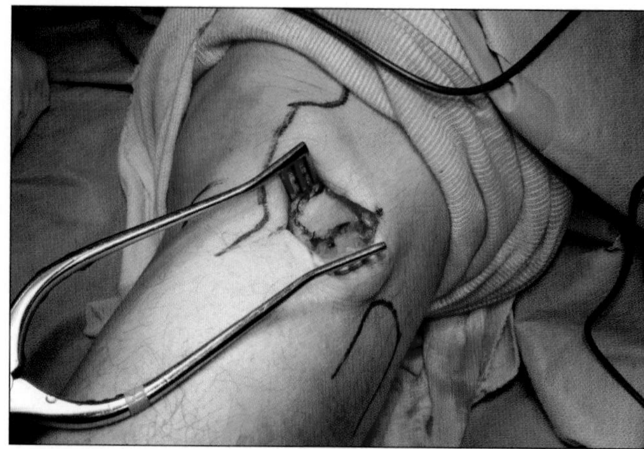

FIGURE 3

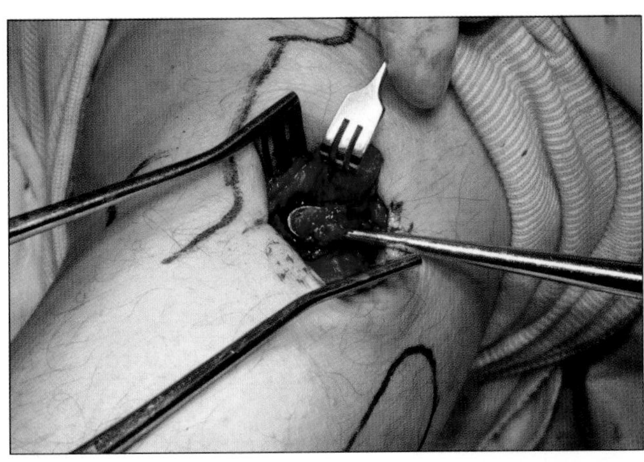

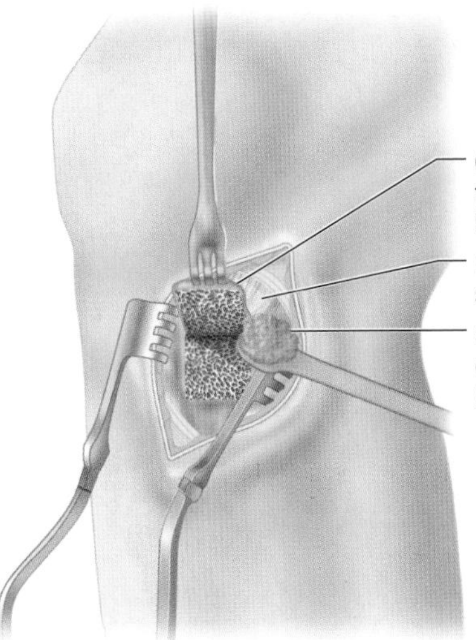

A B

FIGURE 4

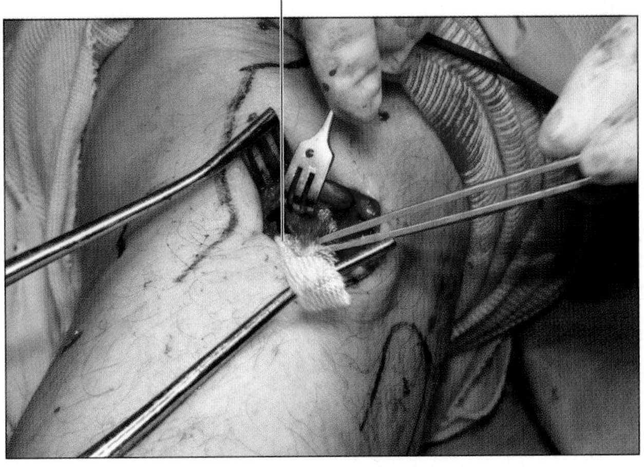

A

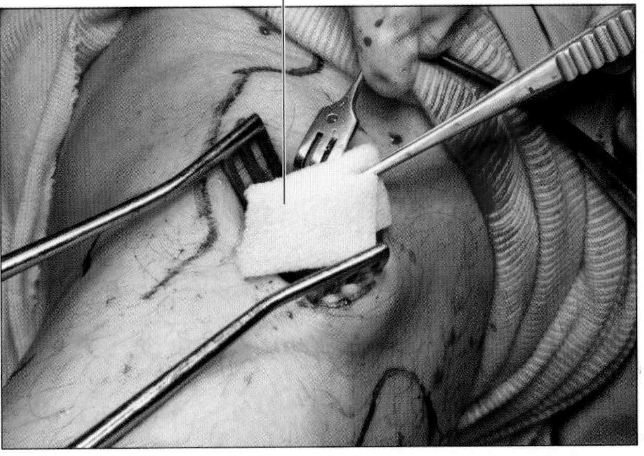

B

FIGURE 5

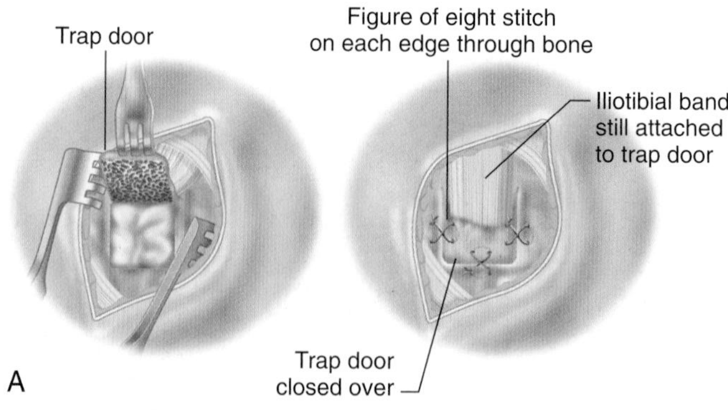

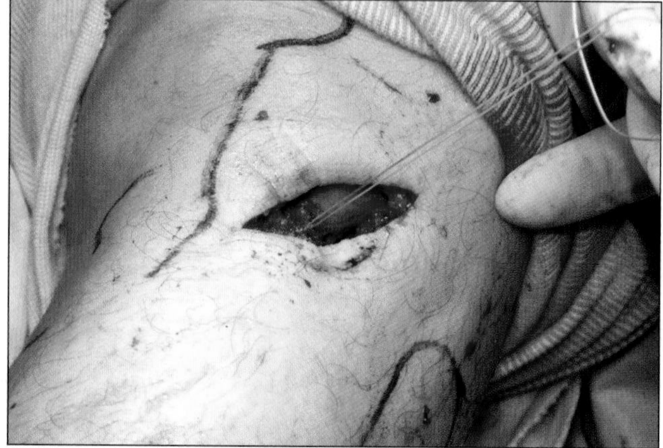

Gerdy's tubercle closed back into place secured with 0 vicryl suture material

FIGURE 6

- The "lid" is then closed and secured back in place using sutures placed on all three sides (Fig. 6A and 6B).
- The subcutaneous tissue and skin are then closed.
- Since the proximal tibia site tends to be at the most proximal portion of the leg splint and is more exposed, the area can be covered with a folded 4 × 4 gauze, which is then covered with liquid adhesive and clear operative incision membrane dressing.

Postoperative Care and Expected Outcomes

- For the most part, this is a safe procedure that yields plentiful graft. Tibial plateau fracture has occurred after proximal tibia donor site.
- Since the splint/cast/cam walker immobilizes the limb, and it (or Tegaderm) covers the site, the site is protected. By the time the foot is healed from the reconstructive procedure, the graft site is ready to progress through physical therapy along with the rest of the limb.

Instrumentation/ Implantation

- A large "soup spoon"–shaped curette is helpful in removing the cancellous graft from the donor site.

Controversies

- Graft "helper": The graft can be mixed with a potentially bioactive material, such as bone morphogenetic protein (BMP), if desired. If a putty form of BMP is used, the putty can be placed first and the graft stuffed in after. The putty BMP holds the graft flakes in place.
- The donor site can be backfilled with allograft or graft substitute, if desired.

Evidence

Alt V, Meeder PJ, Seligson D, Schad A, Atienza C. The proximal tibia metaphysis: a reliable donor site for bone grafting? Clin Orthop Relat Res. 2003;(414):315-21.

This cadaveric study was performed to assess the risk of tibial plateau fracture from eight cadavers in which the cancellous bone was harvested from the proximal tibia. (Level V evidence [cadaveric study])

Alt V, Nawab A, Seligson D. Bone grafting from the proximal tibia. J Trauma. 1999;47:555-7.

This study was a retrospective review of 54 patients who underwent harvesting of the proximal tibia due to fresh fractures with primary grafting and nonunions. Follow-up averaged 26.4 weeks. Outcome was determined by clinical examination and patient subjective assessment. (Level IV evidence [case series])

Geideman W, Early JS, Brodksy J. Clinical results of harvesting autogenous cancellous graft from the ipsilateral proximal tibia for use in foot and ankle surgery. Foot Ankle Int. 2004;25:451-5.

This study was a retrospective review of 155 patients who underwent a foot or ankle procedure utilizing the ipsilateral proximal tibia as the donor site for autogenous cancellous graft. Outcome was determined by clinical examination and patient subjective assessment. (Level IV evidence [case series])

O'Keefe RM, Riemer BL, Butterfield SL. Harvesting of autogenous cancellous bone graft from the proximal tibial metaphysis: a review of 230 cases. J Orthop Trauma. 1991;5:469-74.

This study was a retrospective review of 260 patients who underwent proximal tibia bone graft harvesting for lower extremity fractures or nonunions. Follow-up averaged 20.4 months. Outcome was determined by clinical examination and patient subjective assessment. (Level IV evidence [case series])

Whitehouse MR, Lankester BJ, Winson IG, Hepple S. Bone graft harvest from the proximal tibia in foot and ankle arthrodesis surgery. Foot Ankle Int. 2006;27:913-6.

This study was a retrospective review of 148 cases using autogenous cancellous bone graft from the proximal tibia. At minimum, follow-up was at least 3 months. Outcome was determined by patient subjective assessment and clinical examination. (Level IV evidence [case series])

PROCEDURE 58

Anterior Leg Compartment Release for Exertional Compartment Syndrome

Andrew K. Sands

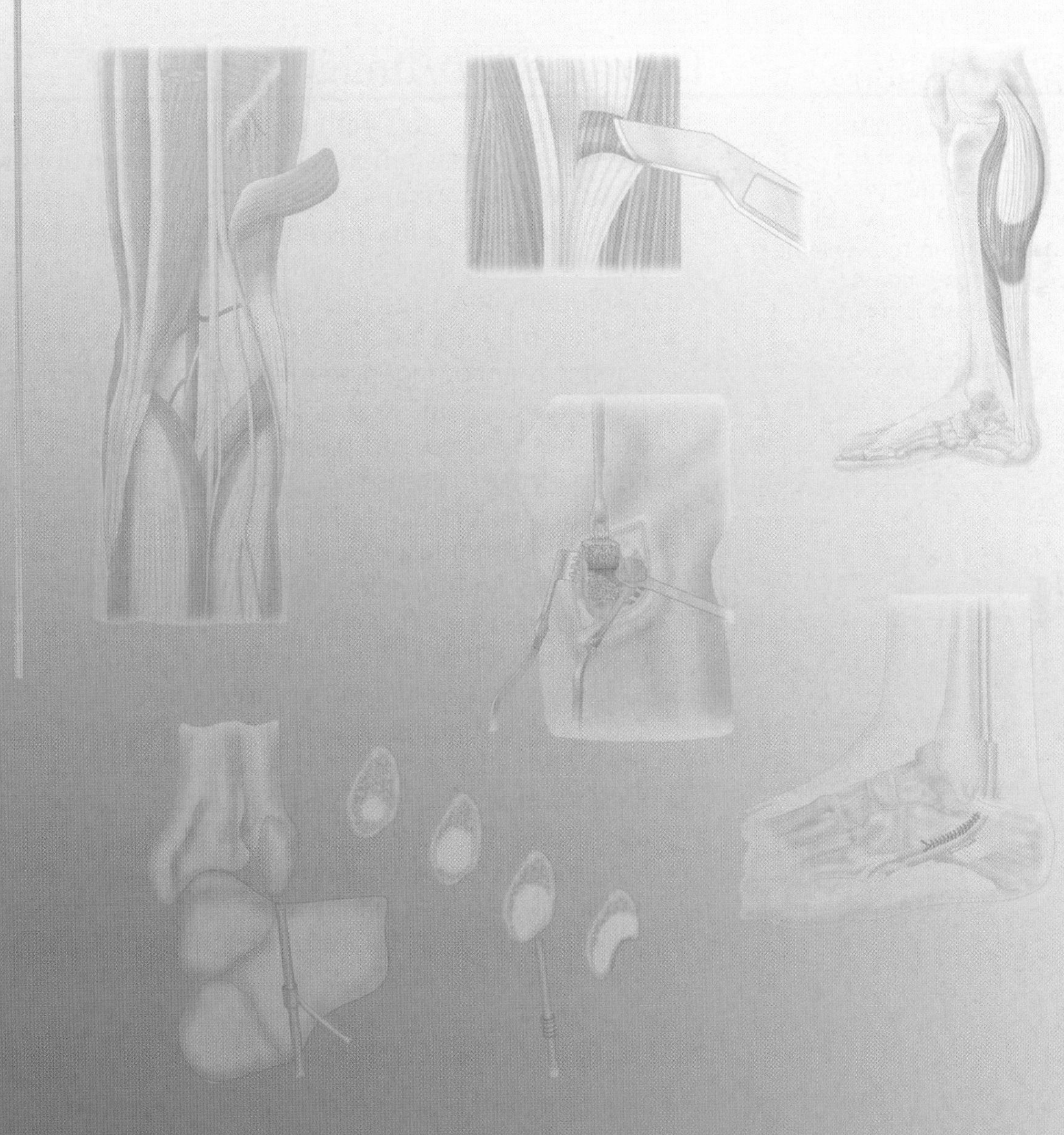

Andrew K. Sands would like to acknowledge the assistance of Edmund Choi, MD with this chapter.

Indications

- Pain in the leg localized to the anterolateral area.
- This is a diagnosis of exclusion (other entities must be eliminated before this diagnosis is considered)
- It is often part of the wastebasket diagnosis of "shin splints," which can be stress fractures, periostitis, or exertional compartment syndrome. One has to exclude mass effects from tumors in the leg or vascular disease/malformations. Trauma also has to be excluded.

Treatment Options

- Physical therapy can often decrease symptoms. If the anterior compartment is overwhelmed by a tight calf (overloaded trying to overcome the equinus contracture), aggressive calf stretching can help.
- However, nonoperative treatment rarely eliminates the pain in a true anterior exertional compartment syndrome.

Examination/Imaging

- The symptoms start with exertion and increase with activity. Whereas a normal person may be able to exercise at a certain level for a certain amount of time, someone with this entity notes severe pain sooner during exercise with much longer time to resolution after exercise.
- The leg may not be abnormal at rest. However, if the patient is encouraged to exercise in the examination room (or sent out to run around the block), the leg becomes swollen and painful. The anterior compartment is tense on palpation. The pain is often accompanied by dysesthesias into the ankle and foot.
- A pressure monitor can be used to confirm the diagnosis. An indwelling wick catheter can be used if desired to graph the pressure of the compartment over time. Often this is a bilateral condition.
- If there is an associated equinus contracture, it may cause the anterior compartment to over-pull against the tight calf.
- Radiographs of the leg can be used to rule out stress fracture of the tibia.
- Magnetic resonance imaging can show masses within the leg that might be causing symptoms, or periostitis or stress fractures or other abnormalities of the marrow.

Surgical Anatomy

- The anterior compartment of the leg comprises the tibialis anterior, extensor digitorum longus, extensor hallucis longus, and peroneus tertius (Fig. 1).
- The anterior tibial artery and deep peroneal nerve travel superficial to the interosseous membrane, between the tibialis anterior and extensor hallucis longus.

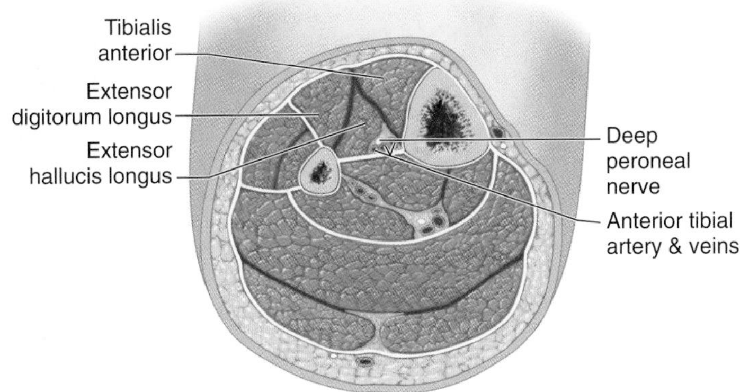

FIGURE 1

- Refer to the information on equinus contracture release (see Procedure 56) if this is being done in conjunction with anterior release.

Positioning

- The patient is supine with an ipsilateral bump. Exposure from the foot to the knee is needed

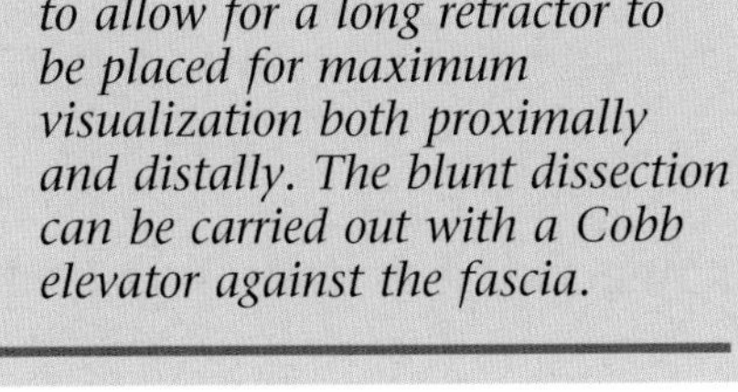

PEARLS

- *Make a sufficiently long incision to allow for a long retractor to be placed for maximum visualization both proximally and distally. The blunt dissection can be carried out with a Cobb elevator against the fascia.*

Portals/Exposures

- The anterior compartment of the leg is approached 8 cm distal to the tibial tubercle and 4 cm lateral to the tibial crest (Fig. 2). The incision is carried straight through the subcutaneous tissue to the fascia, which is then incised, exposing the underlying muscle belly.

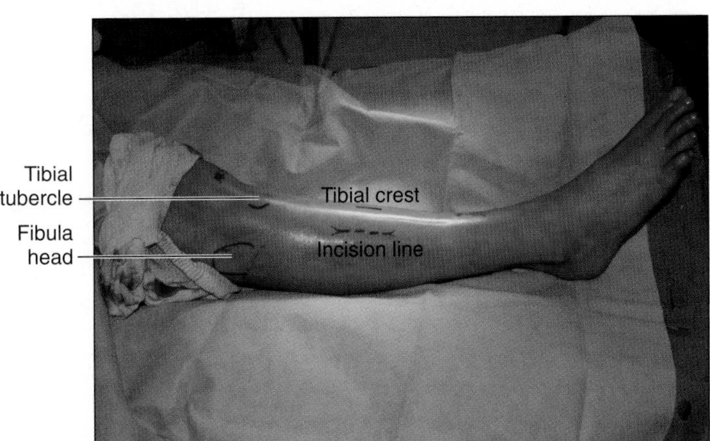

FIGURE 2

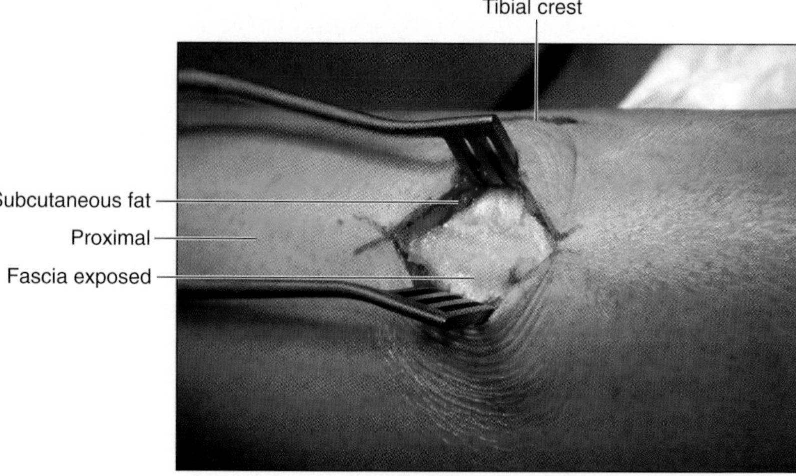

FIGURE 3

Controversies

- Small incision for cosmesis can lead to a higher chance of numb patches from damage to sensory nerves.

- Subcutaneous and subfascial dissection are carried out to visualize the fascia (Fig. 3). This helps protect the small sensory nerves coming out from the fascia into the skin. This will prevent numb patches of the leg.
- The release must be made for the full extent of the fascia both proximal and distal to the ankle extensor retinaculum.

Procedure

Step 1: Calf Lengthening

- If the calf lengthening is needed, it is done first (see Procedure 56).

Step 2: Dissecting the Fascia

- The fascia is incised the length of the incision (Fig. 4).

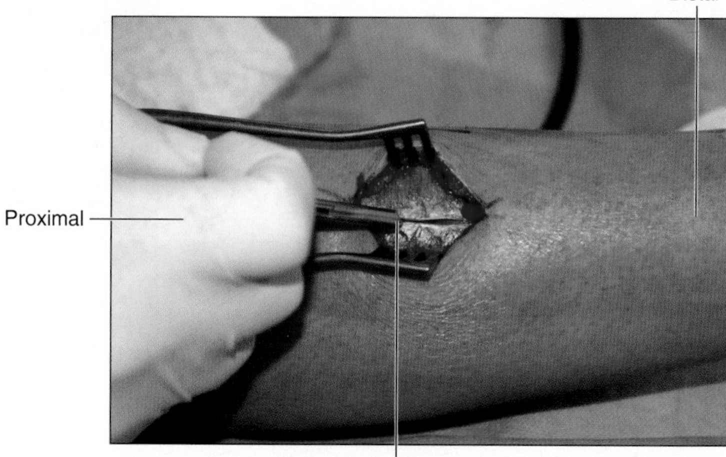

FIGURE 4

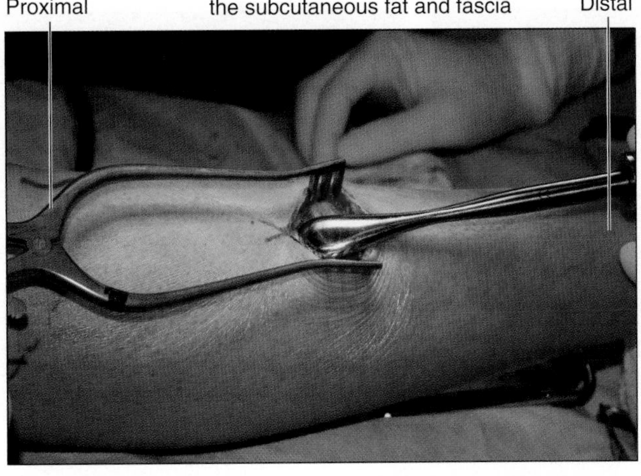

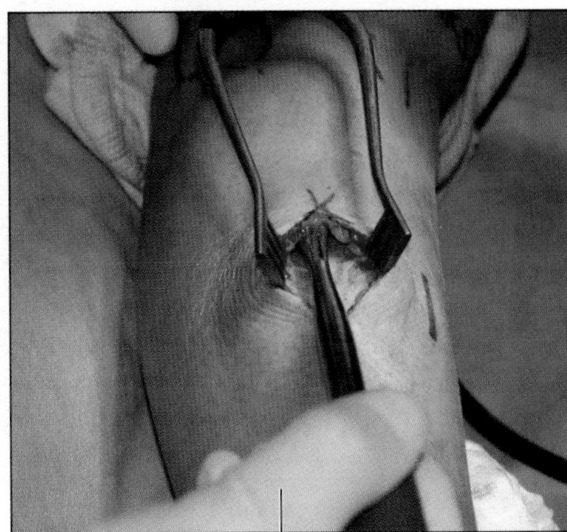

FIGURE 5

Instrumentation/ Implantation

- The subcutaneous dissection can be performed using a Cobb elevator along with a long-bladed retractor such as an oral surgery tongue retractor.
- Also useful is a plastic surgery face-lift lighted long-bladed retractor.

- An elevator is used to carefully elevate the subcutaneous tissue off of the fascia, taking care to avoid sensory branches (Fig. 5A and 5B).
- Once the dissection is carried proximally and distally, the fascia can be divided with a long Mayo scissors.
- A long-bladed retractor helps visualize the space (Fig. 6). Care is taken to avoid injury to the underlying muscle bellies.

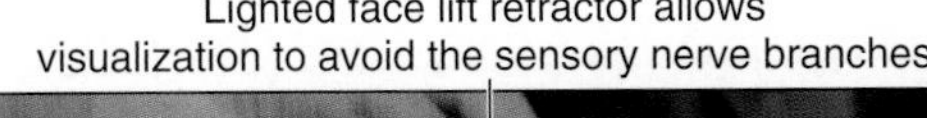

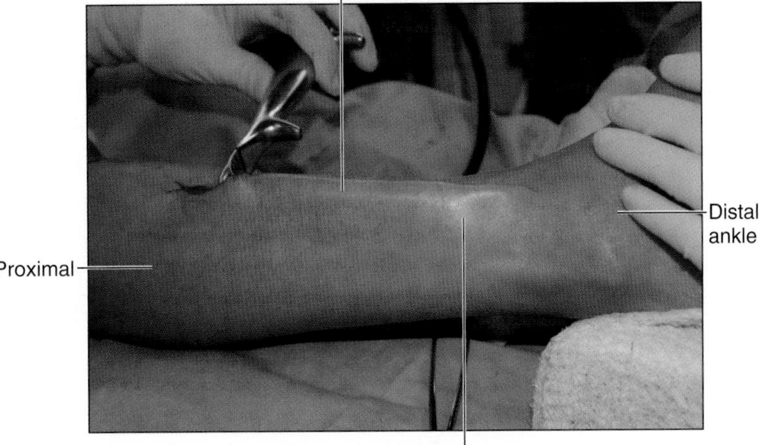

FIGURE 6

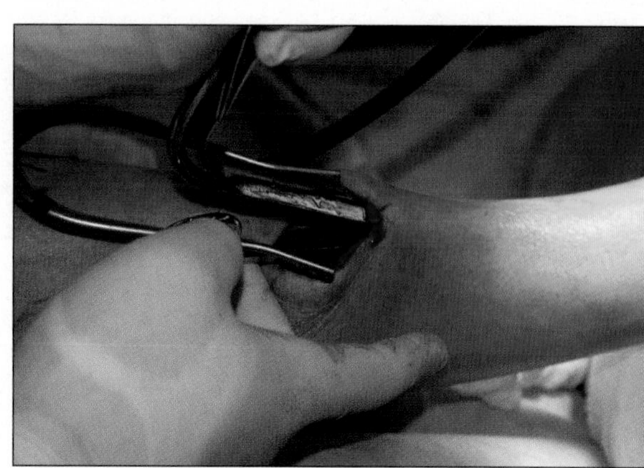

A Inserting Mayo scissors to carefully incise the fascia while both superficial and deep areas are visualized

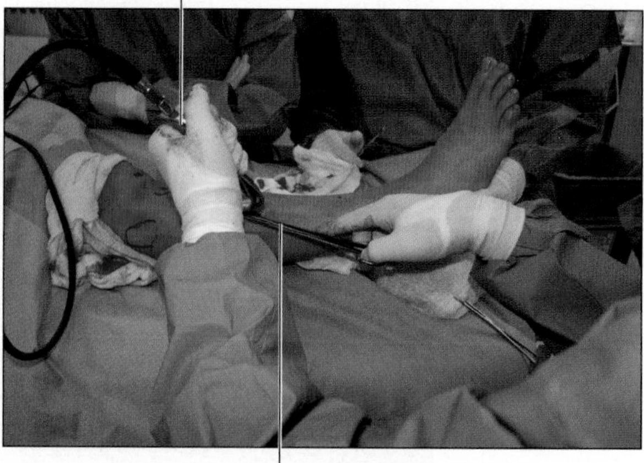

B

FIGURE 7

- The blades can be split with one above and one below the fascia. The fascia can then be divided under direct visualization along the axis of the leg (Fig. 7A and 7B).

Step 3: Wound Closure

- The subcutaneous tissue is closed with 0 braided and 2-0 absorbable suture, and the skin is closed with a running everting mattress suture of 3-0 rapidly absorbable monofilament suture.
- The fascia is not closed over the muscle bellies.

Pearls

- *Direct visualization of the subcutaneous space can help prevent damage to the small branches of the sensory nerves, which traverse the space from the fascia to the skin.*

Pitfalls

- *Failure to directly visualize the subcutaneous space, and a small incision, can lead to numb patches on the anterior lateral leg.*

Postoperative Care and Expected Outcomes

- The patient is placed into a three-sided splint with the leg at 90° for 2 weeks.
- The first postoperative visit is at 2 weeks. The sutures are checked and left in place to self-dissolve, and therefore minimize scarring by helping to disperse the forces that spread the wound.
- If a calf lengthening has been done, a night ankle "L" splint is used for sleep. Otherwise, physical therapy is started immediately and activity is progressed to normal as tolerated.

Evidence

Edmundsson D, Toolanen G, Sojka P. Chronic compartment syndrome also affects nonathletic subjects: a prospective study of 63 cases with exercise-induced lower leg pain. Acta Orthop. 2007;78:136-42.

This study was a retrospective review of 57 patients treated with fasciotomies for chronic exertional compartment syndrome. Outcome was assessed subjectively. (Level IV evidence [case series])

Hislop M, Tierney P, Murray P, O'Brien M, Mahony N. Chronic exertional compartment syndrome: the controversial "fifth" compartment of the leg. Am J Sports Med. 2003;31:770-6.

This study was an anatomic study to delineate the deep posterior compartment. (Level V evidence)

Howard JL, Mohtadi NG, Wiley JP. Evaluation of outcomes in patients following surgical treatment of chronic exertional compartment syndrome in the leg. Clin J Sports Med. 2000;10:176-84.

This study was a retrospective cohort review of 62 consecutive patients treated with fasciotomies. Outcome was determined by patient questionnaires. (Level III evidence [retrospective cohort])

Mouhsine E, Garofalo R, Moretti B, Gremion G, Akiki A. Two minimal incision fasciotomy for chronic exertional compartment syndrome of the lower leg. Knee Surg Sports Traumatol Arthrosc. 2006;14:193-7.

This study was a case series of 18 consecutive athletes treated with double-incision decompressive fasciotomy. Follow-up was 2 years, and outcome was determined by subjective assessment. (Level IV evidence [case series])

Raikin SM, Rapuri VR, Vitanzo P. Bilateral simultaneous fasciotomy for chronic exertional compartment syndrome. Foot Ankle Int. 2005;12:1007-11.

This study was a review of 16 patients with simulataneous bilateral lower extremity fasciotomies. Follow-up averaged 16.4 months. Outcome was determined by patient return to sports participation, subjective pain, and numbness. (Level IV evidence [case series])

Rorabeck CH, Fowler PJ, Nott L. The results of fasciotomy in the management of chronic exertional compartment syndrome. Am J Sports Med. 1988;16:224-7.

This study was a retrospective review of 25 patients with compartment release in either the anterior, anterior/posterior, or deep posterior compartments. Outcome was determined by patient satisfaction. (Level IV evidence [case series])

Schepsis AA, Gill SS, Foster TA. Fasciotomy for exertional anterior compartment syndrome: is lateral compartment release necessary? Am J Sports Med. 1999;27:430-5.

This prospective study examined anterior release alone versus anterior and lateral compartment releases. Outcome was determined by return to full sports by the two groups. (Level II evidence [prospective cohort])

Slimmon D, Bennell K, Brukner P, Crossley K, Bell SN. Long-term outcome of fasciotomy with partial fasciectomy for chronic exertional compartment syndrome of the lower leg. Am J Sports Med. 2002;30:581-8.

This study was a retrospective cohort study of 50 patients who underwent a fasciotomy with partial fasciectomy. Follow-up averaged 51 months. Outcome was determined by subjective assessment. (Level III evidence [retrospective cohort])

Styf JR, Korner LM. Chronic anterior-compartment syndrome of the leg: results of treatment by fasciotomy. J Bone Joint Surg [Am]. 1986;68:1338-47.

This study was a retrospective review of 19 patients treated by anterior compartment releases. Follow-up averaged 25 months. Outcome was determined by subjective assessment and intramuscular pressures. (Level IV evidence [case series])

INDEX

Note: Page numbers followed by f refer to figures.

A

Accessory navicular. *See* Painful accessory navicular
Achilles tendon
anatomy of, 668–670, 669f
insertional degeneration of, 655–665
examination of, 656
imaging of, 656
nonoperative treatment of, 656
surgical treatment of, 656–665
anatomy for, 656–658, 657
calf lengthening in, 661–662, 661f
care after, 664
examination in, 656
exposure in, 658–660, 658f, 659f, 660f, 661f
imaging in, 656
positioning in, 658
tendon reconstruction in, 662–664, 662f, 663f
rupture of, treatment of, 668. *See also* Achilles tendon reconstruction
Achilles tendon bursa, 540, 540f
Achilles tendon reconstruction, 662–664, 662f, 663f
flexor hallucis longus transfer augmentation with, 667–678
anatomy for, 668–670, 669f, 670f
care after, 677
closure in, 677
examination in, 668
exposures for, 670–672, 671f, 672f
fixation augmentation in, 676, 676f
imaging in, 668
indication for, 668
outcomes of, 677
positioning in, 670
suture anchor in, 676, 676f
tendon harvest in, 672, 673f
tendon passage in, 675, 675f
tendon preparation in, 675
tension setting in, 676, 676f
tunnel preparation in, 674, 674f
Anesthetic injection, subtalar joint, 458, 459f
Ankle arthrodesis. *See also* tibiotalocalcaneal arthrodesis; Triple arthrodesis
arthroscopic, 373–380
anatomy for, 375, 375f
care after, 380
débridement in, 377–378, 377f, 378f
guide pin placement in, 378, 379f
imaging in, 374, 374f, 379, 379f
indications for, 374
portals for, 376, 376f
positioning in, 376, 376f
screw placement in, 379, 379f
double plating, 381–394
anatomy for, 383–385, 383f, 384f
care after, 391–392
cartilage removal in, 387, 387f
closure in, 391
examination in, 382
exposure for, 385, 386f
fluoroscopic check in, 390, 390f
graft in, 390, 391f
imaging in, 382, 383f, 392, 392f
indications for, 382
Kirschner wire insertion in, 388, 388f
lateral plate fixation in, 388, 389f
medial plate fixation in, 388, 389f
positioning in, 385
tibial screw fixation in, 388, 389f
failed arthroplasty treatment with, 341–357
allograft for, 348–349, 348f, 349f, 355
anatomy for, 343, 343f
care after, 356
closure in, 355, 355f
dressing in, 355, 355f
examination for, 342
exposure for, 344–346, 345f, 346f
imaging in, 342, 350, 350f
implant removal for, 346, 346f
indications for, 342
outcomes of, 356
positioning in, 344, 344f
screw placement in, 350–354, 351f, 352f, 353f, 354f
subchondral drilling in, 347, 347f
Ankle arthrodesis (*Continued*)
ring/multiplanar external fixation for, 359–372
anatomy for, 361–362, 362f
care after, 372
cartilage removal in, 364, 364f
dual arthrotomy technique in, 363, 363f
exposure for, 363–364, 363f
external fixator assembly in, 366–370, 366f, 367f, 368f
graft in, 364, 364f
half-pin placement in, 369–370, 369f, 370f
imaging in, 360–361
indications for, 360, 361f
physical examination in, 360
positioning in, 363, 363f
provisional pinning in, 365, 365f
talar wire placement in, 370, 371f
thin wire placement in, 367–369, 367f, 368f, 369f
thin wire safe zones in, 362, 362f
tibiotalar joint compression in, 370–372, 371f
Ankle arthroplasty, total. *See* Total ankle arthroplasty
Ankle impingement, anterior. *See* Anterior ankle impingement
Ankle laxity/instability
lateral, 472
Brostrom procedure for. *See* Brostrom procedure
examination of, 472, 473f, 482, 483f, 510–511
failed ligament repair in, 497–507
examination in, 498–499, 499f
salvage repair for, 497–507
anatomy in, 499–500, 499f
care after, 506–507
examination in, 498–499, 499f
exposure in, 500, 500f, 501, 501f
indications for, 498
positioning in, 500
retinaculum fixation in, 506, 506f
semitendinosus graft passage in, 504, 504f
semitendinosus graft placement in, 502, 502f

Ankle laxity/instability (*Continued*)
semitendinosus graft tightening in, 505, 505f
tunnel creation in, 503, 503f, 504, 505f
fourth extensor digitorum communis tendon reconstruction for. *See* Fourth extensor digitorum communis tendon ligament reconstruction
imaging of, 472, 473f, 482, 510–511
plantaris autograft reconstruction for. *See* Plantaris autograft ligament reconstruction
medial
examination of, 522–523, 523f
ligament reconstruction for, 521–536
anatomy for, 524, 525f
care after, 534
examination in, 522, 523f
exposure in, 526, 526f
imaging in, 522–523
indications for, 522
lateral ankle ligament, 532, 533f
lateral lengthening calcaneal osteotomy in, 532–534, 533f, 534f
outcomes of, 534, 535f
positioning in, 524, 525f
posterior tibial tendon reconstruction in, 532
superficial deltoid ligament, 527–531, 527f, 528f, 529f, 530f, 531f
in type I deltoid rupture, 527–529, 527f, 528f
in type II deltoid rupture, 527–529, 527f, 528f
in type III deltoid rupture, 531, 531f
Anterior ankle impingement
arthroscopic treatment of, 615–620
anatomy in, 616, 617f
care after, 620
débridement in, 618, 619f
examination in, 616
imaging in, 616, 617f
indications for, 616
portals in, 618, 619f
positioning in, 616, 617f
smoothing in, 620
examination of, 616
imaging of, 616, 617f
nonoperative treatment of, 616
Anterior drawer test
in lateral ankle instability, 472, 473f
in medial ankle instability, 522
Anterior leg compartment release, 729–735
anatomy for, 730–731, 731f
calf lengthening in, 732. *See also* Calf lengthening
closure in, 734
Anterior leg compartment release (*Continued*)
examination in, 730
exposure in, 731–732, 731f, 732f
fascial dissection in, 732–734, 732f, 733f, 734f
indications for, 730
positioning in, 731
Anterior talofibular ligament, 474, 474f, 499–500, 499f, 511, 511f
Anterior tibiofibular ligament, 484, 485f
Arthritis
ankle, 396, 397f
tibiotalocalcaneal arthrodesis for. *See* Tibiotalocalcaneal arthrodesis
valgus deformity with. *See* Valgus ankle osteoarthritis
varus deformity with. *See* Varus ankle
forefoot, 88, 89f
reconstruction for. *See* Forefoot reconstruction
great toe, 76, 77f
metatarsophalangeal joint arthrodesis for. *See* Metatarsophalangeal joint arthrodesis
Arthrodesis
ankle. *See* Ankle arthrodesis
first tarsometatarsal joint. *See* Modified "Lapidus" procedure
great toe metatarsophalangeal joint. *See* Metatarsophalangeal joint arthrodesis
midfoot. *See* Charcot-Marie-Tooth disease, midfoot arthrodesis in; Charcot-Marie-Tooth disease, midfoot osteotomy and arthrodesis in
tibiocalcaneal, 336–337, 337f
tibiotalar, 334–335, 334f, 335f, 336f
tibiotalocalcaneal. *See* Tibiotalocalcaneal arthrodesis
triple. *See* Triple arthrodesis
Arthroplasty, total. *See* Total ankle arthroplasty
Arthroscopy
great toe. *See* Hallux, arthroscopy of
subtalar. *See* Subtalar joint, arthroscopy of

B

Böhler's angle, 576, 577f
Bone graft
in accessory navicular fusion, 272, 272f
Bone graft (*Continued*)
in ankle arthrodesis, 348–349, 348f, 349f, 355, 364, 364f
in calcaneal fracture treatment, 584, 584f
in lateral calcaneal lengthening osteotomy, 626, 627f
in modified "Lapidus" procedure, 42–43
mosaicplasty. *See* Mosaicplasty with bone-periosteum graft
proximal tibia. *See* Proximal tibial bone graft
in triple arthrodesis, 651
Bone scan
in Charcot neuroarthropathy, 222
of sesamoid bone, 182
Brachymetatarsalgia, 164, 164f
metatarsal lengthening for. *See* Metatarsal lengthening
Brostrom procedure, modified, 471–480, 482
anatomy for, 474, 474f
anterior talofibular ligament in, 476, 477f
calcaneofibular ligament in, 478, 478f
capsule opening in, 476, 476f, 477f
care after, 480
Dwyer closing wedge osteotomy with, 472, 474
examination in, 472, 473f
exposure for, 474, 475f
imaging in, 472, 473f
peroneal tendon sheath opening in, 476, 476f
positioning in, 474
retinaculum dissection in, 474, 475f
suture placement in, 479, 479f
Bunionette deformity
anatomy of, 103, 103f
correction of, 102, 102f. *See also* Fifth metatarsal osteotomy
imaging of, 102, 102f
Bursa
Achilles tendon, 540, 540f
retrocalcaneal, 540, 540f
Bursography, in Haglund's deformity, 549, 549f

C

Calcaneal fracture, 557–574
articular surfaces in, 560, 561f
comminuted, 560, 561f
constant fragment in, 560
examination of, 558, 576
imaging of, 558, 559f, 576–578, 577f, 578f
nonoperative treatment of, 558, 577
open reduction and internal fixation of, 558–574
anatomy for, 558–560, 559f, 561f
care after, 572
closure in, 570–571, 571f

Calcaneal fracture (*Continued*)
exposure in, 562, 562f
extensile lateral incision for, 575–588
anatomy in, 579, 579f
bone graft in, 584, 584f
care after, 585
closure in, 585
contraindications to, 576
examination in, 576
exposure in, 580–581, 580f
imaging in, 576–578, 577f, 578f
indications for, 576
Kirschner wires in, 581, 582, 583f
marking in, 580, 580f
plate and screw placement in, 584, 584f
positioning in, 580, 580f
Schanz pin in, 582, 582f
fluoroscopy in, 564, 565f, 566, 566f
Kirschner wire placement in, 564, 564f, 565f
malreduction with, 564, 565f
outcomes of, 572, 572f
peroneal tendon dislocation repair with, 568–570, 568f, 569f, 570f
plate and screw placement in, 566–568, 566f, 567f, 568f
positioning in, 561
reduction technique in, 563–566, 563f, 564f, 565f, 566f
Schanz pin in, 564, 564f, 565
Calcaneal osteotomy
in cavovarus correction, 204–206, 205f, 206f, 207f
in Haglund's deformity, 552, 552f
lateral. *See* Lateral calcaneal lengthening osteotomy
Myerson's, 622
in valgus ankle treatment, 414, 415f, 423–424, 423f, 424f, 425f
in varus ankle treatment, 599–600, 599f
Calcaneofibular ligament, 474, 474f, 484, 485f, 499f, 500, 511f, 512
Calf lengthening, 709–719
adhesions with, 717
anatomy for, 711–712, 711f
care after, 717–718
closure in, 717
deep vein injury with, 717
examination in, 710–711
exposure in, 712–713
gastrocnemius release in, 716, 716f, 717f
preparation for, 713–715, 713f, 714f, 715f
imaging in, 711
indications for, 710
overlengthening with, 718
positioning in, 712
Calf lengthening (*Continued*)
strength after, 718
sural nerve injury with, 717
Cartilage, structure of, 432, 433f
Charcot-Marie-Tooth disease
arthropathy in, 238–240, 238f, 239f, 240f
cavovarus correction in, 195–215
anatomy for, 202, 202f
calcaneal osteotomy in, 204–206, 205f, 206f, 207f
care after, 214–215
claw toe correction with, 198, 198f, 212, 213f
Cole osteotomy in, 210–212, 211f, 213f
exposure for, 203–204, 203f, 204f
fascial division in, 208, 208f
flexor digitorum longus tenotomy in, 212, 213f
imaging in, 200, 201f, 214, 214f
indications for, 196, 197
metatarsal osteotomy in, 208–210, 209f, 210f
nerve block for, 203, 203f
outcome of, 215, 215f
peroneal tendon transfer in, 206, 207f
positioning in, 203
Coleman block test in, 198, 198f
examination in, 196–200, 196f, 197f, 198f, 200f, 219–220, 221f, 238–240, 238f, 239f
flexibility evaluation in, 199
gait evaluation in, 199
imaging in, 199, 200, 201f, 220–222, 221f, 238–240, 239f, 240f
midfoot arthrodesis in, 237–244
anatomy for, 240
care after, 243
closure after, 243
contraindications to, 238
examination before, 238–239, 238f, 239f
exposure for, 240, 241f
imaging in, 238–240, 239f, 240f
indications for, 238
Kirschner wire insertion for, 241, 243f
positioning in, 240
preparation for, 241
reduction for, 241–243
screw insertion for, 242, 242f
midfoot osteotomy and arthrodesis in, 218–234
anatomy for, 223–225
bony anatomy for, 223
care after, 234
examination in, 219–220, 221f
exposure for, 225–227, 225f, 226f, 227f
external fixation in, 232–233, 233f
imaging in, 220–221, 221f
indications for, 219
Charcot-Marie-Tooth disease (*Continued*)
outcomes of, 234
planning for, 227
plate application in, 231f, 232
principles of, 227–228
screw insertion in, 230–231, 231f
soft tissue anatomy for, 223
transpedal wedge resection in, 228–230, 228f, 229f, 230f
neuroarthropathy in, 218–219
classification of, 224, 224f
differential diagnosis of, 222
examination of, 219–220, 238–240, 238f, 239f
imaging of, 220–222, 221f, 239–240, 239f, 240f
vs. infection, 222
natural history of, 219
nonoperative treatment of, 222
pathogenesis of, 218
staging of, 225, 225f
strength evaluation in, 199
upper extremity in, 196, 196f
Cheilectomy, 66–73
anatomy for, 68, 68f
capsule incision for, 70, 70f
care after, 73
examination in, 66–67, 67f
exposure for, 69, 69f
imaging in, 67–68, 67f
indications for, 66
metatarsal head reshaping for, 71, 72f
Moberg procedure with, 66, 72–73, 73f
osteophyte removal for, 70–71, 71f
phalangeal osteotomy with, 66
positioning in, 69
range of motion check for, 72
Chevron osteotomy, modified. *See* Modified chevron osteotomy
Chondromalacia, hallux, 160
Claw toe correction, in Charcot-Marie-Tooth disease, 198, 198f, 212, 213f
Common peroneal nerve, 700–701, 701f
Computed tomography
in ankle arthrodesis, 342
in calcaneal fracture, 558, 559f, 578, 578f
in cuboid fracture, 288, 289f
in double plating ankle arthrodesis, 382
in failed total ankle arthroplasty, 326, 327f
in flatfoot, 624, 630
in medial ankle instability, 522
in osteoarthritis, 396
of sesamoid bone, 182, 183f
of subtalar joint, 460, 460f
in talar osteochondral lesion, 446, 446f
in valgus ankle, 410
in varus ankle, 591

Cuboid fracture, 288, 289f
open reduction and internal fixation of, 287–295
anatomy for, 290, 291f
care after, 294
distractor for, 292, 292f
exposure for, 290, 291, 291f
imaging in, 288, 289f
indications for, 288
lateral cortex in, 292–293, 292f
plate placement in, 293, 293f, 294f
positioning in, 290
Schanz pin in, 292, 292f
sural nerve in, 290

D

Deltoid ligament, 524, 525f
rupture of, 522–523, 523f. *See also* Ankle laxity/instability, medial
Deviated lesser toe
examination of, 136, 137f
metatarsal shortening (Weil) osteotomy for. *See* Metatarsal shortening (Weil) osteotomy
radiography of, 136, 137f
Double heel-rise test, 622, 623f

E

Electromyography
in footdrop, 700
in tarsal tunnel syndrome, 605
Equinus contracture
calf lengthening for. *See* Calf lengthening
examination of, 710–711
imaging of, 711
Exertional compartment syndrome
anterior leg compartment release for. *See* Anterior leg compartment release
examination of, 730
nonoperative therapy in, 730
Exosectomy. *See* Haglund's deformity, exosectomy for

F

Fibula osteotomy, 421–422, 421f, 422f
Fifth metatarsal osteotomy, 101–109
anatomy for, 103, 103f
capsulotomy imbrication in, 108, 108f
care after, 108–109, 108f
closure in, 108, 108f
exposure for, 104, 104f
imaging in, 102, 102f, 109, 109f
indications for, 102

Fifth metatarsal osteotomy (*Continued*)
L-shaped capsulotomy in, 105, 105f, 108, 108f
lateral eminence resection in, 105, 105f
lateral prominence resection in, 107–108, 107f
positioning in, 104
saw blade passage in, 106, 107f
screw insertion in, 106, 107f
Flatfoot
Evans' osteotomy for, 622
examination of, 622, 623f, 630
Hansen's calcaneocuboidal interposition arthrodesis for, 622
imaging of, 622–624, 623f, 630, 631f
lateral calcaneal lengthening osteotomy for. *See* Lateral calcaneal lengthening osteotomy
Myerson's calcaneal medial sliding osteotomy for, 622
nonoperative treatment of, 630
triple arthrodesis for. *See* Triple arthrodesis
Flexor hallucis longus tendon, 670, 670f
transfer of. *See* Achilles tendon reconstruction, flexor hallucis longus transfer augmentation with
Footdrop
examination of, 700
posterior tibial tendon transfer for. *See* Posterior tibial tendon transfer
Forefoot reconstruction, 87–99
anatomy for, 90, 90f
bone smoothing in, 93, 93f
care after, 98–99
closed osteoclasis in, 94
examination in, 88, 89f
exposure for, 90, 91, 91f
extensor digitorum longus division in, 91, 91f
fifth metatarsal neck cut in, 94, 95f
great toe MTP joint fusion in, 97, 97f
imaging in, 88, 89f, 98, 98f
indications for, 88
Kirschner wire insertion in, 96, 96f
metatarsal division in, 92, 92f
metatarsal excision in, 93, 93f, 94, 95f
positioning in, 90
proximal phalanx in, 85f, 92, 92f, 94, 95f
resection arthroplasty in, 97
results of, 99, 99f
Fourth extensor digitorum communis tendon ligament reconstruction, 509–519
anatomy for, 511–512, 511f
anterior talofibular ligament exposure for, 513, 513f

Fourth extensor digitorum communis tendon ligament reconstruction (*Continued*)
anterior talofibular ligament reconstruction in, 514–517, 515f, 516f
care after, 518
examination in, 510–511
exposures for, 512–513, 512f
graft harvest for, 514, 514f
graft site preparation for, 514
imaging in, 510–511
indications for, 510
positioning in, 512
retained anchors in, 514, 518f
Fracture
calcaneal. *See* Calcaneal fracture
cuboid. *See* Cuboid fracture
Jones'. *See* Proximal fifth metatarsal fracture
Lisfranc/tarsometatarsal. *See* Lisfranc/tarsometatarsal injury
proximal fifth metatarsal. *See* Proximal fifth metatarsal fracture
sesamoid bone, 182, 183f. *See also* Sesamoid bone(s), internal fixation of

G

Gastrocnemius-soleus complex, 656–658, 657, 711, 711f
Gastrocnemius tendon, release of, 661–662, 661f, 716, 716f, 717f. *See also* Calf lengthening
preparation for, 713–715, 713f, 714f, 715f
Great toe. *See* Hallux

H

Haglund's deformity, 547–556
arthroscopic treatment of, 554–556
anatomy for, 550, 550f
care after, 556
portals for, 554, 555f
positioning in, 551
resection in, 554–555, 555f
conservative treatment of, 538, 548
endoscopic calcaneoplasty for, 538
examination of, 538, 539f, 548
exosectomy for, 537–546
Achilles tendon detachment in, 545
anatomy for, 540, 540f
care after, 545
closure in, 545
débridement in, 544
examination in, 538, 539f
exposure in, 541–543, 541f, 542f, 543f
fluoroscopy in, 544, 545f

Haglund's deformity (*Continued*)
imaging in, 538–539, 539f
indications for, 538
positioning in, 540–541, 541f
resection in, 544, 544f
imaging of, 538–539, 539f, 548–549, 549f
open treatment of
Achilles tendon débridement in, 554, 554f
anatomy for, 550, 550f
calcaneal osteotomy in, 552, 552f
care after, 556
examination in, 548
exposures for, 551, 551f
imaging in, 548–549, 549f
positioning in, 551, 551f
resection in, 552–553, 553f
Hallux. *See also* Hallux rigidus; Hallux valgus; Hallux varus
anatomy of, 7, 7f, 68, 68f, 155–156, 155f, 156f
arthritis of, 76, 77f
metatarsophalangeal joint arthrodesis for. *See* Metatarsophalangeal joint arthrodesis
shoes for, 76
arthroscopy of, 153–161
anatomy for, 155–156, 155f, 156f
at anteromedial portal, 159, 159f
care after, 160–161
in chondromalacia, 160
examination before, 154–155, 154f
examination protocol for, 158–160, 159f
indications for, 154
instruments for, 159
magnetic resonance imaging before, 154, 154f
at medial portal, 159, 159f
in osteophyte removal, 160
portals for, 157–158, 157f, 158f
positioning in, 157, 157f
in sesamoid evaluation, 160
capsular-ligamentous injury of. *See* Turf toe
chondromalacia of, 160
innervation of, 7, 7f
osteophytes of, 160
sesamoid bone of. *See* Sesamoid bone
vascular anatomy of, 7, 7f
Hallux rigidus
cheilectomy for. *See* Cheilectomy
examination of, 66–67, 67f
grades of, 68
imaging of, 67–68, 67f
shoes for, 68
Hallux valgus
examination of, 5, 5f, 22, 36, 48, 49f
imaging of, 6, 6f, 22–23, 23f, 36, 48, 49f
modified chevron osteotomy for. *See* Modified chevron osteotomy
Hallux valgus (*Continued*)
modified "Lapidus" procedure for. *See* Modified "Lapidus" procedure
proximal long oblique (Ludloff) first metatarsal osteotomy for. *See* Proximal long oblique first metatarsal osteotomy
scarf osteotomy for. *See* Scarf osteotomy
Hallux varus, 19, 143–152
examination of, 144, 145f
imaging of, 144, 145f
nonsurgical treatment of, 144
surgical treatment of, 144–152
abductor hallucis tendon release in, 147, 147f
anatomy for, 144, 145f
capsular closure in, 150, 151f
capsule division in, 147, 147f
care after, 151–152
Endobutton and Fiberwire passage in, 148–150, 148f, 149f, 150f
examination in, 144, 145f
exposure in, 144, 145f, 146, 146f
fluoroscopy after, 150, 151f
guidewire placement in, 148, 148f
imaging in, 144, 145f, 152, 152f
indications for, 144
positioning in, 144
Hindfoot deformity, triple arthrodesis for. *See* Triple arthrodesis
HINTEGRA prosthesis. *See* Total ankle arthroplasty, three-component design (HINTEGRA prosthesis) for

I

Impingement, ankle, anterior. *See* Anterior ankle impingement
Interdigital nerve fibrosis. *See* Morton's neuroma

J

Jones' fracture. *See* Proximal fifth metatarsal fracture

K

Kager's fat pad, 538

L

Lachman's test, in deviated lesser toe, 136, 137f
"Lapidus" procedure, modified. *See* Modified "Lapidus" procedure
Lateral calcaneal lengthening osteotomy, 621–628
anatomy for, 624, 624f
care after, 628
examination in, 622, 623f
exposure for, 625, 625f
fluoroscopy in, 626, 627f
graft in, 626, 627f
imaging in, 622–624, 623f
indications for, 622
Kirschner wires in, 626, 626f
osteotomy technique in, 626, 626f, 627
positioning in, 625
soft tissue procedures with, 628
Lateral closing wedge osteotomy, for varus ankle, 596–598, 597f, 598f
Lisfranc/tarsometatarsal injury
imaging of, 246, 247f
open reduction and internal fixation in, 245–256
anatomy for, 248
care after, 255
closure for, 254
dorsolateral exposure for, 249f, 250
dorsomedial exposure for, 248, 249f
exposure for, 248–250, 249f
first tarsometatarsal fracture reduction in, 252, 253f
imaging in, 246, 247f, 255
medial exposure for, 250, 250f
positioning in, 248
screws in, 254, 255
second tarsometatarsal fracture reduction in, 250–252, 251f, 252f
third to fifth tarsometatarsal fracture reduction in, 253–254, 253f, 254f
Ludloff first metatarsal osteotomy. *See* Proximal long oblique (Ludloff) first metatarsal osteotomy

M

Magnetic resonance imaging
in Achilles tendon degeneration, 656
in Achilles tendon reconstruction, 668
in anterior ankle impingement, 616
in Charcot-Marie-Tooth disease, 222, 240, 240f
in cuboid fracture, 288
in exertional compartment syndrome, 730
in flatfoot, 624, 630
in Haglund's deformity, 538–539, 539f, 549, 549f
of hallux, 154, 154f

Magnetic resonance imaging (*Continued*)
- in lateral ankle laxity, 472
- in medial ankle instability, 523
- in Morton's neuroma, 123
- in osteoarthritis, 374, 396
- in osteochondral lesion, 432, 433f
- in peroneal tendon subluxation-dislocation, 690, 691f
- in peroneal tendon tear, 681
- of sesamoid bone, 182
- of subtalar joint, 460, 460f
- in talar avascular necrosis, 361
- in talar osteochondral lesion, 444, 445f
- in tarsal tunnel syndrome, 605, 605f
- in total ankle arthroplasty, 302
- in turf toe, 114, 114f
- in valgus ankle osteoarthritis, 410

Medial column hypermobility, modified "Lapidus" procedure for, 36. *See also* Modified "Lapidus" procedure

Medial opening wedge osteotomy, for varus ankle, 600–601, 600f, 601f

Metatarsal fracture, fifth. *See* Proximal fifth metatarsal fracture

Metatarsal lengthening, 163–180
- anatomy for, 165–166, 165f, 166f
- care after, 176
- contraindications to, 164
- corticotomy in, 173–175, 173f, 174f, 175f
- distraction in, 176–179, 176f, 177f, 178f, 179f
- exposure for, 166
- first (distal) pin placement in, 167–169, 167f, 168f, 169f
- floating pin placement in, 170, 172f
- imaging in, 176–179, 177f, 178f, 179f
- indications for, 164, 164f
- intermediate pin placement in, 170, 171f, 172f
- positioning in, 166
- proximal pin placement in, 170, 171f, 172f

Metatarsal osteotomy, in cavovarus correction, 208–210, 209f, 210f

Metatarsal shortening (Weil) osteotomy, 135–142
- anatomy for, 138, 139f
- care after, 141, 142
- examination in, 136
- exposure for, 138, 139f
- imaging in, 136, 137f
- indications for, 136
- oblique cuts in, 104f, 138–140, 139f
- positioning in, 138
- screw placement in, 140, 141f

Metatarsophalangeal joint
- first
  - arthrodesis of. *See* Metatarsophalangeal joint arthrodesis
  - capsular-ligamentous injury of. *See* Turf toe
- lesser, deviated, metatarsal shortening (Weil) osteotomy for. *See* Metatarsal shortening (Weil) osteotomy

Metatarsophalangeal joint arthrodesis, 75–86
- anatomy for, 76, 77f
- articular surface cuts for, 79, 79f
- capsule elevation for, 78, 79f
- care after, 84–85
- examination in, 76
- exposure for, 78, 78f
- flat cuts for, 82
- imaging in, 76, 77f, 85, 85f
- indications for, 76
- Kirschner wire placement for, 83, 83f, 84
- ligament division for, 78, 79f
- outcome of, 85
- plate for, 83–84, 84f
- positioning in, 76
- reaming for, 79–82, 80f, 81f, 82f
- toe positioning in, 82–84, 83f

Midfoot osteotomy. *See* Charcot-Marie-Tooth disease, midfoot osteotomy and arthrodesis in

Moberg procedure, 66, 72–73, 73f

Modified chevron osteotomy, 3–20
- adductor attachment release for, 11, 11f
- anatomy for, 7, 7f
- capsule incision for, 10, 10f
- capsule rupture for, 12, 13f
- capsule tightening for, 16, 17f
- care after, 18–20, 19f
- closing wedge phalangeal osteotomy with, 18, 18f
- complications for, 19–20
- examination in, 5–6, 5f
- exposures for, 8, 8f
- imaging in, 6, 6f
- indications for, 4
- lateral capsule exposure for, 10
- lateral capsule perforation for, 12, 12f
- medial eminence excision for, 9, 9f, 10f
- medial metatarsal smoothing for, 16, 17f
- metatarsal head displacement for, 14, 15f
- osteotomy marking for, 13–14, 13f, 14f
- pin assessment for, 15, 15f
- positioning in, 8
- vs. proximal osteotomy, 4
- sagittal groove exposure for, 8–9, 9f

Modified chevron osteotomy (*Contineud*)
- screw placement for, 14, 15f, 16–18, 16f
- sesamoid exposure for, 11, 11f
- shoe wear after, 18
- transverse metatarsal ligament division for, 12, 12f

Modified "Lapidus" procedure, 35–45
- adhesion release for, 42, 43f
- anatomy for, 37–38, 37f, 38f
- bone grafting for, 42–43
- capsule incision for, 39, 39f
- care after, 43–44
- deformity reduction for, 42
- drills for, 42
- examination in, 36
- exposures for, 38–39, 39f
- fusion for, 40–43, 41f, 43f
- imaging in, 36
- indications for, 36
- osteotomy cuts for, 40, 41f
- outcomes of, 44
- pocket hole for, 40, 40f
- positioning in, 38
- screw placement for, 42, 43f
- towel bump for, 38

Morton's neuroma, 121–126
- anatomy of, 123, 123f
- anesthetic injection in, 123, 128
- examination of, 122, 122f, 128
- imaging of, 122–123
- nonsurgical treatment of, 123, 128
- recurrent, 127–134
  - nonsurgical treatment of, 128
  - revision surgery for, 127–134
    - anatomy for, 129, 129f
    - care after, 134
    - closure in, 132–133, 133f
    - examination in, 128
    - exposure for, 130, 130f
    - fascial division in, 130, 131f
    - indications for, 128
    - nerve transection in, 131–132, 131f, 132f
    - normal nerve identification in, 130, 131f
    - positioning in, 129
- surgical treatment of, 123–126
  - anatomy for, 123, 123f
  - care after, 126
  - exposures for, 124, 124f
  - indications for, 122
  - positioning in, 123
  - technique of, 125, 125f

Mosaicplasty with bone-periosteum graft, 443–455
- anatomy for, 446, 447f
- anterior talofibular ligament in, 448, 449f
- arthroscopy in, 450
- care after, 453, 453f
- closure in, 452, 452f
- drilling in, 450, 451f
- examination in, 444
- exposure in, 448, 449f
- graft harvest in, 450, 451f

Mosaicplasty with bone-periosteum graft (*Continued*)
  graft insertion in, 450, 451f
  imaging in, 444–446, 445f, 446f, 453, 453f
  indications for, 444
  lateral approach to, 448
  medial approach to, 448, 449f
  positioning in, 447

N

Navicular, accessory. *See* Painful accessory navicular
Neuroma, Morton's. *See* Morton's neuroma
Nutcracker injury. *See* Cuboid fracture

O

OATS procedure, 431–441
  anatomy for, 432, 433f
  arthroscopy before, 434, 435f
  care after, 440
  core creation in, 436–437, 437f
  exposure for, 434, 434f
  graft in, 437, 438–440, 438f, 439f, 440f
  imaging in, 432, 433f
  indications for, 432
  inspection in, 434–436, 435f, 436f
  medial malleolar osteotomy in, 436
  positioning in, 434, 434f
  sizing rod in, 436, 437f
Os trigonum, 466, 466f
  débridement of, 465
Osteoarthritis, ankle
  imaging of, 396, 397f
  tibiotalocalcaneal arthrodesis for. *See* Tibiotalocalcaneal arthrodesis
  valgus deformity with. *See* Valgus ankle osteoarthritis
  varus deformity with. *See* Varus ankle
Osteochondral lesion
  ankle
    imaging of, 432, 433f
    OATS procedure for. *See* OATS procedure
  talar
    anatomy for, 446, 447f
    examination of, 444
    imaging of, 444–446, 445f, 446f
    mosaicplasty for. *See* Mosaicplasty with bone-periosteum graft
Osteophytes, hallux, 160
Osteotomy
  calcaneal. *See* Calcaneal osteotomy; Lateral calcaneal lengthening osteotomy
  Chevron, modified. *See* Modified chevron osteotomy
  Evans', 622
Osteotomy (*Continued*)
  fibular, 421–422, 421f, 422f
  fifth metatarsal. *See* Fifth metatarsal osteotomy
  first metatarsal. *See* Proximal long oblique (Ludloff) first metatarsal osteotomy
  metatarsal shortening. *See* Metatarsal shortening (Weil) osteotomy
  midfoot. *See* Charcot-Marie-Tooth disease, midfoot osteotomy and arthrodesis in
  scarf. *See* Scarf osteotomy
  tarsometatarsal. *See* Modified "Lapidus" procedure
  tibial, 414, 414f, 416–420, 417f, 418f, 419f, 420f, 421f
  Weil. *See* Metatarsal shortening (Weil) osteotomy

P

Painful accessory navicular, 258, 259f, 268, 268f, 269, 269f
  fusion procedure in, 267–275
    anatomy for, 269, 269f
    bone débridement in, 271–272, 271f, 272f
    bone graft in, 272, 272f
    care after, 274–275, 275f
    guidewire in, 273, 273f
    imaging in, 268, 268f, 274, 275f
    incision for, 270, 270f
    indications for, 268
    navicular-accessory piece junction in, 271, 271f
    positioning in, 269
    posterior tibial tendon sheath exposure in, 270, 270f
    screw in, 273–274, 274f
  Kidner procedure in, 258–275
    accessory navicular excision in, 263, 263f
    anatomy for, 258–259, 259f
    care after, 266
    examination in, 258
    exposure for, 260–261, 260f, 261f
    flexor digitorum longus tendon transfer with, 264, 265f
    imaging in, 258, 259f
    indications for, 258
    positioning in, 260
    posterior tibial tendon sheath exposure for, 262, 262f
    predrilling in, 263, 263f
    screw insertion in, 264, 264f, 265f
Peroneal nerve, 700–701, 701f
Peroneal tendon subluxation-dislocation, 689–698
  examination of, 690
  imaging of, 690, 691f
  nonsurgical treatment of, 690
Peroneal tendon subluxation-dislocation (*Continued*)
  surgical treatment of, 690–698
    anatomy for, 690–691, 691f
    care after, 697
    drilling in, 694, 695f
    exposure in, 692
    groove deepening in, 694, 695f
    outcomes of, 697
    periosteal flap in, 693, 693f, 696, 696f
    peroneus brevis excision in, 694, 694f
    positioning in, 692, 692f
    retromalleolar groove assessment in, 692, 693f
    side-to-side repair in, 692, 693f
    suture placement in, 696, 696f
    tunnel creation in, 696
Peroneal tendon tear
  débridement and repair of, 679–687
    anatomy for, 681–682, 681f, 682f
    care after, 686
    closure in, 685
    complications of, 686
    examination in, 680
    exposure in, 683–684, 683f
    imaging in, 680–681
    indications for, 680
    positioning in, 682
    retinaculum procedures in, 685
    suture placement in, 684, 684f, 685f
  examination of, 680
  imaging of, 680–681
Peroneal tendon transfer, in cavovarus correction, 206, 207f
Pes planoabductovalgus, modified "Lapidus" procedure for. *See* Modified "Lapidus" procedure
Plantar neuroma. *See* Morton's neuroma
Plantaris autograft ligament reconstruction, 481–496
  alternative autograft harvest in, 490
  anatomy for, 484, 485f
  arthroscopy in, 486, 486f
  autograft harvest in, 488–489, 488f, 489f
  care after, 493–494
  examination in, 482, 483f
  exposure for, 486, 487f
  indications for, 482
  lateral ankle preparation in, 487, 487f
  lateral ankle reconstruction in, 490–492, 490f, 491f, 492f, 493f
  outcomes of, 494
  portals for, 486, 486f
  positioning in, 484, 485f
Posterior tibial tendon transfer, 699–708
  anatomy for, 700–701, 701f

Posterior tibial tendon transfer (*Continued*)
care after, 707
closure in, 707
contraindications to, 700
drill hole in, 704, 705f
examination in, 700
imaging in, 700
incisions for, 702–704, 703f
indications for, 700
outcomes of, 707
positioning in, 701
tendon passage in, 704–706, 705f, 706f
Posterior tibialis muscle, 701, 701f
Pre-Achilles fat pad, 538
Proximal fifth metatarsal fracture, 278, 278f
open reduction and internal fixation of, 277–285
anatomy for, 279, 279f
care after, 285
drill for, 280, 281f
exposure for, 280, 280f
guide pin placement in, 280, 281f, 282
imaging in, 278, 278f, 285, 285f
indications for, 278, 278f
osteotomy with, 284
outcomes of, 285, 285f
positioning in, 279
screw for, 283–284, 283f, 284f
tap for, 280–282, 281f, 282f
Proximal long oblique (Ludloff) first metatarsal osteotomy, 47–64
anatomy for, 48, 50f
callus formation after, 64, 64f
care after, 63–64
closure for, 62, 62f
contraindications to, 48
cuts for, 55–58, 57f
dorsal first web space incision for, 48, 50f
examination in, 48, 49f
exposures for, 48, 50
fluoroscopy for, 58, 59f
imaging in, 48, 49f, 63–64, 63f, 64f
indications for, 48
lateral release for, 51–52, 51f, 52f, 53f
medial capsulorrhaphy for, 60–62, 61f
medial capsulotomy for, 52, 53f
medial eminence resection for, 54, 54f
medial midaxial longitudinal approach for, 50, 50f
osteotomy marking for, 54, 55f
outcome of, 63–64, 63f, 64f
overcorrection with, 60
positioning in, 48
screws for, 56–58, 57f, 59f
undercorrection with, 60, 62
Proximal tibial bone graft, 721–727
anatomy for, 722, 723f
Proximal tibial bone graft (*Continued*)
bone morphogenetic protein with, 726
care after, 726
donor site preparation in, 724, 724f
exposure in, 722–723, 723f
harvest in, 724–726, 725f, 726f
indications for, 722
positioning in, 722
Pump bump, 538, 539f. *See also* Haglund's deformity

R

Radiography
of accessory navicular, 258, 259f, 268, 268f
in Achilles tendon degeneration, 656
in Achilles tendon reconstruction, 668
in ankle arthrodesis, 342
in anterior ankle impingement, 616, 617f
in arthroscopic ankle arthrodesis, 374, 374f
in brachymetatarsalgia, 164, 164f
in bunionette deformity, 102, 102f
in calcaneal fracture, 558, 559f, 576–577, 577f
in Charcot-Marie-Tooth disease, 200, 201f, 220–222, 221f, 238–240, 239f
in cuboid fracture, 288, 289f
in deviated lesser toe, 136, 137f
in double plating ankle arthrodesis, 382, 383f, 392, 392f
in equinus contracture, 711
in exertional compartment syndrome, 730
in failed total ankle arthroplasty, 326, 327f, 334, 334f
in fifth metatarsal osteotomy, 109, 109f
in flatfoot, 622, 623f, 630, 631f
in footdrop, 700
in forefoot reconstruction, 98, 98f
in great toe metatarsophalangeal joint arthrodesis, 76, 77f
in Haglund's deformity, 538, 539f, 548–549, 549f
in hallux rigidus, 67–68, 67f
in hallux valgus, 6, 6f, 22–23, 23f, 36, 48, 49f
in hallux varus, 144, 145f, 152, 152f
in lateral ankle laxity, 472, 473f, 510–511
in Lisfranc/tarsometatarsal injury, 246, 247f
in medial ankle instability, 522
in metatarsal lengthening, 176–179, 177f, 178f, 179f
in metatarsophalangeal joint arthrodesis, 85, 85f
in modified chevron osteotomy for hallux valgus, 18, 19f
Radiography (*Continued*)
in osteoarthritis, 396, 397f
in peroneal tendon subluxation-dislocation, 690, 691f
in peroneal tendon tear, 680
in proximal fifth metatarsal fracture, 278, 278f, 285, 285f
in proximal long oblique (Ludloff) first metatarsal osteotomy, 63–64, 63f, 64f
in retrocalcaneal bursitis, 548–549, 549f
in revision total ankle arthroplasty, 326, 327f, 337–339, 338f, 339f
in rheumatoid disease, 88, 89f
in scarf osteotomy, 33, 33f
of sesamoid bone, 182, 183f
of subtalar joint, 459, 459f
in talar osteochondral lesion, 444, 445f
in tarsal tunnel syndrome, 604
in total ankle arthroplasty, 300–302, 301f, 322, 322f
in triple arthrodesis, 644, 644f, 651, 651f
in turf toe, 113–114, 113f
in valgus ankle, 410, 411f
in varus ankle, 590, 590f
Radionuclide imaging, in valgus ankle osteoarthritis, 410
Retrocalcaneal bursa, 540, 540f
Retrocalcaneal bursitis, 548–549, 549f
Rheumatoid disease
forefoot, 90, 90f
reconstruction for. *See* Forefoot reconstruction
great toe, 76, 77f
metatarsophalangeal joint arthrodesis for. *See* Metatarsophalangeal joint arthrodesis
imaging of, 88, 89f
Ring/multiplanar external fixation. *See* Ankle arthrodesis, ring/multiplanar external fixation for
Romberg test, 510

S

Scarf osteotomy, 21–34
anatomy for, 24, 24f
bandage for, 32, 32f
bone hook for, 26, 27f
capsule incision for, 26, 26f
care after, 33
closure of, 31–32, 31f, 32f
cuts for, 28–29, 29f
examination in, 22
exposure for, 24, 25f
exsanguination for, 24, 25f
imaging in, 22–23, 23f, 33, 33f
indications for, 22
Kirschner guidewire for, 26, 27f

Scarf osteotomy (*Continued*)
ligament release for, 28, 28f
osteotomy stabilization for, 29–31, 30f
positioning in, 24
redundant-bone smoothing for, 31, 31f
Reese guide for, 29, 29f
screw fixation for, 30, 30f
sutures for, 31–32, 31f, 32f
troughing with, 29, 33, 33f
Z-osteotomy marking for, 26, 27f
Sciatic nerve, 700–701, 701f
Sesamoid bone(s)
anatomy of, 184–185, 184f
arthroscopic evaluation of, 160
biomechanics of, 185, 185f
bipartite, 182, 184
bone scan of, 182
excision of, 182, 184
internal fixation of, 181–192
anatomy for, 184–185, 184f
arthrotomy in, 188, 189f
care after, 188, 190–191
examination in, 182, 183f
vs. excision, 182, 184
exposure for, 186, 187f
imaging in, 182, 183f
indications for, 182
outcome of, 190–191, 190f, 191f
pain after, 188, 190
positioning in, 185
screw placement in, 188, 189f
technique of, 188–191, 189f
multipart, 184
in turf toe, 118
Shoes
in great toe arthritis, 76
in hallux rigidus, 68
in hallux valgus, 18
in rheumatoid disease, 90
Single-photon emission computed tomography
in double plating ankle arthrodesis, 382
in failed total ankle arthroplasty, 328
in osteoarthritis, 396
in total ankle arthroplasty, 302, 302f
Sprain. *See* Ankle laxity/instability
Standing test, 522, 523f
Stieda's process, 466, 466f
débridement of, 465
Subtalar joint
anatomy of, 460–461, 461f
anesthetic injection into, 458, 459f
arthroscopy of, 457–469
anatomy for, 460–461, 461f
care after, 468
diagnostic, 464–467, 465f, 466f, 467f
indications for, 458
lateral approach to, 462–463, 463f
portals for, 462–464, 463f, 464
positioning in, 462, 462f
Subtalar joint (*Continued*)
posterior approach to, 463–464, 463f
examination of, 458
imaging of, 459–460, 459f, 460f
Superficial deltoid ligament rupture repair
type I, 527–529, 527f, 528f
type II, 527, 529–531, 529f, 530f, 531f
type III, 527, 531, 531f
Sural nerve, 711f, 712
injury to, 717

T

Talar tilt test, 482, 483f
Talus, osteochondral lesions of, 444–446, 445f, 446f
mosaicplasty for. *See* Mosaicplasty with bone-periosteum graft
Tarsal tunnel syndrome, 603–613
electromyography in, 605
examination in, 604
imaging in, 604–605, 605f
nonoperative treatment in, 604
surgical treatment in, 603–613
abductor hallucis in, 611, 611f
anatomy for, 606–607, 606f
care after, 612
closure in, 612
examination in, 604
exposure in, 608, 608f
flexor retinaculum in, 606f, 607
imaging in, 604–605, 605f
incisions in, 608, 609f
indications for, 604
lesion excision in, 609, 609f
nerve release in, 609–610, 610f
outcomes of, 612
plantar nerve in, 606f, 607, 611, 611f
positioning in, 607
Tarsometatarsal corrective osteotomy and fusion. *See* Modified "Lapidus" procedure
Tibial bone graft. *See* Proximal tibial bone graft
Tibial nerve, 700–701, 701f
Tibial osteotomy, 414, 414f, 416–420, 417f, 418f, 419f, 420f, 421f
Tibial spur. *See* Anterior ankle impingement
Tibiocalcaneal arthrodesis, 336–337, 337f
Tibiotalar arthrodesis, 334–335
graft in, 334, 335f
imaging before, 334, 334f
plate in, 335, 335f, 336f
Tibiotalocalcaneal arthrodesis, retrograde intramedullary nail for, 395–406
anatomy for, 398, 398f, 399f
anterior exposure for, 400–401, 400f
Tibiotalocalcaneal arthrodesis, retrograde intramedullary nail for (*Continued*)
care after, 405
closure in, 404
contraindications to, 396
débridement in, 403
examination in, 396
exposure for, 400–402, 400f, 401f, 402f
imaging in, 396, 397f
indications for, 396
lateral exposure for, 401, 401f
nail insertion in, 403, 403f
plantar exposure for, 402, 402f
positioning in, 400
screw placement in, 404, 404f
subtalar exposure for, 401, 401f
Total ankle arthroplasty
revision, 325–340. *See also* Ankle arthrodesis; Tibiotalocalcaneal arthrodesis
anatomy for, 328–329, 328f, 329f
bone resection in, 332, 333f
care after, 337–339, 338f, 339f
closure in, 333
examination in, 326
exposure for, 330, 331f
imaging in, 326–328, 327f, 337–339, 338f, 339f
implant insertion in, 332
indications for, 326, 332
positioning in, 330
talar trial in, 332, 333f
tibiocalcaneal arthrodesis after, 336–337, 337f
tibiotalar arthrodesis after, 334–335, 334f, 335f, 336f
three-component design (HINTEGRA prosthesis) for, 299–323
anatomy for, 303–305, 303f, 304f
care after, 322
closure in, 320, 321f
cyst removal in, 316, 317f
dressing for, 320, 321f
examination in, 300
exposure for, 304–305, 305f
fluoroscopy in, 315–316, 315f, 320, 320f
imaging in, 300–302, 301f, 302f, 322, 322f
implant insertion in, 318–321, 318f–319f
indications for, 300
positioning in, 304
splint for, 320, 321f
talar resection in, 308–313, 309f, 311f, 313f, 316, 316f
talar trial in, 314–315, 314f, 316, 317f
tibial resection in, 306–308, 306f, 307f
tibial trial in, 314f, 315

Triple arthrodesis, 643–652
anatomy for, 644–646, 645f, 646f
axial incision in, 648
bone graft in, 651
care after, 651
exposure in, 646–648, 647f, 648f
fixation in, 650
imaging in, 644, 644f, 651, 651f
indications for, 644
joint surface preparation in, 649, 649f
lateral incision in, 648, 648f
medial incision in, 646, 646f
Ollier incision in, 648
positioning in, 646
single medial approach for, 629–641
Achilles tendon in, 638
anatomy in, 630–632, 631f, 632f
bone matrix/graft in, 634, 635f
calcaneocuboid joint in, 634
care after, 640
closure in, 638–639, 639f
dressing in, 639, 639f
examination in, 630
exposure in, 632, 633f
fixation technique in, 636–638, 636f, 637f
fluoroscopy in, 638, 638f
imaging in, 630, 631f
indications for, 630
Kirschner wires in, 633, 634, 635f, 637, 638f
positioning in, 632
reduction in, 636
screws in, 637, 637f, 638f
sinus tarsi preparation in, 634, 635f
subtalar joint preparation in, 634, 635f
talonavicular joint preparation in, 633, 633f
Turf toe
anatomy of, 114–115, 114f, 115f
examination of, 113–114, 113f
grade of, 112
imaging of, 113–114, 113f, 114f
mechanism of, 112, 112f
nonoperative treatment of, 113
Turf toe (*Continued*)
repair of, 112–119
anatomy for, 114–115, 114f, 115f, 117f
care after, 118–119, 119f
closure in, 118
defect location in, 116, 117f
examination in, 113–114, 113f
exposure for, 116, 116f
imaging in, 113–114, 113f, 114f
indications for, 112
positioning in, 115
sesamoid diastasis in, 118
suture anchors in, 118
sutures for, 117, 117f

U

Ultrasonography, in Haglund's deformity, 539, 539f

V

Valgus ankle osteoarthritis
fusion for, 410
imaging of, 410, 411f
realignment surgery for, 407–429
anatomy for, 410–413, 411f, 412f, 413f
arthroscopy in, 416, 416f
calcaneal osteotomy in, 414, 415f, 423–424, 423f, 424f, 425f
care after, 426
examination in, 410
exposure in, 414–415, 414f, 415f
extremity shortening with, 420
failure of, 427
fibula in, 420, 421f
fibula osteotomy in, 421–422, 421f, 422f
forefoot supination correction in, 425
heel cord release in, 426
imaging in, 410, 411f, 419, 419f, 421f
indications for, 408
Valgus ankle osteoarthritis (*Continued*)
outcomes of, 426–427
positioning in, 413, 413f
tibial osteotomy in, 414, 414f, 416–420, 417f, 418f, 419f, 420f, 421f
zigzag deformity and, 420, 420f
stage I, 408, 409f
stage II, 408, 409f
stage III, 408, 409f
total ankle replacement for, 410
Varus ankle, 589–602
conservative treatment of, 590
examination of, 590
imaging of, 590–591, 590f
osteotomy for, 589–602
anatomy in, 591–592, 591f, 592f
anterior approach to, 592, 593, 593f, 594–595, 595f
calcaneal, 592, 594, 599–600, 599f
care after, 601
examination in, 590
exposures for, 594–595, 595f
imaging in, 590–591, 590f
indications for, 590
lateral approach to, 591, 591f, 592, 594
lateral closing wedge, 596–598, 597f, 598f
medial approach to, 592, 592f, 593f, 594
medial opening wedge, 600–601, 600f, 601f
positioning in, 592–593, 593f

W

Weil osteotomy. *See* Metatarsal shortening (Weil) osteotomy

Z

Z-osteotomy, calcaneal, for varus ankle, 599–600, 599f